Stedman's
RADIOLOGY
WORDS

FOURTH EDITION

INCLUDES
NUCLEAR MEDICINE
& OTHER IMAGING

To MTs around the world

—Pat Forbis, Editor

Stedman's

RADIOLOGY
WORDS

FOURTH EDITION

INCLUDES
NUCLEAR MEDICINE
& OTHER IMAGING

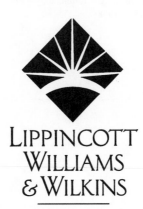

LIPPINCOTT
WILLIAMS
& WILKINS

Publisher: Julie K. Stegman
Series Managing Editor: Trista A. DiPaula
Managing Editor: Heather A. Rybacki
Art Program Project Manager: Jennifer Clements
Assistant Production Manager: Kevin Iarossi
Typesetter: Peirce Graphic Services, LLC.
Printer & Binder: Malloy Litho, Inc.

Printed in the United States of America

Fourth Edition, 2004

Library of Congress Cataloging-in-Publication Data

Stedman's radiology words : includes nuclear medicine & other imaging.—4th ed.
    p. ; cm.
  Includes bibliographical references.
  ISBN 0-7817-4410-5 (alk. paper)
  1. Radiology—Terminology. 2. Radiography, Medical—Terminology. 3. Diagnosis, Radioscopic—Terminology. 4. Diagnostic imaging—Terminology. 5. Radioisotope scanning—Terminology.
    [DNLM: 1. Diagnostic Imaging—Terminology—English. WN 15 S812 2003] I. Stedman, Thomas Lathrop, 1853–1938.
RC78.A3S74 2003
616.07'57'014—dc21   2003004777

                                            03
12 3 4 5 6 7 8 9 10

Contents

Acknowledgments

An important part of our editorial process is the involvement of medical language specialists and other health professionals—as advisors, reviewers, and/or editors.

We extend special thanks to Pat Forbis and Patricia Lee White, CMT, for editing the manuscript and helping to resolve many difficult questions. We are grateful to the members of our Editorial Advisory Board, including Deborah Dale Barrett; Norma Braunstein; Janell DeMello, MLS; Cheryl Hammel, RN CMT; Anna Majoras, CMT; Roxanne Nevenner; Patricia O'Brien-Giglia, CMT; Vicki Runnels; and Dee Ann Thomas, who were instrumental in shaping the direction of this revision. They shared their valuable judgment, insight, and perspective.

We also extend our gratitude to Katharine Boggess, CMT, and Tammy Meissner for revising and developing the appendices; to R. Jo-Ann Clarke, Anna Majoras, CMT, and Roxanne Nevenner for their assistance with the anatomical illustrations; to Patricia O'Brien-Giglia, CMT, and the transcription staff at H. Lee Moffitt Cancer Center & Research Institute for their contributions to the Common Radiation Oncology Terms appendix; and to Jeanne R. Bock, CRS, MT, and Andrea Linderman for their exceptional research skills.

Our appreciation goes to the following reviewers who helped to enhance the A-to-Z content for this edition, including Ellen Atwood; Sue Bartolucci, CMT; Katharine Boggess, CMT; R. Jo-Ann Clarke; Sherry G. Crawford, CMT; L. Fahnestock; Elizabeth Willard Gorsline, CMT; Vicki Hawhee, CMT; Kathy Hess, CMT; Robin Koza; Kathy Kresge, CMT; Tammy Meissner; Kathy Quakenbush, CMT; Lauri C. Rebar, CMT; and Jenifer F. Walker, MA. Thanks also go to Helen Littrell for performing the final prepublication review.

As always, Barb Ferretti played an integral role in the process by reviewing the content files for format, updating the manuscript, and providing a final quality check. Special thanks also go to L. Fahnestock and Kathy Cadle for their assistance working with the manuscript.

As with all our *Stedman's* word references, this resource incorporates the suggestions and expertise of our many contacts in the medical community. Thanks to all of our advisory board participants, reviewers, and editors; AAMT meeting attendees; and others who have written us with requests and comments—keep talking, and we'll keep listening.

.

Editor's Preface

My thanks to the talented and dedicated staff of Lippincott Williams & Wilkins and Stedman's for providing me the opportunity to edit the fourth edition of *Stedman's Radiology Words*. Special thanks go to Heather Rybacki for her leadership and support. Stedman's staff is committed to meeting the needs of medical transcriptionists and others who are involved with the language of medicine. Thanks also to Patty White, CMT, and the individuals named on the *Acknowledgments* page for their commitment to creating a quality product.

The practice of radiology has surely evolved more over the past few years than most medical specialties. New technologies have given rise to new tests, procedures, and instruments, thus creating a broad vocabulary that crosses all medical specialties and often incorporates their specific terminology.

Stedman's radiology lexicon has grown beyond what will reasonably fit between the covers of a single wordbook. It was therefore necessary to dedicate the 4th edition to terms most closely related to radiology, imaging, and nuclear medicine. While other specialty terms, such as drugs, anatomy, and surgery, are touched upon as they relate to radiology and medical imaging, other reference materials should be used for more comprehensive coverage in these areas. The result of these changes is a revised, refreshed edition that is rich with current imaging terminology.

All suggestions for additions or improvements are welcome, and it is easily done by filling out the card inside the back cover and mailing or faxing it to Stedman's. You may prefer to access www.stedmans.com and send an e-mail using the "Got a Good Idea?" link.

Pat Forbis, Editor

Publisher's Preface

Stedman's Radiology Words (Includes Nuclear Medicine and Other Imaging), Fourth Edition, offers an up-to-date, authoritative reference for the wordsmiths of the healthcare professions—medical transcriptionists, medical editors and copyeditors, health information management personnel, court reporters, medical coders, and the many other users and producers of medical documentation.

With the rapid rate of technological advancement, we realized the need to develop a comprehensive reference that reflects the changes that have taken place within radiology, nuclear medicine, and imaging since the Third Edition published. With this revised edition, we have focused on incorporating new developments in technology, including thorough coverage of the equipment and contrast materials used in imaging today, as well as techniques, procedures, tests, and phrases.

Stedman's Radiology Words, Fourth Edition, provides users with tens of thousands of words and phrases encompassing various aspects of imaging and nuclear medicine, including: diagnostic, therapeutic, and interventional radiology; abdominal, chest, gastrointestinal, genitourinary, and skeletal imaging; CT, MRI, PET, and SPECT imaging; mammography, ultrasonography, x-ray, neuroradiology, roentgenology, investigational radiology, radiographics, and radiologic technology terminology; as well as various contrast materials. Users will also find terms for diagnostic and therapeutic procedures, new techniques, and equipment names, plus abbreviations with their expansions. The appendix sections provide labeled anatomical illustrations, contrast media and other related materials, sample reports, and common terms by procedure.

This compilation of more than 100,000 entries, fully cross-indexed for quick access, was built from a base vocabulary of approximately 66,000 medical words, phrases, abbreviations, and acronyms. The extensive A-Z list was developed from the lexicon of *Stedman's Medical Dictionary, 27th Edition,* and supplemented by terminology found in current medical literature (please see list of References on page xvii).

We at Lippincott Williams & Wilkins strive to provide you with the most up-to-date and accurate word references available. Your use of this word book will prompt new editions, which we will publish as often as updates and revisions justify. We welcome your suggestions for improvements, changes, corrections, and additions—whatever will make this *Stedman's* product more useful to you. Please complete the postpaid card at the back of this book and send your recommendations care of "Stedman's" at Lippincott Williams & Wilkins.

Explanatory Notes

Medical transcription is an art as well as a science. Both approaches are needed to correctly interpret the dictation of a physician, whose language is a product of education, training, and experience. This variety in medical language means that there are several acceptable ways to express certain terms, including jargon. *Stedman's Radiology Words, Fourth Edition,* seeks to reflect current usage of medical language and provides variant spellings and phrasings for many terms. These elements, in addition to complete cross-indexing, make *Stedman's Radiology Words, Fourth Edition,* a valuable resource for determining the validity of terms as they are encountered.

Alphabetical Organization

Alphabetization of main entries is letter by letter as spelled, ignoring punctuation, spaces, prefixed numbers, Greek letters, or other characters. For example:

hydrops
hydropyonephrosis
5-hydroxyindoleacetic acid (5-HIAA)
Hypaque
Hypaque-76 imaging agent

In subentry alphabetization, the abbreviated singular form or the spelled-out plural form of the noun main entry word is ignored.

Format and Style

All main entries are in **boldface** to expedite locating a sought-after term, to enhance distinction between main entries and subentries, and to relieve the textual density of the pages.

Irregular plurals and variant spellings are shown on the same line as the singular or preferred form of the word. For example:

index, indices

mammoplasty, mammaplasty

Hyphenation

As a rule of style, multiple eponyms (e.g., Mears-Rubash approach) are hyphenated. Also, hyphens have been added between a manufacturer and one or more eponyms (e.g., Vital-Metzenbaum dissecting scissors). Please note that in many cases, hyphenation is a question of style, not of accuracy, and thus is a matter of choice.

Possessives

Possessive forms have been dropped in this reference for the sake of consistency and conformance with the guidelines of the American Medical Association (AMA), American Association for Medical Transcription (AAMT), and other groups. Please note, however, that in many cases, retaining the possessive, like hyphenating, is a question of style, not of accuracy, and thus is a matter of choice. To form the possessive of a word, simply add the apostrophe or apostrophe "s" to the end of the word.

Cross-indexing

The word list is in an index-like main entry-subentry format that contains two combined alphabetical listings:

(1) A *noun* main entry-subentry organization, which is typical of the A-Z section of medical dictionaries like *Stedman's:*

image
    acoustic i.
    delayed phase i.

table
    binary opacity t.
    radionuclide t.

(2) An *adjective* main entry-subentry organization, which lists words and phrases as you hear them. The main entries are the adjectives or modifiers in a multiword term. The subentries are the nouns around which the terms are constructed and to which the adjectives or modifiers pertain:

magnetic
    m. anisotropy
    m. dipole

bright
    b. echo
    b. signal intensity

This format provides the user with more than one way to locate and identify a multiword term. For example:

gradient
    diastolic g.

diastolic
    d. gradient

assessment
    sonographic a.

sonographic
    s. assessment

It also allows the user to see together all terms that contain a particular descriptor, as well as all types, kinds, or variations of a noun entity. For example:

fracture
    abduction f.
    basal neck f.
    f. bracing

valve
    v. area
    atrioventricular nodal v.
    v. attenuation

Wherever possible, abbreviations are separately defined and cross-referenced. For example:

BI-RADS
    Breast Imaging Reporting and Data System

breast
    B. Imaging Reporting and Data System (BI-RADS)

system
    Breast Imaging Reporting and Data S. (BI-RADS)

To avoid duplication, phrases that include commonly used imaging abbreviations, such as MRI, are only listed with the abbreviated phrase. For example, "cine magnetic resonance imaging" will be listed as "cine MRI." At the main entry for "magnetic resonance imaging," you will be referred to the abbreviated phrase for additional listings, as indicated below:

imaging
>　magnetic resonance i. (MRI) (See MRI)

Multiple Descriptors

Often, a single medical term can be referred to in many different ways, creating a number of synonyms in medical language; for example, Addison disease, Addison syndrome, and Addison phenomenon can be used interchangeably. To avoid duplication, terms that can take multiple descriptors are listed only once in the manuscript; similar listings can be found at the main entry:

machine (*See* device, scanner, system, unit)

References

In addition to the manufacturers' literature we gather at various medical meetings, scientific reports from hospitals, and the lists of our MT Editorial Advisory Board members (from their daily transcription work), we used the following resources in the development of *Stedman's Radiology Words, Fourth Edition*.

Books

The AAMT Book of Style, 2nd Edition. Modesto, CA: AAMT, 2002.

Billups, NF. American Drug Index 2003, 47th Edition. St. Louis, Missouri: Facts & Comparisons, 2002.

Dorland's Radiology/Oncology Word Book for Medical Transcriptionists. Philadelphia: WB Saunders, 2001.

Drake E. Sloane's Medical Word Book, 4th Edition. Philadelphia: WB Saunders, 2002.

Drake E, Drake R. Drake and Drake Pharmaceutical Word Book 2002. Philadelphia: WB Saunders, 2002.

Freeman LM. Nuclear Medicine Annual 2001. Philadelphia: Lippincott Williams & Wilkins, 2001.

Kandarpa K, Aruny JE. Handbook of Interventional Radiologic Procedures, 3rd Edition. Philadelphia: Lippincott Williams & Wilkins, 2002.

Keats TE, Sistrom C. Atlas of Radiologic Measurement, 7th Edition. St. Louis, MO: Mosby, 2001.

Miller WT, Miller WT Jr. Field Guide to the Chest X-Ray. Baltimore: Lippincott Williams & Wilkins, 1999.

Silverman PM, ed. Multislice Computed Tomography: A Practical Approach to Clinical Protocols. Philadelphia: Lippincott Williams & Wilkins, 2002.

Grainger RG, Allison DJ, Adam A, Dixon AK. Grainger & Allison's Diagnostic Radiology: A Textbook of Medical Imaging, 4th Edition. Vols 1–3. London: Churchill Livingstone, 2001.

Lance LL. Quick Look Drug Book 2003. Baltimore: Lippincott Williams & Wilkins, 2003.

Stedman's Medical Dictionary, 27th Edition. Baltimore: Lippincott Williams & Wilkins, 2000.

Stedman's Radiology Words, 3rd Edition. Baltimore: Lippincott Williams & Wilkins, 2000.

Van Heertum RL, Tikofsky RS. Functional Cerebral SPECT and PET Imaging, 3rd Edition. Philadelphia: Lippincott Williams & Wilkins, 2000.

Vera Pyle's Current Medical Terminology, 8th Edition. Modesto, CA: Health Professions Institute, 2000.

Wahl RL, Buchanan JW. Principles and Practice of Positron Emission Tomography. Philadelphia: Lippincott Williams & Wilkins, 2002.

Images

Agur, AMR, Lee, MJ. *Grant's Atlas of Anatomy, 10th Edition*. Baltimore: Lippincott Williams & Wilkins, 1999.

Hardy, Neil O. Westport, CT. From *Stedman's Medical Dictionary, 27th Edition*. Baltimore: Lippincott Williams & Wilkins, 2000.

MediClip Human Anatomy 1–3, CD-ROM. Baltimore: Lippincott Williams & Wilkins.

Senkarik, Mikki. San Antonio, TX. From *Stedman's Medical Dictionary, 27th Edition*. Baltimore: Lippincott Williams & Wilkins, 2000.

Journals

American Journal of Neuroradiology. Oak Brook, IL: American Society of Neuroradiology, 2002.

American Journal of Roentgenology. Leesburg, VA: American Roentgen Ray Society, 2002.

Clinical Nuclear Medicine. Philadelphia: Lippincott Williams & Wilkins, 2001–2002.

Contemporary Diagnostic Radiology. Baltimore: Lippincott Williams & Wilkins, 2001–2002.

Investigative Radiology. Philadelphia: Lippincott Williams & Wilkins, 2001–2002.

JAAMT. Modesto, CA: American Association for Medical Transcription, 2001–2002.

Journal of Computer Assisted Tomography. Philadelphia: Lippincott Williams & Wilkins, 2001–2002.

Journal of Thoracic Imaging. Philadelphia: Lippincott Williams & Wilkins, 2001–2002.

Journal of Vascular and Interventional Radiology. Philadelphia: Lippincott Williams & Wilkins, 2001–2002.

Journal of Women's Imaging. Philadelphia: Lippincott Williams & Wilkins, 2001–2002.

Latest Word. Philadelphia: Saunders, 1999–2002.

Perspectives on the Medical Transcription Profession. Modesto, CA: Health Professions Institute, 1999–2002.

Radiographics. Oak Brook, IL: Radiological Society of North America, 2001–2002.

Radiologic Technology. Albuquerque, NM: American Society of Radiologic Technologists, 2001–2002.

The Radiologist. Philadelphia: Lippincott Williams & Wilkins, 2001–2002.

Radiology. Richmond, VA: Radiological Society of North America, Inc., 2002.

Topics in Magnetic Resonance Imaging. Philadelphia: Lippincott Williams & Wilkins, 2001–2002.

Ultrasound Quarterly. Philadelphia: Lippincott Williams & Wilkins, 2001–2002.

Websites

http://radiology.rsnajnls.org

http://www.ajnr.org

http://www.amershamhealth.com

http://www.bms.com

http://www.bracco.com

http://www.carpe-edatum.com

http://www.diagnosticimaging.com

http://www.drugs.com

http://www.egal.com

http://www.ezem.com

http://www.gemedicalsystems.com

http://www.hpisum.com/terms.html

http://www.iatrics.com

http://www.imageanalysis.com

http://www.link.springer.de

http://www.mallinckrodt.com

http://www.mtdesk.com

http://www.neurophysics.com

http://www.radiographics.org

A
    A level of the esophagus
    A point
    A ring of esophagus
    A scan
A1-A5 segments of anterior cerebral artery
AA
    acetabular anteversion
    anaplastic astrocytoma
    ascending aorta
AAA
    abdominal aortic aneurysm
AAI
    atrial inhibited
    axial acetabular index
        AAI rate-responsive mode
AAL
    anterior axillary line
AAOS acetabular abnormalities classification
Aaron sign
AAS
    acute abdominal series
AASA
    acetabular sector angle
abandonment
        mode a.
abapical pole
ABBI
    advanced breast biopsy instrumentation
        ABBI system
Abbott artery
abbreviated injury scale (AIS)
ABC
    aneurysmal bone cyst
    aortic-brachiocephalic
    argon beam coagulator
abciximab
abdomen
        distended a.
        flat plate of a.
        gasless a.
abdominal
    a. abscess
    a. adenopathy
    a. adhesion
    a. air collection
    a. aorta
    a. aorta thrombosis
    a. aortic aneurysm (AAA)
    a. aortic artery
    a. aortic coarctation
    a. aortic plexus
    a. aortography

    a. apron
    a. blunt trauma
    a. canal
    a. carcinosis
    a. cavity
    a. circumference (AC)
    a. collection of fluid
    a. compression cylinder
    a. content
    a. CT scan
    a. distention
    a. ectopic pregnancy
    a. fat
    a. fibromatosis
    a. fissure
    a. fistula
    a. fluid wave
    a. gas
    a. girth
    a. great vessel
    a. heart
    a. hemorrhage
    a. heterotaxia
    a. hysterectomy
    a. inflammation
    a. kidney
    a. left ventricular assist device (ALVAD)
    a. lymph node
    a. muscle deficiency syndrome
    a. paracentesis
    a. pseudotumor
    a. raphe
    a. ring
    a. roentgenography
    a. sac
    a. series
    a. situs inversus
    a. situs solitus
    a. sonography
    a. space
    a. splenosis
    a. stoma
    a. ultrasound
    a. vascular accident
    a. vertebra
    a. view
    a. visceral arteriography
    a. viscus
    a. wall calcification
    a. wall defect
    a. wall desmoid tumor
    a. wall hernia
abdominogenital

abdominopelvic
a. actinomycosis
a. cavity
a. mass
a. viscus
abdominoscrotal
abdominothoracic
abdominovaginal
abdominovesical
abducens
abducted and externally rotated (ABER)
abduction
a. fracture
a. position
a. stress test
abduction-external rotation fracture
abductor
a. digiti quinti (ADQ)
a. digiti quinti muscle
a. digiti quinti tendon
a. hallucis muscle
a. hallucis tendon
a. pollicis brevis (APB)
a. pollicis brevis muscle
a. pollicis brevis tendon
a. pollicis longus (APL)
a. pollicis longus tendon
abductovalgus
hallux a.
abductus
pes a.
ABE
anatomy-based extraction
ABER
abducted and externally rotated
aberrant
a. band
a. bone marrow
a. bundle
a. ganglion
a. intrahepatic bile duct
a. pancreas
a. papilla
a. right subclavian artery
a. spleen
a. tissue
a. umbilical stomach
a. vascular channel
a. venous drainage
a. vessel
aberration
chromatid-type a.
intersegmental a.
intraventricular a.
ventricular a.
ab-externo laser sclerotomy

ABI
ankle-brachial index
ability
cardiac pumping a.
ab-interno laser sclerotomy
Ablatherm HIFU system
ablation
acetic acid injectable for tumor a.
Amazr radiofrequency catheter a.
ethanol a.
image-guided radiofrequency tumor a.
laser uterosacral nerve a. (LUNA)
microwave a.
percutaneous radiofrequency catheter a.
radioactive iodine a.
radiofrequency a. (RFA)
radiofrequency catheter a. (RFCA)
radiofrequency thermal a.
radiopharmaceutical a.
saline-enhanced RF tissue a.
6-a., 14-a. scheme
small-volume tissue a.
soft tissue a.
stereotactic a.
thermal a.
total a.
transaortic radiofrequency a.
transapical endocardial a.
transcatheter a.
transseptal radiofrequency a.
transurethral needle a. (TUNA)
tumor a.
ultrasound-guided percutaneous interstitial laser a.
Urolase fiber laser a.
ablative laser therapy
abluminal
AbMap electrophysiologic imaging system
abnormal
a. adherence of placenta
a. bright signal
a. cisterna magna
a. dimensions of cardiac chamber
a. ejection fraction response
a. esophageal fold
a. esophageal peristalsis
a. heart chamber dimension
a. lung opacity
a. lung pattern
a. ossification
a. peristaltic esophagus
a. placental size
a. position of foot
a. small bowel fold

a. tissue
a. tracer accumulation
a. tracking
a. tubular function
a. umbilical cord attachment
abnormality
accumulation a.
arch of aorta a.
bony a.
bulbar a.
caliceal a.
cardiopulmonary a.
congenital a.
congruent signal intensity a.
definitive a.
drug-induced brain a.
dyskinetic segmental wall
  motion a.
facial a.
fetal a.
focal limb a.
focal metabolic a.
focal wall motion a.
focal white matter signal a.
functional a.
gestational sac a.
global wall motion a.
gray matter a.
gyral a.
high-signal a.
hyperkinetic segmental wall
  motion a.
hypokinetic segmental wall
  motion a.
ileocecal valve a.
interstitial a.
intracranial vascular a.
labeling a.
left ventricular regional wall
  motion a.
limb reduction a.
mesenchymal a.
microcirculation a.
migration a.
mucosal a.
obstructive a.
osseous a.
paraspinal a.
perfusion a.
pulmonary interstitial a.
regional perfusion a.
restrictive a.

rostrocaudal extent signal a.
screening-detected a.
segmental bronchus perfusion a.
snowman a.
soft tissue a.
spinal cord injury without
  radiographic a. (SCIWORA)
stellate a.
structural a.
subsegmental perfusion a.
torsion a.
tracer a.
ultrastructural a.
urachal a.
vascular a.
vertebral border a.
vertebral endplate a.
vessel wall a.
wall motion a. (WMA)
white matter a.
abnormally thin skull
aborad
aboral direction
abortive neurofibromatosis
above diaphragm (AD)
above-knee amputation (AKA)
above-selected threshold (AST)
ABPA
allergic bronchopulmonary aspergillosis
ABR
artery bronchus ratio
Abrahams sign
Abrams biopsy needle
abrasion
cortical a.
subperiosteal cortical a.
abrasor
Abrikosov tumor
abruption
placental a.
abrupt vessel closure
abscess
abdominal a.
actinomycotic brain a.
acute a.
anaerobic lung a.
anular a.
aortic anulus a.
appendiceal a.
Aspergillus cerebral a.
atheromatous a.
bilateral iliopsoas a.

NOTES

abscess *(continued)*
 bone a.
 brain a.
 breast a.
 Brodie metaphyseal a.
 cerebral a.
 chronic breast a.
 cold breast a.
 cold spine a.
 collar-button a.
 crypt a.
 cuff a.
 daughter a.
 deep interloop a.
 deep pelvic a.
 diverticular a.
 a. drainage catheter
 encapsulated brain a.
 enteroperitoneal a.
 epidural a.
 extradural a.
 a. formation
 frontal a.
 gallbladder wall a.
 growth plate a.
 hepatic a.
 horseshoe a.
 iliac fossa a.
 iliopsoas a.
 interloop a.
 intermesenteric a.
 intersphincteric a.
 intraabdominal a.
 intradural a.
 intrahepatic a.
 intramesenteric a.
 intraosseous a.
 intraperitoneal a.
 intrascrotal a.
 ischiorectal a.
 kidney a.
 lacunar a.
 liver a.
 lung a.
 mediastinal a.
 metaphyseal a.
 midpalmar a.
 Nocardia brain a.
 orbital a.
 ovarian a.
 Paget a.
 pancreatic a.
 paracolic a.
 parapharyngeal a.
 pararectal a.
 pararenal a.
 paraspinal a.

 parotid a.
 partial pericardial a.
 pelvic a.
 perianal a.
 periappendiceal a.
 pericecal a.
 pericholecystic a.
 pericolic a.
 pericolonic a.
 perihepatic a.
 perinephric a.
 perinephritic a.
 perirectal a.
 perirenal a.
 peritoneal a.
 pharyngeal a.
 phlegmonous a.
 postchemoembolization liver a.
 Pott a.
 premasseteric space a.
 prostate a.
 psoas a.
 pulmonary a.
 pulp a.
 pulpal a.
 pyogenic brain a.
 pyogenic liver a.
 renal a.
 retropharyngeal a.
 scrotal a.
 soft tissue a.
 space of Retzius a.
 spinal epidural a. (SEA)
 splenic a.
 sternal a.
 subaponeurotic a.
 subdiaphragmatic a.
 subdural a.
 subgaleal a.
 subhepatic a.
 subperiosteal a.
 subphrenic a.
 subungual a.
 testicular a.
 thecal a.
 thenar space a.
 thyroid a.
 tuboovarian a.
 ventral epidural a.
 walled-off a.
Abscession drainage catheter
abscessogram
abscissa
abscission needle
absconsio
abscopal effect

absence
    congenital pericardial a.
    a. of haustral marking
    a. of innominate line
    limb a.
    a. of outer end of clavicle
    partial pericardial a.
    a. of primary peristalsis
    a. seizure
    a. of spleen
    a. of uptake
    a. of vascular marking

absent
    a. aortic knob
    a. bow-tie sign
    a. bronchial cartilage
    a. diaphragm sign
    a. greater sphenoid wing
    a. kidney
    a. kidney outline
    a. lower esophageal sphincter
    relaxation
    a. peripheral vein
    a. peristalsis
    a. radiotracer uptake
    a. runoff
    a. valve
    a. ventricle

absolute
    a. artery dimension
    a. blood flow
    a. curative resection
    a. dose intensity (ADI)
    a. efficiency
    a. emission probability
    a. granulocyte count
    a. linearity
    a. noncurative resection

absolute-peak efficiency calibration
absorbance
absorbed
    a. dose (AD)
    a. dose range
    a. fraction

absorbent
    a. gland
    a. vessel

absorptiometer
    single-energy x-ray a. (SXA)
absorptiometry
    dual-energy x-ray a. (DEXA,
    DXA)
    dual-photon a. (DPA)
    morphometric x-ray a.
    single-photon a. (SPA)

absorption
    a. atelectasis
    bone radiation a.
    broad-beam a.
    a. cavity
    a. coefficient
    electromagnetic a.
    external a.
    interstitial a.
    laser energy a.
    a. line
    photoelectric a.
    radiofrequency a.
    radioiron oral a.
    a. of radionuclide
    ratio of photoelectric to
        Compton a.
    a. spectrophotometer
    a. unsharpness
    a. x-ray spectrum

abut
abutment
abutting
AC
    abdominal circumference
    acromioclavicular
    alcoholic cirrhosis
    anterior commissure
    aortic closure
    AC 3 plate reader

ACA
    anterior cerebral artery
ACAD
    atherosclerotic carotid artery disease
acalculia
acalculous cholecystitis
acallosal
acanthiomeatal line
acanthocytosis
acantholysis
acanthopelvis
acanthopelyx, acanthopelvis
acanthosis
    glycogenic a.
    a. nigricans
acanthotic
acardia
ACAT
    automated computed axial tomography

NOTES

ACBE
    air-contrast barium enema
accelerated
    a. atherosclerosis
    a. fractionation
    a. particle
    a. peristalsis
    a. phase
    a. phase gain
    a. silicosis
acceleration
    fetal growth a.
    flow a.
    growth a.
    a. index (AI)
    a. map
    a. time (AT)
accelerator
    alpha particle a.
    dual-energy linear a.
    electron linear a.
    a. factor
    high-energy bent-beam linear a.
    linear a. (LINAC)
    a. mass spectrometry (AMS)
    Microtron a.
    modified linear a.
    particle a.
    Philips linear a.
    racetrack microtron a.
    Siemens Mevatron 74 linear a.
    University of Florida linear a.
    Varian a.
Accel stopcock
accentuation
    a. of marking
    paramagnetic enhancement a.
access
    arterial a.
    central venous a.
    femoral a.
    jugular venous a.
    a. loop
    a. set
accessory
    a. adhesion molecule
    a. atlantoaxial ligament
    a. atrium
    BabyFace 3D surface rendering a.
    a. blood supply
    a. breast
    a. canal
    a. cephalic vein
    a. communicating tendon
    a. cusp
    a. diaphragm
    a. digit

    extravasation detection a.
    a. fissure
    a. hemiazygos vein
    a. hemidiaphragm
    a. hepatic duct
    a. hepatic vein
    a. lobe
    a. lymph node
    a. middle cerebral artery
    a. multangular bone
    a. muscle
    a. nasal cartilage
    a. navicular bone
    a. nerve
    a. organ
    a. ossicle
    a. ossification center
    a. pancreas
    a. pancreatic duct
    a. placenta
    a. process
    a. right renal artery
    a. right uterine artery
    a. saphenous vein
    a. sesamoid bone
    a. sign colon
    a. sinus
    a. spleen
    a. thyroid gland
    a. tubercle
    a. ureteral bud
    a. vertebral vein
accident
    abdominal vascular a.
    cardiovascular a. (CVA)
    cerebrovascular a. (CVA)
accidental
    a. correction
    a. intradural injection
accompanying vein
accordion
    a. fold
    a. sign
    a. vertebra
accordion-shaped pleat
accreta
    placenta a.
Accuclot D-dimer assay
Accucore II biopsy needle
accuDEXA
    a. bone densitometer
    a. bone mineral density assessment
      system
AccuLase excimer laser
accumulation
    a. abnormality
    abnormal tracer a.

dependent extracellular fluid a.
fluid a.
a. of gas
intratumoral a.
nonspecific a.
parenchymal tracer a.
a. phase
radiotracer a.
residual urine a.
Thorotrast a.
tracer a.
AccuProbe
accuracy calibrator
AccuView computer workstation
ACD
annihilation coincidence detection
anterior capsular distance
ACE
angiotensin-converting enzyme
ACE inhibition renography
ACE inhibition scintigraphy
acervuloma
acetabula (*pl. of* acetabulum)
acetabular
a. anteversion (AA)
a. bone
a. cavity
a. cup
a. depth
a. depth-to-femoral head diameter
(AD/FHD)
a. fossa
a. head index (AHI)
a. index
a. labrum
a. line
a. posterior wall fracture
a. protrusion
a. reconstruction plate
a. residual dysplasia
a. rim fracture
a. roof
a. sector angle (AASA)
a. shell
acetabular-prosthetic interface
acetabulum, pl. **acetabula**
cartilaginous a.
deep-shelled a.
os a.
Y-shaped a.
acetazolamide
a. challenge brain SPECT imaging

a. dual-isotope image
a. renography
a. vasodilator test
acetazolamide-enhanced SPECT
**acetic acid injectable for tumor
ablation**
acetrizoate
meglumine a.
a. sodium
Acetrizoate contrast agent
acetylated
acetylation
acetylator
ACF
anterior cervical fusion
ACG
angiocardiogram
angiocardiography
apex cardiogram
achalasia
cricopharyngeal a.
a. of esophagus
megaesophagus of a.
primary a.
secondary a.
ureteral a.
vigorous a.
acheiria
achievable
as low as reasonably a. (ALARA)
Achiever balloon dilatation catheter
Achilles
A. bursa
A. densitometer
A. tendon
A. tendon rupture
A. tendon shortening
A. tendon xanthoma
acholangic biliary cirrhosis
achondrogenesis
achondroplasia
achondroplastic dwarfism
achoresis
acid
ametriodinic a.
amidotrizoic a.
benzoic a.
chenodeoxycholic a.
deoxyribonucleic a. (DNA)
diethylenetriaminepentaacetic a.
(DTPA)
dimer captosuccinic a. (DMSA)

NOTES

acid *(continued)*
  dimethyl iminodiacetic a. (DIDA)
  dimethylsuccinic a.
  ethylenediamine tetramethylene
    phosphonic a. (EDTMP)
  ^{18}F-fluoro-6-thia-heptadecanoic a.
    (FTHA)
  ^{18}F-labeled fatty a.
  flavone acetic a. (FAA)
  free fatty a. (FFA)
  gadolinium diethylenetriamine
    pentaacetic a. (Gd-DTPA)
  gadolinium
    tetraazacyclododecanetetraacetic a.
    (Gd-DOTA)
  gadopentetic a.
  gadoxetic a. (Gd-EOB-DTPA)
  gamma-aminobutyric a. (GABA)
  glucoheptonate a. (GHA)
  hepatoiminodiacetic a. (HIDA)
  homovanillic a. (HVA)
  hydroxyethylidene-1,1-
    diphosphonic a. (HEDP)
  5-hydroxyindoleacetic a. (5-HIAA)
  ^{123}I heptadecanoic a.
  iobenzamic a.
  iocarmic a.
  iocetamic a.
  iodine-123 iodophenyl
    pentadecanoic a. (IPPA)
  iodoalphionic a.
  iodopanoic a.
  iodophenyl pentadecanoic a. (IPPA)
  iopanoic a.
  iothalamic a.
  ioxaglic a.
  long-chain fatty a.
  low-dose folic a.
  meclofenamic a.
  mefenamic a.
  metrizoic a.
  nonesterified fatty a. (NEFA)
  okadaic a.
  ophenoxic a.
  palmitic a.
  paraaminobenzoic a.
  paraaminohippuric a.
  paraaminosalicylic a. (PAS)
  para-isopropyl-iminodiacetic a.
    (PIPIDA)
  a. peptic ulcer
  phenoxyacetic a.
  polylactic a. (PLA)
  a. reflux
  ribonucleic a. (RNA)
  ^{99m}Tc-labeled iminodiacetic a.
  technetium-99m diethylenetriamine
    pentaacetic a. (^{99m}Tc-DTPA)
  technetium-99m dimer
    captosuccinic a.
  tetraazacyclododecanetetraacetic a.
    (DOTA)
  trichloroacetic a.
  triiodobenzoic a.
  (V)-dimer captosuccinic a. (DMSA)
acidophilic
  a. adenoma
  a. pituitary tumor
acid-Schiff-positive
acinar
  a. adenocarcinoma
  a. collapse
  a. nodule
  a. pancreatic cell carcinoma
  a. pattern
  a. sarcoidosis
  a. tuberculosis
acinarization
acini (*pl. of* acinus)
acinic
  a. cell adenocarcinoma
  a. cell carcinoma
  a. cell tumor
acinous adenoma
acinus, pl. acini
ACIS
  automated cellular imaging system
ACIST contrast delivery injection
  system
Ackerman criteria for osteomyelitis
Ackrad balloon-bearing catheter
ACL
  anterior cruciate ligament
aclasis
  diaphyseal a.
  tarsoepiphyseal a.
ACM
  automated cardiac flow measurement
  ACM ultrasound
ACoA, AcomA
  anterior communicating artery
Acoma portable x-ray machine
acoprosis
acoustic
  a. artifact
  a. canal
  a. crest
  a. cyst
  a. enhancement
  a. gel
  a. imaging
  a. impedance
  a. interface

a. lens
a. meatus
a. nerve
a. nerve sheath tumor
a. neuroma
a. papilla
a. penetration
a. pressure
a. pressure amplitude
a. quantification
a. reflection method
a. response technology
a. schwannoma
a. shadow
a. trauma
a. tubercle
a. velocity
a. vesicle
a. wave
a. window

acousticofacial
a. crest
a. ganglion

AC-PC
anterior commissure-posterior
commissure
AC-PC line
AC-PC plane

ACPL
antibody-conjugated paramagnetic
liposome

AcQsim CT simulator

acquired
a. acroosteolysis
a. adult Fanconi syndrome
a. aortic valve stenosis
a. atelectasis
a. bronchiectasis
a. cystic kidney disease
a. epidermoid
a. fragility
a. hepatic cyst
a. hepatocerebral degeneration
a. hydrocephalus
a. immunodeficiency syndrome
(AIDS)
a. intestinal lymphangiectasis
a. left ventricle aneurysm
a. megacolon
a. mitral stenosis
a. occupational lung disease
a. porencephaly

a. radiation resistance
a. renal cystic disease
a. spinal stenosis
a. tracheobronchomalacia
a. unilateral hyperlucent lung
a. urethral diverticulum

acquisition
alternated delay a. (ADA)
biphasic a.
cine a.
combined dynamic 2D and bolus-
chase 3D a.'s
continuous volumetric a.
data a.
3D fast low-angle shot a.
2D fast spin-echo a.
3D fast spin-echo a.
3D FLASH a.
double-helix a.
dynamic a.
electronic picture a.
elliptical centric a.
fast spin-echo a.
first-pass a.
FLASH a.
four-slice a.
gradient a.
image a.
interleaved image a.
long axis a.
a. matrix
multiple gated a. (MUGA)
multiple overlapping thin-slab a.
(MOTSA)
multiple slice a.
multiple thin slab a. (MTSA)
multisection multirepetition a.
multislice a.
off-axis rotational a.
a. optimization
polarity-altered spectral-selective a.
primary digital a.
reduced a.
segmented k-space data a.
sequential image a.
short axis a.
signal a.
simultaneous multislice a.
small-voxel a.
spirometric a.
a. technique
a. time

NOTES

acquisition *(continued)*
    T1-weighted a.
    volume a.
    volumetric a.
    whole-brain a.
    a. window
ACR
    ACR rate
    ACR teleradiology standard
acrania
Acrel ganglion
acridine orange
acrocephalosyndactyly,
  acrocephalosyndactylia
    Pfeiffer a.
    Saethre-Chotzen a.
acrodermatitis enteropathica
acrodysostosis
acrofacial
acrokeratosis
acromegaly
acromelia
acromelic
    a. dwarfism
    a. dysplasia
acromesomelic dysplasia
acromial
    a. angle
    a. articular surface
    a. bone
    a. slope
    a. spur
acromiale
    os a.
acromicria
acromioclavicular (AC)
    a. articulation
    a. injury classification
    a. joint
    a. joint disk
    a. joint separation
    a. ligament
    a. space
acromiocoracoid ligament
acromiohumeral
    a. distance
    a. interval (AHI)
acromion
    hooked a.
    a. process
acromutilation
acroosteolysis
    acquired a.
acroosteosclerosis
acropachy
    thyroid a.
acropachyderma

acropectorovertebral dysplasia
acrosomal vesicle
acrosyndactyly
acrylic
    a. microsphere
    a. syringe shield
ACS
    ACS balloon catheter
    ACS OTW Photon coronary
      dilatation catheter
ACS-grade pyridine
ACS-NT
    Gyroscan A.-N.
ACTH-producing tumor
actinic
    a. granuloma
    a. ray
    a. reticuloid
actinium emanation
actinomycetes
    thermophilic a.
actinomycosis
    abdominopelvic a.
    retroperitoneal a.
actinomycotic brain abscess
action
    phase-specific a.
    a. space
activated
    a. atom
    a. partial thromboplastin time
    a. voxel cluster
activation
    a. analysis
    compensatory cortical a.
    a. factor
    a. pattern
    PMC a.
    premotor coret a.
    region of a.
activation-induced uncoupling of
  cerebral oxygen
activation-sequence mapping
activator
    alteplase recombinant tissue
      plasminogen a.
    recombinant tissue plasminogen a.
    tissue-type plasminogen a.
active
    a. biplanar MR imaging guidance
    a. congestion
    a. duodenal ulcer
    a. emptying fraction
    a. hyperemia
    a. infiltrate
    a. mode
    a. osteomyelitis

a. parenchymal disease
a. precordium
a. shielding
a. shimming

activity

a. assessment
background a.
biliary excretion bowel a.
blood pool a.
body background a.
bone morphogenetic a.
brain a.
colonic a.
cortical a.
crossover of a.
decreased a.
dihydropyrimidine dehydrogenase a.
electrical a.
extrapulmonary a.
increased tracer a.
lung/heart ratio of thallium 201 a.
mast cell-enhancing a.
normalized to plasma a.
osseous a.
osteoblastic a.
peak parenchymal a.
peristaltic a.
physiologic high a.
problematic abdominal a.
radiotracer a.
reflux a.
retained cortical a. (RCA)
scatter a.
slow-wave a.
specific a.
time-to-peak a.
tracer a.
ventricular ectopic a. (VEA)

actuator

linear a.

AcuNav ultrasound catheter
acupuncture laser
Acuson

A. 128 apparatus
A. computed sonography
A. 128 Doppler ultrasound
A. 128EP imager
A. 128EP scanner
A. linear array transducer
A. 5-MHz linear array
A. transvaginal sonography

A. V5M multiplane transesophageal echocardiographic transducer
A. XP 10 scanner
A. 128 XP transducer
A. 128XP ultrasound system

acute

a. abdominal obstruction
a. abdominal series (AAS)
a. abscess
a. alveolar hypoperfusion
a. alveolar infiltrate
a. aortic pathology
a. atelectasis
a. avulsion fracture
a. berylliosis
a. central cord syndrome
a. cerebellar hemispheric lesion
a. cerebral infarct imaging
a. cerebrovascular insufficiency
a. chest syndrome
a. cholecystitis
a. compartment syndrome
a. compression triad
a. coronary insufficiency
a. cortical necrosis
a. diffuse bacterial nephritis
a. diffuse interstitial fibrosis
a. disseminated encephalomyelitis (ADEM)
a. diverticulitis
a. eosinophilic pneumonia
a. erosive gastritis (AEG)
a. esophagitis
a. extrinsic allergic alveolitis
a. focal bacterial nephritis
a. glomerulonephritis
a. heart failure
a. hematogenous osteomyelitis (AHO)
a. hemodynamic overload
a. hemorrhagic leukoencephalitis
a. hepatitis
a. hydrocephalus
a. hydronephrosis
a. interstitial lung edema
a. interstitial nephritis (AIN)
a. interstitial pneumonia (AIP)
a. interstitial pneumonitis
a. intramural hematoma
a. ischemic brain infarct
a. juvenile cirrhosis
a. lethal carditis

NOTES

acute *(continued)*
- a. lymphoblastic lymphoma
- a. lymphocytic leukemia
- a. marginal branch
- a. mediastinal widening
- a. mesenteric ischemia
- a. myelofibrosis
- a. myeloid leukemia
- a. myocardial infarct
- a. native kidney tubular necrosis
- a. nonhemorrhagic infarct
- a. nonsuppurative ascending cholangitis
- a. obstructive cholangitis
- a. on chronic fracture
- a. pancreatitis
- a. peptic ulcer
- a. phase of inflammation
- a. pleurisy
- a. posttraumatic myelopathy
- a. pulmonary edema
- a. radiation injury
- a. radiation pneumonitis
- a. radiation syndrome
- a. renal failure (ARF)
- a. renal infarct
- a. renal transplant tubular necrosis
- a. renal vein thrombosis
- a. respiratory distress syndrome (ARDS)
- a. respiratory failure (ARF)
- a. retroviral syndrome
- a. sclerosing hyaline necrosis (ASHN)
- a. silicoproteinosis
- a. sinusitis
- a. splenic tumor
- a. sprain
- a. stretch injury
- a. subarachnoid hemorrhage
- a. subdural hematoma
- a. suppurative ascending cholangitis
- a. suppurative pyelonephritis
- a. suppurative sialadenitis
- a. suppurative thyroiditis
- a. testicular torsion
- a. thromboembolic pulmonary arterial hypertension
- a. transverse myelitis
- a. traumatic aortic injury (ATAI)
- a. tubular necrosis (ATN)
- a. vertebral collapse

AcuTect imaging agent
acutely symptomatic scrotum
ACV
- adaptive cardio volume
- ACV reconstruction

acyanotic congenital heart disease
AD
- above diaphragm
- absorbed dose
- Alzheimer disease
- aortic diameter

ADA
- alternated delay acquisition

ADAC MCD Vertex Plus MCD gamma camera
adactyly, adactylia
adamantinoma of long bone
adamantinomatous craniopharyngioma
Adamkiewicz
- arteria radicularis magna of A.
- A. artery

Adams-Stokes syndrome
adapted standard mammography unit
adapter
- ventricle impedance a.
- VIA 7991 ventricle impedance a.

adaptic detector configuration
adaptive
- a. cardiac volume reconstruction
- a. cardio volume (ACV)
- a. carpus
- a. correction
- a. focusing technology (AFT)
- a. hyperplasia
- a. hypertrophy

ADC
- apparent diffusion coefficient
- ADC decline
- ADC map
- ADC quantization error

ADCav value
Addison
- A. disease
- A. point

add-on
- A.-o. Bucky direct x-ray detector
- A.-o. Bucky image acquisition system
- A.-o. Bucky radiographer detector image
- a.-o. stereotactic unit
- a.-o. technique

adducted thumb
adduction
- a. fracture
- a. frame
- a. to neutral
- a. position
- a. stress

adductor
- a. canal
- a. hallucis

a. hallucis tendon
a. hiatus
a. insertion avulsion syndrome
a. longus
a. magnus
a. magnus muscle
a. muscle strain
a. pollicis
a. pollicis brevis tendon
a. sweep of thumb
a. tubercle
adductus
metatarsus a.
pes a.
true metatarsus a. (TMA)
ADEM
acute disseminated encephalomyelitis
adenitis
cervical lymph node tuberculous a.
mesenteric a.
sclerosing a.
adenoacanthoma
endometrial a.
adenocarcinoma
acinar a.
acinic cell a.
ampullary a.
bronchiolar a.
cervical a.
colloid a.
cystic a.
distal rectal a. (DRA)
ductal pancreatic a.
duct cell a.
duodenal a.
endometrial secretory a.
exophytic a.
gastrointestinal tract a.
giant cell a.
hepatoid a.
infiltrating a.
intraluminal a.
kidney a.
lung a.
medullary-type a.
metastatic a.
mucinous a.
mucin-producing a.
nonmucinous a.
pancreatic ductal a.
papillary serous a.
poorly differentiated a. (PDA)

renal a.
scirrhous infiltrating a.
secretory a.
serous a.
a. in situ
small bowel a.
stomach a.
ulcerating a.
urinary bladder a.
a. of uterus
vulvar adenoid cystic a.
adenocystic carcinoma
adenofibroma
adenofibromyoma
adenography
adenohypophyseal
adenohypophysis
adenoid
a. cystic carcinoma parotitis
a. cystic lung carcinoma
a. squamous cell carcinoma
a. tonsil
a. tumor
adenoidal-nasopharyngeal ratio (AN)
adenoleiomyofibroma
adenolipoma
adenolymphoma
adenoma
acidophilic a.
acinous a.
adnexal a.
adrenal a.
adrenocortical a.
apocrine a.
autonomous thyroid a.
basal cell a.
basophilic brain a.
benign oxyphilic a.
bile duct a. (BDA)
a. of breast
bronchial a.
bronchoalveolar cell a.
bronchogenic a.
Brunner gland a.
carcinoma ex pleomorphic a.
carotid sheath a.
colloid a.
colonic a.
colorectal a.
cortical a.
cutaneous a.
cystic a.

NOTES

adenoma *(continued)*
 ductal a.
 ectopic parathyroid a.
 embryonal a.
 eosinophilic brain a.
 fetal a.
 fibroid a.
 a. fibrosum
 flat a.
 follicular thyroid a.
 Fuchs a.
 functioning pituitary a.
 gallbladder a.
 giant villous a.
 glycoprotein-secreting a.
 gonadotroph cell a.
 gonadotropin-secreting a.
 growth hormone-producing a.
 hepatic a.
 hepatocellular a.
 Hürthle cell a.
 intraspinal a.
 kidney a.
 lactating a.
 Leydig cell a.
 liver cell a.
 macrocystic a.
 malignant pleomorphic a.
 a. malignum
 mediastinal a.
 microcystic a.
 mucinous a.
 multifocal autonomic a.
 nephrogenic bladder a.
 a. of nipple
 nonfunctioning pituitary a.
 nonhyperfunctioning adrenal a.
 oncocytic thyroid a.
 oxyphilic a.
 pancreatic macrocystic a.
 pancreatic microcystic a.
 papillary cystic a.
 parathyroid a. (PA)
 parotid pleomorphic a.
 Pick tubular a.
 pituitary a.
 pleomorphic lung a.
 polypoid a.
 prostatic a.
 proximal tubular a.
 renal cortical a.
 retrotracheal a.
 sebaceous a.
 a. sebaceum
 sessile a.
 small bowel a.
 solitary a.

 suprasellar a.
 sweat duct a.
 testicular tubular a.
 thyroid a.
 thyrotroph cell a.
 toxic a.
 tubulovillous colon a.
 villotubular a.
 villous a.
 well-differentiated a.
adenoma-associated calcification
adenomatoid
 a. malformation
 a. odontogenic tumor
adenomatosis
adenomatous
 a. goiter
 a. hyperplasia
 a. polyp (AP)
adenomyoma
adenomyomatosis
adenomyosarcoma
adenomyosis
 diffuse a.
 ureteral a.
 uterine a.
adenopapillomatosis
 gastric a.
adenopathy
 abdominal a.
 axillary a.
 bilateral hilar a.
 cervical a.
 hemorrhagic mediastinal a.
 hilar a.
 mediastinal a.
 mesenteric a.
 metastatic a.
 paratracheal a.
 postinflammatory a.
 pulmonary a.
 reticulation with hilar a.
 retrocrural a.
 retroperitoneal a.
 sandwich configuration a.
 secondary axillary a.
 thoracic a.
 tuberculous mediastinal a.
 widespread hyperattenuating
  mediastinal a.
adenosarcoma
 breast a.
Adenoscan imaging agent
adenosine
 echocardiogram a.
 a. echocardiography
 a. stress imaging

a. stress imaging agent
a. triphosphate
adenosis
breast a.
microglandular a.
radiation-induced sclerosing a.
sclerosing a.
adenovirus pneumonia
adequate
a. cardiac output
a. contention
a. coronary perfusion
a. stroke volume
AD/FHD
acetabular depth-to-femoral head
diameter
adherence factor
adherent
a. pericardium
a. placenta
a. profundus tendon
a. thrombus
adhesed
adhesion
abdominal a.
attic a.
band-like a.
fibrous pleural a.
inflammatory a.
intraarticular a.
pericardial diaphragmatic a.
peritendinous a.
pleuropericardial a.
pleuropulmonary a.
subacromial bursal a.
subdeltoid bursal a.
adhesive
a. arachnoiditis
a. atelectasis
a. capsulitis
a. ileus
a. inflammation
a. platelet
tissue a.
ADI
absolute dose intensity
atlantodens interval
adiabatic
a. demagnetization
a. demagnetization in the rotating
frame (ADRF)
a. fast passage (AFP)

a. fast scanning technique
a. off-resonance spin locking
a. rapid passage (ARP)
a. slice-selective radiofrequency
pulse
adiadochokinesia
adipiodone
adipose
a. fold
a. fossa
a. ligament
a. tissue
a. tumor
adiposogenital dystrophy
aditus
a. ad antrum
a. pelvis
adjacent
a. edema
a. field x-ray dosimetry
a. organ
a. voxel
adjunctive therapy
adjustment
Bonferroni a.
adjuvant
a. analgesic drug
a. chronotherapy
a. radiation
a. therapy
adjuvanticity
admaxillary gland
admedial
admedian
administration
competitive iron a.
contrast a.
drug a.
intralymphatic radioactivity a.
intraperitoneal drug a.
vasodilator a.
admixture lesion
adnexa
ocular a.
transposed a.
adnexal
a. adenoma
a. carcinoma
a. condition
a. cyst
a. embryo

NOTES

adnexal *(continued)*
   a. metastasis
   a. torsion
adolescent
   a. hallux valgus
   a. idiopathic scoliosis (AIS)
ADPKD
   autosomal dominant polycystic kidney
   disease
ADQ
   abductor digiti quinti
adrenal
   a. adenoma
   a. angiography
   a. artery
   bilateral large a.
   a. calcification
   a. capsule
   a. carcinoma
   a. cortex
   a. cyst
   a. cystic mass
   a. failure
   a. ganglioneuroma
   a. gland
   a. hematoma
   a. hemorrhage
   a. hyperplasia
   a. imaging
   a. incidentaloma
   a. insufficiency
   a. lesion
   a. medulla
   a. medullary disease
   a. metastasis
   a. myelolipoma
   a. neuroblastoma
   a. paraganglioma
   a. pheochromocytoma
   a. pseudocyst
   a. scan
   a. scintigraphy
   a. tuberculosis
   a. tumor
   a. vein
   a. venography
adrenal-to-spleen ratio (ASR)
adrenocortical
   a. adenoma
   a. carcinoma
   a. hyperfunction
   a. hyperplasia
   a. macrocyst
   a. neoplasm
   a. secretion
   a. tumor
adrenocorticotropin microadenoma

adrenogenital syndrome
adrenogram
adrenoleukodystrophy
adrenoleukodystrophy-
   adrenomyeloneuropathy (ALD-AMN)
ADRF
   adiabatic demagnetization in the rotating
   frame
Adrian-Crooks cassette
ADR Ultramark 4 ultrasound
Adson maneuver
adsorption
   competitive a.
adsternal
adult
   a. coarctation
   a. dose
   a. polycystic kidney disease
   a. progeria
   a. respiratory distress syndrome
   (ARDS)
   a. T-cell lymphoma
adult-type III TIE fracture
adumbration
advanced
   a. breast biopsy instrumentation
   (ABBI)
   a. cardiac mapping
   a. multiple-beam equalization
   radiography (AMBER)
   A. NMR Systems scanner
   a. real-time motion analysis
   (ARTMA)
   a. vessel analysis (AVA)
advancement
   frontoorbital a.
   vastus medialis a. (VMA)
Advantage Workstation 3.1
AdvanTeq II TENS unit
Advantx-E Legacy system
Advantx LC+ cardiovascular imaging
   system
adventitia of artery
adventitial
   a. fibroplasia
   a. tissue
adventitious bursa
adverse effect
adynamic
   a. ileus
   a. intestinal obstruction
adynamic/paralytic ileus
AE amputation
Aeby
   A. muscle
   A. plane

AEC
> automatic exposure control
> AEC technique

AEG
> acute erosive gastritis

AEGIS sonography management system

AER
> apical ectodermal ridge

aerated tissue

aeration
> regional differences in a.

aerobilia

aerocele

AeroChamber

aerodigestive
> a. carcinoma
> a. fistula
> a. tract

aerophagia

aerosol
> radioactive a.
> technetium-99m DTPA a.
> a. ventilation scan

aerosolized
> a. ^{99m}Tc DTPA imaging agent

AESOP
> automatic endoscopic system for optimal
> positioning
> AESOP Hermes-Ready system

Aestiva/5 MRI anesthesia machine

AF
> amnionic fluid
> aortic flow
> arcuate fasciculus

A-FAIR
> arrhythmia-insensitive flow-sensitive
> alternating inversion recovery
> A-FAIR imaging

AFBG
> aortofemoral bypass graft

affect
> pseudobulbar a.

afferent
> a. digital nerve
> a. loop
> a. loop syndrome
> a. lymph vessel
> a. nerve lesion
> a. view

AFI
> amnionic fluid index

AFP
> adiabatic fast passage

African
> A. Burkitt lymphoma
> A. Kaposi sarcoma

AFROC
> alternative-free response receiver
> operating characteristic

AFT
> adaptive focusing technology

afterglow

afterload
> increased ventricular a.
> left ventricular a.

afterloader
> Fletcher a.
> Henschke a.
> ^{192}I high-dose-rate remote a.
> Nucletron MicroSelectron/LDR
> remote a.

afterloading
> a. brachytherapy
> high-dose-rate remote a.
> a. radiation
> a. tandem and ovoid
> a. technique

AG
> angular gyrus

aganglionic
> a. bowel
> a. megacolon
> a. segment

aganglionosis
> skip a.

Agatston
> A. calcium scoring method
> A. score

AGC
> anatomically graduated component

AGE
> angle of greatest extension

age
> anatomical a.
> biologic a.
> bone a. (BA)
> chronologic a.
> delayed bone a.
> fetal a.
> gestational a. (GA)
> indeterminate a.
> large for gestational a.

age-indeterminate infarct

NOTES

agenesis
> Bayne classification of radial a.
> callosal a.
> corpus callosum a.
> gallbladder a.
> liver a.
> lumbosacral a.
> lung a.
> partial corpus callosum a.
> pulmonary artery a.
> renal a.
> sacral a.
> thymic a.
> unilateral pulmonary a.
> uterine a.
> vaginal a.
> vermian a.

agenetic
> a. fracture
> a. porencephaly

agent (*See* contrast, material, medium)
> ^{18}F estradiol imaging a.
> ^{18}F fludeoxyglucose imaging a.
> ^{18}F fluorodeoxyglucose imaging a.
> ^{18}F fluoro-DOPA imaging a.
> ^{18}F fluoroisonidazole imaging a.
> ^{18}F fluorotamoxifen imaging a.
> ^{18}F L-DOPA imaging a.
> ^{18}F N-methylspiperone imaging a.
> ^{18}F spiperone imaging a.
> Acetrizoate contrast a.
> AcuTect imaging a.
> Adenoscan imaging a.
> adenosine stress imaging a.
> aerosolized ^{99m}Tc DTPA imaging a.
> air imaging a.
> Altropane radioimaging a.
> AMI 121, 227 contrast a.
> amidotrizoic acid contrast a.
> Amipaque imaging a.
> Amiscan imaging a.
> Angio-Conray imaging a.
> Angiografin imaging a.
> AngioMARK contrast a.
> antifibrin antibody imaging a.
> antimyosin monoclonal antibody imaging a.
> Apomate radiopharmaceutical imaging a.
> baby formula with ferrous sulfate contrast a.
> Baricon imaging a.
> barium sulfate imaging a.
> Baro-CAT imaging a.
> Barosperse imaging a.
> benzamide imaging a.
> Biliscopin imaging a.

> Bilopaque imaging a.
> Biloptin imaging a.
> bioreductive a.
> bis-Gd-MP imaging a.
> blood oxygenation level-dependent contrast a.
> blood pool contrast a.
> bone marrow a.
> bromodeoxyuridine imaging a.
> bromophenol blue imaging a.
> ^{45}Ca imaging a.
> ^{11}C acetate imaging a.
> calcium-45 imaging a.
> calcium ipodate imaging a.
> carbon imaging a.
> Cardiolite imaging a.
> cardioselective a.
> ^{11}C butanol imaging a.
> ^{11}C carfentanil imaging a.
> CEA-Scan imaging a.
> Ceretec radioisotope imaging a.
> cerium silicate imaging a.
> cesium chloride imaging a.
> ^{11}C flumazenil imaging a.
> CheeTah radiopaque contrast a.
> chelating a.
> Cholebrine imaging a.
> Choletec radionuclide imaging a.
> Cholografin meglumine imaging a.
> chromated ^{51}Cr serum albumin imaging a.
> chromium imaging a.
> ^{11}C imaging a.
> ^{11}C-labeled cocaine imaging a.
> ^{11}C-labeled fatty acid imaging a.
> Clariscan imaging a.
> ^{11}C N-methylspiperone imaging a.
> ^{11}C nomifensine imaging a.
> Combidex MRI contrast a.
> CO_2-negative imaging a.
> Conray 30, 43, 400 imaging a.
> contrast a.
> copper imaging a.
> copper-zinc superoxide dismutase imaging a.
> ^{11}C raclopride imaging a.
> ^{11}C thymidine imaging a.
> ^{64}Cu imaging a.
> ^{67}Cu imaging a.
> ^{62}Cu PTSM imaging a.
> ^{64}CU-TETA-octreotide imaging a.
> Cu/Zn-SOD imaging a.
> cyanoacrylate imaging a.
> cyanocobalamin imaging a.
> Cysto-Conray II imaging a.
> Cystografin-Dilute imaging a.
> DaTSCAN imaging a.

denatured ^{99m}Tc-RBC imaging a.
a. detection imaging
deuterium imaging a.
dextrose 5% in water imaging a.
d,1-HMPAO imaging a.
diatrizoate meglumine imaging a.
diatrizoate sodium imaging a.
diethylenetriaminepentaacetic acid
  imaging a.
Digibar 190 contrast a.
dihydroxyphenylalanine imaging a.
Dionosil imaging a.
dispersing a.
dodecafluoropentane imaging a.
DOPA imaging a.
Dopascan radiopharmaceutical
  imaging a.
DTPA imaging a.
Dy-DTPA-BMA imaging a.
dysprosium HP-DO3A imaging a.
echo contrast a.
echo-enhancing a.
EchoGen ultrasound imaging a.
Echovist imaging a.
EDTMP imaging a.
effervescent a.
Eovist contrast a.
Ethiodol imaging a.
etidronate disodium imaging a.
Evans blue imaging a.
exametazime imaging a.
extracellular contrast a.
extravasated contrast a.
extravasation of contrast a.
E-Z Cat Dry contrast a.
Feridex IV MRI contrast a.
ferucarbotran MR imaging a.
feruglose contrast a.
ferumoxide imaging a.
ferumoxsil imaging a.
ferumoxtran imaging a.
Fibrimage diagnostic imaging a.
fluorine imaging a.
fluorocarbon-based ultrasound
  contrast a.
fluorodeoxyglucose imaging a.
^{18}F sodium fluoride imaging a.
FS-069 sterile injectable sonography
  contrast a.
furosemide imaging a.
gadobenic acid imaging a.
gadobutrol imaging a.

gadodiamide imaging a.
gadofosveset trisodium imaging a.
gadolinium-based contrast a.
gadolinium chelate imaging a.
gadolinium oxide imaging a.
Gadolite oral suspension contrast a.
gadopentetate contrast a.
gadopentetate dimeglumine
  imaging a.
gadoterate meglumine imaging a.
gadoteridol imaging a.
gadoversetamide imaging a.
gallium imaging a.
gallium-67 tumor imaging a.
Gastrografin imaging a.
GastroMARK oral imaging a.
Gastroview imaging a.
Gastrovist imaging a.
Gd-BOPTA/Dimeg imaging a.
Gd-BOPTA imaging a.
    gadobenate dimeglumine
Gd-DTPA PGTM imaging a.
Gd-DTPA with mannitol contrast a.
Gd-enhanced imaging a.
Gd-EOB-DTPA imaging a.
Gd-HP-DO3A imaging a.
Gd-153 imaging a.
glomerular filtration a.
glucagon imaging a.
glucarate imaging a.
gold AU-198 imaging a.
GSA imaging a.
hand-agitated imaging a.
hematoporphyrin derivative
  photosensitizing a. (HpD)
hepatobiliary contrast a.
Hepatolite imaging a.
Hexabrix imaging a.
high-density barium imaging a.
high-osmolar contrast a. (HOCA)
Hippuran imaging a.
Histoacryl embolic a.
holmium imaging a.
human serum albumin imaging a.
HumaSPECT imaging a.
hybrid MRI imaging a.
hydrogen peroxide imaging a.
hydrophilic contrast a.
hydrosoluble contrast a.
hyoscine butylbromide imaging a.
Hypaque-Cysto imaging a.
Hypaque-76 imaging a.

NOTES

agent *(continued)*

Hypaque Meglumine imaging a.
Hypaque-M imaging a.
Hypaque Sodium imaging a.
hyperpolarized ^{3}He imaging a.
hyperpolarized ^{129}Xe imaging a.
Imagent GI, US imaging a.
imaging a.
ImmuRAID antibody imaging a.
imodoacetic acid imaging a.
indium imaging a.
indocyanine green imaging a.
inhaled oxygen imaging a.
^{111}In pentetreotide imaging a.
intercalating a.
intratumoral a.
intravenous microbubble contrast a.
iobitridol imaging a.
iocetamic acid imaging a.
iodamine imaging a.
iodinated imaging a.
iodine-123-MIBG radioactive
 imaging a.
iodine-131-MIBG radioactive
 imaging a.
iodipamide meglumine imaging a.
iodized oil imaging a.
5-iodo-2-deoxyuridine imaging a.
Iodo-gen imaging a.
iodohippurate sodium imaging a.
Iodotope imaging a.
iohexol imaging a.
ionic paramagnetic imaging a.
iopamidol imaging a.
Iopamiron 310, 370 imaging a.
iopanoic acid imaging a.
iopentol nonionic imaging a.
iophendylate imaging a.
iopromide nonionic imaging a.
iosefamic acid imaging a.
iothalamate meglumine imaging a.
iothalamate sodium imaging a.
iotroxic acid imaging a.
ioversol imaging a.
ioxaglate meglumine imaging a.
ioxaglate sodium imaging a.
ioxilan imaging a.
ioxithalamic acid contrast a.
ipodate calcium imaging a.
ipodate sodium imaging a.
ipodic acid contrast a.
iridium imaging a.
Isovue-200, -250, -300, -370
 imaging a.
Isovue-M 200, 300 imaging a.
Isovue nonionic imaging a.

kinase C antiglioma monoclonal
 antibody imaging a.
Kinevac imaging a.
LeukoScan imaging a.
LeuTech radiolabeled imaging a.
Levovist imaging a.
ligand a.
Lipiodol myelographic imaging a.
Lipiodol Ultra Fluid imaging a.
lipophilic imaging a.
liquid embolic a.
liver-specific MRI contrast a.
long-scale imaging a.
low-osmolar contrast a. (LOCA)
L-tyrosine imaging a.
lymphangiographic imaging a.
Lymphazurin imaging a.
LymphoScan imaging a.
macroaggregated albumin
 imaging a.
macromolecular imaging a.
Macrotec imaging a.
magnetic resonance receptor a.
magnetite albumin imaging a.
Magnevist imaging a.
mangafodipir trisodium a.
manganese-containing contrast a.
manganese imaging a.
mannitol and saline imaging a.
MD-Gastroview imaging a.
meglumine iodipamide imaging a.
meglumine iotroxate imaging a.
methiodal sodium imaging a.
methyl methacrylate imaging a.
metrizamide imaging a.
metrizoate imaging a.
microbubble-based contrast a.
mineral oil imaging a.
monoclonal antibody imaging a.
monodisperse iodinated
 macromolecular blood pool a.
MS-325 contrast a.
MultiHance imaging a.
myelographic imaging a.
Myoscint imaging a.
Myoview imaging a.
naloxone imaging a.
nanoparticulate imaging a.
negative contrast imaging a.
NeoSpect diagnostic imaging a.
NeoTect imaging a.
Neurolite imaging a.
neurotrophic imaging a.
nicotinamide imaging a.
nimodipine imaging a.
Niopam imaging a.
NIR contrast a.

nitrogen-13 ammonia imaging a.
no-carrier-added ^{18}F imaging a.
nofetumomab diagnostic imaging a.
nonionic iodinated contrast a.
nonionic paramagnetic contrast
  imaging a.
nonnephrotoxic contrast a.
novel a.
occluding a.
OctreoScan 111 radioactive
  imaging a.
Octreotide imaging a.
oil emulsion imaging a.
Omnipaque 140, 180, 240, 300,
  350 imaging a.
Omniscan imaging a.
OncoScint CR/OV breast
  imaging a.
Optiray 10, 240, 300, 320, 350
  imaging a.
Optison sterile injectable
  sonography contrast a.
Oragrafin calcium imaging a.
Oragrafin sodium imaging a.
oral contrast imaging a.
Oxilan imaging a.
oxygen imaging a.
palladium imaging a.
Pantopaque imaging a.
paramagnetic contrast a.
particulate embolic a.
pentagastrin imaging a.
pentavalent DMSA imaging a.
pentetic acid imaging a.
pentetreotide imaging a.
peppermint oil imaging a.
peptide imaging a.
perflubron imaging a.
perfluorocarbon imaging a.
perfusion a.
Persantine imaging a.
phenobarbital imaging a.
phosphoric acid imaging a.
phosphorus imaging a.
PMT imaging a.
polidocanol sclerosing a.
polymerizing a.
potassium imaging a.
ProHance imaging a.
propyliodone imaging a.
ProstaScint monoclonal antibody
  imaging a.

pulmonary perfusion MRI
  contrast a.
radioactive cancer-specific
  targeting a.
radioactive isotope imaging a.
radiolabeled MoAb imaging a.
radiopaque imaging a.
radiopharmaceutical a.
radioprotective a.
radiotherapeutic a.
recombinant thyrotropin contrast a.
  (rTSH)
renal cortical isotope scanning a.
Renografin-60 imaging a.
Renotec imaging a.
Renovist II imaging a.
Renovue-Dip imaging a.
Renovue-65 imaging a.
residual imaging a.
reticuloendothelial imaging a.
rhenium imaging a.
RIGScan CR49 imaging a.
rose bengal ^{131}I radioactive a.
rubidium chloride imaging a.
Rubratope-57 imaging a.
samarium imaging a.
satumomab pendetide imaging a.
sclerosing a.
selenium imaging a.
^{75}Se selenomethionine radioactive a.
sestamibi imaging a.
Sethotope radioactive imaging a.
SH U 508A contrast a.
sincalide imaging a.
Sinografin imaging a.
SmartPrep imaging a.
sodium and/or methylglucamine
  diatrizoate contrast a.
sodium bicarbonate imaging a.
sodium chloride imaging a.
sodium diatrizoate imaging a.
sodium iodide ring imaging a.
sodium iodohippurate imaging a.
sodium iothalamate imaging a.
sodium ipodate imaging a.
sodium meglumine ioxaglate
  contrast a.
sodium metrizoate acid contrast a.
sodium pertechnetate imaging a.
sodium tyropanoate imaging a.
solidifying a.
somatostatin imaging a.

NOTES

agent *(continued)*
Sonazoid contrast a.
sonicated dextrose albumin
imaging a.
SonoRx oral ultrasound contrast a.
sorbitol 70% imaging a.
sprodiamide imaging a.
stool-tagging a.
strontium-89 imaging a.
sucrose polyester imaging a.
sulfobromophthalein imaging a.
sulfur colloid imaging a.
superparamagnetic iron oxide blood
pool a.
superparamagnetic iron oxide
imaging a.
tantalum imaging a.
targeted contrast a.
^{99m}Tc aggregated albumin
imaging a.
^{99m}Tc albumin colloid imaging a.
^{99m}Tc albumin microspheres
imaging a.
^{99m}Tc biciromab imaging a.
^{99m}Tc bicisate imaging a.
^{99m}Tc dimer captosuccinic acid
imaging a.
^{99m}Tc disofenin imaging a.
^{99m}Tc exametazime imaging a.
^{99m}Tc furifosmin imaging a.
^{99m}Tc-galactosyl human serum
albumin imaging a.
^{99m}Tc glucarate imaging a.
^{99m}Tc gluceptate imaging a.
^{99m}Tc GSA imaging a.
^{99m}Tc human serum albumin
imaging a.
^{99m}Tc-labeled cerebral perfusion
imaging a.
^{99m}Tc lidofenin imaging a.
^{99m}Tc mebrofenin imaging a.
^{99m}Tc medronate imaging a.
^{99m}Tc mertiatide imaging a.
^{99m}Tc microaggregated albumin
imaging a.
^{99m}Tc-N-NOEt neutral myocardial
perfusion imaging a.
^{99m}Tc oxidronate imaging a.
^{99m}Tc pentetate calcium trisodium
imaging a.
^{99m}Tc pentetate sodium imaging a.
^{99m}Tc polyphosphate imaging a.
^{99m}Tc pyrophosphate imaging a.
^{99m}Tc sestamibi imaging a.
^{99m}Tc sodium pertechnetate
imaging a.
^{99m}Tc succimer imaging a.

^{99m}Tc sulfur colloid imaging a.
^{99m}Tc teboroxime imaging a.
^{99m}Tc tetrofosmin imaging a.
teboroxime imaging a.
Techneplex imaging a.
TechneScan HDP, MAA, MAG3,
PYP imaging a.
technetium imaging a.
Telepaque imaging a.
teratogenicity of contrast a.
thallium imaging a.
thallous chloride imaging a.
TheraSeed imaging a.
thorium dioxide imaging a.
Thorotrast imaging a.
tissue-specific imaging a.
Tomocat imaging a.
triiodinated imaging a.
Tyropaque imaging a.
Ultravist 150, 240, 300, 370
contrast a.
uniphasic imaging a.
uranium imaging a.
Urografin imaging a.
urokinase imaging a.
Urovist Cysto imaging a.
Urovist Meglumine imaging a.
Urovist Sodium imaging a.
USPIO imaging a.
Varibar oral contrast a.
vasodilating a.
Verluma diagnostic imaging a.
Visipaque 270, 320 contrast a.
water-soluble iodinated imaging a.
water-soluble nonionic imaging a.
xenon imaging a.
xylenol orange imaging a.
age-related change
AGF
angle of greatest flexion
Agfa
A. ADC 70 storage phosphor
system
A. CR, PACS system
A. LR 3300 laser imager
A. Medical scanner
agger nasi
aggregated
a. lymphatic follicle
a. sludge
aggregation
nuclear a.
aggregometer
aggregometry
aggressive
a. angiomyxoma
a. infantile fibromatosis

a. interstitial infiltrate
a. malignancy
a. perivascular infiltrate
aggressiveness
bone tumor a.
aging gut
AGL
anterior glenoid labrum
agnogenic
a. myeloid metaphysis
a. myeloid metaplasia
agonal clot
agranular leukocyte
agretope
agyria pachygria complex
ahaustral
AHI
acetabular head index
acromiohumeral interval
apnea-hypopnea index
Ahmed glaucoma valve
AHO
acute hematogenous osteomyelitis
AHQ
amnionic head quotient
AHR
airway hyperreactivity
AHS
Alpers-Huttenlocher syndrome
AI
acceleration index
AI 5200 diagnostic ultrasound
AICA
anterior-inferior cerebellar artery
anterior-inferior cerebral artery
anterior-inferior communicating artery
Aicardi syndrome
AICD
automatic implantable cardioverter-
defibrillator
AICS
artery of inferior cavernous sinus
AIDS
acquired immunodeficiency syndrome
A. cholangitis
A. encephalopathy
AIDS-related esophagitis
AIN
acute interstitial nephritis
AIOD
aortoiliac occlusive disease

AIP
acute interstitial pneumonia
air
ambient a.
a. arthrography
a. block
a. bolus
bowel loop a.
a. bronchogram
a. cavity
a. cisternography
a. collection
colonic a.
a. conditioner lung
a. contrast study
a. contrast view of the stomach
a. crescent
a. crescent sign
a. cyst
a. cystogram
a. density
a. dose
a. embolus
a. encephalography
a. enema fluoroscopic imaging
a. esophagram
a. exchange
a. expansion
extraalveolar a. (EAA)
extraluminal a.
flail a.
free intraperitoneal a.
free peritoneal a.
a. gap
a. hunger
a. imaging agent
a. inflation
a. injection
inspired a.
a. insufflation
a. interface
intracranial a.
intraluminal a.
intramural colonic a.
intraorbital a.
intraperitoneal a.
a. kerma
a. leak
a. leak complication
a. luminogram
mediastinal a.
a. monitor

NOTES

air *(continued)*
    a. myelography
    a. plasma spray hydroxyapatite
    a. plethysmography
    a. pocket
    a. pyelography
    retrocrural a.
    retroperitoneal a.
    a. sac
    subcutaneous a.
    transradiant a.
    a. trapping
    a. vesicle
air/bone/tissue boundary
airborne transmission
air-containing neck mass
air-contrast
    a.-c. barium enema (ACBE)
    a.-c. imaging
    a.-c. view
air-core magnet
air-driven artificial heart
air-filled
    a.-f. cyst
    a.-f. loop
    a.-f. lung
air-filtration system
airflow obstruction disease (AOD)
air-fluid
    a.-f. level
    a.-f. line
air-gap
    a.-g. radiography
    a.-g. technique
AIRIS II MR system
air-kerma
    a.-k. rate constant
    a.-k. strength
airless
    a. lung
    a. mass
air–soft tissue interface
airspace, air-space
    a. consolidation
    a. disease
    a. edema
    a. enlargement
    lung-a.
    a. nodule
    a. opacity
    retrosternal a.
    terminal a.
    volumetry of ventilated a.
air-trapping zone
airway
    a. anatomy
    asthmatic a.

    bronchiectatic a.
    a. constriction
    dilated small a.
    a. embryology
    esophageal obturator a.
    a. fluoroscopy
    a. hyperreactivity (AHR)
    hypertonic a.
    increased a.
    large a.
    mucoid plugging of a.
    mucus-filled small a.
    a. narrowing
    a. obstruction
    oropharyngeal a.
    a. pattern
    a. pressure
    a. pressure release ventilation
    a. resistance (Raw)
    a. responsiveness
    small a.
    a. tree
    a. tuberculosis
AIS
    abbreviated injury scale
    adolescent idiopathic scoliosis
Aitken
    A. acromioclavicular injury
      classification
    A. classification of epiphyseal
      fracture
    A. femoral deficiency
AIVV
    anterior internal vertebral vein
AJCC-UICC
    A.-U. mediastinal lymph node
      classification
AKA
    above-knee amputation
Akerlund deformity
akinesis
    inferior wall a.
akinetic
    a. left ventricle
    a. segment
    a. segmental wall motion
AL
    anterolateral
ala, pl. **alae**
    collagenous perivascular a.
    a. cristae galli
    sacral a.
Alagille syndrome
alanine-silicone pellet
Alanson amputation
alar
    a. bone

a. cartilage
a. chest
a. dysgenesis
a. fold
a. ligament
a. plate
a. process
a. spine
ALARA
as low as reasonably achievable
ALARP
as low as readily practicable
alba
linea a.
Albarran gland
Albers-Schönberg position
Albert position
Albini nodule
Albinus muscle
Albrecht bone
Albright
A. hereditary osteodystrophy
A. syndrome
Albright-McCune-Sternberg syndrome
albumin
chromium CR 51 serum a.
Evans blue a.
galactosyl human serum a. (GSA)
Gd-DTPA-labeled a.
human serum a. (HSA)
I-labeled macroaggregated a.
iodinated human serum a. (IHSA)
iodinated I-131 aggregated a.
iodinated I-125 serum a.
iodinated I-131 serum a.
macroaggregated a. (MAA)
microaggregated a.
neogalactosyl a.
perfluorocarbon-exposed sonicated
dextrose a. (PESDA)
radioactive iodinated serum a.
(RISA)
radioiodinated serum a. (RISA)
technetium-99m
minimicroaggregated a.
ALCL
anaplastic large cell lymphoma
Alcock
A. canal
A. test
alcohol
polyvinyl a. (PVA)

alcoholic
a. cirrhosis (AC)
a. fatty liver
a. fibrosis
a. heart
a. liver disease (ALD)
a. pneumonia
ALD
alcoholic liver disease
ALD-AMN
adrenoleukodystrophy-
adrenomyeloneuropathy
aldehyde
formic a.
Alder constitutional granulation anomaly
Alder-Reilly anomaly
Alderson anthropomorphic phantom
aldolase
aldosterone-producing carcinoma
aldosterone-secreting carcinoma
Alexander
A. disease
A. view
alexandrite laser
Alexa 1000 system
algebraic reconstruction technique
(ART)
algorithm
annealing a.
bioeffects a.
bone a.
bone-detail a.
Canny edge detection a.
Clarkson scatter-summation a.
clustering a.
cone-beam reconstruction a.
contour-following a.
Cooley-Tukey a.
correlation a. (CR)
decryption a.
defuzzification a.
3D elastic subtraction a.
design rule check a.
digital image processing a.
DIP a.
document-recognition a.
DRC a.
3D reconstruction a.
3D surface detection a.
dual-lookup table a.
edge-enhanced error diffusion a.
elastic subtraction a.

NOTES

algorithm *(continued)*
    encryption a.
    Feldkamp a.
    filtered back-projection a.
    fringe thinning a.
    fully automated segmentation a.
    fuzzy clustering a.
    geometric optimization a.
    high spatial frequency
      reconstruction a.
    high spatial resolution a.
    histogram equalization a.
    image reconstruction a.
    image restoration a.
    interpolation a.
    iterative a.
    K-means clustering a.
    least square a.
    lossy a.
    mapping a.
    maximum intensity projection a.
    maximum likelihood a.
    memory-intensive a.
    MIP a.
    neural evaluation a.
    pixel-oriented a.
    quantizer-design a.
    radix-two a.
    Ramesh and Pramod a.
    reconstruction a.
    regridding a.
    restoration a.
    Shinnar-LeRoux a.
    SSD a.
    thresholding a.
    Z-interpolation a.
ALH
    atypical lobular hyperplasia
aliased flow
aliasing
    a. artifact
    image a.
    temporal a.
Alibert-Bazin syndrome
alignment
    anatomic a.
    angular a.
    bony a.
    Cooley-Tukey a.
    field a.
    a. of fracture fragment
    a. and registration of 3D image
    rotational a.
    torsion a.
    transverse plane a.
    vertebral body a.

alimentary
    a. canal
    a. tract
    a. tract calcification
alkalinity
    Engel a.
Alken-Marberger nephroscope
allantoic
    a. circulation
    a. cyst
    a. vesicle
allergic
    a. bronchopulmonary aspergillosis
    (ABPA)
    a. granulomatosis
    a. pneumonia
    a. reaction
    a. sinusitis
allergy
    iodine a.
Allis sign
Allman classification
allocation
    bit-rate a.
    a. of treatment
allocortex
alloesthesia
allogeneic, allogenic
    a. bone marrow transplant
    a. peripheral cell transplant
allograft
    aortic a.
    bone a.
    bone-chip a.
    renal a.
alloimmune disease
allowed beta transition
alloxan-Schiff reaction
All-Tronics scanner
ALN
    axillary lymph node
alobar holoprosencephaly
Aloka
    A. color Doppler real-time 2D
    blood flow imaging with cine
    memory
    A. imaging
    A. linear ultrasound
    A. sector ultrasound
    A. SSD-1700 transducer
    A. SSD ultrasound system
    A. ultrasound linear scanner
    A. ultrasound sector scanner
Alouette amputation
Alpers-Huttenlocher syndrome (AHS)
alpha
    a. chamber

a. cradle
a. decay
a. frequency band
a. particle
a. particle accelerator
a. particle bombardment
a. radiation
a. ray
a. sigmoid loop
a. threshold
a. tocopherol

alpha-M²
radiolabeled peptide a.-M.

Alpha 21064 microprocessor workstation
alpha-particle emitter
Alpine hunter's cap deformity
ALPSA
anterior labroligamentous periosteal
sleeve avulsion
ALPSA lesion

alta
patella a.
A. reconstruction rod
A. tibial/humeral rod

Altaire
alteplase recombinant tissue plasminogen activator
alteration
bilateral a.
hemodynamic a.
metabolic a.

altered
a. aortic contour
a. blood flow
a. mediastinal contour

alternans
pulsus a.
strabismus convergens a.

alternated delay acquisition (ADA)
alternating
a. calculus
a. current
a. hemifield stimulation
a. sinus

alternative-free response receiver operating characteristic (AFROC)
alternator
film a.

altitudinal hemianopsia
Altman classification
Altropane radioimaging agent
ALT ultrasound system

altus
calcaneus a.

alumina
aluminum
a. ion breakthrough test
a. pneumoconiosis

ALVAD
abdominal left ventricular assist device

alveodental ridge
alveolar
a. atrophy
a. basal cell carcinoma
a. bone fracture
a. border of mandible
a. bronchiole
a. canal
a. clouding
a. collapse
a. consolidation
a. consolidative process
a. crest
a. dead space
a. dilatation
a. distention
a. duct
a. duct emphysema
a. echinococcosis
a. ectasia
a. epithelial hyperplasia
a. foramen
a. gland
a. hemorrhage
a. hydatid
a. hypersensitivity
a. infection
a. infiltrate
a. instability
a. lung disease
a. microlithiasis
a. mucosal carcinoma
a. overdistention
a. overventilation
a. pattern
a. paucity
a. pneumonia
a. point
a. pressure
a. proteinosis
a. pulmonary edema
a. rhabdomyosarcoma
a. ridge
a. sac

NOTES

alveolar *(continued)*
  a. sarcoidosis
  a. septal inflammation
  a. septal necrosis
  a. septum
  a. soft-part sarcoma (ASPS)
  a. supporting bone
  a. ventilation (VA)
  a. volume
alveolar-capillary block
alveolarization
alveoli (*pl. of* alveolus)
alveolingual groove
alveolitis
  acute extrinsic allergic a.
  chronic diffuse sclerosing a.
  chronic extrinsic allergic a.
  chronic fibrosing a.
  cryptogenic fibrosing a.
  desquamative fibrosing a.
  diffuse sclerosing a.
  extrinsic allergic a.
  fibrosing cryptogenic a.
  mural fibrosing a.
  subacute extrinsic allergic a.
alveolobuccal groove
alveolodental canal
alveologram
alveololabial groove
alveolus, pl. **alveoli**
  pulmonary a.
alvine calculus
alymphocytosis
alymphoplasia
Alzheimer disease (AD)
AM
  arterial malformation
Am
  americium
²⁴¹Am
  americium-241
amastia
amaurosis
  central a.
  cerebral a.
  a. fugax
  uremic a.
Amazr radiofrequency catheter ablation
AMBER
  advanced multiple-beam equalization
  radiography
ambient
  a. air
  a. segment of posterior cerebral
  artery
  a. wing of the quadrigeminal
  cistern

ambiguous genitalia
ambilevous
AMBRI
  atraumatic, multidirectional, bilateral
  radial instability
ambulatory
  a. equilibrium angiocardiography
  a. equilibrium angiography
  a. Holter echocardiography
AME
  AME bone growth stimulator
  AME PinSite shield
amelanotic tumor
ameloblastic
  a. adenomatoid tumor
  a. carcinoma
  a. fibroma
  a. fibrosarcoma
  a. sarcoma
ameloblastoma of the jaw
amelogenesis imperfecta
amentia
American
  A. Medical Association Ligament
  Injury Classification System
  A. Shared-CuraCare scanner
  A. Spinal Cord Injury Association
  classification
americium (Am)
  a. radioactive source
americium-241 (²⁴¹Am)
ameroid occluder
ametriodinic acid
AMI 121, 227 contrast agent
amiculum, pl. **amicula**
  a. of olive
amidotrizoic
  a. acid
  a. acid contrast agent
aminobutyrate
  gamma a.
amiodarone
  a. liver
  a. lung
Amipaque imaging agent
Amiscan imaging agent
AML
  angiomyolipoma
Ammon horn
ammonia
  anhydrous a.
ammonium excretion
amniocentesis
  therapeutic a.
amniography
amnioinfusion

amnion
    a. ring
    a. rupture
    a. rupture sequence
amnionic, amniotic
    a. band
    a. band syndrome
    a. cavity
    a. duct
    a. fluid (AF)
    a. fluid embolus
    a. fluid index (AFI)
    a. fluid volume
    a. fold
    a. head quotient (AHQ)
    a. inclusion cyst
    a. membrane
    a. raphe
    a. sac
    a. sheet
amnionicity
A-mode
    amplitude modulation
    A-m. display
    A-m. echocardiography
    A-m. encephalography
    A-m. scan
amorphous
    a. fetus
    a. high signal intensity
    a. selenium
    a. selenium plate
    a. silicon
    a. silicon filmless digital x-ray
      detection technology
amosite
Amoss sign
amp
    low-pressure mercury arc a.
ampere
amphiarthrodial
amphiarthrosis
amphibole asbestos
amphoric echo
amphoteric dipolar ion
Amplatz
    A. Anchor System
    A. angiography needle
    A. Clot Buster
    A. dilator set
    A. Goose Neck snare
    A. left coronary catheter

    A. radiolucent handle
    A. right coronary catheter
    A. Super Stiff catheter
    A. Super Stiff guidewire
    A. technique
    A. Teflon sheath
    A. thrombectomy device
Amplatzer septal occluder device
amplification
    multiscale image detail contrast a.
      (Musica)
amplifier
    buffer a.
    gradient a.
    image a.
    linear a.
    log a.
    nuclear pulse a.
    pulse a.
    servo power a.
    Servox a.
    voltage a.
amplitude
    acoustic pressure a.
    a. asymmetry
    deformation a.
    gradient a.
    a. image
    a. imaging
    a. modulation (A-mode)
    output a.
    peak a.
    a. of phase encoding
    pressure a.
    septal a.
ampulla, pl. **ampullae**
    a. chyli
    duodenal a.
    a. duodeni
    hepatopancreatic a.
    a. hepatopancreatica
    a. membranacea anterior
    a. ossea anterior
    a. ossea posterior
    phrenic a.
    rectal a.
    a. recti
    a. of semicircular canal
    a. tumor
    a. of Vater
ampullar pregnancy

NOTES

ampullary
a. adenocarcinoma
a. aneurysm
a. carcinoma
a. crest
a. stenosis
amputated-foot view
amputation
above-knee a. (AKA)
AE a.
Alanson a.
Alouette a.
Beclard a.
below-knee a.
Berger interscapular a.
Bier a.
Boyd ankle a.
Bunge a.
Burgess below-knee a.
button toe a.
Callander a.
Carden a.
chop a.
Chopart hindfoot a.
circular supracondylar a.
closed flap a.
congenital a.
digital a.
femoral head a.
fetal a.
fingertip a.
fishmouth a.
forearm a.
Guyon a.
Hey a.
interscapulothoracic a.
Jaboulay a.
Kirk distal thigh a.
Le Fort a.
Lisfranc a.
midthigh a.
nonreplantable a.
one-stage a.
Pirogoff a.
ray a.
replantable a.
supramalleolar open a.
Syme ankle disarticulation a.
Teale a.
transcarpal a.
transcondylar a.
translumbar a.
transmetatarsal a. (TMA)
traumatic a.
two-stage a.
Vladimiroff-Mikulicz a.

AMS
accelerator mass spectrometry
Amsterdam dwarfism
Amstutz classification
AMT-25-enhanced
A.-e. MR imaging
amu
atomic mass unit
amygdala
a. of cerebellum
a. volume
amygdaline
amygdalofugal pathway
amygdaloid
a. area
a. fossa
a. nuclear complex
a. tubercle
amylaceum, pl. **amylacea**
corpus a.
amyloid
a. deposit
a. tumor
amyloidoma
amyloidosis
chronic renal failure a.
CNS a.
GI tract a.
heart a.
hereditary a.
idiopathic a.
immunocytic a.
kidney a.
lung a.
a. of multiple myeloma
orbital a.
primary a.
pulmonary a.
renal a.
secondary a.
senile a.
skeletal a.
splenic a.
urethral a.
amyloidotic cardiomyopathy
amyotonia congenita
AN
adenoidal-nasopharyngeal ratio
anacrotic notch
anaerobic lung abscess
anal
a. atresia
a. bulge
a. canal
a. cleft
a. column
a. crypt

a. disk
a. fascia
a. fissure
a. fistula
a. intermuscular septum
a. intersphincteric groove
a. manometry
a. orifice
a. pit
a. plate
a. protrusion
a. stenosis
a. stricture
a. vein
a. verge
analeptic enema
analgesic nephropathy
analog, analogue
a. computations
dysprosium a.
halogenated thymidine a.
a. photo
pyrimidine a.
radiolabeled estrogen a.
a. rate meter
^{99m}Tc-labeled phosphate a.
technetium-99m IDA a.
analogous
analysis, pl. **analyses**
activation a.
advanced real-time motion a.
(ARTMA)
advanced vessel a. (AVA)
basic volume image a.
bayesian a.
5-bromodeoxyuridine a.
cephalometric a.
CEqual quantitative a.
Cerenkov scintillation a.
clinicopathological a.
compartmental a.
computer-aided image a.
computer-assisted joint motion a.
correlation a.
cue-based image a.
deconvolutional a.
deformation-based hippocampal
segmentation and shape a.
diagnostic efficacy a.
digital frequency a.
direct immunofluorescence a.
discriminant a.

Doppler spectral a.
Doppler waveform a.
duplex ultrasound a.
eigenvector a.
electrooculographic a.
fast Fourier spectral a.
field-fitting a.
fission track a.
focal and diffuse lung texture a.
folding potential a.
footprint a.
Fourier a.
fractal a.
fractional volumetric a.
frequency a.
gamma spectrometric a.
high-definition three-dimensional a.
image display and a. (IDA)
intracardiac pressure waveform a.
iodine-131 outcome a.
isotope dilution a.
kinetic parameter a.
late effect a.
least square a.
linear regression a.
liquid scintillation a.
multielemental neutron activation a.
multivariant regressional a.
myocardial texture a.
neutron activation a.
nuclide a.
phase a.
planar thallium with quantitative a.
pole figure texture a.
power spectral a. (PSA)
prospective a.
pulse height spectral a.
quadratic discriminant a. (QDA)
qualitative a.
quantitative a.
radiometric a.
range-gated Doppler spectral
flow a.
rate a.
recursive partitioning a.
regression a.
residual stress a.
roentgen stereophotogrammetric a.
(RSA)
Sassouni a.
saturation a.
sensitivity a.

NOTES

analysis *(continued)*
    signal sonographic feature a.
    slope blot a.
    sonographic feature a.
    spectral a.
    S-phase a.
    stepwise regression a.
    thin film a.
    three-dimensional a.
    time-action a.
    volume a.
    volumetric a.
    x-ray diffraction a.
analytic reconstruction
analyzer
    automated biochemical a.
    automated cerebral blood flow a.
    ChromaVision digital a.
    Dow hollow fiber a.
    Gammex RBA-5 radiation beam a.
    Medigraphics a.
    multichannel a. (MCA)
    platelet function a. (PFA)
    pulse-height a. (PHA)
    single-channel a. (SCA)
anaphylactic reaction
anaphylactoid reaction
anaplasia
    cancer cell a.
    cerebellar a.
anaplastic
    a. astrocytoma (AA)
    a. cerebral glioma
    a. ependymoma
    a. large cell lymphoma (ALCL)
    a. mixed oligoastrocytoma
    a. plasmacytoma
    a. thyroid carcinoma
    a. tumor
anastomosis, pl. anastomoses
    arterial brain a.
    arteriovenous a. (AVA)
    Baffe a.
    bidirectional cavopulmonary a.
    biliary-enteric a.
    Billroth I, II a.
    cobra-head a.
    coiling of a.
    colocolic a.
    colorectal a.
    embryonic a.
    end-to-side biliary-enteric a.
    extradural a.
    Glenn a.
    hepatojejunal a.
    heterocladic a.
    Hofmeister a.

    Horsley a.
    ileal pouch-anal a.
    ileorectal a. (IRA)
    ileotransverse colon a.
    intercavernous a.
    J-shaped a.
    Kocher a.
    Kugel a.
    laser-assisted microvascular a.
    left internal mammary artery a.
    leptomeningeal a.
    LIMA a.
    portosystemic a.
    splenorenal a.
    stenotic esophagogastric a.
    Sucquet-Hoyer a.
    tracheal a.
    ureteroureteral a.
anastomotic
    a. aneurysm
    a. arch
    a. arterial circle
    a. dehiscence
    a. disruption
    a. hemorrhage
    a. leakage
    a. pseudoaneurysm
    a. site
    a. stenosis
    a. stoma
    a. stricture
    a. ulcer
    a. vein
anastomy
    donor-recipient a.
anatomic
    a. alignment
    a. axis
    a. barrier
    a. bile duct variant
    a. brain classification
    a. configuration
    a. dead space
    a. distribution
    a. esophageal vestibule
    a. fracture
    a. genu valgus
    a. image
    a. landmark
    a. localization
    a. marker
    a. moment erratum
    a. neck
    a. overlay
    a. plane
    a. position
    a. reduction

a. resolution
a. root
a. shunt flow
a. snuffbox
a. variability
a. variation
anatomical age
anatomically
a. dominant
a. graduated component (AGC)
anatomopathologic study
anatomy
airway a.
anomalous a.
arterial a.
basal ganglia a.
breast a.
bronchopulmonary lung segment a.
bulbourethral gland a.
carpal bone a.
cochlear a.
computational a.
coronary artery a.
craniovertebral junction a.
cross-sectional lung segment a.
Daseler-Anson classification of
    plantaris muscle a.
distorted a.
endometrial a.
facial nerve a.
hepatic artery a.
inner ear a.
internal auditory canal a.
kidney a.
left-dominant coronary a.
lobar breast a.
Lowsley lobar a.
maxillary nerve a.
medullary venous a.
neck-space a.
normal planar MR a.
ovarian a.
pituitary gland a.
plantar compartmental a.
prostate a.
radiologic a.
renal vascular a.
right dominant coronary a.
Saltzman a.
scrotal a.
sectional segmental a.
segmental liver a.

small bowel fold a.
stapedial nerve a.
superior orbital fissure a.
teardrop pelvic a.
temporal bone a.
thoracic spine a.
trigeminal nerve a.
umbilical cord a.
uterine a.
vascular kidney a.
vascular renal a.
venous a.
zonal prostate a.
zonal uterine a.
anatomy-based extraction (ABE)
anatomy-oriented colon segmentation
    (AOCS)
anchor
Mitek bone a.
a. plate
traction a.
anchoring
a. tendon
a. villus
anconal, anconeal
anconeus muscle
anconoid
Ancure
ancyroid, ankyroid
a. cavity
Anderson-Hutchins tibial fracture
Andren method
androblastoma
androgen-independent prostate
    carcinoma
androgen-producing tumor
android pelvis
anechoic
a. area
a. center
a. cyst
a. fluid
a. fluid collection
a. lesion
a. mantle
a. mass
a. thrombus
anembryonic pregnancy
anemic infarct
anencephaly
aneroid manometry
aneuploid cell line

NOTES

AneuRx
  A. bifurcated stent-graft system
  A. endograft
  A. stent
  A. stent-graft
aneurysm
  abdominal aortic a. (AAA)
  AcomA a.
  acquired left ventricle a.
  ampullary a.
  anastomotic a.
  aortic arch a.
  aortic sinus a.
  aortoiliac a.
  arterial a.
  arteriosclerotic intracranial a.
  arteriosclerotic thoracoabdominal
    aortic a.
  arteriovenous pulmonary a.
  ascending aortic a.
  aspergillotic a.
  atherosclerotic aortic a.
  atrial septal a.
  axillary a.
  bacterial a.
  basilar artery a.
  basilar tip a.
  bifurcation a.
  bland aortic a.
  brachiocephalic arterial a.
  brain a.
  bulging a.
  calcified wall of a.
  cardiac ventricle a.
  carotid artery a.
  carotid-ophthalmic a.
  cavernous sinus a.
  cavity of a.
  celiac artery a.
  cerebral a.
  circumscript a.
  cirsoid a.
  clinoid a.
  clip ligation of a.
  clipping of a.
  coating of a.
  coiling of a.
  communicating artery a.
  compound a.
  congenital aortic sinus a.
  congenital arteriosclerotic a.
  congenital cerebral a.
  congenital intracranial a.
  congenital left ventricular a.
  congenital pulmonary artery a.
  congenital renal a.
  contained leak of aortic a.

  coronary artery a.
  coronary vessel a.
  cranial a.
  cylindroid a.
  degenerative aortic a.
  de novo a.
  dilatation of a.
  dissecting abdominal a.
  dissecting aortic a.
  dissecting basilar artery a.
  dissecting intracranial a.
  distal aortic arch a.
  dome of a.
  Dorendorf sign of aortic arch a.
  Drummond sign of aortic a.
  ductal a.
  ductus arteriosus a.
  ectatic a.
  eggshell border of a.
  embolic a.
  extracerebral a.
  extracranial a.
  false a.
  feeding artery of a.
  fenestration of dissecting a.
  fundus of a.
  fusiform a.
  Galen vein a.
  giant brain a.
  giant saccular a.
  giant serpentine a.
  hepatic artery a.
  hernial a.
  hunterian ligation of a.
  Hunt-Kosnik classification of a.
  iliac artery a.
  induced thrombosis of aortic a.
  infected a.
  inflammatory aortic a.
  infrarenal abdominal aortic a.
  innominate a.
  internal carotid artery a.
  intracerebral a.
  intracranial a. (ICA)
  intracranial berry a.
  intracranial saccular a.
  intramural coronary artery a.
  juxtarenal aortic a.
  kidney a.
  late false a.
  lateral a.
  leaking abdominal aortic a.
  left ventricular a.
  lower basilar a.
  luetic aortic a.
  malignant bone a.
  miliary a.

mirror image a.
mixed a.
M1 segment a.
mural a.
mycotic aortic a.
mycotic brain a.
mycotic intracranial a.
neck of a.
neoplastic a.
nodular a.
orbital a.
oval a.
pararenal aortic a.
pelvic a.
perforating a.
popliteal artery a.
portal vein a.
posterior communicating artery a.
postinfarction ventricular a.
Pott a.
precursor sign to rupture of a.
prerenal aortic a.
prerupture of a.
P2 segment a.
pulmonary arteriovenous a.
pulmonary artery compression
  ascending aortic a.
racemose a.
Rasmussen mycotic a.
rebleeding of a.
a. remnant neck
renal artery a.
ruptured a.
sac of a.
sacciform a.
saccular cerebral a.
sacral a.
serpentine a.
sinus of Valsalva a.
slow-flowing giant saccular a.
spindle-shaped a.
splanchnic a.
splenic artery a.
spontaneous infantile ductal a.
spurious a.
subclavian a.
subvalvular a.
supraclinoid carotid a.
suprarenal aortic a.
suprarenal extension of a.

suprasellar a.
syphilitic aortic a.
thoracic aortic a.
thoracoabdominal aortic a.
thrombosed giant vertebral artery a.
thrombotic a.
trapping of a.
traumatic intracranial a. (TICA)
true aortic a.
true heart a.
true ventricular a.
tubular a.
uterine cirsoid a.
varicose a.
varix of a.
venous a.
ventricular septal a.
verminous a.
wide-neck carotid cavernous a.
windsock a.
a. with simple shape
worm a.
aneurysmal
a. bone cyst (ABC)
a. clip
a. coil
a. dilation
a. dissection
a. fundus
a. hematoma
a. hemorrhage
a. neck
a. ostium
a. outpouching
a. proportion
a. rupture
a. sac
a. vein
a. wall
a. wall calcification
a. wall gas
a. widening of aorta
aneurysmogram
aneurysmography
**AngeLase combined mapping-laser
  probe**
angel-wing sign
Anger scintillation camera
angioarchitecture
angioblastic lymphadenopathy

NOTES

angioblastoma
>bone a.
>cord a.

angiocardiogram (ACG)

angiocardiography (ACG)
>ambulatory equilibrium a.
>biplane a.
>equilibrium radionuclide a.
>exercise radionuclide a.
>first-pass radionuclide exercise a.
>gas a.
>gated radionuclide a.
>intravenous a.
>radionuclide a.
>rapid biplane a.
>retrograde a.
>right-sided a.
>selective a.
>transseptal a.
>venous a.

Angiocath Autoguard Shielded IV catheter

angiocatheter

angiocentric
>a. immunoproliferative disorder
>a. immunoproliferative lesion
>a. lymphoproliferative lesion

angiocholitis

Angio-Conray imaging agent

angio-CT
>superselective a.-CT

angiodynography

angiodysplasia
>a. of colon
>colonic a.

angioedema

angiofibroblastic
>a. hyperplasia
>a. proliferation
>a. tendinosis

angiofibroma
>juvenile nasopharyngeal a. (JNPA)

Angioflow meter system

angiofollicular
>a. lymph node hyperplasia
>a. and plasmacytic polyadenopathy

angiogenesis
>a. gene delivery
>a. tumor

angiogenic factor

Angiografin imaging agent

angiogram (*See* angiography)
>balloon occlusion pulmonary a.
>biplane left ventricular a.
>control a.
>digital subtraction a.
>digital subtraction pulmonary a.

dynamic subtraction magnetic resonance a.
>fluorescein a.
>flush a.
>interventional vascular a.
>overview a.
>projection a.
>radionuclide a. (RNA)
>radionuclide cerebral a.
>spinal a.
>volume-rendered MR a.

angiographic
>a. blush
>a. catheter
>a. corkscrew artery
>a. finding
>a. guidewire
>a. muscle mass index
>a. occlusion
>a. system for unlimited rolling field-of-views (angioSURF)
>a. target
>a. targeting
>a. Teflon dilator

angiographically
>a. occult intracranial vascular malformation (AOIVM)
>a. occult vascular malformation (AOVM)
>a. occult vessel
>a. visualized vascular malformation (AVVM)

angiography
>adrenal a.
>ambulatory equilibrium a.
>aortic arch a.
>axial a.
>basilar a.
>biliary a.
>biplane a.
>black blood magnetic resonance a.
>blood pool radionuclide a.
>blush of dye on a.
>brain capillary a.
>breath-hold contrast-enhanced three-dimensional MR a.
>bronchial a.
>Brown-Dodge method for a.
>cardiac-gated MR a.
>carotid a.
>catheter a.
>cavernous brain a.
>celiac a.
>cerebral a.
>CO_2 a.
>computed tomographic a. (CTA)

computerized tomographic hepatic a. (CTHA)
contrast a.
contrast-enhanced magnetic resonance a. (CE-MRA)
contrast-enhanced MR a.
coronary electron beam a.
CT a.
cut-film a.
cystic duct a.
3D contrast-enhanced MR a.
3D coronary magnetic resonance a.
3DFT magnetic resonance a.
2DFT time-of-flight MR a.
3D gadolinium-enhanced magnetic resonance a.
3D helical CT a.
diagnostic a.
digital celiac trunk a.
digital rotational a. (DRA)
digital subtraction a. (DSA)
digital subtraction rotational a.
3D inflow MR a.
directional color a. (DCA)
dobutamine thallium a.
3D phase-contrast magnetic resonance a.
3D rotational a.
dual-detector helical CT a.
3D volume-rendering CT a.
dynamic tagging magnetic resonance a.
EBCT IV a.
ECG-synchronized digital subtraction a.
edge-detection a.
elastic subtraction spiral CT a.
electrocardiogram-synchronized digital subtraction a.
electron beam a. (EBA)
emission a.
Epistar subtraction a.
equilibrium radionuclide a.
femoral runoff a.
femorocerebral catheter a.
first-pass radionuclide a. (FPRNA)
fluorescein a.
FluoroPlus a.
four-vessel cerebral a.
four-vessel multiple projection biplane a.

frameless stereotactic digital subtraction a.
functional magnetic resonance a. (fMRA)
gadolinium-enhanced elliptically reordered three-dimensional MR a.
gadoterate-enhanced digital subtraction a.
gated blood pool a.
gated equilibrium radionuclide a.
gated nuclear a.
helical computed tomographic a. (HCTA)
helical CT a.
hepatic a.
a. imaging
indocyanine green a.
innominate a.
intercostal artery a.
internal carotid a.
interventional a.
intraarterial digital subtraction a. (IADSA)
intraarterial stereotactic digital subtraction a.
intracranial MR a.
intraoperative digital subtraction a. (IDSA)
intravenous digital subtraction a. (IVDSA)
intravenous fluorescein a. (IVFA)
intravenous renal a.
intravenous stereotactic digital subtraction a.
left coronary a. (LCA)
left ventricular a.
low-field MR a.
magnetic resonance a. (MRA)
magnetic resonance digital subtraction a. (MRDSA)
magnification a.
mesenteric a.
minimum basis set magnetic resonance a. (MBS-MRA)
multigated a.
multiple projection biplane a.
multislab magnetic resonance a.
noncardiac a.
nonselective a.
nontriggered phase-contrast MR a.
nuclear a.
occlusion a.

NOTES

angiography *(continued)*
orbital a.
orthogonal view on a.
pancreatic a.
PC MR a.
peripheral MR a.
phase-contrast a.
postangioplasty a.
postembolization a.
postoperative a.
posttourniquet occlusion a.
preoperative a.
pulmonary artery wedge a.
pulmonary magnetic resonance a.
  (PMRA)
pulmonary vein wedge a.
quantitative coronary a. (QCA)
radionuclide a.
renal a.
resistive index a.
rest-and-exercise-gated nuclear a.
right coronary a. (RCA)
rotational a. (RA)
scintigraphic a.
segmented k-space time-of-flight
  MR a.
Seldinger a.
selective arterial magnetic
  resonance a.
selective presaturation MR a.
selective venous magnetic
  resonance a.
single-plane a.
sitting-up view a.
spinal cord a.
stereotactic cerebral a.
subtraction a.
superselective a.
Tagarno 3SD cine projector for a.
therapeutic a.
thoracic a.
three-compartment wrist a.
three-dimensional digital
  subtraction a. (3D-DSA)
three-dimensional magnetic
  resonance a. (3D MRA)
three-vessel multiple projection
  biplane a.
time-of-flight magnetic resonance a.
  (TOF-MRA)
transfemoral cerebral a.
transseptal a.
transvenous digital subtraction a.
tumor blush on a.
two-dimensional magnetic resonance
  digital subtraction a. (2D
  MRDSA)

ultrafast 3D MR digital
  subtraction a.
velocity encoding on brain MR a.
venous brain a.
vertebral a.
visceral a.
angioimmunoblastic
a. lymphadenopathy
a. lymphadenopathy-like T-cell
  lymphoma
angioinfarction
angioinvasion
AngioJet
A. thrombectomy device
A. Xpeedior catheter
angioleiomyoma
angiolipofibroma
angiolipoma
epidural a.
mediastinal a.
angiolithic
a. degeneration
a. sarcoma
angiolymphangioma
angiolymphoid hyperplasia
angioma, pl. **angiomata**
arterial a.
arteriovenous interhemispheric a.
capillary a.
cavernous a.
cutaneous a.
encephalic a.
extracerebral cavernous a.
extraosseous a.
intracranial cavernous a.
intradermal a.
a. lymphaticum
pulmonary a.
a. serpiginosum
spider a.
superficial a.
telangiectatic a.
venous a.
AngioMARK contrast agent
Angiomat
A. 3000, 6000 contrast delivery
  system
A. ILLUMENA injector system
angiomata (*pl. of* angioma)
angiomatoid
a. malignant fibrous histiocytoma
a. tumor
angiomatosis
cystic bone a.
diffuse skeletal a.
encephalotrigeminal a.
epithelioid a.

leptomeningeal a.
meningofacial a.
a. of retina
retinal a.
retinocerebellar a.
visceral a.
angiomatous
a. disease
a. lymphoid hamartoma
a. nasal polyp
a. syndrome
angiomyofibroma
angiomyolipoma (AML)
hepatic a.
kidney a.
renal a.
angiomyoma
angiomyosarcoma
angiomyxoma
aggressive a.
umbilical cord a.
angioneuromyoma
angioneurotic edema
angioosteohypertrophy syndrome
angiopathy
cerebral amyloid a.
angioplastic meningioma
angioplasty
excimer laser coronary a. (ELCA)
infrainguinal percutaneous
transluminal a.
laser-assisted balloon a. (LABA)
percutaneous transluminal a. (PTA)
percutaneous transluminal
coronary a. (PTCA)
percutaneous transluminal renal a.
(PTRA)
peripheral excimer laser a. (PELA)
peripheral laser a.
a. sheath
smooth excimer laser coronary a.
(SELCA)
transluminal balloon a.
venous a.
vessel reshaping by a.
angiopneumography
AngiOptic microcatheter
AngioRad radiation system
angioreticuloendothelioma of heart
angioreticuloma
spine a.

angiosarcoma
bone a.
breast a.
cavernous a.
a. of heart
hepatic a.
liver a.
parosteal soft tissue a.
spleen a.
angioscintigraphy
angioscopic guidance
Angio-Seal
hemostatic puncture closure device
carrier tube
hemostatic puncture closure device
system
angiosome
AngioSURF system
angiotensin-converting enzyme (ACE)
angiotherapy
vasoocclusive a. (VAT)
angiotomomyelography
angiotropic large cell lymphoma
angitis-granulomatosis disorder
angle
acetabular sector a. (AASA)
acromial a.
anorectal a. (ARA)
antegonial a.
anterior angulation a.
anterior talocalcaneal a.
a. of anteversion
arch a.
basal a.
Baumann a.
Beatson combined ankle a.
beta a.
bimalleolar a.
blunting of costovertebral a.
blurring of costophrenic a.
board a.
Boehler a.
Böhler a.
Bragg a.
brain tumor at cerebellopontine a.
C a.
calcaneal inclination a.
calcaneal pitch a.
calcaneoplantar a.
capital epiphysis a.
capitolunate a.
cardiodiaphragmatic a.

NOTES

angle *(continued)*
cardiohepatic a.
cardiophrenic a.
carinal a.
carpal wrist a.
carrying a.
CCD a.
central collodiaphyseal a.
cephalic a.
cephalometric a.
cerebellopontine a. (CPA)
Clarke arch a.
clivus-canal a.
Cobb scoliosis a.
Codman a.
condylar a.
congruence a.
costal a.
costolumbar a.
costophrenic a.
costosternal a.
costovertebral a. (CVA)
CP a.
craniofacial a.
craniovertebral a.
a. of declination of metatarsal
distal articular set a. (DASA)
distal metatarsal articular a.
  (DMMA)
Doppler a.
dorsiflexion a. (DFA)
dorsoplantar talometatarsal a.
dorsoplantar talonavicular a.
Drennan metaphyseal-epiphyseal a.
duodenojejunal a.
Ebstein a.
a. electron (UE)
epigastric a.
Ernst a.
exposure a.
fan a.
femoral torsion V a.
femorotibial a. (FTA)
Ferguson a.
first-fifth intermetatarsal a.
first metatarsal a.
first-second intermetatarsal a.
flip a.
focal spot-to-film a.
foot-progression a. (FPA)
Frankfort mandibular incisor a.
Garden a.
gastroesophageal a.
Gissane a.
gonial a.
Graf alpha a.
a. of greatest extension (AGE)

a. of greatest flexion (AGF)
hallux dorsiflexion a. (DFA)
hallux interphalangeus a. (HIA)
hallux valgus a. (HVA)
hallux valgus interphalangeus a.
hepatic a.
hepatorenal a.
Hibbs metatarsocalcaneal a.
Hilgenreiner epiphyseal a.
His a.
incident a.
a. of inclination of urethra
a. of incongruity
increased carrying a.
infrasternal a.
a. of insonation
interbronchial a. (IA)
intercarpal a.
intermetatarsal a. (IMA)
kite a.
Konstram a.
lateral divergence a. (LDA)
lateral patellofemoral a.
lateral plantar metatarsal a.
lateral talocalcaneal a.
lateral talometatarsal a.
lateral tarsometatarsal a.
Laurin a.
Lewis a.
Lippman-Cobb a.
Louis a.
Ludovici a.
Ludwig a.
lumbar facet a.
lumbosacral joint a.
magnetization precession a.
mandibular a.
Meary metatarsotalar a.
medial a.
mediolateral radiocarpal a.
Merchant a.
metaphyseal-diaphyseal a.
metaphyseal-epiphyseal a.
metatarsal a.
metatarsocalcaneal a.
metatarsotalar a.
metatarsus adductus a.
metatarsus primus varus a.
  (MPVA)
Mikulicz a.
navicular to first metatarsal a.
neck shaft a.
nidus a.
nutation a.
obliterated costophrenic a.
occipitocervical a.
a. of orientation

patellofemoral a.
Pauwel a.
pelvic femoral a.
phase a.
phrenopericardial a.
Pirogoff a.
plantar metatarsal a.
pontine a.
posterior urethrovesical a. (PUVA)
precession a.
proximal articular set a. (PASSA)
psoas shadow a.
pulse flip a.
Q a.
QRST a.
radiocarpal a.
Ranke a.
resting forefoot supination a.
a. of rib
Rolando a.
rotation a.
sacrohorizontal a.
sacrovertebral a.
scapular a.
set a.
slip a.
sphenoid a.
spinographic a.
splenic a.
splenorenal a.
sternal a.
sternoclavicular a.
subcarinal a. (SA)
substernal a.
subtalar a.
sulcus a.
surgical a.
talar tilt a.
talocalcaneal a.
talocrural a.
Talo horizontal a.
talometatarsal a.
talonavicular a.
tarsometatarsal a.
thigh-foot a. (TFA)
tibiocalcaneal a.
tibiofemoral a. (TFA)
tibiotalar a.
tip a.
tracheal bifurcation a.
tracheobronchial a.
transmalleolar axis-thigh a.

transmetatarsal-thigh a.
urethral a.
urethrovesical a. (UVA)
valgus carrying a.
a. variation resolution
varus metatarsophalangeal a.
venous brain a.
venous neck a.
vertebrophrenic a.
vertical-center-anterior a.
vesicourethral a.
wedge isodose a.
Welcher basal a.
Welcker a.
Wiberg a.
Wiltze a.
xiphoid a.

angled
a. craniocaudal view
a. Glidewire
a. pleural tube
a. slice
angled-tip catheter
Angle-Iron skull immobilizer
angles of trigone
Angström
A. law
A. unit
angular
a. alignment
a. artery
a. bolster
a. curvature
a. deformity
a. deviation
a. frequency
a. gyrus (AG)
a. momentum
a. notch
a. process of orbit
a. sampling
a. vein
a. velocity
angularis
a. body
incisura a.
a. sulcus
angulated
a. catheter
a. fracture
a. lesion
a. segment

NOTES

angulation
   anterior a.
   bowel loop a.
   caudal-cranial a.
   cephalic a.
   coronal a.
   cranial a.
   craniocaudal needle a.
   forefoot a.
   gantry a.
   kyphotic a.
   palmar a.
   posttraumatic a.
   spinal a.
   a. of spine
   valgus a.
   varus a.
   volar a.
angulator
angulus of stomach
anhaustral colonic gas pattern
anhydrous ammonia
ani
aniline carcinoma
anisotrophy
anisotropic
   a. 3D imaging
   a. resolution
   a. rotation
   a. tissue
   a. volume study
anisotropically
   a. rotational diffusion (ARD)
   a. rotational diffusion imaging
anisotropy
   brain diffusion a.
   curvature a.
   decreased diffusion a.
   diffusional a.
   a. factor
   fractional a. (FA)
   magnetic a.
   a. map
anisura
ankle
   athlete's a.
   a. bone
   disk of a.
   eccentric axis of rotation of the a.
   eversion of a.
   fused a.
   a. fusion
   a. instability
   a. inversion injury
   inversion injury of a.
   a. joint
   a. joint complex

   laciniate ligament of a.
   a. mortise
   a. mortise axis
   a. mortise fracture
   a. mortise widening
   neuropathic a.
   a. swelling
   synthetic graft bypass to a.
   a. systolic pressure
   tailor's a.
   transmalleolar a.
   twisted a.
ankle-arm
   a.-a. index
   a.-a. pressure
ankle-brachial
   a.-b. index (ABI)
   a.-b. pressure measurement
   a.-b. pressure ratio
ankylosing
   a. hyperostosis
   a. spondylitis
ankylosis
   bony a.
   extracapsular a.
   false a.
   fibrous a.
   intracapsular a.
   joint a.
   ligamentous a.
   shoulder a.
   spurious a.
   vertebral a.
ankyroid (*var. of* ancyroid)
anlage, pl. **anlagen**
   cartilaginous a.
   pancreatic dorsal a.
   ventral pancreatic a.
ANMR Insta-scan MR scanner
Ann Arbor classification
annealing
   a. algorithm
   simulated a.
annihilation
   a. coincidence detection (ACD)
   a. photon
   a. radiation
   a. reaction
annotated imaging
annotation
annular (*var. of* anular)
ano
   fissure in a.
   fistula in a.
anococcygeal
   a. body

a. ligament
a. raphe
anodal block
anode
molybdenum a.
a. ray
rhodium a.
rotating a.
stationary a.
a. tube
a. tube reloading
tungsten a.
anode-cathode axis
anodontia
anogenital
a. band
a. raphe
anomalad
Robin a.
anomalous
a. anatomy
a. branching
a. bronchus
a. craniovertebral junction
a. development
a. distribution
a. insertion
a. left coronary artery
a. left pulmonary artery
a. muscle
a. origin
a. origin of artery
a. pathway
a. pulmonary venous connection
a. pulmonary venous return
a. right subclavian artery
a. vessel
anomaly, pl. **anomalies**
Alder constitutional granulation a.
Alder-Reilly a.
anorectal a.
aortic arch a.
associated a.
atlas a.
atrioventricular junction a.
axis a.
back-angle a.
bell-clapper a. (BCA)
cardiac a.
cardiovascular a.
cervical rib a.
cloacal a.

conjoined nerve root a.
conotruncal congenital a.
cranial a.
craniofacial a.
craniovertebral a.
Cruveilhier-Baumgarten a.
cutaneous vascular a.
double-inlet ventricle a.
duplication a.
Ebstein a.
extracardiac a.
fast-flow vascular a.
fetal cardiac a.
fetal chest a.
fetal CNS a.
fetal gastrointestinal a.
fetal heart a.
fetal neck a.
fetal urinary tract a.
Freund a.
gastrointestinal fetal a.
genitourinary a.
heart a.
intracranial leptomeningeal
vascular a.
jugular bulb a.
kidney a.
limb reduction a.
May-Hegglin a.
Michel a.
migrational a.
Mondini a.
müllerian duct a.
multiple congenital anomalies
(MCA)
numerary renal a.
occipitoatlantoaxial a.
presacral a.
radial ray a.
renal a.
rotation a.
segmentation a.
Shone a.
slow-flow vascular a.
spinal a.
structural a.
Taussig-Bing a.
tricuspid valve a.
Uhl a.
Undritz a.
urachal a.
urinary tract a.

NOTES

anomaly *(continued)*
    uterine duplication a.
    in utero detection of cardiac a.
    vascular a.
    vena cava a.
    venous a.
    vertebral segmentation a.
    Zahn a.
anonymous vein
anophthalmia
anorectal
    a. angle (ARA)
    a. anomaly
    a. atresia
    a. dysgenesis
    a. fistula
    a. junction (ARJ)
    a. line
    a. lymph node
    a. malformation
    a. manometry
    a. ring
    a. tuberculosis
anorectum
anovaginal fistula
anovular ovarian follicle
anoxia
    brain a.
    cerebral a.
    perinatal a.
anoxic
    a. encephalopathy
    a. ischemia
Anrep effect
ansa, pl. **ansae**
    a. of Vieussens
anserine
    a. bursa
    a. bursitis
anserinus
    pes a.
anteater nose
antebrachial
    a. fascia
    a. vein
antebrachium
antecedent sign
antecolic
antecubital
    a. fossa
    a. space
    a. vein
ante fenestram fissula
anteflexed uterus
anteflexion

antegonial
    a. angle
    a. notch
antegrade
    a. aortography
    a. bile flow
    a. blood flow
    a. cystography
    a. diastolic flow
    a. fast pathway
    a. femoral artery catheterization
    a. filling of vessel
    a. perfusion
    a. perfusion pressure measurement (APPM)
    a. pressure study
    a. puncture
    a. pyelography
    a. pyelography imaging
    a. refractory period
    a. transluminal balloon dilatation
    a. ureteral stenting
    a. urography
    a. venography
antepartum hemorrhage
anteprostatic gland
anterior
    a. abdominal wall
    ampulla membranacea a.
    ampulla ossea a.
    a. angulation
    a. angulation angle
    a. aspect
    a. atlas arch
    a. atrial myocardial bundle
    a. axillary line (AAL)
    a. band
    a. band of colon
    a. basal bronchus
    a. border
    a. border of heart
    a. bowing of sternum
    a. bowing tibia
    a. capsular distance (ACD)
    a. capsular shift
    a. cardiac vein
    a. central beaking
    a. central indentation
    a. cerebral artery (ACA)
    a. cerebral artery crawling under the skull
    a. cervical fusion (ACF)
    a. choroidal artery
    a. clear space
    a. colliculus
    a. column fracture
    a. column of spine

a. commissure (AC)
a. commissure-posterior commissure (AC-PC)
a. communicating artery (ACoA, AcomA)
a. communicating artery complex
a. communicating artery distribution infarct
a. compartment syndrome
a. condylar canal
a. condyloid foramen
a. cord syndrome
a. coronary plexus
a. corpus
a. corticospinal tract
a. cruciate deficit of knee
a. cruciate ligament (ACL)
a. cruciate ligament injury
a. current (AC) generator
a. curvature
a. cusp
a. cutaneous branch
a. descending artery
a. dislocation
a. drawer sign
a. epidural fat
a. exenteration
a. fascicular block
a. feet view
a. fibular ligament
a. fontanelle
a. fornix of vagina
a. glenoid labrum (AGL)
a. gray column
a. gray column of cord
a. horn
a. horn cell disease
a. horn of spinal cord
a. humeral line
a. hypothalamus
a. iliac crest
a. impingement syndrome
a. inferior tibiofibular ligament
a. intercostal artery
a. interhemispheric cistern
a. interhemispheric fissure
a. internal vertebral vein (AIVV)
a. internodal pathway
a. internodal tract of Bachmann
a. interventricular groove
a. intervertebral disk
a. joint capsule thickening

a. jugular vein
a. junction line
a. labral avulsion
a. labral disruption
a. labroligamentous periosteal sleeve avulsion (ALPSA)
a. labroligamentous periosteal sleeve avulsion lesion
a. leaflet prolapse
a. maxillary spine
a. median fissure
a. mediastinal compartment
a. mediastinal mass
a. mediastinum
a. meningeal artery
a. metatarsal arch
a. midbody of corpus callosum
a. motion of posterior mitral valve leaflet
a. myocardial infarct
a. oblique position
a. osteophyte
a. palatine foramen
a. palatine suture
a. papillary muscle (APM)
a. pararenal space (APS)
a. parietal lesion
a. pillar of fauces
a. precordium
a. predominance
a. projection
a. pulmonary plexus
a. recess of ischiorectal fossa
a. rectus fascia
a. rectus sheath
a. sacral foramen
a. sacral meningocele
a. sagittal diameter (ASD)
scalenus a.
a. scalloping of vertebra
a. semicircular canal
a. semilunar valve
a. septal myocardial infarct
serratus a. (SA)
a. spinal artery
a. spinal artery syndrome
a. spinal ligament calcification
a. spine fusion (ASF)
a. spinocerebellar tract
a. spinothalamic tract
a. spur
a. surface of pancreas

NOTES

anterior *(continued)*
    a. synchondrosis intraoccipital
    a. talar dome
    a. talocalcaneal angle
    a. talofibular ligament (ATF)
    a. tarsal tunnel syndrome
    a. temporal branch of posterior
      cerebral artery
    a. terminal vein (ATV)
    a. thalamotomy
    a. thoracic meningocele
    a. tibial artery
    a. tibial bowing
    a. tibial compartment
    tibialis a.
    a. tibial subluxation
    a. tibial tendon
    a. tibiofibular ligament
    a. tibiotalar ligament
    a. tip of temporal lobe
    a. tracheal displacement
    a. tracking
    a. tricuspid valve leaflet
    a. urethra
    a. urethral injury
    a. vertebral body margin
    a. wall antral ulcer
    a. wall motion
    a. wall myocardial infarct
    a. wedging
anterior-inferior
    a.-i. cerebellar artery (AICA)
    a.-i. cerebral artery (AICA)
    a.-i. communicating artery (AICA)
    a.-i. iliac spine
anterior-posterior
    a.-p. flow direction
    a.-p., posterior-anterior view
anterior/posterior
anterior-superior iliac spine (ASIS)
anterior-to-posterior sagittal canal
  diameter
anteroapical
    a. defect
    a. trabecular septum
anterobasal segment
anterochiasmatic lesion
anterofundal placenta
anterograde
    a. block
    a. peristalsis
anteroinferior
    a. corner fracture
    a. dislocation
    a. myocardial infarct
    a. triangular fragment
anterolateral (AL)

    a. abdominal wall
    a. aspect
    a. compression fracture
    a. fontanelle
    a. groove
    a. gutter
    a. impingement
    a. impingement syndrome
    a. myocardial infarct
    a. rotary knee instability
    a. segment
    a. surface
    a. system
    a. white matter of cord
anterolisthesis
anteromedial
    a. superior humeral head impaction
    a. surface
anteromedian groove
anteroposterior (AP)
    a. aspect
    a. axis
    a. diameter
    a. dimension
    a. film
    a. iliac spine
    a. lordotic projection
    a. position
    a. talocalcaneal (APTC)
    a. tube
    a. view
anteroseptal
    a. commissure
    a. myocardial infarct
antetorsion
    femoral a.
anteversion
    acetabular a. (AA)
    angle of a.
    femoral a.
    Magilligan technique for measuring
      neutral a.
anteverted uterus
anthracosilicosis
anthracosis
anthracotic material
anthrax
    a. exposure
    inhalation a.
    a. pneumonia
anthrocotic tuberculosis
anthropoid pelvis
anthropologic baseline
anthropometric imaging
anthropometry
    3D surface a.
anthropomorphic baseline

antiaggregation
antialiasing technique
antibody
    a. half-life
    a. labeling
    radiolabeled a.
    ^{99m}Tc-labeled antigranulocyte a.
antibody-conjugated paramagnetic
    liposome (ACPL)
antibody-labeled circulating granulocyte
anti-CEA
    radiolabeled a.-C.
anticoagulant bleed
anticoagulant-related bleed
anticoagulation
anticoincidence circuit
antiestrogen radiologic therapy
antiferromagnetism
antifibrin
    a. antibody imaging
    a. antibody imaging agent
    a. scintigraphy
antigen expression
antigen-modulated mini-stem cell
    transplant
antigravity muscle
antiidiotypic affinity chromatography
antimesenteric
    a. border
    a. border of distal ileum
    a. fat pad
antimesocolic side of cecum
antimyosin monoclonal antibody imaging
    agent
antineutrino
antiparticle
antiproton
antiradial technique
antiscatter grid
antisense oligonucleotide
antisiphon device
antitragohelicine fissure
antitubercular therapy
Antopol-Goldman lesion
antra (*pl. of* antrum)
antral
    a. beaking
    a. edema
    a. gastritis
    a. G-cell hyperplasia
    a. mucosal diaphragm
    a. mucosal thickening

    a. padding
    a. polyp
    a. pouch
    a. sphincter
    a. stasis
    a. stenosis
    a. stomach narrowing
    a. stricture
    a. ulcer
    a. web
antrochoanal polyp
antroduodenal motility
antropyloric
    a. canal
    a. muscle thickness (APT)
antrum, pl. **antra**
    aditus ad a.
    cardiac a.
    a. cardiacum of Highmore
    gastric a.
    Highmore a.
    Malacarne a.
    mastoid a.
    maxillary a.
    prepyloric a.
    pyloric a.
    retained gastric a.
    a. of stomach
    Willis a.
anular, annular
    a. abscess
    a. appearance
    a. array
    a. array transducer
    a. calcification
    a. constricting lesion
    a. detector
    a. dilatation
    a. disk bulge
    a. disruption
    a. epiphysis
    a. esophageal stricture
    a. fiber
    a. fibrosis
    a. foreshortening
    a. fracture
    a. hypoplasia
    a. lamellae
    a. ligament
    a. ligament of trachea
    a. pancreas
    a. phased-array hyperthermia

NOTES

anular *(continued)*
    a. placement
    a. placenta
    a. rim of cartilage
    a. tear
    a. tear classification
    a. tear extent
    a. tear pattern
anuloaortic ectasia
anulospiral organ
anulus, anulus
    aortic valve a.
    atrioventricular a.
    bulging a.
    calcified a.
    a. fibrosus
    fissure of a.
    friable a.
    mitral valve of a.
    a. ovalis
    periphery of the a.
    posterior a.
    pulmonary valve a.
    redundant scallop of posterior a.
    septal tricuspid a.
    tricuspid valve a.
    valve a.
    Vieussens a.
    Zinn a.
anus
    ectopic a.
    imperforate a.
    levator a.'s
anvil bone
AO
    aorta
    aortic opening
        AO ankle fracture classification
        AO classification of ankle fracture
        AO tension band
AO/AC
    aortic valve opening to aortic valve
    closing ratio
AOCS
    anatomy-oriented colon segmentation
AOD
    airflow obstruction disease
AO-Danis-Weber ankle fracture
classification
AOIVM
    angiographically occult intracranial
    vascular malformation
aorta, pl. **aortae (AO)**
    abdominal a.
    aneurysmal widening of a.
    ascending a. (AA)
    ascending hypoplasia of a.

bifurcation of a.
biventricular origin of a.
biventricular transposed a.
brachiocephalic trunk of a.
calcified a.
central a.
cervical a.
coarctation of a.
descending thoracic a.
dextropositioned a.
dilated descending a.
distal a.
D-malposition of a.
double arch a.
double-barrel a.
draped a.
dynamic a.
ectasia of a.
elongated a.
feminine a.
Hodgson aneurysmal dilatation of
  the a.
infantile coarctation of a.
infrarenal abdominal a.
intramural hematoma of a.
juxtaductal coarctation of a.
kinked a.
L-malposition of a.
native a.
occlusion a.
overriding a.
pericardial a.
porcelain a.
postductal coarctation of a.
proximal a.
pseudocoarctation of a.
recoarctation of a.
reconstruction of a.
retroesophageal a.
reversed coarctation of a.
small feminine a.
stenosis of a.
supraceliac a.
supradiaphragmatic a.
symptomatic coarctation of a.
terminal a.
thoracic a.
thoracoabdominal a.
tortuous a.
transposed a.
tulip bulb a.
uncoiling ascending a.
uncoiling descending a.
unwinding of a.
ventral a.
widening of a.
wide tortuous a.

aorta-left ventricular fistula
aorta-right ventricular fistula
aortic

a. allograft
a. anulus abscess
a. aperture
a. arch
a. arch aneurysm
a. arch angiography
a. arch anomaly
a. arch atresia
a. arch calcification
a. arch interruption
a. arch lesion
a. arch malformation
a. arch obstruction
a. atherosclerosis
a. attenuation
a. bifurcation
a. body tumor
a. bulb
a. button
a. cannulation
a. cartilage
a. closure (AC)
a. coarctation
a. cuff
a. cusp
a. cusp separation
a. deviation
a. diameter (AD)
a. dilation
a. dissection
a. distensibility
a. elongation
a. flow (AF)
a. flow volume
a. foramen
a. gland
a. graft infection
a. hiatus
a. idiopathic necrosis
a. impedance
a. incisura
a. inflammation
a. inflow
a. insult
a. intimal dehiscence
a. intramural hematoma
a. isthmus
a. kinking
a. knob

a. knuckle
a. lumen
a. lymph node
a. motion artifact
a. nipple
a. nipple sign
a. node metastasis
a. notch
a. opening (AO)
a. opening of heart
a. orifice   —
a. ostium
a. outflow gradient
a. outflow obstruction
a. override
a. oxygen saturation
a. paravalvular leak
a. penetrating ulcer
a. plexus
a. prominence
a. pseudoaneurysm
a. pullback
a. reconstruction
a. regurgitation (AR)
a. root
a. root cineangiography
a. root diameter
a. root dilatation
a. root dimension
a. root echocardiography
a. root homograft
a. root pressure
a. root ratio
a. root replacement
a. runoff
a. rupture
a. sac
a. sclerosis
a. segment
a. septal defect
a. septum
a. shag
a. sinotubular junction
a. sinus aneurysm
a. sinus to right ventricle fistula
a. spindle
a. stenosis (AS)
a. stiffness
a. stump blowout
a. thromboembolism
a. thrombosis
a. tract complex hypoplasia

NOTES

aortic *(continued)*
    a. transsection
    a. tube graft
    a. valve (AoV)
    a. valve anulus
    a. valve area (AVA)
    a. valve atresia
    a. valve calcification
    a. valve deformity
    a. valve echocardiography
    a. valve endocarditis
    a. valve gradient (AVG)
    a. valve lesion
    a. valve nodule
    a. valve obstruction
    a. valve opening
    a. valve opening to aortic valve
      closing ratio (AO/AC)
    a. valve peak instantaneous
      gradient
    a. valve pressure gradient
    a. valve replacement (AVR)
    a. valve sinus
    a. valve thickening
    a. valvular disease (AVD)
    a. valvular incompetence
    a. valvular insufficiency
    a. vasa vasorum
    a. vent suction line
    a. vestibule of ventricle
    a. wall thickening
    a. window
    a. window node
    a. wrap
aortic-brachiocephalic (ABC)
    a.-b. injury
aortic-enteric fistula
aortic-left ventricular tunnel
aorticopulmonary *(var. of*
  aortopulmonary)
aorticorenal
    a. ganglion
    a. graft
aortitis
    infectious a.
    luetic a.
    a. syndrome
    Takayasu a.
aortobifemoral reconstruction
aortobiliac bypass
aortocaval fistula
aortocoronary valve
aortoduodenal fistula
aortoenteric fistula
aortoesophageal fistula
aortofemoral
    a. arteriography

    a. bypass graft (AFBG)
    a. runoff
aortogastric
aortogram
    arch a.
    transbrachial arch a.
aortography
    abdominal a.
    antegrade a.
    arch a.
    ascending a.
    balloon occlusive a.
    biplanar a.
    catheter a.
    contrast a.
    countercurrent a.
    digital subtraction a.
    flush a.
    a. imaging
    intravenous a.
    lumbar a.
    postangioplasty a.
    preembolization a.
    renal a.
    retrograde femoral a.
    retrograde transaxillary a.
    retrograde transfemoral a.
    retrograde translumbar a.
    selective visceral a.
    supravalvular a.
    thoracic arch a.
    translumbar a. (TLA)
    ultrasonic a.
    venous a.
    visceral a.
aortoiliac
    a. aneurysm
    a. bypass graft
    a. inflow assessment
    a. inflow system
    a. obstruction
    a. occlusive disease (AIOD)
    a. stenosis
    a. thrombosis
aortoiliofemoral artery
aortojejunal fistula
aortomegaly
    diffuse a.
aortoplasty
    balloon a.
    patch-graft a.
    posterior patch a.
    subclavian flap a.
    a. with patch graft
aortopulmonary, aorticopulmonary
    a. fenestration
    a. fistula

a. mediastinal stripe
a. septal defect
a. septum
a. trunk
a. window
a. window mass
aortosclerosis
aortoseptal continuity
aortosigmoid fistula
aortovelography
transcutaneous a. (TAV)
aortoventriculoplasty
AoV
aortic valve
AOVM
angiographically occult vascular
malformation
AP
adenomatous polyp
anteroposterior
AP inversion stress vagina view
AP malleolar bisection
AP projection
AP supine portable view
apallic syndrome
APC-3, APC-4 collimator
ape hand of syringomyelia
ape-like hand
aperiodic
a. complex
a. functional MR imaging
a. wave
aperistalsis
esophageal a.
aperistaltic
a. distal ureteral segment
a. esophagus
aperta
spina bifida a.
apertura, pl. **aperturae**
a. externa canaliculi cochleae
a. pelvis inferior
a. pelvis superior
a. piriformis
a. sinus frontalis
aperture
aortic a.
coded-image a.
a. diaphragm
superior thoracic a.
apex, pl. **apices**
a. beat

a. of bladder
cardiac a.
a. cardiogram (ACG)
a. cordis
displaced left ventricular a.
duodenal bulb a. (DBA)
external ring a.
a. of femur
a. of fibula
F point of cardiac a.
a. of head of patella
a. of the heart
Koch triangle a.
left ventricular a.
lung a.
orbital a.
petrous a.
a. of petrous portion of temporal
bone
A. Plus excimer laser
a. of prostate
right ventricular a. (RVA)
sternal a.
systolic retraction of a.
uptilted cardiac a.
ventricular a.
APEX 409, 415 camera
aphalangia
apheresis catheter
aphtha, pl. **aphthae**
aphthoid
a. ulcer
aphthous stomach ulcer
apical
a. aspect
a. atelectasis
a. bronchus
a. canaliculus
a. cap
a. capping
a. cap sign
a. complex
a. corn
a. defect
a. duodenal ulcer
a. ectodermal ridge (AER)
a. fenestration
a. five-chamber view
echocardiography
a. foramen
a. gland
a. granuloma

NOTES

apical *(continued)*
   a. hypokinesis
   a. hypoperfusion
   a. impulse
   a. infiltrate
   a. lesion
   a. ligament
   a. lordotic projection
   a. lordotic view
   a. lymph node
   a. myocardial infarct
   a. notch
   a. petrositis
   a. pleural thickening
   a. pneumonia
   a. posterior artery
   a. process
   a. scarring
   a. segment
   a. short-axis slice
   a. and subcostal four-chambered
     view
   a. surface of heart
   a. suture
   a. thinning
   a. tissue
   a. two-chamber view
     echocardiography
   a. wall
   a. wall motion
   a. window
apical-lateral wall myocardial infarct
apically directed chest tube
apices (*pl. of* apex)
apicoposterior
   a. bronchus
   a. segment
apiculate waveform
aplasia
   bilateral semicircular canal a.
   cerebellar a.
   cochlea a.
   a. of deep vein
   deep venous a.
   lung a.
   Michel a.
   pulmonary a.
   radial a.
aplastic uterus
APLD
   automated percutaneous lumbar
   diskectomy
APM
   anterior papillary muscle
apnea-bradycardia ratio
apnea-hypopnea index (AHI)

apocrine
   a. adenoma
   a. carcinoma
   a. cyst
   a. metaplasia
   a. sweat gland
Apogee
   A. CX100, CX200
     echocardiography system
   A. RX400 diagnostic ultrasound
     system
Apollo DXA bone densitometry system
Apomate radiopharmaceutical imaging agent
aponeurosis
   bicipital a.
   digital a.
   epicranial a.
   external oblique a.
   flexor carpi ulnaris a.
   internal oblique a.
   palmar a.
   plantar a.
   tendon a.
aponeurotic
   a. band
   a. fibroma
   a. portion of diaphragm
   a. tendon
   a. triangle
   a. troika
apophyseal, apophysial
   a. fracture
   a. injury
   a. joint
   a. lesion
   a. point
   a. pouch
apophysis, pl. **apophyses**
   bone lesion a.
   calcaneal a.
   fragmentation of a.
   a. of Rau
   rim a.
   ring a.
apophysitis
   calcaneal a.
   iliac a.
apoplexy
   cerebellar a.
   delayed pineal a.
   mesenteric a.
   pineal a.
   pituitary a.
   postpartum pituitary a.
   pulmonary artery a.
   pulmonary vein a.

apoptic
  a. body
  a. nuclear fragment
aporic gland
apotentiality
  cerebral a.
APP
  average pixel projection
AP-PA
  A.-P. skull block
  A.-P. skull immobilizer
apparatus
  Acuson 128 a.
  electrooculogram a.
  extensor a.
  Hilal embolization a.
  Jaquet a.
  juxtaglomerular a. (JGA)
  mitral a.
  oculomotor a.
  stereotactic a.
  valvular a.
  vestibular a.
  zero time of the x-ray a.
apparent
  a. diffusion coefficient (ADC)
  a. paramagnetism
  a. volume of distribution (Vd)
appearance
  anular a.
  apple-core a.
  apple-peel a.
  applesauce a.
  asymmetric target a.
  ball-in-hand a.
  banding a.
  batwing a.
  beaded necklace a.
  beaked a.
  beaten brass a.
  beaten silver a.
  beaver-tail a.
  bilaminar a.
  bird-like a.
  blade-of-grass a.
  blown-out a.
  bone-within-bone a.
  bubble-like a.
  bull-neck a.
  bull's eye a.
  bunch-of-grapes a.
  butterfly a.

candle dripping a.
catheter tip hockey-stick a.
cauliflower a.
chisel-like truncated a.
Christmas tree a.
cobblestone a.
cobra-head a.
cobweb a.
cockscomb a.
coffee-bean a.
coiled spring a.
collar-button a.
colonic lead-pipe a.
corkscrew a.
cottage loaf a.
cotton ball a.
cotton-wool a.
crabmeat-like a.
crazy paving a.
cystic a.
double-bubble a.
double-bulb a.
double-halo a.
drooping lily a.
drumstick a.
dumbbell a.
duodenal teardrop a.
echogenic a.
Erlenmeyer flask a.
feathery a.
featureless a.
figure-8 a.
fine-speckled a.
fish flesh a.
fishnet a.
flame a.
frayed-string a.
frog-like a.
frond-like a.
ground-glass a.
hair-on-end a.
hammered-brass a.
hammered-silver a.
heterogeneous a.
hole-within-hole a.
holly leaf a.
homogeneous a.
Honda sign a.
honeycomb a.
horseshoe a.
hot-cross bun a.
ill-defined a.

NOTES

appearance *(continued)*
  inverse comma a.
  inverted-T a.
  irregular tapered a.
  isodense a.
  jail-bar a.
  jelly-belly a.
  kernel-of-corn a.
  lace-like a.
  leafless tree a.
  light bulb a.
  lobulated saccular a.
  lollipop tree a.
  Mickey Mouse a.
  mixed-echo a.
  molar tooth a.
  moth-eaten a.
  mottled a.
  multiseptate a.
  mushroom a.
  Neptune trident a.
  nodular a.
  nodule-in-a-nodule a.
  onion peel a.
  onionskin a.
  owl's eye a.
  pancake a.
  panda a.
  partial tubular a.
  picket fence a.
  picture frame a.
  plug-like a.
  polka-dot a.
  popcorn-like a.
  pruned-tree a.
  pseudopost Billroth I a.
  pseudotumor a.
  punched-out a.
  radial scar-like mammographic a.
  railroad track a.
  reticulogranular a.
  ring-like a.
  rounded a.
  rugger jersey a.
  saber-shin a.
  sandwich a.
  sausage-shaped a.
  sawtooth a.
  scalloped a.
  scottie dog a.
  septate a.
  serpentine a.
  serrated a.
  shading a.
  shell-of-bone a.
  smooth tapered a.
  snake's head a.
  soap-bubble a.
  spade-like a.
  spiderweb a.
  spiral a.
  spongy a.
  stacked-coin a.
  stained-glass a.
  stepladder a.
  stippled a.
  string-of-beads a.
  string-of-pearls a.
  sunburst a.
  sun-ray a.
  Swiss Alps a.
  Swiss cheese a.
  tam-o-shanter a.
  target a.
  teardrop a.
  thumbprint a.
  tram-track a.
  tree-in-winter bile duct a.
  trefoil a.
  trilaminar a.
  trilayer a.
  twisted small bowel ribbon a.
  ventricle batwing a.
  wafer-like a.
  walking-stick a.
  waterfall a.
  web-like a.
  well-defined a.
  whirlpool a.
  whorled a.
  windsock a.
  wine glass a.
  wormy a.
  yin-yang a.
  zebra stripe a.

appendage
  atrial a.
  cecal a.
  coccygeal a.
  epiploic a.
  left atrial a. (LAA)
  left auricular a. (LAA)
  right atrial a. (RAA)
  testicular torsion a.
  truncated atrial a.
  vermicular a.
  wide-based, blunt-ended, right-sided, atrial a.

appendiceal
  a. abscess
  a. carcinoma
  a. intussusception
  a. mass
  a. stump

appendices (*pl. of* appendix)
appendicolith (*var. of* appendolith)
appendicolithiasis (*var. of*
  appendolithiasis)
appendicular
  a. bone mass measurement
  a. lymph node
  a. skeleton
  a. vein
appendiculare
  skeleton a.
appendix, pl. appendices
  cecal a.
  double a.
  ensiform a.
  a. of epididymis
  epiploic a.
  a. epiploica
  filiform a.
  Morgagni a.
  a. mucocele
  paracecal a.
  perforated gangrenous a.
  retrocecal a.
  retroileal a.
  a. rupture
  subcecal a.
  a. testis
  a. of ventricle of larynx
  vermicular a.
  vermiform a.
  vesiculosa a.
  xiphoid a.
appendolith, appendicolith
appendolithiasis, appendicolithiasis
apperceptive mass
apple-core
  a.-c. appearance
  a.-c. carcinoma
  a.-c. lesion
  a.-c. tumor
apple-peel
  a.-p. appearance
  a.-p. appearance of GI tract
  a.-p. bowel
  a.-p. syndrome
applesauce appearance
application
  infradiaphragmatic a.
  interstitial radioelement a.
  intracavitary radioelement a.

  ribbon a.
  surface radioelement a.
**application-specific integrated circuit
  (ASIC)**
applicator
  beam-therapy a.
  beta-ray a.
  Burnett a.
  colpostat a.
  Henschke seed a.
  intracavitary afterloading a.
  LITT a.
  Mick seed a.
  Nucletron a.
  small LITT a.
  ^{90}Sr-loaded eye a.
  standard LITT a.
  Syed-Puthawala-Hedger
    esophageal a.
  tandem a.
  Wang a.
APPM
  antegrade perfusion pressure
    measurement
apposing articular surface
apposition
  bone-to-bone a.
  bony a.
  close a.
  fracture in close a.
  a. of leaflet
  margin of a.
approach
  axillofemoral a.
  bipediculate a.
  brachial artery a.
  direct transtorcular a.
  endovascular embolization
    femoral a.
  femoral artery a.
  femoral venous a.
  mask-based a.
  organ-sparing treatment a.
  particle a.
  pencil-beam a.
  posterior retrocrural a.
  posterior transcaval a.
  pterional transsylvian a.
  retrograde femoral arterial a.
  skull-base a.
  unipediculate a.

NOTES

approximation
Born a.
apron
abdominal a.
lead-rubber a.
quadriceps a.
a. shield
APS
anterior pararenal space
APT
antropyloric muscle thickness
attached proton test
automatic peak tracking
APTC
anteroposterior talocalcaneal
AQP4 expression
aquagenic
AquariusBLUE 3D imaging
AquariusNET 2D/3D medical imaging server
AquaSens FMS 1000 fluid monitoring system
aqueduct
cerebral a.
cochlear a.
a. compression
forking of sylvian a.
gliosis of sylvian a.
mesencephalon a.
midbrain a.
Monro a.
a. stenosis
sylvian a.
a. of Sylvius
ventricular a.
vestibular a.
aqueductal
a. CSF stroke volume
a. forking
a. jet
a. obstruction
a. occlusion
a. stenosis
aqueous
a. solution
a. vein
Aquilion plus V-detector CT scanner
AR
aortic regurgitation
atrial rate
ARA
anorectal angle
arabinsylguanosine triphosphate
arachnodactilia
arachnodactyly CHD
arachnoid
a. brain cyst

a. canal
a. diverticulum
a. fibrosis
a. granulation
a. granulation calcification
a. loculation of the spine
pia a.
a. retrocerebellar pouch
a. space
a. spine cyst
a. of uncus
a. villi obstruction
a. villus
arachnoidal
a. foramen
a. gliomatosis
arachnoidea mater encephali
arachnoiditis
adhesive a.
cystic a.
fibrosing a.
Arantius
A. canal
A. ligament
A. nodule
nodulus A.
A. ventricle
arborescens
lipoma a.
arborescent
arborization
a. block
cervical mucus a.
a. of duct
a. pattern
pulmonary a.
arborize
arboroid
arc
bregmatolambdoid a.
nasobregmatic a.
nasooccipital a.
pulmonary a.
a. radiotherapy
reflex a.
a. ring
a. therapy
a. welder's lung
arcade
collateral a.
a. of Frohse
Frohse ligamentous a.
gastroepiploic a.
mitral a.
septal a.
Struthers a.

subpleural pulmonary a.
superficialis a.
Arcelin view
arch
anastomotic a.
a. angle
anterior atlas a.
anterior metatarsal a.
a. of aorta abnormality
aortic a.
a. aortogram
a. aortography
articular a.
atlas a.
azygous a.
a. bar
a. of bone
carpal a.
cervical aortic a.
chimney-shaped high aortic a.
circumflex retroesophageal a.
congenital interruption of aortic a.
coracoacromial a.
cortical kidney a.
deep a.
distal aortic a.
double aortic a.
ductal a.
embryonic aortic a.
embryonic branchial a.
a. of fauces
first branchial a.
flattened a.
a. of foot
fourth branchial a.
a. fracture
Hapad metatarsal a.
hemal a.
high a.
Hillock a.
hyoid a.
hypochordal a.
hypoplastic aortic a.
keystone of calcar a.
a. length index
longitudinal a.
lung a.
medial a.
midaortic a.
mural a.
neural vertebral a.
osseocartilaginous a.

osseoligamentous a.
palmar arterial a.
plantar arterial a.
posterior metatarsal a.
posterior neural a.
posterior turn of the aortic a.
pubic a.
retroesophageal a.
right aortic a.
right-sided a.
Riolan a.
a. rupture
second branchial a.
subpubic a.
superciliary a.
superficial palmar arterial a.
target a.
tarsal a.
third branchial a.
tortuous aortic a.
transverse aortic a.
vertebral a.
Zimmerman a.
zygomatic a.
arched crest
archenteric canal
archicortex
arching of mitral valve leaflet
architectural
a. alterations of bone
a. distortion
a. disturbance
a. effacement
a. pattern
a. symmetry
architecture
bony a.
brain a.
disorganized a.
ductal a.
foot a.
hepatic a.
internal a.
intestinal villous a.
intranodal a.
lobular a.
lung a.
microstructural a.
mural a.
trabecular a.
archival system
arciform vein

NOTES

Arco classification
arcuate
- a. artery
- a. complex
- a. crest
- a. eminence
- a. fasciculus (AF)
- a. fiber involvement
- a. ligament
- a. movement
- a. nucleus
- a. uterus
- a. vein
- a. vessel

arcuatus
- pes a.
- talipes a.
- uterus a.

ARD
anisotropically rotational diffusion
ARDS
acute respiratory distress syndrome
adult respiratory distress syndrome
area
- a. of abnormal density
- amygdaloid a.
- anechoic a.
- aortic valve a. (AVA)
- arrhythmogenic a.
- Bamberger a.
- bare a.
- body surface a. (BSA)
- Broca a.
- Brodmann a. 32
- callosal a.
- cardiac frontal a.
- cluster of radiolucent a. (CORLA)
- cortical motor a.
- cross-sectional a. (CSA)
- denervated a.
- a. of denudation
- echo-free a.
- echo-poor a.
- effective balloon-dilated a. (EBDA)
- fat-density a.
- fractional a.
- a. gastrica
- gastrohepatic bare a.
- Gorlin formula for aortic valve a.
- Gorlin formula for mitral valve a.
- Hatle method to calculate mitral valve a.
- hilar a.
- hot a.
- hyperechoic a.
- hypodense a.
- hypoechoic a.

hypometabolic a.
a. of increased radiolabeling
infraclavicular a.
infrahilar a.
ischemic a.
lenticular a.
a. of lucency
luminal a.
lytic a.
metabolically inert a.
midsternal a.
mitral regurgitant signal a.
mitral valve a. (MVA)
motor a.
olfactory a.
parietal association a.
parietooccipital a.
parietotemporal a.
peak a.
periaortic a.
perihilar a.
periportal a.
pharyngeal a.
photon-deficient a.
photopenic a.
postcricoid a.
premotor a.
proliferation a.
a. prostrema
proximal isovelocity surface a. (PISA)
puboischial a.
pulmonary valve a.
pulmonic a.
punched-out a.
radiodensity a.
radiolucent a.
rarefied a.
regurgitant orifice a. (ROA)
retrocardiac a.
retroperitoneal a.
retrosternal a.
Rolando a.
sclerotic a.
scrotal a.
septal a.
skip a.
sonolucent a.
speech a.
stenosis a.
subglottic a.
subhepatic a.
suprapubic a.
transverse cranial a.
tricuspid valve a.
a. under the curve (AUC)
valve a.

water density a.
watershed a.
Wernicke a.
xiphopubic a.
zygomaticomalar a.
area/hemidiameter variation
area-length method for ejection fraction
Arelin method
areola of bone
areolar
a. connective tissue
a. plane
ARF
acute renal failure
acute respiratory failure
ArF excimer laser
argentaffinoma
argon
a. beam coagulator (ABC)
a. laser
a. laser trabeculectomy (ATL)
argon/krypton laser
argon-pumped dye laser
Argus camera
arhinencephaly
ARJ
anorectal junction
arm
Leyla a.
linebacker's a.
outrigger a.
Pinpoint stereotactic a.
scanning a.
Armanni-Ebstein lesion
arm-down image
arm-lung time
armored heart
arms-up positioning
arm-up image
Arnold
A. canal
A. convolution
Arnold-Chiari
A.-C. deformity
A.-C. malformation
A.-C. syndrome
aromatic solvent-induced shift (ASIS)
ARP
adiabatic rapid passage
ARPKD
autosomal recessive polycystic kidney
disease

arrangement
string-of-pearls nuclear a.
array
Acuson 5-MHz linear a.
anular a.
cartesian reference coordinate
voxel a.
coil a.
convex linear a.
detector a.
electrode a.
gate a.
high-density linear a.
linear electrode a.
linear phased a.
9- to 5-MHz convex a.
multiple coil a.
NMR quadrature detection a.
parallel a.
a. processor
silicon diode a.
symmetric phased a.
thin-film transistor a.
voxel a.
arrest
circulatory a.
electrical circulatory a.
epiphyseal a.
flow a.
growth plate a.
intermittent sinus a.
a. reaction
sinus a.
transient sinus a.
arrested circulation
arrhenoblastoma
arrhinencephaly
arrhythmia
a. circuit
a. mapping system
venography-related a.
arrhythmia-insensitive
a.-i. flow-sensitive alternating
inversion recovery (A-FAIR)
a.-i. flow-sensitive alternating IR
arrhythmic myocardial infarct
arrhythmogenic
a. area
a. border zone
a. myocardial tissue ablation
catheter
a. right ventricular cardiomyopathy

NOTES

arrhythmogenic *(continued)*
    a. right ventricular dysplasia (ARVD)
Arrow
    A. catheter
    A. Fischell Evan Needle
    A. PICC line
ArrowFlex sheath
arrowhead-shaped
arrowhead sign
Arrow-Trerotola percutaneous thrombectomy device
ART
    algebraic reconstruction technique
    ART transducer
artefact *(var. of* artifact)
arteria, pl. **arteriae**
    a. lusoria
    a. radicularis anterior magna
    a. radicularis magna of Adamkiewicz
arterial
    a. access
    a. anatomy
    a. aneurysm
    a. angioma
    a. avulsion
    a. blockage
    a. brachiocephalic trunk
    a. brain anastomosis
    a. brain displacement
    a. branch
    a. bulb
    a. bypass graft
    a. calcification
    a. canal
    a. cannulation
    a. capillary
    a. circle
    a. circle of Willis
    a. collateral
    a. cone
    a. cutoff
    a. deficiency pattern
    a. degenerative disease
    a. dilatation
    a. dilatation and rupture
    a. dimension
    a. duct
    a. embolus
    a. endothelium
    a. fenestration
    a. flow-phase image
    a. gland
    a. groove
    a. hemorrhage
    a. hyperemia

    a. hypertension
    a. hypotension
    a. infusion
    a. insufficiency
    a. intima
    a. invasion
    a. kinking
    a. ligament
    a. linear density
    a. lumen
    a. malformation (AM)
    a. narrowing
    a. nephrosclerosis
    a. obstruction
    a. occlusion
    a. opacification
    a. oxygen saturation
    a. patency
    a. peak systolic pressure
    a. phase
    a. plaque
    a. port catheter system
    a. portography
    a. pseudoaneurysm
    a. pulsatility
    a. pulsation artifact
    a. puncture site closure device
    a. return
    a. runoff
    a. sclerosis
    a. scrotum supply
    a. segment
    a. sheath
    a. spasm
    a. steal
    a. stenosis
    a. sump effect
    a. thrombosis
    a. tonus
    a. topography
    a. tree
    a. varix
    a. vein
    a. wall
    a. wall dissection
    a. wall thickness
    a. waveform
arterial-arterial fistula
arterialization
    hypervascular a.
    a. of venous blood
arterial-portal fistula
arteries *(pl. of* artery)
arteriobiliary fistula
arteriocapillary sclerosis
arteriococcygeal gland
arteriogenic impotence

arteriogram
arteriography
    abdominal visceral a.
    aortofemoral a.
    axillary a.
    balloon occlusion a.
    bilateral carotid a.
    biplane pelvic a.
    biplane quantitative coronary a.
    brachial a.
    brachiocephalic a.
    bronchial a.
    carotid cerebral a.
    catheter a.
    celiac a.
    cerebral a.
    cine coronary a.
    completion a.
    contrast a.
    coronary a.
    cortical kidney a.
    CT a.
    delayed phase of a.
    digital subtraction a. (DSA)
    documentary a.
    femoral runoff a.
    four-vessel a.
    hepatic a.
    infrahepatic a.
    intraoperative a.
    ipsilateral antegrade a.
    Judkins coronary a.
    longitudinal a.
    lumbar a.
    mesenteric a.
    operative a.
    pancreatic a.
    pelvic a.
    percutaneous femoral a.
    peripheral a.
    postdilatation a.
    proximity a.
    pulmonary a.
    quantitative coronary a. (QCA)
    renal a.
    retrograde a.
    ring blush on cerebral a.
    runoff a.
    selective cerebral a.
    selective coronary a.
    selective visceral a.
    Sones selective coronary a.

    spinal a.
    spiral computed tomography a.
      (SCTA)
    splenic a.
    subclavian a.
    superior mesenteric a.
    transfemoral a.
    vertebral a.
    visceral a.
    wedge a.
    x-ray a. (XRA)
arteriohepatic dysplasia
arteriolar
    a. ischemic ulcer
    a. narrowing
    a. necrosis
    a. resistance
    a. sclerosis
arteriole
    reactive a.
arteriole-capillary-venous bed
arteriolovenular bridge
arteriomyomatosis
arteriopathy
    plexogenic pulmonary a.
arterioportobiliary fistula
arterioportography
    computed tomography with a.
      (CTAP)
arteriorenal
arteriosclerosis
    calcific a.
    cerebral a.
    coronary a.
    generalized a.
    hyaline a.
    hypertensive a.
    idiopathic pulmonary a. (IPA)
    infantile a.
    intimal a.
    kidney a.
    medial a.
    Mönckeberg a.
    a. obliterans (ASO)
    obliterative a.
    obscuration a.
    obstructing embolus a.
    peripheral a.
    presenile a.
    pulmonary a.
    renal a.
    senile a.

NOTES

arteriosclerotic
    a. cardiovascular disease (ASCVD)
    a. deposit
    a. heart disease (ASHD)
    a. intracranial aneurysm
    a. kidney
    a. occlusive disease
    a. peripheral vascular disease
    a. plaque
    a. thoracoabdominal aortic
      aneurysm
arteriosinusoidal penile fistula
arteriostenosis
arteriosum
    cor a.
    ligamentum a.
arteriosus
    calcified ductus a.
    ductus a.
    embryonic truncus a.
    patent ductus a. (PDA)
    persistent ductus a.
    persistent truncus a. (PTA)
    premature closure of ductus a.
    pseudotruncus a.
    railroad track ductus a.
    reversed ductus a.
    silent patent ductus a.
    truncus a.
arteriovascular calcification
arteriovenous (AV)
    a. anastomosis (AVA)
    a. brain malformation
    a. colon malformation
    a. cord malformation
    a. fistula (AVF)
    a. fistula transplant
    a. hemangioma
    a. interhemispheric angioma
    a. kidney malformation
    a. malformation (AVM)
    a. malformation nidus
    a. pressure gradient
    a. pulmonary aneurysm
    a. shunt imaging
    a. varix
arteritis, pl. arteritides
    carotid artery a.
    cranial granulomatous a.
    luetic a.
    Takayasu a.
    temporal granulomatous a.
artery, pl. arteries
    A1-A5 segments of anterior
      cerebral a.
    Abbott a.
    abdominal aortic a.

aberrant right subclavian a.
accessory middle cerebral a.
accessory right renal a.
accessory right uterine a.
Adamkiewicz a.
adrenal a.
adventitia of a.
ambient segment of posterior
  cerebral a.
angiographic corkscrew a.
angular a.
anomalous left coronary a.
anomalous left pulmonary a.
anomalous origin of a.
anomalous right subclavian a.
anterior cerebral a. (ACA)
anterior choroidal a.
anterior communicating a. (ACoA,
  AcomA)
anterior descending a.
anterior-inferior cerebellar a.
  (AICA)
anterior-inferior cerebral a. (AICA)
anterior-inferior communicating a.
  (AICA)
anterior intercostal a.
anterior meningeal a.
anterior spinal a.
anterior temporal branch of
  posterior cerebral a.
anterior tibial a.
aortoiliofemoral a.
apical posterior a.
arcuate a.
ascending frontoparietal a.
ascending pharyngeal a.
atrial circumflex a.
atrioventricular node a. (AVNA)
auricular a.
axillary a.
azygos anterior cerebral a.
basal cerebral a.
basal perforating a.
basilar a.
beading of a.
bifurcation of anterior
  communicating a.
bifurcation of internal carotid a.
blocked a.
brachial a.
brachiocephalic a.
branch of a.
bronchial a.
a. bronchus ratio (ABR)
buckled innominate a.
bulbourethral a.
calcarine a.

calcific a.
callosomarginal a.
candelabra a.
cannulated a.
caroticotympanic a.
carotid a.
cavernous segment of internal
  carotid a.
C1-C5 segment of internal
  carotid a.
celiac branch a.
central a.
cerebellar a.
cerebellolabyrinthine a.
cerebral a.
cervical segment of internal
  carotid a.
CF a.
choroidal pericallosal a.
circumflex coronary a.
circumflex groove a.
colic a.
collateral circulation in compression
  of a.
common carotid a. (CCA)
common femoral a.
common hepatic a.
common iliac a.
common peroneal a.
communicating a.
complete transposition of great a.
congenital absence of pulmonary a.
congenital aneurysm of
  pulmonary a.
congenitally corrected transposition
  of the great a.
contralateral a.
conus a.
a. of the conus medullaris
corduroy a.
corkscrew appearance of hepatic a.
coronary a.
corrected transposition of great a.
cortical a.
costocervical a.
course of a.
cremasteric a.
CX a.
cystic a.
deep a.
deferential a.
deltoid branch of posterior tibial a.

descending septal a.
dextrotransposition of great a.
diagonal branch of a.
a. diameter
dilated pulmonary a.
diminutive interlobar right
  pulmonary a.
dissection of a.
distal circumflex marginal a.
dominant left coronary a.
dominant right coronary a.
dorsal a.
Drummond marginal a.
ductus deferens a.
duodenal a.
duplex ultrasound carotid a.
dural a.
dynamic entrapment of vertebral a.
eccentric coronary a.
ectatic carotid a.
elastic recoil of a.
en passage feeder a.
a. entrapment
epicardial coronary a.
ethmoidal a.
external carotid a. (ECA)
external iliac a.
extracranial vertebral a.
extradural a.
facial a.
falx a.
familial fibromuscular dysplasia
  of a.
feeder a.
feeding branch of a.
femoral a.
femoropopliteal a.
fenestration of the basilar a.
first diagonal branch a.
first obtuse marginal a.
FP a.
friable a.
frontal a.
frontopolar a.
fusiform narrowing of a.
gastric a.
gastroduodenal a.
gastroepiploic a.
gonadal a.
helicine a.
hepatic a.
Heubner a.

NOTES

artery *(continued)*

high left main diagonal a.
hilar a.
horizontal segment of middle
  cerebral a.
hyaloid a.
hypogastric a.
idiopathic dilated pulmonary a.
ileocolic a.
iliac a.
iliofemoral a.
a. of inferior cavernous sinus
  (AICS)
inferior epigastric a.
inferior mesenteric a. (IMA)
infragastric infragenicular
  popliteal a.
infrageniculate popliteal a.
innominate a.
insular segment of middle
  cerebral a.
intercostal a.
interlobar a.
intermediate coronary a.
internal aberrant carotid a.
internal carotid a. (ICA)
internal iliac a.
internal mammary a. (IMA)
internal pudendal a.
internal thoracic a. (ITA)
intraacinar pulmonary a.
intracavernous internal carotid a.
intracerebral a.
intracranial vertebral a.
invisible main pulmonary a.
ipsilateral downstream a.
Kugel a.
a. of labyrinth
labyrinthine a.
lacrimal a.
left anterior descending a.
left atrioventricular groove a.
left circumflex coronary a.
left common carotid a.
left common femoral a.
left coronary a. (LCA)
left descending a. (LDA)
left gastric a.
left internal carotid a. (LICA)
left internal mammary a. (LIMA)
left main coronary a. (LMCA)
left pulmonary a. (LPA)
lenticulostriate a.
leptomeningeal a.
lingual a.
lumbar a.
main pulmonary a. (MPA)

mainstem coronary a.
major aorticopulmonary collateral a.
mammary a.
marginal branch of left circumflex
  coronary a.
marginal branch of right
  coronary a.
marginal circumflex a.
maxillary a.
medial plantar a.
median sacral a.
medullary a.
meningeal a.
meningohypophyseal a.
mesencephalic a.
mesenteric a.
middle cerebral a. (MCA)
middle meningeal a.
M1-M5 segment of middle
  cerebral a.
multiple aortopulmonary
  collateral a. (MAPCA)
musculophrenic a.
narrowing of a.
native coronary a.
nodular induration of temporal a.
obtuse marginal coronary a.
occipital a.
occlusion of a.
OM a.
omphalomesenteric a.
opercular segment of middle
  cerebral a.
operculofrontal a.
ophthalmic a.
origin of a.
a. ostium
ovarian a.
overriding great a.
pancreaticoduodenal a.
paracentral a.
paramalleolar a.
paramedian thalamic a.
paramedian thalamopeduncular a.
parietal middle cerebral a.
parietooccipital branch of posterior
  cerebellar a.
partial transposition of great a.
patency of a.
peduncular segment of superior
  cerebellar a.
pelvic a.
penile a.
a. of Percheron
perforating a.
pericallosal a.
perimedial renal fibroplasia a.

periosteal a.
peripancreatic a.
peroneal a.
persistent primitive trigeminal a.
persistent sciatic a.
petrous segment of internal
  carotid a.
pharyngeal a.
phrenic a.
pipestem a.
plantar metatarsal a.
plaque-containing a.
pontine a.
popliteal a.
posterior aorta transposition of
  great a.
posterior cerebral a. (PCA)
posterior choroidal a.
posterior circumflex humeral a.
posterior communicating a. (PCA,
  PCoA)
posterior descending a. (PDA)
posterior-inferior cerebellar a.
  (PICA)
posterior intercostal a.
posterior parietal a.
posterior spinal a.
posterior temporal a.
posterior tibial a.
posterolateral spinal a.
posttemporal middle cerebral a.
P1-P4 segment of posterior
  cerebral a.
precentral a.
precommunicating segment of
  anterior cerebral a.
precommunicating segment of
  posterior cerebral a.
prefrontal a.
premammillary a.
primitive acoustic a.
primitive hypoglossal a.
primitive trigeminal a. (PTA)
profunda femoris a.
proper hepatic a. (PHA)
proximal anterior descending a.
proximal anterior tibial a.
proximal circumflex a.
proximal digital a.
proximal left anterior descending a.
proximal popliteal a.
pterygoid a.

pulmonary a. (PA)
quadrigeminal segment of posterior
  cerebral a.
radial digital a.
radicular a.
radiculomedullary a.
radiculospinal a.
radiomedullary a.
ramus intermedius a.
ramus medialis a.
recanalized a.
a. reconstitution
reconstitution of blood flow in a.
reconstitution via profunda a.
redundant carotid a.
renal a.
reperfused a.
resilient a.
retinal a.
retroesophageal right subclavian a.
right coronary a. (RCA)
right descending pulmonary a.
  (RDPA)
right femoral a.
right ileocolic a.
right inferior epigastric a.
right internal iliac a.
right internal jugular a.
right ovarian a.
right pulmonary a. (RPA)
right ventricular branch of right
  coronary a.
Riolan a.
rolandic a.
scalp branch of external carotid a.
sclerotic coronary a.
segmental branch of a.
septal perforator a.
shared coronary a.
side-by-side transposition of
  great a.
single umbilical a.
sinoatrial node a.
sinus nodal a.
a. spectrum
spermatic a.
spinal a.
splenial branch of posterior
  cerebral a.
splenic a. (SA)
stapedial a.
stenotic coronary a.

NOTES

artery *(continued)*
   subclavian a.
   subcostal a.
   subscapular a.
   sudden blockage of coronary a.
   sulcocommissural a.
   superdominant left anterior
    descending a.
   superficial external pudendal a.
   superficial femoral a. (SFA)
   superficial temporal a.
   superior bronchial a.
   superior cerebellar a. (SCA)
   superior epigastric a.
   superior genicular a.
   superior intercostal a.
   superior mesenteric a. (SMA)
   superior pulmonary a.
   superior thyroid a.
   supernormal a.
   supraclinoid segment of internal
    carotid a.
   supraorbital a.
   supratrochlear a.
   surgically corrected transposition of
    the great a.
   takeoff of a.
   telencephalic ventriculofugal a.
   temporal a.
   temporooccipital a.
   terminal segment of posterior
    cerebral a.
   testicular a.
   thalamocaudate a.
   thalamogeniculate a.
   thalamoperforating a.
   thoracoacromial a.
   thoracodorsal a.
   thrombosed intraaortic a.
   thrombotic pulmonary a. (TPA)
   thyrocervical trunk of subclavian a.
   thyroid a.
   tibial a.
   translocation of coronary a.
   transposition of great a. (TGA)
   trifurcation of a.
   truncal a.
   twig of a.
   ulnar digital a.
   umbilical a. (UA)
   uterine a.
   ventriculofugal a.
   vertebral a. (VA)
   vertebrobasilar a.
   vidian a.
   visceral a.
   weakened a.
   a. of Willis
artery-aortic velocity ratio
artery-like pattern of enhancement
artery-vein-nerve bundle
arthrempyesis
arthritic talonavicular change
arthritis, pl. **arthritides**
   a. arthrogram
   Bekhterev a.
   Cedell-Magnusson classification
    of a.
   cystic rheumatoid a.
   degenerative a.
   destructive brucellar a.
   facet joint a.
   gouty a.
   hand/wrist a.
   inflammatory bowel disease a.
   juvenile rheumatoid a. (JRA)
   Kellgren a.
   lunohamate a.
   metatarsophalangeal joint a.
   mixed rheumatoid and
    degenerative a.
   a. mutilans
   pancarpal destructive a.
   reactive a.
   Reiter syndrome a.
   rheumatoid a.
   septic a.
   a. syphilitica deformans (ASD)
   systemic juvenile rheumatoid a.
   traumatic a.
   tuberculous a.
**ArthroCare Coblation-based cosmetic
  surgery system**
arthrodesed digit
arthrodial cartilage
arthrogram
   arthritis a.
arthrography
   air a.
   coronal computed tomographic a.
    (CCTA)
   CT a.
   double-contrast a.
   Gordon-Brostrom single-contrast a.
   a. imaging
   indirect MR a.
   joint a.
   magnetic resonance a.
   opaque a.
   saline-enhanced MR a.
   single-contrast a.
   temporomandibular joint a.

three-compartment a.
vacuum a.
arthrogryposis multiplex congenita
arthroosteitis
pustulotic a.
arthropathy
Charcot a.
crystal deposition a.
dialysis a.
facet a.
gouty a.
Jaccoud a.
neuropathic a.
pyrophosphate a.
rotator cuff a.
urate a.
arthrophyte
arthroplasty
total knee a. (TKA)
arthropneumoradiography
ArthroProbe laser system
arthropyosis
arthroscintigraphy
arthroscopic decompression
arthroscopy
second-look a.
arthrosis
crystal-induced a.
a. deformans
degenerative a.
spiral a.
arthrotomography
contrast computed a.
a. of shoulder
articular
a. arch
a. calculus
a. capsule
a. cartilage
a. cartilage attenuation
a. cartilage degeneration
a. cartilage violation
a. cartilage volume
a. cortex
a. crest
a. derangement
a. disk
a. eminence
a. erosion
a. facet
a. fluid
a. fossa

a. fragment
a. gout
a. hand disorder
a. instability
intercarpal a.
a. labrum
a. lamella
a. lamella of bone
a. mass separation fracture
a. meniscus
a. metaplasia
a. network
a. pillar fracture
a. pit
a. process
a. process of vertebra
a. rheumatism
a. surface
a. tubercle
a. tubercle of temporal bone
a. vascular circle
a. wrist disorder
articularis
meniscus a.
articulated skeleton
articulating surface
articulation
acromioclavicular a.
atlantoaxial a.
calcaneocuboid a.
carpometacarpal a.
carporadial a.
condylar a.
congruent a.
costovertebral a.
DIP a.
disturbance of a.
femoral a.
fixation a.
humeroradial a.
humeroulnar a.
intercarpal a.
intermetacarpal a.
interphalangeal a.
interval a.
joint a.
metacarpophalangeal a.
occipitocervical a.
patellofemoral a.
PIP a.
pisotriquetral a.
posterior membrane a.

NOTES

articulation *(continued)*
    proximal interphalangeal joint a.
    radiocapitellar a.
    radiocarpal a.
    radiohumeral a.
    radiolunate a.
    radioscaphoid a.
    radioulnar a.
    sacroiliac a.
    scapuloclavicular a.
    subluxation a.
    subtalar a.
    talocalcaneal a.
    talocalcaneonavicular a.
    talonavicular a.
    tarsometatarsal a.
    thorax a.
    tibiofibular a.
    triquetropisiform a.
    zygapophyseal a.
artifact, artefact
    acoustic a.
    aliasing a.
    aortic motion a.
    arterial pulsation a.
    asymmetric a.
    attenuation a.
    barium a.
    baseline a.
    beam-hardening a.
    beam-like a.
    black boundary a.
    black comet a.
    blooming a.
    blur a.
    bone-hardening a.
    bounce-point a.
    bowel gas a.
    brace a.
    breast a.
    breathing a.
    broadband noise detection error a.
    bulk susceptibility a.
    calibration failure a.
    catheter impact a.
    catheter tip motion a.
    catheter tip position a.
    catheter whip a.
    center line a.
    central point a.
    chastity ring a.
    chemical shift a.
    clothing a.
    coin a.
    color Doppler twinkling a.
    comet-tail a.
    computer-generated a.

construction a.
corduroy a.
crescent a.
crinkle a.
cross-talk effect a.
crown a.
crush a.
CSF pulsation a.
data-clipping detection error a.
data spike detection error a.
DC offset a.
developer a.
direct current offset a.
dirty film a.
double-exposure drift a.
eddy current a.
eddy ringing a.
edge-boundary a.
edge misalignment a.
edge ringing a.
a. effect
effusion a.
end-pressure a.
entry slice phenomenon a.
equipment a.
external a.
eyebrow ring a.
faulty radiofrequency shielding a.
ferromagnetic a.
fingerprint mark a.
flow effect a.
flow-induced a.
flow-related a.
fluid-flow a.
fog a.
foreign material a.
gaseous oxygen a.
geophagia a.
ghosting a.
glass eye a.
glove phenomenon a.
hair a.
half-moon a.
hardening a.
hot-spot a.
a. image
image postprocessing error a.
imbalance of gain a.
imbalance of phase a.
india ink a.
intensifying screen a.
intravascular stent a.
iron overload a.
kink a.
kissing a.
large clothing a.
large susceptibility a.

lettering a.
linear a.
lip ring a.
low attenuation pulsation a.
low signal intensity a.
magic angle effect a.
magnetic susceptibility a.
main magnetic field
  inhomogeneity a.
mercury a.
metallic a.
micrometallic a.
minus-density a.
mirror-image a.
misregistration a.
mitral regurgitation a.
moiré fringes a.
mosaic a.
motion a.
movement a.
muscle a.
navel ring a.
nipple ring a.
noise spike a.
nose ring a.
orbit a.
out-of-slice a.
overlying attenuation a.
pacemaker a.
pacing a.
paramagnetic a.
partial volume effect a.
patient motion a.
pellet a.
phase discontinuity a.
phase-encoding motion a.
phase-shift a.
pica a.
pick-off a.
plus-density a.
popliteal artery pulsation a.
a. pronunciation
propagation speed a.
pseudofracture a.
pulsation a.
quadrature phase detector a.
radiofrequency overflow a.
radiofrequency spatial distribution
  problem reconstruction a.
range ambiguity a.
reconstruction a.
respiratory motion a.

reticulation a.
reverberation a.
ring-down a.
roller mark a.
scintigraphy a.
screen craze a.
side lobe a.
signal drop-out a.
skin crease a.
skin fold a.
skin lesion a.
slice overlap a.
slice profile a.
spatial misregistration a.
spatial offset image a.
split image a.
stairstep a.
star a.
stent-related a.
stimulated echo a.
streak a.
streak-like a.
subcutaneous injection of
  contrast a.
summation shadow a.
superimposition a.
suppression of heart pulsation a.
surgical a.
susceptibility a.
swallowing a.
swamp-static a.
T a.
T1-contamination a.
temporal instability a.
tongue stud a.
tree a.
truncation band a.
twinkling a.
velocity a.
venetian blind a.
view insufficiency a.
voluming a.
wheelchair a.
white noise a.
wraparound ghosting a.
wrinkle a.
zebra stripe a.
zero-fill a.
zipper a.
artifactitious
artifactual gap

NOTES

artificial
a. cardiac valve
a. fracture
a. heart
a. lumen narrowing
a. lung
a. neural network
a. pleural effusion procedure
a. pneumothorax
a. radioactivity
ARTMA
advanced real-time motion analysis
ARTMA virtual patient technology
Artoscan
A. MRI imaging
A. MRI scanner
A. MRI system
ARVD
arrhythmogenic right ventricular dysplasia
Arvidsson dimension-length method for ventricular volume
aryepiglottic
a. cyst
a. fold
a. fold carcinoma
a. fold neurofibroma
a. fold width
arytenoid
a. cartilage
a. sparing
arytenoidal articular surface
AS
aortic stenosis
as
as low as readily practicable (ALARP)
as low as reasonably achievable (ALARA)
asbestos
amphibole a.
blue a.
a. body
brown a.
chrysotile a.
crocidolite a.
a. exposure
a. fiber
a. pleural plaque
serpentine a.
white a.
asbestos-induced pleural fibrosis
asbestosis
pulmonary a.
asbestos-related
a.-r. lung carcinoma
a.-r. mesothelioma

a.-r. pleural disease
a.-r. pleural effusion
a.-r. pleural thickening
A-scan
A.-s. imaging
A.-s. ultrasound
ascendant follicle
ascending
a. aorta (AA)
a. aorta dilatation
a. aorta hypoplasia
a. aortic aneurysm
a. aortography
a. cholangitis
a. colon
a. contrast MR phlebogram
a. contrast phlebography
a. contrast phlebography imaging
a. contrast venography
a. frontal convolution
a. frontoparietal (ASFP)
a. frontoparietal artery
a. hypoplasia of aorta
a. lumbar vein
a. medullary vein thrombosis
a. parietal convolution
a. parietal gyrus
a. pharyngeal artery
a. process
a. pyelography
a. ramus of ischium
a. tract
a. urography
Ascent guiding catheter
Aschoff
A. node
A. nodule
Aschoff-Tawara node
ascites
chylous a.
a. due to bile leak
fetal a.
gelatinous a.
massive a.
neonatal a.
pancreatic a.
urine a.
ascitic fluid
ASCVD
arteriosclerotic cardiovascular disease
atherosclerotic cardiovascular disease
ASD
anterior sagittal diameter
arthritis syphilitica deformans
atrial septal defect
Aselli pancreas
aseptic necrosis

ASF
   anterior spine fusion
ASFP
   ascending frontoparietal
ASH
   asymmetric septal hypertrophy
ASHD
   arteriosclerotic heart disease
Asherson syndrome
Ashhurst-Bromer classification of ankle fracture
Ashhurst fracture classification system
ash leaf patch
Ashman
   A. index
   A. phenomenon
ASHN
   acute sclerosing hyaline necrosis
ASIC
   application-specific integrated circuit
      ASIC circuit
ASIS
   anterior-superior iliac spine
   aromatic solvent-induced shift
Askin thoracopulmonary neuroepithelial tumor
Ask-Upmark kidney
ASO
   arteriosclerosis obliterans
   atherosclerosis obliterans
asoma
aspect
      anterior a.
      anterolateral a.
      anteroposterior a.
      apical a.
      axial a.
      dorsal a.
      dorsolateral a.
      dorsoplantar a.
      inferior a.
      infrapatellar a.
      lateral a.
      lordotic a.
      medial a.
      mediolateral a.
      mesial a.
      plantar a.
      posterior a.
      posterolateral a.
      proximal a.
      superior a.

      superolateral a.
      ventral a.
Aspen
   A. digital ultrasound system
   A. sonography unit
aspergilloma
aspergillosis
   allergic bronchopulmonary a. (ABPA)
   bronchopulmonary a.
   chronic necrotizing a.
   invasive pulmonary a. (IPA)
   necrotizing a.
   noninvasive a.
   primary a.
   pulmonary a.
   saprophytic a.
   semiinvasive a.
aspergillotic
   a. aneurysm
   a. granuloma
***Aspergillus* cerebral abscess**
asphyxia
   fetal a.
   perinatal a.
asphyxial renal trauma
asphyxia-related renal necrosis
asphyxiating
   a. thoracic dysplasia
   a. thoracic dystrophy
aspiration
   barium a.
   a. biopsy
   a. biopsy needle
   breast cyst a.
   CT-guided needle a.
   endoscopic ultrasound-guided fine needle a. (EUS-FNA)
   fine-needle a.
   meconium a.
   a. of ova
   pleural fluid a.
   a. pneumonia
   a. pneumonitis
   pulmonary a.
   tracheal a.
   transbronchial needle a. (TBNA)
   transtracheal a.
   ultrasonic a.
   ultrasound-guided cyst a.
   ultrasound-guided transthoracic needle a.

NOTES

aspirator
Cavitron Ultrasonic Surgical A. (CUSA)
Sonocut ultrasonic a.
Aspire continuous imaging system
asplenia syndrome R
asplenic
ASPS
alveolar soft-part sarcoma
ASPVD
atherosclerotic peripheral vascular disease
ASR
adrenal-to-spleen ratio
assay
Accuclot D-dimer a.
Clauss a.
erythropoietin a.
immunofluorimetric a.
radiometric a.
renal vein renin a.
assembly
linear array-hydrophone a.
assessment
activity a.
aortoiliac inflow a.
BFM arm impairment a.,
Brunnstrom-Fugl-Meyer arm
impairment a.
diagnostic and therapeutic
technology a.
Doppler a.
hemodynamic a.
indicator dilution method of
perfusion a.
invasive a.
in vivo stereologic a.
lumen a.
myocardial function a.
noninvasive a.
qualitative a.
quantitative Doppler a.
real-time a.
regional wall motion a.
sonographic a.
transmetallation a.
ultrasonic a.
vascular a.
assimilation
atlantooccipital a.
a. pelvis
assist
intraaortic balloon a.
assistance
fluoroscopic a.
Assmann
A. focus
A. tuberculous infiltrate

associated
a. anomaly
a. imaging characteristic
a. sequestrum
association
a. cortex of parietal lobe
a. fiber
VATER a.
AST
above-selected threshold
astatine (At)
asterixis
asteroid body
asthmatic
a. airway
a. bronchitis
a. pneumonia
astragalar bone
astragalocalcanean bone
astragalocrural bone
astragaloscaphoid bone
astragalotibial bone
astragalus
aviator's a.
a. bone
fracture of a.
astroblastoma
astrocytic
a. gliosis
a. hamartoma
a. proliferation
a. tumor
astrocytoma
anaplastic a. (AA)
calcified a.
cerebellar a.
cerebral a.
chiasmatic-hypothalamic pilocytic a.
CNS juvenile pilocytic a.
a. cord
cystic pilocytic a.
desmoplastic infantile a.
gemistocytic a.
giant cell a.
high-grade infiltrative a.
infiltrative a.
juvenile orbital pilocytic a.
juvenile pilocytic a. (JPA)
low-grade a.
macrocystic pilocytic cerebellar a.
microcystic pilocytic cerebellar a.
multifocal anaplastic a.
orbital juvenile pilocytic a.
pilocytic a.
piloid a.
protoplasmic a.
radiation-treated a.

retinal a.
solid pilocytic a.
subependymal giant cell a.
supratentorial a.
temporoinsular a.
well-differentiated a.
astroglial tumor
asymmetric
a. appearance time
a. artifact
a. bile duct
a. breast density
a. closure of cusp
a. data sampling
a. echo
a. intrauterine growth retardation
a. IUGR
a. limb uptake
a. lung opacity
a. negative T-wave
a. pulmonary congestion
a. septal hypertrophy (ASH)
a. target appearance
a. thorax
asymmetrical signal change
asymmetry
amplitude a.
congestive a.
facial a.
focal a.
frontal horn a.
hypertrophic a.
interhemispheric a.
left-right a.
limb-length a.
narrowing a.
septal a.
skull a.
thoracic a.
asymptomatic
a. coarctation
a. gallstone
a. hydrocephalus
a. hypertrophy
asynchronous transfer mode (ATM)
asynergic myocardium
asynergy
infarct-localized a.
left ventricular a.
regional a.
segmental a.
asystolic pause

AT
acceleration time
At
astatine
ATAI
acute traumatic aortic injury
atavistic epiphysis
ataxia telangiectasia
atelectasis
absorption a.
acquired a.
acute a.
adhesive a.
apical a.
band of a.
basilar a.
bibasilar discoid a.
bronchopulmonary a.
chronic a.
cicatricial a.
compressive a.
confluent areas of a.
congenital a.
congestive a.
dependent a.
discoid a.
disk-like a.
initial a.
lobar resorption a.
lobular a.
lower pulmonary lobe a.
middle pulmonary lobe a.
nonobstructive a.
obstructive a.
passive a.
patchy a.
peripheral parenchymal a.
plate-like a.
postobstructive a.
postoperative resorption a.
primary a.
reabsorption a.
relaxation a.
resorption a.
resorptive a.
rounded a.
secondary a.
segmental resorption a.
slowly developing a.
streak of a.
subsegmental bibasilar a.

NOTES

atelectasis *(continued)*
    subsegmental lower lobe a.
    upper pulmonary lobe a.
atelectatic
    a. asbestos pseudotumor
    a. lung
atelosteogenesis
ATF
    anterior talofibular ligament
atherectomy
    directional coronary a. (DCA)
    extraction catheter a.
    percutaneous a.
    percutaneous coronary rotational a.
     (PCRA)
    peripheral directional a.
    retrograde a.
    rotational a. (RA)
    rotational coronary a. (RCA)
    Simpson a.
    transcutaneous extraction catheter a.
    transluminal a.
AtheroCath
    DVI Simpson A.
atheroembolic renal disease
atheroembolism
atherogenesis
atherolysis
    ultrasonic a.
atherolytic
atheroma
    carotid bifurcation a.
    coral reef a.
    a. molding
    protruding a.
    resection of mobile aortic arch a.
atheromatosis
atheromatous
    a. abscess
    a. debris
    a. degeneration
    a. embolus
    a. lesion
    a. material
    a. plaque
    a. stenosis
    a. ulcer
atherosclerosis
    accelerated a.
    aortic a.
    carotid a.
    coronary a.
    extracranial carotid artery a.
    fatty streak a.
    fibrous plaque a.
    intimal a.
    intracranial carotid artery a.

    juxtarenal aortic a.
    native a.
    a. obliterans (ASO)
    pararenal aortic a.
    premature a.
    virulent a.
atherosclerotic
    a. aortic aneurysm
    a. aortic ulcer
    a. calcification
    a. cardiovascular disease (ASCVD)
    a. carotid artery disease (ACAD)
    a. change
    a. debris
    a. fatty streak
    a. lesion
    a. narrowing
    a. occlusive syndrome
    a. peripheral vascular disease
     (ASPVD)
    a. plaque
    a. stenosis
atherostenosis
atherothrombotic brain infarct
athlete
    a. ankle
    A. GT coronary guidewire
    a. heart
    a. pseudonephritis
Atkin epiphyseal fracture
ATL
    argon laser trabeculectomy
    ATL HDI 5000 color Doppler
    ATL HDI 3000, 3500, 4000, 5000
    ultrasound system
    ATL Mark 600 real-time sector
    scanner
    ATL Neurosector real-time scanner
    ATL Ultramark 8, 9
atlantal ligament
Atlantis SR IVUS catheter
atlantoaxial
    a. articulation
    a. instability
    a. interval
    a. joint
    a. relationship
    a. rotary displacement
    a. rotary fixation
    a. separation
    a. subluxation
atlantodens interval (ADI)
atlantodental
atlantomastoid
atlantooccipital
    a. assimilation
    a. dislocation

a. fusion
a. joint
a. junction
a. membrane
a. separation
atlantoodontoid
atlas
a. anomaly
a. arch
bifid a.
A. 2.0 diagnostic ultrasound system
a. facet
a. fracture
Greulich and Pyle a.
a. matching
a. occipitalization
a. odontoid distance
rachischisis of a.
split a.
standard a.
transverse ligament of a.
ATM
asynchronous transfer mode
ATM mode
atmospheric pressure
ATN
acute tubular necrosis
autonomous thyroid nodule
atom
activated a.
Bohr a.
excited a.
ionized a.
labeled a.
nuclear a.
radioactive a.
recoil a.
stripped a.
tagged a.
atomic
a. absorption spectrophotometry
a. absorption spectroscopy
a. energy
a. mass unit (amu)
a. volume
atomization
atonic
a. esophagus
a. ureter
a. urinary bladder
atony, atonia
chronic gastric a.

collecting system a.
gastric a.
intestinal a.
renal collecting system a.
sphincter a.
stomach a.
urinary bladder a.
atopic
atopy
atraumatic
a., multidirectional, bilateral radial instability (AMBRI)
a. occlusion of vessel
atresia
anal a.
anorectal a.
aortic arch a.
aortic valve a.
bile duct a.
biliary a.
bowel a.
bronchial a.
choanal a.
colonic a.
congenital biliary a.
congenital intestinal a.
congenital laryngeal a.
diffuse aortic a.
duodenal a.
esophageal a.
external auditory canal a.
extrahepatic biliary a. (EBA)
familial a.
ileal a.
infundibular a.
inner ear a.
intestinal congenital a.
intrahepatic a. (IHA)
intrahepatic biliary a.
laryngeal a.
mitral valve a.
nasopharyngeal a.
phenobarbital biliary a.
prepyloric a.
pulmonary artery a.
pulmonary valve a.
pulmonary vein a.
pulmonic a.
small bowel a.
tricuspid valve a.
urethral a.

NOTES

atresia *(continued)*
  valvular a.
  ventricular a.
atresic
atretic
  a. aortic segment
  a. ovarian follicle
  a. segment
  a. tube
atria *(pl. of atrium)*
atrial
  a. activation time
  a. appendage
  a. appendage juxtaposition
  a. bigeminal rhythm
  a. canal
  a. cannulation
  a. circumflex artery
  a. complex
  a. cuff
  a. disk
  a. diverticulum of brain
  a. dome
  a. echo
  a. ectopic automatic tachycardia
  a. electrogram
  a. emptying volume
  a. fetal flutter
  a. fibrillation
  a. focus
  a. infarct
  a. inhibited (AAI)
  a. irritability
  a. isomerism
  a. kick
  a. mesenchymoma
  a. myxoma
  a. ostium primum defect
  a. partition
  a. pressure
  a. rate (AR)
  a. septal aneurysm
  a. septal defect (ASD)
  a. septal defect occlusion
  a. septal resection
  a. septostomy
  a. septum
  a. situs
  a. situs solitus
  a. standstill
  a. systole
  a. thrombosis
  a. transposition
atrialized ventricle
atrial-phase volumetric function
atriocaval junction
atriofascicular tract

atriography
  contrast left a.
  negative contrast left a.
atrio-His
  a.-H. bypass tract
  a.-H. fiber
  a.-H. pathway
atriohisian
atrioventricular (AV)
  a. anulus
  a. band
  a. block
  a. bundle
  a. canal
  a. canal defect
  a. connection
  a. gradient
  a. groove
  a. groove branch
  a. junction
  a. junction anomaly
  a. nodal bypass tract
  a. nodal node mesothelioma
  a. nodal orifice
  a. nodal ostium
  a. nodal reentry tachycardia
  a. nodal rhythm
  a. nodal septal defect
  a. nodal septum
  a. nodal valve
  a. node
  a. node artery (AVNA)
  a. node of His
  a. opening of His
  a. septal defect (AVSD)
  a. sulcus
  a. time
  a. trunk
atrium, pl. atria
  accessory a.
  common a.
  a. dextrum cordis
  giant left a.
  high right a. (HRA)
  left a. (LA)
  low right a. (LRA)
  low septal right a.
  maximal volume of left a.
  nontrabeculated a.
  oblique vein of left a.
  a. pulmonale
  pulmonary a.
  respiratory a.
  right a. (RA)
  shunt with normal left a.
  single a.
  a. sinistrum

a. sinistrum cordis
stenosing ring of left a.
thin-walled a.
trabeculated a.
ventricular a.

atrophic

a. brain lesion
a. breast
a. cirrhosis
a. degeneration
a. emphysema
a. fracture
a. gastritis
a. inflammation
a. kidney
a. nonunion
a. pyelonephritis
a. thrombosis
a. villus

atrophie

a. blanch
a. noire

atrophied ovary

atrophy

alveolar a.
back pressure a.
bone a.
brachial a.
brain a.
brown a.
cerebellar a.
cerebral surface a.
compensatory a.
compression a.
cord a.
cortical a.
degenerative a.
denervation a.
divopontocerebellar a.
dorsum sellae a.
eccentric a.
focal a.
frontotemporal a.
gastric a.
hemisphere a.
hippocampal a.
Hoffmann a.
interstitial a.
kidney a.
lesser a.
lobar lung a.
multiple system a.

olivopontocerebellar a.
optic nerve a.
pancreatic a.
parenchymatous a.
physiologic a.
postinflammatory renal a.
postischemic a.
postmenopausal uterine a.
postobstructive renal a.
primary optic a.
radiation-induced cerebral a.
reflux a.
renal reflux a.
seminal vesicle a.
small bowel folds a.
spinal cord a.
spinal muscular a. (SMA)
subacute denervation a.
subcortical Sudeck osteoporotic a.
Sudeck a.
sulcal a.
temporal horn a.
vascular villous a.
villous a.

attached proton test (APT)

attachment

abnormal umbilical cord a.
biopsy-guided a.
capsular a.
central rhomboid a.
cerebellar a.
commissural a.
dural a.
epicardial a.
fibroosseous a.
fibrous a.
Hudson a.
intimate a.
lateral pterygoid tendinous a.
ligamentous a.
meniscocapsular a.
meniscofemoral a.
meniscotibial a.
mesenteric a.
Pearson a.
peritoneal a.
tendinous a.
tendon-to-bone a.
tentorium cerebelli a. (TCA)
vascular pterygoid a.

attack

transient ischemic a. (TIA)

NOTES

attenuate
attenuated
    a. cortical surface
    a. dura
    a. image
    a. intercarpal articular cartilage
    a. ligament
    a. lumen
attenuating
attenuation
    aortic a.
    articular cartilage a.
    a. artifact
    beam a.
    breast a.
    a. coefficient
    a. compensation
    a. correction
    decreased a.
    diaphragmatic a.
    diffuse low a.
    digital beam a.
    a. effect
    expiratory a.
    focal a.
    gamma ray a.
    ground-glass a.
    hemidiaphragm a.
    a. imaging
    increased a.
    inhomogeneous a.
    a. level
    linear a.
    low a.
    a. measurement
    near-water a.
    nonuniform a.
    photon a.
    a. scan
    signal a.
    tendon a.
    theophylline a.
    a. threshold
    ultrasonic a.
    a. value
    valve a.
    x-ray a.
attenuation-based on-line modulation of
   the tube current
attenuation-corrected image
attenuation-correction coefficient
attenuator
attic
    a. adhesion
    a. cholesteatoma
    a. recess
    a. temporal bone

attitude
    fetal a.
attritional
    a. pattern change
    a. tear
attrition rupture of tendon
ATV
    anterior terminal vein
atypical
    a. aortic valve stenosis
    a. benign fibrous histiocytoma
    a. brain teratoma
    a. bronchial pneumonia
    a. carcinoid
    a. chondrocyte
    a. ductal hyperplasia
    a. epithelium
    a. finding
    a. interstitial pneumonia
    a. lobular breast hyperplasia
    a. lobular hyperplasia (ALH)
    a. measles pneumonia
    a. medullary carcinoma
    a. meningioma
    a. primary pneumonia
    a. regenerative hyperplasia
    a. renal cyst
    a. subisthmic coarctation
    a. tuberculosis
    a. verrucous endocarditis
    a. vessel colposcopic pattern
AUC
    area under the curve
^{198}Au colloid
auditory
    a. canal
    a. capsule
    a. cartilage
    a. cortex
    a. ganglion
    a. pit
    a. plate
    a. process
    a. tube
    a. vein
    a. vesicle
Auerbach
    myenteric plexus of A.
Auer body
Auger
    A. effect
    A. electron
Auger-electron emitter
augmentation
    bladder a.
    a. mammoplasty

mechanical a.

thiol a.

augmented

a. breast

a. cardiac output

a. filling

a. filling of right ventricle

a. pressure colostogram

a. stroke volume

aura

A. desktop laser

A. Laser helical scanner

uncinate a.

auricle

left a.

right a.

auricular

a. artery

a. canaliculus

a. cartilage

a. complex

a. fissure

a. ganglion

a. ligament

a. line

a. lymph node

a. muscle

a. notch

a. point

a. surface

a. triangle

a. tubercle

a. vein

auriculoventricular groove

Aurora

A. dedicated breast MRI system

A. diode-based dental laser system

A. diode soft-tissue laser

A. MR breast imaging system scanner

auscultatory finding

Aussies-Isseis unstable scoliosis

Austin Flint phenomenon

Auth Rotablator atherectomy catheter

autoattenuation correction method

autocancellation

AutoCAT intraaortic balloon pump

autocorrelation function

Autocorrelator

autoerythrocyte sensitization syndrome

autofluorescence

autofluoroscope

digital a.

autofusion

autogenous

a. bone

a. vein

a. vein bypass graft

autograft

bridge a.

double a.

autohistoradiograph

autoimmune

a. phenomenon

a. response

a. sialadenitis

autoinjector

autologous

a. blood clot

a. bone marrow rescue

a. bone marrow transplant

a. labeled leukocyte

a. patch graft

a. pericardium

a. stem-cell transplantation

a. vein graft

a. white cell localization

automated

a. airway tree segmentation method

a. angle-encoder system

a. biochemical analyzer

a. biopsy gun

a. biopsy system

a. border detection by echocardiography

a. cardiac flow measurement (ACM)

a. cardiac flow measurement ultrasound

a. cellular imaging system (ACIS)

a. cerebral blood flow analyzer

a. computed axial tomography (ACAT)

a. gamma counter

a. Hough transform

a. infusion system

a. large-core breast biopsy

2.1-mm a. biopsy needle

a. percutaneous lumbar diskectomy (APLD)

a. polyp detection

a. quantification

NOTES

automatic
> a. bladder
> a. collimator
> a. endoscopic system for optimal positioning (AESOP)
> a. exposure control (AEC)
> a. extraction
> a. implantable cardioverter-defibrillator (AICD)
> a. lumen edge segmentation
> a. motion correction
> a. peak tracking (APT)
> a. spring-loaded biopsy device

automaticity
> sinus node a.

automotility factor
autonephrectomy
autonomic
> a. denervation
> a. insufficiency
> a. nerve block
> a. nervous system
> a. plexus

autonomous
> a. thyroid adenoma
> a. thyroid nodule (ATN)

autoparenchymatous metaphysis
autoprescanning
autoradiogram
autoradiograph
autoradiographic
> a. localization
> a. technique

autoradiography
> quantitative track etch a.

autoregressive moving average
autoregulation of cerebral blood flow
autosomal
> a. dominant polycystic kidney disease (ADPKD)
> a. recessive polycystic kidney disease (ARPKD)

autosomal-dominant benign form of osteopetrosis
AutoSPECT
autosplenectomy
autostereoscopic
autotomogram
autotomographic
autotomography
autotopagnosia
autotransformer formula
auxiliary
> a. CT tabletop
> a. ventricle

AV
> arteriovenous

atrioventricular
> AV node
> AV Wenckebach heart block

AVA
> advanced vessel analysis
> aortic valve area
> arteriovenous anastomosis

availability
> PET measurement of dopamine receptor a.

avascular
> a. bone necrosis
> a. brain mass
> a. cortical infarction necrosis
> a. femoral head necrosis
> a. fibrocartilage
> a. kidney mass
> a. necrosis (AVN)
> a. necrosis lunate
> a. renal mass
> a. tarsal scaphoid necrosis
> a. vertebral body necrosis

avascularity
AVD
> aortic valvular disease

AVE bridge stainless steel balloon-expandable stent
Avellis syndrome
Avera breast imaging system
average
> autoregressive moving a.
> a. diffusivity histogram
> a. gradient number
> number of signal a. (NSA)
> a. pixel projection (APP)
> a. positron energy
> signal a.
> spatial average-pulse a. (SAPA)
> spatial average-temporal a. (SATA)
> spatial peak-temporal a. (SPTA)
> time-weighted a.

averaging
> motion a.
> partial volume a.
> spike a.
> volume a.

AVF
> arteriovenous fistula
> spinal dural AVF

AVG
> aortic valve gradient

aviator's astragalus
avis
> calcar a.

Aviva mammography system
AVM
> arteriovenous malformation

intradural spinal AVM
pial AVM
AVM radiotherapy
AVN
avascular necrosis
AVNA
atrioventricular node artery
Avogadro
A. constant
A. law
A. number (Λ)
A. postulate
Avotec
A. MR-compatible headphones
A. MR-compatible liquid crystal display goggles
AVR
aortic valve replacement
AVSD
atrioventricular septal defect
avulse
avulsed
a. fracture fragment
a. ligament
a. retinaculum
avulsion
anterior labral a.
anterior labroligamentous periosteal sleeve a. (ALPSA)
arterial a.
bony humeral a.
a. chip fracture
coracoid tip a.
epiphysis a.
iatrogenic a.
lumbar root a.
nail plate a.
peroneus longus muscle a.
spinal nerve root a.
spinous process a.
a. stress fracture
testicular artery a.
traumatic a.
venous a.
avulsive cortical irregularity
AVVM
angiographically visualized vascular malformation
A-wave pressure
awl
Mark II Kodros radiolucent a.
axes (*pl. of* axis)

axial
a. acetabular index (AAI)
a. angiography
a. aspect
a. BMD center with agreed joint protocol
a. breath-hold gradient-echo cine magnetic resonance imaging
a. carpal dislocation
a. celloidin section
a. cineangiography
a. compression fracture
a. compression injury
a. dimension
a. echo planar diffusion weighted imaging
a. fat-suppressed T2-weighted image
a. grade echo imaging
a. gradient echo image
a. hiatal hernia
horizontal long a. (HLA)
a. joint dissection
a. left anterior oblique ventriculogram
a. loading injury
a. load teardrop fracture
a. load three-part, two-plane fracture
a. localizer
a. manual traction test
multiecho a.
a. multiplanar reformation technique
a. musculature
a. neuritis
a. orientation
a. osteomalacia
a. plane
a. plane imaging
a. plate
a. projection
a. proton-density-weighted image
a. radiograph
a. resolution
a. rotation
a. scan
a. sesamoid view
a. single shot fast spin-echo
a. skeleton
a. slice
a. spin density
a. surface
a. transabdominal image

NOTES

axial *(continued)*
    a. transverse tomography
    a. T1-SE protocol
    a. 0.2T T1-weighted spin-echo
      imaging
    a. unenhanced CT scan
    a. wall
    a. weight loading
axiale
    skeleton a.
axilla, pl. **axillae**
axillary
    a. adenopathy
    a. aneurysm
    a. arteriography
    a. artery
    a. cavity
    a. fascia
    a. fossa
    a. hematoma
    a. line
    a. lymphadenopathy
    a. lymph node (ALN)
    a. muscle
    a. node involvement
    a. node metastasis
    a. plexus
    a. pouch
    a. projection
    a. sheath
    a. space
    a. sweat gland
    a. tail of Spence
    a. tail view
    a. triangle
    a. tumor downstaging
    a. ultrasonography
    a. vein
    a. vein traumatic thrombosis
    a. vessel
axillary-axillary bypass graft
axillary-brachial bypass graft
axillary-femoral bypass graft
axillary-femorofemoral bypass graft
axillobifemoral bypass graft
axillofemoral approach
axillosubclavian vein thrombosis
axiolabiolingual plane
axiomesiodistal plane
axipetal
axis, pl. **axes**
    anatomic a.
    ankle mortise a.
    anode-cathode a.
    a. anomaly
    anteroposterior a.
    basibregmatic a.

    basicranial a.
    bimalleolar foot a.
    a. body
    bowel a.
    carpal axes
    celiac a.
    condylar a.
    coordinate a.
    cortical hinge a.
    craniocaudal a.
    craniospinal a.
    distal reference a. (DRA)
    enteroinsular a.
    femoral shaft a.
    a. fracture
    a. of heart
    horizontal long a.
    HPA a.
    hypothalamic-pituitary a.
    hypothalamic-pituitary-adrenal a.
    hypothalamic-pituitary-gonadal a.
    hypothalamoneurohypophyseal a.
    leg a.
    a. ligament
    long a.
    longitudinal a.
    mechanical a.
    metatarsal a.
    normal a.
    pendulous reference a. (PRA)
    renal a.
    single a.
    spinal a.
    subtalar a.
    T a.
    transcondylar a. (TCA)
    transporionic a.
    vertical a.
    vertical-long a.
    weightbearing a.
    X a.
    Y a.
    Z a.
axon
    obliquely oriented a.
axonal
    a. cylinder
    a. shearing
    a. transport impairment
axonopathic neurogenic thoracic outlet
    syndrome
Ayerza syndrome
azotemic osteodystrophy
azygoesophageal
    a. line
    a. recess
azygogram

azygography
azygos
- a. anterior cerebral artery
- a. artery of vagina
- a. blood flow
- a. continuation
- a. continuation of inferior vena cava
- a. fissure
- a. hematoma cap
- a. lobe of lung
- a. lymph node
- nodus arcus venae a.
- a. vein
- a. vein distention
- a. vein enlargement

azygous arch
Azzopardi tumor

NOTES

B

B level of the esophagus
B ring of esophagus
B scan

B₀

B-19036 chelate
B6 bronchus sign
BA

bone age

Ba

point Ba

BabyFace 3D surface rendering accessory
baby formula with ferrous sulfate contrast agent
babyPAC ventilator
Baccelli sign of pleural effusion
Bachmann

anterior internodal tract of B.
B. bundle

bacillary embolus
back

b. crease
b. pressure atrophy
b. projection
b. stroke volume

back-angle anomaly
backbleeding
backfire fracture
backflow

b. of blood
pyelolymphatic b.
pyelorenal b.
pyelotubular b.
pyelovenous b.
venous b.

backflux
background (BKG)

b. activity
b. count
b. density
b. erase
b. radiation
b. slowing
b. subtraction
b. subtraction technique

back-knee deformity
backlit digitizer
backrush of blood into left ventricle
backscatter

b. of blood
b. electron
b. factor (BSF)
b. peak

backscattered radiation

back-to-back configuration
backup of blood
backward

b. curvature
b. flow
b. heart failure

backwash ileitis
bacterial

b. aneurysm
b. cholangitis
b. endocarditis
b. ependymitis
b. epiglottitis
b. nephritis
b. osteomyelitis
b. pneumonitis
b. sinusitis
b. toxin

badge

film b.
ring b.

BAE

bronchial artery embolization

Baehr-Lohlein lesion
Baer plane
Baerveldt glaucoma drainage implant
Baeyer-Villiger oxidation
Baffe anastomosis
baffled tunnel
baffle leak
BaFT

barium meal and follow through

Bäfverstedt syndrome
bag

b. of bagassosis
balloon b.
bile b.
Tedlar b.

bagassosis

bag of b.

BAI

basion axial interval

Baillinger

inner stripe of B.

bail-lock knee joint
baja

patella b.

baker's leg
BAK interbody fusion system
balance

mass b.

balanced

b. circulation
b. fast-field-echo pulse
b. gradient

balanced *(continued)*
  b. hemivertebra
  b. ischemia
  b. pneumoperitoneum
balanced-gradient technique
balancing subdural hematoma
bald gastric fundus
Balint syndrome
Balkan
  B. fracture frame
  B. nephritis
  B. nephropathy
ball
  b. catcher view
  b. of foot
  keratin urinary tract b.
  kidney fungus b.
  lung fungus b.
  B. method
  mobile fat b.
  myelin b.
  renal fungus b.
  sludge b.
ball-and-socket
  b.-a.-s. ankle mortise
  b.-a.-s. epiphysis
  b.-a.-s. joint
ball-catcher projection
ballerina-foot pattern
ball-in-hand appearance
ballistic
  b. injury
  b. material
ballistocardiography
ball-occluder valve
balloon
  b. aortoplasty
  b. atrial septostomy
  b. bag
  Bardex b.
  barium enema retention b.
  Blue Max high-pressure b.
  b. bronchoplasty
  b. catheter fenestration
  b. catheterization
  b. cholangiogram
  b. counterpulsation
  cutting b.
  b. dilatation
  b. dilator
  b. dissector
  b. embolectomy catheter
  b. epiphysis
  b. expulsion imaging
  high-pressure Blue Max b.
  b. inflation
  kissing b.

low-compliance, fixed diameter b.
  b. mitral valvoplasty
nondetachable b.
  b. occlusion arteriography
  b. occlusion pulmonary angiogram
  b. occlusion tolerance test
  b. occlusive aortography
percutaneous intraaortic b.
PET b.
pressure-detachable silicone b.
  b. proctogram
  b. PTA catheter
  b. pump
radiofrequency b.
rectal b.
  b. remodeling
scintigraphic b.
self-sealing latex b.
  b. tamponade
  b. test occlusion
  b. test occlusion imaging
  b. topography
  b. tuboplasty
Ultrathin Diamond b.
USCI PET b.
  b. valvotomy
waist in b.
windowed b.
7 (x) 40 mm percutaneous
  transluminal angioplasty b.
ballooned
  b. floor of ventricle
  b. sella
ballooning
  b. degeneration
disk b.
  b. mitral cusp
  b. of vertebral interspace
balloon-occluded
  b.-o. arterial infusion
  b.-o. transvenous obliteration
balloon-shaped heart
balloon-tipped angiographic catheter
ball-tip microcatheter
ball-type valve
ball-valve
  b.-v. obstruction
  b.-v. thrombus
  b.-v. tumor
Baló concentric sclerosis
BALT
  bronchus-associated lymphoid tissue
Bamberger area
Bamberger-Marie disease
bamboo spine
b-amyloid senile plaque

banana
    b. fracture
    b. sign
banana-shaped uterine cavity
Bancaud phenomenon
band
    aberrant b.
    alpha frequency b.
    amnionic b.
    anogenital b.
    anterior b.
    AO tension b.
    aponeurotic b.
    b. of atelectasis
    atrioventricular b.
    b. of Broca
    Broca diagonal b.
    calf b.
    Clado b.
    conduction b.
    constriction b.
    dark Mach b.
    dense metaphyseal b.
    b. of density
    b. of deossification
    echogenic b.
    external b.
    fascial b.
    fibroelastic b.
    fibromuscular b.
    fibrous b.
    free band of colon b.
    Gennari b.
    H b.
    Harris b.
    b. heterotopia
    His b.
    Hunter-Schreger b.
    hypoechoic b.
    iliotibial b.
    intercaval b.
    internal b.
    intratesticular b.
    IT b.
    Ladd b.
    Lane b.
    lateral b.
    longitudinal b.
    low signal intensity fibrous b.
    low signal intensity peripheral b.
    lucent b.
    Mach b.
    Maissiat b.
    Marlex b.
    Meckel b.
    mesocolic b.
    metaphyseal lucent b.
    moderator b.
    negative Mach b.
    omental b.
    parenchymal fibrous b.
    parenchymal lung b.
    Parham-Martin b.
    parietal b.
    peritoneal b.
    posterior tracheal b.
    pretendinous b.
    radiofrequency saturation b.
    Reil b.
    saturation b.
    scar b.
    septal b.
    septomarginal b.
    septum b.
    serpiginous b.
    silicone elastomer b.
    Simonart b.
    spatial presaturation b.
    tendinous b.
    b. tenodesis
    tracheal b.
    transverse b.
    valence b.
    vascular b.
    walking saturation b.
    Z b.
bandaletta
bandbox resonance
bandelette
banding
    b. appearance
    halftone b.
band-like
    b.-l. adhesion
    b.-l. margin
    b.-l. shadow
bandpass filter
Bankart
    B. dislocation
    B. fracture
    B. lesion
Bannayan-Riley-Ruvalcaba syndrome
Banti syndrome

NOTES

BAP
    brightness area product
bar
    arch b.
    Bill b.
    bony b.
    cartilaginous b.
    cecal b.
    congenital b.
    coracoclavicular b.
    cricopharyngeal b.
    b. defect
    fibrous b.
    hyoid b.
    median b.
    parallel-line-equal-space b.
    Passavant b.
    physeal b.
    PLES b.
    unsegmented vertebral b.
barber chair position
Bard
    B. CPS system
    B. percutaneous cardiopulmonary support system
    B. rotary atherectomy device
Bardex
    B. balloon
    B. Lubricath catheter
Bardinet ligament
bare area
Baricon imaging agent
baritosis
barium
    b. artifact
    b. aspiration
    b. bolus
    double tracking of b.
    b. enema (BE)
    b. enema imaging
    b. enema retention balloon
    b. enema through colostomy
    b. enema with air contrast
    b. esophagram
    flocculation of b.
    b. fluoride
    b. fluorochloride
    b. follow-through examination
    fragmentation of b.
    high-density b.
    holdup in flow of b.
    hydrophilic nonflocculating b.
    b. injection
    b. injection through colostomy
    b. lead sulfate
    b. meal

    b. meal and follow through (BaFT)
    b. meal study
    b. mixture
    b. pill
    b. platinocyanoide
    b. pneumoconiosis
    pocketing of b.
    b. powder
    b. radiography
    reflux of b.
    residual b.
    retained b.
    retention of b.
    b. segmentation
    b. strontium sulfate
    b. sulfate (BaSO4)
    b. sulfate contrast medium
    b. sulfate imaging agent
    b. suspension
    b. swallow
    b. swallow imaging
    b. titanate
    b. vaginography
barium-based fecal tagging
barium-filled colon
barium-impregnated poppet
barium-sulfate impregnated shunt
barium-water esophagram
barked injury
Barkow ligament
Barlow
    B. hip instability test
    B. syndrome
Baro-CAT imaging agent
baroreceptor
    b. bulb
    carotid bulb b.
Barosperse imaging agent
barotrauma
    intrapulmonary b.
    pulmonary b.
barrel chest
Barré-Lieou syndrome
barreling distortion
barrel-shaped
    b.-s. lesion
    b.-s. stone
Barrett
    B. epithelium
    B. esophagus
    B. ulcer
barrier
    anatomic b.
    b. beam
    blood-brain b. (BBB)
    blood-spinal cord b. (BSCB)

blood-thymus b.
contrast absorption b.
incompetent blood-brain b.
radiation b.
Bart abdominoperipheral angiography unit
Barth hernia
Bartholin
B. duct
B. gland
Barton fracture
Barton-Smith fracture
Bartter syndrome
basal
b. angle
b. arachnoid cistern
b. bone
b. cell adenoma
b. cell carcinoma
b. cell nevus syndrome
b. cell papilloma
b. cerebral artery
b. chorda
b. descent
b. extension
b. ganglia anatomy
b. ganglia calcification
b. ganglia of cerebellum
b. ganglia echogenic focus
b. ganglia hematoma
b. ganglia infarct
b. ganglion
b. ganglionic change
b. hypodense ganglia lesion
b. joint
b. joint of thumb
b. lamella
b. layer
b. neck fracture
b. nucleus
b. perforating artery
b. placenta vein
b. plate
b. ridge
b. segmental bronchus
b. short-axis slice
b. short-axis view
b. skull fracture
b. sphincter
b. surface
b. tuberculosis

b. vein of Rosenthal (BVR)
b. zone
bascule
cecal b.
base
b. of bladder
b. of brain
cranial b.
b. deficit
b. density
Dycal b.
b. of finger
b. fog
b. of heart
invagination skull b.
lung b.
b. of metacarpal
orbital b.
b. of phalanx
b. projection
respiratory disturbance of acid b.
b. of skull (BOS)
b. of skull foramen
b. of thumb
b. of toe
ulcer b.
b. view
baseball
b. bat shape
b. finger
b. finger fracture
b. pitcher's elbow
b. shoulder
Basedow goiter
baseline
anthropologic b.
anthropomorphic b.
b. artifact
b. of bulb
b. chest x-ray
b. correction
b. mammography
radiographic b.
Reid b. (RBL)
reproducible b.
return to b.
b. tenting
b. view
bases (*pl. of* basis)
basial
basialis
basibregmatic axis

NOTES

basic
    b. cycle length (BCL)
    b. drive cycle length (BDCL)
    b. volume image analysis
basicervical fracture
basicranial axis
basicranium
basilar
    b. angiography
    b. artery
    b. artery aneurysm
    b. artery bifurcation
    b. artery ectasia
    b. artery insufficiency
    b. artery syndrome
    b. atelectasis
    b. block skull positioner
    b. cartilage
    b. cistern
    b. crest
    b. femoral neck fracture
    b. fibrosis
    b. groove
    b. impression
    b. intracerebral hemorrhage
    b. invagination
    b. line
    b. occlusion
    b. part of occipital bone
    b. pleural scarring
    b. plexus
    b. pneumonitis
    b. pneumothorax
    b. predominance
    b. process
    b. projection
    b. reticular opacity
    b. sinus
    b. skull fracture
    b. spine
    b. sulcus
    b. suture
    b. tip aneurysm
    b. vertebra
    b. zone infiltrate
basilic vein
basin
    positive node b.
basioccipital bone
basiocciput
    b. hypoplasia
    b. tumor
basion
    b. axial interval (BAI)
    b. dens interval (BDI)
basipharyngeal canal
basis, pl. bases

    b. imaging with selective inversion-prepared
    b. pontis
basisphenoid bone
basivertebral
    b. vein
    b. venous complex
basket
    b. cell
    b. guidewire
basket-like calcification
basket-weave pattern
BaSO4
    barium sulfate
basophilic, basophil
    b. brain adenoma
    b. leukocyte
    b. series
basovertical projection
BAT
    B-mode acquisition and targeting
    bolus arrival time
    BAT system
Bateman classification of full-thickness tears
Batson
    B. plexus
    B. vertebral brain system
battledore placenta
Battle sign
batwing
    b. appearance
    b. configuration
    b. configuration of ventricle
    b. distribution
    b. edema
    b. formation
    b. lung consolidation
    b. shadow
Baudelocque diameter
Bauer Temno biopsy needle
Bauhin valve
Baumann angle
Baumgarten recess
bauxite
    b. fibrosis of lung
    b. pneumoconiosis
bayesian
    b. analysis
    b. calculation
    b. formula
    b. image estimation (BIE)
    b. technique
Bayes theorem
Bayle granulation
Bayler-Pinneau method
Bayliss effect

B

Baylor total artificial heart
Bayne
    B. classification
    B. classification of radial agenesis
bayonet
    b. deformity
    b. dislocation
    b. fracture
    b. fracture position
    b. leg
bayoneting of fracture fragment
Bazex syndrome
BBB
    blood-brain barrier
    BBB breakdown
BBBB
    bilateral bundle-branch block
BBC muscle
BBD
    benign breast disease
BBR
    bundle-branch reentry
BBS
    benign biliary obstruction
BCA
    bell-clapper anomaly
B-cell
    B.-c. monocytoid lymphoma
    B.-c. tumor
BCI
    bicaudate index
BCL
    basic cycle length
BD
    below diaphragm
BDA
    bile duct adenoma
B-D bone marrow biopsy needle
BDCL
    basic drive cycle length
BDI
    basion dens interval
BDM
    border detection method
BE
    barium enema
beach chair position
bead
    immunomagnetic b.
    methyl methacrylate b.
    packed b.

    Sephadex b.
    targeting b.
bead-chain
    b.-c. cystogram
    b.-c. cystography
beaded
    b. bile duct
    b. bronchus
    b. ductal dilatation
    b. hepatic duct
    b. necklace appearance
    b. pancreatic duct
    b. rib
    b. septal thickening
    b. septum sign
    b. ureter
beading
    b. of artery
    rosary b.
    b. of vessel
beak
    dorsal talar b.
    b. fracture
    b. ligament
    b. sign
beaked
    b. appearance
    b. cervicomedullary junction
    b. pelvis
    b. vertebra
beaking
    anterior central b.
    antral b.
    central b.
    b. of head of talus
    inferior b.
    talar b.
    talonavicular b.
    tectal b.
beak-like
    b.-l. configuration
    b.-l. narrowing
    b.-l. osteophyte formation
beak-shaped nose
Beall valve
BEAM
    brain electrical activity mapping
beam
    b. attenuation
    barrier b.
    blended b.
    broad b.

NOTES

beam *(continued)*
  cobalt-60 b.
  cone b.
  coplanar b.
  CT scanner b.
  b. current
  b. diffraction
  electron b.
  b. energy
  b. eye view (BEV)
  b. eye view dosimetry
  fan b.
  b. filtration
  flattening filter b.
  gaussian mode profile laser b.
  b. geometry
  b. hardening
  helium ion b.
  b. intensity
  intensity-modulated photon b.
  laser b.
  lateral opposed b.
  b. limitation
  lucite b.
  megavoltage treatment b.
  b. monitor
  monochromatic x-ray b.
  multifield b.
  narrow b.
  neutron b.
  noncoplanar therapy b.
  open b.
  parallel-opposed b.'s
  b. pattern
  pencil electron b.
  pion b.
  primary b.
  proton b.
  b. quality comparison
  radiation b.
  b. restrictor
  b. shaper
  sound b.
  b. splitter
  b. steering
  b. therapy
  useful b.
  wedged-pair b.
  x-ray b.
beam-bending magnet
beam-hardening
  b.-h. artifact
  b.-h. effect
beam-like artifact
beam-modifying device
beam-splitter
beam-splitting mirror

beam-therapy applicator
bear
  b. claw ulcer
  b. paw hand
beat
  apex b.
  ectopic b.
  escape b.
  inferolateral displacement of
    apical b.
  ventricular capture b. (VCB)
  ventricular ectopic b. (VEB)
  ventricular premature b. (VPB)
  ventricular pseudoperfusion b.
beaten
  b. brass appearance
  b. brass skull
  b. silver appearance
  b. silver appearance of skull
Beath view
Beatson
  B. combined ankle angle
  B. combined ankle length
beat-to-beat variability
beaver-tail appearance
Beck triad
Beckwith-Wiedemann syndrome
Beclard
  B. amputation
  B. hernia
Béclére
  B. method
  B. position
becquerel (Bq)
Becton Dickinson FAC scan
BED
  bioeffect dose
  biologically equivalent dose
bed
  arteriole-capillary-venous b.
  bladder b.
  draining lymphatic b.
  gallbladder b.
  hepatic b.
  ipsilateral jugular lymphatic b.
  liver b.
  lumpectomy b.
  peritubular vascular b.
  portal vascular b.
  primary tumor b.
  prostatic b.
  pulmonary vascular b.
  b. of rib
  skeletal b.
  stomach b.
  tumor b.
  vascular b.

Bednar tumor
bedroom fracture
bedside radiography
beer
    b. heart
    B. law
Beevor sign
Behnken unit
Behr syndrome
BEI
    butanol-extractable iodine
Bekhterev
    B. arthritis
    B. layer
Bell
    B. brachydactyly
    B. phenomenon
bell-and-clapper deformity
bell-clapper anomaly (BCA)
Bellini
    duct of B.
    B. ligament
    papillary duct of B.
bellomedullary
bell-shaped thorax
belly
    bubble of the b.
    b. of muscle
below diaphragm (BD)
below-knee amputation
Benassi
    B. method
    B. position
bend
    dorsal b.
    hand-shaped b.
    knee-like b.
bending fracture
Bends asbestos pleurisy
benediction posture
Benedict-Talbot body surface area
    method
beneficial atrial septal defect
bengal
    I-labeled rose b.
benign
    b. adrenal mass
    b. asbestos-related pleural disease
    b. Bergman ossicle
    b. biliary obstruction (BBS)
    b. biliary stricture
    b. breast calcification

    b. breast disease (BBD)
    b. cerebellar ectopia
    b. chondroblastoma
    b. conal cyst
    b. congenital Wilms tumor
    b. cortical defect
    b. duct ectasia
    b. duodenal tumor
    b. fetal hamartoma
    b. fibrous bone lesion
    b. fibrous bone tumor
    b. fibrous histiocytoma
    b. gastric ulcer
    b. infiltrate
    b. intracranial hypertension
    b. intraductal papilloma
    b. lung tumor
    b. lymphadenopathy
    b. lymphoepithelial lesion
    b. lymphoepithelial parotid tumor
    b. lymphoma of rectum
    b. lymphoproliferative lesion
    b. meningeal fibrosis
    b. mesenchymoma
    b. mesothelioma
    b. metastasizing leiomyoma
    b. mixed tumor parotitis
    b. neoplasm
    b. nephrosclerosis
    b. node
    b. osteoblastoma
    b. osteochondroma
    b. ovarian tumor
    b. oxyphilic adenoma
    b. papillary stenosis
    b. peptic stricture
    b. pleural fibroma
    b. prostatic hyperplasia (BPH)
    b. prostatic hypertrophy (BPH)
    b. sclerosing ductal proliferation
    b. small bowel tumor
    b. subdural effusion
    b. teratoid mediastinum tumor
    b. teratoma
    b. thymoma
    b. tracheobronchial stenosis
    b. urethral tumor
    b. vascular lesion
benign-appearing pattern
Benink tarsal index
Bennett
    B. comminuted fracture

NOTES

Bennett *(continued)*
    B. dislocation
    B. lesion
Benoist penetrometer
bent-knee pelvic tilt
benzamide imaging agent
benzocaine
benzoic
    b. acid
    b. acid contrast medium
bEPI
    blipped echo planar imaging
Berdon syndrome
Berenstein catheter
Berger interscapular amputation
Bergman
    B. fiber
    B. sign
Bergonie-Tribondeau law
beriberi heart
berkelium
Berman angiographic catheter
Bernard canal
Bernard-Horner syndrome
Bernard-Soulier syndrome
Berndt-Hardy talar dome classification
Bernoulli
    B. effect
    B. equation
Bernstein catheter
Berry
    B. aneurysm rupture
    B. ligament
Bertel
    B. method
    B. position
Bertillon cephalometer
Bertin
    column of B.
    B. ligament
    septum of B.
Bertolotti syndrome
berylliosis
    acute b.
    chronic b.
beryllium
    b. granuloma
    b. mammography x-ray tube
    window
best-guess technique
beta
    b. angle
    b. decay
    b. detection
    b. emission
    b. emitter
    b. particle

b. radiation
b. ray
b. transition
Beta-Cath system
beta-emitting isotope
beta-ray
    b.-r. applicator
    b.-r. ophthalmic plaque therapy
    b.-r. spectrometer
betatron
Bethesda unit
Beuren syndrome
BEV
    beam's eye view
    billion electron volt
beveled
    b. electron beam cone
    b. margin
    b. needle
bezoar
BFI
    bifrontal index
B_O field inhomogeneity
B_O field variation
BFM
    Brunnstrom-Fugl-Meyer
    BFM arm impairment assessment
BGO
    $Bi_4Ge_3O_{12}$
    bismuth germanate
    BGO crystal
BH4 precursor
Biad
    B. camera
    B. SPECT imaging system
Biafine RE
Bianchi nodule
bias
    lead-time b.
    length-time b.
    minimizing b.
    overdiagnostic b.
    selection b.
    self-selection b.
    time-to-treatment b.
biatrial
    b. hypertrophy
    b. myxoma
biaxial
BIB
    biliointestinal bypass
bibasally
bibasilar
    b. bronchopneumonia
    b. discoid atelectasis
Bible printer's lung
bicameral uterus

bicanalicular sphincter
BICAP unit
bicaudate
    b. index (BCI)
    b. ratio
bicaval cannulation
biceps
    b., brachialis, coracobrachialis
      muscles
    b. brachialis tendon
    b. brachii tendon
    b. femoris muscle
    b. femoris tendon
    short head of b.
biceps-labral complex
bicerebral infarct
Bichat
    B. canal
    B. foramen
    B. ligament
    B. membrane
bicipital
    b. aponeurosis
    b. bursitis
    b. fascia
    b. groove
    b. rib
    b. synovial sheath
    b. tendon
    b. tendon sheath
    b. tuberosity
bicisate
bicollis
    bicornis b.
    bicornuate b.
bicommissural aortic valve
biconcave
    b. deformity
    b. depression
    b. disk
biconcavity
bicondylar
    b. T-shaped fracture
    b. Y-shaped fracture
biconvex
bicornis
    b. bicollis
    b. uterus
bicornuate
    b. bicollis
    b. uterus
bicoronal synostosis

bicortical
    b. iliac bone
    b. screw
bicristal diameter
bicuspid
    b. aortic valve
    b. atrioventricular valve
    b. valvular aortic stenosis
bicycle
    b. ergometer
    b. exercise radionuclide
      ventriculogram
    b. spoke fracture
Bid-Gd mesoporphyrine
bidirectional
    b. cavopulmonary anastomosis
    b. interface
    b. shunt
BIE
    bayesian image estimation
Biello criterion
Bielschowsky stain
Bier amputation
Bierman needle
biexponential fitting of the left
  ventricular curve
bifascicular bundle branch block
bifemoral graft
bifid
    b. aortic branch
    b. atlas
    b. biceps tendon
    b. pelvis
    b. pons
    b. precordial impulse
    b. rib
    b. thumb deformity
    b. ureter
bifida
    spina b.
bifidum
    cranium b.
bifocal manipulation with distraction
biforate uterus
bifrontal
    b. index (BFI)
    b. oligodendroglioma
bifurcate
bifurcated ligament
bifurcating branch
bifurcatio, pl. bifurcationes
    b. carotidis

NOTES

bifurcation
    b. aneurysm
    b. of anterior communicating artery
    b. of aorta
    aortic b.
    basilar artery b.
    carotid artery b.
    common bile duct b.
    common carotid artery b.
    b. graft
    hepatic duct b.
    iliac b.
    b. of internal carotid artery
    b. lesion
    b. lymph node
    middle cerebral artery b.
    patent b.
    pulmonary artery b.
    pulmonary trunk b.
    tracheal b.
    b. of trunk
    ureteral bud b.
$Bi_4Ge_3O_{12}$ (BGO)
Bigelow ligament
bigeminal
    b. pattern
    b. pregnancy
Bigliani
    B. classification
    B. and Morrison method
bihemispheral insult
biischial diameter
bilaminar
    b. appearance
    b. zone
bilateral
    b. alteration
    b. anterior chest bulge
    b. arachnoid cyst
    b. breast coil
    b. bronchogram
    b. bundle-branch block (BBBB)
    b. carotid arteriography
    b. carotid stenosis
    b. choroid plexus cyst
    b. consolidation
    b. cortical necrosis
    b. diaphragmatic elevation
    b. diffuse increased uptake
    b. ductal ectasia
    b. dysplasia epiphysealis
      hemimelica
    b. elevation of diaphragm
    b. fetal chest mass
    b. hallux valgus
    b. hilar adenopathy
    b. hydrocephalus

    b. hyperlucent lung
    b. iliac crest
    b. iliopsoas abscess
    b. incomplete ureteral injury
    b. infarct
    b. interstitial pulmonary infiltrate
    b. intrafacetal dislocation
    b. invasive lobular carcinoma
    b. juxtafoveal telangiectasis
    b. large adrenal
    b. large kidney
    b. left-sidedness
    b. lesion
    b. locked facets
    b. lower lobe pneumonia
    b. myocutaneous graft
    b. narrowing of urinary bladder
    b. obstruction
    b. occlusion
    b. orbital frontal cortex
    b. pleural tube
    b. reduction of tracer uptake
    b. renal mass
    b. right-sidedness
    b. semicircular canal aplasia
    b. small kidney
    b. striopallidodentate calcinosis
    b. superior parietal hypometabolism
    b. superior vena cava
    b. symmetry
    b. upper lobe cavitary infiltrate
    b. vagotomy effect
bilaterality
bilaterally symmetric
bile
    b. bag
    b. capillary
    concentrated b.
    b. concretion
    b. duct
    b. duct adenoma (BDA)
    b. duct atresia
    b. duct carcinoma
    b. duct cystadenoma
    b. duct dilatation
    b. duct dyskinesia
    b. duct filling defect
    b. duct gas
    b. duct imaging
    b. duct infundibulum
    b. duct lumen
    b. duct multiple hamartoma
    b. duct narrowing
    b. duct pressure
    b. duct proliferation
    b. duct scan
    b. duct stone

b. duct stricture
b. encrustation
b. extravasation
b. flow
b. flow obstruction
gastric reflux of b.
b. lake
b. leakage
lithogenic b.
b. papilla
b. plug
b. pulmonary embolus
b. reflux
b. reflux gastritis
b. stasis
b. tree
bileaflet valve
bile-tagged 3D magnetic resonance colonography
bilharzial
b. carcinoma
b. granuloma
bilharziasis
cardiopulmonary b.
protopulmonary b.
biliary
b. angiography
b. atresia
b. calculus
b. canal
b. cirrhosis
b. cirrhotic liver
b. colic
b. cystadenoma
b. decompression
b. dilatation
b. drainage
b. drainage catheter
b. duct
b. dyskinesia
b. dyssynergia
b. endoprosthesis
b. excretion bowel activity
b. fistula
b. hypoplasia
b. lithotripsy
b. manometry
b. microhamartoma
b. mud
b. obstruction syndrome
b. passage
b. piecemeal necrosis

b. plexus
b. saturation index
b. sludge
b. stent
b. stricture
b. structure
b. system
b. tract
b. tract carcinoma
b. tract CT scan imaging
b. tract disease
b. tract obstruction
b. tract stone
b. tree
b. tree compression
b. tree gas
b. tree obstruction
biliary-cutaneous fistula
biliary-duodenal
b.-d. fistula
b.-d. pressure gradient
biliary-enteric
b.-e. anastomosis
b.-e. fistula
biliary-to-bowel transit
Biligram
bilinear rotation decoupling (BIRD)
bilioenteric fistula
biliointestinal bypass (BIB)
biliopancreatic
b. bypass
b. diversion
b. shunt
bilious bronchial pneumonia
bilirubinate stone
Biliscopin imaging agent
Bilivistan
Bill bar
billion electron volt (BEV)
billowing
b. mitral valve
b. mitral valve prolapse
Billroth
B. I, II anastomosis
B. I, II gastroduodenostomy
B. I, II gastrojejunostomy
bilobate placenta
bilobed
b. configuration
b. gallbladder
b. mass
b. polypoid lesion

NOTES

bilobulation
bilocular
    b. disk
    b. stomach
    b. uterus
biloculare
    cor b.
biloma
    b. in the gallbladder fossa
    intrahepatic b.
    subphrenic b.
Bilopaque imaging agent
Biloptin imaging agent
bimalleolar
    b. angle
    b. ankle fracture
    b. foot axis
bimastoid line
bimodal slice select (BOSS)
bimolecular
binarized image
binary
    b. digit
    b. image
    b. imaging
    b. opacity table
    b. similarity coefficient
bind
    ^{99m}Tc Ceretec b.
binding
    b. energy
    ionic b.
    receptor b.
    b. site
Bing-Horton syndrome
binned
binning
    projection b.
binocular stereoscope
Binswanger
    B. disease
    B. encephalopathy
bioabsorbable
    b. Dexon suture
    b. sheath-delivered vascular device
bioassay
    erythropoietin b.
biocavity laser
biodegradable
    b. implant
    b. magnetic microcluster
    b. stent
bioeffect
    b. dose (BED)
    thermal b.
bioeffects algorithm
biograph molecular imaging system

bioimpedance
    needle-tip b.
biologic
    b. age
    b. half-life
    b. window
biological
    b. osteosynthesis
    b. tissue valve
biologically equivalent dose (BED)
biology
    radiation b.
biomagnetometer
    Magnes b.
biomarker
biomechanical
    b. imbalance
    b. stress
biomechanically normal spine
biomechanics of limb-length discrepancy
biomedical radiography
biometry
    fetal b.
    longitudinal ultrasonic b.
biomicroscopy
    slit-lamp b.
    ultrasound b. (UBM)
biomodulator
biomolecular reaction
bionucleonic
biophysical
    b. limitation
    b. profile score (BPS)
BioPince needle
biopotential
    induced b.
bioprosthesis
    ProCol vascular b.
biopsy
    aspiration b.
    automated large-core breast b.
    blind b.
    bone marrow b.
    breast b.
    computerized tomography-guided
     needle b.
    core needle b.
    CT-directed b.
    CT-guided needle b.
    CT-guided percutaneous b.
    CT-guided transsternal core b.
    curved needle b.
    excisional b.
    fetal liver b.
    fetal skin b.
    fine-needle aspiration b.
    guided b.

B

interactive MR-guided b.
intramedullary tumor b.
large-core ultrasound-guided b.
Monopty core b.
MRI-guided breast b.
b. needle
needle b.
needle-guided excisional b.
needle-localized breast b. (NLBB)
percutaneous transhepatic
  endoluminal biliary b.
percutaneous transhepatic liver b.
placenta b.
point-in-space stereotactic b.
sentinel node localization and b.
skeletal b.
StereoGuide stereotactic needle
  core b.
stereotactic breast b.
stereotactic core needle b. (SCNB)
stereotactic percutaneous needle b.
stereotactic vacuum-assisted b.
stereotaxic core needle b.
systematic ultrasound-guided b.
transbronchial lung b.
b. transducer
transjugular liver b. (TLB)
transthoracic needle aspiration b.
  (TTNAB)
ultrasound-guided anterior subcostal
  liver b.
ultrasound-guided core b.
ultrasound-guided large core-
  needle b.
ultrasound-guided stereotactic b.
ultrasound-guided vacuum-assisted b.
vacuum-assisted b.
vacuum-assisted core b.
ventricular endomyocardial b.
biopsy-guided attachment
Biopsys mammotome
bioptome
Biopty
B. biopsy gun
B. cut needle
bioreductive agent
Biosense-guided LMR
Biosound AU3, AU4, AU5 system
BioSpec
B. MR imaging system
B. MR imaging system scanner
bioterrorism exposure

BioZ system
biparietal
b. bossing
b. diameter (BPD)
b. lesion
b. plane
b. suture
biparietotemporal hypometabolism
bipartite
b. fracture
b. patella
b. sesamoid bone
b. uterus
bipartition
facial b.
bipedal lymphangiography
bipediculate approach
bipennate muscle
bipenniform muscles of hand
biperforate
biphasic
b. acquisition
b. breast tumor
b. contrast-enhanced helical CT
b. CT
b. curve
b. helical CT scan
b. injection protocol
b. magnetic resonance (BP MR)
biplanar
b. aortography
b. MR imaging guidance
b. transducer
biplane
b. angiocardiography
b. angiography
b. axial film
b. cineangiography
b. cinefluorography
b. DSA unit
b. fluoroscopy
b. left ventricular angiogram
b. orthogonal view
b. pelvic arteriography
b. pelvic oblique study
b. projection
b. quantitative coronary
  arteriography
b. radiograph
b. screening
b. sector probe
b. sector scanner

NOTES

biplane *(continued)*
- b. system
- b. transesophageal echocardiography
- b. ventriculogram

bipolar
- b. gradient
- b. hip replacement
- b. lead
- b. pacemaker

BI-RADS
Breast Imaging Reporting and Data System

biramous

BIRD
bilinear rotation decoupling

bird
- b. breeder's lung
- b. eye view
- b. fancier's lung
- b. handler's lung
- b. nest filter
- b. nest lesion

bird-beak
- b.-b. configuration or narrowing
- b.-b. esophagus
- b.-b. taper at esophagogastric junction

bird-cage
- b.-c. coil designed for wrist imaging
- b.-c. head coil
- b.-c. resonator
- b.-c. splint

bird-headed dwarfism

bird-like appearance

birefringent

birhinal phantosmia

birth canal

bisacodyl tannex

bisacromial diameter

bisagittal ridge

bisection
AP malleolar b.

biseptate

bisferious pulse rhythm

bis-gadolinium-mesoporphyrine (bis-Gd-MP)

bis-Gd-MP
bis-gadolinium-mesoporphyrine
bis-Gd-MP imaging agent

bismethylamide
gadolinium diethylenetriamine pentaacetic acid b. (Gd-DTPA-BMA)

bismuth
- b. contrast medium
- b. germanate-68
- b. injection

bismuth-germanate detector (BGO)

1,4-bis(5-phenyloxazol-2-yl)benzene

bispinous diameter

bistephanic

bistratal

bit CT

bite
- b. jumping
- b. plane

bitemporal diameter

bitewing (BW)
- b. film
- b. radiograph

bit-rate allocation

bituberous diameter

bivalve

biventricular
- b. assist device (BVAD)
- b. configuration
- b. enlargement
- b. hypertrophy
- b. origin of aorta
- b. support (BVS)
- b. transposed aorta

bizarre
- b. parosteal osteochondromatous proliferation
- b. subparosteal osteochondromatous proliferation

Björk-Shiley heart valve

BKG
background

black
- b. blood magnetic resonance angiography
- b. blood technique
- b. blood T2-weighted inversion-recovery MR imaging
- b. boundary artifact
- b. comet artifact
- b. echo writing
- b. epidermoid
- b. faceted stone
- b. hole
- b. lung
- b. lung disease
- b. star breast lesion
- b. and white (BW)

black-dot heel

Blackett-Healy method

Blackfan-Diamond syndrome

bladder
apex of b.
atonic urinary b.
b. augmentation

automatic b.
base of b.
b. bed
bilateral narrowing of urinary b.
b. capacity
b. carcinoma
centrally uninhibited b.
contracted b.
b. contractility study
b. contusion trauma
b. distention
b. diverticulitis
b. diverticulum
b. dome
b. dysfunction
b. endometriosis
b. exstrophy
b. flap hematoma
flat-top b.
b. floor
b. fundus
b. hemorrhage
hourglass b.
hypertrophic b.
b. hypertrophy
hypotonic b.
b. incontinence
intraperitoneal rupture of b.
kidneys, ureters, b. (KUB)
b. laceration
b. map
neck of b.
b. neck contracture
b. neck position
b. outlet obstruction
papilloma of b.
pear-shaped urinary b.
b. perforation
b. pheochromocytoma
refluxing spastic neurogenic b.
b. rupture
sensory paralytic b.
shrunken b.
smooth-walled b.
b. stasis
b. stone
teardrop b.
thickened b.
transurethral resection of b.
trigone of b.
b. tumor
uninhibited b.

urinary blunt trauma b.
uvula of b.
b. volume
b. wall
b. wall calcification
b. wall thickness
BladderManager ultrasound device
bladder-prostate rhabdomyosarcoma
BladderScan ultrasound
blade
    b. bone
    b. of grass sign
    b. plate
blade-of-grass
    b.-o.-g. appearance
    b.-o.-g. osteolysis
Blake pouch
Blalock shunt
Blalock-Taussig shunt
blanch
    atrophie b.
Blancophor, blankophor
Blancophor FFG, SV solution
bland
    b. aortic aneurysm
    b. embolus
    b. infarct
Bland-Garland-White syndrome
blankophor (*var. of* Blancophor)
blank scan
blank-to-trues ratio
blast chest
blastic
    b. lesion
    b. metastasis
    b. metastatic prostate carcinoma
    b. phase
    b. transformation
    b. variant
blastocytoma
blastoma
    parenchymal b.
    pleuropulmonary b.
bleb
    emphysematous b.
    oval aneurysm with b.
    ruptured emphysematous b.
    subpleural b.
Bleck metatarsus adductus classification
bleed
    anticoagulant b.
    anticoagulant-related b.

NOTES

bleed (continued)
    herald b.
    intraparenchymal b.
    subcapsular b.
    technetium-99m pertechnetate GI b.
    technetium-99m sulfur colloid
      GI b.
    tumor-related spontaneous b.
bleeding
    first-trimester b.
    gastrointestinal b.
    hepatic b.
    b. into brain parenchyma
    intracystic b.
    intrapericardial b.
    b. lesion
    perirenal b.
    b. point
    b. polyp
    renal anticoagulant-related b.
    b. scintigraphy
    b. site
    splenic b.
    b. ulcer
    b. uterus
blended
    b. beam
    b. beam technique
blennorrhagic swelling
blepharoncus
Blesovsky syndrome
Blessig cyst
blind
    b. biopsy
    b. dimple
    b. enema
    b. foramen
    b. gut
    b. intestine
    b. loop syndrome
    b. percutaneous puncture of
      subclavian vein
    b. pouch syndrome
    b. segment
    b. upper esophageal pouch
blink mode
blipped echo planar imaging (bEPI)
blister
    bone b.
    fracture b.
blistering lesion
Bloch
    B. equation
    B. scale
block
    air b.
    alveolar-capillary b.

    anodal b.
    anterior fascicular b.
    anterograde b.
    AP-PA skull b.
    arborization b.
    atrioventricular b.
    autonomic nerve b.
    AV Wenckebach heart b.
    bifascicular bundle branch b.
    bilateral bundle-branch b. (BBBB)
    bone b.
    bundle-branch heart b.
    celiac ganglion b.
    celiac plexus b.
    Cerrobend b.
    cervical, skull, and shoulder b.
    complete atrioventricular b. (CAVB)
    complete congenital heart b.
    complete fetal heart b.
    complete heart b. (CHB)
    conduction b.
    congenital heart b.
    congenital symptomatic AV b.
    CT-guided superior hypogastric
      plexus b.
    custom shielding b.
    deceleration-dependent b.
    b. detector
    divisional b.
    donor heart-lung b.
    dual lateral skull b.
    entrance b.
    exit b.
    false bundle-branch b.
    fascicular b.
    filler b.
    first-degree AV b.
    first-degree heart b.
    fixed third-degree AV b.
    heart b.
    high-grade AV b.
    incomplete atrioventricular b.
      (IAVB)
    incomplete heart b.
    incomplete left bundle-branch b.
      (ILBBB)
    incomplete right bundle-branch b.
      (IRBBB)
    inflammatory heart b.
    infra-His b.
    intermittent third-degree AV b.
    interventricular b.
    intraatrial b.
    intra-His b.
    intranodal b.
    intravenous b.
    intraventricular b. (IVB)

B

intraventricular conduction b.
intraventricular heart b.
inverted-Y b.
ipsilateral bundle-branch b.
irregular b.
left anterior fascicular b. (LAFB)
left anterior hemiblock b.
left bundle-branch b. (LBBB)
mantle b.
midline mucosa-sparing b.
b. motor task
mucosa-sparing b.
multiple b.
b. paradigm
paroxysmal AV b.
partial heart b.
periinfarction b.
pixel b.
posterior fascicular b.
pseudo-AV b.
retrograde b.
right bundle-branch b. (RBBB)
second-degree AV b.
second-degree heart b.
simple b.
sinoatrial b. (SAB)
sinoatrial exit b.
sinus node exit b.
subarachnoid nerve b.
subarachnoid phenol b.
suprahisian b.
sympathetic b.
third-degree AV b.
third-degree heart b.
transient AV b.
transmission b.
trifascicular b.
unidirectional b.
unifascicular b.
ventricular b.
ventriculoatrial b.
b. vertebra
vesicular b.
Wenckebach AV b.
Wilson b.
8 x 8-pixel b.
blockage
arterial b.
bronchus b.
pulmonary artery b.
ventricular catheter b.

blocked
b. artery
b. bronchus
b. pleurisy
b. shunt tube
b. vertex field
blocker's exostosis
blocking factor
Blom-Singer tracheoesophageal fistula
blood
arterialization of venous b.
backflow of b.
backscatter of b.
backup of b.
b. channel
b. clearance half-time
b. clot
deoxygenated b.
egress of b.
epidural b.
extravasated b.
b. flow
b. flow extraction fraction
b. flow imaging
b. flow measurement
b. flowmetry
b. flow pattern
b. flow redistribution
b. flow reserve
b. flow response
b. flow study
b. flow velocity
hydrostatic pressure of b.
hyperattenuated b.
b. inflow
intracerebral b.
intraparenchymal b.
intraventricular b.
b. leak
left-to-right shunting of b.
marked shunting of b.
mixed venous b.
occult b.
b. oxygenation level-dependent (BOLD)
b. oxygenation level-dependent contrast agent
b. oxygenation level-dependent effect
b. oxygen level-dependent contrast imaging

NOTES

103

blood *(continued)*
    b. oxygen level-dependent fMRI method
    parenchymal b.
    b. patch
    b. perfusion
    b. perfusion monitor (BPM)
    peripheral b.
    periportal tracking of b.
    b. plate thrombus
    b. pool
    b. pool activity
    b. pool contrast agent
    b. pool imaging
    b. pool phase
    b. pool radionuclide angiography
    b. pool radionuclide cardioangiography
    b. pool radionuclide echocardiography
    b. pool radionuclide scan
    b. pool scintigraphy
    b. pressure
    b. pressure response
    right-to-left shunting of b.
    shunted b.
    b. sludge
    splanchnic b.
    subdural b.
    upstream b.
    vascular b.
    venous b.
    b. vessel
    b. vessel invasion
    b. vessel kinking
    b. vessel thermography
    b. vessel tumor
    b. viscosity reduction
    b. volume
    b. volume per minute
blood-brain
    b.-b. barrier (BBB)
    b.-b. barrier disruption
blood-clotting mechanism
blood-containment needle
blood-filled bone sponge
bloodless
    b. fluid
    b. zone of necrosis
blood-spinal cord barrier (BSCB)
blood-thymus barrier
blood-to-fat contrast ratio
blood-to-myocardium
    b.-t.-m. contrast ratio
    b.-t.-m. contrast of TrueFISP
blood-tumor-barrier leakage

blooming
    b. artifact
    b. focal spot
    signal b.
Blount
    B. disease
    B. tibia vara
blow-in fracture
blowing pneumothorax
blown-out appearance
blow-on-blow
blowout
    aortic stump b.
    bone lesion b.
    b. bone lesion
    b. fracture
    b. lesion of posterior vertebral element
    b. view projection
blue
    b. asbestos
    B. Max high-pressure balloon
    B. Max high-pressure reinforced polyethylene balloon catheter
    b. rubber-bleb nevus syndrome
blueberry muffin syndrome
blue-digit syndrome
blue-toe syndrome
Blumberg sign
Blumenbach
    B. clivus
    B. plane
Blumensaat line
Blumenthal lesion
Blumer rectal shelf
blunt
    b. border of lung
    b. chest trauma
    b. gastrointestinal trauma
    b. injury
    b. pancreatic trauma
    b. trauma gallbladder
    b. trauma kidney
blunted
    b. ejection fraction
    b. mucosal fold
    b. posterior sulcus
blunt-end sialogram needle
blunting
    caliceal b.
    costophrenic angle b.
    b. of costovertebral angle
    haustral b.
    b. of valve
blur
    b. artifact
    focal spot b.

geometric b.
motion b.
object-plane b.
blurred-image tomogram
blurring
    b. of aortic knob
    b. of costophrenic angle
    b. of disk margin
    radial b.
    radiographic b.
blurting
blush
    angiographic b.
    choroid plexus b.
    cortical b.
    b. of dye on angiography
    kidney papillary b.
    marrow b.
    myocardial b.
    physiologic uterine b.
    pregnancy-induced uterine b.
    renal parenchymal b.
    tumor b.
    vascular b.
BMC
    bone mineral content
BMD
    bone mineral density
BMIPP SPECT scan imaging
B-mode
    B-m. acquisition and targeting
      (BAT)
    B-m. brightness modulation scan
    B-m. display
    B-m. echocardiography
    B-m. echography
    B-m. imaging
    longitudinal B-m.
    pseudocolor B-m.
    B-m. ultrascan
    B-m. ultrasonography
BMP
    bone marrow pressure
BMS
    bulk magnetic susceptibility
board
    b. angle
    immobilizer b.
    right-angled isosceles triangle b.
boat-shaped heart
Bochdalek
    B. foramen

B. gap
B. hernia
B. muscle
body
    angularis b.
    anococcygeal b.
    apoptic b.
    asbestos b.
    asteroid b.
    b. atomic number
    Auer b.
    axis b.
    b. background activity
    b. box plethysmography
    b. burden
    calcific round b.
    calcified pineal b.
    cancer b.
    carotid b.
    caudate b.
    b. cavity
    coccygeal b.
    b. coil
    b. coil imaging
    b. composition measurement
    compressed b.
    b. contour orbit
    dense b.
    diffuse low signal replacement of
      the vertebral b.
    elementary b.
    embryoid b.
    enlargement of vertebral b.
    b. of epididymis
    esophageal b.
    b. of femur
    ferruginous b.
    flat vertebral b.
    foreign b. (FB)
    free b.
    b. of gallbladder
    geniculate b.
    glenoid labral ovoid b.
    b. glomus
    b. habitus
    H-shaped vertebral b.
    b. interface
    intraarticular loose b.
    intraluminal foreign b.
    intraocular foreign b.
    intravascular foreign b.
    juxtarestiform b.

NOTES

body *(continued)*
  ketone b.
  lamellar b.
  lateral geniculate b.
  loose intraarticular b.
  Luys b.
  malpighian b.
  mamillary b.
  b. mass index
  Masson b.
  medial geniculate b.
  metallic foreign b. (MFB)
  Michaelis-Gutmann b.
  Mott b.
  multilaminar b.
  b. of nail
  navicular b.
  nonradiopaque foreign b.
  no-threshold b.
  opaque foreign b.
  ossified b.
  osteochondral loose b.
  osteochondrotic loose b.
  pacchionian b.
  b. of the pancreas
  pearly b.
  pharmacoradiologic disimpaction of
    esophageal foreign b.
  Pick b.
  picture frame pattern of
    vertebral b.
  pineal b.
  psammoma b.
  radiopaque foreign b.
  restiform b.
  retained foreign b.
  rhinencephalic mamillary b.
  rice joint b.
  Russell b.
  scalloping of margin of
    vertebral b.
  b. scanning
  b. of scapula
  scapular b.
  Schaumann b.
  Schiller-Duval b.
  b. section radiography
  b. section radiography imaging
  Seidelin b.
  small vertebral b.
  squared vertebral b.
  b. stalk
  b. of the stomach
  b. surface area (BSA)
  b. surface area calculation
  b. surface Laplacian mapping
    (BSLM)

  b. surface potential mapping
  Symington b.
  threshold b.
  thyroid psammoma b.
  tracheobronchial foreign b.
  trapezoid b.
  uterine b.
  b. of uterus
  Verocay b.
  b. of vertebra
  vesalianum of vertebral b.
  b. wall
  Weibel-Palade b.
  b. weight
  Zuckerkandl b.
body-coil-based contrast-enchanced MRA
body-coil MRI
Boehler angle
Boerhaave syndrome
boggy
  b. synovitis
  b. synovium
Bogros space
Böhler angle
Bohr
  B. atom
  B. effect
  B. equation
  B. magneton
  B. radius
  B. theory
BOLD
  blood oxygenation level-dependent
  BOLD contrast functional MRI
  BOLD contrast imaging
  BOLD effect
  BOLD signal
  BOLD time course change
BOLD-fMRI
bolster
  angular b.
  breast b.
  b. finger
  knee arthrography b.
Bolton
  B. plane
  B. point
  B. triangle
Bolton-nasion
  B.-n. line
  B.-n. plane
Boltzmann
  B. distribution
  B. equation
bolus
  air b.
  b. arrival time (BAT)

barium b.
CARE b.
b. challenge imaging
b. challenge test
b. chase
b. chase technique
contrast b.
b. contrast enhancement
b. dose
dynamic b.
electron b.
intravenous b.
b. intravenous injection
marshmallow b.
b. passage perfusion measurement
radioactive b.
simple b.
special b.
b. tagging
test b.
b. timing
tracer b.
b. tracking
b. transit
water b.
bolus-chase stepping-table 3D MRA
bombard
bombardment
alpha particle b.
end of saturated b. (EOSB)
neutron b.
bond
iodine I-131 iodine PVP b.
valence b.
wedge b.
bone (os)
b. abscess
accessory multangular b.
accessory navicular b.
accessory sesamoid b.
acetabular b.
acromial b.
adamantinoma of long b.
b. age (BA)
b. age imaging
b. age ratio
alar b.
Albrecht b.
b. algorithm
b. allograft
alveolar supporting b.
b. angioblastoma

b. angiosarcoma
ankle b.
anvil b.
apex of petrous portion of
  temporal b.
arch of b.
architectural alterations of b.
areola of b.
articular lamella of b.
articular tubercle of temporal b.
astragalar b.
astragalocalcanean b.
astragalocrural b.
astragaloscaphoid b.
astragalotibial b.
astragalus b.
b. atrophy
attic temporal b.
autogenous b.
basal b.
basilar part of occipital b.
basioccipital b.
basisphenoid b.
bicortical iliac b.
bipartite sesamoid b.
blade b.
b. blister
b. block
bowed long b.
breast b.
bregmatic b.
brittle b.
bundle b.
calcaneal b.
calvarial b.
b. canaliculus
cancellated b.
candle-wax appearance of b.
cannon b.
b. capillary hemangioma
capitate b.
b. carcinoma
carpal navicular b.
cartilage b.
cavalry b.
b. cement
b. center
central b.
chalky b.
cheek b.
chevron b.
b. chip

NOTES

B

bone (*continued*)
b. chloroma
b. coccidioidomycosis
coccygeal b.
coccyx b.
coffin b.
compact b.
condylar part of occipital b.
continuity of b.
b. contusion
convoluted b.
b. core
b. cortex
cortical b.
corticocancellous b.
costal b.
coxal b.
cranial b.
cribriform b.
b. crisis
cubital b.
cuboid b.
cuneiform b.
dancer's b.
dead b.
b. debris
b. demineralization
dense structure of b.
b. densitometer
b. densitometry
b. density imaging
b. density measurement
b. density study
depression of nasal b.
dermal b.
detecting Down syndrome by
 ultrasound of the nose b.
devitalized allogeneic b.
devitalized portion of b.
diastasis of cranial b.
dimple of b.
displaced fragment of b.
dorsal talonavicular b.
b. dysplasia
b. dystrophy
eburnated b.
b. echinococcosis
b. end
endochondral b.
entrapped plantar sesamoid b.
epactal b.
epihyal b.
epihyoid b.
epiphysis b.
epipteric b.
episternal b.
erosion of epiphyseal b.

ethmoid b.
exoccipital b.
exoccipital part of occipital b.
b. expansion
facial b.
femoral b.
fencer's b.
b. fibrosarcoma
fibular sesamoid b.
first cuneiform b.
b. fixation device
b. fixation plate
flank b.
b. flap
flat b.
b. formation
b. formation cloaca
fourth turbinated b.
b. fracture
fracture running length of b.
b. fragment
frontal b.
Goethe b.
gracile b.
b. graft
greater multangular b.
great toe sesamoid b.
growth center of b.
b. growth stimulator
hallux sesamoid b.
hamate b.
b. hardening
heel b.
heterotopic b.
hip b.
b. histology
b. histomorphometry
hollow b.
hooked b.
humeral b.
hyoid b.
hyperplastic b.
b. hypertrophy
iliac cancellous b.
immature b.
b. implant
b. implantation cyst
incisive b.
incomplete fracture of b.
incus b.
b. infarct
infected b.
inferior turbinated b.
inflammation of b.
b. ingrowth
b. injury radiation
inner table of frontal b.

innominate b.
intermaxillary b.
intermediate cuneiform b.
interparietal b.
b. interstice
intracartilaginous b.
intrachondral b.
intramembranous b.
irregular b.
ischial b.
b. island
jaw b.
knuckle b.
lacrimal b.
b. lacuna
lamellar b.
lateral part of occipital b.
lateral sesamoid b.
b. length imaging
b. length study
lenticular b.
lentiform b.
b. lesion apophysis
b. lesion blowout
b. lesion epiphysis
b. lesion of the rib
b. and limb growth velocity ratio
lingual b.
b. lipoma
long b.
long axis of b.
lunate b.
lunocapitate b.
luxated b.
b. lymphoma
malar b.
malignant fibrous histiocytoma
  of b. (MFH-B)
malleolus b.
marble b.
b. marrow
b. marrow agent
b. marrow biopsy
b. marrow boundary
b. marrow depression
b. marrow edema
b. marrow edema pattern on MR
  imaging
b. marrow embolus
b. marrow fibrosis
b. marrow hypoplasia
b. marrow infiltrate

b. marrow lesion
b. marrow lymphoid hyperplasia
b. marrow microenvironment
b. marrow myeloid precursor
b. marrow pressure (BMP)
b. marrow purging
b. marrow relapse
b. marrow rescue
b. marrow scan
b. marrow scintigraphy
b. marrow stroma
b. marrow toxicity
b. marrow transplant
b. mastocytosis
mastoid b.
b. maturation
mature b.
maxillary b.
medial cuneiform b.
medial sesamoid b.
medullary b.
membrane of b.
mesocuneiform b.
metacarpal b.
b. metastasis
metatarsal b.
b. microarchitecture
middle cuneiform b.
middle turbinate b.
b. mineral content (BMC)
b. mineral content imaging
b. mineral content study
b. mineral density (BMD)
b. mineral immobilization
b. mineralization
morcellized b.
b. morphogenetic activity
mortise of b.
multangular b.
nasal b.
navicular b.
b. neck
necrotic b.
b. neoplasm
Nicoll b.
occipital b.
odontoid b.
omovertebral b.
orbicular b.
orbital b.
orbitosphenoidal b.
os calcis b.

NOTES

bone *(continued)*

osteonal b.
osteopenic b.
osteoporosis of b.
osteoporotic b.
b. overdevelopment
b. oxalosis
Paget disease of b.
pagetoid b.
palatine b.
parietal b.
b. particle
pedal b.
pelvic b.
perichondral b.
periosteal b.
periotic b.
peroneal b.
petrosal b.
petrous temporal b.
phalangeal b.
phantom b.
b. phase image
b. phase imaging
b. pinhole
Pirie b.
pisiform b.
b. plug
pneumatic b.
pole of scaphoid b.
porous b.
postsphenoid b.
posttraumatic atrophy of b.
postulnar b.
b. powder
preinterparietal b.
premaxillary b.
presphenoid b.
primitive b.
proliferation of b.
prominence of b.
pterygoid b.
pubic b.
b. pulley
pyramidal b.
quadrilateral b.
b. quantitative CT (BQCT)
radial b.
b. radiation absorption
Recklinghausen disease of b.
refractured b.
b. remodeling
replacement b.
b. resorption
reticulated b.
rider's b.
ring-of-b.

rudimentary b.
sacral b.
b. sarcoidosis
scaphoid b.
scapular b.
b. scintiscan imaging
sclerosed temporal b.
b. screw
scroll b.
second cuneiform b.
b. seeker
semilunar b.
septal b.
sesamoid b.
b. shaft
shank b.
shin b.
short b.
sieve b.
b. sliver
solid b.
sphenoid b.
sphenoidal turbinated b.
splintered b.
spoke b.
spongy b.
b. spur
squamous part of frontal b.
squamous part of occipital b.
squamous part of temporal b.
stirrup b.
b. strut
subchondral b.
subperiosteal new b.
b. substance
b. substitute
superior turbinated b.
supernumerary sesamoid b.
supracollicular spike of cortical b.
suprainterparietal b.
supraoccipital b.
suprapharyngeal b.
suprasternal b.
supreme turbinate b.
b. surface
b. survey
sutural b.
b. syphilis
tail b.
talus b.
target b.
tarsal b.
temporal b.
thick b.
thigh b.
thoracic b.
tibia b.

tibial sesamoid b.
trabecular b.
trabeculated b.
trapezium b.
trapezoid b.
triangular b.
triquetral b.
b. tuberculosis
tuberculous b.
tubular b.
b. tumor
b. tumor aggressiveness
tumor-bearing b.
b. tumor matrix
b. tumor scalloping
turbinate b.
b. turnover
tympanic b.
ulnar b.
ulnar sesamoid b.
unciform b.
b. unloading
upper jaw b.
vascular b.
vesalian b.
vomer b.
weightbearing b.
b. window
wing of sphenoid b.
wormian b.
woven b.
wrist triquetrum b.
b. xanthogranuloma
xiphoid b.
zygomatic b.
bone-air interface
bone-chip allograft
bone-detail algorithm
bone-forming
  b.-f. bone tumor
  b.-f. sarcoma
bone-hardening artifact
bone-implant interface
bonelet
bone-on-bone contact
bone-tendon-bone graft
bone-tendon exposure
bone-to-bone apposition
bone-within-bone
  b.-w.-b. appearance
  b.-w.-b. vertebra
Bonferroni adjustment

bonnet
  gluteal b.
bony
  b. abnormality
  b. alignment
  b. ankylosis
  b. apposition
  b. architecture
  b. bar
  b. bridge
  b. callus
  b. callus formation
  b. change
  b. coalition
  b. contusion
  b. cortex interruption
  b. decompression
  b. defect
  b. deformity
  b. degeneration
  b. deposit
  b. destruction
  b. disruption
  b. eburnation
  b. encroachment
  b. enlargement
  b. erosion
  b. excrescence
  b. exostosis
  b. fossa
  b. fusion
  b. glenoid marrow fat
  b. glenoid rim
  b. healing
  b. heart
  b. humeral avulsion
  b. hyperostosis
  b. island
  b. labyrinth
  b. lysis
  b. necrosis
  b. nonunion
  b. orbit
  b. osteophyte
  b. overgrowth
  b. pelvis
  b. plate
  b. process
  b. projection from vertebra
  b. proliferation
  b. prominence
  b. protuberance

B

NOTES

bony *(continued)*
    b. rarefaction
    b. reabsorption
    b. remodeling
    b. ridge
    b. sclerosis
    b. semicircular canal
    b. sequestrum
    b. shadow
    b. skeleton
    b. skull landmark
    b. spicule
    b. spurring
    b. stability
    b. structure
    b. suture
    b. thoracic cage
    b. thorax
    b. tissue
    b. trabecular injury
    b. trabecular pattern
    b. tuft of finger
    b. union
    b. vertebra projection
boomerang tendon
BOOP
    bronchiolitis obliterans with organizing
    pneumonia
Boorman classification of gastric
carcinoma
boost
    brachytherapy b.
    b. dose
    electron-beam b.
    GK-SRS b.
    interstitial b.
    b. therapy
booster heart
boot-shaped heart
boot-top fracture
border
    anterior b.
    antimesenteric b.
    cardiac b.
    ciliated b.
    corticated b.
    crescentic b.
    b. detection method (BDM)
    diaphragmatic b.
    echocardiographic automated b.
    gradually tapering b.
    heart b.
    inferior b.
    interosseous b.
    irregular b.
    lateral b.
    left sternal b. (LSB)

    lobulated b.
    lower sternal b. (LSB)
    medial b.
    mediastinal b.
    mesenteric b.
    midleft sternal b.
    overhanging b.
    peripheral b.
    posterior b.
    rounded convex b.
    scalloped b.
    scapulovertebral b.
    sclerotic b.
    serpiginous low signal intensity b.
    shagging of cardiac b.
    shaggy heart b.
    smooth b.
    spiculated b.
    sternal b.
    sternocleidomastoid muscle b.
    straight anterior vertebral b.
    superior b.
    tapering b.
    thin b.
    upper sternal b.
    well-defined b.
    b. zone
borderline
    b. cardiomegaly
    b. heart size
    b. malignancy
    b. normal
Borell and Fernström method
Borg scale of treadmill exertion
Born
    B. approximation
    B. method
boron
    b. counter
    b. neutron capture
BOS
    base of skull
Bosniak classification
BOSS
    bimodal slice select
boss
    carpal b.
    parietal b.
bossa
bosselated
    b. stone
    b. surface
bosselation
bossing
    biparietal b.
    frontal b.
    occipital b.

B

Bosworth
    B. bone peg insertion
    B. fracture
Botallo
    B. duct
    B. foramen
    B. ligament
both-bone fracture
both-column fracture
botryoid
    b. rhabdomyosarcoma
    b. sarcoma
Böttcher canal
Bouchard
    B. disease
    B. node
bougienage technique
Bouillaud disease
bounce-point artifact
bouncing
    ligamentous b.
bound
    Cramer-Rao minimum variance b.
    (CR-MVB)
    b. electron
boundary
    air/bone/tissue b.
    bone marrow b.
    b. edge
    horizontal b.
    b. layer
    tumor b.
bouquet
    fixed shaped coplanar or nonplanar
    radiation beam b.
Bourgery ligament
Bourneville disease
Bourneville-Pringle disease
boutonnière
    b. deformity
    b. dislocation
Bouveret syndrome
Bovero muscle
bovine heart xenograft
Bowditch effect
bowed
    b. legs
    b. long bone
    b. micromelia
bowel
    aganglionic b.
    apple-peel b.

b. atresia
b. axis
b. and bladder dysfunction
b. caliber
b. carcinoma
b. content
b. continuity
corkscrew appearance of small b.
dead b.
dilated dry small b.
dilated fetal b.
dilated loops of b.
dilated wet small b.
distal small b.
b. distention
echogenic fetal b.
fixed segment of b.
fluid-filled loop of b.
free-floating loop of b.
functional immaturity of b.
b. gangrene
b. gas
b. gas artifact
b. gas pattern
herniated b.
hoop-shaped loops of b.
b. incontinence
b. infarct
b. intussusception
ischemic b.
kinked b.
large b.
b. loop
b. loop air
b. loop angulation
b. loop dilatation
b. loop fixation
b. lumen
b. migration
b. motion
b. movement
b. mucosa
multiple loops of small b.
multiple stenotic lesions of
  small b.
b. necrosis
normal caliber b.
b. obstruction
b. perforation
b. peristalsis
pleating of small b.
b. preparation

NOTES

bowel *(continued)*
> proximal small b.
> b. pseudoobstruction
> ribbon b.
> b. secretion
> b. serosal endometrial implant
> b. shock
> small b.
> b. sound
> b. spasm
> b. stenosis
> b. stoma
> strangulated b.
> b. wall
> b. wall hematoma
> b. wall penetration

bowing
> anterior tibial b.
> b. deformity
> b. fracture
> b. of mitral valve leaflet
> b. of tendon

bowleg
bowler's
> b. hat sign
> b. thumb

Bowman
> B. capsule
> B. disk
> B. muscle
> B. space

bowstring
> b. sign
> b. tear

bowstringing
bow-tie sign
box
> carpal b.
> ligamentous b.
> mammographic view b.
> shadow b.
> view b.

box-and-whisker plot
boxer's
> b. elbow
> b. fracture

box-like cardiomegaly
Boyd
> B. ankle amputation
> B. formula
> B. perforating vein
> B. type II fracture

Boyden
> B. sphincter
> B. test meal

Boyd-Griffin trochanteric fracture classification

Bozzolo sign
BP
> bronchopleural
> bronchopulmonary
> bypass
>> BP fistula
>> Imagent BP
>> BP MR

BPD
> biparietal diameter
> bronchopulmonary dysplasia

BPFM
> bronchopulmonary foregut malformation

BPH
> benign prostatic hyperplasia
> benign prostatic hypertrophy

BPM
> blood perfusion monitor

BPS
> biophysical profile score
>> fetal BPS

Bq
> becquerel

BQCT
> bone quantitative CT

brace artifact
bracelet
> ^{89}Sr b.

brachia (*pl. of* brachium)
brachial
> b. arteriography
> b. artery
> b. artery approach
> b. artery compression
> b. artery cuff pressure
> b. artery end-diastolic pressure
> b. artery peak systolic pressure
> b. artery pulse pressure
> b. atrophy
> b. fascia
> b. lymph node
> b. plexus
> b. plexus birth injury
> b. plexus compression
> b. plexus infiltrate
> b. plexus neuritis
> b. plexus tendon
> b. vein

brachial-basilar insufficiency
brachialis tendon
brachicephaly
brachii
> triceps b.

brachiocephalic
> b. arterial aneurysm
> b. arteriography
> b. artery

b. artery stenting
b. artery thrombolysis
b. branch
b. ischemia
b. lymph node
b. trunk
b. trunk of aorta
b. vein
b. vessel
brachiocubital
brachioradialis
b. muscle
b. tendon
brachium, pl. **brachia**
b. of colliculus
b. conjunctivum
b. pontis
Bracht-Wachter lesion
brachycephalic head shape
brachycephaly
brachydactyly
Bell b.
Christian b.
Mohn-Wriedt b.
brachymetatarsia
brachypellic pelvis
brachytelephalangic type of cystic fibrosis
brachytherapy
afterloading b.
b. boost
endovascular b.
episcleral plaque b.
b. implant removal
interstitial b.
intracavitary application b.
intraluminal b.
IOHDR b.
permanent b.
remote afterloading b. (RAB)
Ultraseed b.
vascular b.
bracing
fracture b.
bradyphemic
bradyphrenia
Bragard sign
Bragg
B. angle
B. curve
B. equation
B. ionization peak

B. law
B. peak radiosurgery
B. spectrometer
Bragg-Gray cavity
braided diagnostic catheter
brain
b. abscess
b. activation study
b. activity
b. anatomy classification
b. aneurysm
b. anoxia
b. architecture
atrial diverticulum of b.
b. atrophy
base of b.
b. bridging vein
Broca motor speech area of b.
buckling cortical b.
b. calcification hemangioma
b. candle dripping
b. capillary angiography
b. carcinoma
b. cavernoma
b. concussion
b. contusion
b. cyst
b. death
b. degeneration
b. diffusion anisotropy
dura mater of b.
b. dysfunction
b. dysgerminoma
b. edema
edematous b.
b. electrical activity mapping (BEAM)
eloquent area of b.
b. empyema
b. ependymoma
b. fissure
b. function
b. geography
b. hamartoma
b. hematoma
b. homeostasis
horseshoe configuration of b.
b. imaging radiopharmaceutical
b. incidentaloma
b. infarct
inflammation of b.
insular region of b.

NOTES

brain *(continued)*
   b. ischemia
   b. laceration
   left b.
   b. lesion
   b. lipoma
   b. lymphoma
   b. mantle
   b. mass
   b. mass in jugular foramen
   meninges of b.
   b. metastasis
   b. paragonimiasis
   b. parenchyma
   b. perfusion
   b. perfusion reserve
   b. perfusion scintigraphy
   b. perfusion SPECT
   b. plasticity
   b. proton magnetic resonance
    spectroscopy
   b. region vesicle
   right b.
   sagging b.
   b. scan
   b. scan imaging
   b. shrinkage
   silent area of b.
   smooth b.
   softening of b.
   split b.
   b. stem
   b. stenosis hemorrhage
   b. structure
   b. substance
   b. surface matching technique
   b. swelling
   b. tissue herniation
   b. tuber
   b. tuberculoma
   b. tumor
   b. tumor at cerebellopontine angle
   b. tumor classification
   unicameral b.
   Virchow-Robin space of b.
   b. volume
   b. water content
   water on the b.
   watershed zone in the b.
   wet b.
   b. window
brain-core gradient
BrainLAB VectorVision neuronavigation
  system
brainstem
   b. compression
   b. demyelination

   b. displacement
   b. edema
   b. encephalitis
   b. ependymoma
   b. glioma
   b. hemorrhage
   b. infarct
   b. ischemia
   b. lesion
   b. pyramidal tract
   reticular formation of the b.
   b. reticular formation
   tegmentum of b.
brain-to-background ratio
BrainVoyager interactive software
braking radiation
branch
   acute marginal b.
   anterior cutaneous b.
   arterial b.
   b. of artery
   atrioventricular groove b.
   bifid aortic b.
   bifurcating b.
   brachiocephalic b.
   bronchial b.
   bronchus b.
   cardiac b.
   caudal b.
   circumflex b.
   collateral b.
   cortical b.
   cutaneous lateral b.
   b. decay
   diagonal b.
   digital b.
   distal b.
   dorsal b.
   feeding b.
   first major diagonal b.
   first septal perforator b.
   geniculate b.
   inferior cardiac b.
   inferior wall b.
   intrahepatic portal vein b.
   large obtuse marginal b.
   left bundle b.
   marginal b.
   midmarginal b.
   motor b.
   muscular b.
   musculophrenic b.
   nonlingular b.
   obtuse marginal b. (OMB)
   paired parietal b.
   paired visceral b.
   pancreatic duct b.

perforating b.
phalangeal b.
b. point
posterior descending b.
posterior intercostal b.
posterior ventricular b.
premamillary b.
proper digital nerve b.
pruning of pancreatic duct b.
pudendal b.
b. pulmonary artery stenosis
ramus intermedius artery b.
ramus medialis artery b.
right bundle b.
second diagonal b.
segmental renal artery b.
septal perforating b.
side b.
sinoatrial b.
subcostal b.
subsegmental renal artery b.
sulcocommissural b.
superior phrenic b.
thalamoperforating b.
unpaired parietal b.
unpaired visceral b.
b.'s of vein
ventral b.
ventricular b.

branched
    b. calculus
    b. chain

branchial
    b. cartilage
    b. cleft cyst
    b. cleft development
    b. duct
    b. efferent column
    b. fistula
    b. pouch
    b. sinus

branching
    anomalous b.
    b. calcification
    b. centrilobar opacity
    b. decay
    b. fraction
    b. line
    b. linear structure
    mirror-image brachiocephalic b.
    b. pattern
    b. ratio

right aortic arch with mirror
    image b.
b. tubular structure
Brasdor method
Brasfield scoring system
Braun
    B. canal
    B. tumor
Braune muscle
Braunwald-Cutter valve
Braunwald sign
bread-and-butter
    b.-a.-b. heart
    b.-a.-b. pericarditis
bread loaf technique
breadth
    photopeak b.
breakdown
    BBB b.
breakthrough
    normal perfusion pressure b.
    b. vasodilation
    b. visualization
breast
    b. abscess
    accessory b.
    adenoma of b.
    b. adenosarcoma
    b. adenosis
    b. anatomy
    b. angiosarcoma
    b. artifact
    atrophic b.
    b. attenuation
    augmented b.
    b. biopsy
    b. bolster
    b. bone
    b. cancer risk factor
    b. cancer screening
    B. cancer system 2100
    b. carcinoma
    central solitary papilloma b.
    b. coil
    compression of b.
    b. cyst
    b. cyst aspiration
    cystic disease of b.
    b. degeneration
    b. edema
    b. embryology
    fascia of b.

NOTES

breast *(continued)*
b. fat necrosis
b. fibroadenolipoma
b. fibroadenoma
b. fibroadenomatosis
fibrocystic b.
b. fibrosis
b. hamartoma
b. hematoma
b. hyperplasia
B. Imaging Reporting and Data System (BI-RADS)
b. lesion
b. lipofibroadenoma
b. lipoma
lobule b.
b. localizer
b. lymphoma
b. mammographic technique
b. metastasis
b. microcalcification
Miraluma nuclear scan of b.
b. mucocele
b. neoplasm
b. papilloma
b. parenchyma
b. phyllode tumor
b. pneumocystography
b. popcorn calcification
prepubertal female b.
b. prosthesis rupture
b. pseudolymphoma
radiographic-dense b.
round cancer of the b.
b. sarcoma
b. shadow
shoemaker's b.
b. skin thickening
b. sonography
stromal pattern of b.
tail of b.
b. thrombophlebitis
b. tissue
b. tissue displacement
b. traction
b. trigger point
b. ultrasound
variocele tumor of b.
breastbone
breaststroker's knee
breath-hold
b.-h. cine-MR
b.-h. contrast-enhanced MRI
b.-h. contrast-enhanced three-dimensional MR angiography
b.-h. fast-recovery fast SE pulse sequence

b.-h. fast spin-echo image
b.-h. gradient-recalled echo sequence
b.-h. MR cholangiography
b.-h. scanning
b.-h. segmented k-space gradient-echo imaging
b.-h. technique
b.-h. T1-weighted gradient echo imaging
b.-h. T1-weighted MP-GRE MR imaging
b.-h. ungated imaging
b.-h. velocity-encoded cine MR imaging
breathing
b. artifact
b. feedback
breath pentane measurement
breech presentation
breeder reactor
bregma
bregmatic
b. bone
b. fontanelle
bregmatolambdoid arc
bregmatomastoid suture
Bremer
B. AirFlo Vest
B. Halo Crown system
bremsstrahlung
b. process
b. radiation
b. scan
Brenner tumor
Breschet canal
Brescia-Cimino
B.-C. fistula
B.-C. graft
Breslow classification
Brett sun
Breuerton view of hand
breve
vinculum b.
Brevi-Kath epidural catheter
brevis
abductor pollicis b. (APB)
coxa b.
extensor carpi radialis b. (ECRB)
extensor digitorum b. (EDB)
extensor pollicis b.
flexor digiti minimi b.
flexor digiti quinti b.
flexor digitorum b.
flexor hallucis b. (FHB)
flexor pollicis b.
palmaris b.

split peroneus b.
b. tendon

bridge
arteriolovenular b.
b. autograft
bony b.
b. circuit
interthalamic b.
intraductal b.
loop ostomy b.
mucosal b.
muscular b.
myocardial b.
nasal b.
osseous b.
osteophytic b.
portal-to-portal b.
skin b.
transphyseal bone b.
ventral b.
Wheatstone b.

bridged loop-gap resonator

bridging
b. callus
b. defect
b. necrosis
b. osteophyte
physeal bony b.

bright
b. contrast enhancement
b. cystic focus
b. echo
b. fatty marrow
b. layer
b. pixel value
b. signal
b. signal intensity

bright-field imaging

brightly
b. echogenic focus
b. increased renal parenchymal
echogenicity

brightness
b. area product (BAP)
b. gain
b. mode
b. modulation
b. modulation scan

brightness-time curve

bright-signal-intensity tumor

Brilliance 109 MP PC monitor

brim
pelvic b.
b. of the pelvis
quadrilateral b.
b. sign

brimstone liver

brisement therapy

brisk wall motion

Brissaud syndrome

Brite Tip 5F–10F guiding catheter

British thermal unit

brittle
b. bone
b. bone disease

broad
b. beam
b. fascia
b. ligament
b. ligament hernia
b. ligament pregnancy
b. maxillary ridge

broadband
b. noise detection error artifact
b. transducer

broad-based
b.-b. disk protrusion
b.-b. polyp

broad-beam
b.-b. absorption
b.-b. scattering

Broadbent-Bolton plane

broadening
dipolar b.
quadripolar signal b.
spectral b.

Broca
B. area
band of B.
B. convolution
B. diagonal band
B. gyrus
B. index
B. motor speech area of brain
B. pudendal pouch
B. region

Brödel
B. avascular line
B. bloodless line of incision

NOTES

Broden
- B. position
- B. view

Broders tumor index classification
Brodie
- B. bursa
- B. disease
- B. knee
- B. ligament
- B. metaphyseal abscess

Brodmann
- B. area 32
- B. cytoarchitectonic field

broken bough pattern
bromide
- perfluorooctyl b. (PFOB)

brominated oil
bromine-76 bromospirone
brominized oil contrast medium
bromodeoxyuridine
- 5-b. analysis
- b. imaging agent
- b. labeling index

bromophenol blue imaging agent
bromospirone
- bromine-76 b.

bronchi (*pl. of* bronchus)
bronchial
- b. adenoma
- b. angiography
- b. anular cartilage
- b. arteriography
- b. artery
- b. artery embolization (BAE)
- b. atresia
- b. branch
- b. bud
- b. calculus
- b. caliber
- b. carcinoid tumor
- b. carcinoma
- b. cleft cyst
- b. collateral circulation
- b. cuff sign
- b. dehiscence
- b. diameter
- b. dilatation
- b. distortion
- b. erosion
- b. fracture
- b. groove
- b. inflammation
- b. kinking
- b. lumen
- b. mucocele
- b. mucosa
- b. obstruction

- b. polyp
- b. provocation imaging
- b. provocation testing
- b. reactivity
- b. rupture
- b. septum
- b. sinus
- b. smooth muscle spasm
- b. spur
- b. stenosis
- b. stenting
- b. stricture
- b. tract
- b. tree
- b. tube
- b. vein
- b. vessel
- b. wall thickening

bronchiectasis
- acquired b.
- capillary b.
- central b.
- congenital b.
- cylindrical b.
- cystic b.
- distal b.
- dry b.
- follicular b.
- fusiform b.
- polynesian b.
- postinfectious b.
- recurrent b.
- reversible b.
- saccular b.
- b. traction
- tuberculous b.
- tubular b.
- varicose b.

bronchiectasis-ethmoid sinusitis
bronchiectatic
- b. airway
- b. cyst
- b. pattern

bronchiolar
- b. adenocarcinoma
- b. carcinoma
- b. dilatation
- b. edema
- b. emphysema
- b. narrowing
- b. obstruction

bronchiole
- alveolar b.
- conducting b.
- irreversible narrowing of b.
- lobular b.
- membranous b.

respiratory b.
terminal b.
tree-in-bud b.
bronchiolectasis
traction b.
bronchioli (*pl. of* bronchiolus)
bronchiolitis
cellular b.
constrictive b.
diffuse aspiration b.
exudative b.
b. fibrosa obliterans
follicular b.
b. obliterans with organizing
pneumonia (BOOP)
obliterative b.
pediatric b.
proliferative b.
respiratory b.
smoker's b.
vesicular b.
bronchioloalveolar carcinoma
bronchiolocentric
bronchiolus, pl. **bronchioli**
bronchitis
asthmatic b.
follicular b.
irritant b.
bronchoadenitis
bronchoalveolar
b. carcinoma
b. cell adenoma
bronchoarterial bundle
bronchobiliary fistula
bronchocavernous
bronchocavitary fistula
bronchocele
bronchocentric
b. granulomatosis
b. inflammatory infiltrate
bronchoconstriction
exercise-induced b.
isocapnic hyperventilation-induced b.
bronchoconstrictor
bronchocutaneous fistula
bronchodilation, bronchodilatation
bronchodilator effect
bronchoesophageal fistula
bronchogenic
b. adenoma
b. carcinoma
b. duplication cyst

bronchogram
air b.
bilateral b.
Cope method b.
fiberoptic b.
fluid-filled b.
b. imaging
mucinous b.
mucous b.
scattered air b.
Swiss cheese air b.
tantalum b.
unilateral b.
bronchography
Cope-method b.
percutaneous transtracheal b.
broncholith
broncholithiasis
bronchomalacia
bronchomediastinal lymph trunk
bronchomotor effect
bronchoplasty
balloon b.
bronchoplegia
bronchopleural (BP)
b. fistula
bronchopleuropneumonia
bronchopneumonia
bibasilar b.
hemorrhagic b.
hypostatic b.
inhalation b.
b. pattern
subacute b.
tuberculous b.
bronchopneumonitis
bronchopulmonary (BP)
b. aspergillosis
b. atelectasis
b. dysplasia (BPD)
b. fistula
b. foregut
b. foregut malformation (BPFM)
b. lung segment anatomy
b. lymph node
b. marking
b. neoplasm
b. segment
b. sequestration
bronchoradiography
bronchorrhea

NOTES

bronchoscopy
    fiberoptic b. (FOB)
    virtual b. (VB)
bronchosinusitis
bronchospasm
    paradoxical b.
bronchospastic effect
bronchostaxis
bronchostenosis
bronchotracheal
bronchovascular
    b. anatomy cross-section
    b. bundle
    b. marking
    b. pattern
bronchovesicular marking
bronchus, pl. **bronchi**
    anomalous b.
    anterior basal b.
    apical b.
    apicoposterior b.
    basal segmental b.
    beaded b.
    b. blockage
    blocked b.
    b. branch
    cardiac segmental b.
    contracted b.
    depression of left mainstem b.
    dilated b.
    distended central bronchi
    ectatic b.
    edematous b.
    epiarterial b.
    extrapulmonary b.
    fractured b.
    granulomatous inflammation of b.
    hyparterial b.
    inferior lobe b.
    inflamed b.
    intermediate b.
    b. intermedius
    intrapulmonary b.
    inverted-T appearance mainstem b.
    lateral basal segmental b.
    left main stem b.
    left primary b.
    lingular b.
    lobar b.
    mainstem b.
    major b.
    medial basal segmental b.
    medium-sized b.
    middle lobe b.
    mucoid impaction of b.
    nonlingular branch of upper
      lobe b.

    normal-appearing b.
    posterior basal segmental b.
    primary left b.
    primary right b.
    principal b.
    right lobe b.
    right mainstem b.
    right primary b.
    secondary b.
    secretion-filled b.
    segmental b.
    b. sign
    b. stem
    subapical b.
    subsegmental b.
    superior lobe b.
    superior segmental b.
    tracheal b.
bronchus-associated lymphoid tissue (BALT)
bronchus-to-pulmonary artery ratio
bronzed sclerosing encephalitis
bronze liver
Brooker periarticular heterotopic ossification classification
Brooke tumor
Broselow-Luten Pediatric System
brow-down
    b.-d. position
    b.-d. projection
    b.-d. skull view
brown
    b. asbestos
    b. atrophy
    b. cell cyst
    b. edema
    b. fat origin
    b. induration of lung
    b. tumor
    b. tumor of hyperparathyroidism
Brown-Dodge method for angiography
brownian water motion
Brown-Roberts-Wells (BRW)
    B.-R.-W. CT stereotactic guide
    B.-R.-W. frame
    B.-R.-W. stereotactic system
    B.-R.-W. technique
Brown-Séquard
    B.-S. lesion
    B.-S. syndrome
brow presentation
brow-up
    b.-u. position
    b.-u. projection
    b.-u. skull view
brucellar
    b. myositis

b. osteomyelitis
b. synovitis
Bruch gland
Bruck disease
Brücke muscle
Brudzinski sign
Bruel-Kjaer
B.-K. ultrasound
B.-K. ultrasound scanner
Brugada syndrome
Bruker
B. AMX 300 NMR spectrometer
B. console
B. CSI Omega MR system
B. minispec measuring device
B. PC-10 relaxometer
B. scanner
B. TC-10 relaxometer
Brunner
B. gland
B. gland adenoma
B. gland hyperplasia
B. gland hypertrophy
Brunnstrom-Fugl-Meyer (BFM)
B.-F.-M. arm impairment
assessment
brush
Castaneda thrombolytic b.
Cragg thrombolytic b.
BRW
Brown-Roberts-Wells
BRW CT stereotaxic guide
BRW stereotactic system
Bryant
B. sign
B. triangle
BSA
body surface area
B-scan imaging
BSCB
blood-spinal cord barrier
BSF
backscatter factor
BSLM
body surface Laplacian mapping
bubble
b. of the belly
encapsulated gas b.
free gas b.
Garren-Edwards gastric b.
gas b.
gastric air b.

GEG b.
intragastric b.
microscopic air b.
b. oxygenator
b. sign
stomach b.
bubble-like appearance
bubbling lesion
bubbly
b. bone lesion
b. bulb
b. lung
b. opacity
b. pattern
bubonulus
bucca, pl. **buccae**
buccal
b. cavity
b. groove
b. mucosa
b. mucosal carcinoma
b. shelf
b. space
b. space infection
b. surface
buccinator
b. crest
b. lymph node
buccogingival ridge
buccolingual plane
bucconeural duct
buccopharyngeal fascia
Buck
B. extension
B. fascia
bucket-handle
b.-h. meniscus tear
b.-h. pattern of fracture
b.-h. pelvic fracture
Buckland-Wright macroradiography
buckle
b. fracture
wire-fixation b.
buckled innominate artery
buckling
b. cortical brain
innominate artery b.
bucky
chest b.
B. diaphragm
B. digital x-ray device
B. film

NOTES

bucky *(continued)*
    B. grid
    oscillating B.
    B. ray
    B. tomogram
    B. view
bud
    accessory ureteral b.
    bronchial b.
    capillary b.
    dorsal pancreatic b.
    end b.
    limb b.
    ureteral b.
    vascular b.
    ventral pancreatic b.
Budd
    B. cirrhosis
    B. syndrome
Budd-Chiari syndrome
Budge
    ciliospinal center of B.
budgerigar fancier's lung
**Budin-Chandler anteversion
    determination**
Budin joint
buffalo
    b. hump
    B. malleolar rule
buffer amplifier
Buford complex
Buhl desquamative pneumonia
bulb
    aortic b.
    arterial b.
    baroreceptor b.
    baseline of b.
    bubbly b.
    carotid b.
    dehiscent jugular b.
    dental b.
    duodenal b.
    end b.
    heart b.
    high jugular b. (HJB)
    inferior jugular vein b.
    internal jugular b.
    b. of occipital horn of lateral
      ventricle
    olfactory b.
    b. of penis
    b. of posterior horn of lateral
      ventricle
    sinovaginal b.
    superior jugular vein b.
    b. ureterography
    b. of vein

bulbar
    b. abnormality
    b. intracerebral hemorrhage
    b. peptic ulcer
    b. ridge
    b. septum
    b. swelling
    b. tract
bulbi
    b. muscle
    phthisis b.
bulbocavernosus muscle
bulbocavernous gland
bulbosity
bulbospongiosus muscle of penis
bulbourethral
    b. artery
    b. gland
    b. gland anatomy
    b. gland lesion
bulbous
    b. configuration
    b. costochondral junction
    b. enlargement
    b. stump
    b. urethra
bulbus cordis
bulge
    anal b.
    anular disk b.
    bilateral anterior chest b.
    disk b.
    epiphrenic b.
    inguinal b.
    late systolic b.
    palpable presystolic b.
    parasternal b.
    precordial b.
    suprasternal b.
bulging
    b. aneurysm
    b. anulus
    b. dura
    b. fontanelle
    b. lung fissure
    b. precordium
bulk
    b. laxative
    b. magnetic susceptibility (BMS)
    b. magnetization vector
    mediastinal b.
    muscle b.
    b. susceptibility artifact
bulky tumor
bulla, pl. **bullae**
    emphysematous b.

ethmoidal b.
b. formation
bullet
hollow-point b.
b. kit culture medium
metallic track of b.
stabilizing b.
tripoint b.
bullet-shaped vertebra
Bull method
bull-neck appearance
bullosa
concha b.
junctional epidermolysis b.
bullous
b. disorder
b. edema
b. edema of bladder wall
b. emphysema
b. emphysema of intestine
b. lung disease
bull's
b. eye appearance
b. eye configuration
b. eye deformity
b. eye image
b. eye imaging
b. eye lesion
b. eye polar map
b. eye technique
b. eye view
bump
hip b.
inion b.
runner's b.
splenic b.
bumper fracture
bunamiodyl
bunch-of-grapes appearance
bundle
aberrant b.
anterior atrial myocardial b.
artery-vein-nerve b.
atrioventricular b.
Bachmann b.
b. bone
bronchoarterial b.
bronchovascular b.
central bronchovascular b.
common b.
fascicular b.
fiberoptic b.

Flechsig b.
b. function
Gierke respiratory b.
Gowers b.
His b.
intercostal neuromuscular b.
James b.
Keith sinoatrial b.
b. of Kent accessory bypass fiber
Kent-His b.
Mahaim b.
main b.
middle perforating collagen b.
neurovascular b.
Pick b.
Probst callosal b.
Schultze b.
sinoatrial b.
b. of Stanley Kent
Thorel b.
vascular b.
b. of Vicq d'Azyr
bundle-branch
b.-b. heart block
b.-b. reentry (BBR)
Bunge amputation
bunion formation
bunk-bed fracture
Bunsen-type valve
Burdach
column of B.
burden
body b.
maximum permissible body b.
tumor b.
Burger scalene triangle
Burgess below-knee amputation
buried tonsil
Burke-type metaphyseal dysplasia
Burkhalter-Reyes method of phalangeal fracture
Burkitt-like lymphoma
Burkitt lymphoma
burn
b. boutonnière deformity
radiation b.
x-ray b.
burned-out
b.-o. colon
b.-o. mucosa
b.-o. tabes

B

NOTES

burned-out *(continued)*
    b.-o. tumor
    b.-o. tumor of testis
Burnett
    B. applicator
    B. BiDirectional TMJ device
    B. cylinder
burning
    selective hole b.
burnout
    detail b.
Burns ligament
Burrow vein
bursa, pl. **bursae**
    Achilles b.
    adventitious b.
    anserine b.
    Brodie b.
    calcaneal b.
    coracoid b.
    deltoid b.
    b. exostotica
    b. of Fabricius
    Fleischmann b.
    flexor b.
    gastrocnemius b.
    gastrocnemius-semimembranosus b.
    iliopsoas b.
    infrapatellar b.
    interligamentous b.
    intermediate b.
    intermetatarsophalangeal b.
    intraligamentous b.
    intratendinous b.
    ischiogluteal b.
    lateral epicondylar b.
    Luschka b.
    MCL b.
    medial epicondylar b.
    Monro b.
    olecranon b.
    omental b.
    patellar b.
    pes anserine b.
    plantar b.
    popliteus b.
    premalleolar b.
    prepatellar b.
    radial b.
    retrocalcaneal b.
    semimembranosus b.
    semimembranosus-tibial collateral
      ligament b.
    subacromial b.
    subacromial-subdeltoid b.
    subdeltoid b.
    subgluteus maximus b.

    subgluteus medius b.
    submetatarsal b.
    subscapular b.
    subtendinous b.
    superficial tendo-Achilles b.
    suprapatellar b.
    synovial b.
    tendo-Achilles b.
    tibial collateral ligament b.
    trochanteric b.
    ulnar b.
bursal
    b. calcification
    b. flap
    b. fluid
    b. inflammation
    b. osteochondromatosis
    b. sac
bursitis
    anserine b.
    bicipital b.
    calcaneal b.
    calcific b.
    chronic retrocalcaneal b.
    cubital b.
    iliopsoas b.
    infracalcaneal b.
    intermetatarsal b.
    intermetatarsophalangeal b.
    intertubercular b.
    ischial b.
    ischiogluteal b.
    olecranon b.
    patellar b.
    pes anserinus b.
    posterior calcaneal b.
    prepatellar b.
    pseudotrochanteric b.
    radiohumeral b.
    retrocalcaneal b.
    SA-SD b.
    septic b.
    subacromial b.
    subacromial-subdeltoid septic b.
    subcoracoid b.
    subdeltoid b.
    Tornwaldt b.
    trochanteric b.
bursography
bursolith
burst
    b. fracture
    b. injury
    respiratory b.
burst-forming unit
bursting
    b. dislocation

b. fracture
b. pressure
Buschke-Löwenstein tumor
Buster
Amplatz Clot B.
butanol-extractable iodine (BEI)
Butcher staging classification
butterfly
b. appearance
b. breast shadow
b. coil
b. configuration
b. distribution
b. fracture
b. fracture fragment
b. glioblastoma
b. glioma
b. lesion
b. lymphoma
b. pattern
b. pattern of infiltrate
b. vertebra
butterfly-wing vertebra
Butterworth filter
button
aortic b.
duodenal b.
full-thickness Carrel b.
Kistner tracheal b.
patellar b.
b. procedure
b. sequestrum eosinophilic
granuloma
b. sequestrum skull
subdural b.
b. toe amputation
tracheal B b.
buttoned device
buttonhole
b. deformity

b. fracture
b. mitral stenosis
b. opening
radiopaque wire of
counteroccluder b.
b. rupture
b. tear
buttressing
medial femoral b.
buttress plate
butyral
polyvinyl b. (PVB)
BV2 needle
BVAD
biventricular assist device
BVR
basal vein of Rosenthal
BVS
biventricular support
BW
bitewing
black and white
bypass (BP)
aortobiliac b.
biliointestinal b. (BIB)
biliopancreatic b.
b. circuit
extracranial-intracranial b.
b. failure
b. graft
iliofemoral crossover b.
jejunoileal b. (JIB)
byproduct material
byssinosis
bystander effect
byte mode
B-zone small lymphocytic lymphoma

NOTES

C
  carbon
  coulomb
    C angle
    C loop of duodenum
    C scan
    C sign
    C-to-E amplitude of mitral valve
^{11}C
  carbon-11
    ^{11}C acetate imaging agent
    ^{11}C butanol imaging agent
    ^{11}C carbon monoxide
    ^{11}C carfentanil imaging agent
    ^{11}C deoxyglucose
    ^{11}C flumazenil imaging agent
    ^{11}C imaging agent
    ^{11}C L-159
    ^{11}C L-884
    ^{11}C L-methylmethionine
    ^{11}C lumazenil
    ^{11}C methionine
    ^{11}C methoxystaurosporine
    ^{11}C N-methylspiperone imaging agent
    ^{11}C N-methylspiroperidol
    ^{11}C nomifensine imaging agent
    ^{11}C palmitate
    ^{11}C palmitic acid radioactive
    ^{11}C raclopride imaging agent
    ^{11}C thymidine imaging agent
^{12}C
  carbon-12
^{13}C
  carbon-13
^{14}C
  carbon-14
    ^{14}C lactose breath test
C-150 LXP EBT scanner
C1-C5 segment of internal carotid artery
C-60 teletherapy
Ca
  calcium
^{47}**Ca, Ca-47**
  calcium-47
^{45}**Ca, Ca-45**
  calcium-45
    ^{45}Ca imaging agent
CAAS
  cardiovascular angiography analysis system
    CAAS QCA system

CABBS
  computer-assisted blood background subtraction
CABG
  coronary artery bypass graft
cable
    FlexStrand c.
Cabrol composite graft procedure
CABS
  coronary artery bypass surgery
CAC
  coronary artery calcification
CACG
  cineangiocardiogram
CACS
  coronary artery calcium score
    CACS threshold
CAD
  computer-aided detection
  computer-aided diagnosis
cadaveric renal transplant
CAD-evaluated mammogram
cadmium (Cd)
    c. iodide detector
CADx SecondLook system
Caffey
    C. hyperostosis
    C. syndrome
Caffey-Kempe syndrome
cage
    bony thoracic c.
    Faraday c.
    Harms c.
    metallic c.
    osseocartilaginous thoracic c.
    threaded fusion c. (TFC)
CAH
  congenital adrenal hyperplasia
caisson disease
Cajal
    nucleus of C.
cake
    c. kidney
    omental c.
calcaneal
    c. apophysis
    c. apophysitis
    c. articular surface
    c. avulsion fracture
    c. bone
    c. bursa
    c. bursa inflammation
    c. bursitis
    c. displaced fracture
    c. inclination angle

C

calcaneal *(continued)*
   c. pitch
   c. pitch angle
   c. process
   c. spur
   c. stress fracture
   c. tendon
   c. tubercle
   c. tuberosity
calcanei (*pl. of* calcaneus)
calcaneocavus
   c. foot
   pes c.
   talipes calcaneus c.
   talipes cavus c.
calcaneoclavicular ligament
calcaneocuboid
   c. articulation
   c. joint
   c. ligament
calcaneofibular ligament (CFL)
calcaneonavicular
   c. coalition
   c. ligament
calcaneoplantar angle
calcaneotibial
   c. fusion
   c. ligament
calcaneovalgocavus
calcaneovalgus
   c. flatfoot
   pes c.
calcaneovarus deformity
calcaneus, pl. calcanei
   c. altus
   c. deformity
   pes c.
   sulcus calcanei
   talipes c.
   tendo c.
   thalamic fracture of c.
calcar
   c. avis
   c. femorale
   c. pedis
   pivot of c.
calcareous
   c. degeneration
   c. deposit
   c. infiltrate
   c. metastasis
   c. renal calculus
calcarine
   c. artery
   c. cortex
   c. fissure
   c. sulcus

calciferous canal
calcific
   c. arteriosclerosis
   c. artery
   c. bicuspid valvular stenosis
   c. bursitis
   c. cochleitis
   c. density
   c. diskitis
   c. matrix
   c. myonecrosis
   c. round body
   c. senile aortic valvular stenosis
   c. shadow
   c. spur
   c. tendonitis
calcificans
   chondrodysplasia c.
   chondroplasia c.
   liponecrosis macrocystica c.
   liponecrosis microcystica c.
calcification
   abdominal wall c.
   adenoma-associated c.
   adrenal c.
   alimentary tract c.
   aneurysmal wall c.
   anterior spinal ligament c.
   anular c.
   aortic arch c.
   aortic valve c.
   arachnoid granulation c.
   arterial c.
   arteriovascular c.
   atherosclerotic c.
   basal ganglia c.
   c. of basal ganglion
   basket-like c.
   benign breast c.
   bladder wall c.
   branching c.
   breast popcorn c.
   bursal c.
   calcium phosphate c.
   cardiac c.
   carotid artery c.
   cartilage c.
   casting breast c.
   cerebral c.
   chicken-wire c.
   choroid plexus c.
   clustered c.
   coarse c.
   conglomerate c.
   coronary artery c. (CAC)
   costal cartilage c.
   curvilinear c.

dentate nuclei c.
dermal breast c.
diffuse abdominal c.
disk c.
dural c.
dystrophic soft tissue c.
eggshell breast c.
eggshell nodal c.
falx c.
female genital tract c.
fetal intraabdominal c.
fine c.
fingertip c.
flaky c.
flocculent focus of c.
focal alimentary tract c.
focus of c.
free body c.
genital tract c.
glial tumor c.
granular c.
gyriform c.
habenular commissure c.
heart valve c.
hepatic c.
idiopathic pleural c.
inadequate calvarial c.
inadequate cranial c.
intervertebral cartilage c.
intervertebral disk c.
intraabdominal c.
intraabdominal fetal c.
intracardiac c.
intracranial physiologic c.
intraductal c.
intraocular c.
intratumoral c.
involutional breast c.
inwardly displaced c.
irregular c.
isolated clustered c.'s
kidney c.
laminated c.
layering c.
ligamentous c.
c. line
linear c.
liver c.
lobular breast c.
lung popcorn c.
lymph node eggshell c.
male genital tract c.

malignant breast c.
medial collateral ligament c.
medullary c.
meniscus-shaped c.
mesenteric c.
metastatic soft tissue c.
milk-of-calcium c.
mitral ring c.
mitral valve c.
Mönckeberg c.
mottled c.
mulberry-type c.
multiple pulmonary c.
myocardial c.
c. of myocardium
needle-shaped breast c.
neoplastic c.
node c.
normal c.
oyster-pearl breast c.
pancreatic c.
paraarticular c.
paraspinal c.
parentheses-like c.
parietal pericardial c.
pathologic intracranial c.
pearl-like breast c.
Pellegrini-Stieda c.
periarticular c.
pericardial c.
periductal c.
peritendinous c.
periventricular c.
phlebolith-like c.
pineal gland c.
plaquing c.
pleomorphic c.
pleural c.
popcorn c.
poppy seed-like c.
postbiopsy eggshell c.
postradiation c.
premature c.
psammomatous c.
pulmonary c.
punctate c.
railroad track c.
renal c.
retroperitoneal c.
rice-like muscle c.
ring-and-arc c.
ring apophysis c.

NOTES

C

calcification *(continued)*
    rod-shaped c.
    scrotal c.
    sebaceous gland c.
    secondary c.
    secretory c.
    sella turcica c.
    semilunar c.
    skin c.
    snowflake-like c.
    splenic c.
    stippled c.
    subanular c.
    suprasellar mass c.
    sutural c.
    target c.
    teacup breast c.
    teacup-shaped c.
    thrombus c.
    thyroid adenoma c.
    tramline cortical c.
    tram-track ductus arteriosus c.
    tram-track gyral c.
    tram-track renal cortical necrosis c.
    tumoral c.
    urinary bladder wall c.
    valvular leaflet c.
    vascular abdominal c.
    venous c.
    visceral pericardial c.
    wall c.
calcified
    c. amorphous tumor
    c. anulus
    c. aorta
    c. aortic valve
    c. astrocytoma
    c. brain mass
    c. cartilage
    c. cysticercus granuloma
    c. density structure
    c. ductus arteriosus
    c. fetus
    c. fibroadenoma
    c. fibroid
    c. fibroma
    c. free fragment
    c. intracranial mass
    c. kidney mass
    c. lesion
    c. lung nodule
    c. lymph node
    c. medullary defect
    c. myocardial tuberculoma
    c. nodularity
    c. ovarian metastases
    c. pericardial cyst

    c. pericardium
    c. pineal body
    c. pineal gland
    c. plaque
    c. renal mass
    c. sclerosis
    c. sequestra of low signal intensity
    c. thrombus
    c. wall of aneurysm
calciform lobe
calcifying
    c. Malherbe epithelioma
    c. metastasis
calcinosis
    bilateral striopallidodentate c.
    c. circumscripta
    cutis c.
    generalized c.
    interstitial c.
    tumoral c.
calcis
    os c.
    trigonum c.
calcium (Ca)
    c. bile soap
    c. debris
    c. hydroxyapatite
    c. hydroxyapatite deposition disease
    c. infiltrate
    intracardiac c.
    c. ion
    c. ipodate imaging agent
    c. layering
    liquid c.
    c. metabolism
    milk of c.
    c. phosphate calcification
    c. pyrophosphate deposition disease (CPPD)
    c. pyrophosphate dihydrate crystal deposition
    c. pyrophosphate dihydrate deposition disease
    c. pyrophosphate dihydrate hand
    c. salt deposit
    c. scoring
    sedimented c.
    c. sign
    c. tungstate
calcium-45 (^{45}Ca, Ca-45)
    c. imaging agent
calcium-47 (^{47}Ca, Ca-47)
calcium/oxyanion-containing particle
calculated
    c. clearance time
    c. image
    c. resistance

calculation
 bayesian c.
 body surface area c.
 Cerenkov c.
 contrast-to-noise c.
 gap c.
 magnitude c.
 Monte Carlo c.
 multiplane dosage c.
 radiation dosimetry c.
 signal-to-noise c.
 spectrophotometric c.
 velocity c.
 volume implant c.
calculi (*pl. of* calculus)
calculogram
calculography
calculous
 c. cholecystitis
 c. cirrhosis
calculus, pl. **calculi**
 alternating c.
 alvine c.
 articular c.
 biliary c.
 branched c.
 bronchial c.
 calcareous renal c.
 cat's eye c.
 coral c.
 cystic c.
 cystine c.
 decubitus c.
 dendritic c.
 echogenic c.
 encysted c.
 gallbladder c.
 gastric hemic c.
 gonecystic c.
 hemic c.
 hemp seed c.
 hepatic c.
 impacted c.
 indigo c.
 intestinal c.
 intrahepatic biliary c.
 joint c.
 kidney c.
 lacteal c.
 lucent c.
 lung c.
 mammary c.

 matrix c.
 metabolic c.
 mulberry c.
 nephritic c.
 noncalcareous renal c.
 nonopaque c.
 obstructive c.
 opaque c.
 pancreatic c.
 pocketed c.
 primary vesical c.
 prostatic c.
 radiopaque vesical c.
 renal c.
 salivary c.
 spermatic c.
 staghorn c.
 Steinstrasse c.
 stomach c.
 stone-like c.
 struvite c.
 submandibular duct c.
 urate c.
 ureteral c.
 urethral c.
 uric acid c.
 urinary bladder c.
 urinary tract c.
 urostealith c.
 vesicle c.
 xanthic c.
Caldani ligament
Caldwell
 C. method
 C. occipitofrontal view
 C. position
 C. projection
Caldwell-Moloy classification
calf, pl. **calves**
 c. band
 c. vein thrombosis
caliber
 bowel c.
 bronchial c.
 internal c.
 luminal c.
 medium c.
 modest c.
 narrow c.
 normal bladder c.
 spinal cord c.
 tracheal c.

NOTES

caliber *(continued)*
    vessel c.
    wide c.
calibrate
calibrated leak
calibration
    absolute-peak efficiency c.
    catheter c.
    cross c.
    E-dial c.
    c. factor
    c. failure artifact
    film density c.
    c. method
calibrator
    accuracy c.
    digital isotope c.
    dose c.
    isotope c.
    radioisotope c.
caliceal
    c. abnormality
    c. blunting
    c. clubbing
    c. dilatation
    c. diverticulum
    c. nephrostolithotomy
    c. system
calices (*pl. of* calix)
caliectasis
    focal c.
    localized c.
californium (Cf)
californium-252 (^{252}**Cf**)
calipers
    restraint c.
calix, calyx, pl. **calices**
    cupping of the c.
    major c.
    minor c.
    renal c.
    spider-like c.
    c. tube
Callander amputation
callosal
    c. agenesis
    c. area
    c. dysgenesis
    c. formation
    c. gyrus
    c. lesion
    c. sulcus
callosomarginal
    c. artery
    c. fissure
callosum
    anterior midbody of corpus c.

    corpus c.
    genu of corpus c.
    isthmus of corpus c.
    posterior midbody of corpus c.
    rostral body of corpus c.
    rostrum of corpus c.
    splenium of corpus c.
callous
callus
    bony c.
    bridging c.
    central c.
    definitive c.
    c. deposit
    endosteal c.
    ensheathing c.
    external c.
    exuberant c.
    florid c.
    c. formation
    fracture c.
    intermediate c.
    permanent c.
    provisional c.
    tumoral c.
    c. weld
Calot triangle
calvaneovalgus
    pes c.
calvaria, pl. **calvariae**
    external table of c.
    internal table of c.
calvarial
    c. bone
    c. echogenicity
    c. fracture
Calvé
    septal cusp of C.
    C. vertebra plane
Calvé-Legg-Perthes disease
Calvé-Perthes disease
calves (*pl. of* calf)
calyx (*var. of* calix)
CAM
    computer-assisted myelography
camera
    ADAC MCD Vertex Plus MCD
      gamma c.
    Anger scintillation c.
    APEX 409, 415 c.
    Argus c.
    Biad c.
    CerASPECT c.
    CID c.
    Cidtech c.
    cine c.
    Circon video c.

crystal gamma c.
data c.
Digirad gamma c.
DSI c.
dual-head coincidence c.
dual single-crystal gamma c.
electron diffraction c.
Elscint APEX 409-AG ECT c.
Elscint APEX 009 Precursor c.
Elscint dual-detector cardiac c.
Elscint Dual-Head Helix c.
four-head c.
gamma c.
gantry-free gamma c.
GE 400AC/T;STAR II c.
GE gamma c.
Genesys c.
GE Neurocam c.
GE single-detector SPECT-
  capable c.
GE Starcam single-crystal
  tomographic scintillation c.
Haifa c.
Helix c.
Hitachi SPECT 2000H-40 c.
hybrid PET/SPECT c.
infrared c.
integral uniformity scintillation c.
isocon c.
Israel c.
large field of view gamma c.
Medx c.
multicrystal gamma c.
multiformat c.
multiple-headed gamma c.
nuclear medicine c.
Orthicon c.
Picker c.
pinhole c.
Pixsys FlashPoint c.
positron scintillation c.
radioisotope c.
radionuclide c.
R&F c.
rotating gamma c.
Scanditronix 1024-7B c.
Scinticore multicrystal
  scintillation c.
scintillation c.
Shimadzu HeadTome Set-031 c.
Siemens gamma c.

Siemens Orbiter large-field-of-
  view c.
single-head rotating gamma c.
SKYLight gantry-free nuclear
  medicine gamma c.
slip-ring c.
Sopha DSX1 c.
SOPHY c.
SP6 c.
Starcam c.
Strichman SME-810 c.
Technicare c.
Toshiba GGA 9300 c.
Trionix c.
Trionix-Triad c.
triple-head gamma c.
variable-angle gamma c.
Vertex c.
video display c.
Vision c.
cameral fistula
Cameron method
Campbell ligament
Camper
  C. chiasma
  C. fascia
  C. ligament
  C. line
Camp grid cassette
camptocormia
camptodactyly
camptomelic dysplasia
Camurati-Engelmann disease
CAMV
  congenital anomaly of mitral valve
canal
  abdominal c.
  accessory c.
  acoustic c.
  adductor c.
  Alcock c.
  alimentary c.
  alveolar c.
  alveolodental c.
  ampulla of semicircular c.
  anal c.
  anterior condylar c.
  anterior semicircular c.
  antropyloric c.
  arachnoid c.
  Arantius c.
  archenteric c.

NOTES

canal *(continued)*
    Arnold c.
    arterial c.
    atrial c.
    atrioventricular c.
    auditory c.
    basipharyngeal c.
    Bernard c.
    Bichat c.
    biliary c.
    birth c.
    bony semicircular c.
    Böttcher c.
    Braun c.
    Breschet c.
    calciferous c.
    caroticotympanic c.
    carotid c.
    carpal c.
    caudal c.
    central spinal c.
    cerebrospinal c.
    cervical c.
    cervicoaxillary c.
    ciliary c.
    Civinini c.
    Cloquet c.
    cochlear c.
    common atrioventricular c.
    complex atrioventricular c.
    condylar c.
    condyloid c.
    connecting c.
    Corti c.
    Cotunnius c.
    craniopharyngeal c.
    crural c.
    Cuvier c.
    c. decompression
    deferent c.
    diploic c.
    Dorello c.
    Dupuytren c.
    endocervical c.
    endometrial fluid in c.
    ethmoid c.
    eustachian c.
    facial nerve c.
    fallopian c.
    femoral medullary c.
    Ferrein c.
    flexor c.
    Fontana c.
    galactophorous c.
    ganglionic c.
    Gartner c.
    gastric c.

    genital c.
    gray horns in spinal c.
    greater palatine c.
    gubernacular c.
    Guyon c.
    gynecophoric c.
    Hannover c.
    haversian c.
    hemal c.
    Henle c.
    Hensen c.
    Hering c.
    hernia c.
    Hirschfeld c.
    His c.
    Huguier c.
    Hunter c.
    Huschke c.
    hyaloid c.
    hydrops c.
    hypoglossal c.
    iliac c.
    incisive c.
    inferior dental c.
    infraorbital c.
    inguinal c.
    interfacial c.
    internal auditory c.
    intersacral c.
    intestinal c.
    intramedullary c.
    Jacobson c.
    Kovalevsky c.
    lacrimal c.
    Lambert c.
    lateral semicircular c.
    Löwenberg c.
    lumbar spinal c.
    lumbosacral c.
    lymphatic c.
    mandibular c.
    marrow c.
    mastoid c.
    maxillary c.
    medullary c.
    mental c.
    Müller c.
    musculotubal c.
    narrowing of spinal c.
    nasal c.
    nasolacrimal c.
    nasopalatine c.
    neural c.
    neurenteric c.
    notochordal c.
    Nuck c.
    olfactory c.

optic c.
orbital c.
palatine c.
palatomaxillary c.
palatovaginal c.
paraurethral c.
parturient c.
pelvic c.
pericardioperitoneal c.
persistent common
  atrioventricular c.
petrous carotid c.
pharyngeal c.
pleural c.
pleuropericardial c.
pleuroperitoneal c.
pneumoenteric c.
portal c.
posterior semicircular c.
principal artery of pterygoid c.
pterygoid c.
pterygopalatine c.
pudendal c.
pulmoaortic c.
pulp c.
pyloric c.
recurrent c.
Reichert c.
Rivinus c.
Rosenthal c.
sacculocochlear c.
sacculoutricular c.
sacral c.
Santorini c.
c. of Scarpa
Schlemm c.
scleral c.
semicircular c.
c. septum
sheathing c.
small internal auditory c.
sphenopalatine c.
sphenopharyngeal c.
spinal cord c.
c. stenosis
Stensen c.
Stilling c.
c. of stomach
subsartorial c.
Sucquet-Hoyer c.
supraorbital c.
target c.

tarsal c.
temporal c.
Theile c.
tibial medullary c.
tight spinal c.
tubal c.
tubotympanic c.
umbilical c.
uniting c.
urogenital c.
uterine c.
uterocervical c.
uterovaginal c.
utriculosaccular c.
vaginal c.
ventricular c.
Verneuil c.
vertebral c.
vesicourethral c.
vestibular c.
vidian c.
Volkmann c.
vomerine c.
vomerorostral c.
vomerovaginal c.
vulvouterine c.
widened optic c.
zygomaticofacial c.
zygomaticotemporal c.
**Canale-Kelly talar neck fracture
  classification**
canalicular
  c. duct
  c. sphincter
canaliculus, pl. **canaliculi**
  apical c.
  auricular c.
  bone c.
  cochlear c.
  haversian c.
  innominate c.
canalization
Canavan disease
Canavan-van Bogaert-Bertrand disease
cancellated bone
cancellation
  fat-water signal c.
  phase c.
cancellous
  c. bone chip
  c. hematopoietic marrow
  c. osteoid osteoma

NOTES

cancellous (*continued*)
   c. screw
   c. tissue
cancer (*See* carcinoma)
   c. body
   c. cell anaplasia
   c. embolus
   c. of unknown primary (CUP)
cancerization
   field c.
cancriform
cancroid
candela
   c. lithotripsy
   C. 405-nm pulsed dye laser
candelabra
   c. artery
   sylvian c.
candida
   c. enteritis
   c. esophagitis
candle
   c. drip disk
   c. dripping appearance
   c. wax dripping
candle-flame osteolysis
candle-guttering
candle-wax appearance of bone
caniocervical junction
cannon
   c. bone
   C. point
Cannon-Boehm point
cannula
   Fluoro Tip c.
   indwelling c.
   metallic tip c.
   ultrasonic lithotripter c.
cannulated
   c. artery
   c. central vein
   percutaneously c.
cannulation
   aortic c.
   arterial c.
   atrial c.
   bicaval c.
   direct caval c.
   endoscopic retrograde pancreatic
     duct c.
   left atrial c.
   ostial c.
   retrograde c.
   selective c.
   single-cannula atrial c.
   subselective c.
   two-stage venous c.

   venoarterial c.
   venous c.
   venovenous c.
Canny edge detection algorithm
Canon scanner
Cantelli sign
canthomeatal line
canthus, pl. **canthi**
   outer c.
Cantlie line
Cantor tube
Cantrell
   pentalogy of C.
cap
   apical c.
   azygos hematoma c.
   cartilaginous c.
   duodenal c.
   fibrous c.
   hilar c.
   left pleural apical hematoma c.
   phrygian c.
   c. plate
   pleural apical hematoma c.
   pyloric c.
   thin fibrous c.
capacious vein
capacitative calcium entry
capacitor
   MOS c.
capacitive
   c. interaction
   c. reactance
capacity
   bladder c.
   closing c.
   cranial c.
   decreased vital c.
   diffusing c.
   dye-binding c. (DBC)
   functional bladder c.
   functional residual c.
   gastric c.
   limited oxidative c.
   lung c.
   residual volume/total lung c.
     (RV/TLC)
   respiratory c.
   secretory c.
   total lung c.
   urinary bladder c.
   vasodilatory c.
   vital c. (VC)
Capener
   triangle of C.
capillary, pl. **capillaries**
   c. angioma

arterial c.
bile c.
c. blockade perfusion C-mode scan
c. blood flow
c. blood volume
c. bronchiectasis
c. bud
c. congestion
continuous c.
c. density
c. embolus
c. endothelium
c. filling
c. filling time
c. hemangioblastoma
c. hemangioendothelioma
c. hemangioma
c. hemorrhage
c. hydrostatic pressure
c. lake
c. leak
c. leak syndrome
c. loop
lymph c.
c. lymphangioma
c. lymphatic space invasion
c. malformation
Meigs c.
c. perfusion
c. permeability
c. pneumonia
c. pulsation
c. refill
ruptured c.
sinusoidal c.
c. telangiectasia
telangiectasia brain c.
c. tube
c. valve
c. vein
venous c.
c. vessel
c. wall
c. wedge pressure
capillary-lymphatic malformation (CLM)
capita (*pl. of* caput)
capital
    c. epiphysis (CE)
    c. epiphysis angle
    c. epiphysis angle of Wiberg
    c. extension
    c. femoral epiphysis

c. flexor
c. fragment
capitate
    c. bone
    c. facet
    c. fracture
    c. hamate joint
    c. soft spot
capitella
capitellar fracture
capitellum
    humeral c.
capitis
    fovea c.
capitolunate
    c. angle
    c. joint
capitular
    c. epiphysis
    c. process
capitulum, pl. capitula
    c. costae
    c. fibulae
    c. humeri
    c. mandibula
    c. radiale humeri fracture
    c. ulnae
Caplan
    C. nodule
    C. syndrome
capping
    apical c.
    c. cyst
capsular
    c. attachment
    c. contracture
    c. drop lesion
    c. imbrication
    c. infarct
    c. insertion
    c. ligament
    c. plane
    c. reefing
    c. space
    c. thickening
    c. thrombosis
capsule
    adrenal c.
    articular c.
    auditory c.
    Bowman c.
    cartilage c.

C

NOTES

capsule *(continued)*
cricoarytenoid articular c.
cricothyroid articular c.
dorsal c.
external c.
facet joint c.
fatty renal c.
fibrous renal c.
Gerota c.
Given imaging capsule/M2A c.
glenoid labrum c.
Glisson c.
hepatic c.
hypointense fibrous c.
internal c.
joint c.
limb of anterior c.
liver c.
medial carpal c.
metatarsophalangeal c.
organ c.
otic c.
plantar c.
posterolateral c.
prostate c.
redundant c.
renal c.
rim of c.
Sitzmarks c.
splenic c.
suprasellar c.
talonavicular c.
thyroid c.
tissue c.
tumor c.
volar c.
wrist c.
capsulitis
adhesive c.
capsulocaudate infarct
capsulolabral complex
capsuloma
capsuloperiosteal envelope
capsuloputaminal infarct
capsuloputaminocaudate infarct
Captopril-enhanced renal scintigraphy
Captopril renogram
Captopril-stimulated renal imaging
capture
boron neutron c.
cross-section c.
electron c.
gamma ray c.
K c.
resonance c.
caput, pl. capita

c. cecum
c. medusae
carbogen radiosensitizer
Carbomedics valve
carbon (C)
c. dioxide (CO_2)
c. dioxide generator
c. dioxide laser
double-bonded c.
c. fiber-reinforced plastic
c. imaging agent
c. metabolism
carbon-11 (^{11}C)
carbon-12 (^{12}C)
carbon-13 (^{13}C)
c. spectroscopy
carbon-14 (^{14}C)
carbuncle
renal c.
Carcassonne ligament
carcinogenesis
radiation c.
carcinoid
atypical c.
colorectal c.
c. GI tract
c. syndrome
thymic c.
c. tumor
carcinoma, pl. carcinomata, carcinomas
acinar pancreatic cell c.
acinic cell c.
adenocystic c.
adenoid cystic lung c.
adenoid squamous cell c.
adnexal c.
adrenal c.
adrenocortical c.
aerodigestive c.
aldosterone-producing c.
aldosterone-secreting c.
alveolar basal cell c.
alveolar mucosal c.
ameloblastic c.
ampullary c.
anaplastic thyroid c.
androgen-independent prostate c.
aniline c.
apocrine c.
appendiceal c.
apple-core c.
aryepiglottic fold c.
asbestos-related lung c.
atypical medullary c.
basal cell c.
bilateral invasive lobular c.
bile duct c.

bilharzial c.
biliary tract c.
bladder c.
blastic metastatic prostate c.
bone c.
Boorman classification of gastric c.
bowel c.
brain c.
breast c.
bronchial c.
bronchiolar c.
bronchioloalveolar c.
bronchoalveolar c.
bronchogenic c.
buccal mucosal c.
cavitary squamous cell c.
cavitating c.
cecal c.
cerebriform c.
cholangiocellular c.
chorionic c.
choroid plexus c.
clay pipe c.
colloid c.
colon c.
colorectal c.
comedo-basal cell c.
conjugal c.
contact c.
corpus c.
cortisol-producing c.
cribriform c.
cylindrical c.
cylindromatous c.
cystic renal cell c.
dendritic c.
differentiated c. (DC)
distal bile duct c. (DBDC)
ductal papillary c.
ductal in situ breast c.
duct cell c.
embryonal cell c.
encephaloid c.
c. en cuirasse
endobronchial c.
endometrial c.
endometrioid ovarian c.
epidermal c.
epidermoid lung c.
epiglottic c.
epithelial-myoepithelial c.
epithelial ovarian c.

esophageal c.
ethmoid sinus c.
exophytic c.
c. ex pleomorphic adenoma
extensive intraductal c. (EIC)
extrahepatic bile duct c.
extrapulmonary small cell c.
fallopian tube c.
false cord c.
fibrolamellar hepatocellular c.
FIGO stage c.
flat colorectal c.
focal lobular c.
follicular thyroid c.
gallbladder c.
gastric remnant c.
gastric stump c.
gastroesophageal junction c.
gastrointestinal c.
gelatinous c.
genital c.
genitourinary c.
giant cell lung c.
gingival c.
glandular c.
glans c.
glottic c.
granulosa cell c.
hard palate c.
head and neck c.
hepatic c.
hepatobiliary c.
hepatocellular c.
hereditary nonpolyposis colorectal c.
  (HNPCC)
hormone-receptor negative c.
hormone-resistant prostate c.
hyopharyngeal c.
hypernephroid c.
hypervascular hepatocellular c.
hypopharyngeal c.
infantile embryonal c.
infiltrating ductal c.
infiltrating esophageal c.
infiltrating lobular c.
inflammatory breast c. (IBC)
intracystic breast c.
intraductal c. (IDC)
intraductal papillary c.
intrahepatic biliary c.
invasive breast c.
invasive lobular c.

C

NOTES

141

carcinoma *(continued)*

jugular node metastatic c.
juvenile embryonal c.
known primary c.
Kulchitsky cell c. (KCC)
large cell neuroendocrine c. (LCNEC)
large cell undifferentiated c.
laryngeal c.
lenticular c.
leptomeningeal c.
linitis plastica c.
lobular c.
locoregional breast c.
lung c.
mammographically occult c.
maxillary sinus c.
medullary breast c.
medullary thyroid c.
meibomian gland c.
melanotic c.
Merkel cell c.
mesometanephric c.
metachronous transitional cell c.
metaplastic c.
metastatic urothelial c.
micropapillary c.
missed bronchogenic c.
mucin-hypersecreting c.
mucinous breast c.
mucin-producing c.
mucoepidermoid c.
mucous c.
multicentric basal cell c.
multicentric invasive lobular c.
multifocal breast c.
multifocal invasive lobular c.
nasopharyngeal c. (NPC)
nasopharyngeal squamous cell c.
necrotic renal cell c.
neuroendocrine small-cell c.
nevoid basal cell c.
node-negative c.
node-positive c.
noncalcified c.
non-small cell lung c. (NSCLC)
oat cell c.
occult papillary c.
occult thyroid c.
osteoid c.
ovarian c.
Paget c.
palpatory T-stage prostate c.
pancreatic c.
papillary breast c.
papillary renal cell c.
papillary serous c.

papillary thyroid c.
paranasal sinus c.
parathyroid c.
perforating colorectal c.
periampullary c.
pharyngeal wall c.
pigmented basal cell c.
piriform sinus c.
platinum-resistant ovarian c.
polypoid c.
postcricoid c.
posterior pharyngeal wall c.
preinvasive c.
prickle cell c.
primary hepatocellular c.
primary intraosseous c.
primary neuroendocrine small-cell c.
prostate c.
prostatic c.
pulmonary squamous cell c.
radiation-induced c.
rectal c.
rectosigmoid c.
renal c.
resectable colorectal c.
retinoblastoma hereditary human c.
retromolar trigone c.
salivary gland c.
scar c.
schistosomal bladder c.
schneiderian c.
scirrhous breast c.
sclerosing basal cell c.
sclerosing hepatic c. (SHC)
sebaceous c.
secretory c.
serous c.
sessile nodular c.
sigmoid c.
signet ring cell c.
c. simplex
sinonasal c.
c. in situ
skin c.
small bowel c.
small-cell cribriform c.
small-cell lung c. (SCLC)
small-cell undifferentiated c.
small intestine c.
small round cell c.
soft palate c.
solid circumscribed breast c.
solid and papillary pancreatic c.
spiculated c.
splenic flexure c.
sporadic colorectal c.
string cell c.

stump c.
subareolar c.
subglottic c.
superficial basal cell c.
superficial depressed c.
superficial spreading esophageal c.
superficial spreading stomach c.
supraglottic c.
suture line c.
sweat gland c.
synchronous transitional cell c.
telangiectatic c.
terminal c.
testicular c.
testis c.
thymic c.
thyroid c.
tongue c.
tonsil c.
tonsillar c.
trabecular c.
transitional cell c. (TCC)
transitional kidney cell c.
transitional urinary bladder cell c.
transition ureteral cell c.
transverse colon c.
tripartite duodenal c.
tubular breast c.
typical medullary c.
ulcerative esophageal c.
undifferentiated nasopharyngeal c.
unresectable colorectal c.
urachal c.
ureteral c.
urothelial c.
uterine cervix c.
uterine corpus c.
uterine papillary serous c. (UPSC)
vaginal c.
varicoid esophageal c.
verrucous c.
villous c.
vocal cord c.
vulvar c.
vulvovaginal c.
Walker c.
wolffian duct c.
carcinomatosa
carcinomatosis
lymphangitic c.
lymphatic c.

peritoneal c.
c. peritonei
carcinomatosum
carcinomatous
c. cavitary metastasis
c. implant
c. myelopathy
c. myopathy
c. neuromyopathy
c. subacute cerebellar degeneration
carcinosarcoma
embryonal c.
esophageal c.
renal c.
Walker c.
carcinosis
abdominal c.
carcinostatic
Carden amputation
cardia
crescent of c.
gastric c.
patulous c.
cardiac
c. anomaly
c. antrum
c. apex
c. atrial shunt
c. blood pool imaging
c. border
c. branch
c. calcification
c. catheterization
c. catheterization imaging
c. chamber
c. cirrhosis
c. compression
c. congestion
c. contractility
c. creep
c. decompensation
c. decompression
c. decortication
c. denervation
c. diameter
c. dilatation
c. effusion
c. failure
c. fibroma
c. fibrosarcoma
c. filling pressure
c. fossa

NOTES

cardiac *(continued)*
c. frontal area
c. ganglion
c. gating
c. gating compensation
c. hamartoma
c. hemangioma
c. hydatidosis
c. hypertrophy
c. hypokinesis
c. impression
c. impression on liver
c. incisura
c. index (CI)
c. infarct
c. insufficiency
c. inversion
c. irritability
c. ischemia
c. laminography
c. lipoma
c. long axis view
c. lymphangioma
c. mapping
c. margin
c. mogul
c. monitor
c. MRI
c. muscle
c. muscle fiber
c. muscle inflammation
c. myocyte
c. myxoma
c. node
c. notch
c. oblique reformatting
c. obstruction
c. orifice
c. osteosarcoma
c. output (CO, Q)
c. output echocardiography
c. output measurement
c. output video densitometry
c. overload
c. perforation
c. PET
c. phase
c. plexus
c. polyp
c. position
c. positron emission tomography imaging
c. pulmonary edema
c. pulse duplicator
c. pumping ability
c. radiography
c. radiography imaging
c. recovery
c. reserve
c. rhabdomyoma
c. rhabdomyosarcoma
c. rupture
c. sarcoidosis
c. sarcoma
c. scan
c. scintigraphy
c. scintigraphy ejection fraction
c. segment
c. segmental bronchus
c. series
c. shadow
c. shape
c. shock
c. short axis view
c. shunt detection
c. silhouette
c. silhouette enlargement
c. situs invertus
c. situs solitus
c. skeleton
c. sling
c. standstill
c. steady state
c. stomach
c. tamponade
c. teratoma
c. thrombosis
c. tumor
c. valve
c. valve mucoid degeneration
c. valvular lesion
c. vasculature
c. vein
c. ventricle aneurysm
c. ventriculography
C. View probe
c. volume
c. waist
c. wall motion
c. wall motion imaging

cardiac-gated
c.-g. MR angiography
c.-g. PGSE sequence
c.-g. respiration
c.-g. study

cardinal
c. event
c. finding
c. ligament
c. point
c. sign
c. vein

cardioangiography
    blood pool radionuclide c.
    retrograde c.
CardioBeeper CB-12L cardiac monitor
cardiochalasia
cardiocutaneous syndrome
Cardio Data MK3 Holter scanner
cardiodiaphragmatic angle
cardioesophageal (CE)
    c. junction
cardiogenesis
cardiogenic
    c. embolic stroke
    c. embolus
    c. plate
    c. pulmonary edema
    c. shock heart
cardiogram
    apex c. (ACG)
    derived value on apex c. (dD/dt)
    ultrasonic c. (UCG)
cardiographic
cardiography
    M-mode c.
    radionuclide c.
    ultrasonic c.
cardiohepatic
    c. angle
    c. triangle
cardiohepatomegaly
cardioinhibitory response
cardiokymography (CKG)
Cardiolite
    C. imaging agent
    C. scan imaging
    technetium-tagged C.
    C. Tl-201
cardiomediastinal shadow
cardiomegaly
    borderline c.
    box-like c.
    funnel-like c.
    globular c.
    iatrogenic c.
cardiomotility
cardiomyopathic degeneration
cardiomyopathy
    amyloidotic c.
    arrhythmogenic right ventricular c.
    concentric hypertrophic c.
    congenital dilated c.
    congestive c.

    constrictive c.
    degenerative c.
    diabetic c.
    diffuse symmetric hypertrophied c.
    dilated c. (DCM)
    end-stage c.
    familial hypertrophic c. (FHC)
    Friedreich ataxic c.
    hypertrophic c. (HCM)
    hypertrophic obstructive c. (HOC, HOCM)
    idiopathic dilated c. (IDC)
    idiopathic restrictive c.
    infantile c.
    infectious c.
    infiltrative c.
    ischemic congestive c.
    left ventricular c.
    metabolic c.
    nonischemic congestive c.
    nonobstructive c.
    obliterative c.
    obstructive hypertrophic c.
    peripartum dilated c.
    postmyocarditis dilated c.
    postpartum c.
    restrictive c.
    right-sided c.
    right ventricular c.
    tachycardia-induced c.
    toxic c.
cardionecrosis
cardiophrenic
    c. angle
    c. junction
    c. right-angle mass
cardiopneumatic
cardioptosis
    Wenckebach c.
cardiopulmonary
    c. abnormality
    c. bilharziasis
    c. disease
    c. edema
    c. insufficiency
    c. support system
cardiopyloric
cardiorenal disease
cardiorespiratory sign
cardiorrhexis
cardioscan
Cardioscint

NOTES

145

cardiosclerosis
CardioSEAL occluder
cardioselective agent
cardiospasm
cardiosplenic syndrome
cardiosynchronous stimulation
cardiothoracic
    c. index
    c. ratio (CT, CTR)
    c. trauma
cardiothymic
    c. shadow
    c. silhouette
cardiothyrotoxicosis
cardiotocogram
cardiotocography imaging
cardiotopometry
cardiovalvular
cardiovascular
    c. accident (CVA)
    c. angiography analysis system
      (CAAS)
    c. anomaly
    c. computed tomographic scanner
      (CVCT)
    c. disease (CD, CVD)
    c. imaging technique
    c. malformation
    c. pressure
    c. radioisotope scan and function
      imaging
    c. radiology
    c. renal disease
    c. shadow
    c. shunt
    c. silhouette
    c. system
cardioverter-defibrillator
    automatic implantable c.-d. (AICD)
cardiovolume
    multislice c. (MSCV)
carditis
    acute lethal c.
    Lyme c.
CARE bolus
Carey-Coons soft stent biliary
  endoprosthesis
carina, pl. carinae
    mainstem c.
    sharp c.
    c. of trachea
carinal
    c. angle
    c. angle narrowing
    c. lesion
Carleton spot

C-arm
    C-a. DSA system
    C-a. fluoroscopic control
    C-a. fluoroscopy
    MINI 6000 C-a.
    C-a. portable x-ray unit
Carman sign
Carnesale-Stewart-Barnes hip dislocation
  classification
Carnett sign
Carney
    C. syndrome
    C. triad
Carnoy solution
Caroli disease
caroticocavernous fistula
caroticoclinoid ligament
caroticojugular spine
caroticotympanic
    c. artery
    c. canal
carotid
    c. angiography
    c. artery
    c. artery aneurysm
    c. artery arteritis
    c. artery bifurcation
    c. artery calcification
    c. artery disease
    c. artery dissection trauma
    c. artery ischemia
    c. artery kinking
    c. artery occlusion
    c. artery plaque
    c. artery stenosis
    c. artery stenting
    c. atherosclerosis
    c. atherosclerotic disease
    c. bifurcation atheroma
    c. blowout syndrome
    c. body
    c. body tumor
    c. bulb
    c. bulb baroreceptor
    c. canal
    c. cerebral arteriography
    c. circulation
    c. cistern
    c. compression tonography
    c. disobliteration
    c. distribution TIA
    c. duct
    c. duplex imaging
    c. duplex study
    c. duplex ultrasound
    c. ejection time
    c. endarterectomy (CEA)

external c.
c. foramen
c. ganglion
c. gland
c. groove
c. hemorrhage
internal c.
c. lumen
c. occlusive disease
c. phonoangiography
c. plaque hematoma
c. plexus
c. pulse peak
c. pulse tracing
c. pulse upstroke
c. revascularization endarterectomy
  stent trial
c. sheath
c. sheath adenoma
c. shudder
c. sinus
c. sinus hypersensitivity
c. sinus imaging
c. sinus syndrome (CSS)
c. siphon
c. sonography
c. space
c. space mass
c. string sign
c. sulcus
c. triangle
c. tubercle
c. vein
c. velocity
c. wall
carotid-carotid venous bypass graft
carotid-cavernous
  c.-c. fistula (CCF)
  c.-c. fistula occlusion
  c.-c. sinus fistula
carotid-dural fistula
carotidis
  bifurcatio c.
carotid-jugular fistula
carotid-ophthalmic aneurysm
carotid-subclavian transposition
carpal
  c. arch
  c. articular surface
  c. axes
  c. bone anatomy
  c. bone stress fracture

c. boss
c. box
c. canal
c. coalition
c. content ratio
c. deviation
c. groove
c. height index
c. height ratio
c. navicular
c. navicular bone
c. navicular fracture
c. row
c. scaphoid bone fracture
c. tunnel
c. tunnel projection
c. tunnel syndrome
c. tunnel view
c. wrist angle
Carpentier-Edwards ring
Carpentier ring
carpet
  c. lesion
  c. lesion of colon
  c. polyp
carpi (*pl. of* carpus)
carpometacarpal
  c. articulation
  c. fusion
  c. joint (CMC)
  c. joint fracture
  c. ligament
carpophalangeal joint
carporadial articulation
carpotarsal osteolysis
carpus, pl. **carpi**
  adaptive c.
  cuneiform bone of c.
  carpi radialis brevis tendon
  carpi radialis longus tendon
  ulnar translocation of the c.
carrier
  c. added radionuclide
  c. free radionuclide
  ^{67}Ga GABA uptake c.
  c. protein
  radionuclide c.
  c. tube
carrier-free
  c.-f. isotope
  c.-f. radioisotope

C

NOTES

carrier-free *(continued)*
    c.-f. separation
    c.-f. separation process
carrier-mediated transport system
Carrington disease
carrot-shaped trachea
Carr-Purcell (CP)
    C.-P. sequence
Carr-Purcell-Meiboom-Gill (CPMG)
    C.-P.-M.-G. sequence
carrying angle
Carter equation
Carter-Rowe view
cartesian
    c. reference coordinate system
    c. reference coordinate voxel array
cartilage
    absent bronchial c.
    accessory nasal c.
    alar c.
    anular rim of c.
    aortic c.
    arthrodial c.
    articular c.
    arytenoid c.
    attenuated intercarpal articular c.
    auditory c.
    auricular c.
    basilar c.
    c. bone
    branchial c.
    bronchial anular c.
    c. calcification
    calcified c.
    c. capsule
    ciliary c.
    circumferential c.
    conchal c.
    connecting c.
    corniculate c.
    costal intraarticular c.
    cricoid c.
    cricothyroid c.
    cuneiform c.
    delayed gadolinium-enhanced
      magnetic resonance imaging of c.
      (dGEMRIC)
    elastic c.
    c. endplate
    ensiform c.
    epiglottic c.
    epiphyseal c.
    facet c.
    falciform c.
    fibroelastic c.
    fibrous c.
    flaking of c.

    floating c.
    free flap of c.
    c. hair hypoplasia
    hyaline articular c.
    interarticular c.
    c. island
    c. joint space
    c. lacuna
    laryngeal c.
    lip-like projection of c.
    loss of elasticity of c.
    c. matrix
    ossified c.
    osteoarthritic c.
    patellofemoral articular c.
    physeal c.
    pitted c.
    pulmonary c.
    quadrangle c.
    rim of c.
    roughened c.
    scored c.
    semilunar c.
    shelling off of c.
    softening of c.
    sternal c.
    c. stroma
    swelling of c.
    tag of c.
    talar dome articular c.
    thinned c.
    thyroid c.
    tracheal c.
    triradiate c.
    unossified c.
    xiphoid c.
    Y c.
    yellow c.
cartilage-capped exostosis
cartilage-containing giant cell tumor
cartilage-forming bone tumor
cartilaginous
    c. acetabulum
    c. anlage
    c. bar
    c. cap
    c. cap of phalangeal head
    c. degeneration
    c. disk
    c. endplate
    c. epiphysis
    c. growth plate
    c. growth plate disorder
    c. hamartoma
    c. joint surface
    c. lesion
    c. metaplasia

c. node
c. nodule
c. ring
c. septum
c. soft-tissue tumor
c. synchondrosis
c. tissue
c. viscerocranium
CARTO EP navigation system
cartographic projection
cartwheel fracture
Carvallo sign
Cary-Coon biliary stent
CAS
coronary artery scan
coronary artery spasm
CAS imaging
cascade
diagnostic c.
gamma c.
c. stomach
c. system
time-dependent metabolic c.
caseating granuloma
caseous
c. necrosis
c. pneumonia
Casser
C. ligament
C. muscle
casserian
c. ligament
c. muscle
cassette
Adrian-Crooks c.
Camp grid c.
Curix film screen c.
film screen c.
CAST
computer automated scan technology
Castaneda thrombolytic brush
casting breast calcification
Castleman
C. disease
C. lymphoma
CAT
computerized axial tomography
catamenial pneumothorax
catapophysis
cataract
radiation c.
catarrhal pneumonia

catastrophe
vascular c.
catecholamine-producing tumor
catechol-O-methyltransferase
catenary system
cathartic colon
catheter
abscess drainage c.
Abscession drainage c.
Achiever balloon dilatation c.
Ackrad balloon-bearing c.
ACS balloon c.
ACS OTW Photon coronary
dilatation c.
AcuNav ultrasound c.
Amplatz left coronary c.
Amplatz right coronary c.
Amplatz Super Stiff c.
Angiocath Autoguard Shielded
IV c.
angiographic c.
c. angiography
AngioJet Xpeedior c.
angled-tip c.
angulated c.
c. aortography
apheresis c.
arrhythmogenic myocardial tissue
ablation c.
Arrow c.
c. arteriography
Ascent guiding c.
Atlantis SR IVUS c.
Auth Rotablator atherectomy c.
balloon embolectomy c.
balloon PTA c.
balloon-tipped angiographic c.
Bardex Lubricath c.
Berenstein c.
Berman angiographic c.
Bernstein c.
biliary drainage c.
Blue Max high-pressure reinforced
polyethylene balloon c.
braided diagnostic c.
Brevi-Kath epidural c.
Brite Tip 5F–10F guiding c.
c. bursting pressure
c. calibration
Caud-A-Kath c.
central venous c. (CVC)
c. cholangiogram

NOTES

catheter *(continued)*

cholangiography c.
Cobra 2 c.
cobra-shaped c.
c. coiling sign
conductance c.
Conquest balloon dilatation c.
contrast-filled c.
Cook-Cope type loop c.
Cope loop c.
Cordis Brite Tip 5F–10F
  guiding c.
cutting balloon c.
Dawson-Mueller drainage c.
Derek Harwood-Nash c.
directional atherectomy c.
double lumen central venous c.
drainage c.
EchoMark c.
eight-lumen manometric c.
electrothermal c.
endoscopic retrograde
  cholangiopancreatography c.
Envoy 6F guiding c.
Epimed spring guide c.
Equinox occlusion balloon c.
ERCP c.
c. exit site
external biliary drainage c.
FasTracker c.
c. fixation
Flexima biliary drainage c.
Flexi-Tip ureteral c.
fluid-filled c.
Fogarty balloon embolectomy c.
8-French guiding c.
9-French guiding c.
gastrojejunostomy c.
gastrostomy c.
Greenfield c.
Grollman pigtail c.
Groshong distal-valve c.
Grüntzig balloon dilatation c.
H1 c.
Headhunter c.
helium-filled balloon c.
hemodialysis c.
Hickman tunneled indwelling c.
hockey-stick c.
H/S Elliptosphere balloon c.
HSG c.
Hydrolyser hydrodynamic
  thrombectomy c.
hydrophilic-coated guiding c.
hysterosalpingography c.
ILUS c.
Imager II c.

c. impact artifact
impeller basket c.
implantable access c.
indwelling Foley c.
Infuse-a-Port c.
infusion c.
c. insertion
Insyte Autoguard Shielded IV c.
internal/external c.
intraarterial chemotherapy c.
Intracath c.
intraluminal ultrasound c.
intravascular ultrasound c.
IVUS c.
jejunostomy c.
Judkins left coronary c.
Judkins right coronary c.
jugular c.
c. kinking
Kumpe c.
large-bore c.
LifeJet c.
Maglinte c.
Malecot nephrostomy c.
c. mapping
MediPort c.
Medi-tech c.
Medtronic c.
Mercator atrial high-density
  array c.
Mewissen infusion c.
micromanometer-tipped c.
MicroMewi multiple sidehole
  infusion c.
c. migration
Motarjeme c.
multiaccess c.
multielectrode c.
multipurpose c.
multi-sideport infusion c.
Navarre c.
Navi-Star ablation c.
Nd:YAG laser c.
neodymium:yttrium-aluminum-garnet
  laser c.
NephroMax balloon c.
nephrostomy c.
nondetachable balloon c.
nylon c.
Oasis triple-lumen c.
c. obstruction
Omni Flush 3F, 4F, 5F c.
Omni Selective 0-3 c.
OneStep paracentesis drainage c.
Opticath c.
Opti-Flow dialysis c.

OptiQue c.
Oracle MegaSonics c.
Oracle Micro Plus c.
Oracle PTCA c.
PASV c.
PE c.
percutaneous cavity drainage c.
percutaneous cholecystotomy c.
peripherally inserted central c.
 (PICC)
peritoneal dialysis c.
pigtail c.
c. placement
polyethylene c.
polypropylene c.
Proforma c.
PU c.
PulseSpray/PRO infusion c.
PVC c.
quantum Monorail balloon c.
Raaf Cath vascular c.
Rapid Transit c.
Resolve non-locking draining c.
Ring biliary drainage c.
rotatable pigtail c.
Royal Flush 4F pigtail c.
Rusch c.
Saf-T-Intima integrated IV c.
Schneider Guider c.
self-retaining Cope loop pigtail c.
c. sheath
Sidewinder c.
Simmons c.
Simpson directional atherectomy c.
single-curved Cobra c.
Softouch c.
Soft-Tip c.
Soft Torque uterine c.
Soft-Vu angiographic c.
solid-state manometry c.
Sonicath Ultra imaging c.
Stimucath continuous nerve
 block c.
straight end-hole c.
straight side-hole c.
sump drainage c.
Swan-Ganz balloon c.
Tamp c.
Teflon c.
temporary pacing c.
Temp Tip drainage c.
Tenckhoff c.

thin-walled c.
c. tip
c. tip hockey-stick appearance
c. tip motion
c. tip motion artifact
c. tip position
c. tip position artifact
Torcon blue c.
Tracker 10 c.
Tracker Excel c.
transducer-tipped c.
TRAX c.
tunneled c.
Ultra ICE 9F/9 MHz c.
Uni-Fuse infusion c.
Van Aman pulmonary pigtail c.
Van Sonnenberg sump c.
Vaxcel peripherally inserted c.
ventriculography c.
visceral c.
water-infusion c.
c. whip artifact
c. with preformed curves
Z-MED balloon c.
catheter-borne sector transducer
catheter-delivered platinum coil
catheter-directed
 c.-d. extremity thrombolysis
 c.-d. fenestration
 c.-d. interventional procedure
 c.-d. thrombolytic therapy
 c.-d. urokinase
catheter-induced
 c.-i. coronary artery spasm
 c.-i. embolus
 c.-i. pulmonary artery hemorrhage
 c.-i. subclavian vein thrombosis
 c.-i. thromboembolization
catheterization
 antegrade femoral artery c.
 balloon c.
 cardiac c.
 high brachial artery c.
 interventional c.
 left axillary artery c.
 left heart c.
 retrograde femoral artery c.
 right heart c.
 Seldinger c.
 superior petrosal sinus c.
 superselective mesenteric artery c.
catheter-securing technique

NOTES

catheter-skin interface
catheter-tissue contact
cathode
    c. glow
    c. ray
    c. ray tube (CRT)
CathTrack catheter locator system
cation
    paramagnetic c.
cat phantom
cat's
    c. eye calculus
    c. tail configuration
cauda, pl. caudae
    c. equina
    c. equina compression
    c. equina syndrome (CES)
caudad projection
Caud-A-Kath catheter
caudal
    c. branch
    c. canal
    c. direction
    c. flexure
    c. ligament
    c. pharyngeal complex
    c. pons
    c. projection
    c. regression
    c. regression syndrome
    c. sheath
    c. tilt
    c. vertebra
    c. view
caudal-cranial angulation
caudalward
caudate
    c. body
    c. lobe
    c. lobe of liver
    c. nucleus
    c. process
    c. vein
    c. volume
caudocranial
    c. projection
    c. tangential view
caudothalamic groove
cauliflower appearance
cauliflower-shaped filling defect
caustic esophagitis
cava
    azygos continuation of inferior
      vena c.
    bilateral superior vena c.
    collapsed inferior vena c.
    duplicated inferior vena c.

    inferior vena c. (IVC)
    infrahepatic vena c.
    juxtarenal c.
    membranous obstruction of inferior
      vena c.
    paired inferior vena c.
    persistent left inferior vena c.
    persistent left superior vena c.
    redirection of inferior vena c.
    retrohepatic vena c.
    sinus of vena c.
    superior bilateral vena c.
    superior vena c. (SVC)
    suprahepatic vena c.
    transposition of inferior vena c.
    vena c.
cavagram
    inferior vena c.
caval
    c. filter
    c. fold
    c. lymph node
    c. opening
    c. tourniquet
    c. valve
cavalry bone
CAVB
    complete atrioventricular block
cavernoma
    brain c.
    portal vein c.
cavernosa
cavernosogram
cavernosography
    corpora c.
cavernosometry
cavernous
    c. angioma
    c. angiosarcoma
    c. brain angiography
    c. brain hemangioma
    c. groove
    c. lymphangioma
    c. malformation
    c. plexus
    c. portal vein transformation
    c. portion
    c. segment of internal carotid
      artery
    c. sinus
    c. sinus aneurysm
    c. sinus fistula
    c. sinus lesion
    c. sinus meningioma
    c. sinus syndrome
    c. tissue
    c. transfer of portal vein

c. transformation of portal vein
c. tumor
c. urethra
caviar lesion
cavitary
    c. dilatation
    c. fluid
    c. infiltrate
    c. lung lesion
    c. mass
    c. metastasis
    c. prostatitis
    c. pulmonary lesion
    c. small bowel lesion
    c. space
    c. squamous cell carcinoma
    c. tuberculosis
cavitate
cavitating
    c. carcinoma
    c. lung metastasis
    c. lung nodule
    c. neoplasm
    c. pattern
    c. pneumonia
cavitation
    collapse c.
    crescent of c.
    lobar c.
    pulmonary c.
    stable c.
    transient c.
**Cavitron Ultrasonic Surgical Aspirator
  (CUSA)**
cavity
    abdominal c.
    abdominopelvic c.
    absorption c.
    acetabular c.
    air c.
    amnionic c.
    ancyroid c.
    c. of aneurysm
    axillary c.
    banana-shaped uterine c.
    body c.
    Bragg-Gray c.
    buccal c.
    chest c.
    cleavage c.
    coexistent c.
    cotyloid c.

cranial c.
crown c.
dome-shaped roof of pleural c.
embryonic abdominal c.
endometrial c.
epidural c.
funnel-shaped c.
glenoid c.
grape-skin lung c.
greater sac of peritoneal c.
intraperitoneal c.
joint c.
lesser sac of peritoneal c.
lung c.
marrow c.
Meckel c.
medullary c.
midcarpal joint c.
miniature uterine c.
multiple thin-walled lung c.
nasal c.
orbital c.
pericardial c.
peritoneal c.
pleural c.
popliteal c.
pulmonary c.
resection c.
retroperitoneal c.
sac-like c.
septum pellucidum c.
sigmoid c.
sinonasal c.
sinus c.
Stafne idiopathic bone c.
subarachnoid c.
subchondral cystic c.
subdural c.
surgically created resection c.
synovial c.
syringohydromyelic c.
syrinx c.
thin-walled lung c.
thoracic c.
trigeminal c.
tubular c.
tympanic c.
uterine c.
ventricular c.
c. volume
c. wall
cavoatrial junction

NOTES

cavogram
cavography
cavopulmonary connection
cavovalgus
    pes c.
    talipes c.
cavovarus
    c. deformity
    pes c.
cavum
    c. septum pellucidum
cavus
    c. deformity
    global c.
    local c.
    pes c.
    posttraumatic c.
    talipes c.
Cayler syndrome
CBCL
    cutaneous B-cell lymphoma
CBD
    common bile duct
CBDE
    common bile duct exploration
CBF
    cerebral blood flow
CBFV
    coronary blood flow velocity
CBI
    convergent beam irradiation
CBT
    corticobulbar tract
CBV
    cerebral blood volume
CBV/CBF
    cerebral blood volume to cerebral blood
     flow ratio
C-C
    convexoconcave
     C-C heart valve
cc
    cubic centimeter
CCA
    common carotid artery
CCAM
    congenital cystic adenomatoid
     malformation
CCD
    central collodiaphyseal
    charge-coupled device
     CCD angle
     CCD detector
     CCD photodetector
CCF
    carotid-cavernous fistula

CCRT
    computer-controlled conformal radiation
     therapy
CCT
    cranial computed tomography
CCTA
    coronal computed tomographic
     arthrography
CD
    cardiovascular disease
    cluster of differentiation
    coincidence detection
    color Doppler
    Crohn disease
Cd
    cadmium
CDFI
    color-coded Doppler flow imaging
CDH
    congenital dislocation of hip
CDI
    color Doppler imaging
CDR
    computed dental radiography
CDRPan digital x-ray system
CDS
    color Doppler sonography
CDUS
    color Doppler ultrasound
CE
    capital epiphysis
    cardioesophageal
     CE angle of Wiberg
     CE junction
CEA
    carotid endarterectomy
CEA-Scan
    CEA-S. diagnostic imaging
    CEA-S. imaging agent
cebocephaly
ceca (*pl. of* cecum)
cecal
    c. appendage
    c. appendix
    c. bar
    c. bascule
    c. carcinoma
    c. deformity
    c. filling defect
    c. fold
    c. foramen
    c. hernia
    c. ileus
    c. recess
    c. serosa
    c. sphincter

c. thickening
c. volvulus
cecocutaneous fistula
cecostomy
percutaneous c.
CECT
contrast enhanced computed tomography
cecum, pl. ceca
antimesocolic side of c.
caput c.
coned c.
conical c.
c. diameter
kidney-shaped distended c.
c. mobile
subhepatic c.
Cedell
C. fracture
C. fracture of talus
Cedell-Magnusson
C.-M. arthritis classification
C.-M. classification of arthritis
Ceelen-Gellerstedt syndrome
CE-FAST
contrast-enhanced Fourier-acquired
steady state
CE-FAST scan
Celestin tube
celiac
c. angiography
c. arteriography
c. artery aneurysm
c. artery compression syndrome
c. axis
c. axis occlusion
c. axis syndrome
c. branch artery
c. disease
c. ganglion
c. ganglion block
c. lymph node
c. lymph node metastasis
c. plexus
c. plexus block
c. plexus neurolysis, endoscopic
ultrasound-guided
c. trunk
celiacography
celiectasia
celioma
celiomesenteric trunk
celioscopy

celiotomy
cell
basket c.
cerebellar granule c.
chromium-heated red blood c.
encroaching endothelial c.
epithelial c.
ethmoid air c.
glomerular mesangial c.
homophilic Purkinje c.
human aortic smooth muscle c.
^{111}In-labeled white blood c.
Kulchitsky c.
morula-like epithelial c.
Onodi c.
pluripotential bronchial epithelial
stem c.
c. polarization
polygonal elongate c.
c. preparation bone marrow uptake
protein-nucleic acid synthesis in
tumor c.
RAEL c.
red blood c. (RBC)
Rieder c.
Schwann c.
tagged red c.
tanned red c. (TRC)
technetium-tagged red blood c.
totipotential stem c.
c. tumor
white blood c. (WBC)
Zimmerman c.
cella medix index
cell-dose threshold
celloidin section
CellSeek technology
cellular
c. binding site
c. bronchiolitis
c. embolus
c. fibroadenoma
c. tumor
cellule formation
cellulitis
iodine-131-induced c.
orbital c.
celomic
c. metaphysis
c. pouch
CEM
central extensor mechanism

NOTES

155

Cemax/Icon PACS system
cement
    bone c.
    c. line
    c. mantle
    radiopaque bone c.
    residual c.
cemental
    c. dysplasia
    c. fracture
cementation
cementifying fibroma
cementinoma
cementoblastoma
cementoma
    gigantiform c.
cementoosseous dysplasia
cementoossifying fibroma
cementosis
cementum
CE-MRA
    contrast-enhanced magnetic resonance
    angiography
Cencit surface scanner
Centauri Er:YAG dental laser system
center
    accessory ossification c.
    anechoic c.
    bone c.
    cortical c.
    diaphyseal c.
    elbow bone c.
    emetic c.
    enlargement with low-density lymph
      node c.
    epileptogenic c.
    epiphyseal fetal bone c.
    epiphyseal ossification c.
    femoral ossification c.
    fetal epiphyseal bone c.
    c. line artifact
    lucent c.
    ossification c.
    ovoid ossification c.
    swallowing c.
    tibial tubercle ossification c.
    vertebral body ossification c.
    window c.
center-edge angle of Wiberg
center-to-center distance
centigray (cGy)
centimeter (cm)
    cubic c. (cc)
central
    c. airway disease
    c. amaurosis
    c. aorta

c. aortic pressure
c. artery
c. axis depth dose
c. beaking
c. blood volume
c. bone
c. bronchiectasis
c. bronchovascular bundle
c. caged ball occluder valve
c. caged disk occluder valve
c. callus
c. canal stenosis
c. cavity of cerebrum
c. cementifying fibroma
c. cerebellar fissure
c. cervical cord syndrome
c. channel
c. chondrosarcoma
c. collodiaphyseal (CCD)
c. collodiaphyseal angle
c. dislocation
c. extensor mechanism (CEM)
c. fat signal intensity
c. fatty hilum
c. fibrosarcoma
c. fracture
c. groove
c. gyrus
c. hemorrhagic component
c. herniation
c. high-signal intensity stripe
c. hilar structure
c. horn
c. indentation
c. intraluminal saturation stripe
c. intrasubstance signal intensity
c. lung distance (CLD)
c. lymph node
c. medullary bone lesion
c. necrosis
c. nervous system (CNS)
c. nervous system tumor
c. neurocytoma
c. neurofibromatosis
c. nidus of high-intensity marrow
c. ossifying fibroma
c. osteosarcoma
c. pancreatic lesion scar
c. perineal tendon
c. pit
c. placenta previa
c. pneumonia
c. point artifact
c. pontine
c. pontine myelinolysis
c. ray (CR)
c. rhomboid attachment

c. sacral line (CSL)
c. sinus lipomatosis
c. solitary papilloma breast
c. spinal canal
c. spinal cord syrinx
c. spinal stenosis
c. splanchnic venous thrombosis (CSVT)
c. sulcus
c. tegmental tract (CTT)
c. tendon diaphragm
c. vein
c. venous access
c. venous catheter (CVC)
c. venous drainage
c. venous line position
c. venous obstruction
c. venous pressure (CVP)
c. venous pressure line
c. vertebral osteomyelitis
centralis
fovea c.
centrally
c. ordered phase encoding
c. uninhibited bladder
centriacinar emphysema
centriciput
centrifugation
discontinuous density gradient c.
centrilobar opacity
centrilobular
c. congestion
c. distribution
c. emphysema
c. lesion
c. micronodule
c. necrosis
c. region of liver
c. shadow
centroblast
centroblastic lymphoma
centrocyte-like type
centrocytic lymphoma
centrocytoid
centroid
endocardial c.
epicardial c.
floating endocardial c.
floating epicardial c.
myocardial c.
centroid-based maximum intensity projection

centromere
centrum
c. commune
c. ovale
c. semiovale
c. semiovale pattern
cephalad-caudad direction
cephalad direction
cephalhematoma (*var. of* cephalohematoma)
cephalic
c. angle
c. angulation
c. flexure
c. index
c. pole
c. presentation
c. presentation of fetus
c. tilt view
c. triangle
c. vein
c. ventricle
cephalization of blood flow
cephalized vessel
cephalocaudad length
cephalocele
occipital c.
oral c.
sincipital c.
cephalofacial proportionality
cephalogram imaging
cephalohematocele
cephalohematoma, cephalhematoma
parietal c.
cephalomedullary nail fracture
cephalometer
Bertillon c.
cephalometric
c. analysis
c. angle
c. radiograph
cephalometry
radiographic c.
ultrasonic c.
cephalopelvic
c. disproportion (CPD)
c. disproportion index
cephalopelvimetry
cephalostat
cephalosyndactyly
Vogt c.
CEqual quantitative analysis

NOTES

CerASPECT
    C. camera
    C. system
ceratocricoid ligament
cerebella (*pl. of* cerebellum)
cerebellar
    c. anaplasia
    c. aplasia
    c. apoplexy
    c. artery
    c. astrocytoma
    c. atrophy
    c. attachment
    c. cortex
    c. cystic mass
    c. degeneration
    c. diaschisis
    c. ectopia
    c. epidermoid
    c. fiber
    c. folia
    c. gliosarcoma
    c. granule cell
    c. hemisphere
    c. hemorrhage
    c. heterotopia
    c. hypoperfusion
    c. hypoplasia
    c. infarct
    c. notch
    c. pathway
    c. peduncle
    c. peg
    c. sarcoma
    c. syndrome
    c. tonsil
    c. tract
    c. uvula
    c. vermis
    c. view
    c. volume
cerebelli
    falx c.
    gyrus c.
    mediastinum c.
    tentorium c.
    vallecula c.
cerebellolabyrinthine artery
cerebellomedullary cistern
cerebelloolivary degeneration
cerebellopontine
    c. angle (CPA)
    c. angle meningioma
    c. angle tumor
    c. cistern
    c. cisternography
    c. recess

cerebelloretinal
    c. hemangioblastoma
    c. hemangioblastomatosis
cerebellum, pl. **cerebella**
    amygdala of c.
    basal ganglia of c.
    dentate nucleus of c.
    fetal c.
    flocculonodular lobe of c.
    Gowers bundle in c.
    inverse c.
    midline c.
    petrosal c.
    towering c.
cerebra (*pl. of* cerebrum)
cerebral
    c. abscess
    c. amaurosis
    c. amyloid angiopathy
    c. aneurysm
    c. angiography
    c. anoxia
    c. apotentiality
    c. aqueduct
    c. arterial circle
    c. arteriography
    c. arteriosclerosis
    c. arteriovenous fistula
    c. arteriovenous malformation
    c. artery
    c. artery infarct
    c. artery stenosis
    c. astrocytoma
    c. blood flow (CBF)
    c. blood flow study
    c. blood vessel
    c. blood volume (CBV)
    c. blood volume to cerebral blood
        flow ratio (CBV/CBF)
    c. blood volume map
    c. calcification
    c. circulation
    c. circulation time
    c. commissure
    c. congestion
    c. contrast medium
    c. contusion
    c. convexity
    c. convolution
    c. cortex
    c. cortical gyral pattern
    c. CT venography
    c. cyst
    c. death
    c. dominance
    c. dysfunction
    c. edema

c. embolism
c. fat embolus
c. fissure
c. flexure
c. flow image technique
c. gammography
c. gigantism
c. glioma
c. gyri interdigitation
c. hemiatrophy
c. hemidecortication
c. hemisphere
c. hemorrhage
c. herniation
c. hypoperfusion
c. hypotension
c. inflammatory disease
c. infundibulum
c. ischemia
c. ischemic event
c. lesion
c. lymphoma
c. malformation classification
c. mantle
c. metabolic oxygen consumption
c. metabolic rate of oxygen (CMRO$_2$)
c. metabolism
c. metastasis
c. microarteriovenous malformation (micro-AVM)
c. microembolism
c. neuroblastoma
c. nodule
c. operculum
c. palsy pathological fracture
c. parenchyma
c. peduncle
c. perfusion pressure (CPP)
c. perfusion SPECT imaging
c. perfusion SPECT scan
c. perfusion study
c. pneumoencephalography
c. pneumography
c. pneumonia
c. porosis
c. radionecrosis
c. revascularization
c. ridge
c. salt wasting
c. scintigraphy
c. shunt

c. sinovenous occlusion
c. sinusography
c. SPECT
c. steal syndrome
c. sulcus
c. surface
c. surface atrophy
c. thrombophlebitis
c. toxoplasmosis
c. vascular microlattice
c. vasculature
c. vasoreactivity
c. vasospasm
c. vein
c. venous sinus
c. venous thrombosis
c. ventricle
c. ventricular shunt connector
c. ventriculography
c. vesicle
c. Whipple disease
c. white matter hypoplasia
c. xenon-enhanced blood flow (X-CBF)

cerebri
choana c.
commotio c.
contusio c.
falx c.
fornix c.
gliomatosis c.
gyri c.
hypophysis c.
mediastinum c.
pseudotumor c. (PTC)

cerebriform carcinoma
cerebritis
sinusitis c.
cerebrohepatorenal syndrome (CHRS)
cerebromacular degeneration (CMD)
cerebromeningeal intracerebral hemorrhage
cerebropontocerebellar pathway
cerebroside lipidosis
cerebrospinal
c. canal
c. fluid (CSF)
c. fluid circulation
c. fluid-containing lesion
c. fluid diversion
c. fluid fistula
c. fluid flow measurement

NOTES

cerebrospinal *(continued)*
    c. fluid flow waveform
    c. fluid leak
    c. fluid obstruction
    c. fluid pathway
    c. fluid shunt function
    c. fluid volume
cerebrotendinous xanthomatosis
cerebrovascular
    c. accident (CVA)
    c. aneurysmal clip
    c. insufficiency
    c. insult
    c. malformation
    c. occlusive disease
    c. stroke
cerebrum, pl. cerebra
    central cavity of c.
    cistern of lateral fossa of c.
    cortex of c.
    degenerative disease in c.
    c. demyelination
    first ventricle of c.
    great vein of c.
    lateral ventricle of c.
    second ventricle of c.
    third ventricle of c.
Cerenkov
    C. calculation
    C. count
    C. counter
    C. measurement
    C. radiation
    C. radiation production
    C. scintillation analysis
Ceretec
    C. brain imaging
    C. radioisotope imaging agent
    ^{99m}Tc C.
cerium-doped lutetium oxyorthosilicate (LSO)
cerium silicate imaging agent
ceroid gallbladder granuloma
Cerrobend block
cervical
    c. adenocarcinoma
    c. adenopathy
    c. aorta
    c. aortic arch
    c. canal
    c. cord
    c. cord lesion
    c. CSF systole
    c. CT
    c. disk
    c. disk disease
    c. disk herniation

c. disk syndrome
c. dysplasia
c. enlargement
c. esophagostomy
c. esophagus
c. eversion
c. facet dislocation
c. fascia
c. flexure
c. flush
c. fusion of spine
c. ganglion
c. heart
c. interbody fusion
c. intraepithelial neoplasm
c. length
c. loop
c. lordosis
c. lordotic curvature
c. lymph node tuberculous adenitis
c. magnetic resonance phlebography (CMRP)
c. meningocele
c. mover ligament
c. mucus arborization
c. muscle
c. musculature
c. myelography
c. nerve root
c. neural foramen
c. osteophyte
c. outlet
c. pain syndrome
c. paratracheal lymph node
c. pleura
c. plexus
c. polyp
c. pregnancy
c. rest
c. rib
c. rib anomaly
c. rib syndrome
c. sarcoma
c. segment of internal carotid artery
c. sinus
c. skull pillow
c., skull, and shoulder block
c. spine curve
c. spine dens view
c. spine fracture
c. spine fusion
c. spine injury
c. spine spondylosis
c. spondylotic myelopathy (CSM)
c. spondylotic radiculopathy
c. stenosis

c. stroma
c. structure
c. synostosis
c. synspondylism
c. syringomyelia
c. thymic cyst
c. triangle
c. tumor
c. vein
c. vertebra
c. vesicle
cervices (*pl. of* cervix)
cervicitis
cervicoaxillary canal
cervicocerebral
cervicocranium
cervicography
cervicomedullary
c. junction
c. kink
cervicooccipital fusion
cervicothoracic
c. ganglion
c. junction
c. sagittal scout image
cervicothoracolumbar
cervicotrochanteric fracture
cervigram
cervix, pl. **cervices**
cockscomb appearance of c.
double c.
incompetent c.
c. uteri
uterine c.
CES
cauda equina syndrome
cesium
c. chloride imaging agent
c. implant
c. iodide input phosphor
c. iodide scintillator
c. needle
c. with barium 137m
cesium-137 (^{137}Cs, Cs-137)
Cestan-Chenais syndrome
cestodic tuberculosis
Cf
californium
^{252}Cf
californium-252
CF artery

CFD
color-flow Doppler
CFI
color-flow imaging
CFL
calcaneofibular ligament
C-flex stent
CFR
coronary flow reserve
CGI
common gateway interface
CGR biplane angiographic system
cGy
centigray
CH20 Kernal and slim 2 profile
Chaddock sign
chain
branched c.
c. cystogram
c. cystourethrography
heavy c.
image c.
internal mammary lymphatic c.
J c.
jugulodigastric c.
c. of lakes deformity
Markov c.
obturator nodal c.
sympathetic c.
chalasia
chalky bone
challenge
solid bolus c.
chamber
abnormal dimensions of cardiac c.
alpha c.
cardiac c.
cloud c.
c. compression
defective communication between
    cardiac c.'s
c. dilatation
c. enlargement
false aneurysmal c.
c. of heart
hydraulic c.
infundibular c.
ion c.
ionization c.
irradiation c.
left atrial c.
left ventricular c.

NOTES

C

chamber *(continued)*
    multiwire proportional c.
    personal ionization c.
    pocket c.
    reduced compliance of c.
    reentrant well c.
    right atrial c.
    right ventricular c.
    rudimentary outlet c.
    rudimentary ventricular c.
    spark c.
    c. volume
    well-type ionization c.
    Wilson cloud c.

Chamberlain
    C. line
    C. procedure

Chamberlain-Towne view

champagne
    c. glass iliac wing
    c. glass pelvis
    c. glass ureter

champagne-bottle legs

chance
    c. equivalent
    C. spinal fracture

change
    age-related c.
    arthritic talonavicular c.
    asymmetrical signal c.
    atherosclerotic c.
    attritional pattern c.
    basal ganglionic c.
    BOLD time course c.
    bony c.
    consolidative c.
    cystic c.
    deep gray matter nucleus c.
    degenerative osseous c.
    drug-induced brain c.
    dystrophic c.
    E:A c.
    epithelial degenerative c.
    fibrocystic c.
    fibrotic c.
    fMRI signal c.
    focal degenerative c.
    high-signal-intensity ischemic c.
    hydropic c.
    interstitial c.
    interval c.
    ischemic c.
    lytic c.
    marrow signal c.
    mural c.
    myxoid degenerative c.
    nonspecific c.

    osteoarthritic c.
    papillary apocrine c.
    parenchymal c.
    paroxysmal c.
    pathophysiologic c.
    pelvicaliceal c.
    pleural c.
    polyneuropathy, organomegaly,
      endocrinopathy, monoclonal
      gammapathy, skin c.'s (POEMS)
    postbiopsy c.
    postsurgical c.
    posttherapy c.
    postthoracotomy c.
    precancerous c.
    prediverticular c.
    preslip c.
    proliferative c.
    pulmonary parenchymal c.
    radiation-induced c.
    radiation-related ischemic c.
    reciprocal c.
    residual interstitial c.
    residual limb-shaped c.
    roentgenographic c.
    senescent c.
    senile c.
    serial c.
    signal c.
    spinal endplate c.
    spondylitic c.
    spongiform c.
    stenotic c.
    vasomotor c.

changer
    Elema roll-film c.
    film c.
    Franklin c.
    Puck film c.
    rapid film c.
    Sanchez-Perez cassette c.
    Schonander film c.
    serial film c.

channel
    aberrant vascular c.
    blood c.
    central c.
    collateral venous c.
    deep venous c.
    dentate output c.
    enlarged vascular c.
    false c.
    gastric c.
    haversian c.
    Lambert c.
    lymphatic c.
    pancreaticobiliary common c.

pyloric c.
c. pyloric ulcer
thread-and-streaks vascular c.
true c.
vascular c.
chaotic heart
Chaoul
C. therapy
C. voltage x-ray tube
Chaput
C. fracture
C. tubercle
characteristic
alternative-free response receiver
operating c. (AFROC)
associated imaging c.
contrast transfer c.
c. curve
echo c.
c. emission
excitatory pulse c.
c. finding
generator c.
pathognomonic imaging c.
c. radiation
receiver operating c. (ROC)
signal c.
suspension c.
tip dispersion c.
c. x-ray
characterization
tissue c.
charcoal
dextran-coated c.
Charcot
C. arthropathy
C. chondroma
C. cirrhosis
C. deformity
C. foot
C. fracture
C. joint
C. spine
C. triad
Charcot-Bouchard intracerebral microaneurysm
Charcot-Marie-Tooth (CMT)
C.-M.-T. disease
charge
homogeneous positive c.

charge-coupled
c.-c. device (CCD)
c.-c. device scanner
charged-particle radiosurgery
charge-injection device (CID)
chart
Segre c.
x-ray tube rating c.
Chassaignac muscle
Chassard-Lapiné
C.-L. position
C.-L. projection
C.-L. view
chastity ring artifact
Chauffard point
chauffeur's fracture
Chausse
C. III projection
third projection of C.
C. view
Chaussier
C. line
C. projection
C. view
CHB
complete heart block
CHD
common hepatic duct
congenital heart defect
congenital heart disease
arachnodactyly CHD
oligemia-related cyanotic CHD
plethora-related cyanotic CHD
check
design rule c. (DRC)
Check-Flo sheath
Checkmate system
checkrein
c. deformity
c. ligament
check-valve
c.-v. mechanism
c.-v. sheath
Chédiak-Steinbrinck-Higashi syndrome
cheek bone
cheese
c. handler's lung
c. washer's lung
cheese-wiring
cheesy pneumonia
CheeTah radiopaque contrast agent
cheirolumbar

C

NOTES

cheiromegaly
cheirospasm
chelate
  B-19036 c.
  Cr-HIDA c.
  gadolinium c.
  Gd-HIDA c.
chelating agent
chelonian pneumonia
chemical
  c. dosimeter
  c. peritonitis
  c. pleurodesis
  c. pneumonia
  c. pneumonitis
  c. potential energy
  c. pulmonary edema
  c. ray
  c. shift
  c. shift artifact
  c. shift imaging (CSI)
  c. shift imaging technique
  c. shift ratio
  c. shift reference
  c. shift selective suppression
    technique
  c. shift spatial offset
chemically-induced
  c.-i. dynamic nuclear depolarization
    (CIDNP)
  c.-i. dynamic nuclear polarization
chemical-selective
  c.-s. fat-saturation imaging
  c.-s. fat-saturation MR
chemiluminescence
chemisorb
chemisorption
chemistry
  nuclear c.
  radiation c.
  radiopharmaceutical c.
chemodectoma
  chest c.
chemoembolization
  hepatic c.
  therapeutic c.
  transarterial c. (TACE)
  transcatheter arterial c. (TACE)
  transcatheter hepatic arterial c.
  transcatheter oily c.
Chemo-Port vascular access system
chemotherapy
  CT-guided intraarterial c.
chemotoxic reaction
chemsat fat suppression
chenodeoxycholic acid

Chen-Smith
  C.-S. image coder
Cherenkov effect
cherubism
CHESS method
chest
  alar c.
  barrel c.
  blast c.
  c. bucky
  c. cavity
  c. chemodectoma
  cobbler's c.
  cylindrical c.
  dirty c.
  c. empyema
  expiratory c.
  c. film
  flail c.
  c. fluke lung
  c. fluoroscopy
  foveated c.
  funnel c.
  globular c.
  hollow c.
  hourglass c.
  jail-bar c.
  keeled c.
  c. lead
  narrow c.
  paralytic c.
  phthinoid c.
  pigeon c.
  pneumonectomy c.
  pterygoid c.
  c. radiology
  symmetric c.
  tetrahedron c.
  c. tube
  c. view
  c. wall
  c. wall hamartoma
  c. wall lateral xeromammogram
  c. wall lesion
  c. wall mesenchymoma
  c. wall neuroblastoma
  c. wall paradoxical motion
  c. wall retraction
  c. wall rhabdomyosarcoma
  c. wall trauma
  c. x-ray (CXR)
chevron
  c. bone
  c. fracture
  c. fusion

CHF
congenital hepatic fibrosis
congestive heart failure
CHI
closed head injury
Chiari
C. formation
C. I–II malformation
C. I–IV lesion
Chiari-associated syringomyelia
chiasm
c. of digit of hand
optic c.
chiasma
Camper c.
cistern of c.
chiasmal
c. compression
c. lesion
chiasmata, pl. **chiasma**
chiasmatic
c. cistern
c. defect
c. groove
chiasmatic-hypothalamic pilocytic astrocytoma
chiasmaticus
sulcus c.
Chiba
C. needle
C. percutaneous cholangiogram
chicken-wire calcification
Chilaiditi
C. sign
C. syndrome
childhood
c. diskitis
c. fracture
c. osteomyelitis
c. rhabdomyosarcoma
Child-Pugh classification
CHILD syndrome
chimera
radiation c.
chimney-shaped high aortic arch
Chinese fluke liver
chin-occiput piece
chip
bone c.
cancellous bone c.
corticocancellous bone c.
c. fracture

chisel fracture
chisel-like truncated appearance
chloride
^{111}In c.
magnesium c.
manganese c.
polyvinyl c. (PVC)
stannous c.
strontium-89 c.
thallium-201 c.
Tl-201 c.
triphenyltetrazolium c. (TTC)
chloriodized oil
chlormerodrin accumulation test
chlormerodrin-cysteine complex
chloroma
bone c.
gastric c.
c. granulocytic sarcoma
kidney c.
choana cerebri
choanal
c. atresia
c. polyp
chocolate
c. cyst
c. joint effusion
cholangiectasis
extrahepatic c.
cholangiocarcinoma
extrahepatic c.
hilar c.
intrahepatic c.
peripheral c. (PCC)
Cholangiocath
cholangiocatheter
cholangiocellular carcinoma
cholangiodrainage
cholangiodysplastic pseudocirrhosis
cholangiofibromatosis
cholangiogram
balloon c.
catheter c.
Chiba percutaneous c.
common duct c.
contrast selective c.
cystic duct c.
drip infusion c. (DIC)
endoscopic retrograde c. (ERC)
fine-needle transhepatic c. (FNTC)
intraoperative c.
intravenous c. (IVC)

C

NOTES

cholangiogram (continued)
    magnetic resonance c. (MRC)
    operative c.
    percutaneous transhepatic c. (PTC,
     PTCA, PTHC)
    retrograde c.
    serial c.
    single-shot MR c.
    transhepatic c. (THC)
    transjugular c.
    T-tube c. (TTC)
cholangiography
    breath-hold MR c.
    c. catheter
    computed tomographic c.
    cystic duct c.
    delayed operative c.
    direct percutaneous transhepatic c.
    drip infusion c. (DIC)
    endoscopic c. (ERC)
    c. imaging
    intraoperative c.
    intravenous c.
    percutaneous hepatobiliary c.
    percutaneous transhepatic c. (PTHC)
    postoperative c.
    transabdominal c.
    T-tube c.
cholangiohepatitis
    Oriental c.
cholangiolithiasis
cholangiopancreatography
    endoscopic percutaneous c.
    endoscopic retrograde c. (ERCP)
    kinematic MR c.
    magnetic resonance c. (MRCP)
cholangioscopy
    contrast-enhanced virtual MR c.
cholangiotomogram
cholangiovenous communication
cholangitic biliary cirrhosis
cholangitis
    acute nonsuppurative ascending c.
    acute obstructive c.
    acute suppurative ascending c.
    AIDS c.
    ascending c.
    bacterial c.
    chronic nonsuppurative
     destructive c.
    fibrous obliterative c.
    intrahepatic sclerosing c.
    nonsuppurative ascending c.
    nonsuppurative destructive c.
    primary sclerosing c.
    progressive suppurative c.
    pyogenic c.

    recurrent pyogenic c.
    sclerosing c.
    secondary sclerosing c.
    septic c.
    suppurative ascending c.
Cholebrine imaging agent
cholecystectomy
    endoscopic laser c.
cholecystenteric fistula
cholecystitis
    acalculous c.
    acute c.
    calculous c.
    chronic c.
    emphysematous c.
    gangrenous c.
    gaseous c.
    lipid c.
    perforated c.
    c. with cholelithiasis
    xanthogranulomatous c.
cholecystocholangiography
cholecystocholangitis
cholecystocholedochal fistula
cholecystocolic fistula
cholecystocutaneous fistula
cholecystoduodenal
    c. fistula
    c. ligament
cholecystoduodenocolic
    c. fistula
    c. fold
cholecystoenteric fistula
cholecystogram
    Graham-Cole c.
    oral c. (OCG)
cholecystography
    intravenous c.
    oral c.
    post fatty meal c.
cholecystokinetic food
cholecystokinin cholescintigraphy
cholecystolithiasis
cholecystomegaly
cholecystopaque
cholecystopathy
cholecystoptosis
cholecystosis
    hyperplastic c.
cholecystosonography
cholecystostomy
    percutaneous transhepatic c.
    ultrasound-guided percutaneous c.
choledochal
    c. cyst
    c. sphincter
choledochal-colonic fistula

choledochocele
choledochocholedochostomy
choledochoduodenal
    c. fistula
    c. junctional stenosis
choledochofiberscope
    Olympus CHF-BP30
    transduodenal c.
choledochogram
choledochograph
choledochography
choledochojejunostomy stricture
choledocholithiasis
choledochopancreatic ductal junction
choledochoscope
choledochoscopy
    percutaneous c.
choledochostomy
choledochous duct
cholegraphy
cholelith, chololith
cholelithiasis
    cholecystitis with c.
cholelithoptysis
cholescintigraphy
    cholecystokinin c.
    radionuclide c.
    sincalide c.
cholescintography
cholestasis, cholestasia
    intrahepatic c.
cholestatic liver disease
cholesteatoma
    attic c.
    congenital c.
    ear c.
    GU tract c.
    inflammatory c.
    pars flaccida c.
    pars tensa c.
    primary acquired c.
    primary CNS c.
    primary temporal bone c.
    secondary acquired c.
cholesterinosis, cholesterolosis,
  cholesterosis
cholesterol
    c. debris
    c. ear cyst
    c. ear granuloma
    c. embolus
    c. gallbladder polyp

    c. gallstone
    I-labeled c.
cholesterol-based scintigraphy
cholesterol-containing brain lesion
cholesterolosis (*var. of* cholesterinosis)
cholesterosis (*var. of* cholesterinosis)
Choletec radionuclide imaging agent
cholioangiopancreatography
Cholografin meglumine imaging agent
chololith (*var. of* cholelith)
chondral
    c. defect
    c. fracture
    c. fragment
chondrification
chondritis
chondroblastic osteosarcoma
chondroblastoma
    benign c.
    c. straddling
chondrocalcinosis
    familial c.
chondrocyte
    atypical c.
    c. degeneration
    epiphyseal c.
    regenerative c.
chondrodiastasis
chondrodysplasia
    c. calcificans
    Jansen-type metaphyseal c.
    McKusick-type metaphyseal c.
    metaphyseal c.
    c. punctata
    Schmid-like metaphyseal c.
chondrodystrophia
    c. calcificans congenita
    c. fetalis
chondrodystrophy
chondroectodermal dysplasia
chondrofibroma
chondrogenic tumor
chondrogladiolar
chondroid
    c. matrix
    c. syringoma
    c. tissue
chondroid-origin tumor
chondroitin sulfate iron colloid-enhanced
  MRI
chondrolipoma

C

NOTES

chondrolysis
  posttraumatic c.
chondroma
  Charcot c.
  extraskeletal c.
  joint c.
  juxtacortical c.
  soft tissue c.
chondromalacia
  c. patella
  patellar c.
  ulnar c.
  c. with fibrillation
  c. with surface fraying
chondromanubrial
chondromatosis
  Henderson-Jones c.
  secondary c.
  synovial c.
chondromatous hamartoma
chondromyofibroma
chondromyxoid fibroma (CMF)
chondromyxoma
chondromyxosarcoma
chondronecrosis
chondroosteodystrophy
chondrophyte
chondroplasia calcificans
chondroporosis
chondrosarcoma
  central c.
  endosteal c.
  exostotic c.
  extraskeletal mesenchymal c.
  juxtacortical c.
  malignant c.
  mesenchymal c.
  myxoid extraskeletal c.
  parosteal c.
  peripheral c.
chondrosarcomatosis
chondrosteoma
chondrosternal junction
chondroxiphoid ligament
chop amputation
Chopart
  C. fracture
  C. fracture-dislocation
  C. hindfoot amputation
  C. joint
chopper
  McIlwain tissue c.
Chopper-Dixon fat suppression imaging
Choquet fuzzy integral
choracobrachialis

chord
  contiguous parallel c.
  multiple c.'s
chorda, pl. **chordae**
  basal c.
  cleft c.
  commissural c.
  first-order c.
  c. magna
  second-order c.
  strut c.
  third-order c.
chordal rupture
chordate
chordocarcinoma
chordoepithelioma
chordoma
  clivus c.
  sacral c.
  sacrococcygeal c.
  sphenooccipital c.
  spinal c.
  vertebral c.
chordosarcoma
chorioallantoic placenta
chorioamnionic
  c. elevation
  c. separation
chorioangioma
choriocarcinoma
  esophageal c.
  gestational c.
  ovarian c.
  primary ovarian c.
  testicular c.
choriodecidua
choriodecidual reaction
chorionic
  c. carcinoma
  c. disk
  c. gonadotropin
  c. sac
  c. tissue
chorionicity
choristoma
  middle ear c.
  renal c.
choroid
  c. glomera
  c. plexus
  c. plexus blush
  c. plexus calcification
  c. plexus carcinoma
  c. plexus cyst
  c. plexus hemorrhage
  c. plexus neoplasm
  c. plexus papilloma

c. point
c. vein
choroidal
  c. fissure
  c. hemangioma
  lateral posterior c. (LPCh)
  medial posterior c. (MPCh)
  c. neovascularization (CNV)
  c. osteoma
  c. pericallosal artery
choroidal-hippocampal fissure complex
choroidea
  tela c.
choroideum
  glomus c.
Choron
Christian brachydactyly
Christmas tree appearance
chromaffin
  c. paraganglioma
  c. tumor
chromated ^{51}Cr serum albumin imaging agent
chromatic spectrum
chromatid-type aberration
chromatogram
chromatographic-fluorometric technique
chromatographic separation
chromatography
  antiidiotypic affinity c.
  DEAE-Sephadex A-25 c.
  gas-liquid phase c. (GLPC)
  high-performance liquid c.
  high-performance size-exclusion c.
  high-pressure liquid c.
  ion-exchange c.
ChromaVision digital analyzer
chromic phosphate suspension
chromium (Cr)
  c. CR 51 serum albumin
  c. imaging agent
  c. phosphate
chromium-heated red blood cell
chromium:yttrium-aluminum-garnet
  erbium c.-a.-g. (ErCr:YAG)
chromophobe
  kidney carcinoma c.
  pituitary adenoma c.
chromoscopy time
chronic
  c. abdominal inflammation
  c. airway obstruction

c. alveolar infiltrate
c. atelectasis
c. atrophic duodenitis
c. atrophic pyelonephritis
c. berylliosis
c. breast abscess
c. calcifying pancreatitis
c. cerebral ischemia
c. cholecystitis
c. communicating hydrocephalus
c. constrictive state
c. diffuse confluent lung opacity
c. diffuse reticulation
c. diffuse sclerosing alveolitis
c. diverticulitis
c. duodenal ileus
c. edema
c. esophagitis
c. extrinsic allergic alveolitis
c. fibrosing alveolitis
c. fibrosing mesenteritis
c. fissure
c. functional instability
c. gastric atony
c. gastritis
c. glomerulonephritis
c. heart failure
c. hemodynamic overload
c. hepatitis
c. hereditary nephritis
c. hydronephrosis
c. hypertrophic emphysema
c. idiopathic intestinal pseudoobstruction (CIIP)
c. ileus duodenum
c. infantile hyperostosis
c. insufficiency of vein
c. interstitial pneumonia
c. interstitial salpingitis
c. interstitial simulating airspace lung disease
c. irritation
c. ischemic brain infarct
c. ligament complex laxity
c. ligamentous injury
c. lung thromboembolism
c. lymphedematous limb
c. lymphocytic leukemia
c. lymphocytic thyroiditis
c. mesenteric ischemia (CMI)
c. multifocal ill-defined lung opacity

NOTES

chronic *(continued)*
   c. myeloid leukemia
   c. necrotizing aspergillosis
   c. nonsuppurative destructive
   cholangitis
   c. obstructive emphysema
   c. obstructive lung disease (COLD)
   c. obstructive pancreatitis
   c. obstructive pulmonary disease
   (COPD)
   c. obstructive uropathy
   c. overuse syndrome
   c. parenchymal hemorrhage
   c. partial epilepsy
   c. passive congestion
   c. peptic ulcer
   c. periaortitis
   c. peripheral arterial disease
   (CPAD)
   c. phase
   c. pleurisy
   c. pneumonitis
   c. posttraumatic aortic
   pseudoaneurysm
   c. pulmonary emphysema (CPE)
   c. recurrent dislocation
   c. recurrent multifocal osteomyelitis
   c. recurrent sialadenitis
   c. renal failure (CRF)
   c. renal failure amyloidosis
   c. renal infarct
   c. renal vein thrombosis
   c. reserve flow
   c. respiratory decompensation
   c. retrocalcaneal bursitis
   c. sclerosing osteomyelitis
   c. simple silicosis
   c. sinusitis
   c. sprain
   c. subdural hematoma (CSDH)
   c. subperitoneal sclerosis
   c. tamponade
   c. testicular torsion
   c. tuberculous emphysema
   c. ulcerative colitis (CUC)
   c. venous insufficiency
   c. venous stasis
chronologic age
chronotherapy
   adjuvant c.
chronotropic incompetence
chronotropy
CHRS
   cerebrohepatorenal syndrome
CHRYS CO$_2$ laser
chrysotile asbestos
Churg-Strauss syndrome

chyle
   c. cistern
   effused c.
   c. leak
   c. vessel
chyli
   ampulla c.
   cisterna c.
chyliferous vessel
chylocele
   nonfilarial c.
chyloma
chylomediastinum
chylopericardium
chylothorax
   postoperative c.
chylous
   c. ascites
   c. effusion
   c. fistula
   c. leakage
CI
   cardiac index
   confidence interval
   continuous imaging
Ci
   curie
cicatricial
   c. atelectasis
   c. kidney
   c. stricture
cicatrizing
CID
   charge-injection device
   CID camera
CIDNP
   chemically-induced dynamic nuclear
   depolarization
Cidtech camera
cigarroa formula
CIIP
   chronic idiopathic intestinal
   pseudoobstruction
ciliaris
   zonula c.
ciliary
   c. canal
   c. cartilage
   c. ganglionic plexus
   c. ligament
   c. ring
   c. vein
ciliated border
ciliospinal center of Budge
Cimino
   C. AV shunt
   C. dialysis shunt

cine
  c. acquisition
  c. camera
  c. coronary arteriography
  c. CT
  c. CT imaging
  c. CT scan
  c. CT scanner
  c. film
  c. fistulogram
  c. gradient-echo MR imaging
  c. gradient-echo sequence
  c. gradient magnetic resonance
    imaging
  c. left ventriculogram
  c. loop
  c. magnetic resonance function
    image
  c. magnetic resonance tagging
  C. Memory with color flow
    Doppler imaging
  c. mode
  c. MRI
  parallel c.
  c. phase contrast imaging
  c. projector
  c. raw data
  c. study
  velocity-encoded c. (VEC)
  c. view
  c. view imaging
  c. view in MUGA scan
cineangiocardiogram (CACG)
cineangiocardiography
cineangiogram
  ventricular c.
cineangiography
  aortic root c.
  axial c.
  biplane c.
  coronary c.
  radionuclide c.
  selective coronary c.
cinearteriography
  Judkins selective left coronary c.
cine-based viewing
cinebronchogram
cinecardioangiography
cinedefecogram
cinedensigraphy
cine-encoded image
cineesophagogram

cine-FFE breath-hold sequence
cinefluorography
  biplane c.
cinefluoroscopy
  valve c.
cine-gated imaging
cine-loop
cinematography
cinematoradiography
cinemicrography
cine-mode display
cine-MR
  breath-hold c.-MR
cinepharyngoesophagogram
cinephlebography
cineportography
cineradiographic view
cineradiography imaging
cinereum
  tuber c.
cineroentgenofluorography
cineroentgenography
cineurography
cineventriculogram
cineventriculography
cingulate
  c. gyrus
  c. herniation
  c. sulcus
cingulum, pl. **cingula**
cipher
  transposition c.
circadian
  c. continuous infusion
  c. pattern
  c. periodicity
  c. variation
circle
  anastomotic arterial c.
  arterial c.
  articular vascular c.
  cerebral arterial c.
  c. of confusion
  c. loop biliary drainage
  c. of Vieussens
  c. of Weber
  c. of Willis
  c. wire nephrostomy
Circon video camera
circuit
  anticoincidence c.

NOTES

171

circuit *(continued)*
    application-specific integrated c. (ASIC)
    arrhythmia c.
    ASIC c.
    bridge c.
    bypass c.
    coincidence c.
    doubly broadband triple-resonance NMR probe c.
    macroreentrant c.
    magnetic c.
    magnetoresistive sensor c.
    microreentrant c.
    phototube output c.
    quad resonance NMR probe c.
    reentry c.
    shunting c.
    triple-resonance NMR probe c.

circular
    c. dichroism spectroscopy
    c. fold
    c. lesion
    c. muscle
    c. plane
    c. polarization wave
    c. polarized volume head coil
    c. sinus
    c. supracondylar amputation
    c. syncytium

circularly polarized coil
circulating blood volume
circulation
    allantoic c.
    arrested c.
    balanced c.
    bronchial collateral c.
    carotid c.
    cerebral c.
    cerebrospinal fluid c.
    codominant c.
    c. collapse
    collateral mesenteric c.
    compensatory c.
    cutaneous collateral c.
    derivative c.
    devoid of c.
    c. disturbance
    extracardiac collateral c.
    extracorporeal c.
    extracranial carotid c.
    extracranial cerebral c.
    c. failure
    fetal c.
    greater c.
    high-impedance c.
    intervillous c.

    intraaneurysmal flow c.
    intracranial c.
    Korotkoff test for collateral c.
    microvascular c.
    peripheral c.
    persistent fetal c.
    placental c.
    portosystemic collateral c.
    posterior fossa c.
    pulmonary arterial c.
    reduced c.
    c. shock
    spiderweb c.
    c. stasis
    systemic arterial c.
    thebesian c.
    thoracoabdominal venous collateral c.
    c. time (CT)
    uteroplacental c.
    venous c.
    vertebrobasilar c.
    c. volume

circulator
    sequential c.
circulatory
    c. arrest
    c. compromise
    c. embarrassment
    c. impairment
circumaortic left renal vein
circumaxillary
circumcaval ureter
circumduction
circumduction-adduction shoulder maneuver
circumference
    abdominal c. (AC)
    femur length to abdominal c.
    fetal abdominal c.
    c. of fetal head
    fetal head c.
    fetal thoracic c.
    head c. (HC)
    thoracic c. (TC)
circumferential
    c. cartilage
    c. echo-dense layer
    c. extremity coil
    c. fibrocartilage
    c. fracture
    c. lamella
    c. narrowing
    c. shortening
    c. thickening
    c. venous stenosis

circumflex
> c. branch
> c. coronary artery
> c. groove artery
> humeral c.
> left c. (LCF, LCX)
> c. retroesophageal arch
> c. system
> c. vein
> c. vessel

circummarginate placenta
circummesencephalic cistern
circumscribed
> c. edema
> c. infiltrate
> c. lesion
> c. margin
> c. mass
> c. nodule
> c. pleurisy

circumscripta
> calcinosis c.
> myositis ossificans c.
> osteoporosis c.

circumscript aneurysm
circumvallate papilla
circumventricular organ
cirrhosis
> acholangic biliary c.
> acute juvenile c.
> alcoholic c. (AC)
> atrophic c.
> biliary c.
> Budd c.
> calculous c.
> cardiac c.
> Charcot c.
> cholangitic biliary c.
> congestive c.
> Cruveilhier-Baumgarten c.
> cryptogenic c.
> decompensated alcoholic c.
> diffuse c.
> end-stage c.
> fatty c.
> focal biliary c.
> frank c.
> glabrous c.
> Hanot c.
> hepatic c.
> hypertrophic c.
> Indian childhood c.

> juvenile c.
> liver c.
> macrolobular c.
> medionodular c.
> metabolic c.
> microlobular c.
> micronodular c.
> multilobular c.
> nutritional c.
> obstructive biliary c.
> periportal c.
> pipestem c.
> porta c.
> posthepatic c.
> postnecrotic c.
> primary biliary c.
> progressive familial c.
> pulmonary c.
> secondary biliary c.
> septal c.
> stasis c.
> Todd c.
> toxic c.
> unilobular c.
> vascular c.

cirrhosis-related fibrosis
cirrhotic
> c. gastritis
> c. inflammation
> c. liver
> c. nodule

cirsoid
> c. aneurysm
> c. placenta

cistern
> ambient wing of the
>   quadrigeminal c.
> anterior interhemispheric c.
> basal arachnoid c.
> basilar c.
> carotid c.
> cerebellomedullary c.
> cerebellopontine c.
> c. of chiasma
> chiasmatic c.
> chyle c.
> circummesencephalic c.
> crural c.
> c. effacement
> great c.
> increased basilar c.
> c. indium

C

NOTES

cistern *(continued)*
>> interpeduncular c. (IPC)
>> c. isotope
>> c. of lamina terminalis
>> c. of lateral fossa of cerebrum
>> mesencephalic c.
>> opticochiasmatic c.
>> c. oxygen
>> parasellar c.
>> c. of Pecquet
>> perimesencephalic c.
>> pontine c.
>> posterior c.
>> prepontine c.
>> quadrigeminal plate c.
>> c. radioisotope
>> subarachnoid c.
>> suprasellar subarachnoid c.
>> sylvian c.
>> c. of Sylvius
>> terminal c.
>> trigeminal c.

cisterna
>> c. chyli
>> c. magna
>> c. magna effacement

cisternal
>> c. herniation
>> c. puncture
>> c. space

cisternogram
>> CT c.
>> metrizamide CT c.

cisternography
>> air c.
>> cerebellopontine c.
>> computed tomography c.
>> CT c.
>> gas CT c.
>> c. imaging
>> isotopic c.
>> Katzman infusion of radionuclide c.
>> metrizamide computed tomography c. (MCTC)
>> oxygen c.
>> Pantopaque c.
>> radioisotope c.
>> radionuclide c.

cisternomyelography

citrate
>> clomiphene c.
>> fentanyl c.
>> ferrous c.
>> gallium-67 c.
>> gallium Ga 57 c.
>> manganese c.

CIVI
>> continuous intravenous infusion

Civinini
>> C. canal
>> C. ligament

CJD
>> Creutzfeldt-Jakob disease

CKG
>> cardiokymography
>> CKG imaging

C-labeled
>> ^{11}C-labeled cocaine
>> ^{11}C-labeled cocaine imaging agent
>> ^{11}C-labeled fatty acid imaging agent

^{11}C-labeled

Clado
>> C. band
>> C. ligament
>> C. point

clamshell double umbrella occluder

Clariscan imaging agent

Clarke
>> C. arch angle
>> C. column

Clarke-Hadefield syndrome

Clark malignant melanoma classification

Clarkson scatter-summation algorithm

classical
>> c. nephroblastoma
>> c. osteosarcoma
>> c. scattering

classic carpal tunnel view

classification
>> AAOS acetabular abnormalities c.
>> acromioclavicular injury c.
>> Aitken acromioclavicular injury c.
>> AJCC-UICC mediastinal lymph node c.
>> Allman c.
>> Altman c.
>> American Spinal Cord Injury Association c.
>> Amstutz c.
>> anatomic brain c.
>> Ann Arbor c.
>> anular tear c.
>> AO ankle fracture c.
>> AO-Danis-Weber ankle fracture c.
>> Arco c.
>> Bayne c.
>> Berndt-Hardy talar dome c.
>> Bigliani c.
>> Bleck metatarsus adductus c.
>> Bosniak c.
>> Boyd-Griffin trochanteric fracture c.
>> brain anatomy c.

brain tumor c.
Breslow c.
Broders tumor index c.
Brooker periarticular heterotopic
  ossification c.
Butcher staging c.
Caldwell-Moloy c.
Canale-Kelly talar neck fracture c.
Carnesale-Stewart-Barnes hip
  dislocation c.
Cedell-Magnusson arthritis c.
cerebral malformation c.
Child-Pugh c.
Clark malignant melanoma c.
CNS anomaly c.
CNS tumor c.
Colonna hip fracture c.
congenital heart disease c.
Copeland-Kavat metatarsophalangeal
  dislocation c.
Couinaud c.
Danis-Weber ankle fracture c.
D'Antonio acetabular c.
DeBakey aortic c.
Delbet hip fracture c.
Denis c.
Dickhaut-DeLee discoid meniscus c.
distance-based block c.
Essex-Lopresti calcaneal fracture c.
Evans intertrochanteric fracture c.
Fielding-Magliato subtrochanteric
  fracture c.
fracture c.
Fränkel spinal cord injury c.
Freeman calcaneal fracture c.
Fries score for rheumatoid
  arthritis c.
Frykman distal radius fracture c.
Galassi arachnoidal cyst c.
Garden femoral neck fracture c.
Gawkins talar neck fracture c.
Gertzbein seatbelt injury c.
Glasscock-Jackson c.
Goldsmith & Woodburne c.
Graf hip dysplasia c.
Grantham femur fracture c.
Gumley seatbelt injury c.
Gustilo-Anderson tibial plafond
  fracture c.
Hahn-Steinthal capitellum
  fracture c.
Hansen fracture c.

Hardy-Clapham sesamoid c.
Herbert-Fisher fracture c.
Hinchey c.
Hohl tibial condylar fracture c.
Holdsworth spinal fracture c.
Hughston Clinic injury c.
Hunt-Kosnik c.
Hyams grading of
  esthesioneuroblastoma c.
Jahss dislocation c.
Jones c.
Judet epiphyseal fracture c.
Kalamchi-Dawe congenital tibial
  deficiency c.
Kazangia and Converse facial
  fracture c.
Kernohan brain tumor c.
Key-Conwell pelvic fracture c.
Kiel non-Hodgkin lymphoma c.
Kilfoyle condylar fracture c.
Kimura c.
King-Moe c.
Kistler subarachnoid hemorrhage c.
Klatskin tumor c.
Kocher-Lorenz capitellum
  fracture c.
Kostuik-Errico spinal stability c.
Kyle fracture c.
Lauge-Hansen ankle fracture c.
Mason radial fracture c.
Mazur ankle evaluation c.
McCabe-Fletcher c.
McLain-Weinstein spinal tumor c.
Melone distal radius fracture c.
Merland perimedullary arteriovenous
  fistula c.
Meyer-McKeever tibial fracture c.
Michels c.
Milch elbow fracture c.
Mink-Deutsch c.
Mitchell c.
Modic disk abnormality c.
mulberry-type c.
Müller humerus fracture c.
multiaxial c.
Neer-Horowitz humerus fracture c.
Neviaser frozen shoulder c.
Newman radial fracture c.
Nurick spondylosis c.
NYHA congestive heart failure c.
O'Brien radial fracture c.
Ogden epiphyseal fracture c.

NOTES

classification *(continued)*
Olerud and Molander fracture c.
osteoarthritis grading c.
Ovadia-Beals tibial plafond
    fracture c.
Papile c.
Pauwel femoral neck fracture c.
percentage c.
pineal gland tumor c.
Pipkin femoral fracture c.
pneumoconiosis c.
Poland epiphyseal fracture c.
Potter c.
primary CNS tumor c.
Rappaport c.
Ratliff avascular necrosis c.
REAL c.
REAL c.
rickets c.
Riemann c.
Riordan club hand c.
Riseborough-Radin intercondylar
    fracture c.
Robson staging c.
Rockwood acromioclavicular
    injury c.
Rowe calcaneal fracture c.
Rowe-Lowell fracture-dislocation c.
Ruedi-Allgower tibial plafond
    fracture c.
Runyon c.
Russell-Rubinstein cerebrovascular
    malformation c.
Salter-Harris growth plate injury c.
Salter-Harris-Rang epiphyseal
    fracture c.
Schatzker fracture c.
Shelton femur fracture c.
Smith sesamoid position c.
Snyder c.
soft tissue lesion c.
Sorbie calcaneal fracture c.
Stanford aortic dissection c.
Steinberg c.
Steinbrocker rheumatoid arthritis c.
Steinert epiphyseal fracture c.
Steward-Milford fracture c.
talocalcaneal index c.
Thompson-Epstein femoral
    fracture c.
Todani c.
Tronzo intertrochanteric fracture c.
Trunkey fracture c.
Vostal radial fracture c.
Watanabe discoid meniscus c.
Watson-Jones tibial tubercle
    avulsion fracture c.

Werner c.
WHO c.
Wiberg patellar types c.
Wilkins radial fracture c.
Winquist-Hansen femoral fracture c.
Wiseman c.
Wolfe breast carcinoma c.
Working Formulation c.
World Health Organization c.
clasticus
conus c.
Claude syndrome
claudication of jaw
Clauss
C. assay
C. method
claustrum, pl. **claustra**
clavicle
absence of outer end of c.
penciling of the distal c.
clavicular
c. birth fracture
c. facet
c. head of sternocleidomastoid
c. notch
c. osteitis condensans
clavipectoral
c. fascia
c. triangle
clavus
interdigital c.
clawfoot deformity
clawhand deformity
clawtoe deformity
clay
c. pipe carcinoma
c. shoveler's fracture
Claybrook sign
CLD
central lung distance
clean shadow
cleansing enema
clear
c. cell neoplasm of ovary
c. cell sarcoma
enemas until c.
c. zone
clearance
c. curve
c. half-time
isotope c.
multicompartment c.
multiple-sample c.
c. phase ventilation scan
radioactive xenon c.
radioaerosol c.

renal c.
single-sample c.
ClearView CO$_2$ laser
cleavage
c. cavity
c. fracture
plane of c.
c. tear
cleaved cell lymphoma
Cleaves
C. method
C. position
cleaving
plaque c.
cleft
anal c.
c. chorda
coronal c.
c. face syndrome
facial c.
first visceral c.
full-thickness c.
gill c.
Hahn c.
intergluteal c.
interinnominoabdominal c.
intranuclear c.
intravertebral body vacuum c.
lateral facial c.
median facial c.
median lip c.
meniscal c.
midline longitudinal pontine c.
c. mitral valve
neural arch c.
pudendal c.
radiolucent c.
retrosomatic c.
spinal cord c.
c. spine
splenic c.
synaptic c.
vacuum c.
ventricular c.
c. vertebra
cleidocranial
c. dysostosis
c. dysplasia
Cleland ligament
Clements-Nakayama position
clenched fist view
Cleopatra view

Clerc-Levy-Cristico
C.-L.-C. syndrome
climbing fiber
clinical
c. complete response
c. correlation
c. feature
c. parameter
c. partial response
c. target volume (CTV)
clinicopathological analysis
clinodactyly
factitious c.
traumatic c.
clinoid
c. aneurysm
c. ligament
c. process
clinoparietal line
clip
aneurysmal c.
cerebrovascular aneurysmal c.
c. ligation of aneurysm
sternal c.
clip-editing plane
clipping
c. of aneurysm
ureteric c.
clival meningioma
clivus, pl. **clivi**
Blumenbach c.
c. chordoma
c. meningioma tumor
c. metastasis
clivus-canal angle
CLM
capillary-lymphatic malformation
cloaca, pl. **cloacae**
bone formation c.
cloacal
c. anomaly
c. exstrophy
c. formation
c. malformation
c. plate
cloaking
perivascular c.
perosteal c.
clock cycle
clockwise whirlpool sign
clomiphene citrate

NOTES

C

cloning
    subtraction c.
clonogen number
C loop
    duodenal C l.
Cloquet
    C. canal
    C. fascia
    hyaloid canal of C.
    C. inguinal lymph node
    C. ligament
close apposition
closed
    c. conducting loop
    c. core transformer
    c. dislocation
    c. exstrophy
    c. flap amputation
    c. fontanelle
    c. fracture
    c. head injury (CHI)
    c. pneumothorax
    c. reduction
    c. spinal dysraphism
closed-break fracture
closed-fist configuration
closed-loop intestinal obstruction
closed-mouth view
close-space thin-section scanning
close-up view
closing
    c. capacity
    c. slope
    c. velocity
    c. volume
closure
    abrupt vessel c.
    aortic c. (AC)
    c. device
    growth center c.
    incomplete c.
    native aortic valve c.
    physeal c.
    premature valve c.
    sandwich patch c.
    Stanford type B dissection c.
    threatened vessel c.
    tricuspid valve c.
    valve c.
    velopharyngeal c.
clot
    agonal c.
    autologous blood c.
    blood c.
    internal c.
    intramural c.
    isoechoic c.

    c. maceration
    marantic c.
    mural c.
    passive c.
    plastic c.
    preformed c.
    c. removal by laser thrombolysis
    c. retraction
    subarachnoid c.
    subdural c.
clot-filled lumen
clothesline injury
clothing artifact
cloud
    c. chamber
    electron c.
clouding
    alveolar c.
cloudy
    c. sinus
    c. swelling of heart
cloverleaf
    c. deformity
    c. plate
    c. skull
cloverleaf-shaped lumen
Cloward bone graft
clubbed
    c. finger
    c. penis
clubbing
    caliceal c.
clubfoot deformity
clubhand deformity
club-shaped conus
cluneal nerve
cluster
    activated voxel c.
    c. of differentiation (CD)
    grape-like c.
    c. of grapes lung
    K-means c.
    microcalcification c.
    c. of radiolucent area (CORLA)
clustered
    c. calcification
    c. data
clustering algorithm
Clutton painful joint
clysis
Clysodrast
CM
    contrast medium
        iodinated intravascular C.
cm
    centimeter
        3/6-cm 3D GDC

2-mm/3-cm coil
2-mm/6-cm coil
CMC
carpometacarpal joint
CMD
cerebromacular degeneration
corticomedullary differentiation
[11]C-methionine
[11]C-m. PET scan
[11]C-m. positron emission
tomography (MET-PET)
CMF
chondromyxoid fibroma
CMI
chronic mesenteric ischemia
CMJ
corticomedullary junction
CMJ imaging
CMOS
complementary metal oxide
semiconductor
CMR
congenital mitral regurgitation
CMRO$_2$
cerebral metabolic rate of oxygen
CMRP
cervical magnetic resonance
phlebography
CMS
compliance matching stent
CMT
Charcot-Marie-Tooth
CMV encephalitis
CNR, C/N
contrast-to-noise ratio
CNS
central nervous system
CNS amyloidosis
CNS anomaly classification
CNS cortical hamartoma
CNS empyema
CNS fibromuscular dysplasia
CNS ghost tumor
CNS juvenile pilocytic astrocytoma
CNS multifocal tumor
CNS teratoma
CNS toxoplasmosis
CNS tumor classification
CNV
choroidal neovascularization
CO
cardiac output

CO$_2$
carbon dioxide
CO_2 angiography
CO_2 cylinder
CO_2 generator
CO_2 insufflation
CO_2 laser
CO_2 retention
Co
cobalt
[57]Co
cobalt-57
[58]Co
cobalt-58
[60]Co
cobalt-60
COACH syndrome
coadaptation
coagulation
disseminated intravascular c. (DIC)
microwave tumor c.
c. necrosis
coagulator
argon beam c. (ABC)
coagulopathy
intravascular consumption c.
coal
c. macule
c. miner's lung
c. tar
c. worker's lung
c. worker's pneumoconiosis (CWP)
coalesce
coalescence
coalescent granuloma
coalition
bony c.
calcaneonavicular c.
carpal c.
fibrous c.
intercarpal c.
lunate-triquetral c.
Minaar classification of c.
osseous c.
talocalcaneal c.
target c.
tarsal c.
c. view
coanalgesic
coaptation point
coapted leaflet

NOTES

coarctation
  abdominal aortic c.
  adult c.
  c. of aorta
  aortic c.
  asymptomatic c.
  atypical subisthmic c.
  congenital isthmic c.
  infantile c.
  isthmic c.
  juxtaductal aortic c.
  localized c.
  postductal aortic c.
  preductal aortic c.
  reversed c.
  c. syndrome
  thoracic aortic c.
coarcted segment
coarse
  c. bronchovascular marking
  c. calcification
  c. injection
  c. linear opacity
  c. lung reticulation
  c. microcalcification
  c. nodularity
  c. pattern
  c. reticular opacity
coarsening
coat hanger osteochondroma
coating of aneurysm
Coats disease
coaxial
  c. micropuncture needle set
  c. sheath cut-biopsy needle
  c. steering
coaxially
  pass c.
cobalt (Co)
  c. alloy stent
  c. 60 beam therapy unit
  c. megavoltage machine
  c. pneumopathy
  radioactive c.
  c. radioactive source
cobalt-57 (^{57}Co)
cobalt-58 (^{58}Co)
cobalt-60 (^{60}Co)
  c. beam
  c. gamma knife radiosurgical
    treatment
**cobalt-chromium-molybdenum alloy
  metal implant**
**cobalt-chromium-tungsten-nickel alloy
  metal implant**
Cobb
  C. measurement

  C. measurement of scoliosis
  C. method
  C. method of measuring kyphosis
  C. scoliosis angle
  C. syndrome
cobbler's chest
cobblestone
  c. appearance
  c. appearance of bile duct
  c. appearance of the colon
  c. appearance duodenum
  c. appearance eosinophilic
    gastroenteritis
  c. appearance esophagus
  c. appearance lymphoma
  c. appearance stomach
  c. degeneration
  c. ileum
  c. lissencephaly
  c. mucosa
  c. pattern
  c. sign
cobblestoning
Cobra 2 catheter
cobra-head
  c.-h. anastomosis
  c.-h. appearance
  c.-h. effect
  c.-h. ureter
cobra-shaped catheter
cobweb
  c. appearance
  c. pattern
cocaine
  ^{11}C-labeled c.
coccidioidoma
coccidioidomycosis
  bone c.
  disseminated c.
  latent c.
  lung c.
  Posadas-Wernicke c.
  primary c.
  progressive c.
  secondary c.
coccygeal
  c. appendage
  c. body
  c. bone
  c. ganglion
  c. gland
  c. ligament
  c. plexus
  c. sinus
  c. spine
  c. vertebra

c. vestige
c. whorl
coccygeopubic diameter
coccygeus
vortex c.
coccyx, pl. **coccyges**
c. bone
c. fracture
coccyx
cochlea, pl. **cochleae**
c. aplasia
single-cavity c.
cochleae
apertura externa canaliculi c.
cochlear
c. anatomy
c. aqueduct
c. canal
c. canaliculus
c. duct
c. implant
c. labyrinth
c. lesion
c. nerve
c. otosclerosis
c. recess
c. root
cochleariform process
cochlearis
stria vascularis ductus c.
cochleate uterus
cochleitis
calcific c.
ossifying c.
Cockayne syndrome
cocking injury
cock-robin position
cockscomb
c. appearance
c. appearance of cervix
c. papilloma
cock-up deformity
Co-Cr-Mo alloy metal implant
Co-Cr-W-Ni alloy implant metal
cocurrent flow-related enhancement
COD
computerized optical densitometry
CoDe
coincidence detection
Code and Carlson radiograph
coded-aperture imaging
coded-image aperture

coder
Chen-Smith image c.
ICS c.
improved c. (ICS)
codfish
c. deformity
c. vertebra
Codivilla extension
Codman
C. angle
C. Medos programmable valve
C. sign
C. triangle
C. tumor
codominant
c. circulation
c. vessel
coefficient
absorption c.
apparent diffusion c. (ADC)
attenuation c.
attenuation-correction c.
binary similarity c.
c. conversion
correlation c.
curve fit c.
diffusion c.
effective mass attenuation c.
Fourier c.
linear absorption c.
linear attenuation c.
mass absorption c.
mass attenuation c.
Ostwald solubility c. (Λ)
partition c.
Pearson correlation c.
reflection c.
Spearman correlation c.
stiffness c.
uniform attenuation c.
c. of variation (c.v.)
viscosity c.
coeur en sabot
coexistent
c. cavity
c. intravoxel fat and water
coffee
c. grounds material
c. worker's lung
coffee-bean appearance
coffin bone
Cogan lid twitch sign

NOTES

cognitive
    c. fMRI
    c. functional MR imaging
cogwheel sign
coherence
    multiple quantum c.
    phase c.
coherent
    C. CO2 surgical laser
    c. scattering
    steady-state c.
    C. UltraPulse 5000C laser
coil
    aneurysmal c.
    c. array
    bilateral breast c.
    bird-cage head c.
    body c.
    breast c.
    butterfly c.
    catheter-delivered platinum c.
    circularly polarized c.
    circular polarized volume head c.
    circumferential extremity c.
    c. closure of coronary artery
      fistula
    collagen-filled interlocking
      detachable c.
    conventional head c.
    coupled array c.
    crossed c.
    custom-curved c.
    DCS-10, DCS-18 mechanically
      detachable platinum c.
    dedicated phased-array c.
    c. delivery
    c. deposition
    detachable platinum c.
    detector c.
    double breast c.
    electrically detachable c.
    embedding of stent c.
    c. embolization
    endoanal c.
    endoesophageal MRI c.
    endorectal c.
    endoscopic quadrature
      radiofrequency c.
    endovaginal c.
    endovascular c.
    extremity c.
    fat-suppressed body c.
    field-profiling c.
    flexible radiofrequency c.
    flexible surface c.
    four element phased array c.
    free fibered c.

GDC-10 soft c.
Gianturco occlusion c.
Gianturco-Wallace-Anderson c.
Gianturco-Wallace-Chuang c.
Gianturco wool-tufted wire c.
Golay c.
gonion gradient c.
Gore 1.5T torso array MRI
  surface c.
gradient sheet c.
Guglielmi detachable c. (GDC)
head c.
Helmholtz c.
high-speed gradient c.
immediately detachable c.
interlocking detachable c. (IDC)
c.'s of intestine
intrarectal c.
intravascular c.
in vitro evaluation of c.
linearly polarized c.
liver c.
c. loading
local c.
local gradient c.
Maxwell c.
mechanically detachable platinum c.
Medrad Mrinnervu endorectal colon
  probe c.
c. migration
2-mm/3-cm c.
2-mm/6-cm c.
3 mm × 6 cm interlocking
  detachable c.
4 mm × 8 cm interlocking
  detachable c.
modified bird-cage c.
MRCP using HASTE with a
  phased array c.
multiply tuned c.
neck c.
opposed loop-pair quadrature
  NMR c.
orthogonal radiofrequency c.
parallel data acquisition c.
pelvic phased-array c.
phased-array surface c.
phased-array torso c.
planar circular c.
platinum c.
posterior neck surface c.
c. protrusion
proximal c.
quadrature body c.
quadrature cervical spine c.
quadrature radiofrequency
  receiver c.

quadrature terminal latency
  surface c.
quadrature transmit/receive head c.
radiofrequency c.
radiofrequency transmitter-receiver c.
receive-only circular surface c.
receiver c.
RF c.
right ventricular c.
saddle c.
c. selection
send-receive phased-array
  extremity c.
sensing c.
c. sensitive encoding
shielded gradient c.
shim c.
shoulder surface c.
solenoid surface c.
stainless steel c.
steel c.
Stylet esophageal MRI c.
surface c.
Surgi-Vision MRI c.
switchable c.
three-axis gradient c.
thrombogenic c.
Tornado c.
torso phased-array c. (TPAC)
transmit-receive c.
transmitter c.
two-element phased-array c.
c. vascular stent
volume c.
whole-volume c.
wool c.
wrist quadrature phased-array
  surface c.
2 (x) 3, 4, 5, 6 fibered Guglielmi
  detachable c.

coiled
  c. spring appearance
  c. spring pattern
  c. spring sign

coiling
  c. of anastomosis
  c. of aneurysm

coil-to-vessel diameter

coin
  c. artifact
  fracture en c.
  c. lesion

c. lesion of lung
c. test

coincidence
  c. circuit
  counting c.
  c. detection (CD, CoDe)
  c. detection mode
  c. detection positron emission
    tomography
  c. detection scan
  c. event
  c. imaging
  c. imaging scanner
  loss c.
  sum peak c.

coincidence-resolving window
coincidence-summing correction
coin-on-edge vertebra
Coiter muscle
Colapinto
  C. needle
  C. sheath

Colbert method
COLD
  chronic obstructive lung disease

cold
  c. breast abscess
  c. defect
  c. defect renal scintigraphy
  c. lesion
  c. nodule thyroid
  c. quartz lamp germicidal lamp
  c. spine abscess
  c. spot
  c. spot myocardial imaging
  c. thyroid nodule

colectasia
coli
  elastin deposition in taeniae c.
  familial polyposis c.
  haustra c.
  melanosis c.
  pneumatosis c.

colic
  c. artery
  biliary c.
  c. impression
  c. omentum
  c. plexus
  renal c.
  c. sphincter

NOTES

colic *(continued)*
 c. surface
 c. vein
colitis
 chronic ulcerative c. (CUC)
 Crohn c.
 focal c.
 fulminant c.
 fulminating ulcerative c.
 granulomatous transmural c.
 ischemic c.
 myxomembranous c.
 c. polyposa
 pseudomembranous c.
 radiation-induced c.
 regional c.
 single-stripe c. (SSC)
 transmural c.
 ulcerative c. (UC)
 c. ulcerosa gravis
collagen
 c. defect type I, II
 c. fiber separation
 c. fibril
 c. fragmentation
 c. plug
 c. tissue proliferation
collagen-filled interlocking detachable coil
collagenosis
 mediastinal c.
collagenous
 c. perivascular ala
 c. structure
 c. tissue
collapse
 acinar c.
 acute vertebral c.
 alveolar c.
 c. cavitation
 circulation c.
 jugular venous pressure c.
 scapholunate advanced c. (SLAC)
 scapholunate arthritic c.
 subchondral c.
 vertebral body c.
collapsed
 c. distal ileum
 c. inferior vena cava
 c. lobe
 c. lung
 c. lung field
 c. subpectoral implant
collapsing cord sign
collar
 implant c.
 periosteal bone c.

 periportal c.
 c. sign
collarbone
collar-button
 c.-b. abscess
 c.-b. appearance
 c.-b. chest lesion
 c.-b. ulcer
collateral
 c. arcade
 arterial c.
 c. blood flow
 c. blood supply
 c. branch
 c. circulation in compression of artery
 developed c.
 c. edema
 c. eminence
 c. fissure
 gastroesophageal c.
 c. hyperemia
 c. ligament
 c. ligament of knee
 c. mesenteric circulation
 portosystemic c.
 c. sulcus
 c. system
 tributary c.
 c. trigone
 venous c.
 c. venous channel
 c. vessel
collateralization
collecting
 c. system
 c. system atony
 c. system filling defect
 c. system opacification
 c. tube
 c. tubule
 c. venous pouch
 c. vessel
collection
 abdominal air c.
 air c.
 anechoic fluid c.
 complex fluid c.
 c. of contrast material
 crescentic c.
 EAA c.
 extraalveolar air c.
 extraaxial fluid c.
 extracerebral fluid c.
 fluid c.
 gas c.
 hypoechoic fluid c.

intratendinous fluid c.
list mode data c.
mottled gas c.
pancreatic fluid c.
periarticular fluid c.
pericholecystic fluid c.
perifascial fluid-like c.
perinephric fluid c.
peripancreatic fluid c.
pleural fluid c.
posttraumatic subcapsular hepatic
  fluid c.
retrocerebellar CSF c.
saccular c.

collective paramagnetism
Colles
C. fascia
C. fracture
C. ligament
Collet-Sicard syndrome
colli
fibromatosis c.
pterygium c.
vertebrae c.
collicular fracture
colliculus, pl. **colliculi**
anterior c.
brachium of c.
facial c.
fused colliculi
inferior c.
plicae colliculi
posterior c.
seminal c.
superior c.
Collier sign
collimated slice width
collimating system
collimation
c. CT
detector c.
dynamic multileaf c.
electronic c.
c. imaging
lead c.
narrow c.
c. scanning
c. scintillation detector
secondary c.
tertiary c.
c. width

collimator
APC-3, APC-4 c.
automatic c.
converging c.
converging-hole c.
diverging c.
dual-shaped c.
Eureka c.
c. exchange effect
fan-beam c.
focusing c.
heart-shaped c.
c. helmet
high-resolution c.
high-resolution, fan-beam c.
high-resolution multileaf c.
LEAP c.
LEUHR fan beam c.
LEUHR parallel-hole c.
Leur-par c.
long-bore c.
low-energy c.
medium-energy c.
Micro-Cast c.
multihole c.
multileaf c. (MLC)
multirod c.
parallel-hole medium sensitivity c.
pinhole c.
c. plugging pattern
c. scattering
single-hole c.
slant hole c.
slit c.
thick-septa c.
thin-septa c.
triple-leaf c.
ultrahigh-resolution, parallel-hole c.
colliquative necrosis
collision
c. detecting
elastic c.
c. tumor
collodiaphyseal
central c. (CCD)
colloid
c. adenocarcinoma
c. adenoma
^{198}Au c.
c. carcinoma
c. cyst
c. cystadenoma

NOTES

185

C

colloid *(continued)*
    c. cystic tumor
    c. cyst of third ventricle
    c. degeneration
    c. goiter
    minimicroaggregated albumin c.
    c. oncotic pressure (COP)
    radioactive c.
    radiogold c.
    c. shift
    c. shift on scan
    sulfur c.
    ^{99m}Tc sulfur c.
    TechneScan Sulfur C.
    technetium-99m antimony
      trisulfide c.
    technetium-99m minimicroaggregated
      albumin c.
    technetium-sulfur c.
colloidal
    c. brain cyst
    c. chromic phosphorus
    c. sulfur
    c. suspension
colobomatous cyst
colocolic
    c. anastomosis
    c. fistula
    c. intussusception
colocutaneous fistula
colography
    CT c.
Colombo count
colon
    accessory sign c.
    angiodysplasia of c.
    anterior band of c.
    ascending c.
    barium-filled c.
    burned-out c.
    c. carcinoma
    carpet lesion of c.
    cathartic c.
    cobblestone appearance of the c.
    coned-down appearance of c.
    Crohn disease of c.
    c. cutoff sign
    c. cyst duplication
    descending c.
    distal c.
    double-tracking c.
    c. duplication
    epithelial c.
    fecal-filled c.
    free band of c.
    giant c.

hepatodiaphragmatic interposition
    of c. (HDIC)
hypoganglionosis of c.
iliac c.
inflammation of c.
intramural air in c.
irritable c.
jejunization of c.
c. kinking
knuckle of c.
lateral reflection of c.
left c.
c. margin
mesosigmoid c.
midsigmoid c.
pelvic c.
perisigmoid c.
proximal c.
c. pseudostricture
right c.
sigmoid c.
spastic c.
c. stenting
thumbprinting appearance of the c.
transverse c.
colonic
    c. activity
    c. adenoma
    c. adenomatous polyp
    c. air
    c. angiodysplasia
    c. apple-core lesion
    c. atresia
    c. carpet lesion
    c. dilatation
    c. distention
    c. diverticular hemorrhage
    c. diverticulitis
    c. diverticulosis
    c. diverticulum
    c. duplication cyst
    c. evacuation
    c. filling defect
    c. fistula
    c. flexure
    c. gas composition
    c. hamartomatous polyp
    c. haustra
    c. ileus
    c. interposition
    c. involvement of endometriosis
    c. lead-pipe appearance
    c. loop
    c. motility
    c. mucosal excretion
    c. myenteric plexus
    c. narrowing

c. necrosis
c. neoplasm
c. obstruction
c. perforation
c. pit
c. pseudoobstruction
c. saddle lesion
c. spasm
c. stricture
c. transit time
c. ulcer
c. urticaria pattern
c. varix
c. volvulus

colonization
saprophytic c.

Colonna hip fracture classification

colonography
bile-tagged 3D magnetic resonance c.
computed tomographic c. (CTC)
CT c.
MR c.
Virtual CT c.
volume-rendered CT c.

colonoscope
Olympus CF-1T100L c.
Olympus CF-200Z c.

colonoscopy
virtual c.

colony-forming unit

coloproctitis

coloptosis

color
c. amplitude imaging
c. Doppler (CD)
c. Doppler imaging (CDI)
c. Doppler recording
c. Doppler signal
c. Doppler sonography (CDS)
c. Doppler twinkling artifact
c. Doppler ultrasound (CDUS)
c. duplex interrogation
c. duplex ultrasound
c. encoded brain MR imaging
c. gain
c. kinesis
c. power transcranial Doppler sonography
c. power transcranial Doppler ultrasound
c. space conversion

c. space interpolation
c. space interpolator
c. spectrum
c. velocity imaging
c. void

color-coded
c.-c. Doppler flow imaging (CDFI)
c.-c. duplex sonography
c.-c. duplex ultrasound
c.-c. pulmonary blood flow imaging
c.-c. real-time sonography
c.-c. real-time ultrasound

colorectal (CR)
c. adenoma
c. anastomosis
c. cancer endoscopy
c. carcinoid
c. carcinoma
c. duplication
c. hemorrhage
c. lymphoma
c. mucosa
c. polyp

color-flame scale

color-flow
c.-f. Doppler (CFD)
c.-f. Doppler imaging
c.-f. Doppler real-time 2D blood flow imaging
c.-f. Doppler sonography
c.-f. duplex imaging
c.-f. duplex scan
c.-f. imaging Doppler echocardiography
c.-f. mapping

color-flow imaging (CFI)

colorimetric
c. color reproduction
c. test

color-scale image

coloscopy
endocervical canal c.

colosigmoid resection

colostogram
augmented pressure c.

colostomy
barium enema through c.
barium injection through c.
fecal diversion c.

colovaginal fistula

colovesical fistula

NOTES

C

colpocele
colpocephaly
colpoptosis
colposcopy
colpostat applicator
column
    anal c.
    anterior gray c.
    c. of Bertin
    branchial efferent c.
    c. of Burdach
    Clarke c.
    contrast medium c.
    corrugated air c.
    dye c.
    extraction c.
    c. extraction method
    Gowers c.
    head of barium c.
    intermediolateral gray c.
    Lissauer c.
    c. mode sinogram image
    c. of Morgagni
    Quick Spin Sephadex G-50 c.
    renal c.
    thoracolumbar spine c.
    variceal c.
    vertebral c.
    weighted spin-echo c.
columnar-lined esophagus
columnar metaphysis
columnization of contrast material
column-mode sinogram imaging
Colyte bowel preparation
Combidex MRI contrast agent
combination
    c. flow and pressure load
    molybdenum-molybdenum target
      filter c. (Mo-Mo)
    molybdenum-rhodium target filter c.
      (Mo-Rh)
    rhodium-rhodium target filter c.
      (Rh-Rh)
    target-filter c.
combined
    c. anatomic registration
    c. dynamic 2D and bolus-chase
      3D acquisitions
    c. flexion-distraction injury and
      burst fracture
    c. leukocyte-marrow imaging
    c. multisection diffuse-weighted and
      hemodynamically weighted echo-
      planar MR
    c. Myoscint/thallium imaging
    c. pregnancy
    c. radial-ulnar-humeral fracture

    c. ^{99m}Tc-DMSA and ^{99m}Tc-DTPA
      scanning
    c. thallium-Tc-HMPAO imaging
    c. transmission-emission scintiphoto
    c. ventilation-perfusion scintigraphy
comb sign
comedo
    c. necrosis
    c. pattern
comedo-basal cell carcinoma
comedomastitis
comedo-type DCIS
comet-tail
    c.-t. artifact
    c.-t. artifact gallbladder
    c.-t. sign
comitans
    vena c.
comma-shaped
    c.-s. crus
    c.-s. duodenum
commemorative sign
commencement of vessel
comminuted
    c. bursting fracture
    c. intraarticular fracture
    c. teardrop fracture
commission
commissural
    c. attachment
    c. chorda
    c. function
    c. leaflet
    c. point
commissure
    anterior c. (AC)
    anterior commissure-posterior c.
      (AC-PC)
    anteroseptal c.
    cerebral c.
    fused c.
    gray c.
    mitral valve c.
    posterior c. (PC)
    scalloped c.
    tectum c.
    temporal limb of the anterior c.
    valve c.
    vestigial c.
    white matter c.
common
    c. atrioventricular canal
    c. atrium
    c. basal vein
    c. bile duct (CBD)
    c. bile duct bifurcation
    c. bile duct diverticulum

c. bile duct exploration (CBDE)
c. bile duct obstruction
c. bile duct spontaneous perforation
c. bile duct stone
c. bile duct stricture
c. bundle
c. cardinal vein
c. carotid artery (CCA)
c. carotid artery bifurcation
c. carotid plexus
c. cavity phenomenon
c. duct cholangiogram
c. duct dilatation
c. dural sac
c. extensor tendinosis
c. facial vein
c. femoral artery
c. femoral vein
c. gall duct
c. gateway interface (CGI)
c. hepatic artery
c. hepatic duct (CHD)
c. iliac artery
c. iliac lymph node
c. peroneal artery
c. pulmonary vein stenosis
c. synovial flexor sheath
c. tendinous ring
c. tendon

commotio cerebri
commune
centrum c.
crus c.
mesenterium c.
persistent ostium atrioventriculare c.

communicating
c. artery
c. artery aneurysm
c. cavernous ectasia
c. cyst
c. fistula
c. hydrocephalus
c. syringomyelia
c. vein
c. vein incompetence

communication
cholangiovenous c.
fistulous gas c.
interatrial c.
macrofistulous arteriovenous c.

Medical Ultrasound Three-Dimensional Portable Advanced C.'s (MUSTPAC)
peritoneopleural c.
pleuroperitoneal c.

communis
extensor digitorum c. (EDC)

community-acquired pneumonia
Comolli sign
compact
c. bone
c. island
c. osteoma

companion
c. lymph node
c. shadow
c. vein

comparative value
comparison
beam quality c.
c. film
histopathologic c.
c. view
yield c.

compartment
anterior mediastinal c.
anterior tibial c.
deep posterior c.
distal radioulnar joint c.
extensor c.
extracellular c.
extradural c.
extravascular c.
fifth c.
fourth c.
iliopsoas c.
infracolic c.
infratentorial c.
lateral c.
medial c.
midcarpal c.
patellofemoral c.
peribronchovascular interstitial c.
perirenal c.
plantar c.
posterior c.
posterolateral c.
posteromedial c.
radiocarpal c.
sixth c.
superficial posterior c.
supracolic c.

NOTES

compartment *(continued)*
    supramesocolic c.
    c. syndrome
    vascular c.
    wrist extensor c.
compartmental
    c. analysis
    c. modeling
    c. radioimmunoglobulin therapy
compartmentalization
COMPASS stereotactic system
compensated
    c. composite spin-lock pulse
    c. congestive heart failure
    c. hydrocephalus
compensating filter
compensation
    attenuation c.
    cardiac gating c.
    depth c.
    flow c. (FC)
    gradient c.
    respiratory c.
    scatter c.
    second-order c.
    section-select flow c.
    supratentorial flow c.
    time-gain c.
    velocity c.
compensator
    multivane intensity modulation c. (MIMIC)
    scattering foil c.
    tissue deficit c.
compensatory
    c. atrophy
    c. capillary filling
    c. circulation
    c. cortical activation
    c. deformity
    c. emphysema
    c. enlargement
    c. enlargement of ventricle
    c. hyperplasia
    c. lobe hyperexpansion
    c. mechanism
    c. nodular kidney hypertrophy
    c. pause
competence of ureterovesical junction
competent ileocecal valve
competitive
    c. adsorption
    c. inhibition
    c. iron administration
complementary
    c. hypertrophy

    c. metal oxide semiconductor (CMOS)
    c. spatial modulation of magnetization (CSPAMM)
complete
    c. anatomic cure
    c. atrioventricular block (CAVB)
    c. atrioventricular dissociation
    c. bladder emptying
    c. bowel obstruction
    c. congenital heart block
    c. dislocation
    c. duplication
    c. fetal heart block
    c. fracture
    c. heart block (CHB)
    c. myelography
    c. nerve lesion
    c. occlusion
    c. placenta previa
    c. situs inversus
    c. small bowel malrotation
    c. stent expansion
    c. stress/rest study
    c. tear
    c. transposition of great artery
    c. vascular stasis
completed stroke
completion arteriography
complex, pl. **complexes**
    agyria pachygria c.
    amygdaloid nuclear c.
    c. anatomic relationship
    ankle joint c.
    c. anorectal fistula
    anterior communicating artery c.
    aperiodic c.
    apical c.
    arcuate c.
    atrial c.
    c. atrioventricular canal
    auricular c.
    basivertebral venous c.
    biceps-labral c.
    c. breast cyst
    Buford c.
    capsulolabral c.
    caudal pharyngeal c.
    chlormerodrin-cysteine c.
    choroidal-hippocampal fissure c.
    complex blocking c.
    compound dislocation c.
    c. conjugate
    Dandy-Walker c.
    discoligamentous c.
    Eisenmenger c.
    epispadia exstrophy c.

c. extraperitoneal rupture
fabellofibular c.
fibrocartilage c.
c. fluid collection
foot-ankle c.
frontonasal dysplasia
  malformation c.
gadolinium c.
gallium-transferrin c.
gastrocnemius-soleus c.
gastroduodenal artery c.
Ghon c.
Ghon-Sachs c.
growth plate c.
hallux sesamoid c.
hallux valgus-metatarsus primus
  varus c.
hindfoot joint c.
hippocampal-amygdaloid c.
hypoperfusion c.
hypovolemic c.
inferior glenohumeral ligament
  labral c. (IGLLC)
inverted-Y c.
Kirklin meniscal c.
labral capsular c.
labrum-ligament c.
lateral collateral ligament c.
ligamentous c.
limb-body wall c.
Lutembacher c.
mantle c.
mastoid c.
medial collateral ligament c.
  (MCLC)
mesenteric adenitis-ileitis c.
metal chelate c.
Michaelis c.
multiform ventricular c.
c. myxoma
nipple-areolar c.
ostiomeatal c.
outer anular/posterior longitudinal
  ligament c.
oxidized c.
pelvic mass c.
c. periosteal reaction
preintegration c.
primary c.
pulmonary sling c.
Ranke c.
renal sinus c.

respiratory chain c. I–VI
c. sclerosing lesion
sesamoid c.
shoulder labral capsular c.
c. simple fracture
sling ring c.
c. solid and cystic mass
subluxation c.
c. subtraction
superior olivary c.
syndesmotic ligament c.
tibiocalcaneal joint c.
transluminal coronary artery
  angioplasty c.
transposition c.
triangular fibrocartilaginous c.
  (TFCC)
VATER c.
ventricular premature c. (VPC)
vertebrobasilar c.
c. of vessel
VIII nerve c.
von Meyenburg c.
zygomaticomaxillary c.

compliance
craniospinal c.
lung c.
c. matching stent (CMS)
reduced pulmonary c.

complicated
c. dislocation
c. fracture
c. myoma
c. pneumoconiosis
c. renal cyst
c. scleroderma
c. silicosis

complication
air leak c.
nonfetal c.

component
anatomically graduated c. (AGC)
central hemorrhagic c.
cystic c.
dispersive c.
extensive intraductal c. (EIC)
extracellular matrix c.
frequency c.
irregularly layered astrocytic c.
irregularly layered neuronal c.
markedly accentuated pulmonic c.
mitral c.

NOTES

191

component *(continued)*
    obstructive c.
    secretory c.
    solid c.
composite
    c. aortic valve
    c. fracture
    c. pulse
    c. signal
composition
    colonic gas c.
    hydropic c.
    renal stone mineral c.
compound
    c. aneurysm
    c. comminuted fracture
    c. complex fracture
    c. dislocation
    c. dislocation complex
    lipophilic c.
    PET c.
    c. pregnancy
    c. presentation
    radiolabeled c.
    reference c.
    c. skull fracture
    thorium c.
    titanium c.
    unsaturated c.
compressed body
compressibility and phasicity study
compression
    aqueduct c.
    c. atrophy
    biliary tree c.
    brachial artery c.
    brachial plexus c.
    brainstem c.
    c. of breast
    cardiac c.
    cauda equina c.
    chamber c.
    chiasmal c.
    coned-down spot c.
    contrecoup c.
    cord c.
    c. device
    external pneumatic calf c.
    extrinsic bladder c.
    fingerprint image c.
    c. flexion injury
    c. fracture
    image c.
    interfragmental c.
    intrinsic c.
    irreversible c.
    lossless image data c.

    lossy image data c.
    magnification and spot c.
    manual c.
    multiplanar c.
    nerve root c.
    c. neuropathy
    neurovascular c.
    optic nerve c.
    orbital mass c.
    c. paddle
    pancake c.
    plaque c.
    c. plate
    c. plate and screw
    radicular c.
    c. ratio
    real-time c.
    root c.
    c. sonography
    spinal cord c.
    spot c.
    subchondral trabecular c.
    symptomatic metastatic spinal
     cord c.
    c. syndrome
    thermal c.
    c. ultrasonography
    ultrasound-guided
     pseudoaneurysm c.
    vascular esophageal c.
    vascular tracheal c.
    wavelet c.
compressive
    c. atelectasis
    c. edema
    c. hyperextension injury
compromise
    circulatory c.
    respiratory c.
    vascular c.
compromised
    c. flow
    c. pregnancy
    c. ventricular function
Compton
    C. coherent scattering densitometry
    C. edge
    C. effect
    C. electron
    C. interaction
    C. scattering
    C. scattering cross-section
    C. scattering photon
    C. suppression spectrometer
    C. suppression system
    C. wavelength

Compuscan
C. Hittman computerized electrocardioscanner
C. Hittman computerized imaging
computation
analog c.
computational anatomy
computed
c. dental radiography (CDR)
c. ejection fraction
c. myelography
c. radiography (CR)
c. radiology (CR)
c. tomographic angiography (CTA)
c. tomographic cholangiography
c. tomographic colonography (CTC)
c. tomographic cystography
c. tomographic dacryocystography
c. tomographic enteroclysis
c. tomography (CT)
c. tomography cisternography
c. tomography dose index (CTDI)
c. tomography during arterial portography (CTAP)
c. tomography fluoroscopy (CTF)
c. tomography-guided percutaneous radiofrequency denervation of the sacroiliac joint
c. tomography laser mammography (CTLM)
c. tomography scan
c. tomography with arterioportography (CTAP)
c. transmission tomography
c. transmission tomography imaging
computer
c. automated scan technology (CAST)
c. fusion imaging
image reconstruction c.
c. information system
c. method
c. strain-gauge plethysmography (CSGP)
c. subtraction technique
computer-aided
c.-a. detection (CAD)
c.-a. diagnosis (CAD)
c.-a. diagnosis scheme
c.-a. image analysis

computer-assisted
c.-a. blood background subtraction (CABBS)
c.-a. intracranial navigation
c.-a. joint motion analysis
c.-a. myelography (CAM)
c.-a. resection of cerebral arteriovenous malformation
c.-a. stereotactic resection
c.-a. volumetric stereotaxis
computer-controlled conformal radiation therapy (CCRT)
computer-generated
c.-g. artifact
c.-g. image
computerized
c. axial tomography (CAT)
c. cranial tomography
c. fluoroscopy
c. optical densitometry (COD)
c. radiography
c. radiotherapy
c. texture analysis of lung nodules and lung parenchyma
C. Thermal Imaging system
c. tomographic hepatic angiography (CTHA)
c. tomographic holography (CTH)
c. tomography guidance
c. tomography-guided needle biopsy
c. tomography/magnetic resonance (CT/MR)
c. transverse axial image
c. transverse axial tomography (CTAT)
conal
c. cyst
c. papillary muscle
c. septum
c. ventricular septal defect
concatenation of shadows
Concato disease
concave skull disk
concavity
posterior c.
concavoconvex
concealed
c. hemorrhage
c. penis
concentrated bile
concentration
deoxyhemoglobin c.

NOTES

concentration *(continued)*
    directional gradient c. (DGC)
    hypertensive contrast c.
    maximum permissible c.
    methylene diphosphonate (MDP) c.
    organ-specific c.
    Poisson distributed activity c.
    c. of radionuclide
    synaptic dopamine c.
    time-dependent xenon c.
    c. times time (C x T)
concentration-time curve
concentric
    c. anular tear
    c. atherosclerotic plaque
    c. circle technique
    c. contraction
    c. fibroma
    c. heart hypertrophy
    c. hernia
    c. herniation
    c. hourglass stenosis
    c. hypertrophic cardiomyopathy
    c. lamella
    c. lesion
    c. narrowing
    c. pantomography
    c. reduction
concentrica
    encephalitis periaxialis c.
concept
    gooseneck c.
    line integral c.
    no-threshold c.
    ring-of-bone c.
concertina pattern
concha, pl. **conchae**
    c. bullosa
    nasal c.
conchal
    c. cartilage
    c. crest
concomitant
    c. boost radiation therapy
    c. defect
    c. finding
    c. infarct
    c. pneumonia
    c. tracheal injury
concordance
    c. of MR finding
    radiologic-pathologic c.
    situs c.
concordant result
concretion
    bile c.
    fecal c.

concussion
    brain c.
    spinal c.
condensans
    clavicular osteitis c.
condition
    adnexal c.
    grade 0, 2 insonation c.
    insonation c.
    nonfetal uterine c.
    nonthromboembolic c.
conditioned reflex (CR)
conductance catheter
conducting bronchiole
conduction
    c. band
    c. block
    interval intraatrial c.
    nodal c.
    c. ratio
    reciprocating c.
    retrograde ventriculoatrial c.
    ventriculoatrial c.
    zone of slow c.
conductive
    c. development
    c. loop
conductivity
    thermal c.
    tissue c.
    vascular hydraulic c.
conductor
    fiberoptic c.
    c. resistivity
conduit
    detour c.
    ileal c.
    intestinal c.
    nonvalved c.
    right ventricle-pulmonary artery c.
    urinary c.
    c. valve
    ventriculoarterial c.
condylar
    c. angle
    c. articulation
    c. axis
    c. canal
    c. emissary vein
    c. flare
    c. fossa
    c. part of occipital bone
    c. plate
    c. skull hypoplasia
    c. split fracture
    c. translation

condyle
> c. cord
> external c.
> femoral c.
> lateral c.
> mandibular c.
> medial c.
> occipital c.
> tibial c.

condyloid
> c. canal
> c. joint
> c. process

condyloma, pl. **condylomata**
> c. urethra acuminata

cone
> arterial c.
> c. beam
> beveled electron beam c.
> c. disk
> c. epiphysis
> c. of extraocular muscle
> medullary c.
> parenchymal c.
> c. spot compression view
> transvaginal c.

cone-beam
> c.-b. image
> c.-b. reconstruction algorithm

coned
> c. cecum
> c. down

coned-down
> c.-d. appearance of colon
> c.-d. compression view
> c.-d. radiograph
> c.-d. spot compression

CO_2-negative imaging agent
confidence interval (CI)
configuration
> adaptic detector c.
> anatomic c.
> back-to-back c.
> batwing c.
> beak-like c.
> bilobed c.
> biventricular c.
> bulbous c.
> bull's eye c.
> butterfly c.
> cat's tail c.
> closed-fist c.

> Cupid's bow c.
> cylindrical c.
> discoid c.
> dome-and-dart c.
> double-halo c.
> expansile c.
> fishmouth mitral valve c.
> geriatric c.
> globular c.
> Helmholtz c.
> hexagonal c.
> horizontal dipole c.
> horseshoe c.
> hourglass c.
> hybrid detector c.
> inverted-Y c.
> isosceles triangular c.
> left ventricular c.
> lock-washer c.
> mass-like c.
> molar tooth c.
> mosaic detector c.
> multilobular c.
> octagonal c.
> reverse 3 c.
> ring-like c.
> rosary bead c.
> sandwich c.
> sawtooth c.
> scalloped luminal c.
> shepherd's crook c.
> sigmoid-shaped c.
> snowman c.
> stellate c.
> streak-like c.
> surface c.
> swallowtail c.
> T c.
> tentorium keyhole c.
> thoracic cage c.
> tombstone pelvis c.
> triangle c.
> triple-peak cerebellum c.
> unidirectional lead c.
> water-bottle c.
> winged c.
> wooden shoe c.
> Y c.

configurational formula
confinement
> regional tumor c.

NOTES

confluence
>pulmonary c.
>stellate c.
>c. of vascular marking

confluent
>c. areas of atelectasis
>c. consolidation
>c. fibrosis
>c. infiltrate

confocal image

conformal
>c. neutron and photon radiation therapy
>c. radiation therapy (CRT)

confusion
>circle of c.

congenita
>amyotonia c.
>arthrogryposis multiplex c.
>chondrodystrophia calcificans c.

congenital
>c. abnormality
>c. absence of kidney
>c. absence of pulmonary artery
>c. absence of pulmonary valve
>c. absence of thymus
>c. adrenal hyperplasia (CAH)
>c. adrenocortical hyperplasia
>c. adrenogenital syndrome
>c. amputation
>c. aneurysm of pulmonary artery
>c. anomaly of mitral valve (CAMV)
>c. aortic regurgitation
>c. aortic sinus aneurysm
>c. arteriosclerotic aneurysm
>c. atelectasis
>c. bar
>c. biliary atresia
>c. bipartite scaphoid
>c. bronchiectasis
>c. bronchogenic cyst
>c. cardiac tumor
>c. cerebral aneurysm
>c. cholesteatoma
>c. cystic adenomatoid malformation (CCAM)
>c. cystic dilatation
>c. cystic neck lesion
>c. deformity
>c. diaphragmatic hernia
>c. diffuse fibromatosis
>c. dilated cardiomyopathy
>c. dislocation of hip (CDH)
>c. disorder
>c. duodenal obstruction
>c. dysplasia of hip

>c. Finnish nephrosis
>c. fracture
>c. generalized fibromatosis
>c. goiter
>c. heart block
>c. heart defect (CHD)
>c. heart disease (CHD)
>c. heart disease classification
>c. heart malformation
>c. hemiplegia
>c. hepatic cyst
>c. hepatic fibrosis (CHF)
>c. hip dislocation
>c. hip dysplasia
>c. hippocampal sclerosis
>c. hydrocele
>c. hydrocephalus
>c. hydronephrosis
>c. infiltrating lipomatosis of the face
>c. interruption of aortic arch
>c. intestinal atresia
>c. intracranial aneurysm
>c. isthmic coarctation
>c. kidney fibrosarcoma
>c. laryngeal atresia
>c. laxity of ligament
>c. left-sided outflow obstruction
>c. left ventricular aneurysm
>c. leukodystrophy
>c. liver fibrosis
>c. lobar emphysema
>c. lobar hyperinflation
>c. lymphangiectasia of intestine
>c. lymphangiectasis
>c. mediastinal arterial variant
>c. megacalix
>c. megacolon
>c. mesoblastic nephroma
>c. mitral regurgitation (CMR)
>c. muscular dystrophy
>c. nasal mass
>c. pelviureteric junction obstruction
>c. pericardial absence
>c. pneumothorax
>c. polyvalvular dysplasia
>c. pulmonary arteriovenous fistula
>c. pulmonary artery aneurysm
>c. pulmonary valve insufficiency
>c. pulmonary venolobar syndrome
>c. radioulnar synostosis
>c. renal aneurysm
>c. renal hypoplasia
>c. renal osteodystrophy
>c. ring
>c. splenomegaly
>c. stenosis of pulmonary vein

c. stippled epiphysis
c. subpulmonic obstruction
c. symptomatic AV block
c. tracheobiliary fistula
c. tracheobronchomegaly
c. tracheomalacia
c. ureteric obstruction
c. urethral diverticulum
c. urethral stricture
c. vascular-bone syndrome (CVBS)
c. vascular malformation (CVM)
c. vertical talus
c. vesicoureteral reflux

congenitally
c. absent pericardium
c. corrected transposition
c. corrected transposition of the great artery
c. short esophagus

congested
c. kidney
c. pleura

congestion
active c.
asymmetric pulmonary c.
capillary c.
cardiac c.
centrilobular c.
cerebral c.
chronic passive c.
hepatic c.
hypostatic c.
c. index
intravascular c.
passive hepatic c.
passive vascular c.
pulmonary vascular c.
pulmonary venous c. (PVC)
splenic c.
symmetric pulmonary c.
vascular c.
venous heart c.

congestive
c. asymmetry
c. atelectasis
c. brain swelling
c. cardiomyopathy
c. cirrhosis
c. heart failure (CHF)
c. splenomegaly

conglomerate
c. calcification

c. mass
nonspecific c.
c. opacity
c. pulmonary nodule

conglutinating complement absorption test

congruence
c. angle
patellofemoral c.

congruent
c. articulation
c. point
c. reduction
c. signal intensity abnormality

conical
c. cecum
c. heart
c. mass

conjoined
c. cusp
c. nerve root anomaly
c. root sleeve
c. tendon
c. twin

conjugal carcinoma

conjugate
complex c.
c. diameter
c. foramen
c. gradient
c. ligament

conjunctival vein

conjunctivum
brachium c.

connate teeth

connectedness
theory of fuzzy c.

connecting
c. canal
c. cartilage
c. plate
c. tubule

connection
anomalous pulmonary venous c.
atrioventricular c.
cavopulmonary c.
corticocerebellar c.
partial anomalous pulmonary venous c.
partial pulmonary venous c.
rostral c.
slip-in c.

C

NOTES

connection *(continued)*
  total anomalous pulmonary
    venous c.
  ventriculoarterial c.
  wispy c.
connective
  c. tissue
  c. tissue disease
  c. tissue fibrous tumor
  c. tissue neoplasm
  c. tissue proliferation
  c. tissue septum
connector
  cerebral ventricular shunt c.
Conn syndrome
conoid
  c. ligament
  c. process
  c. tubercle
conotruncal congenital anomaly
conoventricular defect
Conquest balloon dilatation catheter
Conrad-Bugg trapping of soft tissue in
  ankle fracture
Conrad-Crosby bone marrow biopsy
  needle
Conradi-Hünermann syndrome
Conradi line
Conray 30, 43, 400 imaging agent
consecutive dislocation
consistency
  glaze c.
console
  Bruker c.
  direct display c. (DDC)
  Siemens Satellite CT evaluation c.
consolidated
  c. infiltrate
  c. lung
consolidation
  airspace c.
  alveolar c.
  batwing lung c.
  bilateral c.
  confluent c.
  dense c.
  discrete area of c.
  exudative c.
  fracture line of c.
  hemorrhage c.
  ill-defined c.
  lobar c.
  lung parenchyma c.
  nonhomogeneous c.
  parenchymal c.
  patchy area of c.
  peripheral c.

  pulmonary c.
  segmental bronchus c.
  solid c.
  symmetric c.
  unilateral c.
consolidative
  c. change
  c. pneumonia
  c. process
conspicuity
constant
  air-kerma rate c.
  Avogadro c.
  coupling c.
  decay c.
  disintegration c.
  equilibrium dissociation c.
  equilibrium dose c.
  c. infusion excretory urogram
  maximum amplitude c.
  c. permeability
  permeability c.
  Planck c.
  radioactive c. (Λ)
  c. tilt wave
  time c.
  transformation c.
  T2 time c.
constellation
  c. of findings
  c. of symptoms
constituent
  plaque c.
constitutional
  c. osteosclerosis
  c. symptom
constricting esophageal lesion
constriction
  airway c.
  c. band
  c. band syndrome
  ductal c.
  hourglass c.
  occult pericardial c.
  postglomerular arteriolar c.
  c. ring
  supraanular c.
  tangential c.
  waist-like c.
constrictive
  c. bronchiolitis
  c. cardiomyopathy
  c. pericarditis
construction artifact
consultation
  curbstone c.

consumption
cerebral metabolic oxygen c.
myocardial oxygen c.
oxygen c. (QO_2)

contact
bone-on-bone c.
c. B-scan ultrasound
c. carcinoma
catheter-tissue c.
c. effect
c. image
c. lateral view
poor screen/film c.
c. radiation therapy
c. radiograph
c. radiotherapy
screen-film c.
stent-vessel wall c.
c. transscleral laser
cytophotocoagulation (CTLC)

contained
c. aneurysmal rupture
c. aortic rupture
c. disk
c. leak
c. leak of aortic aneurysm

contamination
radionuclide c.
venous c.

content
abdominal c.
bone mineral c. (BMC)
bowel c.
brain water c.
digestive tract c.
disk water c.
fat-supressing c.
femoral triangular c.
gastric c.
herniated abdominal c.
homogenous echogenic uterine c.
intestinal c.
intravascular c.
macromolecular c.
overlying bowel c.
retrograde flow of gastric c.
small bowel c.
tissue water c.
venous oxygen c.

contention
adequate c.

contiguous
c. articular surface
c. image
c. interleaved axial section
c. loop
c. organ involvement
c. parallel chord
c. scan
c. segment
c. slice
c. slice MEMP (CSMEMP)
c. supramarginal gyrus
c. ventricular septal defect

continuation
azygos c.

continuity
aortoseptal c.
c. of bone
bowel c.
c. equation
pancreatic-enteric c.

continuous
c. capillary
c. diaphragm sign
c. hyperfractionated accelerated
radiation therapy
c. hyperfractionated accelerated
radiotherapy
c. hyperthermic peritoneal perfusion
c. imaging (CI)
c. intravenous infusion (CIVI)
c. mode
c. scanning
c. scan thermograph
c. volumetric acquisition
c. wave (CW)
c. x-ray spectrum

**continuous-loop exercise
echocardiography**
continuous-wave
c.-w. Doppler echocardiography
c.-w. Doppler imaging
c.-w. Doppler recording
c.-w. Doppler ultrasound system
c.-w. laser system
c.-w. NMR

continuum
Dandy-Walker c.

contour
altered aortic c.
altered mediastinal c.
convex outward c.

NOTES

contour *(continued)*
    Cupid's bow c.
    diaphragmatic c.
    double diaphragm c.
    c. extraction
    irregular hazy luminal c.
    isodose c.
    lobulated c.
    local bulge of kidney c.
    local bulge renal c.
    c. mapping
    patellar c.
    reniform c.
    S c.
    sawtooth irregularity of bowel c.
    scalloping c.
    smooth c.
    undulating c.
    vascular c.
contoured tilting compression mammography
contour-following algorithm
contracted
    c. bladder
    c. bronchus
    c. gallbladder
    c. kidney
    c. pelvis
contractile
    c. function
    c. pattern
    c. reserve
    c. ring dysphagia
    c. stricture
    c. work index
contractility
    cardiac c.
    c. index
    myocardial c.
contraction
    c. band necrosis
    concentric c.
    esophageal c.
    focal myometrial c.
    kissing c.
    myometrial c.
    nodal premature c.
    peristaltic c.
    phasic c.
    premature nodal c. (PNC)
    premature ventricular c. (PVC)
    ring-like c.
    c. stress test (CST)
    uterine c.
    ventricular premature c. (VPC)
    ventricular segmental c.

contracture
    bladder neck c.
    capsular c.
    c. deformity
    Dupuytren c.
    elbow c.
    fixed flexion c.
    flexion c.
    flexion-adduction c.
    gastrocnemius-soleus c.
    hip flexion c.
    ischemic c.
    joint c.
    knee flexion c.
    muscle c.
    myocardial c.
    myostatic c.
    scar c.
    secondary c.
    soft tissue c.
    Volkmann ischemic c.
    web c.
contralateral
    c. artery
    c. hypertrophy
    c. kidney
    c. lung
    c. sign
    c. subtraction technique
    c. vessel
contrast *(See* agent, material, medium)
    c. absorption barrier
    c. administration
    c. agent
    c. angiography
    c. aortography
    c. arteriography
    barium enema with air c.
    c. bolus
    c. computed arthrotomography
    CT scan with c.
    c. data
    c. ductography
    dynamic susceptibility c. (DSC)
    echo c.
    c. echocardiography
    c. enema
    c. enhanced computed tomography (CECT)
    c. enhancement
    c. enhancement of computed tomographic imaging
    c. enhancement pattern
    c. esophagram
    c. extravasation
    image c.
    c. inhomogeneity

c. injection
intraarticular c.
c. laryngography
c. left atriography
c. loading
long-scale c.
c. lymphangiography
magnetization transfer c. (MTC)
c. material
c. material-enhanced scanning
c. material instillation
c. media adverse effect
c. media excretion
c. media-induced nephropathy
c. media leakage
c. media nephrotoxicity
c. medium (CM)
c. medium column
c. medium-induced pulmonary
  vascular hyperpermeability
c. medium washout
near-resonance spin-lock c.
c. opacification
phase c. (PC)
c. precipitation
puddling of c.
radiographic c.
c. radiography
c. resolution
c. selective cholangiogram
c. sensitivity
short scale c.
soft tissue c.
spontaneous echo c.
subject c.
c. subtraction mammography
time-to-peak c. (TPC)
tissue c.
c. to-noise-ratio
c. transfer characteristic
unsharp mask-type c.
c. uptake
c. venography
c. ventriculogram
c. window level
c. window width
contrast-enhanced
c.-e. color Doppler
c.-e. computed tomography
c.-e. CT
c.-e. CT with saline flush
  technique

c.-e. dynamic snapshot
c.-e. echocardiography
c.-e. FAST
c.-e. Fourier-acquired steady state
  (CE-FAST)
c.-e. fundamental imaging
c.-e. magnetic resonance
  angiography (CE-MRA)
c.-e. magnetic resonance imaging
c.-e. MR
c.-e. MRA
c.-e. MR angiography
c.-e. MR image
c.-e. near-infrared laser
  mammography
c.-e. power Doppler
c.-e. radiographic examination
c.-e. T1-GRE imaging
three-dimensional c.-e. (3DCE)
c.-e. transrectal sonography
c.-e. T1-weighted fat-suppressed
  image
c.-e. T1-weighted spin-echo high-
  field-strength MR imaging
c.-e. ultrasound
c.-e. virtual MR cholangioscopy
contrast-enhancing parametric imaging
contrast-filled
c.-f. catheter
c.-f. stomach
contrast-improvement factor
contrast-induced renal failure
contrast-to-noise
c.-t.-n. calculation
contrecoup
c. compression
c. fracture
c. injury
c. mechanism
control
c. angiogram
automatic exposure c. (AEC)
C-arm fluoroscopic c.
dynamic range c. (DRC)
fluoroscopic c.
image c.
locoregional c.
radiofrequency radiographic c.
radiographic c.
radiopharmaceutical quality c.
roentgenographic c.
scintigraphy quality c.

NOTES

control *(continued)*
SPECT quality c.
Spli-Prest negative c.
Spli-Prest positive c.
time-varied gain c.
controlled ventricular response
controller
IMED Gemini PC-2 volumetric c.
contusio cerebri
contusion
bone c.
bony c.
brain c.
cerebral c.
frontal lobe c.
lung c.
myocardial c.
osseous bone c.
c. pneumonia
pontine c.
pulmonary c.
rib c.
soft tissue c.
urinary bladder c.
conus
c. arteriosus medullaris
c. artery
c. branch ostia
c. clasticus
club-shaped c.
c. elasticus
c. eye
c. hypoplasia
c. ligament
c. medullaris lesion
c. medullaris position
c. septum
c. tip
conventional
c. head coil
c. hysterography
c. osteosarcoma
c. planar imaging (CPI)
c. processor
c. pulse sequence
c. radiograph
c. spin-echo imaging
c. study
c. tomography
c. transverse cross-sectional image
c. venography
conventionally fractionated stereotactic radiation therapy
convergence zone
convergent
c. beam irradiation (CBI)

C. color Doppler
c. color Doppler imaging
converging collimator
converging-hole collimator
conversion
coefficient c.
color space c.
c. defect
c. efficiency
c. electron
internal c.
c. ratio
spontaneous c.
thoracofemoral c.
converter
digital-to-analog c. (DAC)
image c.
motion-compensating format c.
multiplying digital-to-analog c. (MDAC)
real-time format c.
scan c.
convex
c. border of stomach
c. linear array
9- to 5-MHz c. array
c. outward contour
c. posterior margin
convexity
cerebral c.
frontocentral c.
c. of the lung
c. meningioma
paratracheal c.
parietal c.
soft tissue c.
convexobasia
convexoconcave (C-C)
c. heart valve
convoluted
c. bone
c. T-cell lymphoma
c. tubule
convolution
Arnold c.
ascending frontal c.
ascending parietal c.
Broca c.
cerebral c.
Gratiolet c.
Heschl c.
c. mask
occipitotemporal c.
Zuckerkandl c.
convolutional
c. differencing
c. impression

c. marking
c. pattern

Cook-Cope type loop catheter

Cook enforcer

coolant

Cooley-Tukey
C.-T. algorithm
C.-T. alignment

Coolidge
C. transformer
C. x-ray tube

cooling
tissue c.

Coopernail sign

Cooper suspensory ligament

coordinate
c. axis
Talairach c.
c.'s for target lesion

coordination
meniscocondylar c.

COP
colloid oncotic pressure

COPD
chronic obstructive pulmonary disease
emphysematous COPD

Cope
C. biopsy needle
C. loop
C. loop catheter
C. loop nephrostomy
C. mandril guidewire
C. method bronchogram
C. point

Copeland-Kavat metatarsophalangeal dislocation classification

Cope-method bronchography

coplanar
c. beam
c. contour point

copper (Cu)
c. filtration
c. imaging agent
c. 7, T intrauterine device
c. wire effect

copper-64 (^{64}Cu)

copper-67 (^{67}Cu)

coprecipitation

coprolith

coprostasis

copy
magnification hard c.

coracoacromial
c. arch
c. ligament
c. process

coracobrachialis

coracoclavicular
c. bar
c. joint
c. ligament
c. space

coracohumeral ligament

coracoid
c. bursa
c. fracture
c. notch
c. process
c. tip avulsion
c. tuberosity

coral
c. calculus
c. reef atheroma
c. thrombus

cord
c. angioblastoma
anterior gray column of c.
anterior horn of spinal c.
anterolateral white matter of c.
astrocytoma c.
c. atrophy
cervical c.
c. compression
condyle c.
c. deformation
dura mater of spinal c.
c. edema
c. embarrassment
ependymoma c.
c. epidural extramedullary lesion
false vocal c.
fibrous c.
hepatic c.
c. intradural extramedullary mass
c. intramedullary lesion
medullary c.
meninges of spinal c.
mucoid degeneration of
  umbilical c.
multiple focal lesions of spinal c.
noncoiled umbilical c.
nuchal c.
posterior gray column of c.
c. presentation

NOTES

cord *(continued)*
    pretendinous c.
    c. prolapse
    prolapse of umbilical c.
    reactive cyst c.
    c. remodeling
    rope-like c.
    rostral spinal c.
    c. sign
    size of spinal c.
    spermatic c.
    spinal c.
    split spinal c.
    straight c.
    c. structure
    c. subarachnoid space ratio
    tethered spinal c.
    thoracic spinal c.
    three-vessel umbilical c.
    transsection of spinal c.
    true vocal c.
    two-vessel umbilical c.
    umbilical c.
    velamentous insertion of c.
    vocal c.
    Weitbrecht c.
    white commissure of spinal c.
cordate pelvis
cordiform pelvis
cordis
    apex c.
    atrium dextrum c.
    atrium sinistrum c.
    C. Brite Tip 5F–10F guiding
      catheter
    bulbus c.
    chordae tendineae c.
    crux c.
    ectopia c.
    C. endovascular system
    fetal ectopia c.
    fossa ovalis c.
    C. injector
    C. multipurpose access port
    C. sheath
    ventriculus c.
    vortex c.
cord-like
    c.-l. mass
    c.-l. trunk
cordocentesis
    therapeutic c.
Cordonnier ureteroileal loop
corduroy
    c. artery
    c. artifact
    c. cloth pattern

core
    c. biopsy needle
    bone c.
    fibrovascular c.
    ischemic c.
    c. needle biopsy
    nitinol wire c.
coregistered
    c. MRI
    c. scan
coregistration
    image c.
    morphological and physiological
      image c.
    c. paradigm
Corinthian stainless steel balloon-
    expandable stent
corkscrew
    c. appearance
    c. appearance of the esophagus
    c. appearance of hepatic artery
    c. appearance of small bowel
    c. pattern
    c. ureter
    c. vessel
CORLA
    cluster of radiolucent area
corn
    apical c.
corneae
    vertex c.
corneal
    c. facet
    c. tube
Cornell protocol
corner
    c. film
    c. fracture
    c. of knee
cornflake esophageal motility study
corniculate
    c. cartilage
    c. tubercle
corniculopharyngeal ligament
cornu, pl. cornua
    c. of sacrum
    c. of uterus
cornual ectopic pregnancy
corona, pl. coronae, coronas
    c. radiata
coronal
    c. angulation
    c. bending view
    c. cleft
    c. cleft vertebra
    c. computed tomographic
      arthrography (CCTA)

c. ECD brain SPECT image
c. FLAIR MRI
c. GRE MR image
c. maximum-intensity projection
c. oblique technique
c. orientation
c. planar image
c. plane
c. proton-density-weighted fast spin-echo image
c. reconstruction
c. reconstruction view
c. scan
c. section
c. slab
c. slice
c. SPIR image
c. suture
c. suture synostosis
c. T1-weighted image
corona radiata
coronary
c. arteriography
c. arteriosclerosis
c. arteriosystemic fistula
c. arteriovenous fistula
c. artery
c. artery anatomy
c. artery aneurysm
c. artery bypass graft (CABG)
c. artery bypass graft patency
c. artery bypass surgery (CABS)
c. artery calcification (CAC)
c. artery calcium score (CACS)
c. artery cameral fistula
c. artery disease
c. artery dominance
c. artery ectasia
c. artery embolus
c. artery of heart
c. artery lesion
c. artery malformation
c. artery ostium
c. artery-pulmonary artery fistula
c. artery to right ventricular fistula
c. artery scan (CAS)
c. artery scan imaging
c. artery spasm (CAS)
c. artery steal syndrome
c. artery stenosis
c. artery of stomach
c. artery tree

c. atherosclerosis
c. blood flow
c. blood flow velocity (CBFV)
c. cineangiography
c. cusp
c. electron beam angiography
c. embolism
c. flow reserve (CFR)
c. groove
c. insufficiency
c. ischemia
c. ligament
c. luminal stenosis
c. node
c. occlusion
c. orifice
c. ostial revascularization
c. ostial stenosis
c. perfusion gradient
c. perfusion pressure
c. plexus
proximal c. (PCS)
c. radiation therapy (CRT)
c. remodeling
c. reserve flow (CRF)
c. sclerosis
c. sinus (CS)
c. sinus CT
c. sinus electrogram
c. sinus os
c. sinus ostium
c. sinus retroperfusion
c. sinus root
c. sinus of Valsalva
c. sinus valve
c. stenosis index (CSI)
c. sulcus
c. tendon
c. thrombosis (CT)
c. vascular resistance
c. vascular resistance index (CVRI)
c. vein
c. vessel aneurysm
c. vessel geometry
c. wedge pressure
coronary-subclavian steal syndrome
coronas (*pl. of* corona)
coronoid
c. fossa
c. of mandibula
c. process

NOTES

coronoid *(continued)*
    c. process fracture
    c. of ulna
Coroskop Plus cardiac angiography system
corpora *(pl. of* corpus*)*
corpulence
corpulent
corpus, pl. corpora
    c. albicans cyst
    c. amylaceum
    anterior c.
    c. callosum
    c. callosum agenesis
    c. callosum dysgenesis
    c. callosum lipoma
    c. callosum ring-enhancing lesion
    c. carcinoma
    corpora cavernosa penis
    corpora cavernosography
    c. cavernosonography imaging
    corpora fornicis
    c. hemorrhagicum
    c. luteum cyst
    c. luteum hematoma
    c. medullare
    corpora restiformia
    c. spongiosum
    c. spongiosum penis
    c. sterni
    c. striatum
    c. uteri
corpuscular radiation
corrected
    c. gradient echo phase imaging
    c. sinus node recovery time
    c. thrombosis in myocardial infarction frame count (CTFC)
    c. transposition of great artery
correction
    accidental c.
    adaptive c.
    attenuation c.
    automatic motion c.
    baseline c.
    coincidence-summing c.
    degree of c.
    3D motion c.
    echo phase c. (EPC)
    fuzzy logic contrast c.
    inhomogeneity c.
    multiilluminant color c.
    on-the-fly random c.
    phase c.
    Picker SPECT attenuation c.
    scatter c.
    second-order c.

    section timing c.
    summing c.
    surface variable-attenuation c.
correlation (CR)
    c. algorithm (CR)
    c. analysis
    clinical c.
    c. coefficient
    false-negative c.
    functional c.
    histologic c.
    histopathologic CT c.
    imaging-anatomic c.
    imaging-pathologic c.
    mammographic-histopathologic c.
    morphological c.
    pathologic c.
    radiologic-anatomic c.
    radiologic-pathologic c.
    c. time
    in vivo c.
correlative
    c. diagnostic imaging
    c. Doppler study
    c. pertechnetate thyroid imaging
Correra line
corresponding ray
Corrigan sign
corrosive
    c. esophagitis
    c. gastritis
corrugated
    c. air column
    c. fat pad surface
Cortenema retention enema
cortex, pl. cortices
    adrenal c.
    articular c.
    auditory c.
    bilateral orbital frontal c.
    bone c.
    calcarine c.
    cerebellar c.
    cerebral c.
    c. of cerebrum
    eloquent c.
    entorhinal c.
    femoral c.
    frontal c.
    frontoparietal parasagittal c.
    increased renal echogenicity c.
    inner adrenal c.
    lymphatic c.
    mesial-frontal c.
    motor c.
    nonolfactory c.
    opercular c.

orbitofrontal c.
ovarian c.
parastriate c.
parietal c.
patchy atrophy of renal c.
perirolandic parietal c.
peristriate c.
perisylvian c.
postrolandic parietal c.
premotor c.
primary auditory c.
primary motor c. (PMC)
primary visual c.
pyramidal layer of cerebral c.
rarefaction of c.
renal c.
renin-angiotensin-dependent outer c.
rolandic c.
sensorimotor c.
somatosensory c.
striate c.
visual c.

Corti
C. canal
C. organ

cortical
c. abrasion
c. activity
c. adenoma
c. artery
c. atrophy
c. blush
c. bone
c. bone infarct
c. bone lesion
c. bone resorption
c. branch
c. center
c. cerebellar degeneration
c. defect
c. deficit
c. desmoid
c. destruction
c. diffusion restriction
c. dysfunction
c. dysplasia
c. flattening
c. fracture
c. fragment
c. gray matter
c. hamartoma
c. hinge axis

c. hyperintensity
c. hyperostosis
c. hypointensity
c. intracerebral hemorrhage
c. ischemia
c. kidney arch
c. kidney arteriography
c. kidney necrosis
c. mapping
c. margin
c. motor area
c. nephrocalcinosis
c. nodular hyperplasia
c. nodule
c. notching
c. osteoid osteoma
c. plate
c. renal cyst
c. rim nephrogram
c. rim sign
c. scalloping
c. scarring of kidney
c. scintigraphy
c. signet ring shadow
c. sulcus
c. thinning
c. thumb
c. tissue
c. transgression
c. tuber
c. vein
c. vein sign
c. vein thrombosis
c. venous reflux
c. white matter
c. window

corticale
cryptostroma c.
corticated border
cortices (*pl. of* cortex)
corticobasal ganglionic degeneration
corticobulbar tract (CBT)
corticocallosal dysgenesis
corticocancellous
c. bone
c. bone chip
c. strut
corticocerebellar connection
corticogram
corticography
corticomedullary
c. differentiation (CMD)

NOTES

corticomedullary *(continued)*
    c. junction (CMJ)
    c. phase
corticopontine tract
corticorubral tract
corticospinal
    c. motor pathway
    c. pathway lesion
    c. tract (CST)
corticosteroid-induced osteoporosis
corticostriatospinal degeneration
cortisol-producing carcinoma
corundum smelter's lung
Corvita endoluminal graft
cosine
    c. curve
    c. transform
cosmic radiation
costa, pl. costae
    c. fluctuans decima
    c. retraction
    costae spuriae
    costae verae
costal
    c. angle
    c. bone
    c. cartilage calcification
    c. facet
    c. groove
    c. intraarticular cartilage
    c. margin
    c. notch
    c. osteoma
    c. part of diaphragm
    c. pit
    c. pleura
    c. pleurisy
    c. process
    c. sulcus
    c. surface
    c. tubercle
    c. tuberosity
costoaxillary vein
costocervical
    c. artery
    c. trunk
costochondral
    c. joint
    c. junction
    c. junction separation
costochondritis
costoclavicular
    c. ligament
    c. line
    c. maneuver
    c. syndrome
    c. test

costocolic
    c. fold
    c. ligament
costodiaphragmatic
    c. margin
    c. recess
    c. recess of pleura
costolateral
costolumbar angle
costomediastinal
    c. recess
    c. sinus
costophrenic (CP)
    c. angle
    c. angle blunting
    c. recess
    c. septal line
    c. sinus
    c. sulcus
costopleural
costosternal angle
costotransverse
    c. foramen
    c. joint
    c. ligament
costovertebral
    c. angle (CVA)
    c. articulation
    c. joint
costoxiphoid ligament
COSY H-1 MR spectroscopy
Cotrel-Dubousset system
cottage loaf appearance
cotton
    C. ankle fracture
    c. ball appearance
    c. fiber embolus
cotton-wool
    c.-w. appearance
    c.-w. spot
Cotunnius canal
cotyloid
    c. cavity
    c. ligament
couch view
cough
    c. fracture of rib
    c. resonance
Couinaud classification
coulomb (C)
    c. force
Coulomb law
Coulter counter
coumarin pulsed dye laser
count
    absolute granulocyte c.
    background c.

Cerenkov c.
Colombo c.
corrected thrombosis in myocardial
 infarction frame c. (CTFC)
c. density
direct liquid scintillation c.
filament-nonfilament c.
noise effective c. (NEC)
out-of-field c.
c. per plane
random c.
c. rate
scattered c.

count-density threshold

counter
automated gamma c.
boron c.
Cerenkov c.
Coulter c.
event c.
gamma ray c.
gamma well c.
Geiger c.
Geiger-Müller c.
ionization c.
proportional c.
radiation c.
scaler c.
scintillation c.
well c.
whole-body c.

countercurrent
c. aortography
c. flow-related enhancement

counteroccluder

counterpulsation
balloon c.
diastolic c.
intraaortic balloon c.
mechanical c.

counterstimulation

counting
c. coincidence
double-label c.
c. rate meter
whole-body c.

coupled array coil

couplet
ventricular premature contraction c.

coupling
c. constant
dipole c.

dipole-dipole c.
dynamic c.
electric quadrupole c.
c. exchange
hyperfine c.
magnetic dipole-dipole c.
scalar c.
spin c.
spin-spin c.
static c.

Cournand arteriography needle
Cournand-Grino angiography needle
course
c. of artery
extracranial c.
midlateral c.
relapsing c.
remitting c.
signal time c.
undulating c.

coursing
c. of gas
c. vessel

Courvoisier
C. gallbladder
C. law
C. sign

Courvoisier-Terrier syndrome
Couvelaire uterus
coverage
interleaved k-space c.
spiral k-space c.

Cowden
C. disease
C. syndrome

cow horn deformity
Cowper
C. gland lesion
C. ligament

COX
cytochrome oxidase
COX deficiency

coxa, pl. **coxae**
c. brevis
c. flexa
c. magna
os coxae
c. plana
c. saltans
c. senilis
c. valga deformity

NOTES

C

coxa *(continued)*
c. vara
c. vara deformity
coxal bone
coxarthrosis
Postel destructive c.
coxitis fugax
Cox sterilizer and incinerator unit
CP
Carr-Purcell
costophrenic
cross polarization
CP angle
CP sequence
CPA
cerebellopontine angle
CPAD
chronic peripheral arterial disease
CPD
cephalopelvic disproportion
CPE
chronic pulmonary emphysema
C-PET scanner
CPI
conventional planar imaging
cpm
cycle per minute
CPMG
Carr-Purcell-Meiboom-Gill
CPMG sequence
CPP
cerebral perfusion pressure
CPPD
calcium pyrophosphate deposition disease
CPPD arthritis of the hand
cps
cycles per second
CR
central ray
colorectal
computed radiography
computed radiology
conditioned reflex
correlation
correlation algorithm
crown-rump length
CR103
OncoScint CR103
Cr
chromium
CR-39 nuclear tract detector
crabmeat-like appearance
crack
c. fracture
hairline c.
cracked-pot resonance

cradle
alpha c.
CT scan c.
Spectrum DG-P pediatric c.
Cragg
C. EndoPro stent-graft
C. FX-wire
C. stent
C. thrombolytic brush
Cramer-Rao minimum variance bound (CR-MVB)
Crampton
C. line
C. muscle
crania (*pl. of* cranium)
cranial
c. aneurysm
c. angled view
c. angulation
c. anomaly
c. base
c. bone
c. capacity
c. cavity
c. computed tomography (CCT)
c. diameter
c. fixation plate
c. flexure
c. fontanelle
c. foramen
c. fossa
c. granulomatous arteritis
c. meningocele
c. nerve
c. nerve involvement
c. nerve neoplasm
c. nerve sheath tumor
c. nerve sign
c. nucleus
c. osteopetrosis
c. ridge
c. root
c. sinus
c. suture
c. synostosis
c. ultrasound
c. vault
c. vertebra
c. vessel
cranii
pneumatocele c.
synchondroses c.
vertex c.
craniocaudal, craniocaudad
c. axis
c. needle angulation

c. projection
c. view
craniocervical junction
craniofacial
c. angle
c. anomaly
c. dysjunction
c. dysjunction fracture
c. dysostosis
c. notch
c. pain syndrome
c. plexiform neurofibroma
c. remodeling
c. synostosis
craniography
craniolacunia
craniomandibular syndrome
craniometric
c. diameter
c. point
cranioorbital deformity
craniopagus twin
craniopharyngeal
c. canal
c. duct
craniopharyngioma
adamantinomatous c.
ectopic c.
nasopharyngeal c.
cranioschisis
craniosclerosis
cranioskeletal dysplasia
craniospinal
c. axis
c. axis radiation therapy
c. compliance
c. hemangioblastoma
craniostenosis, pl. craniostenoses
craniosynostosis, pl. craniosynostoses
c. syndrome
craniotabes
craniotelencephalic dysplasia
craniotomy defect
craniotrypesis
craniovertebral
c. angle
c. anomaly
c. junction
c. junction anatomy
cranium, pl. crania
c. bifidum
fetal c.

split c.
vertex of bony c.
crankshaft phenomenon
crater
ulcer c.
crater-like ulcer
crazy
c. paving appearance
c. paving pattern
Cr-chromate-labeled red cell technique
CRE
cumulative radiation effect
C-reactive protein level
crease
back c.
infragluteal c.
inframammary c.
inguinal c.
stellate c.
creation
percutaneous peritoneovenous
shunt c.
Cree leukoencephalopathy
creep
cardiac c.
diaphragmatic c.
periosteal c.
creeping epithelialization
cremaster
cremasteric
c. artery
c. fascia
crescendo TIA
crescent
air c.
c. artifact
c. of cardia
c. of cavitation
c. of gas
c. hip line
c. sign
crescentic
c. border
c. collection
c. lumen
c. submucosal fold
crescent-in-doughnut sign
crescent-shaped
c.-s. fibrocartilaginous disk
c.-s. glomerulonephritis
cress-correlation technique

NOTES

211

crest
  acoustic c.
  acousticofacial c.
  alveolar c.
  ampullary c.
  anterior iliac c.
  arched c.
  arcuate c.
  articular c.
  basilar c.
  bilateral iliac c.
  buccinator c.
  conchal c.
  deltoid c.
  dental c.
  ethmoidal c.
  falciform c.
  frontal c.
  ganglionic c.
  gingival c.
  gyral c.
  iliac c.
  infundiboventricular c.
  intertrochanteric c.
  posterior iliac c.
  pubic c.
  sacral c.
  supraventricular c. (SVC)
  terminal c.
  tibial c.
  urethral c.
CREST syndrome
Creutzfeldt-Jakob disease (CJD)
crevice
  nonpolar c.
CRF
  chronic renal failure
  coronary reserve flow
Cr-HIDA chelate
cribrate
cribration
cribriform
  c. bone
  c. carcinoma
  c. DCIS
  c. fascia
  c. pattern
  c. plate
  c. process
cricket bat shape
cricoarytenoid articular capsule
cricoesophageal tendon
cricoid cartilage
cricopharyngeal
  c. achalasia
  c. bar
  c. diameter

  c. diverticulum
  c. ligament
  c. sphincter
cricopharyngeus muscle
cricothyreotomy
cricothyroid
  c. articular capsule
  c. cartilage
  c. ligament
  c. membrane
cricotracheal ligament
cri-du-chat syndrome
crimp stop
crinkle artifact
crinkling
  mucosal c.
  patch c.
crisis, pl. **crises**
  bone c.
crisscross heart
crista
  c. galli
  c. pulmonis
  c. supraventricularis
criterion, pl. **criteria**
  Biello c.
  error-sum c.
  interpretive c.
  Jones c.
  morphologic c.
  Nyquist c.
  PIOPED criteria
  radiographic c.
  Schumacher c.
  Schwartz c.
  c. standard
critical
  c. coronary stenosis
  c. dose table
  c. lesion
  c. mass
  c. organ
  c. valvular stenosis
CRL
  crown-rump length
Cr-labeled red blood cell technique
CR-MVB
  Cramer-Rao minimum variance bound
crocidolite asbestos
Crohn
  C. colitis
  C. disease (CD)
  C. disease of colon
  C. duodenitis
  C. granulomatous enteritis
  C. ileitis
  C. ileocolitis

C. jejunitis
C. regional enteritis
Crohn-like lymphoid reaction
Crone-Renkin index of permeability
Cronkhite-Canada syndrome
Cronqvist cranial index
Crookes
C. space
C. tube
cross
c. calibration
c. ligament
c. polarization (CP)
c. section
c. slice
cross-aortic
crossbar symptom of Fränkel
cross-collateralization
cross-correlation technique
cross-ectopic kidney
crossed
c. cerebellar diaschisis
c. coil
c. embolus
crossed-coil design
crossed-fused renal ectopia
cross-filling
crossfire
c. radiation therapy
c. treatment
cross-fogging
crosshatch grid
crossover
c. of activity
femorofemoral c.
cross-pelvic collateral vessel
cross-section
bronchovascular anatomy c.-s.
c.-s. capture
Compton scattering c.-s.
elastic c.-s.
normalized c.-s.
pharynx c.-s.
thigh muscle c.-s.
vertebral c.-s.
cross-sectional
c.-s. area (CSA)
c.-s. area stenosis
c.-s. imaging
c.-s. lung segment anatomy
c.-s. modality
c.-s. pattern

c.-s. plane
c.-s. transverse projection
c.-s. two-dimensional
echocardiography
c.-s. ultrasonographic image
c.-s. zone
crosstable
c. lateral film
c. lateral view (CTLV)
cross-table
c.-t. lateral position
c.-t. lateral projection
c.-t. leg immobilizer
cross-talk effect artifact
cross-union
Crouzon syndrome
CR/OV
crowded dentition
crowding of bronchovascular marking
Crowe pilot point
Crow-Fukase syndrome
crown
c. artifact
c. cavity
halo c.
c. indemnity
c. tubercle
crown-heel length
crown-rump length (CR, CRL)
CRT
cathode ray tube
conformal radiation therapy
coronary radiation therapy
3D CRT
CrTmEr
crucial angle of Gissane
cruciate
c. eminence
c. ligament
c. orientation
cruciatum cruris ligament
cruciform
c. eminence
c. ligament
crunch
mediastinal c.
crural
c. canal
c. cistern
c. cistern widening
c. fascia
c. fossa

NOTES

crural *(continued)*
    c. septum
    c. sheath
    c. triangle
crus, pl. **crura**
    comma-shaped c.
    c. commune
    c. cupula
    c. of the diaphragm
    diaphragmatic c.
    displaced c.
    c. dome
    c. hiatus
    lateral c.
    left c.
    medial c.
    muscular c.
    c. of penis
    c. pericardium
    c. pleura
    right c.
crush
    c. artifact
    c. fracture
    c. injury
    c. kidney
    c. preparation
    c. syndrome
    thoracic c.
crushed
    c. eggshell fracture
    c. tissue
Cruveilhier
    C. fascia
    C. joint
    C. ligament
    C. nodule
    C. ulcer
Cruveilhier-Baumgarten
    C.-B. anomaly
    C.-B. cirrhosis
crux cordis
cryogen
CRYOguide ultrasound guidance system
CryoHit tumor ablation system
cryomagnet
cryoprobe
cryosection
cryostable magnet
crypt
    c. abscess
    anal c.
    enamel c.
    epithelium c.
    ileal c.
    Lieberkühn c.

    Luschka c.
    Morgagni c.
cryptic vascular malformation (CVM)
cryptococcal
    c. meningitis
    c. spondylitis
cryptococcoma
    focal parenchymal c.
cryptococcosis
    intracranial c.
cryptogenic
    c. cirrhosis
    c. fibrosing alveolitis
    c. organizing pneumonia
cryptorchidism
cryptostroma corticale
crystal
    BGO c.
    c. deposition arthropathy
    c. deposition disease
    c. field theory
    c. gamma camera
    pyrophosphate c.
    scintillation c.
CrystalEYES video system
crystal-induced arthrosis
crystalline phosphor detector
crystallogram
crystallography
    x-ray c.
CS
    coronary sinus
^{137}Cs, Cs-137
    cesium-137
    ^{137}Cs point source
CSA
    cross-sectional area
CSDH
    chronic subdural hematoma
CSF
    cerebrospinal fluid
    CSF 14-3-3 isoform
    CSF oscillatory motion
    CSF 14-3-3 protein
    CSF pulsation artifact
    CSF systole length
    CSF ventricular systole
CSF-suppressed T2-weighted 3D MP-RAGE MR imaging
CSGP
    computer strain-gauge plethysmography
CSI
    chemical shift imaging
    coronary stenosis index
    risk-adapted CSI
    CSI spectroscopy

CSL
central sacral line
CSM
cervical spondylotic myelopathy
CSMEMP
contiguous slice MEMP
CSPAMM
complementary spatial modulation of
magnetization
C-spine pseudosubluxation
CSS
carotid sinus syndrome
CST
contraction stress test
corticospinal tract
CSVT
central splanchnic venous thrombosis
CT
cardiothoracic ratio
circulation time
computed tomography
coronary thrombosis
CT angiography
CT arteriography
CT arthrography
CT attenuation value
biphasic CT
biphasic contrast-enhanced helical
CT
bit CT
CT body scanner
bone quantitative CT (BQCT)
CT bone window
CT bone window photography
cervical CT
cine CT
CT cisternogram
CT cisternography
collimation CT
CT colography
CT colonography
contrast-enhanced CT
coronary sinus CT
3D drip infusion cholangiography
CT
CT densitometer
CT densitometry
3D portography using multislice
helical CT
3D processed ultrafast CT
dual-energy CT

dual-isotope single-photon emission
CT
dual-phase CT
dynamic contrast-enhanced CT
electrocardiogram-gated multislice
spiral CT
enhanced CT
expiratory CT
fast dynamic volumetric x-ray CT
helical biphasic contrast-enhanced
CT (HBCT)
helical thin-section CT
high spatial resolution cine CT
CT imaging error
indirect CT
intravascular contrast-enhanced CT
Marconi/Elscint MxTwin CT
CT Max 640 scanner
CT, MR peritoneography
multidetector CT (MDCT)
multidetector helical CT
multidetector-row CT (MDCT)
multiphasic helical CT
multislice CT
CT myelography
noncontrast head CT (NCCT)
non-ECG-assisted multidetector row
CT
nonenhanced CT
CT number
perfusion CT
CT Perfusion 2 software
postmyelography CT
quantitative spirometrically
controlled CT
CT ratio
CT reconstruction image
renal helical CT
CT scan
CT scan cradle
CT scan gantry
CT scanner beam
CT scan with contrast
CT scan with renal stone protocol
CT sialography
single-detector helical CT
single-photon emission CT
single-slice helical CT
slip-ring CT
spiral multidetector CT
spiral volumetric CT
stable Xenon CT

NOTES

CT *(continued)*
    CT stereotactic guide
    surgical simulation CT
    thallium-201 single-photon emission CT
    thin-section CT
    thin-slice CT
    CT tracheobronchography
    triphasic spiral CT
    twin-beam CT
    two-phase helical CT
    ultrafast CT
    CT unit
    Xenon CT
    xenon-enhanced CT
    Z-dependent CT

CTA
    computed tomographic angiography
    helical CTA
    CTA image
    multidetector CTA
    single-detector CTA
    single-slice CTA

CT-aided volumetry

CTAP
    computed tomography arterioportography

CTAT
    computerized transverse axial tomography
    CTAT imaging

CT-based viral tracheobronchoscopy

CTC
    computed tomographic colonography

CTDI
    computed tomography dose index

CT-directed
    CT-d. biopsy
    CT-d. hook-wire localization
    CT-d. puncture

C-telopeptide
    type II collagen C-t.

CT-enteroclysis
    helical CT-e. (HCTE)

CTE:YAG laser

CTF
    computed tomography fluoroscopy

CTFC
    corrected thrombosis in myocardial infarction frame count

CT-guided
    CT-g. intraarterial chemotherapy
    CT-g. needle aspiration
    CT-g. needle biopsy
    CT-g. percutaneous biopsy
    CT-g. percutaneous endoscopic gastrostomy

    CT-g. percutaneous excision
    CT-g. stereotactic surgery
    CT-g. superior hypogastric plexus block
    CT-g. transsternal core biopsy
    CT-g. ultrasound

CTH
    computerized tomographic holography

CTHA
    computerized tomographic hepatic angiography

CTI
    CTI 933/04 ECAT scanner
    CTI 931 PET scanner

CTLC
    contact transscleral laser cytophotocoagulation
    Nd:YAG CTLC

CTLM
    computed tomography laser mammography

CTLV
    crosstable lateral view

CTMM
    metrizamide-assisted computed tomography

CT/MR
    computerized tomography/magnetic resonance

CT/MRI-compatible stereotactic head frame

CT/MRI-defined
    CT/MRI-d. tumor slice image
    CT/MRI-d. tumor volume image

CTR
    cardiothoracic ratio

C-TRAK hand-held gamma detector

CT9000, 9800 scanner

CT/SPECT fusion imaging

CTT
    central tegmental tract

CTV
    clinical target volume

Cu
    copper

^{64}Cu
    copper-64
        ^{64}Cu imaging agent
        ^{64}Cu-TETA-octreotide imaging agent

^{67}Cu
    copper-67
        ^{67}Cu imaging agent

cube vertex

cubic
> c. centimeter (cc)
> c. convolution interpolation
> c. voxel

cubital
> c. bone
> c. bursitis
> c. fossa
> c. lymph node
> c. tunnel
> c. tunnel retinaculum
> c. tunnel syndrome

cubitocarpal
cubitoradial
cubitus
> c. valgus
> c. valgus deformity
> c. varus
> c. varus deformity

cuboid
> c. bone
> c. fracture

cuboidal articular surface
cuboideonavicular ligament
cubonavicular joint
CUC
> chronic ulcerative colitis

cue-based image analysis
cuff
> c. abscess
> aortic c.
> atrial c.
> inflow c.
> musculotendinous c.
> pressure c.
> rectal muscle c.
> right atrial c.
> rotator c.
> suprahepatic caval c.
> vaginal c.

cuffed endotracheal tube
cuffing
> peribronchial c.
> perivascular c.

CUG
> cystourethrogram

cuirasse
> carcinoma en c.
> cor en c.

cul-de-sac
> Douglas c.-d.-s.
> dural c.-d.-s.

Culiner theory
Cullen sign
culpocephaly
culprit
> c. lesion
> c. stenosis
> c. vessel

cumulative
> c. dose
> c. radiation effect (CRE)

cuneatus
> funiculus c.

cuneiform
> c. bone
> c. bone of carpus
> c. cartilage
> c. fracture
> c. fracture-dislocation
> c. joint
> c. lobe
> c. mortise
> c. tubercle

cuneocerebellar tract
cuneocuboid ligament
cuneonavicular ligament
CUP
> cancer of unknown primary

cup
> acetabular c.
> Diogenes c.
> migration of acetabular c.
> prosthetic c.
> retroversion of acetabular c.

cup-and-spill stomach
cupboard
> RF-shielded c.

Cupid's
> C. bow configuration
> C. bow contour

cupola sign
cupping of the calix
^{62}Cu PTSM imaging agent
cupula, pl. cupulae
> crus c.
> diaphragmatic c.
> gas c.
> pleural c.

curbstone consultation
cure
> complete anatomic c.

curie (Ci)

C

NOTES

curie *(continued)*
    C. effect
    C. law
curie-hour
curietherapy
curium
Curix
    C. Capacity Plus film processing system
    C. film screen cassette
    C. Ultra UV-L film
curlicue ureter
curling
    c. esophagus
    C. ulcer
curly toe deformity
Currarino triad
current
    alternating c.
    attenuation-based on-line modulation of the tube c.
    beam c.
    direct c. (DC)
    eddy c.
    gradient drive c.
    ionization c.
    c. leak
    c. line distortion
    pulsating c.
    pulsing c.
    saturation c.
    single-phase c.
    three-phase c.
    tube c.
    unidirectional c.
    unmodulated radiofrequency c.
    variable tube c.
Curry intravascular retriever set
curtain
    subaortic c.
curvature
    angular c.
    c. anisotropy
    anterior c.
    backward c.
    cervical lordotic c.
    dorsal kyphotic c.
    flattening of normal lordotic c.
    gingival c.
    kyphotic c.
    lumbar c.
    radius of c.
    stomach c.
curve
    area under the c. (AUC)
    biexponential fitting of the left ventricular c.

    biphasic c.
    Bragg c.
    brightness-time c.
    catheter with preformed c.'s
    cervical spine c.
    characteristic c.
    clearance c.
    concentration-time c.
    cosine c.
    depth-dose c.
    c. of duodenum
    dye dilution c.
    elimination c.
    c. fit coefficient
    flattening of normal lumbar c.
    flow-time c.
    fractionated dose-survival c.
    Frank-Starling c.
    free induction delay c.
    full-width at half-maximum of lorentzian c.
    gaussian c.
    glow c.
    Harrison c.
    H and D c.
    Hurter and Driffield c.
    indicator dilution c.
    indocyanine dilution c.
    isoclosed c.
    isodose c.
    kinetic c.
    lordotic c.
    lorentzian c.
    loss of sigmoid c.
    lumbar lordotic c.
    lung count c.
    normal lordotic c.
    pulmonary time activity c.
    renal flow c.
    renogram c.
    ROC c.
    sensitometric c.
    sigmoid density c.
    signal intensity time c.
    spline c.
    Starling c.
    stress-strain c.
    superincumbent spinal c.
    thoracic spine c.
    time-activity c.
    time-attenuation c.
    time-density c.
    time intensity c. (TIC)
    ventricular function c.
    videodensity c.
    washout c.

curved
- c. needle biopsy
- c. planar reformation
- c. radiolucent line
- c. reconstruction
- c. vessel

curve-fit

curvilinear
- c. calcification
- c. defect
- c. density
- c. reconstruction
- c. subpleural line
- c. threshold shoulder

CUSA
- Cavitron Ultrasonic Surgical Aspirator

Cushing
- C. disease
- C. phenomenon
- C. syndrome
- C. triad
- C. ulcer

Cushing-Rokitansky ulcer

cushion
- c. defect
- endocardial c.
- foam c.

cusp
- accessory c.
- anterior c.
- aortic c.
- asymmetric closure of c.
- ballooning mitral c.
- conjoined c.
- coronary c.
- c. degeneration
- dysplastic c.
- c. fenestration
- fibrocalcific c.
- fishmouth c.
- fusion of c.
- intact valve c.
- left coronary c.
- left pulmonary c.
- mitral valve c.
- c. motion
- noncoronary c.
- perforated aortic c.
- posterior c.
- prolapse of right aortic valve c.
- pulmonary valve c.
- right coronary c.

- ruptured aortic c.
- semilunar valve c.
- septal c.
- c. shot
- tricuspid valve c.
- valve c.

custom-curved coil

custom-fabricated graft

custom shielding block

cut
- c. and cine film
- high-resolution coronal c.
- off-center c.
- scalpel c.
- tangential c.
- tomographic c.

cutaneous
- c. adenoma
- c. angioma
- c. B-cell lymphoma (CBCL)
- c. collateral circulation
- c. fissure
- c. lateral branch
- c. lymphoscintigraphy
- c. necrotizing venulitis
- c. nodule
- c. pit
- c. pneumocystosis
- c. ridge
- c. T-cell lymphoma
- c. twig
- c. vascular anomaly
- c. vein

cut-film
- c.-f. angiography
- c.-f. technique

cuticular overgrowth

cutis
- atrophia c.
- c. calcinosis
- osteoma c.
- tuberculosis verrucosa c.

cutoff
- arterial c.
- c. sign

cutting
- c. balloon
- c. balloon catheter

Cuvier
- C. canal
- C. duct

NOTES

Cu/Zn-SOD
copper-zinc superoxide dismutase
Cu/Zn-SOD imaging agent
c.v.
coefficient of variation
CVA
cardiovascular accident
cerebrovascular accident
costovertebral angle
CVBS
congenital vascular-bone syndrome
CVC
central venous catheter
CVCT
cardiovascular computed tomographic
scanner
CVD
cardiovascular disease
CVIS imaging system
CVM
congenital vascular malformation
cryptic vascular malformation
CVP
central venous pressure
CVRI
coronary vascular resistance index
CW
continuous wave
C-wave pressure
CWP
coal worker's pneumoconiosis
CX artery
CXR
chest x-ray
C x T
concentration times time
cyanoacrylate imaging agent
cyanocobalamin
c. Co (cobalt)
c. imaging agent
radioactive c.
cyanocobalamin Co 57, 58, 60
cyanotic
c. congenital heart disease
c. kidney
Cyber 170/720
CyberKnife stereotactic radiosurgery
system
Cyberware 3D scanning system
Cybex ergometer
cycle
clock c.
Krebs c.
pentose c.
c. per minute (cpm)
c.'s per second (cps)

c. time
tricarboxylic acid c.
cycle-length window
cyclic
c. adenosine monophosphate
c. guanosine monophosphate
c. guanosine triphosphate
c. idiopathic edema
cycling
phase c.
cyclooxygenased deficiency
cyclopia
cyclops lesion
cyclosporin nephrotoxicity
cyclotron
medical c.
multiparticle c.
negative-ion c.
positive-ion c.
c. radiation
CY color space
cylinder
abdominal compression c.
axonal c.
Burnett c.
CO_2 c.
dome c.
Fletcher-Delclos dome c.
sum of c. (SOC)
vaginal c.
cylindrical
c. bronchiectasis
c. carcinoma
c. chest
c. configuration
c. format
c. map projection
c. projection map
c. thorax
cylindrical-ablation scheme
cylindroid aneurysm
cylindroma
lung c.
c. parotitis
cylindromatous carcinoma
cylindrosarcoma
cyllosis
Cyma line
Cyriax syndrome
cyst
acoustic c.
acquired hepatic c.
adnexal c.
adrenal c.
air c.
air-filled c.
allantoic c.

amnionic inclusion c.
anechoic c.
aneurysmal bone c. (ABC)
apocrine c.
arachnoid brain c.
arachnoid spine c.
aryepiglottic c.
atypical renal c.
benign conal c.
bilateral arachnoid c.
bilateral choroid plexus c.
Blessig c.
bone implantation c.
brain c.
branchial cleft c.
breast c.
bronchial cleft c.
bronchiectatic c.
bronchogenic duplication c.
brown cell c.
calcified pericardial c.
capping c.
cerebral c.
cervical thymic c.
chocolate c.
choledochal c.
cholesterol ear c.
choroid plexus c.
colloid c.
colloidal brain c.
colobomatous c.
colonic duplication c.
communicating c.
complex breast c.
complicated renal c.
conal c.
congenital bronchogenic c.
congenital hepatic c.
corpus albicans c.
corpus luteum c.
cortical renal c.
cysticercus c.
Dandy-Walker c.
daughter c.
decidual c.
dental c.
dentigerous c.
dermoid ovarian c.
dorsal enterogenous c.
duplication c.
echinococcal c.
endodermal c.

endometrial c.
endometriotic c.
enteric duplication c.
enterogenous c.
entrapped ovarian c.
ependymal c.
epidermal inclusion c.
epididymal c.
epidural arachnoid c.
epithelial inclusion c.
esophageal duplication c.
expansile aneurysmal bone c.
extradural arachnoid c.
extraparenchymal c.
false splenic c.
first branchial cleft c.
fluid-filled c.
follicular ovarian c.
foregut c.
functional ovarian c.
ganglion c.
Gartner duct c.
gastric duplication c.
gastrointestinal c.
hemorrhagic corpus luteum c.
hemorrhagic ovarian c.
hepatic c.
honeycomb c.
hydatid heart c.
hydatid lung c.
hydatid mediastinum c.
implantation c.
inclusion c.
interhemispheric c.
interosseous c.
intracranial dermoid c.
intraduodenal choledochal c.
intradural arachnoid c.
intramedullary epidermoid c.
intrameniscal c.
intraneural ganglion c.
intraosseous keratin c.
intraparenchymal c.
intrapulmonary bronchogenic c.
intrasellar Rathke cleft c.
intraspinal dermoid c.
intraspinal enteric c.
intraspinal epidermoid c.
intraspinal neurenteric c.
intratesticular c.
intrathoracic c.
intratumoral c.

NOTES

cyst *(continued)*
    intraventricular cryptococcal c.
    joint c.
    keratin testicular c.
    kidney c.
    Kimura-type choledochal c.
    leptomeningeal arachnoid c.
    lipid c.
    liver c.
    lumbar synovial c.
    lung c.
    luteal c.
    mammary c.
    mediastinal bronchogenic c.
    mediastinal dorsal enteric c.
    mediastinal duplication c.
    meibomian c.
    mesenteric c.
    mesothelial c.
    midline of brain c.
    milk of calcium urinary tract c.
    morgagnian c.
    mucinous c.
    mucous retention c.
    müllerian duct c.
    multilocular renal c.
    multiple pulmonary c.'s
    multiple thyroid c.'s
    myxoid c.
    nabothian c.
    nasolabial c.
    nasopharyngeal mucous retention c.
    neoplastic c.
    neuroenteric c.
    noncommunicating c.
    nonneoplastic c.
    nuchal c.
    odontogenic c.
    oil c.
    omental c.
    omphalomesenteric duct c.
    orbital blood c.
    orbital chocolate c.
    orbital dermoid c.
    ovarian dermoid c.
    ovarian follicular c.
    ovarian image signature c.
    ovarian retention c.
    pancreatic c.
    paraglenoid c.
    paralabral c.
    parameniscal c.
    paramesonephric duct c.
    paraovarian c.
    parapelvic c.
    parapharyngeal space c.
    parathyroid c.

    paratubal serous c.
    paraurethral c.
    parovarian c.
    pelvic chocolate c.
    peribiliary c.
    pericaliceal c.
    pericardial duplication c.
    perineural arachnoid c.
    perineural sacral c.
    peripelvic c.
    peritoneal inclusion c.
    peritumoral c.
    physiologic ovarian c.
    pilonidal c.
    pineal c.
    pituitary c.
    placental septal c.
    pleural c.
    pleuropericardial c.
    c. or polyp
    pontine hydatid c.
    popliteal c.
    porencephalic c.
    posterior fossa c.
    postmenopausal adnexal c.
    posttraumatic oil c.
    posttraumatic spinal cord c.
    primordial tooth c.
    prostatic c.
    pulmonary c.
    pyelogenic c.
    racemose c.
    radicular c.
    Rathke cleft c.
    reactive spinal c.
    rectal duplication c.
    regressed c.
    renal sinus c.
    retention c.
    retrocerebellar arachnoid c.
    retroperitoneal c.
    sacral c.
    c. sclerosis
    sebaceous c.
    secondary archnoid c.
    second branchial cleft c.
    seminal vesicle c.
    septal placenta c.
    serous intraparenchymatous c.
    simple bone c.
    simple breast c.
    simple cortical renal c.
    small bowel duplication c.
    solitary bone c.
    spinal hydatid c.
    splenic epidermoid c.
    subarachnoid c.

subarticular c.
subchondral c.
subcortical c.
subependymal c.
subpleural air c.
syndrome with multiple cortical
  renal c.
synovial c.
synovium-filled degenerative c.
tailgut c.
talar dome c.
Tarlov c.
tarsal c.
tectal c.
tension c.
testicular c.
theca-lutein ovarian c.
thick-walled c.
thin-walled c.
thoracic duct c.
thymic c.
thyroglossal duct c.
thyroid c.
Todani-type c.
Tornwaldt c.
traumatic bone c.
traumatic lipid c.
traumatic lung c.
tunica albuginea c.
umbilical cord c.
unicameral bone c.
unilocular c.
urachal c.
wolffian c.

cystadenocarcinoma
mucinous ovarian c.
ovarian serous c.
pancreatic c.
pseudomucinous c.
serous c.

cystadenofibroma
ovarian c.

cystadenoma
bile duct c.
biliary c.
colloid c.
endometrioid c.
glycogen-rich pancreatic c.
c. lymphomatosum
macrocystic c.
mucinous c.
ovarian c.

pancreas c.
papillary epididymal c.
serous c.
thyroid c.

cystic
c. adenocarcinoma
c. adenoma
c. adenomatoid malformation
c. airspace HRCT
c. appearance
c. arachnoiditis
c. area thyroid
c. artery
c. bone angiomatosis
c. breast disease
c. breast mass
c. bronchiectasis
c. calculus
c. change
c. component
c. degeneration
c. dilatation
c. disease of breast
c. duct angiography
c. duct cholangiogram
c. duct cholangiography
c. duct lumen
c. duct remnant
c. duct remnant stone
c. duct stump
c. endometrial hyperplasia
c. epididymis lesion
c. fibrosis
c. fibrous dysplasia
c. fistula
c. fluid
c. gall duct
c. ganglioglioma
c. glandular hyperplasia
c. glioma
c. goiter
c. hemangioblastoma
c. hyperplasia photomicrograph
c. intracranial fetal lesion
c. intraparenchymal meningioma
c. kidney
c. kidney disease
c. liver lesion
c. lymph node
c. lysis
c. mastoplasia
c. medial necrosis

NOTES

cystic *(continued)*
    c. medionecrosis
    c. mesothelioma
    c. metastasis
    c. myelomalacia
    c. myelopathy
    c. neck hygroma
    c. nephroma
    c. orbital hygroma
    c. osteofibromatosis
    c. ovarian disease
    c. ovary
    c. partially differentiated
    nephroblastoma
    c. pattern
    c. pilocytic astrocytoma
    c. plexus
    c. pneumatosis
    c. polyp
    c. process
    c. pulmonary emphysema
    c. renal cell carcinoma
    c. rheumatoid arthritis
    c. sac
    c. splenic lesion
    c. splenic neoplasm
    c. structure
    c. teratoma
    c. teratomatous mass
    c. tuberculosis
    c. tuberculous osteomyelitis
    c. tumor
    c. vein
    c. wall
cystica
    cystitis c.
    mastitis fibrosa c.
    osteitis fibrosa c.
    pyelitis c.
    pyeloureteritis c.
    ureteritis c.
cystic-choledochal junction
cysticercus
    c. cyst
    c. granuloma
cysticohepatic triangle
cystine
    c. calculus
    c. stone
cystinosis
    nephropathic c.
cystitis
    c. cystica
    emphysematous c.
    interstitial c.
    radiation c.
    tuberculous c.

cystoatrial shunt
cystocarcinoma
cystocele
    protrusion of c.
cystocolpoproctography
Cysto-Conray II imaging agent
cystoduodenal ligament
cystofiberscope
cystofibroma
Cystografin-Dilute imaging agent
cystogram
    air c.
    bead-chain c.
    chain c.
    delayed c.
    double voiding c.
    excretory c.
    postdrainage c.
    radioisotope voiding c.
    radionuclide c.
    radiopharmaceutical voiding c.
    retrograde c. (RC)
    stress c.
    triple-voiding c.
    voiding c.
cystography
    antegrade c.
    bead-chain c.
    computed tomographic c.
    c. imaging
    radionuclide c.
    retrograde c.
    triple-voiding c.
cystoid
cystoma
cystomatous
cystometrography
cystomorphous
cystoplasty
    ileocecal c.
cystopyelography
cystoradiogram
cystoradiography
cystosarcoma phyllodes
cystoscope
cystoscopic urography
cystoscopy
    virtual c.
cystosonography
    echo-enhanced c.
cystostomy
cystoureterogram
cystoureterography
cystourethrogram (CUG)
    lateral c.
    micturating c. (MCU)
    voiding c. (VCU, VCUG)

cystourethrography
>	chain c.
>	expression c.
>	isotope voiding c. (IVCU)
>	micturating c.
>	micturition c.
>	radionuclide voiding c.
>	retrograde c.
>	video c.
>	voiding c. (VCU, VCUG)

cystourethroscopy imaging

cytochrome oxidase (COX)

cytomegalovirus
>	c. encephalitis
>	c. esophagitis

Cytomel suppression

cytometer
>	FACScan flow c.

cytometry
>	DNA flow c.
>	flow c.
>	image c.
>	multicolor flow c.

cytophotocoagulation
>	contact transscleral laser c. (CTLC)

cytophotometry
>	DNA c.

cytoskeletal
>	c. misalignment
>	c. perturbation

cytotoxic
>	c. edema
>	c. edema of the gray matter

C

NOTES

D

D point
D signal

2D

two-dimensional
2D B-mode ultrasound machine
2D color-coded imaging of blood
flow
2D fast spin-echo acquisition
2D filtering process
2D format
2D GRE dynamic protocol
2D IVUS
2D J-resolved 1H MR spectroscopy
2D MRDSA
2D multiplanar reformatted
technique
multislice FLASH 2D
2D portal image registration
2D pulsatility index mapping
2D resistance index mapping
2D spatially selective
radiofrequency pulse
2D time-of-flight technique
2D TOF

3D

three-dimensional
3D acquired/2D reconstructed
3D anatomic data set
3D conformal radiation therapy
3D connect operation
3D contrast-enhanced MR
angiography
3D coronary magnetic resonance
angiography
3D CRT
3D deformation field
3D dose profile
3D echo planar imaging
3D elastic subtraction algorithm
3D endoluminal view
3D endosonography
3D FASTER
3D fast low-angle shot acquisition
3D fast low-angle shot imaging
3D fast spin-echo acquisition
3D fast spin-echo magnetic
resonance imaging
3D field echo acquisition with
short repetition time and echo
reduction (3D FASTER)
3D FLASH acquisition
3D format
3D Fourier transform gradient-echo
sequence with spoiler gradient

3D freehand ultrasound
3D gadolinium-enhanced magnetic
resonance angiography
gadolinium-enhanced subtracted MR
angiography, 3D
3D gadolinium sequence
3D gradient echo (3D GRE)
3D gradient echo acquisition
technique
3D GRE
3D helical CT angiography
3D image reconstruction
3D inflow MR angiography
3D IVUS
3D KWE direct Fourier imaging
3D laparoscope
3D low pass filtering
3D magnetic resonance microscopy
3D magnetic source imaging
3D magnetization-prepared rapid
gradient echo
3D modeling
3D motion correction
3D MRA
3D MRA slab
3D MRI data set
3D-MSI
3D neuroimaging
3D phase-contrast magnetic
resonance angiography
3D physiologic flow pattern
3D plate
3D portography using multislice
helical CT
3D post filtering
3D pre-filtering
3D processed ultrafast computerized
imaging
3D processed ultrafast CT
3D projection reconstruction
imaging
3D proton MR spectroscopy
3D pulse design
3D radiation treatment planning
3D reconstructed target
3D reconstruction
3D reconstruction algorithm
3D reformatting
3D RODEO
3D rotating delivery of excitation
off-resonance
3D rotational angiography
3D RTP
3D shape of neuroanatomic
structure

D

3D *(continued)*

    3D spatial encoding
    3D spoiled gradient-recalled echo sequence
    3D stereotactic surface projection
    3D superficial liposculpture
    3D surface anthropometry
    3D surface detection algorithm
    3D surface digitizer
    3D surface digitizer scanner
    3D surface rendering
    3D technique
    3D time-of-flight magnetic resonance angiographic sequence
    3D transesophageal echocardiographic sequence
    3D transesophageal echocardiography
    3D turbo fluid-attentuated inversion recovery
    3D turbo SE imaging
    3D T1-weighted gradient-echo imaging
    3D ultrasound reconstruction imaging
    3D ultrasound volumetry
    3D VIEWNIX software system
    3D volume
    3D volume-rendering CT angiography
    3D volume-rendering reconstruction image
    3D volume-rendering technique
    3D volume technique

D$_{max}$

    maximum density

d,1-HMPAO imaging agent

Da

    dalton

DAC

    digital-to-analog converter

Dacron-coated microcoil

Dacron-covered stent graft

Dacron stent

dacryoadenitis

dacryocystocele

dacryocystogram

dacryocystography

    computed tomographic d.
    d. imaging
    magnetic resonance d.
    radiopharmaceutical d.

dacryocystorhinostomy

    endoscopic laser d.

dacryoscintigraphy

dactylitis

    tuberculous d.

dagger sign

Dagradi classification of esophageal varix

DAI

    diffuse axonal injury
    DAI in vivo

Dalen-Fuchs nodule

DALM

    dysplasia with associated lesion or mass

dalton (Da)

damage

    drug-induced pulmonary d.
    endothelial d.
    fatigue d.
    focal d.
    hemisphere d.
    hypoxic brain d.
    ischemic brain d.
    physeal d.
    projection fiber d.
    renal vascular d.
    seminiferous tubular d.
    U-fiber d.
    valvular d.
    vascular cord d.

dammed-up cerebrospinal fluid

dampened

    d. obstructive pulse
    d. pulsatile flow
    d. waveform

dampening

    Doppler waveform d.

damping of catheter tip pressure

Damus-Kaye-Stansel (DKS)

    D.-K.-S. procedure

dancer's

    d. bone
    d. foot malformation
    d. fracture

Dance sign

Dandy-Walker

    D.-W. complex
    D.-W. continuum
    D.-W. cyst
    D.-W. deformity
    D.-W. malformation
    D.-W. spectrum
    D.-W. syndrome
    D.-W. variant

dangling choroid plexus

Danis-Weber

    D.-W. ankle fracture classification
    D.-W. fracture

DANTE

    delay alternating with nutation for tailored excitation
    DANTE sequence

DANTE-selective pulse
D'Antonio acetabular classification
DAP
> dose area product

dark
> d. lung
> d. Mach band
> d. pixel value
> d. region
> d. signal intensity
> d. signal intensity rim

darkfield
> d. imaging
> d. microscopy

darkroom error
Darkschewitsch
> nucleus of D.

Darrach-Hughston-Milch fracture
dartoic tissue
dartos muscle
darwinian tubercle
DAS
> data-acquisition system

DASA
> distal articular set angle

Daseler-Anson classification of plantaris muscle anatomy
dashboard fracture
DAT
> symmetric loss of DAT

data, sing. **datum**
> d. acquisition
> d. acquisition time
> d. camera
> cine raw d.
> d. clipping detection error
> clustered d.
> d. collection system
> contrast d.
> emission and transmission d.
> ferrokinetic d.
> functional d.
> mask d.
> radiology outcomes d.
> relaxivity d.
> rotating raw cine d.
> d. set
> d. spike detection error
> d. spike detection error artifact
> stereotactic d.
> transmission d.

> volume rendering of helical CT d.
> volumetric image d.

data-acquisition system (DAS)
data-clipping detection error artifact
dating
> second-trimester gestational d.
> third-trimester gestational d.

DaTSCAN
> D. imager
> D. imaging agent

datum (*sing. of* data)
Daubenton
> D. line
> D. plane

daughter
> d. abscess
> d. cyst
> d. element
> d. isotope
> d. nuclide

David Letterman sign
Davidson shunt
Davies
> D. endocardial fibrosis
> D. endomyocardial fibrosis

Davies-Colley syndrome
da Vinci surgical system
Davis intubated pyelotomy
Dawbarn sign
Dawson finger
Dawson-Mueller drainage catheter
daylight processor
d'Azyr
> bundle of Vicq d.

DBA
> duodenal bulb apex

DBC
> dye-binding capacity

DBDC
> distal bile duct carcinoma

DBM
> demineralized bone matrix

2D B-mode ultrasound
DC
> differentiated carcinoma
> direct current
> > DC offset artifact

DCA
> directional color angiography
> directional coronary atherectomy

DCBE
> double-contrast barium enema

NOTES

DCCF
dural carotid cavernous fistula
3DCE
three-dimensional contrast-enhanced
DCE-MRI
dynamic contrast-enhanced magnetic
resonance imaging
3DCE-T1-MRA
DCIS
ductal carcinoma in situ
comedo-type DCIS
cribriform DCIS
micropapillary DCIS
papillary DCIS
solid DCIS
Van Nuys Prognostic Index for
DCIS
DCM
dilated cardiomyopathy
DCS
distal coronary sinus
**DCS-10, DCS-18 mechanically
detachable platinum coil**
1D-CSI
one-dimensional chemical-shift imaging
DCT
discrete cosine transform
dynamic computed tomography
DDC
direct display console
DDD
double-dose delay
dual-mode, dual-pacing, dual-sensing
dD/dt
derived value on apex cardiogram
DDFP
dodecafluoropentane
DDH
developmental dysplasia of hip
DDREF
dose/dose-rate effective factor
3D-DSA
three-dimensional digital subtraction
angiography
3D-DSA image
DE
dose equivalent
de
de Broglie wavelength
de Lange syndrome
de Morsier syndrome
de Musset sign
de novo aneurysm
de novo lesion
de Quervain disease
de Quervain fracture
de Quervain thyroiditis

deactivation
dead
d. bone
d. bowel
d. space
d. time
d. time loss
d. tissue
DEAE-Sephadex A-25 chromatography
death
brain d.
cerebral d.
early fetal d.
fetal d.
imminent d.
intermediate fetal d.
late fetal d.
quadrant of d.
sudden cardiac d.
DeBakey aortic classification
deblurring technique
debris
atheromatous d.
atherosclerotic d.
bone d.
calcium d.
cholesterol d.
echogenic d.
embolic d.
extraarticular d.
foreign d.
gelatinous d.
grumous d.
intimal d.
intraarticular d.
intraluminal d.
joint d.
layering d.
metallic d.
necrotic d.
particulate d.
thallium d.
debris-fluid level
DEC
direction-encoded color mapping
decade scaler
decalcification
decalcified dorsum sella
decannulation
decay
alpha d.
beta d.
branch d.
branching d.
d. constant
energy d.
d. equation

exponential d.
free-induction d. (FID)
isomeric d.
isotope d.
d. mode
nuclear d.
positron d.
d. product
radioactive d.
repeated free-induction d.
d. scheme
d. series
d. time
decay-activating factor
deceleration-dependent block
deceleration time
decelerative injury
dechondrification
decidua
decidual
d. cyst
d. fissure
d. sac
decidualized endometrium
deciduate placenta
deciduous
decima
costa fluctuans d.
decimalized variance map
decision matrix
decline
ADC d.
declotting
decoding
document image d. (DID)
Viterbi d.
decompensated
d. alcoholic cirrhosis
d. congestive heart failure
decompensation
cardiac d.
chronic respiratory d.
end-stage adult cardiac d.
end-stage fetal cardiac d.
hemodynamic d.
ischemic d.
respiratory d.
ventricular d.
decomposition
linear prediction with singular
value d.
three-level Haar wavelet d.

decompression
arthroscopic d.
biliary d.
bony d.
canal d.
cardiac d.
endoscopic d.
foramen magnum d.
d. of fracture
gastric d.
hydrostatic d.
intestinal d.
microvascular d.
percutaneous transhepatic d.
peripheral nerve d.
portal d.
d. sickness
spinal cord d.
surgical d.
transduodenal endoscopic d.
transpedicular d.
d. tube
tube d.
variceal d.
venous d.
deconditioned exercise response
deconditioning
deconvolution
d. method
d. technique
deconvolutional analysis
decortication
cardiac d.
heart d.
lung d.
decoupling
bilinear rotation d. (BIRD)
decrease
intraluminal attenuation d.
split renal function d.
decreased
d. activity
d. attenuation
d. cerebral blood flow
d. closing velocity
d. diffusion anisotropy
d. distal perfusion
d. E-to-F slope
d. intensity
d. peripheral vascular resistance
d. peristalsis
d. placenta size

D

NOTES

231

decreased *(continued)*
    d. pulmonary vascularity
    d. stroke volume
    d. systemic resistance
    d. thyroid radiotracer uptake
    d. tidal volume
    d. uptake of radiotracer
    d. vital capacity
decrement
    scan d.
decryption algorithm
DecThreads software
decubitus
    d. calculus
    d. film
    d. pad
    d. position
    d. radiograph
    d. ulcer
    d. view
decussate
decussation
dedicated
    d. head scanner
    d. mammography system
    d. PET scanner
    d. phased-array coil
    d. viewer
dedifferentiation
DeeMed
deep
    d. arch
    d. artery
    d. cardiac plexus
    d. collateral ligament
    d. Doppler velocity interrogation
    d. fascia
    d. fascia of penis
    d. gray matter nucleus change
    d. interloop abscess
    d. lymphatic vessel
    d. muscle
    d. myometrial invasion
    d. to the nipple
    d. pelvic abscess
    d. perineal pouch
    d. posterior compartment
    d. roentgen ray therapy
    d. sulcus sign
    d. tumor
    d. vein
    d. vein system of leg
    d. venous aplasia
    d. venous channel
    d. venous incompetence
    d. venous insufficiency (DVI)
    d. venous occlusion
    d. venous thromboembolization
    d. venous thrombosis (DVT)
    d. white ischemia matter
    d. white matter track
deep-seated
    d.-s. lesion
    d.-s. tumor
deep-shelled acetabulum
de-excitation
default display protocol
defecogram
defecography
    dynamic open magnetic
      resonance d.
    open magnetic resonance d.
defect
    abdominal wall d.
    anteroapical d.
    aortic septal d.
    aortopulmonary septal d.
    apical d.
    atrial ostium primum d.
    atrial septal d. (ASD)
    atrioventricular canal d.
    atrioventricular nodal septal d.
    atrioventricular septal d. (AVSD)
    bar d.
    beneficial atrial septal d.
    benign cortical d.
    bile duct filling d.
    bony d.
    bridging d.
    calcified medullary d.
    cauliflower-shaped filling d.
    cecal filling d.
    chiasmatic d.
    chondral d.
    cold d.
    collecting system filling d.
    colonic filling d.
    conal ventricular septal d.
    concomitant d.
    congenital heart d. (CHD)
    conoventricular d.
    contiguous ventricular septal d.
    conversion d.
    cortical d.
    craniotomy d.
    curvilinear d.
    cushion d.
    developmental d.
    discoid filling d.
    duodenal filling d.
    Eisenmenger d.
    endocardial cushion d. (ECD)
    endocardial cushion ventricular
      septal d.

esophageal filling d.
extradural d.
extrinsic filling d.
extrinsic ureteral d.
fetal abdominal wall d.
fibrous cortical d.
fibrous medullary d.
fibrous metaphyseal-diaphyseal d.
field d.
filling d.
fixed intracavitary filling d.
fixed perfusion d.
flap valve ventricular septal d.
focal liver scintigraphic d.
focal plaque-like d.
frond-like filling d.
frontal d.
fusiform d.
fusion d.
gallbladder filling d.
gastric remnant filling d.
global cortical d.
gouge d.
hatchet d.
hernia d.
high d.
Hill-Sachs d. (HSD)
hot d.
incisura d.
inferoapical d.
infracristal ventricular septal d.
infundibular ventricular septal d.
interatrial septal d.
intercalary d.
interventricular septal d. (IVSD)
intraarterial filling d.
intraatrial filling d.
intracavitary filling d.
intraductal breast filling d.
intraluminal filling d.
intramural filling d.
intravascular filling d.
intrinsic filling d.
inverted umbrella d.
ischemic d.
joint capsule d.
junctional cortical d.
junctional parenchymal kidney d.
juxtaarterial ventricular septal d.
juxtatricuspid ventricular septal d.
linear d.

lingular mandibular bony d.
  (LMBD)
lobulated filling d.
lucent d.
luminal d.
lung perfusion d.
luteal phase d.
malaligned atrioventricular septal d.
mapping of d.
mass d.
membranous ventricular septal d.
metaphyseal fibrous d.
monoradicular filling d.
multiple colon filling d.
multiple small bowel filling d.
mural d.
muscular ventricular septal d.
neural tube d. (NTD)
nonexpansile well-demarcated
  multilocular bone d.
nonexpansile well-demarcated
  unilocular bone d.
nonsubperiosteal cortical d.
nonuniform rotational d. (NURD)
obstructive ventilatory d.
open neural tube d.
organification d.
osseous d.
osteocartilaginous d.
osteochondral d. (OCD)
osteophytic d.
ostium primum atrial septal d.
ostium secundum atrial septal d.
pars interarticularis d.
partial atrioventricular canal d.
pear-shaped d.
pericardial d.
perimembranous ventricular
  septal d.
photopenic d.
plaque-like linear d.
plication d.
pneumoenteric d.
polypoid filling d.
porta hepatis d.
postcricoid d.
posteroapical d.
postinfarction ventriculoseptal d.
postoperative skull d.
punched-out bony d.
radial ray d.
radiolucent linear filling d.

D

NOTES

defect *(continued)*
    resolving ischemic neurologic d.
    restrictive ventilatory d.
    reversible ischemic d.
    right ventricular conduction d.
    Roger ventricular septal d.
    scan d.
    scintigraphic perfusion d.
    secundum atrial septal d.
    segmental bone d.
    segmental bronchus d.
    septal d. (SD)
    septation septal d.
    septum transversum d.
    serpiginous luminal filling d.
    sessile filling d.
    single colonic filling d.
    sinus venosus atrial septal d.
    small bowel filling d.
    soft tissue d.
    solitary small bowel filling d.
    spontaneous closure of d.
    stellate d.
    stomach filling d.
    subcortical d.
    subperiosteal cortical d.
    subsegmental perfusion d.
    superior caval d.
    superior marginal d.
    supracristal ventricular septal d.
    Swiss cheese ventricular septal d.
    thyroid organification d.
    thyroid trapping d.
    transient perfusion d.
    trapping thyroid d.
    triangular d.
    trochlear d.
    tumor d.
    type I (supracristal) ventricular
        septal d.
    type II (infracristal) ventricular
        septal d.
    type IV (muscular) ventricular
        septal d.
    ureteral filling d.
    valvular cardiac d.
    venous d.
    ventilation d.
    ventilation-perfusion d.
    ventral hernia d.
    ventricular septal d. (VSD)
    wedge-shaped d.
    wire-related d.

defective
    d. communication between cardiac
        chambers
    d. volume regulation delay
deferens, pl. deferentia
    ductus d.
    vas d.
deferent
    d. canal
    d. duct
deferential
    d. artery
    d. plexus
defibrillation
    rectilinear biphasic waveform for
        external d.
defibrination syndrome
deficiency
    Aitken femoral d.
    COX d.
    cyclooxygenased d.
    photon d.
    proximal focal femoral d. (PFFD)
    RDS-like surfactant d.
    respiratory distress syndrome-like d.
    surfactant d.
deficit
    base d.
    cortical d.
    focal d.
    hand motor d.
    lateralization d.
    posterior column d.
    reversible ischemic neurologic d.
    significant residual d.
    space d.
definition
    ground-glass d.
    loss of d.
    pseudopolyp d.
definitive
    d. abnormality
    d. callus
Definity
    D. injectable suspension
    D. suspension for IV injection
deflation
deflection
    fracture simple and depressed full-
        scale d. (FSD)
    intrinsic d.
deflector
    tip d.
defluorescence
defluxion
deformability

deformable
>d. manipulation
>d. template

deformans
>arthritis syphilitica d. (ASD)
>arthrosis d.
>osteitis d.
>osteochondrodystrophia d.
>ostitis d.
>Paget osteitis d.
>spondylitis d.
>spondylosis d.

deformation
>d. amplitude
>cord d.
>d. posterior plagiocephaly
>shear-strain d.

deformation-based
>d.-b. hippocampal segmentation and shape analysis
>d.-b. surface-rendered image

deformity
>Åkerlund d.
>Alpine hunter's cap d.
>angular d.
>aortic valve d.
>Arnold-Chiari d.
>back-knee d.
>bayonet d.
>bell-and-clapper d.
>biconcave d.
>bifid thumb d.
>bony d.
>boutonnière d.
>bowing d.
>bull's eye d.
>burn boutonnière d.
>buttonhole d.
>calcaneovarus d.
>calcaneus d.
>cavovarus d.
>cavus d.
>cecal d.
>chain of lakes d.
>Charcot d.
>checkrein d.
>clawfoot d.
>clawhand d.
>clawtoe d.
>cloverleaf d.
>clubfoot d.
>clubhand d.

cock-up d.
codfish d.
compensatory d.
congenital d.
contracture d.
cow horn d.
coxa valga d.
coxa vara d.
cranioorbital d.
cubitus valgus d.
cubitus varus d.
curly toe d.
Dandy-Walker d.
digital d.
digitus flexus d.
dinner-fork d.
duodenal bulb d.
endometrial surface d.
equinovalgus d.
equinovarus hindfoot d.
equinus d.
Erlenmeyer flask-like d.
eversion-external rotation d.
femoral head d.
flatfoot d.
flexible spastic equinovarus d.
flexion d.
foot d.
forefoot abduction d.
fracture d.
funnel chest d.
garden spade d.
gastric wall d.
genu valgum d.
genu varum d.
gibbous d.
gooseneck outflow tract d.
gunstock d.
Haglund d.
hallux flexus d.
hallux malleus d.
hallux rigidus d.
hallux valgus d.
hallux varus d.
hammertoe d.
hatchet-head d.
Hill-Sachs d.
hindbrain d.
hindfoot d.
hockey-stick tricuspid valve d.
hourglass d.
humpback d.

D

NOTES

deformity *(continued)*
    Ilfeld-Holder d.
    internal rotation d.
    intrinsic minus d.
    intrinsic plus d.
    J-hook d.
    joint d.
    J-sella d.
    keyhole d.
    Kirner d.
    kleeblatschädel d.
    Klippel-Feil d.
    knock-knee d.
    lanceolate d.
    lobster-claw d.
    Madelung d.
    mallet-finger d.
    mermaid d.
    metatarsus adductocavus d.
    metatarsus adductovarus d.
    metatarsus adductus d.
    metatarsus atavicus d.
    metatarsus latus d.
    metatarsus primus varus d.
    metatarsus varus d.
    Michel d.
    mitral valve d.
    nasal tip d.
    neuropathic midfoot d.
    pannus d.
    parachute mitral valve d.
    pectus carinatum d.
    pectus excavatum d.
    pencil-in-cup d.
    penciling d.
    pencil-like d.
    pencil-point metatarsal d.
    perigastric d.
    pes arcuatus clawfoot d.
    pes cavus clawfoot d.
    pes planovalgus d.
    pes planus d.
    phrygian cap d.
    pigeon-breast d.
    ping-pong ball d.
    pistol-grip femur d.
    planovalgus foot d.
    plantar flexion-inversion d.
    postoperative thoracic d.
    procurvature d.
    pseudo-Hurler d.
    pulmonary valve d.
    recurvatum d.
    reduction d.
    rocker d.
    rocker-bottom foot d.
    rolled edge d.

    rotational d.
    rotoscoliotic d.
    roundback d.
    round shoulder d.
    saber-shin d.
    sandal-gap d.
    scimitar d.
    seal-fin d.
    shepherd's crook d.
    snowman d.
    spastic equinovarus d.
    spastic hindfoot valgus d.
    splayfoot d.
    split foot d.
    spondylitic d.
    Sprengel d.
    static foot d.
    subtrochanteric varus d.
    supination d.
    supratip nasal tip d.
    swan-neck finger d.
    talus foot d.
    thoracic d.
    thumb-in-palm d.
    torsion d.
    trefoil d.
    tricuspid valve d.
    trigger finger d.
    triphalangeal thumb d.
    turned-up pulp d.
    ulnar drift d.
    valgus heel d.
    varus d.
    Velpeau d.
    vertical talus foot d.
    VISI d.
    Volkmann d.
    wasp-tail d.
    wedging d.
    whistling d.
    Whitehead d.
    windblown d.
    windswept d.
defuzzification algorithm
degenerated
    d. fibroadenoma
    d. tissue
    d. uterine leiomyoma
degeneration
    acquired hepatocerebral d.
    angiolithic d.
    articular cartilage d.
    atheromatous d.
    atrophic d.
    ballooning d.
    bony d.
    brain d.

breast d.
calcareous d.
carcinomatous subacute cerebellar d.
cardiac valve mucoid d.
cardiomyopathic d.
cartilaginous d.
cerebellar d.
cerebelloolivary d.
cerebromacular d. (CMD)
chondrocyte d.
cobblestone d.
colloid d.
cortical cerebellar d.
corticobasal ganglionic d.
corticostriatospinal d.
cusp d.
cystic d.
disk d.
Doyne honeycomb d.
dystrophic d.
esophageal d.
facet d.
fatty d.
fibrinous d.
fibroid d.
gliosis-induced microcystic d.
granulovacuolar d.
gray matter d.
heart d.
hepatic d.
hepatocerebral d.
hepatolenticular d.
Holmes cortical cerebellar d.
honeycomb d.
hyaline d.
hydropic d.
hypertensive vascular d.
hypertrophic olivary d.
internal d.
intimal d.
intrameniscal mucoid d.
liquefaction d.
malignant d.
Menzel olivopontocerebellar d.
microcystic d.
mitral valve myxomatous d.
Mönckeberg d.
mucinous d.
mucoid umbilical cord d.
mucous d.
mural d.
muscular d.

myocardial cellular d.
myocardial fibrous d.
myxomatous d.
olivary d.
olivopontocerebellar d. (OPCD)
d. of pancreas
pancreatic d.
paraneoplastic cerebellar d.
parenchymatous cerebellar d.
paving-stone d.
primary progressive cerebellar d.
progressive d.
Regnauld-type great toe d.
renal tubular d.
retinal d.
retrograde d.
rim d.
sclerotic d.
secondary d.
senile d.
spinal d.
spinocerebellar d.
spongiform d.
spongy white matter d.
striatonigral d.
subacute combined spinal cord d.
testicular d.
thyroid d.
trabecular d.
traumatic d.
Wallerian d.
wear-and-tear d.
Zenker d.

degenerative
d. aortic aneurysm
d. arthritis
d. arthrosis
d. atrioventricular node disease
d. atrophy
d. brain disease
d. cardiomyopathy
d. dementia
d. disease in cerebrum
d. disk
d. disk disease
d. horizontal cleavage tear
d. joint disease (DJD)
d. liver
d. microcystic formation
d. narrowing
d. nuclear pattern
d. osseous change

D

NOTES

degenerative *(continued)*
    d. osteoarthritis
    d. spinal instability
    d. spondylolisthesis
    d. spondylosis
    d. spur
    d. spurring
deglutition
    d. disorder
    d. mechanism
    muscle of d.
    d. pneumonia
Degos syndrome
degradable starch microsphere
degradation
    fibrinogen d.
    d. of image
    image quality d.
    motion d.
degraded
    d. liver
    d. photon
degranulation
degree
    d. of correction
    d. of head rotation
    d. of inspiration
    80-d. linear interpolation
    d. of neck obliquity
    noncircularity d.
    45-d. spinal wedge
    55-d. tomography wedge
dehalogenation
dehiscence
    anastomotic d.
    aortic intimal d.
    bronchial d.
    Killian d.
    valve d.
    wound d.
dehiscent jugular bulb
dehydration-induced renal dysfunction
dehydrogenase
    succinate d. (SDH)
DEI
    diffraction-enhanced imaging
deivisum
    pancreatic d.
Dejérine-Roussy
    thalamic syndrome of D.-R.
Dejérine sign
Delarnette scanner
delay
    d. alternating with nutation for
      tailored excitation (DANTE)
    defective volume regulation d.
    double-dose d. (DDD)

    interscan d. (ID)
    intraventricular conduction d.
    phase d.
    postinjection scan d.
    readout d.
    regrowth d.
    regular wedge d.
    regurgitant flow d.
    regurgitant lesion d.
    temporal phase d.
    d. time selection
    transition d. (TD)
    trigger d. (TD)
    upfront d.
delayed
    d. bone age
    d. bone imaging
    d. closure of suture
    d. cystogram
    d. development
    d. excretion of contrast medium
    d. film
    d. fracture union
    d. gadolinium-enhanced magnetic
      resonance imaging of cartilage
      (dGEMRIC)
    d. gastric emptying
    d. hydrocephalus
    d. myelination
    d. operative cholangiography
    d. phase
    d. phase of arteriography
    d. phase image
    d. phase scanning
    d. pineal apoplexy
    d. posttraumatic myelopathy
    d. resolution of pneumonia
    d. rupture spleen
    d. small bowel transit
    d. splenic rupture
    d. transit time
    d. transport of tracer
    d. traumatic intracerebral hematoma
      (DTICH)
    d. traumatic intracerebral
      hemorrhage
    d. unilateral nephrogram
    d. visualization
    d. washout
Delbet
    D. hip fracture classification
    D. sign
deleterious effect
delimitation
delineation
    lumen d.

delivered
> d. by balloon inflation
> d. total dose (DTD)

delivery
> angiogenesis gene d.
> coil d.
> intracavitary d.
> intravascular angiogenesis gene d.
> percutaneous endometrial drug d.
> timed bolus d.
> transcutaneous angiogenesis gene d.
> viral vector d.

Delmege
> D. sign of tuberculosis

Delphian lymph node

delta
> D. 32 digital stereotactic system
> d. ray
> d. sign
> D. 32 TACT three-dimensional
> breast imaging system

DELTAmanager MedImage system

deltoid
> d. branch of posterior tibial artery
> d. bursa
> d. crest
> d. eminence
> d. fascia
> d. ligament
> d. tuberosity

deltoideopectoral
> d. triangle
> d. trigone

deltopectoral
> d. groove
> d. lymph node

demagnetization
> adiabatic d.
> d. field effect

demarcate

demarcation
> d. line
> nidus d.
> shell-like d.

dementia
> degenerative d.
> multiinfarct d.
> subcortical ischemic vascular d.

Demianoff sign

demifacet

demineralization
> bone d.

demineralized
> d. bone matrix (DBM)
> d. bony structure

demise
> embryo d.
> d. of fetus
> imminent d.
> intrauterine d.

demodulator

Demons-Meigs syndrome

demyelinating disease

demyelination
> brainstem d.
> cerebrum d.
> intramedullary d.
> large-fiber d.
> leopard skin d.
> posterior column d.
> postinfectious d.
> segmental d.
> tigroid d.
> white matter d.

demyelinative disorder

DeMyer system of cerebral malformation

denatured
> d. ^{99m}Tc-RBC
> d. ^{99m}Tc-RBC imaging agent

dendritic
> d. calculus
> d. carcinoma
> d. lesion
> d. spine
> d. vegetation

dendrocytoma

denervated area

denervation
> d. atrophy
> autonomic d.
> cardiac d.
> sympathetic d.

Denis
> D. classification
> D. classification of spinal fracture

Dennis tube

Denonvilliers
> D. fascia
> D. ligament

dens
> d. in dente
> d. fracture
> hypoplasia of the d.

D

NOTES

dens *(continued)*
    d. view
    d. view of cervical spine
dense
    d. body
    d. brain mass
    d. cerebral mass
    d. connective tissue
    d. consolidation
    d. echo
    d. enhancing brain lesion
    d. lung lesion
    d. MCA sign
    d. metaphyseal band
    d. rib
    d. scar
    d. structure of bone
densitometer
    accuDEXA bone d.
    Achilles d.
    bone d.
    CT d.
    DEXA dual-energy x-ray
      absorptiometry d.
    DPX-IQ d.
    dual-photon d.
    Expert-XL d.
    Hologic 2000 d.
    Lunar DPX d.
    Lunar Expert d.
    Norland XR26 bone d.
    OsteoView digital bone d.
    pDEXA x-ray peripheral bone d.
    Sahara portable bone d.
    single-photon d.
densitometric measurement
densitometry
    bone d.
    cardiac output video d.
    Compton coherent scattering d.
    computerized optical d. (COD)
    CT d.
    dual-photon d.
    dynamic spiral CT lung d.
    Norland bone d.
    photon d.
    QCT 3000 system for bone d.
    quantitative CT d.
    spirometrically controlled CT
      lung d.
    d. z score
density
    air d.
    area of abnormal d.
    arterial linear d.
    asymmetric breast d.
    axial spin d.

background d.
band of d.
base d.
bone mineral d. (BMD)
calcific d.
capillary d.
count d.
curvilinear d.
diffuse increase in breast d.
diffuse reticular d.
diffuse reticulogranular lung d.
discrete perihilar d.
d. discrimination
double d.
echo d.
echo-spin d.
endoluminal d.
energy flux d.
d. equalization filter
falx increased d.
fat d.
fibroglandular d.
fluid d.
focal asymmetric d.
ground-glass d.
hazy d.
homogeneous soft tissue d.
hydrogen spin d.
ill-defined breast d.
ill-defined multifocal lung d.
increased bone d.
increased splenic d.
inherent d.
integrated optical d. (IOD)
ionization d.
lamellar body d. (LBD)
linear d.
low d.
lung d.
magnetic flux d.
d. matrix theory
maximum d. (D_{max})
metallic d.
minimum pixel d.
mixed fat-water breast lesion d.
mottled d.
multiple pleural d.
near-water d.
nodular d.
optical d. (OD)
patchy area of d.
peak count d.
perihilar d.
photon d.
pleural d.
proton-d.
pulmonary d.

radiographic d.
radiolucent d.
radiopaque d.
reticulogranular pulmonary d.
retroareolar d.
retrocardiac d.
segmental lung d.
soft tissue d.
spicular d.
spin d.
spleen d.
strands of increased d.
streak of increased d.
subareolar breast d.
tissue d.
T-score measurement of bone
  mineral d.
tubular lung d.
urographic d.
variation in d.
water d.
wedge-shaped d.
densography
dental
d. bulb
d. contrast material
d. crest
d. cyst
d. granuloma
d. groove
d. neck
d. polyp
d. radiography
d. radiology
d. ridge
d. root
d. sac
d. scan
d. shelf
d. tubercle
DentaScan
D. imaging
D. multiplanar reformation
dentata
vertebra d.
dentate
d. fascia
d. fissure
d. fracture
d. gyrus
d. ligament
d. line

d. nuclei
d. nuclei calcification
d. nucleus of cerebellum
d. output channel
d. suture
d. suture of skull
dentatoolivary pathway
dentatothalamic tract
dente
dens in d.
denticulate
d. ligament
d. suture
dentiform
dentigerous cyst
dentin
dentinal
d. sheath
d. tubule
dentinogenesis imperfecta
dentition
crowded d.
dentoskeletal relationship
denture-supporting structure
DENT-X intraoral x-ray unit
denudation
area of d.
denutrition
Denver shunt
Denys-Drash tumor
Denys syndrome
deossification
band of d.
6-deoxy-1-galactose
deoxygenated blood
deoxyglucose
^{11}C d.
2-deoxyglucose
2-fluoro -d. (FDG)
deoxyhemoglobin concentration
deoxyribonucleic acid (DNA)
dependence
quadratic d.
relaxation rate frequency d.
solvent water TI frequency d.
dependent
d. atelectasis
d. edema fluid resorption
d. extracellular fluid accumulation
d. lung
d. opacity
d. pouch of Douglas

D

NOTES

dephase-rephase magnitude subtraction technique
dephasing
    d. gradient
    intraluminal d.
    intravoxel d.
    odd-echo d.
    rapid d.
    signal d.
    spin d.
depicted Hounsfield unit
depiction
    magnetic resonance d.
    d. of vasculature
depletion
    intravascular volume d.
deployed stent
deployment
    stent d.
depolarization
    chemically-induced dynamic
      nuclear d. (CIDNP)
    ventricular premature d. (VPD)
deposit
    amyloid d.
    arteriosclerotic d.
    bony d.
    calcareous d.
    calcium salt d.
    callus d.
    endochondral bone d.
    intramuscular hemosiderin d.
    pericardium calcareous d.
deposition
    calcium pyrophosphate dihydrate
      crystal d.
    coil d.
    radiotracer d.
    d. of tracer
depreotide
    ^{99m}TC d.
    technetium-99m d.
depressed
    d. diaphragm
    d. ejection fraction
    d. right ventricular contractile
      function
    d. skull fracture
depression
    biconcave d.
    bone marrow d.
    fragment d.
    hemidiaphragm d.
    iodinated CM-induced cardiac d.
    iodinated contrast material-induced
      cardiac d.
    d. of left mainstem bronchus

    marginal kidney d.
    myocardial d.
    d. of nasal bone
    pacchionian d.
    parasagittal d.
    reciprocal d.
    d. of renal margin
    sinus node d.
    spinal cord d.
    tibial plateau d.
    translucent d.
    ventricular d.
depression-type intraarticular fracture
deprivation dwarfism
depth
    acetabular d.
    d. compensation
    d. dose
    d. dose distribution
    lumbosacral spine d.
    midplane d.
    photon interaction d.
    d. pulse
    d. resolution
    scatterer d.
    signal d.
    skin d.
    target d.
    d. of tumor invasion assessed by
      EUS
depth-dose curve
depth-pulse technique
depth-resolved surface spectroscopy (DRESS)
DER
    dual-energy radiograph
deranged tissue development
derangement
    articular d.
    disk d.
    internal d.
    longitudinal transarticular d.
    painful disk d.
    soft tissue d.
derby hat fracture
Derek Harwood-Nash catheter
derivative
    d. circulation
    pyridone d.
derived value on apex cardiogram (dD/dt)
dermal
    d. bone
    d. breast calcification
    d. duct tumor
    d. sinus tract
dermal–subcutaneous fat interface

dermatoarthritis
  lipoid d.
dermatofibrosarcoma protuberans
dermoid
  mediastinum d.
  monodermal d.
  ovarian d.
  d. ovarian cyst
  d. plug
  spinal d.
  d. tumor
derotate
derotation
DES
  diffuse esophageal spasm
  DES exposure
Desault
  D. dislocation
  D. fracture
descending
  d. aorta dissection
  d. colon
  d. duodenum
  left anterior d. (LAD)
  d. septal artery
  d. thoracic aorta
  d. tract
  d. urography
  d. venography
descent
  basal d.
  epididymal d.
  perineal d.
desert rheumatism
desiccated
desiccation
  disk d.
design
  crossed-coil d.
  3D pulse d.
  factorial d.
  over-the-wire d.
  PORT radiofrequency electrode d.
  pulse d.
  d. rule check (DRC)
  d. rule check algorithm
Desilets-Hoffman introducer
desmectasis
desmocytoma
desmofibromatosis
desmoid
  cortical d.

  d. lesion
  periosteal d.
  subperiosteal d.
  d. tumor
desmoma
desmoplasia
desmoplastic
  d. fibroma
  d. infantile astrocytoma
  d. reaction
  d. response
  d. small round-cell tumor (DSRCT)
desmosis
desmosome
d'Eśpine sign
desquamated epithelial breast
  hyperplasia
desquamative
  d. fibrosing alveolitis
  d. interstitial pneumonia (DIP)
destruction
  bony d.
  cortical d.
  geographic bone d.
  moth-eaten bone d.
  mucosal d.
  pattern of d.
  permeative bone d.
  sellar d.
  temporomandibular joint d.
  d. of tissue
  trabecular d.
destructive
  d. bone lesion
  d. brucellar arthritis
  d. diskovertebral lesion
  d. interference technique
  d. process
  d. spondyloarthropathy
  d. tumor
detachable platinum coil
detail
  d. burnout
  exquisite d.
  fetal d.
  fine d.
  intraluminal d.
  rib d.
  suboptimal d.
detectability
  lesion d.

D

NOTES

243

detecting
    collision d.
    d. Down syndrome by ultrasound of the nose bone
    d. module
detection
    annihilation coincidence d. (ACD)
    automated polyp d.
    beta d.
    cardiac shunt d.
    coincidence d. (CD, CoDe)
    computer-aided d. (CAD)
    d. echocardiography
    edge d. (ED)
    focus d.
    ICP-AES d.
    magnetic resonance d.
    molecular coincidence d. (MCD)
    occult d.
    photooptical d.
    quadrature d.
    radioactivity d.
    radwaste radioactivity d.
    sonographic d.
    d. threshold
    turbidimetric d.
    d. zone
detective quantum efficiency (DQE)
detector
    Add-On Bucky direct x-ray d.
    anular d.
    d. array
    bismuth-germanate d. (BGO)
    block d.
    cadmium iodide d.
    CCD d.
    d. coil
    d. collimation
    collimation scintillation d.
    CR-39 nuclear tract d.
    crystalline phosphor d.
    C-TRAK hand-held gamma d.
    dielectric track d.
    digital amorphous silicon flat-panel d.
    digital x-ray d.
    diode d.
    Doppler ultrasonic blood flow d.
    Doppler ultrasonic velocity d.
    element-specific d.
    flame ionization d.
    flat-plate d.
    gamma probe radiation d.
    gas-filled d.
    GE d.
    Geiger-Müller d.
    glass tract d.

    HPGe d.
    ionization d.
    kinestatic charge d. (KCD)
    NaI d.
    Neoprobe 1000, 1500 portable radioisotope d.
    Neoprobe radioactivity d.
    passive track d.
    Pediatric IngestaScan metal d.
    16-d. PET system
    phase-sensitive d.
    planar d.
    quadrature phase d. (QPD)
    radiation d.
    rature d.
    ring d.
    scintillation d.
    semiconductor d.
    Si (Li) d.
    slot-scanning d.
    sodium iodide d.
    solid-state nuclear track d.
    d. system
    thallium-activated sodium iodine d.
    Thoravision selenium x-ray d.
    tissue-equivalent d.
    Wang-Binford edge d.
    x-ray d.
determinant
    sequential d.
determination
    Budin-Chandler anteversion d.
    d. of lung volume
    particle size d.
    void d.
detorsion
    spontaneous d.
detour conduit
detritus
detrusor
    d. hyperreflexia
    d. instability
    d. muscle
Detsky modified cardiac risk index
detunable elliptic transmission line resonator
deuterium imaging agent
deuterium-tritium generator
deuteron, deuton
Deutschländer disease
devascularization
    paraesophagogastric d.
developed collateral
developer artifact
development
    anomalous d.
    branchial cleft d.

conductive d.
delayed d.
deranged tissue d.
distal bone marrow d.
endocardial cushion d.
interval d.
lymphatic d.
metacarpophalangeal bone
  marrow d.
metatarsophalangeal bone marrow d.
tibia bone marrow d.

developmental
d. defect
d. dysplasia of hip (DDH)
d. groove

Deventer
D. diameter
D. pelvis

deviated mediastinum

deviation
angular d.
aortic d.
carpal d.
fracture d.
left axis d. (LAD)
mean d.
mediastinal d.
needle d.
radial d.
right axis d. (RAD)
rotary d.
septal d.
significant axis d.
standard d.
tracheal d.
ulnar d.
ureter d.
valgus d.
varus d.

device (*See also* machine, scanner,
  system, unit)
abdominal left ventricular assist d.
  (ALVAD)
Amplatzer septal occluder d.
Amplatz thrombectomy d.
AngioJet thrombectomy d.
antisiphon d.
Arrow-Trerotola percutaneous
  thrombectomy d.
arterial puncture site closure d.
automatic spring-loaded biopsy d.
Bard rotary atherectomy d.

beam-modifying d.
bioabsorbable sheath-delivered
  vascular d.
biventricular assist d. (BVAD)
BladderManager ultrasound d.
bone fixation d.
Bruker minispec measuring d.
Bucky digital x-ray d.
Burnett BiDirectional TMJ d.
buttoned d.
CardioBeeper CB-12L cardiac d.
charge-coupled d. (CCD)
charge-injection d. (CID)
closure d.
compression d.
copper 7, T intrauterine d.
directional atherectomy d.
DirectRay direct-to-digital image
  capture d.
Duett arterial puncture site
  closure d.
DynaWell medical compression d.
electrooptical d.
Endostaple d.
external fixation d.
FemoStop compression d.
halo d.
hemostatic puncture closure d.
HiSonic ultrasonic bone conduction
  hearing d.
Hysterocath
  hysterosalpingography d.
Ilizarov d.
implantable vascular access d.
internal fixation d.
intramedullary fixation d.
intraoperative d.
Kendall sequential compression d.
kinematic wrist d.
Laser Lancet laser d.
left ventricular assist d. (LVAD)
lost intrauterine d.
magnetic induction d.
Molteno double plate drainage d.
Molteno single plate drainage d.
MultiDop P, T, X transcranial
  Doppler d.
nail-plate d.
nonferromagnetic positioning d.
Nuclear Magnetic Device Lypoo
  Profile d.
Oasis thrombectomy d.

D

NOTES

device *(continued)*
>Optical Path Difference-Scan optical d.
>OsteoAnalyzer bone densitometry d.
>Palpagraph breast mapping d.
>Perclose arterial closure d.
>percutaneous arterial closure d.
>percutaneous vascular surgical d.
>Pigg-O-Stat pediatric positioning d.
>Prostar XL 8, 10 suture mediated closure d.
>RadStat hemostasis d.
>Rashkind double umbrella d.
>right ventricular assist d. (RVAD)
>scaling d.
>Sideris buttoned double-disk d.
>Sonotron electronic therapeutic d.
>spinal fixation d.
>spot film d.
>stereotactic d.
>superconducting quantum interference d. (SQUID)
>synchronization d.
>Telos radiographic stress d.
>T-fastener d.
>The Closer arterial puncture site closure d.
>thrombectomy d.
>Trak Back pullback d.
>Trerotola thrombectomy d.
>TriSpan aneurysm neck-bride d.
>tube d.
>vascular access d.
>VasoSeal ES, VHD arterial puncture site closure d.
>venous access d.
>ventricular assist d.

device-independent (DVI)

devitalized
>d. allogeneic bone
>d. portion of bone
>d. tissue

devoid of circulation

DEXA
>dual-energy x-ray absorptiometry
>DEXA bone density scan imaging
>DEXA densitometer
>DEXA scan

dexamethasone suppression test imaging

dexter
>cor triatriatum d.

Dexter-Grossman classification of mitral regurgitation

dextrad

dextral

dextran
>Gd-DTPA-labeled d.
>iron d.
>technetium-99m d.

dextran-coated charcoal

dextrocardia

dextroconcave

dextrogastria

dextro loop (D-loop)

dextroposition

dextropositioned aorta

dextrorotary scoliosis

dextrorotoscoliosis

dextroscoliosis

dextrose 5% in water imaging agent

dextrosinistral

dextrotransposition of great artery

dextrotropic

dextroversion of heart

dextrum
>cor d.

DFI
>dye fluorescence index

2D Fourier transform (2DFT)

2D Fourier transformation imaging

DFP
>diastolic filling pressure

DFS
>distraction-flexion staging

DFT
>discrete Fourier transform

2DFT
>two-dimensional Fourier transform
>>2DFT method
>>2DFT time-of-flight MR angiography

3DFT
>three-dimensional Fourier transform
>>3DFT gradient-echo MR imaging
>>3DFT magnetic resonance angiography
>>3DFT volume imaging

DGC
>directional gradient concentration

dGEMRIC
>delayed gadolinium-enhanced magnetic resonance imaging of cartilage

DGHAL
>Doppler-guided hemorrhoid artery ligation

DGR
>duodenogastric reflux

2D gradient-encoded image

DHCT
    dual-phase helical computed tomography
DHS screw
DI
    diagnostic imaging
diabetic
    d. cardiomyopathy
    d. gastroparesis
    d. nephropathy
diacondylar fracture
diagniol
diagnosis, pl. **diagnoses**
    computer-aided d. (CAD)
    prospective investigation of
        pulmonary embolus d. (PIOPED)
    radiologic d.
    roentgenographic d.
    sonographic d.
    ultrasound d.
Diagnost 120
diagnostic
    d. angiography
    d. cascade
    d. efficacy analysis
    d. imaging (DI)
    d. mammography
    d. modality
    d. pneumoperitoneum
    d. pneumothorax
    d. procedure
    d. puncture
    d. radiation
    d. radioiodine scanning (DxRaI)
    d. radiology
    d. radiopharmaceutical
    d. range ultrasound
    d. skull series
    d. teleradiology
    d. and therapeutic technology
        assessment
    d. x-ray camera and imaging
        source
    d. yield
diagonal
    d. branch
    d. branch of artery
    d. conjugate diameter
diagram
    energy level d. (ELD)
    Ladder d.
    marker-channel d.
diagrammatic radiography

dialysis
    d. arthropathy
    d. fistula
    d. shunt
    d. tube
diamagnetic
    d. shift
    d. substance
    d. susceptibility
diamagnetism
    Landau d.
diametaphyseal
diametaphysis
diameter
    acetabular depth-to-femoral head d.
        (AD/FHD)
    anterior sagittal d. (ASD)
    anterior-to-posterior sagittal canal d.
    anteroposterior d.
    aortic d. (AD)
    aortic root d.
    artery d.
    Baudelocque d.
    bicristal d.
    biischial d.
    biparietal d. (BPD)
    bisacromial d.
    bispinous d.
    bitemporal d.
    bituberous d.
    bronchial d.
    cardiac d.
    cecum d.
    coccygeopubic d.
    coil-to-vessel d.
    conjugate d.
    cranial d.
    craniometric d.
    cricopharyngeal d.
    Deventer d.
    diagonal conjugate d.
    film d.
    frontomental d.
    frontooccipital d.
    gestational sac d.
    GS d.
    increased anteroposterior d.
    increment in luminal d.
    inferior longitudinal d.
    intercristal d.
    internal d. (ID)
    internal conjugate d.

NOTES

D

diameter *(continued)*
    intertubercular d.
    left anterior internal d. (LAID)
    left ventricular internal d. (LVID)
    Löhlein d., Loehlein d.
    lumen d.
    maximum anteroposterior d.
    mean sac d. (MSD)
    mentooccipital d.
    mentoparietal d.
    midsagittal d. (MSD)
    minimal luminal d. (MLD)
    minimal port d. (MPD)
    narrow anteroposterior d.
    d. obliqua pelvis
    oblique d.
    occipitofrontal d. (OFD)
    occipitomental d.
    orthonormal d.
    parietal d.
    pelvic d.
    posterotransverse d.
    pyloric d.
    right ventricular internal d. (RVID)
    sacropubic d.
    sagittal canal d. (SCD)
    spinal cord d.
    spleen d.
    stenosis d.
    suboccipitobregmatic d.
    temporal d.
    d. transversa pelvis
    transverse cerebellar d. (TCD)
    transverse pelvic d.
    ureter d.
    valve d.
    vertebromammary d.
    vertical d.
    vessel d.
    yolk sac d.
diametric pelvic fracture
diamniotic pregnancy
Diamond-Blackfan syndrome
diapedesis
diaphanography
diaphragm
    above d. (AD)
    accessory d.
    antral mucosal d.
    aperture d.
    aponeurotic portion of d.
    below d. (BD)
    bilateral elevation of d.
    Bucky d.
    central tendon d.
    costal part of d.
    crus of the d.

    depressed d.
    dome of d.
    duodenal d.
    d. duplication
    elevated d.
    d. embryology
    eventration of the d.
    excursion of the d.
    flattening of d.
    free air under d.
    gastric d.
    inferior vena cava d.
    leaf of d.
    lumbar part of d.
    median arcuate ligament of d.
    muscular crus of d.
    paralysis of d.
    pelvic d.
    polyarcuate d.
    Potter-Bucky d.
    respiratory d.
    sella turcica d.
    sternal part of d.
    sternocostal part of d.
    tenting of d.
    thoracoabdominal d.
    traumatic rupture of the d. (TRD)
    urogenital d.
    vertebral part of d.
diaphragma sella
diaphragmatic
    d. attenuation
    d. border
    d. contour
    d. creep
    d. crus
    d. cupula
    d. dome
    d. echo
    d. elevation
    d. esophageal hiatus
    d. eventration
    d. fascia
    d. hernia
    d. hump
    d. ligament
    d. lymph node
    d. myocardial infarct (DMI)
    d. paralysis
    d. pericardium
    d. pleura
    d. pleurisy
    d. rupture
    d. sarcoma
    d. segment
    d. slip
    d. surface

d. surface of heart
d. surface of liver
diaphyseal, diaphysial
    d. aclasis
    d. bone length ratio
    d. center
    d. cortical mortise
    d. dysplasia
    d. fracture
    d. lesion
    d. ossification
    d. sclerosis
diaphyseal-epiphyseal fusion
diaphysis, pl. **diaphyses**
diaphysitis
    luetic d.
diaplasis
diapositive
diarthrodial intervertebral joint
diarthrosis
diaschisis
    cerebellar d.
    crossed cerebellar d.
    ipsilateral cortical d.
diascope
diascopy
Diasonics
    D. ultrasound
    D. ultrasound scanner
diastasis
    d. of cranial bone
    fracture d.
    d. heart period
    d. of suture
    syndesmotic d.
    tibiofibular d.
diastatic
    d. fracture
    d. lambdoid suture
diastematomyelia
    spinal d.
diastolic
    d. atrial volume
    d. counterpulsation
    d. depolarization phase
    d. depolarization pulse
    d. doming
    d. filling period
    d. filling pressure (DFP)
    d. gating
    d. gradient
    d. heart failure

d. left ventricular index
d. notch impedance
d. overload
d. perfusion pressure
d. perfusion time
d. pressure-time index (DPTI)
d. pseudogating
d. regurgitant velocity
d. reserve
d. velocity ratio
d. zero flow
diastrophic
    d. dwarfism
    d. dysplasia
diathermic
    d. loop
    d. vascular occlusion
diathermy ultrasound
diathesis, pl. **diatheses**
    hypertensive d.
diatrizoate
    meglumine d.
    d. meglumine imaging agent
    methylglucamine d.
    d. sodium imaging agent
diatrizoic acid contrast medium
DIC
    disseminated intravascular coagulation
    drip infusion cholangiogram
    drip infusion cholangiography
dicephalus
dichorionic, dichorial
    d. diamniotic twin pregnancy
dichorionic-diamniotic twin
dichromate
    d. dosimeter
    d. dosimetry
Dickhaut-DeLee discoid meniscus classification
DICOM-3 compatible digital computer format
dicondylar fracture
Dicopac test
dicrotic notch
DID
    document image decoding
DIDA
    dimethyl iminodiacetic acid
didactylism
didelphia
    uterine d.
didelphic uterus

D

NOTES

didelphys
uterine d.
dielectric track detector
diencephalic herniation
diencephalon, pl. **diencephala**
die-punch fracture
DIET
D. fast SE imaging
D. method of fat suppression
diethylenetriaminepentaacetic
d. acid (DTPA)
d. acid imaging agent
Dieulafoy
D. disease
D. lesion
D. vascular malformation
difference
field-echo d.
hemispheric regional
lateralization d.
potential d.
rib-vertebral angle d.
transient hepatic attenuation d.
(THAD)
differencing
convolutional d.
d. fiber
d. filter
differential
d. diagnosis bone lesion
d. diagnostic lung mass feature
d. interference contrast microscopy
renal function d.
scintillation camera linearity d.
scintillation camera uniformity d.
d. signal
d. uniformity
d. uptake ratio
d. washout
differentiated carcinoma (DC)
differentiation
cluster of d. (CD)
corticomedullary d. (CMD)
gray matter-white matter d.
gray-white d.
liposarcomatous d.
nuclear anular d.
difficult-to-treat vascular lesion
diffracting Doppler transducer
diffraction
beam d.
high-resolution d.
high-temperature d.
low-temperature d.
d. pattern

d. peak
x-ray d.
diffraction-enhanced imaging (DEI)
diffuse
d. abdominal calcification
d. adenomyosis
d. aggressive lymphoma
d. aggressive polymorphous
infiltrate
d. airspace disease
d. airspace opacity
d. alveolar interstitial infiltrate
d. aortic atresia
d. aortic dilatation
d. aortomegaly
d. arterial ectasia
d. arteriolar spasm
d. aspiration bronchiolitis
d. axonal injury (DAI)
d. bacterial nephritis
d. bilateral alveolar infiltrate
d. cerebral histiocytosis
d. cirrhosis
d. CNS sclerosis
d. contrast agent distribution
pattern
d. dilation of the esophagus
d. edema
d. emphysema
d. enlargement of the thymus
d. esophageal spasm (DES)
d. fatty liver infiltrate
d. fibrosis type
d. fine lung reticulation
d. gallbladder wall thickening
d. ganglion
d. haziness
d. hepatic enlargement
d. hyperemia
d. idiopathic skeletal hyperostosis
(DISH)
d. increase in breast density
d. infection
d. inflammation
d. intermediate lymphocytic
lymphoma
d. interstitial pulmonary fibrosis
(DIPF)
d. intimal thickening
d. irregularity
d. large-cell lymphoma (DLCL)
d. liver enlargement
d. low attenuation
d. low signal replacement of the
vertebral body
d. lung uptake
d. lymphangioma

d. malformation
d. malignant peritoneal mesothelioma
d. mixed small- and large-cell lymphoma
d. mottling
d. mucosal polyposis
d. myelinoclastic sclerosis
d. narrowing
d. necrosis
d. necrotizing leukoencephalopathy
d. osteosclerosis
d. panbronchiolitis
d. pancreatitis
d. parenchymal lung disease
d. periapical sclerosing osteitis
d. pericarditis
d. perivascular infiltrate
d. pleural thickening
d. pleurisy
d. pneumonia
d. pneumonitis
d. pulmonary alveolar hemorrhage
d. pulmonary neuroendocrine cell hyperplasia
d. reflector
d. reticular density
d. reticulogranular lung density
d. reticulonodular infiltrate
d. sarcomatosis
d. scleroderma
d. sclerosing alveolitis
d. signal hyperintensity
d. skeletal angiomatosis
d. skeletal metastasis
d. small-cell lymphocytic lymphoma
d. spasm of the esophagus
d. spatial distribution
d. spondylosis
d. stenosis
d. subarachnoid hemorrhage
d. symmetric hypertrophied cardiomyopathy
d. synovial lipoma
d. thymic enlargement
d. toxic goiter
d. ulcerative lesion
d. uterine enlargement
d. ventricular hypokinesis
d. white matter injury
diffusible tracer
diffusing capacity

diffusion
anisotropically rotational d. (ARD)
d. anisotropy thresholding
d. characteristics of water
d. coefficient
directional d.
d. encoding strength
d. factor
Fick first law of d.
d. gradient
d. magnetic resonance imaging
molecular d.
d. pulse sequence
restricted d.
restricted water d.
d. scan
spectral d.
d. spectroscopy
spin d.
d. tension (DT)
d. tension imaging (DTI)
d. tensor (DT)
d. tensor imaging (DTI)
d. tensor MR imaging
thermal d.
d. time
translational d.
diffusional anisotropy
diffusion/perfusion snapshot FLASH (DPSF)
diffusion-sensitive sequence
diffusion-sensitizing gradient
diffusion-weighted
d.-w. echo planar imaging
d.-w. image
d.-w. imaging (DWI)
d.-w. MR imaging
d.-w. pulse sequence
d.-w. scanning
diffusivity
mean d.
white matter d.
diffusum
papilloma d.
digastric
d. fossa
d. groove
d. impression
d. line
d. muscle
d. notch
d. triangle

D

NOTES

DiGeorge syndrome
digestive
    d. system
    d. tract
    d. tract content
    d. tube
digestive-respiratory fistula
DIGGEST
    direct imaging of local gradients by
    group echo selection tomography
Digibar 190 contrast agent
Digirad
    D. gamma camera
    D. 2020tc imager
digiscope
    Direx d.
digit
    accessory d.
    arthrodesed d.
    binary d.
    fibroosseous pseudotumor of d.
    flail d.
    photoplethysmographic d.
    replanted d.
    sausage d.
    supernumerary d.
    syndactylization of d.
digital
    d. abdominal radiograph
    D. Add-On-Bucky radiographic
    detector image acquisition system
    d. amorphous silicon flat-panel
    detector
    d. amputation
    d. aponeurosis
    d. artery of foot
    d. artery of hand
    d. autofluoroscope
    d. beam attenuation
    d. branch
    d. celiac trunk angiography
    d. chest imaging
    d. chest imaging system
    d. chest radiograph
    d. deformity
    d. ejection fraction
    D. Equipment system
    d. extensor tendon
    d. flexor tendon
    d. fluorography
    d. fluoroscopy
    d. fossa
    d. free hepatic venography
    d. frequency analysis
    D. Fundus imager
    d. gray scale
    d. holography system

    d. image processing algorithm
    D. Imaging and Communications in
    Medicine interface
    d. imaging processing (DIP)
    d. isotope calibrator
    d. livedo reticularis infarct
    d. mammographic system
    d. mammography
    d. marking
    D. Medical System
    d. neuroma
    D. OsteoView 2000
    d. parabola
    d. plethysmography
    d. process of fat
    d. radiography (DR)
    d. radiography imaging
    d. ray
    d. rectal evacuation
    d. reformatting knee MRI
    d. road mapping
    d. rotational angiography (DRA)
    d. runoff
    d. sampling rate
    d. selenium-based chest imaging
    system
    d. storage
    d. subtraction
    d. subtraction angiogram
    d. subtraction angiography (DSA)
    d. subtraction aortography
    d. subtraction arteriography (DSA)
    d. subtraction film
    d. subtraction mammography
    (DSM)
    d. subtraction pulmonary angiogram
    d. subtraction rotational angiography
    d. subtraction technique
    d. subtraction ventriculogram
    d. tomosynthesis
    D. Traumex system
    d. unraveling
    d. vascular imaging (DVI, DVI
    mode)
    d. vein
    d. videoangiography
    d. video gastrointestinal radiography
    d. x-ray detector
digitalization noise
digitally
    d. fused CT and radiolabeled
    imaging
    d. fused CT and radiolabeled
    monoclonal antibody SPECT
    image
    d. reconstructed radiograph (DRR)
digital-to-analog converter (DAC)

digitate ectasia
digiti (*pl. of* digitus)
    d. manus
    d. quinti proprius tendon
digitization
digitized
    d. contact mammogram
    d. CT slice
    d. film image
    d. spinography
digitizer
    backlit d.
    3D surface d.
    laser d.
    multiple jointed d.
    multisensor structured light
      range d.
    Polhemus 3D d.
digitorum
    extensor d.
**Digitron digital subtraction imaging
system**
Di Guglielmo
    Di G. disease
    Di G. syndrome
**dihydropyrimidine dehydrogenase
activity**
dihydroxyphenylalanine imaging agent
diiodotyrosine
dilacerated tooth root
dilatation, dilation
    alveolar d.
    d. of aneurysm
    antegrade transluminal balloon d.
    anular d.
    aortic root d.
    arterial d.
    ascending aorta d.
    balloon d.
    beaded ductal d.
    bile duct d.
    biliary d.
    bowel loop d.
    bronchial d.
    bronchiolar d.
    caliceal d.
    cardiac d.
    cavitary d.
    chamber d.
    colonic d.
    common duct d.
    congenital cystic d.

cystic d.
diffuse aortic d.
distal ureteral d.
ductal d.
Eder-Puestow d.
esophageal d.
extrahepatic biliary cystic d.
fusiform d.
gaseous d.
gastric d.
hepatic web d.
d. and hypertrophy
idiopathic pulmonary artery d.
idiopathic right atrial d.
intestinal d.
intrahepatic biliary cystic d.
intrahepatic biliary ductal d.
intrahepatic biliary tract d.
intraluminal d.
junctional d.
left ventricular d.
megacolon d.
multiple mural d.
mural d.
myocardial d.
pancreatic duct d.
paradoxical colon d.
pelvicaliceal d.
percutaneous transluminal balloon d.
periportal sinusoidal d.
pharmacologic d.
poststenotic d.
prestenotic d.
probe d.
prognathic d.
proximal esophagitis d.
pulmonary artery d.
pulmonary trunk idiopathic d.
pulmonary valve stenosis d.
rectal d.
respiratory bronchiolar d.
right ventricular d.
saccular d.
stress-induced left ventricular d.
sulcal d.
sulcus d.
d. of sulcus
thickened irregular small bowel
  fold d.
thickened smooth small bowel
  fold d.
tortuous vein d.

D

NOTES

dilatation *(continued)*
　　track d.
　　transient left ventricular d.
　　transluminal d.
　　tubular d.
　　d. of ureter
　　ureteral d.
　　vein d.
　　d. of ventricle
　　ventricular wall d.
　　Virchow-Robin space d.
　　Wirsung d.
dilated
　　d. aortic root
　　d. bile duct
　　d. bowel loop
　　d. bronchus
　　d. cardiomyopathy (DCM)
　　d. collateral vein
　　d. descending aorta
　　d. dry small bowel
　　d. duodenum
　　d. esophagus
　　d. fetal bowel
　　d. gallbladder
　　d. intercavernous sinus
　　d. intrahepatic duct
　　d. loops of bowel
　　d. lymphatic
　　d. mammary duct
　　d. myocardium
　　d. pulmonary artery
　　d. pulmonary trunk
　　d. rete testis
　　d. small airway
　　d. subareolar duct
　　d. ureter
　　d. ventricle
　　d. wet small bowel
dilation *(var. of* dilatation*)*
　　aneurysmal d.
　　aortic d.
　　proximal d.
dilator
　　angiographic Teflon d.
　　balloon d.
　　Teflon fascial d.
　　telescopic aerial d.
dilution
　　isotopic d.
　　ultrasound d.
**DIMAQ integrated ultrasound
　workstation**
dimeglumine
　　gadopentate d.
　　gadopentetate d. (Gd-DTPA)
　　Magnevist gadopentate d.

dimension
　　abnormal heart chamber d.
　　absolute artery d.
　　anteroposterior d.
　　aortic root d.
　　arterial d.
　　axial d.
　　fractal d. (FD)
　　intraluminal d.
　　intrathoracic d.
　　left ventricular diastolic d. (LVdd)
　　left ventricular end-diastolic d.
　　　(LVEDD)
　　left ventricular end-systolic d.
　　　(LVESD)
　　left ventricular internal diastolic d.
　　　(LVIDd, LVIDD)
　　lumbar spine d.
　　luminal d.
　　right ventricular d. (RVD)
　　spleen d.
dimer
　　d. captosuccinic acid (DMSA)
　　Dimer X
　　ethyl cysteinate d. (ECD)
　　ionic hexaiodinated d.
　　^{99m}Tc-ethyl cysteinate d.
　　technetium-99m L-ethyl
　　　cysteinate d. (^{99m}Tc-ECD)
　　technetium-99m ethyl cysteinate d.
dimerization
dimethyl iminodiacetic acid (DIDA)
dimethylsuccinic acid
diminished
　　d. airway perfusion
　　d. lung volume
　　d. marrow signal intensity
　　d. systemic perfusion
diminutive
　　d. interlobar right pulmonary artery
　　d. vessel
dimple
　　blind d.
　　d. of bone
　　pretibial d.
dinner-fork deformity
diode
　　d. detector
　　infrared light-emitting d.
　　d. laser
　　d. measurement
　　PIN d.
　　positive-intrinsic-negative d.
　　Zener d.
diodone
Diodrast
Diogenes cup

Dionosil imaging agent
dioxide
    carbon d. (CO_2)
    radiopaque medium thorium d.
    titanium d.
DIP
    desquamative interstitial pneumonia
    digital imaging processing
    distal interphalangeal
        DIP algorithm
        DIP articulation
        DIP joint
dip
    d. phenomenon
    septal d.
DIPF
    diffuse interstitial pulmonary fibrosis
diphosphate
    dipyridoxal d.
    manganese dipyridoxyl d.
diphosphine
    lipophilic cationic d.
diphosphonate
    methylene d. (MDP)
diploë
diplogram
diploic
    d. canal
    d. vein
diplomyelia
dipolar
    d. broadening
    d. interaction
dipole
    d. coupling
    electric d.
    d. field
    magnetic d.
dipole-dipole
    d.-d. coupling
    d.-d. interaction
    proton electron d.-d.
    d.-d. relaxation rate
diprosopus
dipygus
dipyridamole
    d. echocardiography
    d. echocardiography imaging
    d. handgrip imaging
    d. handgrip test
    d. infusion imaging

    d. technetium-99m-2-methoxy
        isobutyl
    d. technetium-99m-2-methoxy
        isobutyl isonitrile
    d. thallium-201 imaging
    d. thallium-201 scintigraphy
    d. thallium stress imaging
    d. thallium ventriculogram
dipyridoxal diphosphate
direct
    d. caval cannulation
    d. current (DC)
    d. current generator
    d. current offset artifact
    d. digital radiography
    d. display console (DDC)
    d. embolus
    d. Fourier transformation imaging
    d. fracture
    d. imaging of local gradients by
        group echo selection tomography
        (DIGGEST)
    d. immunofluorescence analysis
    d. inguinal hernia
    d. liquid scintillation count
    d. needle puncture
    d. percutaneous transhepatic
        cholangiography
    d. puncture MR phlebogram
    d. puncture phlebography
    d. radiation
    d. radioiodination
    d. ray
    d. slice
    d. splenoportography
    d. transtorcular approach
    d. venography
    d. vision spectroscope
    d. visualization
direct-contact transmission
direction
    aboral d.
    anterior-posterior flow d.
    caudal d.
    cephalad d.
    cephalad-caudad d.
    mediolateral flow d.
    noncollinear d.
    phase-encoding d.
    superior-inferior flow d.
    white matter tract d.

D

NOTES

directional
    d. atherectomy catheter
    d. atherectomy device
    d. color angiography (DCA)
    d. coronary atherectomy (DCA)
    d. diffusion
    d. gradient concentration (DGC)
direction-encoded color mapping (DEC)
director
    grooved d.
DirectRay direct-to-digital image capture device
DirectView CR 900 imaging system
Direx
    D. digiscope
    D. Thermex
    D. Tripter
dirty
    d. acoustic shadowing
    d. chest
    d. fat
    d. film artifact
    d. mass
    d. necrosis
disappearance
    d. frequency
    d. slope
disappearing
    d. bone disease
    d. fetus
disarray
    myocardial d.
disarticulation
    hip d.
disc (*var. of* disk)
discectomy (*var. of* diskectomy)
discernible venous motion
discharge
    periodic synchronous d. (PSD)
    sympathetic d.
    d. tube
discharging tubule
disci (*pl. of* discus)
discitis
discogenic
    d. disease
    d. osteophytes
discogram (*var. of* diskogram)
discography (*var. of* diskography)
discoid
    d. atelectasis
    d. chest mass
    d. configuration
    d. filling defect
    d. kidney
    d. lateral meniscus
    d. shadow

discoligamentous complex
discontinuous
    d. density gradient
    d. density gradient centrifugation
    d. imaging
    d. scanning
discordance
    radiologic-pathologic d.
discordant
    d. finding
    d. nodule thyroid
    d. thyroid nodule
    d. twin
Discovery
    D. LS imaging system
    D. LS, ST^4 PET/CT scanner
discrepancy
    biomechanics of limb-length d.
    leg-length d. (LLD)
    limb-length d. (LLD)
discrete
    d. area of consolidation
    d. area of effusion
    d. bleeding source
    d. cosine transform (DCT)
    d. focal stenosis
    d. Fourier transform (DFT)
    d. hyperintense focus
    d. hyperintense signal intensity
    d. lesion
    d. mass
    d. narrowing
    d. perihilar density
    d. plaque
    d. pulmonary nodule
    d. segment of normal esophagus
    d. subaortic stenosis
    d. subvalvular aortic stenosis (DSAS)
    d. tumor
discriminant analysis
discriminate
discrimination
    density d.
discriminator setting
discus, pl. **disci**
DISE
    driven inversion spin echo
disease (*See* phenomenon, syndrome)
    acquired cystic kidney d.
    acquired occupational lung d.
    acquired renal cystic d.
    active parenchymal d.
    acyanotic congenital heart d.
    Addison d.
    adrenal medullary d.
    adult polycystic kidney d.

airflow obstruction d. (AOD)
airspace d.
alcoholic liver d. (ALD)
Alexander d.
alloimmune d.
alveolar lung d.
Alzheimer d. (AD)
angiomatous d.
anterior horn cell d.
aortic valvular d. (AVD)
aortoiliac occlusive d. (AIOD)
arterial degenerative d.
arteriosclerotic cardiovascular d.
  (ASCVD)
arteriosclerotic heart d. (ASHD)
arteriosclerotic occlusive d.
arteriosclerotic peripheral
  vascular d.
asbestos-related pleural d.
atheroembolic renal d.
atherosclerotic cardiovascular d.
  (ASCVD)
atherosclerotic carotid artery d.
  (ACAD)
atherosclerotic peripheral vascular d.
  (ASPVD)
autosomal dominant polycystic
  kidney d. (ADPKD)
autosomal recessive polycystic
  kidney d. (ARPKD)
Bamberger-Marie d.
benign asbestos-related pleural d.
benign breast d. (BBD)
biliary tract d.
Binswanger d.
black lung d.
Blount d.
Bouchard d.
Bouillaud d.
Bourneville d.
Bourneville-Pringle d.
brittle bone d.
Brodie d.
Bruck d.
bullous lung d.
caisson d.
calcium hydroxyapatite
  deposition d.
calcium pyrophosphate deposition d.
  (CPPD)
calcium pyrophosphate dihydrate
  deposition d.

Calvé-Legg-Perthes d.
Calvé-Perthes d.
Camurati-Engelmann d.
Canavan d.
Canavan-van Bogaert-Bertrand d.
cardiopulmonary d.
cardiorenal d.
cardiovascular d. (CD, CVD)
cardiovascular renal d.
Caroli d.
carotid artery d.
carotid atherosclerotic d.
carotid occlusive d.
Carrington d.
Castleman d.
celiac d.
central airway d.
cerebral inflammatory d.
cerebral Whipple d.
cerebrovascular occlusive d.
cervical disk d.
Charcot-Marie-Tooth d.
cholestatic liver d.
chronic interstitial simulating
  airspace lung d.
chronic obstructive lung d. (COLD)
chronic obstructive pulmonary d.
  (COPD)
chronic peripheral arterial d.
  (CPAD)
Coats d.
Concato d.
congenital heart d. (CHD)
connective tissue d.
coronary artery d.
Cowden d.
Creutzfeldt-Jakob d. (CJD)
Crohn d. (CD)
crystal deposition d.
Cushing d.
cyanotic congenital heart d.
cystic breast d.
cystic kidney d.
cystic ovarian d.
degenerative atrioventricular node d.
degenerative brain d.
degenerative disk d.
degenerative joint d. (DJD)
demyelinating d.
de Quervain d.
Deutschländer d.
Dieulafoy d.

NOTES

disease *(continued)*

diffuse airspace d.
diffuse parenchymal lung d.
Di Guglielmo d.
disappearing bone d.
discogenic d.
disk d.
disseminated d.
diverticular colon d.
Duroziez mitral stenosis d.
end-stage lung d.
end-stage renal d.
Engelmann d.
eosinophilic lung d.
Erb d.
Erdheim-Chester d.
extracolonic d.
extracranial carotid artery
  occlusive d.
extramammary Paget d.
extrathoracic d.
Fahr d.
Fairbank d.
Favre d.
fibrocystic breast d.
fibrocystic lung d.
Flatau-Schilder d.
flax-dresser d.
focal lung d.
focal small-bowel d.
Fong d.
Forestier d.
Freiberg d.
Friedreich d.
Fukuyama congenital muscular d.
  (FCMD)
Gandy-Nanta d.
Garré d.
gastroesophageal reflux d. (GERD)
Gaucher d.
Gee-Herter d.
Gee-Thaysen d.
Gerstmann-Straussler-Scheinker d.
gestational trophoblastic d. (GTD)
Gilchrist d.
Glénard d.
Gorham d.
Graves d.
heart d. (HD)
heavy-chain d.
Heberden d.
hepatic vein d.
hepatic veno-occlusive d.
hepatobiliary d.
hepatocerebral d.
Hirschsprung d. (HD)
Hodgkin d. (HD)

Hodgson d.
Hoffa d.
Horton d.
Hunter d.
Huppert d.
hyaline membrane d. (HMD)
hydroxyapatite deposition d.
  (HADD)
hypertensive cardiovascular d.
hypertensive renal d.
hypertensive vascular d.
idiopathic mural endomyocardial d.
ileocolic d.
immunoproliferative small
  intestine d. (IPSID)
infantile polycystic kidney d.
infectious heart d.
inflammatory bowel d.
interfollicular Hodgkin d.
interstitial fibrotic lung d.
intrasynovial d.
ischemic bowel d.
Jaffe-Lichtenstein d.
Jansen d.
juvenile autosomal recessive
  polycystic d.
juvenile Paget d.
Kahler d.
Kawasaki d.
Keinböck d.
Keshan d.
Kikuchi d.
Kikuchi-Fujimoto d.
Kinnier-Wilson d.
Köhler d.
Krabbe d.
Kugelberg-Welander d.
Kussmaul-Maier d.
kyphoscoliotic heart d.
Legg-Calvé-Perthes d. (LCP)
Leigh d.
leptomeningeal d.
Lichtenstein-Jaffe d.
light chain deposition d. (LCDD)
Ligman-Sacks endocarditis d.
liver hydatid d.
local nodal d.
locoregional d.
maple bark d.
marble bone d.
Marchiafava-Bignami d.
Marie-Bamberger d.
Marie-Strümpell d.
Martin d.
medullary cystic d.
Ménétrier d.
Mèniére d.

mesenteric Weber-Christian d.
metabolic bone d.
metastatic d.
microvascular d.
Mikulicz d.
miliary lung d.
miliary parenchymal d.
Milroy d.
mixed connective-tissue d. (MCTD)
Mondor d.
monostotic Paget d.
moyamoya d.
multicentric Castleman d. (MCD)
multiple gland d.
muscle-eye-brain d.
mushroom picker's d.
neonatal wet lung d.
neurodegenerative d.
Niemann-Pick d.
Nievergelt d.
nodal d.
nodular lung d.
nodular sclerosis Hodgkin d.
nodular thyroid d.
no evidence of d. (NED)
no evidence of recurrent d.
 (NERD)
nonatherosclerotic d.
Norrie d.
obstructive airway d.
obstructive lung d.
obstructive pulmonary d. (OPD)
occlusive cerebrovascular d.
occupational lung d.
Ollier d.
optic chiasm d.
Ormond d.
Osgood-Schlatter d.
Osler d.
osseous metastatic d.
Otto d.
Paas d.
Paget jaw d.
pancreatic d.
pancreaticobiliary d.
Panner d.
Parenti-Fraccaro d.
Pelizaeus-Merzbacher d.
Pellegrini-Stieda d.
pelvic inflammatory d.
peptic ulcer d. (PUD)
pericardial d.

perihilar lung d.
periodontal d.
peripheral airspace d.
peripheral arterial d.
peripheral arterial occlusive d.
 (PAOD)
peripheral lung d.
peripheral vascular d. (PVD)
peripheral vascular occlusive d.
Perthes d.
Peyronie d.
Pfaundler-Hurler d.
Pfeiffer d.
Pick d.
pleural d.
Plummer d.
polycystic kidney d.
polycystic liver d.
polycystic ovarian d. (PCOD)
Pompe d.
popliteal artery occlusive d.
posttransplant coronary artery d.
Pott d.
prediverticular d.
Preiser d.
primary pigmented nodular
 adrenocortical d.
pseudo-Whipple d.
pulmonary embolic septic d.
pulmonary interstitial d.
pulmonary thromboembolic d.
Pyle d.
radiation-induced liver d. (RILD)
ragpicker's d.
reactive airway d. (RAD)
renal cystic d.
renal parenchymal d.
renovascular d.
respiratory bronchiolitis-associated
 interstitial lung d. (RB-ILD)
restrictive lung d.
restrictive myocardial d.
reticulonodular lung d.
reversible airway d.
rheumatic heart d.
rheumatic valvular d.
rheumatoid lung d.
Ribbing d.
Roger d.
Rosai-Dorfman d.
Ruysch d.
sacroiliac d.

NOTES

disease *(continued)*
    Scheuermann d.
    Schilder d.
    Schmid d.
    Schmorl d.
    Sever d.
    Shaver d.
    silo-filler's d.
    Simmond d.
    Sinding-Larsen-Johansson d. (SLJD)
    single-vessel d.
    small bowel d.
    Still d.
    subarachnoid metastatic d.
    subarachnoid space d.
    synchronous d.
    systemic granulomatous d.
    Takayasu d.
    three-vessel coronary d.
    thromboembolic d. (TED)
    thromboembolic lung d.
    thyrocardiac d.
    thyroid d.
    tibial artery d.
    tibioperoneal occlusive d.
    toxic lung d.
    Trevor d.
    Uhl d.
    ulcer d.
    upper lung d.
    upper respiratory tract d.
    valvular d. (VD)
    valvular heart d.
    van Buchem d.
    vanishing bone d.
    Vaquez d.
    variant of Creutzfeldt-Jacob d.
      (vCJD)
    vascular occlusive d.
    venous thromboembolic d. (VTED)
    vertebrobasilar d.
    von Recklinghausen d.
    von Willebrand d.
    Voorhoeve d.
    Warburg d.
    Werdnig-Hoffmann d.
    Westphal-Strümpell d.
    Whipple d.
    white matter d.
    Wilson d.
    Winiwarter-Buerger d.
    Zuska d.
disease-free vessel
DISH
    diffuse idiopathic skeletal hyperostosis
dishpan fracture

DISI
    dorsal intercalated segmental instability
disintegration
    d. constant
    myofibrillar d.
    nuclear d.
    radioactive d.
    d. rate
    spontaneous d.
disintegrator
    electrohydraulic d.
disjointing
disk, disc
    acromioclavicular joint d.
    anal d.
    d. of ankle
    anterior intervertebral d.
    articular d.
    atrial d.
    d. ballooning
    biconcave d.
    bilocular d.
    Bowman d.
    d. bulge
    d. calcification
    candle drip d.
    cartilaginous d.
    cervical d.
    chorionic d.
    concave skull d.
    cone d.
    contained d.
    crescent-shaped fibrocartilaginous d.
    d. degeneration
    degenerative d.
    d. derangement
    d. desiccation
    d. disease
    d. displacement
    distal radioulnar d.
    embryonic d.
    d. of endocardium
    Engelmann d.
    epiphyseal d.
    extruded d.
    d. extrusion
    fibrocartilaginous d.
    fibrous ring of d.
    fixation d.
    d. fragment
    frayed d.
    growth d.
    H d.
    herniated intervertebral d. (HID)
    d. herniation
    hydrodynamic potential of d.
    interarticular d.

d. interspace
intervertebral d.
isotropic d.
kidney d.
d. lesion
locking d.
lumbar d.
lumbosacral d.
magnetic d.
mandibular d.
d. margin
massive herniated d.
d. maturation
midline herniation of d.
Molnar d.
d. morphology
occult residual herniated d.
d. ossification
d. oxygenator
placental d.
d. plication
d. poppet
protruded d.
d. protrusion
rectangular d.
ruptured d.
sequestered d.
d. sequestration
d. space
d. space height
d. space infection
d. space narrowing
spherical d.
sternoclavicular joint d.
tactile d.
temporomandibular joint d.
thoracic d.
thoracolumbar vertebral d.
d. tissue
triangular d.
unilocular d.
vertebral d.
d. water content
Winchester d.
diskectomy, discectomy
automated percutaneous lumbar d.
(APLD)
percutaneous automated d.
same-day microsurgical arthroscopic
lateral-approach laser-assisted
fluoroscopic d.
stereotactic percutaneous lumbar d.

diskitis
calcific d.
childhood d.
juvenile calcific d.
septic d.
disk-like atelectasis
diskogram, discogram
intervertebral d.
intranuclear d.
diskographer
diskographic technique
diskography, discography
diskovertebral
d. infection
d. osteomyelitis
d. spondylitis
disk-shaped bone graft
disk-thecal sac interface
disk-to-magnetic
d.-t.-m. field
d.-t.-m. field orientation
disk-type valve
dislocated
d. hip
d. knee
dislocation
anterior d.
anteroinferior d.
atlantooccipital d.
axial carpal d.
Bankart d.
bayonet d.
Bennett d.
bilateral intrafacetal d.
boutonnière d.
bursting d.
central d.
cervical facet d.
chronic recurrent d.
closed d.
complete d.
complicated d.
compound d.
congenital hip d.
consecutive d.
Desault d.
divergent d.
dysplasia d.
facet d.
fracture d.
frank d.
glenohumeral d.

D

NOTES

dislocation *(continued)*
- Hill-Sachs d.
- hip d.
- hyperextension d.
- incomplete d.
- interfacetal d.
- interphalangeal d.
- irreducible dorsal d.
- isolated d.
- joint d.
- Kienböck d.
- Lisfranc d.
- lunate d.
- midcarpal d.
- milkmaid's elbow d.
- Monteggia d.
- Nélaton d.
- open d.
- partial d.
- d. of patella
- patellar d.
- pathologic d.
- perilunar d.
- perilunate d.
- primitive d.
- radiocarpal d.
- recent d.
- recurrent d.
- rotational d.
- scapholunate d.
- shoulder d.
- simple d.
- Smith d.
- sternoclavicular d.
- subastragalar d.
- subspinous d.
- tibiofemoral joint d.
- tibiotarsal d.
- transradial styloid perilunate d.
- transscaphoid perilunate d.
- traumatic d.
- triquetrolunate d.
- unilateral facet d.
- unilateral interfacetal d.
- unilateral intrafacetal d.
- upward and backward d.
- upward lens d.
- volar d.
- wrist d.

dislodgement
- partial d.

dismutase
- copper-zinc superoxide d. (Cu/Zn-SOD)
- superoxide d.

disobliteration
- carotid d.

disodium
- pamidronate d.

disofenin
- technetium-99m d.

disorder
- angiocentric immunoproliferative d.
- angitis-granulomatosis d.
- articular hand d.
- articular wrist d.
- bullous d.
- cartilaginous growth plate d.
- congenital d.
- deglutition d.
- demyelinative d.
- drug-induced bullous d.
- esophageal functional d.
- esophageal morphologic d.
- esophageal motility d.
- evacuation d.
- functional d.
- gastric motor d.
- infectious pulmonary d.
- intractable bleeding d.
- lymphoproliferative d.
- metabolic bone d.
- migration d.
- motility d.
- myeloproliferative d.
- neurogenic d.
- nonspecific esophageal motility d. (NEMD)
- patellofemoral d.
- posttransplant lymphoproliferative d.
- pulmonary lymphoid d.
- surfactant deficiency d. (SDD)
- systemic d.
- underlying d.

disorganized architecture
dispenser
- film d.

dispersing agent
dispersion
- gradient-induced phase d.
- intravoxel phase d.
- d. mode

dispersive component
disphenoid extraction
displaced
- d. crus
- d. fracture
- d. fracture fragment
- d. fragment of bone
- d. gallbladder
- d. left paraspinal line
- d. left ventricular apex
- d. osteochondral fragment
- d. vertebra

displacement
>anterior tracheal d.
>arterial brain d.
>atlantoaxial rotary d.
>d. of bowel gas
>brainstem d.
>d. of brain vessel
>breast tissue d.
>disk d.
>Ellis Jones peroneal d.
>esophageal d.
>d. field-fitting MR imaging
>hilar d.
>inferior d.
>d. of interhemispheric fissure
>left apex cardiogram, calibrated d. (LACD)
>mediastinum d.
>palmar d.
>d. placentogram (DPG)
>radial epiphyseal d.
>retroperitoneal fat stripe d.
>rotational d.
>superolateral d.
>tracheal d.

display
>A-mode d.
>B-mode d.
>cine-mode d.
>d. coordinate system
>dynamic volume-rendered d.
>image d.
>M-mode d.
>multiparametric color composite d.
>multiplanar d. (MPD)
>real-time d.
>segmentation method for real-time d.
>shaded surface d.
>stack mode d.
>static image d.
>surface shaded d. (SSD)
>d. system
>tile mode d.

disproportion
>cephalopelvic d. (CPD)
>fetal-pelvic d.
>fetal ventricular heart d.
>fiber-type d.
>ventricular d.

disproportionate upper septal thickening
disrupted plaque

disruption
>anastomotic d.
>anterior labral d.
>anular d.
>blood-brain barrier d.
>bony d.
>d. of the cartilaginous synchondrosis
>d. of duct
>epiglottic d.
>facet capsule d.
>ligamentous d.
>myofascial d.
>retinacular d.
>skeletal d.
>superior peroneal retinaculum d.
>supraspinous ligament d.
>trabecular d.
>traumatic aortic d.
>volar radiocarpal ligament d.

dissecans
>osteochondritis d.
>osteochondrosis d.

dissecting
>d. abdominal aneurysm
>d. aortic aneurysm
>d. aortic hematoma
>d. basilar artery aneurysm
>d. intracranial aneurysm
>d. intramural hematoma

dissection
>aneurysmal d.
>aortic d.
>arterial wall d.
>d. of artery
>axial joint d.
>descending aorta d.
>esophageal d.
>extensive d.
>extracapsular d.
>extrapericardial d.
>familial aortic d.
>groin d.
>intimal-medial d.
>medial d.
>sentinel node d.
>sharp d.
>spiral d.
>spontaneous carotid d.
>spontaneous coronary artery d. (SCAD)
>Stanford type B aortic d.

D

NOTES

dissection *(continued)*
    subintimal d.
    thoracic aortic d.
    d. tubercle
    vertebral arterial d.
dissector
    balloon d.
disseminated
    d. CNS histoplasmosis
    d. coccidioidomycosis
    d. disease
    d. inflammation
    d. intravascular coagulation (DIC)
    d. intravascular coagulation
        syndrome
    d. lipogranulomatosis
    d. necrotizing leukoencephalopathy
    d. sclerosis
    d. tuberculosis
dissemination
    hematogenous d.
    lymphogenous d.
    d. pattern
Disse space
dissociation
    complete atrioventricular d.
    electromechanical d. (EMD)
    interference d.
    scapholunate d.
dissociative instability
dissolution of gallstone
distal
    d. acinar emphysema
    d. aorta
    d. aortic arch
    d. aortic arch aneurysm
    d. articular set angle (DASA)
    d. bile duct
    d. bile duct carcinoma (DBDC)
    d. blind stomach
    d. bone marrow development
    d. branch
    d. bronchiectasis
    d. bulbar septum
    d. carpal row
    d. circumflex marginal artery
    d. colon
    d. common bile duct obstruction
    d. convoluted tubule
    d. coronary perfusion pressure
    d. coronary sinus (DCS)
    d. duodenum
    d. esophageal ring
    d. femoral epiphyseal fracture
    d. femur
    d. humoral fracture
    d. ileitis

d. interphalangeal (DIP)
d. interphalangeal joint
d. intestinal obstruction syndrome
d. leak type I
d. leg cross section
d. line of reference (DLR)
d. lobular emphysema
d. metatarsal articular angle
    (DMMA)
d. occlusal distention
d. radial fracture
d. radioulnar disk
d. radioulnar joint (DRUJ)
d. radioulnar joint compartment
d. radioulnar subluxation
d. rectal adenocarcinoma (DRA)
d. reference axis (DRA)
d. runoff
d. runoff vessel
d. segment
d. shift
d. small bowel
d. splenorenal shunt
d. surface
d. tibial physis
d. tibiofibular syndesmosis
d. ureteral dilatation
distalward
distance
    acromiohumeral d.
    anterior capsular d. (ACD)
    atlas odontoid d.
    center-to-center d.
    central lung d. (CLD)
    Doppler-derived stroke d.
    fanning of the interspinous d.
    film tube d.
    flexion interspinous d. (FID)
    focal film d. (FFD)
    focal spot-to-object d.
    focus object d. (FOD)
    focus-skin d. (FSD)
    interarch d.
    intercaudate d.
    interlaminar d.
    internuclear d.
    interopercular d.
    interorbital d.
    interpedicular d.
    interridge d.
    interslice d.
    interspinous d. (ISD)
    interuncal d. (IUD)
    object-film d. (OFD)
    pisoscaphoid d.
    posterior capsular d. (PCD)
    probe-surface d.

source-film d. (SFD)
source-skin d. (SSD)
source-surface d. (SSD)
source-to-image receptor d. (SID)
source-tray d. (STD)
surface d.
target-film d. (TFD)
target-skin d. (TSD)
teardrop d. (TDD)
ulnotriquetral d.
widened teardrop d.

distance-based block classification
distant
d. metastasis
d. spread

distended
d. abdomen
d. central bronchi
d. gallbladder
d. kidney
d. stomach
d. vein

distensibility
aortic d.

distensible
distention, distension
abdominal d.
alveolar d.
azygos vein d.
bladder d.
bowel d.
colonic d.
distal occlusal d.
d. of the esophagogastric region
gaseous d.
gastric d.
hydraulic d.
intestinal d.
jugular venous d.
luminal d.
maximal radiographic d.
passive venous d.
pelvicaliceal d.
postvagotomy small-bowel d.
radiographic d.
d. ratio
rectal d.
ureteral d.
venous d.
vesical d.

distinction
loss of d.

distorted
d. anatomy
d. mucosal fold

distortion
architectural d.
barreling d.
bronchial d.
current line d.
focal d.
geometric d.
image d.
pincushion d.
radiographic pincushion d.
S d.
spiculated d.
Y-shaped d.

distraction
bifocal manipulation with d.
d. of fracture
d. gap
d. hyperflexion injury
joint d.
d. osteogenesis
physeal d.
segment d.
small-step d.
soft tissue d.

distraction-flexion staging (DFS)
distractor
intramedullary skeletal kinetic d.
(ISKD)

distribution
anatomic d.
anomalous d.
apparent volume of d. (Vd)
batwing d.
Boltzmann d.
butterfly d.
centrilobular d.
depth dose d.
diffuse spatial d.
dose d.
gaussian d.
geometric d.
harness-shaped d.
homogeneous susceptibility d.
homogeneous thallium d.
inhomogeneous tracer d.
interstitial lung disease d.
loop d.
lung infiltrate d.
maxwellian d.

D

NOTES

distribution *(continued)*
    mottled d.
    normal variant fluorodeoxyglucose
      uptake d.
    normal whole body
      fluorodeoxyglucose d.
    peribronchial d.
    perivascular d.
    Poisson d.
    radioactivity d.
    rapid d.
    regional myocardial mass d.
    reverse d.
    rim-like calcium d.
    spatial d.
    spatial dose d.
    spectral noise d.
    symmetric d.
    thallium-201 uptake and d.
    trace element d.
    d. transformer
    uniform d.
    unusual marrow d.
distributive shock
disturbance
    architectural d.
    d. of articulation
    circulation d.
disturbed orientation
disuse osteoporosis
diuresis
    d. renogram
    d. urogram
diuretic
    d. radionuclide urography
    d. renal imaging
    d. renal scan
    d. renography
divergent
    d. dislocation
    d. ray projection
    d. spiculated pattern
diverging
    d. collimator
    d. meniscus
diversion
    biliopancreatic d.
    cerebrospinal fluid d.
    urinary d.
    ventriculoperitoneal d.
diversity segment
diverticular
    d. abscess
    d. colon disease
    d. prostatitis
diverticulitis
    acute d.

    bladder d.
    chronic d.
    colonic d.
    Meckel d.
    sigmoid d.
diverticulogram
diverticulosis
    colonic d.
    intramural esophageal d.
    jejunal d.
    tracheal d.
diverticulum
    acquired urethral d.
    arachnoid d.
    bladder d.
    caliceal d.
    colonic d.
    common bile duct d.
    congenital urethral d.
    cricopharyngeal d.
    divisional block d.
    dorsal d.
    ductus d.
    duodenal intraluminal d.
    esophageal d.
    fallopian tube d.
    false d.
    fourth ventricle d.
    functional d.
    gallbladder d.
    Ganser d.
    gastric d.
    giant sigmoid d.
    Graser d.
    hepatic d.
    Hutch d.
    hypopharyngeal d.
    interaorticobronchial d.
    interbronchial d.
    intestinal d.
    intraluminal duodenal d. (IDD)
    intramural d.
    inverted Meckel d.
    jejunal d.
    jejunoileal d.
    juxtapapillary d.
    Kirchner d.
    Kommerell d.
    Kumeral d.
    Meckel d.
    metanephric d.
    midesophageal d.
    Nuck d.
    paraureteral d.
    perforated d.
    periampullary d.
    pharyngoesophageal d.

pulsion d.
pyelocaliceal d.
Rokitansky d.
roofless fourth ventricle d.
sigmoid d.
small bowel d.
stomach d.
thoracic pulsion d.
thoracic root sleeve d.
traction d.
urachal d.
urethral d.
urinary bladder d.
Vater d.
vesical d.
Zenker d.
diverting stoma
divided dose
diving goiter
division
mandibular d.
maxillary d.
ureteral d.
divisional
d. block
d. block diverticulum
divisionary line
divisum
pancreas d.
divopontocerebellar atrophy
Dixon
D. fat-fraction measurement
D. method of phase unwrapping
D. quantitative chemical shift
image
dizygotic twin
DJD
degenerative joint disease
DJF
duodenojejunal flexure
DJJ
duodenojejunal junction
DKS
Damus-Kaye-Stansel
DKS procedure
2D KWE direct Fourier imaging
DLCL
diffuse large-cell lymphoma
limited-stage DLCL
D-loop
dextro loop

ventricular D-loop
D-loop ventricular situs
DLR
distal line of reference
D-malposition of aorta
2D mapping
DMI
diaphragmatic myocardial infarct
DMMA
distal metatarsal articular angle
**2D modified KWE direct Fourier
imaging**
DMPE
DMSA
dimer captosuccinic acid
(V)-dimer captosuccinic acid
^{99m}Tc (V) DMSA
2D multislice
DNA
deoxyribonucleic acid
DNA cytophotometry
DNA flow cytometry
DNA microinjection technique
DNET
dysembryoplastic neuroepithelial tumor
2D NMR
DNP
dynamic nuclear polarization
DNR
dose nonuniformity ratio
DOBI
dynamic optical breast imaging system
DOBI system
dobutamine
d. stress echocardiography (DSE)
d. thallium angiography
DOBV
double-outlet both ventricles
doctrine
Monroe-Kellie d.
documentary arteriography
document image decoding (DID)
document-recognition algorithm
Dodd perforating vein group
dodecafluoropentane (DDFP)
d. imaging agent
Dodge
D. area-length method for
ventricular volume
D. method for ejection fraction
D. principle
Doerner-Hoskins distribution law

D

NOTES

doigt en lornette
dolens
dolichocephalic
dolichocephaly
dolichocolon
dolichoectasia
 vertebrobasilar d.
dolichoesophagus
dolichopellic pelvis
dolichosigmoid
dolichostenomelia
DoLi S extracorporeal shock wave lithotripter
DOLV
 double-outlet left ventricle
domain
 dose rate d.
 extracellular d.
 Fourier d.
 frequency d.
 magnetic d.
 scene d.
 spatial frequency d.
 time d.
dome
 d. of aneurysm
 anterior talar d.
 atrial d.
 bladder d.
 crus d.
 d. cylinder
 d. of diaphragm
 diaphragmatic d.
 d. fracture
 lateral talar d.
 liver d.
 shoulder d.
 talar d.
 weightbearing acetabular d.
dome-and-dart configuration
dome-shaped
 d.-s. heart
 d.-s. roof of pleural cavity
dome-to-neck ratio
dominance
 cerebral d.
 coronary artery d.
 orbitofrontal d.
dominant
 anatomically d.
 d. follicle
 d. hemisphere
 d. hemisphere infarct
 d. hemisphere lesion
 hepatic arterial d.
 d. left coronary artery
 portal venous d.

 d. right coronary artery
 d. vessel
doming
 diastolic d.
 d. of leaflet
 d. of valve
donor
 d. graft
 d. heart
 d. heart-lung block
 d. site
 d. twin
donor-recipient anastomy
DOPA imaging agent
dopaminergic dysfunction
dopamine transporter
Dopascan radiopharmaceutical imaging agent
doped water
DOPING
 double pulse interlaced echo imaging
Doppler
 D. angle
 D. ankle systolic pressure
 D. assessment
 ATL HDI 5000 color D.
 D. blood flow monitor
 D. blood flow velocity signal
 D. blood pressure
 color D. (CD)
 color-flow D. (CFD)
 D. color-flow imaging
 D. color-flow mapping
 D. continuous-wave echocardiography
 contrast-enhanced color D.
 contrast-enhanced power D.
 Convergent color D.
 duplex B-mode D.
 D. effect
 D. equation
 D. flow echocardiographic probe
 D. flow index
 D. flowmeter
 D. flowmetry
 D. flow probe study
 D. flow signal enhancement
 D. frequency shift
 D. frequency spectrum
 D. gain
 gray-scale D.
 high-frequency D. (HFD)
 high pulse repetition frequency D.
 D. insonation
 D. interrogation
 intraoperative D.
 multigate D.

D. ovary signal
periorbital bidirectional D.
pocket D.
power D.
D. pulse
pulsed-wave D.
D. pulsed-wave echocardiography
range-gated pulsed D.
real-time D.
renal D.
D. Resistive Index (DRI)
D. shift frequency
D. shift principle
D. signal enhancement
D. sonography
D. sonography of the SMA
SonoSite pulsed wave D.
spectral D.
D. spectral analysis
D. spectral waveform
D. study of blood flow
D. System 97
D. tissue imaging (DTI)
transcranial D. (TCD)
transcranial color-coded D.
D. tricuspid regurgitation
D. ultrasonic blood flow detector
D. ultrasonic fetal heart monitor
D. ultrasonic velocity detector
D. ultrasonic velocity detector
  segmental plethysmography
D. ultrasonography imaging
D. ultrasound
D. ultrasound segmental blood
  pressure testing
D. venous examination
D. venous imaging
D. VWF
D. waveform analysis
D. waveform dampening
Doppler-derived stroke distance
Doppler-guided hemorrhoid artery
  ligation (DGHAL)
Dorello canal
Dorendorf
D. sign
D. sign of aortic arch aneurysm
dormancy
tumor d.
Dornier
D. compact lithotripter

D. HM3, HM4 lithotripter
D. scanner
Dor reconstruction
dorsal
d. abdominal wall
d. artery
d. artery of penis
d. aspect
d. bend
d. branch
d. capsule
d. decubitus position
d. dermal sinus
d. diverticulum
d. enteric fistula
d. enteric sinus
d. enterogenous cyst
d. induction
d. induction error
d. intercalated segmental instability
  (DISI)
d. interossei
d. kyphotic curvature
d. meningocele
d. metacarpal ligament
d. muscle
d. nerve of penis
d. pancreas
d. pancreatic bud
d. penile vein
d. plate
d. point
d. primary ramus
d. ramus of spinal nerve
d. recumbent position
d. ridge
d. rim
d. rim distal radial fracture
d. root entry zone (DREZ)
d. root entry zone lesion
d. root ganglion (DRG)
d. scapular
d. spinal cord horn
d. spine
d. spinocerebellar tract
d. subaponeurotic space
d. subcutaneous space
d. talar beak
d. talonavicular bone
d. tubercle
d. vertebra
d. view

D

NOTES

dorsal *(continued)*
    d. wing fracture
    d. wrist ligament
dorsalis
    funiculus d.
    d. pedis
    tabes d.
dorsalward
dorsiflexion
    d. angle (DFA)
    d. view
dorsiflexor
dorsispinal vein
dorsoanterior
dorsocephalad
dorsolateral
    d. aspect
    d. tract
dorsomedial
    d. nucleus
    d. thalamotomy
dorsoplantar
    d. aspect
    d. projection
    d. talometatarsal angle
    d. talonavicular angle
    d. view
dorsoposterior
dorsoradial
dorsorostral
dorsosacral position
dorsum
    d. pedis
    d. of penis
    d. sella
    d. sellae atrophy
DORV
    double-outlet right ventricle
dose
    absorbed d. (AD)
    adult d.
    air d.
    d. area product (DAP)
    bioeffect d. (BED)
    biologically equivalent d. (BED)
    bolus d.
    boost d.
    d. calibrator
    central axis depth d.
    cumulative d.
    delivered total d. (DTD)
    depth d.
    d. distribution
    divided d.
    doubling d.
    epilation d.
    d. equivalent (DE)

    d. equivalent radiation
    exit d.
    exposure d.
    ^{67}Ga higher d.
    genetically significant d.
    glandular d.
    gonadal d.
    incremental d.
    d. infiltration
    integral d.
    iodine d.
    isoeffect d.
    d. kernel
    lethal d.
    matched peripheral d. (MPD)
    mean central d. (MCD)
    mean gonad d.
    median lethal d.
    d. nonuniformity ratio (DNR)
    percentage depth d. (PDD)
    radiation adsorbed d. (rad)
    d. rate domain
    reference d.
    scatter d.
    skin d.
    tapering d.
    threshold erythema d.
    tissue tolerance d. (TTD)
    tracer d.
dose-area product meter
dose/dose-rate effective factor (DDREF)
dose-limiting toxicity
dose-surface histogram
dose-time relationship
dose-volume
    d.-v. histogram (DVH)
    d.-v. relationship
dosimeter
    chemical d.
    dichromate d.
    electronic d.
    Gardray d.
    high-dose film d.
    LiF thermoluminescence d.
    pencil d.
    pocket d.
    silicon diode d.
    sucrose d.
    thermoluminescent d. (TLD)
    ultraviolet fluorescent d.
    Victoreen d.
dosimetric penumbra
dosimetrist
dosimetry
    adjacent field x-ray d.
    beam's eye view d.
    dichromate d.

electron d.
four-field x-ray d.
free-radical d.
Fricke d.
high-dose film d.
large-field x-ray d.
LiF thermoluminescence d.
marrow d.
medical internal radiation d.
  (MIRD)
phantom d.
pion d.
polymer d.
radiation d.
radiopharmaceutical d.
single x-ray d.
thermoluminescence d.
transmission d.
x-ray d.

Dos Santos aortography needle
dot
d. scan
subpleural d.
DOTA
tetraazacyclododecanetetraacetic acid
dot-and-dash pattern
Dotter
D. effect
D. tube
dottering effect
double
d. aortic arch
d. aortic arch of Edwards
d. appendix
d. arch aorta
d. autograft
d. breast coil
d. camelback sign of knee
d. cervix
d. coronary orifice
d. decidual sac
d. decidual sac sign
d. density
d. density heart
d. density sign
d. diaphragm sign
d. duct sign
d. emission
d. fracture
d. gallbladder
d. helical CT scan
d. injection

d. inversion recovery sequence
d. kidney
d. label
d. lesion sign
d. line sign
d. lumen
d. lumen central venous catheter
d. outflow
d. outline
d. penis
d. pleurisy
d. pneumonia
d. pulse interlaced echo imaging
  (DOPING)
d. reverse alpha sigmoid loop
d. systolic apical impulse
d. tracking of barium
d. track sign
d. uterus
d. vagina
d. voiding cystogram
d. wall sign
double-arc gallbladder shadow
double-barrel
d.-b. aorta
d.-b. esophagus
d.-b. lumen
double-bleb sign
double-bonded carbon
double-bubble
d.-b. appearance
d.-b. shadow
d.-b. sign
double-bulb appearance
double-channel endoscope
double-contrast
d.-c. arthrography
d.-c. arthrotomography of shoulder
d.-c. barium enema (DCBE)
d.-c. barium meal
d.-c. barium study
d.-c. esophagography
d.-c. eversion examination
d.-c. laryngography
d.-c. radiograph
d.-c. radiography
d.-c. roentgenography
d.-c. technique
d.-c. visualization
double diaphragm contour
double-dose
d.-d. delay (DDD)

D

NOTES

double-dose (continued)
    d.-d. delayed-contrast MRI
    d.-d. gadolinium imaging
double-echo
    d.-e. Broglie wavelength
    d.-e. method
    d.-e. three-point Dixon method fat
    suppression
double-exposed rib
double-exposure drift artifact
double-freeze technique
double-halo
    d.-h. appearance
    d.-h. configuration
    d.-h. sign
double-helical CT imaging
double-helix
    d.-h. acquisition
    d.-h. prostatic stent
double-inlet
    d.-i. left ventricle
    d.-i. single ventricle
    d.-i. ventricle anomaly
double-J ureteral stent
double-label counting
double-lumen
    d.-l. breast implant
    d.-l. endoprosthesis
double-mode steady state
double-mouthed uterus
double-outlet
    d.-o. both ventricles (DOBV)
    d.-o. left ventricle (DOLV)
    d.-o. right ventricle (DORV)
double-phase technetium-99m sestamibi
    imaging
double-pigtail endoprosthesis
double-populated detector ring
double-probe pH study
double-ring
    d.-r. esophageal sign
    d.-r. esophagus
double-spin echo proton spectroscopy
double-spiral CT arterial portography
double-stem silicone lesser MP implant
double-strand scission
double-throw
    single-pole d.-t. (SPDT)
double-tracking colon
double-umbrella technique
double-wire atherectomy technique
doubling dose
doubly broadband triple-resonance
    NMR probe circuit
doughnut
    d. kidney
    d. lesion

    d. magnet
    d. sign
    d. transformer
doughy mass
Douglas
    D. cul-de-sac
    dependent pouch of D.
    D. fold
    D. ligament
    D. rectouterine pouch
Dow
    D. hollow fiber analyzer
    D. method for measuring cardiac
    output
dowager's hump
dowel
    iliac d.
dowel-shaped bone graft
down
    coned d.
    ramp d.
downhill varix
downscatter
downsloping
downstaging
    axillary tumor d.
downstream sampling method
Down syndrome
downward
    d. displacement of apical impulse
    d. slope
    d. vergence
Doyne honeycomb degeneration
DPA
    dual-photon absorptiometry
dP/dt
    peak dP/dt
DPG
    displacement placentogram
2D portal image
DPR
    dynamic planar reconstructor
DPSF
    diffusion/perfusion snapshot FLASH
DPTA
    D. CSF flow study
    ^{99m}Tc-D.
DPTI
    diastolic pressure-time index
DPX-IQ densitometer
DQE
    detective quantum efficiency
DR
    digital radiography
DRA
    digital rotational angiography

distal rectal adenocarcinoma
distal reference axis
dragon pyelogram
drain
external ventricular d. (EVD)
radiopaque d.
retroperitoneal d.
rubber d.
sump d.
drainage
aberrant venous d.
biliary d.
d. catheter
central venous d.
circle loop biliary d.
enteric exocrine d.
external-internal d.
extrapleural d.
gaseous d.
guided d.
imaging guided catheter d.
infradiaphragmatic totally anomalous
pulmonary venous d.
internal biliary d.
intrathoracic catheter d.
pancreatic pseudocyst d.
percutaneous abscess d.
percutaneous antegrade biliary d.
percutaneous biliary d. (PBD)
percutaneous catheter d. (PCD)
percutaneous transhepatic biliary d.
(PTBD)
percutaneous transhepatic
cholangial d. (PTCD)
pulmonary venous d.
spondylodiskitis d.
spontaneous d.
total anomalous pulmonary
venous d. (TAPVD)
transhepatic d.
transvaginal ultrasound-guided d.
tube d.
venous d.
ventricular d.
draining
d. lymphatic bed
d. sinus
d. with venous pressure
drain-out film
draped aorta
Drash syndrome

DRC
design rule check
dynamic range control
DRC algorithm
Drennan metaphyseal-epiphyseal angle
DRESS
depth-resolved surface spectroscopy
Dressler syndrome
DREZ
dorsal root entry zone
DREZ lesion
DRG
dorsal root ganglion
DRI
Doppler Resistive Index
D-ribose
Driffield
Hurter and D. (H and D)
drift
field d.
radial d.
drifting wedge pressure
drill
lithoclast miniature pneumatic d.
drink
effervescent d.
drip
3D d. infusion cholangiography CT
d. infusion cholangiogram (DIC)
d. infusion cholangiography (DIC)
d. infusion pyelography
d. infusion technique
d. infusion urography
dripping
brain candle d.
candle wax d.
driven
d. equilibrium Fourier transform
d. equilibrium Fourier transform
technique
d. inversion spin echo (DISE)
dromedary hump
drooping
d. lily appearance
d. lily sign
d. shoulder
drop
d. finger
d. foot
d. heart
d. metastasis

D

NOTES

drop *(continued)*
    d. shoulder
    d. test for pneumoperitoneum
drop-lock ring
dropped stone
drowned lung
DRR
    digitally reconstructed radiograph
drug
    adjuvant analgesic d.
    d. administration
    d. fraction
    macromolecular d.
    slow-channel blocking d.
    d. tolerance
drug-induced
    d.-i. bone marrow suppression
    d.-i. brain abnormality
    d.-i. brain change
    d.-i. bullous disorder
    d.-i. drug resistance
    d.-i. erythematous lupus
    d.-i. esophagitis
    d.-i. nephrotoxicity
    d.-i. pneumonitis
    d.-i. pulmonary damage
drug-resistant
    d.-r. extratemporal epilepsy
    d.-r. tumor
DRUJ
    distal radioulnar joint
Drummond
    D. marginal artery
    D. sign
    D. sign of aortic aneurysm
drum spur
drumstick
    d. appearance
    d. phalanx
Drusen
    optic nerve D.
dry
    d. bowel preparation
    d. bronchiectasis
    d. heat sterilizer and incinerator
    unit
    d. laser imaging
    d. pleurisy
    d. swallow
dryer system
Drystar dry imager
DryView laser imaging system
DS
    duplex sonography
DSA
    digital subtraction angiography

digital subtraction arteriography
    DSA image
DSAS
    discrete subvalvular aortic stenosis
DSC
    dynamic susceptibility contrast
    DSC MR imaging
DSE
    dobutamine stress echocardiography
2D sequential slice
D-shaped vessel lumen
DSI camera
DSM
    digital subtraction mammography
DSR
    dynamic spatial reconstructor
    DSR scanner
DSRCT
    desmoplastic small round-cell tumor
DT
    diffusion tension
    diffusion tensor
    DT MR imaging
DTD
    delivered total dose
2D technique
DTI
    diffusion tension imaging
    diffusion tensor imaging
    Doppler tissue imaging
DTICH
    delayed traumatic intracerebral hematoma
D-to-E slope
DTPA
    diethylenetriaminepentaacetic acid
    DTPA imaging agent
    ^{111}In DTPA
    DTPA renography
    technetium-99m DMSA, DTPA
    ytterbium-169 DTPA
DTU-215 cardiac digital stimulator
DU
    duplex ultrasound
dual
    d. atrioventricular node pathway
    d. blood supply
    d.-emulsion mammography film
    d. gradient-recalled echo pulse
    sequence
    d. intracoronary scintigraphy
    d. isotope imaging
    d. isotope scanning
    d. lateral hand positioner
    d. lateral skull block
    d. leg immobilizer
    d. lookup table
    d. oblique hand positioner

d. photon
d. plate
d. single-crystal gamma camera
d. transverse linear-array sonogram
d. ventricle
dual-balloon method
dual-coil imaging
dual-contrast study
dual-demand pacing mode
dual-detector helical CT angiography
dual-echo
    d.-e. DIET fast spin-echo imaging
    d.-e. and DT MR imaging
    d.-e. sequence
    d.-e. turbo spin-echo
dual-energy
    d.-e. CT
    d.-e. imaging
    d.-e. linear accelerator
    d.-e. mammography
    d.-e. radiograph (DER)
    d.-e. subtraction
    d.-e. x-ray absorptiometry (DEXA, DXA)
    d.-e. x-ray absorptiometry densitometer
dual-head
    d.-h. coincidence camera
    d.-h. coincidence detection system
    d.-h. SPECT
dual-isotope
    d.-i. single-photon emission CT
    d.-i. SPECT
    d.-i. subtraction technique
    d.-i. TI 201
dual-lookup table algorithm
dual-mode, dual-pacing, dual-sensing (DDD)
dual-phase
    d.-p. CT
    d.-p. helical computed tomography (DHCT)
    d.-p. scan
    d.-p. ^{99m}Tc-sestamibi imaging
dual-photon
    d.-p. absorptiometry (DPA)
    d.-p. densitometer
    d.-p. densitometry
dual-probe rectilinear scanner
dual-sensing
    dual-mode, dual-pacing, d.-s. (DDD)

dual-shaped collimator
dual-tracer imaging
Dubin-Johnson syndrome
Duchenne
    D. muscular dystrophy
    D. sign
duct
    aberrant intrahepatic bile d.
    accessory hepatic d.
    accessory pancreatic d.
    alveolar d.
    amnionic d.
    arborization of d.
    arterial d.
    asymmetric bile d.
    Bartholin d.
    beaded bile d.
    beaded hepatic d.
    beaded pancreatic d.
    d. of Bellini
    bile d.
    biliary d.
    Botallo d.
    branchial d.
    bucconeural d.
    canalicular d.
    carotid d.
    d. cell adenocarcinoma
    d. cell carcinoma
    choledochous d.
    cobblestone appearance of bile d.
    cochlear d.
    common bile d. (CBD)
    common gall d.
    common hepatic d. (CHD)
    craniopharyngeal d.
    Cuvier d.
    cystic gall d.
    deferent d.
    dilated bile d.
    dilated intrahepatic d.
    dilated mammary d.
    dilated subareolar d.
    disruption of d.
    distal bile d.
    duodenal end of dorsal d.
    duodenal end of main d.
    efferent d.
    ejaculatory d.
    endolymphatic d.
    excretory d.
    extrahepatic bile d.

NOTES

D

duct *(continued)*
    extralobular terminal d.
    focally dilated d.
    frontonasal d.
    fusiform widening of d.
    galactophorous d.
    gall d.
    Gartner d.
    genital d.
    hepatic d.
    hypophyseal Rathke d.
    infundibulum of bile d.
    interlobular bile d.
    intrahepatic bile d.
    intralobular terminal d.
    involution of d.
    lacrimal d.
    lactiferous d.
    d. lumen
    lymph d.
    lymphatic d.
    main pancreatic d. (MPD)
    main papillary d. (MPD)
    mammary d.
    middle extrahepatic bile d.
    müllerian d.
    nasofrontal d.
    nasolacrimal d.
    nipple-like common bile d.
    normal caliber d.
    d. obstruction
    omphalomesenteric d.
    pancreatic d.
    paramesonephric d.
    paraurethral d.
    parotid d.
    percutaneous dilatation of biliary d.
    perilobular d.
    preampullary portion of bile d.
    prepapillary bile d.
    prostatic d.
    proximal part of dorsal d.
    pruned-tree-appearance bile d.
    pseudocalculus bile d.
    Rathke d.
    rat-tail common bile d.
    right hepatic d.
    Rivinus d.
    ruptured thoracic d.
    Santorini d.
    solitary dilated d.
    sphincter of bile d.
    spontaneous perforation of common bile d.
    Stensen d.
    subareolar d.
    submandibular d.
    subvesical d.
    terminal bile d.
    thoracic d.
    thyroglossal d.
    Vater d.
    vitelline d.
    Wharton d.
    Wirsung d.
    wolffian d.

ductal
    d. adenoma
    d. aneurysm
    d. arch
    d. architecture
    d. breast microcalcification
    d. carcinoma in situ (DCIS)
    d. constriction
    d. dilatation
    d. ectasia
    d. epithelial hyperplasia
    d. epithelium
    d. pancreatic adenocarcinoma
    d. papillary carcinoma
    d. papilloma
    d. pattern
    d. remnant
    d. in situ breast carcinoma

ductectatic
    d. mucinous cystic neoplasm
    d. mucinous tumor

ductogram
    mammary d.

ductography
    contrast d.
    peroral retrograde pancreaticobiliary d.

duct-penetrating sign
ductular
ductule
ductus, pl. **ductus**
    d. arteriosus
    d. arteriosus aneurysm
    d. arteriosus occlusion
    d. arteriosus patency
    d. deferens
    d. deferens artery
    d. diverticulum
    d. infundibulum
    d. of Kommerell
    recanalized d.
    d. venosus
    d. venosus patency
    window d.

Duett arterial puncture site closure device
Dulcolax bowel preparation

dullness
>left border of cardiac d. (LBCD)
>triangular area of d.

1D ultrasound

dumbbell
>d. appearance
>d. brain mass
>d. lesion
>d. needle
>d. neurofibroma
>d. shape
>d. tumor

dumbbell-shaped shadow

dumbbell-type neuroblastoma

dummy source

dumping
>d. stomach
>d. syndrome

Duncan placenta

Dunlop-Shands view

duodenal
>d. adenocarcinoma
>d. ampulla
>d. artery
>d. atresia
>d. bulb
>d. bulb apex (DBA)
>d. bulb deformity
>d. button
>d. cap
>d. C loop
>d. diaphragm
>d. duplication
>d. end of dorsal duct
>d. end of main duct
>d. erosion
>d. filling defect
>d. fossa
>d. gastrinoma
>d. hernia
>d. hourglass stenosis
>d. impression
>d. intraluminal diverticulum
>d. leiomyosarcoma
>d. ligament
>d. loop
>d. lumen
>d. narrowing
>d. papilla
>d. polyp
>d. segment
>d. sphincter

>d. stricture
>d. stump
>d. sweep
>d. teardrop appearance
>d. terminus
>d. ulcer
>d. ulcer perforation
>d. varix
>d. vein
>d. villus
>d. wall hamartoma
>d. web

duodenal-gastric outlet obstruction

duodeni
>ampulla d.

duodenitis
>chronic atrophic d.
>Crohn d.
>erosive d.
>hemorrhagic d.

duodenobiliary
>d. pressure gradient
>d. reflux

duodenocolic fistula

duodenogastric reflux (DGR)

duodenogastroesophageal reflux

duodenogastroscopy

duodenogram

duodenography
>hypotonic d.
>d. imaging

duodenojejunal
>d. angle
>d. flexure (DJF)
>d. fold
>d. fossa
>d. junction (DJJ)
>d. recess
>d. sphincter

duodenojejunitis

duodenomesocolic fold

duodenopancreatic
>d. fistula
>d. reflux

duodenorenal ligament

duodenoscope
>Olympus JF1T10 d.

duodenum
>chronic ileus d.
>C loop of d.
>cobblestone appearance d.
>comma-shaped d.

D

NOTES

duodenum *(continued)*
  curve of d.
  descending d.
  dilated d.
  distal d.
  d. extrinsic pressure effect
  first portion of d.
  d. inversum
  d. malignant tumor
  d. megabulbus
  mobile d.
  onion-shaped dilatation of d.
  postbulbar d.
  scarified d.
  scarred d.
  second portion of d.
  supravaterian d.
  suspensory muscle of d.
  third portion of d.
  d. water trap
  widened sweep d.
  windsock appearance of d.
Duografin
duplex
  d. B-mode Doppler
  d. B-mode ultrasound
  d. carotid imaging
  d. carotid ultrasound
  d. Doppler imaging
  d. Doppler ultrasound
  d. echocardiography
  d. scanner
  d. screening test
  d. sonography (DS)
  d. ultrasound (DU)
  d. ultrasound analysis
  d. ultrasound carotid artery
  d. ultrasound error
  d. uterus
duplex-pulsed
  d.-p. Doppler sonography
  d.-p. Doppler ultrasound
duplicated
  d. inferior vena cava
  d. renal collecting system
duplication
  d. anomaly
  colon d.
  colon cyst d.
  colorectal d.
  complete d.
  d. cyst
  diaphragm d.
  duodenal d.
  esophageal d.
  foregut d.

  gallbladder d.
  hindgut d.
  incomplete ureteral d.
  inferior vena cava d.
  intestinal d.
  d. of left kidney
  partial ureter d.
  renal d.
  d. of right kidney
  thoracoabdominal d.
  ureteral d.
duplicator
  cardiac pulse d.
DuPont
  D. Cronex x-ray film
  D. scanner
Dupré muscle
Dupuytren
  D. canal
  D. contracture
  D. fracture
  D. sign
dura
  attenuated d.
  bulging d.
  effacement of d.
  lamina d.
  d. mater of brain
  d. mater of spinal cord
  d. mater venous sinus
dural
  d. arachnoid lymphoma
  d. arteriovenous fistula
  d. arteriovenous malformation
  d. artery
  d. attachment
  d. calcification
  d. carotid cavernous fistula (DCCF)
  d. cul-de-sac
  d. ectasia
  d. fold
  d. hematoma
  d. impingement
  d. ossification
  d. root pouch
  d. sac
  d. sac effacement
  d. sheath
  d. sinus occlusion
  d. sinus thrombosis infarct
  d. tail
  d. tear
  d. venous sinus
  d. venous sinus thrombosis
Duran ring
Dürck node

Duret
> D. hemorrhage
> D. lesion

Durham flatfoot

durocutaneous fistula

Duroliopaque

Duroziez
> D. mitral stenosis disease
> D. sign

durum
> heloma d.
> osteoma d.
> papilloma d.

DUS
> dynamic ultrasound of shoulder

Duverney
> D. foramen
> D. fracture
> D. gland
> D. muscle

DVH
> dose-volume histogram

DVI
> deep venous insufficiency
> device-independent
> digital vascular imaging
> DVI mode
> DVI Simpson AtheroCath

DVT
> deep venous thrombosis

dwarfism
> achondroplastic d.
> acromelic d.
> Amsterdam d.
> bird-headed d.
> deprivation d.
> diastrophic d.
> late-onset d.
> lethal d.
> Lorain-Lévi d.
> mesomelic d.
> metatrophic d.
> micromelic d.
> nonlethal d.
> pituitary d.
> renal d.
> Russell-Silver d.
> thanatophoric d.
> Walt Disney d.

dwarf pelvis

dwell position

DWI
> diffusion-weighted imaging

Dwyer correction of scoliosis

DXA
> dual-energy x-ray absorptiometry

DxRaI
> diagnostic radioiodine scanning

Dy
> dysprosium

Dycal base

dyclonine

Dy-DTPA-BMA imaging agent

dye
> d. column
> d. dilution curve
> d. extravasation
> fill-and-spill of d.
> d. fluorescence index (DFI)
> halogenated phenolphthalein d.
> indentation of myelography d.
> indocyanine green d.
> d. injection technique
> d. laser
> d. laser system
> lipophilic d.
> d. punch fracture
> d. reduction spot test
> rose bengal d.
> d. uptake

dye-binding capacity (DBC)

^{166}Dy generator

Dyggve-Melchior-Clausen dysplasia

Dyke-Davidoff-Masson syndrome

Dynabead

dynamic
> d. acquisition
> d. antral scintigraphy
> d. aorta
> d. axial fixator
> d. beat filtration
> d. bolus
> d. bolus tracking technique
> d. computed tomography (DCT)
> d. computerized tomography
> d. conformal therapy
> d. contrast-enhanced CT
> d. contrast-enhanced magnetic
>   resonance imaging (DCE-MRI)
> d. contrast-enhanced MRI
> d. contrast-enhanced subtraction MR
>   imaging

D

NOTES

dynamic *(continued)*
    d. contrast-enhanced subtraction study
    d. coupling
    d. CT scan
    d. emission scan
    d. enhancement
    d. entrapment of vertebral artery
    d. filtering
    d. focusing
    d. ileus
    d. image
    d. lineshape effect
    d. lung
    d. magnetic resonance imaging
    d. multileaf collimation
    d. nuclear polarization (DNP)
    d. open magnetic resonance defecography
    d. optical breast imaging system (DOBI)
    d. pedobarography
    d. planar reconstructor (DPR)
    d. pulmonary hyperinflation
    d. radiation therapy
    d. radionuclide renal scintigraphy
    d. radiotherapy
    d. range
    d. range control (DRC)
    d. renal imaging
    d. scintigraphy imaging
    d. series
    d. snapshot
    d. sonography
    d. spatial reconstructor (DSR)
    d. spiral CT lung densitometry
    d. stabilizer
    d. stereotactic radiosurgery
    d. subaortic stenosis
    d. subtraction magnetic resonance angiogram
    d. supine study
    d. susceptibility contrast (DSC)
    d. susceptibility contrast magnetic resonance imaging
    d. tagging magnetic resonance angiography
    d. ultrasound of shoulder (DUS)
    d. ventilation He-MRI
    d. volume imaging
    d. volume-rendered display
    d. volumetric SPECT
    d. wedge
dynamic-condenser electrometer
dynamic-contrast MRI
dynamite heart
Dynapix

DynaRad portable x-ray system
DynaWell medical compression device
dyne
dynode
dynography
dysarthria clumsy hand syndrome
dysautonomia
    familial d.
dyschezia
dyschondroplasia
dyschondrosteosis
dyschromia
dyscollagenosis
dyscrasic fracture
dysembryoplastic neuroepithelial tumor (DNET)
dysfunction
    bladder d.
    bowel and bladder d.
    brain d.
    cerebral d.
    cortical d.
    dehydration-induced renal d.
    dopaminergic d.
    frontal lobe d.
    hepatocellular d.
    left ventricular d. (LVD)
    lower esophageal sphincter d.
    oropharyngeal d.
    positional d.
    regional myocardial d.
    renal d.
    reversible temporary myocardial d.
    right ventricular d. (RVD)
    salivary gland d.
    sinoatrial node d.
    sinus node d.
    small airway d.
    sphincter d.
    swallowing d.
    testis d.
    valvular d.
    ventilatory d.
    ventricular d.
dysfunctional kidney
dysgenesis
    alar d.
    anorectal d.
    callosal d.
    corpus callosum d.
    corticocallosal d.
    epiphyseal d.
    gonadal d.
    hindbrain d.
    mixed gonadal d.
    ovarian d.
    renal tubular d.

sacral d.
sacrolumbar d.
segmental spinal d. (SSD)
thyroid d.
tubular d.
dysgenetic kidney
dysgerminoma
brain d.
mediastinum d.
ovarian d.
pineal d.
dysjunction
craniofacial d.
dyskeratosis, pl. **dyskeratoses**
kidney d.
dyskinesia, dyskinesis
bile duct d.
biliary d.
regional d.
dyskinetic
d. cerebral palsy
d. segmental wall motion
d. segmental wall motion
abnormality
d. septum
dysmaturity
pulmonary d.
dysmorphism
lobar d.
dysmotile esophagus
dysmotility
esophageal d.
dysmyelination
dysosteogenesis
dysostosis, pl. **dysostoses**
cleidocranial d.
craniofacial d.
epiphyseal d.
mandibulofacial d.
metaphyseal d.
d. multiplex
mutational d.
dysphagia
contractile ring d.
esophageal d.
d. inflammatoria
liquid food d.
d. lusoria
oropharyngeal d.
d. paralytica
postvagotomy d.
preesophageal d.

progressive d.
sideropenic d.
soft food d.
solid food d.
d. spastica
vallecular d.
d. valsalviana
dysplasia
acetabular residual d.
acromelic d.
acromesomelic d.
acropectorovertebral d.
arrhythmogenic right ventricular d.
(ARVD)
arteriohepatic d.
asphyxiating thoracic d.
bone d.
bronchopulmonary d. (BPD)
Burke-type metaphyseal d.
camptomelic d.
cemental d.
cementoosseous d.
cervical d.
chondroectodermal d.
cleidocranial d.
CNS fibromuscular d.
congenital hip d.
congenital polyvalvular d.
cortical d.
cranioskeletal d.
craniotelencephalic d.
cystic fibrous d.
diaphyseal d.
diastrophic d.
d. dislocation
Dyggve-Melchior-Clausen d.
endocardial d.
epiarticular osteochondromatous d.
epiphyseal d.
d. epiphysealis hemimelica
d. epiphysealis multiplex
epiphysealis punctua d.
external auditory canal d.
familial arterial fibromuscular d.
fetal musculoskeletal d.
fibromuscular d.
fibrous temporal bone d.
focal cerebellar d.
focal cortical d.
foot d.
frontonasal d.
hip d.

D

NOTES

dysplasia *(continued)*
    idiopathic diffuse cerebellar d.
    isolated focal cerebellar cortical d.
    Jansen metaphyseal d.
    Joubert focal cerebellar d.
    Kniest d.
    lethal bone d.
    lethal musculoskeletal d.
    mammary d.
    McKusick-type metaphyseal d.
    mesodermal d.
    mesomelic d.
    metaphyseal d.
    metatrophic d.
    Meyer d.
    micromelic d.
    microscopic cortical d.
    Mondini d.
    monostotic fibrous d.
    multicystic d.
    multiple epiphyseal d.
    Namaqualand hip d.
    neuroectodermal d.
    nonlethal d.
    nonsyndromic focal cerebellar d.
    obstructive renal d.
    odontoid d.
    osseous d.
    osteofibrous d.
    periapical cemental d.
    perimedial d.
    periosteal d.
    polyostotic fibrous d.
    polypoid d.
    Potter d.
    progressive diaphyseal d. (PDD)
    pulmonary valve d.
    Pyle d.
    renal artery fibromuscular d.
    retinal d.
    retroareolar d.
    rhizomelic d.
    right ventricular d.
    Scheibe d.
    Schmid-type metaphyseal d.
    septooptic d.
    sheet-like d.
    short limb d.
    skeletal d.
    sphenoid d.
    spondylocostal d.
    spondyloepiphyseal d.
    spondylothoracic d.
    Streeter d.
    tapetoretinal d.
    testis d.
    thanatophoric d.

    thoracic d.
    thymic d.
    transmantle d.
    tricuspid valve d.
    variable cerebral d.
    ventricular d.
    ventriculoradial d.
    d. with associated lesion or mass
        (DALM)
dysplasia-carcinoma sequence
dysplastic
    d. cerebellar gangliocytoma
    d. cusp
    d. kidney
    d. liver nodule
    d. meniscus
    d. pulmonary valve
dysprosium (Dy)
    d. analog
    d. HP-DO3A imaging agent
dysprosium-DTPA
dysprosium-holmium (^{166}Dy-166Ho) in vivo generator
dysraphia
    tectocerebellar d.
dysraphic spine
dysraphism
    closed spinal d.
    occult spinal d.
dysrhythmia of fetal heart
dyssynergia, dyssynergy
    biliary d.
    Ramsay Hunt cerebellar
      myoclonic d.
    regional d.
    segmental d.
dystocia
    fetal d.
    labor d.
    shoulder d.
dystonia
dystonic reaction
dystopia
dystrophic
    d. change
    d. degeneration
    d. soft tissue calcification
dystrophy
    adiposogenital d.
    asphyxiating thoracic d.
    bone d.
    congenital muscular d.
    Duchenne muscular d.
    Fukuyama congenital muscular d.
        (FCMD)
    infantile thoracic d.
    limb-girdle muscular d.

merosin-deficient congenital
  muscular d.
muscular d.
neuraxonal d.

oculopharyngeal d.
reflex sympathetic d.
Sudeck d.
sympathetic d.

NOTES

D

E

E plane
E point of cardiac apex pulse
E point on echocardiography
E point to septal separation
(EPSS)
E sign on x-ray

E₁

prostaglandin E₁

E:A

E:A change
E:A wave ratio

EAA

extraalveolar air
EAA collection

Eagle-Barrett syndrome
ear

e. cholesteatoma
frontal horn Mickey Mouse e.
inner e.
middle e.

early

e. bone scintigraphy
e. echo
e. endovascular treatment
e. fetal death
e. opening of valve
e. osteoarthritis
e. osteomyelitis
e. pneumonitis
e. repolarization pattern
e. segmental opacification
e. stromal invasion
e. systolic peak
e. venous filling

early-phase termination
Eastman Kodak scanner
Easy Wallstent stent
Eaton agent pneumonia
EBA

electron beam angiography
extrahepatic biliary atresia

EBCT

electron-beam computed tomography
EBCT IV angiography
volume-mode EBCT

EBDA

effective balloon-dilated area

EBER
EBIORT

electron-beam intraoperative radiotherapy

EBRT

external beam radiation therapy

Ebstein

E. angle

E. anomaly
E. lesion
E. malformation
E. sign

EBT

electron-beam tomography
EBT scanner

eburnated bone
eburnation

bony e.
trapezium-metacarpal e. (TME)

eburneum

osteoma e.

ECA

external carotid artery

E-CABG

endoscopic coronary artery bypass graft

E.CAM dual-head emission imaging system
ECAT

emission computerized axial tomography
ECAT Reveal PET/CT imaging
system

eccentric

e. atherosclerotic plaque
e. atrophy
e. axis of rotation of the ankle
e. coronary artery
e. enhancing nodule
e. epicenter
e. ledge
e. left ventricular hypertrophy
e. medullary bone lesion
e. monocuspid disk valve
e. narrowing
e. pantomography
e. restenosis lesion
e. stenosis
e. vessel

eccentrically placed lumen
eccentricity index
ecchondroma
Eccocee CS ultrasound system
eccrine angiomatous hamartoma
ECD

endocardial cushion defect
ethyl cysteinate dimer
⁹⁹ᵐTc ECD
⁹⁹ᵐ Technetium L-ethyl cysteinate
dimer
⁹⁹ᵐTc-ECD

ECE

extracapsular extension

ECG, EKG

echocardiogram

E

285

ECG *(continued)*
    echocardiography
    electrocardiogram
    electrocardiography
        ECG trigger
ECG-gated
    ECG-g. multislice
    ECG-g. multislice MR imaging
    ECG-g. spin echo
    ECG-g. spin-echo MR imaging
ECG-synchronized digital subtraction angiography
ECG-triggered, flow-compensated gradient echo image
echinococcal cyst
echinococcosis
    alveolar e.
    bone e.
    liver e.
    lung e.
echo
    amphoric e.
    asymmetric e.
    atrial e.
    bright e.
    e. characteristic
    e. contrast
    e. contrast agent
    e. delay time (TE)
    dense e.
    e. density
    3D gradient e. (3D GRE)
    diaphragmatic e.
    3D magnetization-prepared rapid gradient e.
    driven inversion spin e. (DISE)
    early e.
    ECG-gated spin e.
    endometrial e.
    e. enhancement
    even distribution of e.'s
    fast-field e. (FFE)
    fast spoiled gradient-recalled e. (FSPGR)
    fat-suppressed spin e.
    FID-acquired e.'s (FAcE)
    field e. (FE)
    e. FLASH MR
    fuzzy e.
    generalized interferography using spin echoes and stimulated e.'s (GINSEST)
    generation e.
    gradient-recalled e.
    gradient-refocused e. (GRE)
    gradient-spin e.
    hepatic pattern e.

high-amplitude e.
highly mobile e.
highly reflective e.
homogeneous e.
e. imaging
inhomogeneous e.
internal e.
linear e.
low-amplitude internal e.
low-level e.
magnetization-prepared rapid acquisition gradient e.
median level e.
metallic e.
mirror-like e.
multiplanar gradient-recalled e.
multiple spin e.
navigator e.
offset radiofrequency spin e.
out-of-phase gradient e.
partial saturation spin e.
particulate e.
e. pattern
pencil-beam navigator e.
e. phase correction (EPC)
e. planar readout
pulsed-gradient spin e. (PGSE)
e. ranging
rapid acquisition spin e. (RASE)
rapid gradient e. (RAGE)
e. reflectivity
renal sinus e.
e. rephasing
reverberation e.
RF spin e.
ring-down e.
salvo of e.'s
shower of e.'s
e. signature
simulated e.
single-shot fast spin e. (SSFSE)
sludge-like intraluminal e.
smoke-like e.
solid e.
sonographic e.
e. space
specular e.
spin e.
spin-echo using repeated gradient e.'s
spoiled gradient e. (SGE)
standard single e.
stimulated e. (STE)
supraventricular venous e.
swirling smokelike e.'s
symmetric e.
e. texture

thick e.
e. time (TE)
time of formation of RF spin-echo
when adjusted to be different
from gradient spin-e. (TER)
e. train
e. train echo time (T_E)
turbo gradient-refocused e.
(turboGRE)
T1-weighted spin e.
ultrasonographic e.
ventricular e.
echoaortography
echocardiogram (ECG, EKG)
e. adenosine
e. planar imaging
echocardiographic
e. automated border
e. gating
echocardiography (ECG, EKG)
adenosine e.
ambulatory Holter e.
A-mode e.
aortic root e.
aortic valve e.
apical five-chamber view e.
apical two-chamber view e.
automated border detection by e.
biplane transesophageal e.
blood pool radionuclide e.
B-mode e.
cardiac output e.
color-flow imaging Doppler e.
continuous-loop exercise e.
continuous-wave Doppler e.
contrast e.
contrast-enhanced e.
cross-sectional two-dimensional e.
detection e.
dipyridamole e.
dobutamine stress e. (DSE)
Doppler continuous-wave e.
Doppler pulsed-wave e.
3D transesophageal e.
duplex e.
epicardial Doppler e.
E point on e.
exercise e.
Feigenbaum e.
fetal e.
four-chamber e.

high-pulse repetition frequency
Doppler e.
H-mode e.
hypokinesis on e.
e. imaging
intracardiac e. (ICE)
intracoronary contrast e.
intraoperative cardioplegic
contrast e.
Meridian e.
mitral valve e.
M-mode e.
multiplanar transesophageal e.
myocardial contrast e. (MCE)
myocardial perfusion e.
parasternal long-axis view e.
parasternal short-axis view e.
pharmacologic stress e.
postcontrast e.
postexercise e.
postinjection e.
postmyocardial infarction e.
precontrast e.
preinjection e.
premyocardial infarction e.
pulsed Doppler transesophageal e.
pulsed-wave Doppler e.
real-time e.
resting e.
short axis view e.
stress e.
subcostal short-axis view e.
supine bicycle stress e.
transesophageal e. (TEE)
transthoracic three-dimensional e.
two-chamber e.
two-dimensional e. (TDE)
ultrasound e.
ventricular wall motion e.
Echo-Coat ultrasound biopsy needle
echocolonoscope
echo-dense
e.-d. layer
e.-d. pattern
e.-d. valve
echoencephalogram
echoencephalograph
midline e.
echoencephalography
echoendoscope
FG-36UX scanning e.
linear array e.

NOTES

echoendoscope *(continued)*
  Olympus GF-UM2, GF-UM3 e.
  Olympus GIF-1T10 e.
  Olympus JF-UM20 e.
  Olympus VU-M2 e.
  Olympus XIF-UM3 e.
echo-enhanced cystosonography
echo-enhancer
  pulmonary stable e.-e.
echo-enhancing agent
EchoEye ultrasound imaging system
echo-free
  e.-f. area
  e.-f. central zone
  e.-f. layer
  e.-f. space
echogastroscope
EchoGen-enhanced ultrasound
echogenic
  e. appearance
  e. band
  e. calculus
  e. debris
  e. fetal bowel
  e. focus
  e. intraluminal thrombus
  e. liver
  e. liver metastasis
  e. mass
  e. nodule
  e. noise
  e. periphery
  e. plaque
  e. plug
  e. ring
  e. solid lesion
  e. tumor
echogenicity
  brightly increased renal
    parenchymal e.
  calvarial e.
  focally increased renal e.
  generalized increased liver e.
  increased e.
  internal e.
  normal e.
  parenchymal e.
  periventricular e. (PVE)
  e. scatterer
  ultrasound e.
EchoGen ultrasound imaging agent
echogram
  mitral valve e.
echographer
echographia
echography
  B-mode e.

  ophthalmic biometry by
    ultrasound e.
  transrectal e.
  transvaginal e.
echoic
echoicity
echoing
echolaminography
echolocation
echolucent
  e. pattern
  e. plaque
EchoMark catheter
echonography
echophonocardiography
  M-mode e.
echo-planar
  e.-p. diffusion-weighted imaging
  e.-p. FLAIR imaging
  e.-p. GRE T2*-weighted imagining
  e.-p. image
  e.-p. imaging (EPI)
  e.-p. imaging method
  e.-p. pulse sequence
echo-poor
  e.-p. area
  e.-p. testis
echo-ranging
Echospeed
  E. Signa LX 1.5 T scanner
  E. 1.5T MR machine
echo-speed gradient
echo-spin density
echo-tagging technique
echotexture
  internal e.
  mottled e.
echo-train
  e.-t. length (ETL)
  e.-t. value
Echovist imaging agent
ECI
  Ensemble contrast imaging
Eck fistula
Eclipse
  E. MR System
  E. TENS unit
  E. TMR laser
eclipse effect lung
ECRB
  extensor carpi radialis brevis
    ECRB muscle
ECRL
  extensor carpi radialis longus
    ECRL muscle
ECS
  electrocerebral silence

ECT
    emission computed tomography
ectasia
    alveolar e.
    anuloaortic e.
    e. of aorta
    basilar artery e.
    benign duct e.
    bilateral ductal e.
    communicating cavernous e.
    coronary artery e.
    diffuse arterial e.
    digitate e.
    ductal e.
    dural e.
    gonadal venous e.
    mammary duct e.
    moniliform e.
    renal tubular e.
    saccular e.
    seminiferous tubular e.
    tubular e.
    vascular colon e.
ectatic
    e. aneurysm
    e. aortic valve
    e. bronchus
    e. carotid artery
    e. emphysema
ectocardia
ectodermal groove
ectomesenchyme
ectopia
    benign cerebellar e.
    cerebellar e.
    e. cordis
    crossed-fused renal e.
    longitudinal renal e.
    posterior pituitary gland e.
    testicular e.
    tonsillar e.
    transverse testicular e.
ectopic
    e. ACTH syndrome
    e. anus
    e. beat
    e. bone growth
    e. craniopharyngioma
    e. endometrial tissue
    e. focus
    e. gallbladder
    e. gland

    e. impulse
    e. intraluminal gallstone
    e. kidney
    e. meningioma
    e. ossification
    e. pancreas
    e. parathyroid
    e. parathyroid adenoma
    e. pinealoma
    e. pregnancy (EP)
    e. spleen
    e. testis
    e. thymus
    e. thyroid tissue
    e. ureter
    e. ureterocele
ectopy
ectrodactyly-ectodermal
    e.-e. dysplasia-clefting
    e.-e. dysplasia-clefting syndrome
ECU muscle
ED
    edge detection
EDAMS
    encephaloduroarteriomyosynangiosis
EDAS
    encephaloduroarteriosynangiosis
EDB
    extensor digitorum brevis
        EDB muscle
EDC
    extensor digitorum communis
    ^{99m}Tc-ethyl cysteinate dimer
        EDC muscle
eddy
    e. current
    e. current artifact
    e. current mapping
    e. formation
    e. ringing artifact
edema
    acute interstitial lung e.
    acute pulmonary e.
    adjacent e.
    airspace e.
    alveolar pulmonary e.
    angioneurotic e.
    antral e.
    batwing e.
    bone marrow e.
    brain e.
    brainstem e.

E

NOTES

edema *(continued)*
  breast e.
  bronchiolar e.
  brown e.
  bullous e.
  cardiac pulmonary e.
  cardiogenic pulmonary e.
  cardiopulmonary e.
  cerebral e.
  chemical pulmonary e.
  chronic e.
  circumscribed e.
  collateral e.
  compressive e.
  cord e.
  cyclic idiopathic e.
  cytotoxic e.
  diffuse e.
  e. of epididymis
  fetal scalp e.
  fingerprint e.
  e. fluid
  focal e.
  frank pulmonary e.
  fulminant pulmonary e.
  generalized pulmonary e.
  gravitational e.
  gut e.
  hemorrhagic pulmonary e.
  high-altitude pulmonary e. (HAPE)
  hypervolemic pulmonary e.
  idiopathic e.
  ileocecal e.
  inflammatory e.
  intercellular e.
  interstitial pulmonary e.
  intracompartmental e.
  intraosseous e.
  laryngeal e.
  leg e.
  liver e.
  local e.
  localized e.
  lung e.
  lymphatic e.
  lymphaticovenous secondary e.
  malignant brain e.
  massive ovarian e.
  massive pulmonary hemorrhagic e.
  mediastinal fat e.
  mild e.
  negative image pulmonary e.
  e. neonatorum
  nephrotic e.
  nerve root e.
  neurogenic pulmonary e.
  neuronal cytotoxic e.

  noncardiac pulmonary e.
  noncardiogenic pulmonary e.
  orbital e.
  osmotic e.
  ovarian e.
  paroxysmal pulmonary e.
  passive e.
  patchy e.
  e. pattern
  pericholecystic e.
  pericystic e.
  perihilar e.
  perineoplastic e.
  periorbital e.
  peripheral vasogenic e.
  peritumoral e.
  perivascular e.
  permeability pulmonary e.
  placental e.
  preosteonecrosis marrow e.
  pulmonary e. (PE)
  reactive marrow e.
  reexpansion pulmonary e.
  renal e.
  reperfusion lung e.
  reversible vasogenic e.
  solid e.
  stasis e.
  stomal e.
  subchondral marrow e.
  subcutaneous e.
  subglottic e.
  supraglottic e.
  terminal e.
  testicular posttraumatic e.
  thalamic e.
  trace e.
  transient bone marrow e.
  umbilical cord e.
  unilateral pulmonary e.
  vasogenic e.
  venous e.
  vernal e.
  visceral e.
  white matter e.
edematous
  e. brain
  e. bronchus
  e. gallbladder
  e. kidney
  e. pancreatitis
  e. pleura
  e. tissue
Eder-Puestow dilatation
edge
  boundary e.
  Compton e.

e. detection (ED)
e. effect
e. enhancement
leading e.
ligament reflecting e.
ligament shelving e.
liver e.
e. misalignment artifact
e. packing
patellar e.
e. response function (ERF)
e. ringing
e. ringing artifact
sawtooth e.
e. shadow
shelving e. of Poupart ligament
sternal e.
tentorial e.
ulcer with heaped-up e.'s
edge-boundary artifact
edge-detection
e.-d. angiography
e.-d. procedure
edge-enhanced error diffusion algorithm
edge-region pixel
EDH
epidural hematoma
E-dial calibration
Edison
E. effect
E. fluoroscope
editing
spectral e.
EDL muscle
EDQ muscle
EDR
exposure data recognizer
EDSS
expanded-disability status scale
EDTMP
ethylenediamine tetramethylene
phosphonic acid
EDTMP imaging agent
Edwards
double aortic arch of E.
E. syndrome
EDXRF spectrometer
EEG
electroencephalography
EF
ejection fraction

EFF
electromagnetic focusing field
effaced mucosal fold
effacement
architectural e.
cistern e.
cisterna magna e.
e. of dura
dural sac e.
mesencephalic cistern e.
nerve root sheath e.
pelvocaliceal e.
sulcus e.
ventricle e.
effect
abscopal e.
adverse e.
Anrep e.
arterial sump e.
artifact e.
attenuation e.
Auger e.
Bayliss e.
beam-hardening e.
Bernoulli e.
bilateral vagotomy e.
blood oxygenation level-
dependent e.
Bohr e.
BOLD e.
Bowditch e.
bronchodilator e.
bronchomotor e.
bronchospastic e.
bystander e.
Cherenkov e.
cobra-head e.
collimator exchange e.
Compton e.
contact e.
contrast media adverse e.
copper wire e.
cumulative radiation e. (CRE)
Curie e.
deleterious e.
demagnetization field e.
Doppler e.
Dotter e.
dottering e.
duodenum extrinsic pressure e.
dynamic lineshape e.
edge e.

E

NOTES

effect *(continued)*
    Edison e.
    first-pass e.
    flow-related enhancement e.
    flow void e.
    gastrointestinal adverse e.
    genitourinary adverse e.
    halo e.
    heel e.
    hematocrit e.
    hemispheral mass e.
    hemodynamic e.
    isotope e.
    lag e.
    Laplace e.
    localized mass e.
    Mach band e.
    Macklin e.
    macromolecular hydration e.
    magic angle e.
    magnetization transfer e.
    magnetohydrodynamic e.
    masquerading e.
    mass e.
    methemoglobin e.
    missile e.
    multilog e.
    neurotoxic e.
    nozzle e.
    nuclear Overhauser e.
    osmotic e.
    outflow e.
    Overhauser e.
    oxygen e.
    pacemaker e.
    pad e.
    paramagnetic e.
    phase e.
    phase-shift e.
    photoechoic e.
    photoelectric e.
    photographic e. (PE)
    photonuclear e.
    piezoelectric e.
    pinchcock e.
    postvagotomy e.
    priming e.
    purse-stringing e.
    radiation e.
    radiographic e.
    reservoir e.
    Russell e.
    sausage segment e.
    scalar e.
    side e.
    silver wire e.
    sink e.

    skin e.
    skin-sparing e.
    snowplow e.
    sonic e.
    star e.
    steal e.
    susceptibility e.
    systematic relaxation e.
    T2 dephasing e.
    teratogenic e.
    thermal e.
    time-of-flight e.
    tracheal mass e.
    vagatomy e.
    vasodilatory e.
    Venturi e.
    Volta e.
    Warburg e.
    washboard e.
    wash-in e.
    washout e.
    Wolff-Chaikoff e.
effective
    e. atomic number
    e. balloon-dilated area (EBDA)
    e. focal spot size
    e. half-life
    e. mass attenuation coefficient
    e. path length (EPL)
    e. pulmonary blood flow (EPBF)
    e. pulmonic index
    e. refractory period (ERP)
    e. renal plasma flow (ERFP, ERPF)
    e. section thickness
    e. transverse relation time
effectiveness
    relative biological e. (RBE)
effector/target cell interaction
efferent
    e. arteriolar resistance
    e. digital nerve
    e. duct
    e. ductule of testis
    e. loop
    e. loop obstruction
    e. lymph vessel
    e. view
effervescent
    e. agent
    e. drink
efficacy study
efficiency
    absolute e.
    conversion e.
    detective quantum e. (DQE)
    full-energy peak e.

geometric e.
geometrical e.
intrinsic e.
kidney extraction e.
quantum detection e. (QDE)
valvular e.
window e.
efficient relaxation time
effluents
radioactive e.
effort
inspiratory e.
respiratory e.
shallow inspiratory e.
suboptimal e.
e. thrombosis
ventilatory e.
voluntary e. (VE)
effort-dependent
effused chyle
effusion
e. artifact
asbestos-related pleural e.
Baccelli sign of pleural e.
benign subdural e.
cardiac e.
chocolate joint e.
chylous e.
discrete area of e.
epidural e.
exudative pleural e.
fetal pleural e.
free pleural e.
hemorrhagic pleural e.
inflammatory joint e.
ipsilateral pleural e.
joint e.
Karplus sign of pleural e.
Kellock sign of pleural e.
knee joint e.
large volume joint e.
layering e.
left-sided pleural e.
liquid pleural e.
loculated pleural e.
malignant pleural e.
massive pleural e.
milky e.
moderate-sized volume joint e.
noninflammatory joint e.
parapneumonic e.
pericardial e. (PE)

peritoneal e.
pleural e.
pleuropericardial e.
pseudochylous e.
serofibrinous pericardial e.
serous e.
e. shadow
subdeltoid bursal e.
subdural e.
subpleural e.
subpulmonic e.
taut pericardial e.
transient pleural e.
transudative pleural e.
tuberculous e.
unilateral pleural e.
EFG
electric field gradient
EFW
estimated fetal weight
EG
esophagogastric
Egan mammography
EGD
esophagogastroduodenoscopy
egg-on-its-side heart
egg-shaped orbit
eggshell
e. border of aneurysm
e. breast calcification
e. calcification of lymph node
e. nodal calcification
egress of blood
Egyptian splenomegaly
EHL
electrohydraulic lithotripsy
extensor hallucis longus
Ehlers-Danlos syndrome
EHM
extrahepatic metastasis
EHT
electrohydrothermal electrode
EIC
extensive intraductal carcinoma
extensive intraductal component
eigenvector
e. analysis
principal e.
eight-ball hemorrhage
eighth nerve tumor
eight-lumen manometric catheter

E

NOTES

Eindhoven magnet
einsteinium (Es)
einsteinium-255 (^{255}Es)
Einthoven triangle
EIP muscle
EIS
> electrical impedance scanning
> > EIS spot
> > targeted EIS

Eisenmenger
> E. complex
> E. defect
> E. group
> E. reaction
> E. syndrome

EIT
> electrical impedance tomography

ejaculatory duct
ejection
> e. fraction (EF)
> e. fraction by first-pass technique
> e. phase index
> e. time (ET)

EJV
> external jugular vein

EKG (*var. of* ECG)
> echocardiogram
> echocardiography
> electrocardiogram

Eklund
> E. technique
> E. view

EKY
> electrokymogram

El-Ahwany classification of humeral supracondylar fracture
elastance
> maximum ventricular e.

elastic
> e. cartilage
> e. collision
> e. cross-section
> e. imaging
> e. recoil of artery
> e. scattering spectroscopy
> e. stable intramedullary nailing (ESIN)
> e. subtraction algorithm
> e. subtraction spiral CT angiography

elasticity
elasticum
> pseudoxanthoma e.

elasticus
> conus e.

elastin deposition in taeniae coli
elastofibroma

elastography
> magnetic resonance e. (MRE)

elastomyofibrosis
elastosis
elbow
> baseball pitcher's e.
> e. bone center
> boxer's e.
> e. contracture
> e. coronal scan
> e. extensor tendon
> floating e.
> e. fracture
> golfer's e.
> javelin thrower's e.
> e. joint
> milkmaid's e.
> nursemaid's e.
> reverse tennis e.
> tennis e.
> thrower's e.
> wrestler's e.

ELCA
> excimer laser coronary angioplasty

ELD
> energy level diagram

electric
> e. dipole
> e. field gradient (EFG)
> e. generator
> e. induction
> e. interaction
> e. joint fluoroscopy
> e. joint fluoroscopy imaging
> e. quadrupole coupling
> e. stimulation
> e. syringe

electrical
> e. activity
> e. circulatory arrest
> e. impedance scanning (EIS)
> e. impedance tomography (EIT)
> e. potential energy

electrically
> e. activated implant
> e. detachable coil

electrocardiogram (ECG, EKG)
> resting e.
> signal-averaged e. (SAECG, SaECG)
> e. tracing
> e. trigger

electrocardiogram-gated
> e.-g. MRI
> e.-g. MRI imaging
> e.-g. multislice spiral CT

e.-g. multislice spiral CT of the heart
e.-g. SPECT
e.-g. tomography
electrocardiogram-synchronized digital subtraction angiography
electrocardiographic
    e. gating
    e. trigger method
    e. variant
electrocardiograph triggering
electrocardiography (ECG, EKG)
electrocardiography-gated echo-planar imaging
electrocardiophonogram
electrocardioscanner
    Compuscan Hittman
      computerized e.
electrocautery
    endoluminal radiofrequency e.
    monopolar radiofrequency e.
electrocerebral silence (ECS)
electrocoagulation
    intraluminal e.
electrode
    e. array
    electrohydrothermal e. (EHT)
    esophageal pill e.
    e. monitoring
    monopolar e.
    MRI-compatible e.
    patch e.
    polarographic needle e.
    subcutaneous array e.
electrodesiccation
electrodiagnosis
electrodiagnostic imaging
electroencephalogram
    flat e.
    isoelectric e.
electroencephalography (EEG)
    intracranial e.
    quantitative e. (QEEG)
electrogastrogram
electrogastrograph
electrogram
    atrial e.
    coronary sinus e.
    esophageal e.
    high right atrial e. (HRA)
    His bundle e. (HBE)
    intraatrial e.

    intracardiac e.
    right ventricular e.
    right ventricular apical e.
    RVA e.
    sinus node e.
electrography
electrohydraulic
    e. disintegrator
    e. fragmentation
    e. lithotripsy (EHL)
    e. probe
    e. shockwave lithotripsy
electrohydrothermal electrode (EHT)
electrohysterogram
electrohysterography
electrokymogram (EKY)
electrokymograph
electroluminescent sensitometer
electrolytic reduction
electromagnet
    structured coil e.
electromagnetic (EM)
    e. absorption
    e. blood flow imaging
    e. blood flow study
    e. energy
    e. field
    e. flow probe
    e. focusing field (EFF)
    e. induction
    e. interference (EMI)
    e. interference scan
    e. modeling
    e. radiation
    e. radiation exposure
    e. spectrum
    e. unit (emu)
    e. wave
electromagnetism
electromechanical dissociation (EMD)
electrometer
    dynamic-condenser e.
    vibrating-reed e.
electromotive force (emf)
electromyogram (EMG)
electromyography (EMG)
electron
    angle e. (UE)
    e. arc therapy
    Auger e.
    backscatter e.
    e. beam

E

NOTES

electron *(continued)*
- e. beam angiography (EBA)
- e. beam CT scanner
- e. beam therapy
- e. bolus
- bound e.
- e. capture
- e. cloud
- Compton e.
- conversion e.
- e. diffraction camera
- e. dosimetry
- emission e.
- e. equilibrium loss
- excited e.
- e. flow
- e. flux
- free e.
- e. gun
- internal conversion e.
- K e.
- L e.
- e. linear accelerator
- e. microscopy
- e. multiplier tube
- e. neutrino
- e. orbit
- orbital e.
- oscillating e.
- e. paramagnetic resonance (EPR)
- e. paramagnetic resonance spatial imaging
- positive e.
- e. radiography
- e. radiography imaging
- recoil e.
- secondary e.
- e. spin
- e. spin resonance (ESR)
- e. stream
- e. theory
- transition e.
- e. valence
- e. volt (eV, ev)

electron-beam
- e.-b. boost
- e.-b. computed tomography (EBCT)
- e.-b. CT-derived CAC score
- e.-b. intraoperative radiotherapy (EBIORT)
- e.-b. tomography (EBT)

electron-capture decay mode
electron-dense
electroneuromyography
electronic
- e. atlas of the hippocampus
- e. collimation

- e. dosimeter
- e. independent beam steering
- e. linear array transducer
- e. magnification
- e. picture acquisition
- e. portal imaging
- e. stabilization

electron-photon field matching
electron-positron pair
electrooculogram apparatus
electrooculographic analysis
electrooptical device
electropherogram
electrophilic radioiodination
electrophysiologic mapping
electrophysiology (EP)
electroradiology
electroradiometer
electroretinogram (ERG)
- flicker e.

electroscope
electrospray ionization mass spectroscopy
electrostatic
- e. generator
- e. imaging
- e. imaging system
- e. potential

electrothermal catheter
electrovectorcardiogram
electrovectorcardiography
Elema roll-film changer
element
- blowout lesion of posterior vertebral e.
- daughter e.
- estrogen-response e. (ERE)
- fibroglandular e.
- infiltrative hemorrhagic e.
- inflammatory e.
- 8000-e. linear array CCD scanner
- neoplastic destruction of spinal e.
- parent e.
- picture e.
- radioactive e.
- resolution e.
- e. subluxation
- volume e.
- voxel e.

elementary
- e. body
- e. fracture

element-specific detector
elephant
- e. ears pelvis
- e. trunk graft

elephantiasis neuromatosa

elevated
- e. diaphragm
- e. gradient
- e. leg support
- e. lower esophageal sphincter resting pressure
- e. retinal hamartoma

elevation
- bilateral diaphragmatic e.
- chorioamnionic e.
- diaphragmatic e.
- periosteal e.
- unilateral diaphragmatic e.

elevatus
- hallux e.

ELF
- extremely low frequency

elimination
- e. curve
- e. half-life
- e. kinetics
- pyelography by e.

Ellestad protocol
ellipsoid
- e. joint
- e. lesion
- e. method

elliptic
elliptical
- e. centric acquisition
- e. lumen

ellipticity index
Ellis
- E. Jones peroneal displacement
- E. line
- E. technique for Barton fracture

Ellis-Garland line
Ellis-van Creveld syndrome
Eloesser procedure
elongated
- e. aorta
- e. heart
- e. mass
- e. structure

elongation
- aortic e.
- e. and tortuosity
- e. of ventricle

eloquent
- e. area of brain
- e. cortex

ELPS
- excessive lateral pressure syndrome

Elscint
- E. APEX 409-AG ECT camera
- E. APEX 009 Precursor camera
- E. dual-detector cardiac camera
- E. Dual-Head Helix camera
- E. Excel 905 scanner
- E. MR scanner
- E. Prestige MRI system
- E. Twin CT scanner

elution
elutriation
EM
- electromagnetic

EMA
emanation
- actinium e.
- radium e.
- thorium e.

emanatorium
emanon
emanotherapy
embarrassment
- circulatory e.
- cord e.
- nerve root e.
- respiratory e.

Embden-Meyerhof glycolytic pathway
embedding of stent coil
EmboGold microsphere
embolectomy
- percutaneous e.

emboli (*pl. of* embolus)
embolic
- e. aneurysm
- e. cerebral infarct
- e. debris
- e. event
- e. material
- e. necrosis
- e. obstruction
- e. occlusion
- e. phenomenon
- e. pneumonia
- e. shower
- e. stroke

embolism
- cerebral e.
- coronary e.
- venography-related air e.
- venous e.

E

NOTES

embolization
> bronchial artery e. (BAE)
> coil e.
> fibroid e.
> Guglielmi detachable coil e.
> Lipiodol e.
> N-butyl-2-cyanoacrylate e.
> nontarget e.
> ovarian vein e.
> paradoxical e.
> particulate arterial e.
> platinum coil e.
> polyvinyl alcohol particle e.
> pulmonary artery e.
> spontaneous hemodialysis catheter
>   fracture and e.
> testicular vein e.
> e. transcatheter therapy
> uterine artery e. (UAE)
> uterine fibroid e. (UFE)

embolotherapy
> percutaneous e.

embolus, pl. **emboli**
> air e.
> amnionic fluid e.
> arterial e.
> atheromatous e.
> bacillary e.
> bile pulmonary e.
> bland e.
> bone marrow e.
> cancer e.
> capillary e.
> cardiogenic e.
> catheter-induced e.
> cellular e.
> cerebral fat e.
> cholesterol e.
> coronary artery e.
> cotton fiber e.
> crossed e.
> direct e.
> fat e.
> fibrin platelet e.
> foam e.
> foreign body e.
> hematogenous e.
> infective e.
> intracranial e.
> intraluminal e.
> lymphogenous e.
> massive e.
> e. migration
> miliary e.
> multiple emboli
> obturating e.
> occluding spring e.

> oil e.
> pantaloon e.
> paradoxical cerebral e.
> peripheral e.
> plasmodium e.
> platelet-fibrin e.
> polyurethane foam e.
> prosthetic valve e.
> pulmonary e. (PE)
> pulmonary venous-systemic air e.
> pyemic e.
> recurrent e.
> renal cholesterol e.
> retinal e.
> retrograde e.
> riding e.
> saddle e.
> septic pulmonary e.
> silent cerebral e.
> straddling e.
> submassive pulmonary e.
> therapeutic e.
> thrombus e.
> trichinous e.
> tumor e.
> venous thrombosis e.
> visceral e.

embosphere
> E. microsphere
> e. particle

embryo
> adnexal e.
> e. demise
> e. size

embryogenesis
embryoid body
embryology
> airway e.
> breast e.
> diaphragm e.
> genital tract e.
> reproductive tract e.
> urogenital e.

embryonal
> e. adenoma
> e. carcinosarcoma
> e. cell carcinoma
> e. liver sarcoma
> e. ovary teratoma
> e. rhabdomyosarcoma
> e. tumor
> e. vein

embryonic
> e. abdominal cavity
> e. anastomosis
> e. aortic arch
> e. branchial arch

e. disk
e. organizer
e. ovary
e. period
e. sac
e. truncus arteriosus
e. tumor
e. umbilical vein
embryopathy
warfarin e.
embryotoxon
posterior e.
EMD
electromechanical dissociation
EMED scanner
emetic center
EMF
endomyocardial fibrosis
emf
electromotive force
EMG
electromyogram
electromyography
EMI
electromagnetic interference
EMI brain scanner
EMI CT 500 scanner
EMI 7070 scanner
EMI unit
eminence
arcuate e.
articular e.
collateral e.
cruciate e.
cruciform e.
deltoid e.
facial e.
frontal e.
genital e.
hypothenar e.
iliopectineal e.
iliopubic e.
intercondylar e.
malar e.
medial e.
occipital e.
parietal e.
pyramidal e.
thenar e.
thyroid e.
tibial intercondylar e.

emissary
e. sphenoidal foramen
e. vein
emission
e. angiography
beta e.
characteristic e.
e. computed tomography (ECT)
e. computer-assisted tomography
e. computerized axial tomography (ECAT)
double e.
e. electron
filament e.
gamma e.
e. hepatogram
induced acoustic e.
negatron e.
photoelectric e.
e. probability
radioactive e.
e. range
e. renography
source of e.
spectral e.
stimulated acoustic e. (SAE)
thermonic e.
e. tomography
e. and transmission data
emitter
alpha-particle e.
Auger-electron e.
beta e.
gamma e.
EMP
extramedullary plasmacytoma
emphysema
alveolar duct e.
atrophic e.
bronchiolar e.
bullous e.
centriacinar e.
centrilobular e.
chronic hypertrophic e.
chronic obstructive e.
chronic pulmonary e. (CPE)
chronic tuberculous e.
compensatory e.
congenital lobar e.
cystic pulmonary e.
diffuse e.
distal acinar e.

E

NOTES

emphysema *(continued)*
distal lobular e.
ectatic e.
false e.
focal-dust e.
gangrenous e.
gastric e.
generalized e.
giant bullous e.
glass blower's e.
hypoplastic e.
idiopathic unilobar e.
increased marking of e.
infantile lobar e.
interlobular e.
interstitial intestinal e.
interstitial lung e.
intestinal e.
intramural gastric e.
irregular e.
linear e.
liquefactive e.
lobar e.
localized obstructive e.
lung e.
mediastinal e.
neck e.
necrotizing e.
neonatal cystic pulmonary e.
obstructive e.
orbital e.
oxygen-dependent e.
panacinar e.
panlobular e.
paracicatricial e.
paraseptal e.
pericicatricial e.
perifocal e.
postoperative e.
postsurgical e.
proximal acinar e.
pulmonary interstitial e. (PIE)
pulmonary subcutaneous
   encephalitis e.
restrictive pulmonary e.
scar e.
senile e.
skeletal e.
small-lunged e.
subcutaneous e.
surgical e.
traumatic e.
unilateral lobar e.
vesicular e.
emphysematosa
vaginitis e.

emphysematous
e. bleb
e. bulla
e. cholecystitis
e. COPD
e. cystitis
e. enterocolitis
e. expansion
e. gastritis
e. lung
e. pyelitis
e. pyelonephritis (EPN)
empirical method
empty
e. collapsed lung
e. gestational sac
e. heart
e. sella
e. sella syndrome
e. uterus
emptying
complete bladder e.
delayed gastric e.
gastric e. (GE)
incomplete bladder e.
oropharyngeal e.
e. time
tortuous e.
empyema
brain e.
chest e.
CNS e.
epidural e.
gallbladder e.
Hawkins accordion-type e.
interlobar e.
intracranial e.
latent e.
left-sided e.
loculated e.
metapneumonic e.
pericardial e.
pleural e.
pulsating e.
right-sided e.
spinal e.
subdural e.
synpneumonic e.
thoracic e.
tuberculous e.
E-MRI
extremity MRI
emu
electromagnetic unit
emulsion
e. film
nuclear e.

Emulsoil bowel preparation
en
>en bloc excision
>en bloc resection
>en face
>en face view
>en passage feeder artery

enalaprilat
enalaprilat-enhanced renography
enamel
>e. crypt
>e. lamella

enantiomer
enarthrosis
encapsulated
>e. brain abscess
>e. fat-containing lesion
>e. fluid
>e. gas bubble
>e. mass
>e. neoplasm
>e. radioactive seed
>e. subdural hematoma

encased heart
encasement
>vascular e.
>ventricular e.

encephali
>arachnoidea mater e.

encephalic
>e. angioma
>e. vesicle

encephalitis, pl. encephalitides
>brainstem e.
>bronzed sclerosing e.
>CMV e.
>cytomegalovirus e.
>herpes simplex virus type 1 e.
>HIV e.
>HSV1 e.
>listeria e.
>e. periaxialis concentrica
>postinfectious e.
>primary HIV e.
>subacute e.
>toxoplasmosis e.

encephaloarteriography
encephalocele
>frontoethmoidal e.
>frontosphenoidal e.
>occipital e.
>parietal e.

>sphenoethmoidal e.
>sphenoidal e.
>sphenomaxillary e.
>sphenoorbital e.
>sphenopharyngeal e.
>transethmoidal e.

encephaloclastic
>e. lesion
>e. porencephaly

encephalocystocele
encephaloduroarteriomyosynangiosis (EDAMS)
encephaloduroarteriosynangiosis (EDAS)
encephalodysplasia
encephalogram
encephalograph
encephalography
>air e.
>A-mode e.
>fractional e.
>gamma e.
>positive contrast e.

encephaloid carcinoma
encephalolith
encephaloma
encephalomalacia
>inherited cavernous angioma-related
>>posthemorrhage e.
>macrocystic e.
>microcystic e.
>multicystic e.
>neonate e.

encephalomeningocele
encephalometry
encephalomyelitis
>acute disseminated e. (ADEM)
>enteroviral e.
>postinfectious e. (PIE)

encephalomyelopathy
>subacute necrotizing e.

encephalomyopathy
>mitochondrial e.

encephalopathy
>AIDS e.
>anoxic e.
>Binswanger e.
>HIV e.
>hypertensive e.
>hypoxic ischemic e.
>ischemic e.
>lead e.

E

NOTES

encephalopathy *(continued)*
  subcortical arteriosclerotic e.
  subcortical atherosclerotic e.
encephalotrigeminal
  e. angiomatosis
  e. syndrome
encerclage
enchondral
  e. bone formation
  e. ossification
enchondroma
enchondromatosis
  multiple e.
enchondrosarcoma
encode
  frequency e. (FE, FR)
encoded-Fourier
encoding
  amplitude of phase e.
  centrally ordered phase e.
  coil sensitive e.
  3D spatial e.
  frequency e.
  gradient e.
  one-dimensional phase e.
  ordered phase e.
  phase e. (PE)
  position e.
  reordering of phase e.
  respiratory ordered phase e.
   (ROPE)
  respiratory sorted phase e.
  sensitivity e. (SENSE)
  spatial e.
  wavelet e.
encroaching endothelial cell
encroachment
  bony e.
  foraminal e.
  luminal e.
  soft tissue canal e.
  stenosis e.
encrustation
  bile e.
encryption algorithm
encysted
  e. calculus
  e. pleurisy
end
  e. of atrial systole
  bone e.
  e. bud
  e. bulb
  e. exhalation
  e. expiration
  fimbriated e.
  e. inhalation

  e. organ resistance
  e. plate
  e. point
  e. of saturated bombardment
   (EOSB)
  seen on e.
  e. systole (ES)
endarterectomy
  carotid e. (CEA)
  extraluminal e.
  femoral e.
  e. graft
  surgical e.
  transluminal e.
endarteritis obliterans
end-diastolic
  e.-d. aortic-left ventricular pressure
   gradient
  e.-d. imaging
  e.-d. polar map
  e.-d. pressure-volume relation
  e.-d. velocity measurement
  e.-d. volume
  e.-d. volume index
end-expiratory lung volume
end-fire transducer
end-hole introducer
endoanal
  e. coil
  e. MR imaging
  e. sonography
  e. ultrasound
Endobile
endobiliary stenting
EndoBlade
endobrachyesophagus
endobronchial
  e. carcinoma
  e. hamartoma
  e. Kaposi sarcoma
  e. lesion
  e. metastasis
  e. obstruction
  e. sarcoidosis
  e. tube
  e. tuberculosis
  e. tumor
endocardial, endocardiac
  e. activation mapping
  e. catheter mapping
  e. centroid
  e. cushion
  e. cushion defect (ECD)
  e. cushion development
  e. cushion malformation
  e. cushion ventricular septal defect
  e. dysplasia

e. fibroelastosis
e. fibrosis
e. plaque
e. pressure
e. sclerosis
e. trabeculation
e. volume
endocarditis
aortic valve e.
atypical verrucous e.
bacterial e.
Löffler fibroplastic e.
marantic e.
subacute bacterial e.
thrombotic e.
endocardium
disk of e.
wafer of e.
endocatheter ruler
endocervical
e. canal
e. canal coloscopy
e. mucosa
endochondral
e. bone
e. bone deposit
endochondroma
endocranium
endocrine
e. ablative therapy
e. gland
e. imaging
e. tumor
endocyst
endodermal
e. cyst
e. pouch
e. sinus
e. sinus ovarian tumor
e. sinus testis tumor
endodiascope
endodiascopy
endoergic reaction
endoesophageal MRI coil
endofluoroscopic technique
endofluoroscopy
flexible e.
percutaneous e.
rigid e.
endogenous
e. adenosine contrast medium

e. callus formation
e. lipid pneumonia
Endografin
endograft
AneuRx e.
endoleak
e. graft
type I e. (T1EL)
type II e. (T2EL)
endoluminal
e. density
e. MRI
e. radiofrequency electrocautery
e. sonography
e. view
e. visualization
endolymphatic
e. duct
e. hydrops
e. sac
e. sac tumor
e. stromal myosis
endometria (*pl. of* endometrium)
endometrial
e. adenocanthoma
e. anatomy
e. canal fluid
e. carcinoma
e. cavity
e. cyst
e. echo
e. fluid in canal
e. hyperplasia
e. implant
e. island
e. polyp
e. secretory adenocarcinoma
e. stripe
e. stromal sarcoma
e. surface deformity
e. thickness
endometrioid
e. cystadenoma
e. ovarian carcinoma
e. tumor
endometrioma
endometriosis
bladder e.
colonic involvement of e.
GI tract e.
gynecologic e.
e. interna

E

NOTES

endometriosis *(continued)*
sciatic e.
ureteral e.
endometriotic cyst
endometritis
inflammatory e.
endometrium, pl. **endometria**
decidualized e.
FIGO staging of adenocarcinoma of e.
inactive e.
postmenopausal e.
proliferative phase e.
secretory phase e.
thickened irregular e.
endometry
endomyelography
endomyocardial
e. fibroplasia
e. fibrosis (EMF)
endoneural
endoneurium
end-on vessel
endopelvic fascia
endophlebitis
Endo-P-Probe
endoprobe
rotating e.
single-crystal e.
endoprosthesis
biliary e.
Carey-Coons soft stent biliary e.
double-lumen e.
double-pigtail e.
IntraCoil e.
large-bore bile duct e.
metallic biliary e.
self-expanding metallic e.
VIATORR e.
Wallgraft e.
Wallstent biliary e.
endopyelotomy
percutaneous e.
endorectal
e. coil
e. ileal pouch
e. surface-coil MR imaging
e. ultrasound (ERU, ERUS, EUS)
end-organ response
endosaccular packing
endosalpingosis
endoscope
double-channel e.
Olympus EVIS Q-200V e.
Olympus TJF-100 e.
virtual e.

endoscopic
e. cholangiography (ERC)
e. coronary artery bypass graft (E-CABG)
e. decompression
e. laser
e. laser cholecystectomy
e. laser dacryocystorhinostomy
e. lithotripsy
e. optical coherence tomography (EOCT)
e. percutaneous cholangiopancreatography
e. procedure
e. quadrature radiofrequency coil
e. retrograde cholangiogram (ERC)
e. retrograde cholangiopancreatography (ERCP)
e. retrograde cholangiopancreatography catheter
e. retrograde pancreatic duct cannulation
e. retrograde pancreatography
e. retrograde parenchymography (ERP)
e. sonography
e. surveillance
e. ultrasound (EUS)
e. ultrasound-guided fine needle aspiration (EUS-FNA)
e. washing pipe
endoscopy
colorectal cancer e.
gastrointestinal e.
laser-assisted spinal e. (LASE)
M2A imaging capsule e.
percutaneous e.
upper gastrointestinal e.
virtual arterial e.
endoskeleton
endosonographic image
endosonography
3D e.
hydrogen peroxide-enhanced anal e.
rectal e.
transduodenal e.
transgastric e.
vaginal e.
endosonoscopy
endosseous implant
Endostaple device
endosteal
e. callus
e. chondrosarcoma
e. revascularization
e. scalloping
e. surface

endosteoma
endosteum
endothelia (*pl. of* endothelium)
endothelial
   e. damage
   e. hypoplasia
   e. injury
   e. leukocyte
   e. myeloma
   e. surface
endothelialization
endothelialized vascular graft
endotheliomatous meningioma
endothelium, pl. **endothelia**
   arterial e.
   capillary e.
   pulmonary capillary e.
endothoracic fascia
endothorax
   tension e.
endotracheal (ET)
   e. intubation
   e. tube
endovaginal
   e. coil
   e. sonography
   e. ultrasound (EVUS)
endovascular
   e. aortic graft
   e. brachytherapy
   e. coil
   e. embolization femoral approach
   e. flow wire study
   e. photo acoustic recanalization
   (EPAR)
   e. repair
   e. stent-graft
   e. system
   e. technique
   e. ultrasonography
   e. ultrasound
EndoVasix EPAR laser system
endplate
   cartilage e.
   cartilaginous e.
   hyaline cartilage e.
   e. sclerosis
   vertebral body e.
endpoint
   measurable e.
   stress e.
end-pressure artifact

end-stage
   e.-s. adult cardiac decompensation
   e.-s. cardiomyopathy
   e.-s. cirrhosis
   e.-s. fetal cardiac decompensation
   e.-s. lung disease
   e.-s. renal disease
   e.-s. renal failure (ESRF)
end-systolic
   e.-s. polar map
   e.-s. pressure (ESP)
   e.-s. pressure:end-systolic volume
   e.-s. pressure:end-systolic volume
   ratio (ESP:ESV ratio, ESP:ESV
   ratio)
   e.-s. pressure-volume relation
   e.-s. residual volume
   e.-s. reversal
   e.-s. volume (ESV)
   e.-s. volume index (ESVI)
   e.-s. wall index/end-systolic volume
   ratio
end-to-side biliary-enteric anastomosis
end-viewing transducer
Enecat CT concentrated rectal
  suspension
enema
   air-contrast barium e. (ACBE)
   analeptic e.
   barium e. (BE)
   blind e.
   cleansing e.
   contrast e.
   Cortenema retention e.
   double-contrast barium e. (DCBE)
   full-column barium e.
   Gastrografin e.
   Harris flush e.
   hydrocortisone e.
   hydrogen peroxide e.
   Hypaque e.
   mesalamine e.
   methylene blue e.
   nuclear e.
   opaque e.
   phosphate e.
   phosphosoda e.
   retention e.
   Rowasa e.
   single-contrast barium e.
   small bowel e.

E

NOTES

enema *(continued)*
    therapeutic barium e.
    water-soluble contrast e.
enemas until clear
energetic positron
energy
    atomic e.
    average positron e.
    beam e.
    binding e.
    chemical potential e.
    e. decay
    electrical potential e.
    electromagnetic e.
    e. fluence
    e. flux density
    e. frequency
    gravitational potential e.
    kinetic e.
    laser e.
    e. level
    e. level diagram (ELD)
    low-photon e.
    mechanical potential e.
    nuclear e.
    photon e.
    potential e.
    quadrant e.
    quantum e.
    radiant e.
    radiation e.
    radiofrequency e.
    recoil e.
    e. resolution
    e. spectrum
    e. subtraction
    thermal e.
    e. transfer
    e. transfer process
    treatment e.
    variable e.
    e. wave
    e. wavelength
    e. window
    x-ray e.
enforcer
    Cook e.
Engel alkalinity
Engelmann
    E. disease
    E. disk
engorged
    e. tissue
    e. vein
enhanced
    e. CT
    e. CT scan

    e. glycolysis
    e. imaging
enhancement
    acoustic e.
    artery-like pattern of e.
    bolus contrast e.
    bright contrast e.
    cocurrent flow-related e.
    contrast e.
    countercurrent flow-related e.
    Doppler flow signal e.
    Doppler signal e.
    dynamic e.
    echo e.
    edge e.
    evanescent e.
    exercise-induced contrast e.
    e. factor
    flip-flop e.
    flow-related e.
    focal nodular e.
    gadolinium e.
    gyral brain e.
    heterogeneous isodense e.
    homogeneous e.
    hybrid rapid acquisition with
      relaxation e. (HRARE)
    inhomogeneous contrast e.
    inhomogeneous moderate e.
    internal e.
    isodense e.
    meningeal e.
    microbubble contrast e.
    e. morphology
    multislice flow-related e.
    nodular e.
    nonhomogeneous e.
    nuclear magnetic resonance
      relaxation rate e.
    paradoxical e.
    paramagnetic contrast e.
    parenchymal e.
    e. pattern
    peak of maximum e. (PME)
    peripheral lesion e.
    peritoneal e.
    portal vein e.
    posterior acoustic e.
    proton relaxation e. (PRE)
    pulmonary nodule e.
    punctate e.
    radiation e.
    rapid acquisition with relaxation e.
      (RARE)
    real-time e.
    rim e.
    ring e.

scan with contrast e.
serpentine e.
signal e.
sulcal e.
time-of-flight e.
T2 proton relaxation e. (T2 PRE)
transient peritumoral e.
vascular MR contrast e.

enhancing
e. brain lesion
e. mass
e. nodule
e. ventricular margin

enlarged
e. cardiac silhouette
e. frontal horn
e. gallbladder
e. heart
e. kidney
e. liver
e. presacral space
e. pulmonary vessel
e. thyroid gland
e. vascular channel
e. vertebral foramen
e. vestibular vascular aqueduct
  syndrome

enlargement
airspace e.
azygos vein e.
biventricular e.
bony e.
bulbous e.
cardiac silhouette e.
cervical e.
chamber e.
compensatory e.
diffuse hepatic e.
diffuse liver e.
diffuse thymic e.
diffuse uterine e.
e. of epididymis
epiglottic e.
extraocular muscle e.
gastric fold e.
global renal e.
iliopsoas compartment e.
e. of lacrimal gland
left atrial e. (LAE)
lymph node e.
masseteric e.
mediastinal lymph node e.

optic nerve e.
panchamber e.
papilla of Vater e.
e. of parotid gland
pituitary gland e.
placenta e.
right atrial e. (RAE)
right ventricular e. (RVE)
sella e.
e. of the subarachnoidal space
sulcal e.
thymic e.
e. of uterus
e. of ventricle
ventricular e.
e. of vertebral body
e. of vertebral foramen
e. with low-density lymph node
  center

enostosis
Ensemble contrast imaging (ECI)
ensheathing callus
ensiform
e. appendix
e. cartilage
e. process

eNTEGRA workstation
enteric
e. duplication cyst
e. exocrine drainage
e. fistula
e. plexus
e. stricture

enteric-drained pancreas transplant
enteritis
candida e.
Crohn granulomatous e.
Crohn regional e.
eosinophilic e.
e. follicularis
radiation e.
regional e.

enterobiliary
enterocele sac
enterocleisis
enteroclysis
computed tomographic e.

enterococcus, pl. **enterococci**
enterocolic fistula
enterocolitis
emphysematous e.
granulomatous e.

NOTES

enterocolitis *(continued)*
    Hirschsprung-associated e. (HAEC)
    necrotizing e.
    neutropenic e.
enterocutaneous fistula
enterocystoma
enterocytic processing
enteroenteral fistula
enterogenous cyst
enteroinsular axis
enterolith
enteropathica
    acrodermatitis e.
enteropathy
    exudative e.
    gluten-sensitive e.
    protein-losing e.
    radiation e.
enteropathy-associated T-cell lymphoma
enteroperitoneal abscess
enteroptosis
enteroscope
    Olympus SIF-100 video e.
enteroscopy
    small bowel e. (SBE)
enterospinal fistula
enterourethral fistula
enterovaginal fistula
enterovesical fistula
enteroviral encephalomyelitis
Entero Vu contrast medium
enthesis
enthesitis
enthesopathic transformation
enthesophyte
    plantar calcaneal e.
    subacromial e.
entity
    tumor e.
entorhinal cortex
entrance
    e. block
    e. skin exposure
entrapment
    artery e.
    gas e.
    guidewire e.
    lateral e.
    median nerve e.
    nerve e.
    e. neuropathy
    patellar e.
    posterior interosseous nerve e.
    scar tissue e.
    soft tissue e.
    suprascapular nerve e.
    ulnar nerve e.

entrapped
    e. ovarian cyst
    e. plantar sesamoid bone
EntroEase oral radiopaque contrast medium
entry
    capacitative calcium e.
    e. flap
    e. point
    e. slice phenomenon artifact
    e. tear
    e. zone
envelope
    capsuloperiosteal e.
    fascial e.
    soft tissue e.
    synovial e.
environmental
    e. factor
    e. plutonium
Envoy 6F guiding catheter
enzyme
    angiotensin-converting e. (ACE)
    e. replacement therapy
    e. supplementation therapy
enzyme-multiplied immunoassay technique
EOCT
    endoscopic optical coherence tomography
EOSB
    end of saturated bombardment
eosinophilia
    tumor-associated tissue e.
eosinophilic
    e. brain adenoma
    e. enteritis
    e. granuloma
    e. infiltrate
    e. leukocyte
    e. lung disease
    e. pneumonia
Eovist contrast agent
EP
    ectopic pregnancy
    electrophysiology
    excretory phase
EP2000 electrophysiology imaging system
epactal bone
EPAR
    endovascular photo acoustic recanalization
    EPAR laser system
EPBF
    effective pulmonary blood flow
EPB muscle

EPC
   echo phase correction
ependyma
ependymal cyst
ependymitis
   bacterial e.
   e. granularis
ependymoblastoma
ependymoma
   anaplastic e.
   brain e.
   brainstem e.
   e. cord
   intramedullary e.
   malignant e.
   myxopapillary e.
   spinal cord e.
   subcutaneous sacrococcygeal
      myxopapillary e.
ephemeral pneumonia
EPI
   echo-planar imaging
   spiral EPI (SEPI)
epiarterial bronchus
epiarticular osteochondromatous
   dysplasia
epicardial
   e. attachment
   e. centroid
   e. coronary artery
   e. Doppler echocardiography
   e. Doppler flow sector transducer
   e. fat pad
   e. imaging
   e. implantation
   e. mapping
   e. space
   e. surface
   e. tension
   e. volume
epicardium
epicenter
   eccentric e.
epicolic lymph node
epicondylar
   e. fracture
   e. fracture of humerus
   e. ridge
epicondyle
   humeral e.
   medial e.

epicondylitis
   lateral e.
   medial e.
epicondyloolecranon ligament
Epic ophthalmic 3-in-1 laser
epicortical lesion
epicranial aponeurosis
epidermal
   e. carcinoma
   e. inclusion cyst
   e. ridge
epidermoid
   acquired e.
   black e.
   cerebellar e.
   e. lung carcinoma
   e. mediastinum
   e. spine
   e. tumor
   white e.
epidermoidoma
   incisural e.
   intradural e.
   prepontine white e.
epididymal
   e. cyst
   e. descent
   e. fibrosarcoma
epididymis, pl. epididymides
   appendix of e.
   body of e.
   edema of e.
   enlargement of e.
   inflammation of e.
   interstitial congestion of e.
   e. lesion
   ligament of e.
   lobule of e.
   postvasectomy change in e.
   sinus of e.
   tail of e.
epididymitis
epididymography imaging
epididymoorchitis
epididymovesiculography
epidural
   e. abscess
   e. angiolipoma
   e. anular fibrosis
   e. arachnoid cyst
   e. blood
   e. blood patch

E

NOTES

epidural *(continued)*
- e. cavernous hemangioma
- e. cavity
- e. effusion
- e. empyema
- e. extramedullary lesion
- e. fat
- e. hematoma (EDH)
- e. hemorrhage
- e. implant
- e. infusion
- e. lipoma
- e. lipomatosis
- e. lymphoma
- e. mass
- e. pneumatosis
- e. space
- e. steroid injection
- e. venography
- e. venous plexus

epidurogram

epidurography
- magnetic resonance e.

epigastric
- e. angle
- e. fold
- e. fossa
- e. hernia
- e. lymph node
- e. vein

epigastrium

epiglottic
- e. carcinoma
- e. cartilage
- e. disruption
- e. enlargement
- e. fold
- e. tubercle

epiglottitis
- bacterial e.

epignathus

epihyal
- e. bone
- e. ligament

epihyoid bone

epilarynx

EpiLaser

epilation dose

epilepsy
- chronic partial e.
- drug-resistant extratemporal e.
- extratemporal e.
- idiopathic e.
- structural e.
- temporal lobe e. (TLE)

epileptic focus

epileptogenic
- e. center
- e. focus
- e. lesion
- e. zone

Epimed spring guide catheter

epipericardial ridge

epiphora

epiphrenic bulge

epiphyseal
- e. arrest
- e. cartilage
- e. cartilage plate
- e. chondroblastic growth
- e. chondrocyte
- e. coxa vara
- e. disk
- e. dysgenesis
- e. dysostosis
- e. dysplasia
- e. exostosis
- e. fetal bone center
- e. growth plate
- e. hematopoietic marrow
- e. hyperplasia
- e. hypertrophy
- e. ischemic necrosis
- e. lesion
- e. line
- e. ossification center
- e. osteochondroma
- e. overgrowth
- e. plate fracture
- e. plate injury
- e. slip fracture
- e. slippage
- e. tibial fracture

epiphysealis punctua dysplasia

epiphyseolysis
- femoral head e.
- idiopathic e.
- juvenile e.

epiphysis, pl. **epiphyses**
- anular e.
- atavistic e.
- e. avulsion
- ball-and-socket e.
- balloon e.
- e. bone
- bone lesion e.
- capital e. (CE)
- capital femoral e.
- capitular e.
- cartilaginous e.
- cone e.
- congenital stippled e.

familial avascular necrosis of
  phalangeal e.
femoral capital e.
humeral e.
ossifying e.
osteochondrotic separation of
  epiphysis
Perthes e.
pressure e.
ring e.
slipped capital femoral e. (SCFE)
slipped upper femoral e. (SUFE)
tibial e.
traction e.
epiphysitis
  juvenile e.
  vertebral e.
epiploia
epiploic
  e. appendage
  e. appendix
  e. foramen
epiploica
  appendix e.
epipteric bone
epirenal septum
episcleral
  e. plaque brachytherapy
  e. space
  e. vein
episode
  ischemic e.
  silent ischemic e.
epispadia exstrophy complex
Epistar
  E. perfusion technique
  E. subtraction angiography
episternal bone
epitendineum
epithalamus
epithelia (*pl. of* epithelium)
epithelial
  e. cell
  e. colon
  e. colonic polyp
  e. degenerative change
  e. hyperplasia
  e. inclusion cyst
  e. malignancy
  e. neoplasm
  e. ovarian carcinoma

  e. spleen
  e. tumor
epithelialization
  creeping e.
epithelial-myoepithelial carcinoma
epithelioid
  e. angiomatosis
  e. granuloma
  e. hemangioendothelioma
  e. hemangioma
  e. leiomyoma
  e. malignant mesothelioma
  e. osteosarcoma
  e. sarcoma
epithelioma
  calcifying Malherbe e.
epitheliosis
  infiltrating breast e.
epitheliotropism
epithelium, pl. **epithelia**
  atypical e.
  Barrett e.
  e. crypt
  ductal e.
  normal ovarian surface e. (NOSE)
  papilla of columnar e.
  squamous metaplasia white e.
  surface e.
  tumor of surface e.
  white e.
epithermal neutron
EpiTouch laser
epitrochlear lymph node
epituberculous infiltrate
epitympanic
  e. recess (EPR)
  e. space
epitympanum
EPL
  effective path length
  extensor pollicis longus
  EPL muscle
EPN
  emphysematous pyelonephritis
epoch
  VNS e.
eponychium
epoöphoron
Eppendorf pO$_2$ histograph
EPR
  electron paramagnetic resonance
  epitympanic recess

NOTES

E

311

epsilon̂m
TDE-derived epsilonþ and e.
EPSS
E point to septal separation
eptifibatide
epulofibroma
EQP
equal in intensity
equalization
histogram e.
pressure e.
equalized diastolic pressure
equation
Bernoulli e.
Bloch e.
Bohr e.
Boltzmann e.
Bragg e.
Carter e.
continuity e.
decay e.
Doppler e.
Fick e.
hamiltonian e.
Kety e.
Larmor e.
linear-quadratic e.
modified Bernoulli e.
Nernst e.
Schroedinger e.
Solomon-Bloembergen e.
Stewart-Hamilton e.
Teichholz e.
transformer e.
equilibration
equilibrium
e. dissociation constant
e. dose constant
e. factor
e. magnetization
e. MUGA imaging
e. MUGA scan
e. phase
e. point
radioactive e.
e. radionuclide angiocardiography
e. radionuclide angiocardiography
technique
e. radionuclide angiography
secular e.
state e.
thermal e.
transient e.
e. view
equina
cauda e.
nerve roots of the cauda e.

equinovalgus
e. deformity
pes e.
equinovarus
e. hindfoot deformity
pes e.
talipes e.
Equinox
20-mm E. balloon microcatheter
E. occlusion balloon catheter
equinus
e. deformity
pes e.
equipment
e. artifact
RapidScreen RS-2000 x-ray e.
equivalence
mass energy e.
equivalent
chance e.
dose e. (DE)
meconium ileus e.
total effective dose e. (TEDE)
total organ dose e. (TODE)
e. treatment
equivalent-physical
roentgen e.-p. (REP)
equivocal finding
ER
estrogen-receptor
ER positive
erase
background e.
Erb
E. disease
E. injury
E. point
Erb-Duchenne-Klumpke injury
erbium
e. chromium:yttrium-aluminum-garnet
(ErCr:YAG)
2040 e. SilkLaser
erbium-171
erbium:YAG
e.-YAG infrared laser
ERC
endoscopic cholangiography
endoscopic retrograde cholangiogram
ERCP
endoscopic retrograde
cholangiopancreatography
ERCP catheter
ERCP imaging
ERCP manometry

ErCr:YAG
  erbium chromium:yttrium-aluminum-
    garnet
    ErCr:YAG laser
Erdheim
  E. cystic medial necrosis
  E. tumor
Erdheim-Chester disease
ERE
  estrogen-response element
  external rotation in extension
erect
  e. fluoro spot projection
  e. lateral flexion/extension
    radiograph
  e. position
  e. view
erector spinae
ERF
  edge response function
  external rotation in flexion
ERFP
  effective renal plasma flow
ERG
  electroretinogram
ergometer
  bicycle e.
  Cybex e.
ergonomics
  hands-up e.
Erichsen sign
Erlenmeyer
  E. flask
  E. flask appearance
  E. flask-like deformity
Ernst angle
erosion
  articular e.
  e. of articular surface
  bony e.
  bronchial e.
  duodenal e.
  e. of epiphyseal bone
  focal cartilage e.
  gastric antral e.
  graft-enteric e.
  infraspinatus insertion e.
  linear e.
  marginal e.
  mouse ear e.
  odontoid e.
  osteoclastic e.

  pedicle e.
  plaque e.
  rat-bite e.
  salt-and-pepper duodenal e.
  stomach varioliform e.
  tumor e.
  varioliform e.
erosive
  e. duodenitis
  e. gastritis
  e. gingivitis
  e. osteoarthritis
ERP
  effective refractory period
  endoscopic retrograde parenchymography
ERPF
  effective renal plasma flow
erratum
  anatomic moment e.
error
  ADC quantization e.
  CT imaging e.
  darkroom e.
  data clipping detection e.
  data spike detection e.
  e. diffusion method
  dorsal induction e.
  duplex ultrasound e.
  flow-related phase e.
  generalized compensation for
    resonance offset and pulse
    length e.'s (GROPE)
  Hausdorff e.
  interobserver e.
  intraobserver e.
  isocenter placement e.
  magnification e.
  mean-square e.
  photoreceptor fractional velocity e.
  positioning e.
  preparation e.
  quantization e.
  random e.
  raster spacing e.
  relative e.
  sampling e.
  sensing e.
  size estimation e.
  spatial frequency e.
  systematic e.
error-sum criterion

E

NOTES

ERU
    endorectal ultrasound
      gray-scale ERU
eruption
    rhythmic paradoxical e.
ERUS
    endorectal ultrasound
ERV
    expiratory reserve volume
erythema
    e. of joint
    radiation e.
    e. threshold
erythrocyte
    e. iron turnover
    technetium-99m heat-denatured e.
erythropoietin
    e. assay
    e. bioassay
ES
    end systole
Es
    einsteinium
^{255}Es
    einsteinium-255
Esaote extremity scanner
escalation
escape
    e. of air into lung connective
      tissue
    e. beat
    e. interval
escape-capture rhythm
escape-peak ratio
ESIN
    elastic stable intramedullary nailing
Esophacoil stent
esophageal
    e. achalasia pattern
    e. aperistalsis
    e. apple-core lesion
    e. atresia
    e. balloon technique
    e. body
    e. carcinoma
    e. carcinosarcoma
    e. choriocarcinoma
    e. contraction
    e. degeneration
    e. dilatation
    e. displacement
    e. dissection
    e. diverticulum
    e. duplication
    e. duplication cyst
    e. dysmotility
    e. dysphagia

e. electrogram
e. fibroadenoma
e. filling defect
e. fold
e. functional disorder
e. function imaging
e. graft
e. groove
e. hernia
e. hiatus
e. impression
e. inflammation
e. inlet
e. leiomyoma
e. leiomyomatosis
e. leiomyosarcoma
e. lipomatosis
e. lumen
e. manometry
e. margin serration
e. morphologic disorder
e. motility
e. motility disorder
e. mucosal nodule
e. mucosal ring
e. muscular ring
e. narrowing
e. neoplasm
e. obstruction
e. obturator airway
e. opening
e. peptic stricture
e. perforation
e. peristalsis
e. peristaltic pressure
e. pill electrode
e. plaque
e. plexus
e. pseudosarcoma
e. reflux
e. rupture
e. shiver
e. shunt
e. spasm
e. sphincter relaxation
e. stenosis
e. stent
e. tear
e. transition zone
e. transit time
e. tumor
e. ulcer
e. variceal sclerosis
e. varix
e. vein
e. vestibule

e. web
e. window
esophageal-pleural stripe
esophagectomy
Ivor Lewis e.
transhiatal e.
transthoracic e.
esophagi (*pl. of* esophagus)
esophagitis
acute e.
AIDS-related e.
candida e.
caustic e.
chronic e.
corrosive e.
cytomegalovirus e.
drug-induced e.
herpes e.
HIV e.
peptic e.
pill e.
reflux e. (RE)
Sonnenberg classification of
erosive e.
stasis e.
viral e.
esophagogastrectomy
esophagogastric (EG)
e. fat pad
e. intubation
e. junction
e. orifice
e. region
e. tamponade
esophagogastroduodenoscopy (EGD)
esophagogastrostomy
esophagogram (*var. of* esophagram)
esophagography
double-contrast e.
e. imaging
esophagojejunostomy
esophagorespiratory fistula
esophagoscopy
esophagospasm
esophagostomy
cervical e.
palliative e.
esophagotracheal fistula
esophagram, esophagogram
air e.
barium e.
barium-water e.

contrast e.
pullback e.
radionuclide e.
esophagraphy
esophagus, pl. **esophagi**
abnormal peristaltic e.
achalasia of e.
A level of the e.
aperistaltic e.
A ring of e.
atonic e.
Barrett e.
bird-beak e.
B level of the e.
B ring of e.
cervical e.
cobblestone appearance e.
columnar-lined e.
congenitally short e.
corkscrew appearance of the e.
curling e.
diffuse dilation of the e.
diffuse spasm of the e.
dilated e.
discrete segment of normal e.
double-barrel e.
double-ring e.
dysmotile e.
extrinsic impression of the e.
foamy e.
foreign body in e.
intramural rupture of the e.
long smooth narrowing e.
middle third of thoracic e.
muscular ring e.
nutcracker e.
polypoid lesion of the lower e.
rat-tail e.
rosary beading e.
scleroderma of e.
shaggy e.
shish kabob e.
short-segment Barrett e. (SSBE)
spastic e.
submerged segment of the e.
thoracic e.
tortuous e.
upper thoracic e.
Z-line of e.
ESP
end-systolic pressure

E

NOTES

ESP:ESV ratio
> end-systolic pressure:end-systolic volume ratio

ESR
> electron spin resonance

ESRF
> end-stage renal failure

essential
> e. osteolysis
> e. tumor

Essex-Lopresti
> E.-L. calcaneal fracture classification
> E.-L. joint depression fracture

ester
> iodipamide ethyl e.

esthesioneuroblastoma

esthesioneurocytoma

esthesioneuroepithelioma

estimated fetal weight (EFW)

estimation
> bayesian image e. (BIE)
> fractional moving blood volume e.
> frequency e.
> magnetic resonance volume e.
> stereologic method of volume e.
> volume e.

estradiol

estrogen-producing tumor

estrogen-receptor (ER)
> e.-r. positive

estrogen-response element (ERE)

ESV
> end-systolic volume

ESVI
> end-systolic volume index

ESWL
> extracorporeal shock wave lithotripsy

ET
> ejection time
> endotracheal
> etiology

etching
> track e.

ETF
> extension teardrop fracture

ethanol (EtOH)
> e. ablation
> e. injection

Ethiodane

ethiodized
> e. oil
> e. oil contrast medium

Ethiodol imaging agent

ethmocephaly

ethmoid
> e. air cell

> e. bone
> e. canal
> e. sinus
> e. sinus carcinoma

ethmoidal
> e. artery
> e. bulla
> e. crest
> e. foramen
> e. groove
> e. labyrinth
> e. meningoencephalocele
> e. notch
> e. process
> e. vein

ethmoidolacrimal suture

ethmoidomaxillary suture

ethmovomerine plate

ethyl
> e. cysteinate dimer (ECD)
> ^{18}F-labeled polyfluorinated e.

ethylenediamine tetramethylene phosphonic acid (EDTMP)

ethyliodophenylundecyl contrast medium

etidronate
> e. disodium imaging agent
> rhenium-186 e.
> technetium-99m e.

etiology (ET)
> multifactorial e.'s

etiopathogenetic

ETL
> echo-train length

E-to-F
> E.-to-F. slope
> E.-to-F. slope of valve

E-TOF detecting module

EtOH
> ethanol

ETT
> exercise tolerance test

EU
> excretory urography

euchromatin

eukinesis

Euler number

Eureka collimator

europium-activated barium fluorohalide

EUS
> endorectal ultrasound
> endoscopic ultrasound
> depth of tumor invasion assessed by EUS

EUS-FNA
> endoscopic ultrasound-guided fine needle aspiration

eustachian
>   e. canal
>   e. tonsil
>   e. tube
>   e. valve

eV, ev
>   electron volt

Evac-Q-Kwik bowel preparation

evacuation
>   colonic e.
>   digital rectal e.
>   e. disorder
>   e. pouchography
>   precipitate e.
>   e. proctography

evaluation
>   e. of glucose metabolism
>   e. of mass mammography
>   shunt e.

evanescent enhancement

Evans
>   E. blue albumin
>   E. blue imaging agent
>   E. intertrochanteric fracture
>   classification
>   E. ratio

Evans-D'Angio staging system

EVD
>   external ventricular drain

even distribution of echoes

even-echo rephasing

event
>   cardinal e.
>   cerebral ischemic e.
>   coincidence e.
>   e. counter
>   embolic e.
>   inciting e.
>   ischemic e.
>   main timing e. (MTE)
>   precipitating e.
>   random coincidence e.
>   scattered coincidence e.
>   true e.

eventration
>   e. of the diaphragm
>   diaphragmatic e.

event-related paradigm

eversion
>   e. of ankle
>   cervical e.

>   e. position
>   e. sprain

eversion-external rotation deformity

evidence
>   scintigraphic e.

evolution
>   stroke in e. (SIE)
>   E. XP scanner

evolving
>   e. hematoma
>   e. myocardial infarct

evulsion

EVUS
>   endovaginal ultrasound

Ewald
>   E. node
>   E. test meal

Ewart sign

Ewing
>   E. sarcoma
>   E. sarcoma-Wilms tumor 1 (EWS-
>   WT1)
>   E. tumor

EWS-WT1
>   Ewing sarcoma-Wilms tumor 1

ex
>   ex vacuo ventriculomegaly
>   ex vivo magnetic resonance
>   imaging

ExAblate 2000 ultrasound system

exacerbation

exact framing

exaggerated
>   e. craniocaudal lateral (XCCL)
>   e. craniocaudal view

exametazime imaging agent

examination
>   barium follow-through e.
>   contrast-enhanced radiographic e.
>   Doppler venous e.
>   double-contrast eversion e.
>   first-pass e.
> ^{67}Ga e.
>   gated exercise e.
>   gray-scale e.
>   image-acquisition gated e.
>   limited e.
>   neuroradiologic e.
>   postglucose loading e.
>   proton brain e. (PROBE)
>   reinjection thallium stress e.
>   rest redistribution e.

NOTES

E

examination *(continued)*
    single-voxel proton brain e. (PROBE-SV)
    stress-gated blood pool cardiac e.
    stress-redistribution e.
    stress-rest reinjection e.
    suboptimal e.
    transcranial e.
    transforaminal e.
    unsuppressed e.
    venous Doppler e.
    in vivo e.
    volumetric interpolated breath-hold e. (VIBE)
    whole-body nuclear physical e.

excavation
    saucer-shaped e.

excavatum
    pectus e.

Excelart short-bore MRI
Excel-14 microcatheter
Excelsior microcatheter
excessive
    e. callus formation
    e. lateral pressure syndrome (ELPS)

exchange
    air e.
    coupling e.
    e. guidewire
    half-time of e.
    intestinal gas e.
    narrowing e.
    proton-proton magnetization e.
    pulmonary gas e.
    rapid e. (RX)
    spin e.

excimer
    e. laser
    e. laser coronary angioplasty (ELCA)
    e. laser system
    XeCl e.

excision
    CT-guided percutaneous e.
    en bloc e.
    large loop e.

excisional biopsy
excitation
    delay alternating with nutation for tailored e. (DANTE)
    fast acquisition multiple e.
    e. function
    e. function measurement
    magnetization-prepared rapid gradient echo-water e. (MP-RAGE-WE)

    nonuniform e.
    number of e. (NEX, NOX)
    e. profile
    quadrature e.
    rebound e.
    selective e.
    slice-selective e.
    spatial and chemical-shift encoded e. (SPACE)
    e. spectrum
    supernormal e.
    tailored e.
    tilted optimized nonsaturating e. (TONE)
    uniform TR e.
    variable-angle uniform signal e. (VUSE)
    variable flip-angle e.
    volume-selective e.
    wave of e.

excitation-spoiled fat-suppressed T1-weighted SE image
excitatory
    e. lesion
    e. neurotransmitter
    e. pulse characteristic

excited
    e. atom
    e. electron

excitotoxic
    e. cord injury
    e. mechanism

Excluder stent-graft
exclusion
    subtotal gastric e.

exclusion-HPLC technique
excrescence
    bony e.
    papillary e.

excrescentic thickening of the optic nerve
excretion
    ammonium e.
    colonic mucosal e.
    contrast media e.
    ^{67}Ga e.
    e. pyelography
    uptake and e.
    urinary e.
    e. urography
    vicarious contrast e.

excretory
    e. cystogram
    e. duct
    e. intravenous pyelography
    e. phase (EP)

e. urethrogram drip infusion urography
e. urogram
e. urography (EU)
e. urography imaging

excursion of the diaphragm
exencephaly
exenteration
    anterior e.
    pelvic e.
exercise
    e. echocardiography
    e. first-pass LVEF
    flexion and extension e.'s
    e. image
    e. index
    e. load
    e. LV function
    modified stage e.
    e. myocardial perfusion scintigraphy
    e. radionuclide angiocardiography
    e. radionuclide ventriculogram
    e. renography
    e. strain gauge venous plethysmography
    e. stress-redistribution scintigraphy
    e. thallium scintigraphy
    e. thallium-201 stress imaging
    e. thallium-201 tomography
    e. tolerance test (ETT)
exercise-induced
    e.-i. bronchoconstriction
    e.-i. contrast enhancement
    e.-i. transient myocardial ischemia
exertion
    Borg scale of treadmill e.
exertional rhabdomyolysis
exhalation
    end e.
exit
    e. block
    e. dose
    e. wound
Exner plexus
exocardia
exoccipital
    e. bone
    e. part of occipital bone
exoergic reaction
Exogen
    E. 2000+ low-intensity, ultrasound fracture healing system

E. 2000+ noninvasive ultrasound therapy
E. 2000 SAFHS
exogenous
    e. glucose rate
    e. invasion
    e. lipoid pneumonia
exophthalmic goiter
exophytic
    e. adenocarcinoma
    e. carcinoma
    e. fibroid
    e. neoplasia
exostoses
    hereditary multiple e. (HME)
    hereditary multiple cartilaginous e.
    multiple cartilaginous e.
exostosis, pl. **exostoses**
    blocker's e.
    bony e.
    cartilage-capped e.
    epiphyseal e.
    hypertrophic e.
    impingement e.
    marginal e.
    multiple hereditary exostoses
    osteocartilaginous e.
    pelvic e.
    retrocalcaneal e.
    tackler's e.
    traction e.
    turret e.
exostotica
    bursa e.
exostotic chondrosarcoma
expanded
    e. lung
    e. polytetrafluoroethylene-covered nitinol TIPS stent graft
    e. polytetrafluoroethylene graft
expanded-disability status scale (EDSS)
expanding
    e. cavernous sinus brain lesion
    e. intracranial mass
expansile
    e. aneurysmal bone cyst
    e. aortic segment
    e. configuration
    e. lytic lesion
    e. mass
    e. multilocular bone lesion
    e. osteoblastoma

E

NOTES

expansile *(continued)*
   e. osteolysis
   e. rib lesion
   e. unilocular well-demarcated bone lesion

expansion
   air e.
   bone e.
   complete stent e.
   emphysematous e.
   fluid e.
   infarct e.
   localized e.
   lung e.
   passive chest e.
   peripheral e.
   rapid fluid e.
   stent e.
   uneven air e.

expenditure
   resting energy e.

Expert-XL densitometer

expiration
   end e.
   flow-limited e.
   quantitative CT during e.
   e. view

expiratory
   e. attenuation
   e. chest
   e. computed tomography
   e. CT
   e. film
   e. flow
   e. image
   inspiratory to e.
   e. phase
   e. reserve volume (ERV)
   e. resistance
   e. view

exploration
   common bile duct e. (CBDE)

Explorer X70 intraoral radiography system

explosion fracture

explosive follicular hyperplasia

exponential
   e. decay
   e. kinetics
   e. shape
   e. weighting

exposure
   e. angle
   anthrax e.
   asbestos e.
   bioterrorism e.
   bone-tendon e.

   e. data recognizer (EDR)
   DES e.
   e. dose
   electromagnetic radiation e.
   entrance skin e.
   index of e.
   intraperitoneal e.
   ionizing radiation e.
   magnetic radiation e.
   e. meter
   operator e.
   overcouch e.
   radiation e.
   e. variation
   zero e.

expoSURE

expression
   antigen e.
   AQP4 e.
   e. cystourethrography
   receptor e.
   upregulated AQP4 e.
   e. vector

exquisite detail

exsanguinating hemorrhage

exstrophy
   bladder e.
   cloacal e.
   closed e.
   urinary bladder e.

extended
   e. field of view
   e. pattern

extended-field
   e.-f. irradiation therapy
   e.-f. radiotherapy

extension
   angle of greatest e. (AGE)
   basal e.
   Buck e.
   capital e.
   Codivilla e.
   external rotation in e. (ERE)
   extraaxial e.
   extracapsular e. (ECE)
   extranodal tumor e.
   extrascleral e.
   hilar e.
   e. injury
   e. injury of spine
   internal rotation in e. (IRE)
   intracavitary e.
   medial e.
   metaphyseal e.
   parenchymal e.
   parietal e.
   e. position

radiolucent operating room table e.
subligamentous e.
supradiaphragmatic e.
suprasellar e.
e. teardrop fracture (ETF)
thrombus e.
tumor e.
e. view

extensive
e. anterior myocardial infarct
e. bilateral pneumonia
e. dissection
e. head injury
e. intraductal carcinoma (EIC)
e. intraductal component (EIC)

extensor
e. apparatus
e. carpi radialis brevis (ECRB)
e. carpi radialis brevis muscle
e. carpi radialis brevis tendon
e. carpi radialis longus (ECRL)
e. carpi radialis longus muscle
e. carpi radialis longus tendon
e. carpi ulnaris
e. carpi ulnaris muscle
e. carpi ulnaris sheath
e. carpi ulnaris tendon
e. compartment
e. digiti minimi tendon
e. digiti quinti
e. digiti quinti muscle
e. digiti quinti tendon
e. digitorum
e. digitorum brevis (EDB)
e. digitorum brevis muscle
e. digitorum brevis tendon
e. digitorum communis (EDC)
e. digitorum communis muscle
e. digitorum communis tendon
e. digitorum longus
e. digitorum longus muscle
e. digitorum longus tendon
e. hallucis longus (EHL)
e. hallucis longus muscle
e. hallucis longus tendon
e. indicis
e. indicis proprius muscle
e. indicis proprius tendon
e. mechanism
e. pollicis brevis
e. pollicis brevis muscle
e. pollicis brevis tendon

e. pollicis longus (EPL)
e. pollicis longus muscle
e. pollicis longus tendon
e. quinti tendon
e. retinaculum
ulnar e.

extensor-supinator group

extensus
hallux e.

extent
anular tear e.

exteriorization

externa
theca e.

external
e. absorption
e. acoustic foramen
e. anal sphincter
e. artifact
e. auditory canal atresia
e. auditory canal dysplasia
e. auditory meatus
e. band
e. beam radiation
e. beam radiation therapy (EBRT)
e. beam radiotherapy
e. beam with tandem
e. biliary drainage catheter
e. biliary fistula
e. callus
e. capsule
e. carotid
e. carotid artery (ECA)
e. condyle
e. ear mass
e. ear neoplasm
e. elastic lamina
e. fiducial marker
e. fixation
e. fixation device
e. gamma dose reconstruction
e. heat generating source
e. hemorrhage
e. hernia
e. iliac artery
e. iliac lymph node
e. iliac stenosis
e. inguinal ring
e. jugular vein (EJV)
e. looping technique
e. oblique aponeurosis
e. oblique muscle

NOTES

E

external *(continued)*
    e. os
    e. pneumatic calf compression
    e. pudendal vein
    e. retractor
    e. ring apex
    e. rotation in extension (ERE)
    e. rotation in flexion (ERF)
    e. rotation view
    e. scanning
    e. snapping hip
    e. table of calvaria
    e. tibial torsion
    e. urethral orifice
    e. urethral sphincter
    e. ventricular drain (EVD)
    e. wire fixation
    e. x-ray therapy
external-internal drainage
externum
    os tibiale e.
externus
    obturator e.
extinction phenomenon
extirpation
    e. of saphenous vein
    tumor e.
extraadrenal
    e. chromaffin tissue
    e. paraganglioma
    e. site
extraalveolar
    e. air (EAA)
    e. air collection
extraarachnoid
    e. injection
    e. myelography
extraarticular
    e. debris
    e. fracture
    e. hip fusion
    e. posterior ossification
    e. resection
extraaxial
    e. cavernous hemangioma
    e. CNS lesion
    e. extension
    e. fluid collection
    e. low-attenuation lesion
    e. space
    e. tumor
extracapsular
    e. ankylosis
    e. dissection
    e. extension (ECE)
    e. fracture

    e. ligament
    e. metastasis
extracardiac
    e. anomaly
    e. collateral circulation
    e. focal uptake
    e. mass
extracavitary
    e. infected graft
    e. prosthetic arterial graft
extracellular
    e. compartment
    e. contrast agent
    e. domain
    e. fluid
    e. fluid volume
    e. matrix
    e. matrix component
    e. space
extracerebral
    e. aneurysm
    e. cavernous angioma
    e. fluid collection
    e. hematoma
    e. intracranial glioneural hamartoma
    e. soft tissue uptake
extrachorial placenta
extracolonic
    e. disease
    e. structure
extracompartmental tumor
extracorporeal
    e. circulation
    e. liver
    e. membrane oxygenation
    e. membrane oxygenator
    e. photochemotherapy
    e. shock wave
    e. shock wave lithotripsy (ESWL)
extracranial
    e. aneurysm
    e. carotid artery atherosclerosis
    e. carotid artery occlusive disease
    e. carotid circulation
    e. carotid system
    e. cerebral circulation
    e. cerebral vasculature
    e. course
    e. mass lesion
    e. meningioma
    e. pneumatocele
    e. vertebral artery
    e. vessel
extracranial-intracranial bypass
extraction
    anatomy-based e. (ABE)
    automatic e.

e. catheter atherectomy
e. column
contour e.
disphenoid e.
first-pass thallium e.
fringe skeleton e.
e. generator
e. method
stone e.
vacuum e.
vascular segmentation and e.

extradural
e. abscess
e. anastomosis
e. arachnoid cyst
e. artery
e. brain hematoma
e. compartment
e. defect
e. hemorrhage
e. space
e. tumor
e. venography
e. vertebral plexus
e. vertebral plexus of vein

extraembryonic mesoderm
extrafascial hysterectomy
extragonadal seminoma
extrahepatic
e. bile duct
e. bile duct carcinoma
e. biliary atresia (EBA)
e. biliary cystic dilatation
e. binary obstruction
e. cholangiectasis
e. cholangiocarcinoma
e. lesion
e. metastasis (EHM)
e. portal hypertension
e. portal vein tributary
e. primary malignant tumor
e. stone

extraintestinal
extralobar sequestration
extralobular
e. connective tissue
e. stroma
e. terminal duct

extraluminal
e. air
e. contrast medium
e. endarterectomy

e. gas
e. hemorrhage

extramammary Paget disease
extramedullary
e. compressive lesion
e. hemangioma
e. hematopoiesis
e. involvement
e. plasmacytoma (EMP)
e. tumor

extramural hemorrhage
extraneous material
extranodal
e. follicular lymphoma
e. proliferation
e. site
e. tumor extension

extraoctave fracture
extraocular
e. muscle
e. muscle enlargement

extraoral radiograph
extraosseous
e. angioma
e. Ewing sarcoma
e. mass
e. osteosarcoma
e. uptake

extraovarian mass
extraparenchymal cyst
extrapelvic malignancy
extrapericardial dissection
extraperitoneal
e. bladder rupture
e. fascia
e. fat
e. implant
e. organ

extrapleural
e. drainage
e. hemorrhage
e. mass
e. pneumothorax
e. sign
e. space

extrapolate
extrapolation
half-scan with e. (HE)

extrapontine myelinolysis
extrapulmonary
e. activity
e. bronchus

E

NOTES

extrapulmonary *(continued)*
- e. sequestration
- e. small cell carcinoma
- e. tuberculosis

extrapyramidal
- e. reaction
- e. system
- e. tract

extrarenal renal pelvis
extrascleral extension
extraskeletal
- e. chondroma
- e. mesenchymal chondrosarcoma
- e. osteosarcoma
- e. uptake

extrasphincteric anal fistula
extraspinal neurofibroma
extra stiff guidewire
extrasynovial
extratemporal
- e. epilepsy
- e. structural lesion

extratesticular
- e. lesion
- e. tumor

extrathecal nerve root
extrathoracic
- e. disease
- e. lesion
- e. metastasis
- e. obstruction

extrauterine
- e. gestation
- e. pelvic mass
- e. pregnancy

extravaginal testicular torsion
extravasated
- e. blood
- e. contrast agent

extravasation
- bile e.
- contrast e.
- e. of contrast agent
- e. detection accessory
- dye e.
- fluid e.
- intravascular content e.
- joint fluid e.
- radiopaque fluid e.
- renal transplant urine e.
- secondary e.
- spontaneous urinary e.
- urinary e.

extravascular
- e. compartment
- e. fluid
- e. granuloma

- e. mass
- e. pressure

extraventricular obstructive hydrocephalus
extravesical
- e. infrasphincteric ectopic ureter
- e. opacification

extravital ultraviolet
extremely
- e. low frequency (ELF)
- e. low-frequency field

extreme micromelia
extremity
- e. coil
- e. gigantism
- e. hemangioma
- left lower e. (LLE)
- lower e. (LE)
- e. malformation
- e. MRI (E-MRI)
- e. osteosarcoma
- e. rhabdomyosarcoma
- upper e. (UE)

extrinsic
- e. allergic alveolitis
- e. bladder compression
- e. cellular parameter
- e. esophageal impression
- e. field uniformity
- e. filling defect
- e. foot muscle
- e. impression of the esophagus
- e. intraabdominal inflammation
- e. lesion
- e. ligament
- e. malignant obstruction
- e. neoplasia
- e. sphincter
- e. stomach impression
- e. ureteral defect

extrude
extruded
- e. disk
- e. disk fragment

extrusion
- disk e.
- joint fluid e.

extubate
extubation
exuberant
- e. atheroma formation
- e. callus
- e. granulation tissue
- e. synovium
- e. tumor

exudative
- e. bronchiolitis

e. consolidation
e. enteropathy
e. pleural effusion
e. pleurisy
e. tuberculosis

eye

conus e.
e. exposure limit
fetal e.
hamartoma of the e.
intraconal portion of the e.
e. myositis
e. trauma

eyebrow ring artifact
eye-ear plane
eyelet
rod e.
eyepiece
Huygens e.
eye-view
e.-v. 3D conformal radiation
therapy
E-Z Cat Dry contrast agent
E-Z-EM cut biopsy needle
E-zero offset
E-Z-Paque barium suspension

NOTES

E

F
female
fluorine
    F point of cardiac apex
    F T line
F-19
fluorine-19
^{19}F
fluorine-19
^{18}F, F-18
fluorine-18
    ^{18}F 2-deoxyglucose uptake
    ^{18}F estradiol imaging agent
    ^{18}F FDG-negative imaging
    ^{18}F fludeoxyglucose imaging agent
    ^{18}F fluorodeoxyglucose
    ^{18}F fluorodeoxyglucose imaging agent
    ^{18}F fluoro-DOPA imaging agent
    ^{18}F fluoroisonidazole imaging agent
    ^{18}F fluorotamoxifen imaging agent
    ^{18}F L-DOPA imaging agent
    ^{18}F N-methylspiperone imaging agent
    ^{18}F spiperone imaging agent
f
farad
frequency
F-15 renogram
FA
fractional anisotropy
FAA
flavone acetic acid
Fab
    ^{131}I-labeled monoclonal Fab
fabella
    os f.
fabellae
fabellofibular
    f. complex
    f. ligament
Fabricius
    bursa of F.
FAcE
FID-acquired echoes
face
    congenital infiltrating lipomatosis of the f.
    en f.
    f. presentation
faceless kidney
facet
    f. arthropathy
    articular f.
    atlas f.

bilateral locked f.'s
capitate f.
f. capsule disruption
f. cartilage
clavicular f.
corneal f.
costal f.
f. degeneration
f. dislocation
flat f.
f. fusion
hamate f.
inferior medial f.
f. joint
f. joint arthritis
f. joint capsule
f. joint incongruity
f. joint injection
f. joint vacuum
jumped f.
Lenoir f.
locked f.
lunate f.
occlusal f.
scaphoid f.
squatting f.
superior articular f.
superior costal f.
f. surface of vertebra
f. syndrome
transverse costal f.
f. tropism
facetal imbrication
facetectomy
faceted gallstone
faceting
facial
    f. abnormality
    f. artery
    f. asymmetry
    f. bipartition
    f. bone
    f. cleft
    f. colliculus
    f. eminence
    f. fracture
    f. hemangioma
    f. nerve
    f. nerve anatomy
    f. nerve canal
    f. plane
    f. plexus
    f. root
    f. schwannoma
    f. thickening

F

facial *(continued)*
    f. triangle
    f. vein
faciale
facialis
facioauriculovertebral syndrome
faciostenosis
FACScan
    fluorescence-activated cell sorter
    FACScan flow cytometer
FACSVantage cell sorter
FACT
    focused appendix computed tomography
factitious
    f. clinodactyly
    f. regurgitation
factor
    accelerator f.
    activation f.
    adherence f.
    f. analysis of dynamic series (FADS)
    f. analysis of dynamic study
    angiogenic f.
    anisotropy f.
    automotility f.
    backscatter f. (BSF)
    blocking f.
    breast cancer risk f.
    calibration f.
    contrast-improvement f.
    decay-activating f.
    diffusion f.
    dose/dose-rate effective f. (DDREF)
    enhancement f.
    environmental f.
    equilibrium f.
    filling f.
    Fletcher f.
    gamma f.
    geometry f.
    granulocyte colony stimulating f.
    growth f.
    Hageman f. (HF)
    inciting f.
    incremental risk f.
    intensification f.
    intrinsic f.
    kerma-to-dose conversion f.
    magnification f. (MF)
    Mayneord F f.
    net magnetization f.
    off-axis f. (OAF)
    overrelaxation f.
    peak scatter f.
    protection f.
    quality f. (QF)

    radiation weighting f.
    relative conversion f.
    releasing f.
    rheumatoid f.
    scatter degradation f.
    screen-intensifying f. (IF)
    therapeutic gain f.
    tissue inhomogeneity f.
    tissue weighting f.
    tumor-angiogenesis f.
    wedge f.
factorial design
FADS
    factor analysis of dynamic series
Fahr disease
failed
    f. back surgery syndrome (FBSS)
    f. back syndrome (FBS)
    f. pregnancy
    f. valve
failure
    acute heart f.
    acute renal f. (ARF)
    acute respiratory f. (ARF)
    adrenal f.
    backward heart f.
    bypass f.
    cardiac f.
    chronic heart f.
    chronic renal f. (CRF)
    circulation f.
    compensated congestive heart f.
    congestive heart f. (CHF)
    contrast-induced renal f.
    decompensated congestive heart f.
    diastolic heart f.
    end-stage renal f. (ESRF)
    fetal heart f.
    forward heart f.
    frank congestive heart f.
    fulminant hepatic f. (FHF)
    functional classification of congestive heart f.
    graft f.
    heart f. (HF)
    hepatic f.
    high-output heart f.
    intractable heart f.
    intrauterine cardiac f.
    intrauterine heart f.
    irreversible organ f.
    kidney f.
    left-sided heart f.
    left ventricular f.
    liver f.
    low-output heart f.
    Mamm-Aire heart f.

multiple organ f.
neonatal cardiac f.
neonatal heart f.
ovulatory f.
pituitary f.
posttransplant acute renal f.
prerenal f.
pulmonary f.
refractory congestive heart f.
renal f.
respiratory f.
right-sided heart f.
right ventricular f.
systolic heart f.
time-to-distant f.
time-to-local f.
time-to-treatment f. (TTF)
TIPS f.
ventilatory f.
ventricular f.
failure-free survival
Fairbank disease
falces (*pl. of* falx)
falciform
    f. cartilage
    f. crest
    f. fold
    f. ligament
    f. ligament sign
    f. process
falcine meningioma
falcotentorial meningioma
falcula
falcular
fallen lung sign
fallopian
    f. canal
    f. ligament
    f. pregnancy
    f. tube
    f. tube carcinoma
    f. tube diverticulum
    f. tube mass
    f. tube occlusion
    f. tube recanalization
falloposcopy
Fallot
    pentalogy of F.
    F. syndrome
    F. tetrad
    tetralogy of F. (TOF)
    trilogy of F.

fallout
    radioactive f.
    signal f.
false
    f. aneurysm
    f. aneurysmal chamber
    f. ankylosis
    f. bundle-branch block
    f. channel
    f. colonic obstruction
    f. color scale
    f. cord carcinoma
    f. diverticulum
    f. emphysema
    f. frequency
    f. hypoechogenicity
    f. knot
    f. localizing sign
    f. lumen
    f. pelvis
    f. pregnancy
    f. rib
    f. sac
    f. splenic cyst
    f. steal
    f. suture
    f. vertebra
    f. vocal cord
false-negative
    f.-n. correlation
    f.-n. mammogram
    f.-n. ratio
    f.-n. result
false-positive
    f.-p. ratio
    f.-p. result
falx, pl. falces
    f. artery
    f. calcification
    f. cerebelli
    f. cerebri
    f. fenestration
    f. increased density
familial
    f. adenomatous polyposis (FAP)
    f. adenomatous polyposis syndrome
    f. aortic dissection
    f. arterial fibromuscular dysplasia
    f. atresia
    f. avascular necrosis of phalangeal epiphysis
    f. cavernous malformation

F

NOTES

familial *(continued)*
 f. cerebral ferrocalcinosis
 f. chondrocalcinosis
 f. colorectal polyposis
 f. dysautonomia
 f. fibromuscular dysplasia of artery
 f. gastrointestinal polyposis
 f. goiter
 f. hypertrophic cardiomyopathy (FHC)
 f. hypertrophy (FHC)
 f. intestinal polyposis
 f. intestinal pseudoobstruction
 f. juvenile polyposis
 f. multiple polyposis
 f. myxoma
 f. onychoosteodysplasia
 f. polyposis coli
 f. varicose vein
fan
 f. angle
 f. beam
 f. sign
fan-beam
 f.-b. collimator
 f.-b. formula
 f.-b. projection
 f.-b. reconstruction
Fanconi-Hegglin syndrome
Fanconi syndrome
fanning
 f. of the interspinous distance
 f. of the spinous process
fan-shaped
 f.-s. mesentery
 f.-s. view
FAP
 familial adenomatous polyposis
farad (f)
Faraday
 F. cage
 F. law
 F. shield
 F. shielded resonator
far field
farmer's lung
fascia, pl. fasciae, fascias
 anal f.
 antebrachial f.
 anterior rectus f.
 axillary f.
 bicipital f.
 brachial f.
 f. of breast
 broad f.
 buccopharyngeal f.
 Buck f.

Camper f.
cervical f.
clavipectoral f.
Cloquet f.
Colles f.
cremasteric f.
cribriform f.
crural f.
Cruveilhier f.
deep f.
deltoid f.
Denonvilliers f.
dentate f.
diaphragmatic f.
endopelvic f.
endothoracic f.
extraperitoneal f.
Gerota f.
iliac f.
infraspinous f.
investing f.
Laimer f.
f. lata
lateral conal f.
lateral oblique f.
lateroconal f.
lumbar f.
medial geniculate f.
obturator internus f.
palmar f.
parietal pelvic f.
pelvic f.
perineal f.
pharyngobasilar f.
prepectoral f.
prevertebral f.
psoas f.
quadratus femoris f.
rectal f.
renal f.
retromammary f.
rim of f.
Scarpa f.
Sibson f.
spigelian f.
subcutaneous f.
superficial temporalis f.
superficial temporoparietal f.
supraanal f.
thoracolumbar f.
transversalis f.
umbilicovesical f.
vesical f.
visceral pelvic f.
Waldeyer f.
Zuckerkandl f.
fasciagram

fasciagraphy
fascial
- f. band
- f. envelope
- f. incisor
- f. margin necrosis
- f. plane
- f. rent
- f. sheath
- f. stranding
- f. tract

fascias (*pl. of* fascia)
fascicle
- synovium-lined f.
- tibioligamentous f.
- triquetroscaphoid f.
- triquetrotrapezoid f.

fascicular
- f. block
- f. bundle
- f. sarcoma

fasciculata
- zona f.

fasciculation
- tongue f.

fasciculus, pl. **fasciculi**
- arcuate f. (AF)
- Gowers f.
- lenticular f.
- longitudinal f.
- longitudinalis medialis f.
- mamillothalamic f.
- medial longitudinal f. (MLF)
- occipitofrontal f.
- superior longitudinal f.
- superior occipitofrontal f.

fasciitis
- fulminant f.
- necrotizing f.
- f. ossificans
- palmar f.
- plantar f.
- pseudosarcomatous f.
- scrotal f.

fasciogram
fasciolar gyrus
fascioliasis
fashion
- snapshot f.

fasiculoventricular bypass tract

FAST
- focused abdominal sonography for trauma
- Fourier-acquired steady state
- contrast-enhanced FAST
- FAST pulse sequence
- reduced-acquisition matrix FAST
- RF-spoiled FAST
- FAST technique
- T1-weighted FAST

fast
- f. acquisition multiple excitation
- f. adiabatic trajectory in steady state (FATS)
- f. cardiac phase contrast cine imaging
- f. dynamic volumetric x-ray CT
- f. exchange-cellular suspension
- f. exchange-soft tissue
- f. FLAIR sequence
- f. fluid-attenuation inversion recovery image
- f. Fourier flow (FFF)
- f. Fourier imaging
- f. Fourier projection (FFP)
- f. Fourier spectral analysis
- f. Fourier transform (FFT)
- f. Fourier transform image
- f. fractionation
- f. gradient-echo sequence
- f. imaging with steady-state precession (FISP)
- f. inversion-recovery Fourier transform (FIRFT)
- f. low-angle shot (FLASH)
- f. multiplanar inversion recovry imaging
- f. multiplanar spoiled gradient-recalled imaging
- f. neutron
- f. neutron radiotherapy
- f. PC cine MR sequence with echo-planar gradient
- f. routine production
- f. scan magnetic resonance imaging
- f. short tau inversion recovery
- f. spin-echo (FSE)
- f. spin-echo acquisition
- f. spin-echo black blood imaging
- f. spin-echo and fast inversion recovery imaging
- f. spin-echo MR imaging

F

NOTES

fast *(continued)*
  f. spin-echo T2-weighted image
  f. spin-echo view
  f. spoiled gradient-recalled echo
    (FSPGR)
  f. spoiled gradient-recalled MR
    imaging
  f. STIR
fast-array processor
fast-breeder reactor
Fastcard
FastCine
FASTER
  3D FASTER
    3D field echo acquisition with
      short repetition time and echo
      reduction
fast-field echo (FFE)
fast-FLAIR technique
fast-flow
  f.-f. lesion
  f.-f. malformation
  f.-f. vascular anomaly
fast-neutron radiation therapy
FasTracker catheter
fast-scan magnetic resonance
fast-twitch muscle
fat
  abdominal f.
  f. absorption test
  anterior epidural f.
  bony glenoid marrow f.
  f. density
  f. density mass
  digital process of f.
  dirty f.
  f. embolism syndrome (FES)
  f. embolus
  epidural f.
  extraperitoneal f.
  herniated preperitoneal f.
  intraabdominal f.
  f. island
  isointense background f.
  lipid content of storage f.
  f. lobule
  f. lung herniation
  mediastinal f.
  mesocolonic f.
  f. metabolism
  microvesicular f.
  f. necrosis
  f. pad
  f. pad sign
  parametrial f.
  peribursal f.

  pericolonic f.
  perigastric f.
  perihilar f.
  perinephric f.
  perineural f.
  perirectal f.
  perirenal f.
  f. plane
  posterior epidural f.
  preperitoneal f.
  prerenal f.
  properitoneal f.
  protruding f.
  radiolucent f.
  renal sinus f.
  retrobulbar f.
  retromammary f.
  f. saturation
  f. signal intensity
  f. signal suppression
  f. stranding
  subcutaneous f.
  subdiaphragmatic f.
  subepicardial f.
  f. suppression pulse
  f. suppression technique
  tumoral f.
  ventral epidural f.
fatal dose of radiation
fat-blood
  f.-b. interface (FBI)
  f.-b. interface sign
fat-containing
  f.-c. breast lesion
  f.-c. mass
fat-density
  f.-d. area
  f.-d. line
fat-fluid
  f.-f. density interface
  f.-f. level
fat-fraction measurement
fatigue
  f. damage
  f. fracture
FATS
  fast adiabatic trajectory in steady state
fat-saturated
  f.-s. spin-echo proton density-
    weighted image
  f.-s. T2-weighted fast spin-echo
    image
fat-selective presaturation
fat-spared
  f.-s. area in fatty liver
  f.-s. area in pancreas

fat-suppressed
> f.-s. acquisition with TE and TR times shortened
> f.-s. body coil
> f.-s. 3D spoiled gradient-recall echo imaging
> f.-s. gadolinium-enhanced imaging
> f.-s. spin echo
> f.-s. three-dimensional spoiled gradient-echo FLASH MR imaging
> f.-s. T1-weighted 3D spoiled gradient-echo image
> f.-s. T2-weighted fast spin-echo sequence
> f.-s. T2-weighted FSE technique

fat-suppression pulse sequence
fat-supressing content
fatty
> f. acid metabolism
> f. cirrhosis
> f. degeneration
> f. filum
> f. filum terminale
> f. halo
> f. heart
> f. infiltrate
> f. intima streak
> f. kidney
> f. liver
> f. marrow
> f. meal
> f. meal sonogram (FMS)
> f. meal sonography
> f. mesentery
> f. necrosis
> f. plaque
> f. prostatic tissue
> f. renal capsule
> f. soft tissue tumor
> f. sparing
> f. streak atherosclerosis

fat-water
> f.-w. interface
> f.-w. out of phase
> f.-w. signal cancellation

fat/water
> f. chemical shift imaging
> f. signal separation

fat- and water-suppressed T2-weighted image

fauces
> anterior pillar of f.
> arch of f.

faucial
> f. pillar
> f. tonsil

fault
> sagittal plane f.

faulty
> f. radiofrequency shielding
> f. radiofrequency shielding artifact
> f. union

faveolate
Favre disease
FB
> foreign body

FBI
> fat-blood interface
> FBI sign

FBM
> fetal breathing movement

FBP method
FBS
> failed back syndrome

FBSS
> failed back surgery syndrome

FC
> flow compensation

FCMD
> Fukuyama congenital muscular disease
> Fukuyama congenital muscular dystrophy

FCS
> F. series
> full cervical spine series
> F. view

FD
> fractal dimension

FDDNP PET scan contrast medium
FDG
> ^{18}F-fluoro-2-deoxyglucose
> fluorodeoxyglucose
> 2-fluoro 2-deoxyglucose
> FDG myocardial imaging
> FDG positron emission tomography
> FDG SPECT
> FDG uptake

FDG-blood flow mismatch
FDG-labeled positron imaging
FDG-PET
> ^{18}F-fluorodeoxyglucose positron emission tomography

F

NOTES

FDG-PET (*continued*)
  fluorodeoxyglucose positron emission
    tomography
^{18}**FDG PET scan**
FDG-6-phosphate
FDI
  first digital interosseous
  frequency domain imaging
    FDI ultrasound
FDL muscle
^{18}**FDP PET**
FDQB muscle
FDS muscle
FE
  field echo
  frequency encode
^{52}**Fe**
  iron-52
^{55}**Fe**
  iron-55
^{59}**Fe**
  iron-59
feasibility of image registration
FeatherTouch CO$_2$ laser
feathery
  f. appearance
  f. pattern
feature
  clinical f.
  differential diagnostic lung mass f.
  geriatric f.
  mammographic f.
  mongoloid f.
  proctographic f.
featureless appearance
fecal
  f. concretion
  f. diversion colostomy
  f. fistula
  f. impaction
  f. incontinence
  f. material
  f. obstruction
  f. residue
  f. stone
  f. tumor
fecal-filled colon
fecalith
fecaloid
fecaloma
fecaluria
feces
  impacted f.
  inspissated f.
  semiliquid f.
feculence
feculent

feedback
  breathing f.
  real-time respiratory f.
feeder
  f. artery
  f. vein
feeding
  f. artery of aneurysm
  f. branch
  f. branch of artery
  f. mean arterial pressure (FMAP)
  f. tube
  f. vessel
  f. vessel sign
FEER
  field-echo sequence with even-echo
    rephasing
  field-even echo rephasing
feet (*pl. of* foot)
Fe-Ex orogastric tube magnet
Feigenbaum echocardiography
feign tumor
Feiss line
Feist-Mankin position
Feldkamp algorithm
Fellow
  F. of the American College of
    Nuclear Medicine
  F. of the American College of
    Nuclear Physicians
Felson
  silhouette sign of F.
Felty syndrome
female (F)
  f. genital tract calcification
  f. genital tract rhabdomyosarcoma
  intersex f.
  f. pelvis
  f. pseudohermaphroditism
  f. urethra
feminine aorta
feminization
  testicular f.
feminizing
  f. adrenal tumor
  f. testes syndrome
femora (*pl. of* femur)
femoral
  f. access
  f. antetorsion
  f. anteversion
  f. artery
  f. artery approach
  f. articulation
  f. bone
  f. capital epiphysis
  f. condylar shaving

f. condyle
f. cortex
f. endarterectomy
f. fossa
f. head
f. head amputation
f. head deformity
f. head epiphyseolysis
f. head vascularity
f. hernia
f. intertrochanteric fracture
f. leak
f. ligament
f. medullary canal
f. neck
f. neck fracture
f. nerve
f. ossification center
f. physeal scar
f. plate
f. plexus
f. pulsatility index (FPI)
f. retrotorsion
f. retroversion
f. ring
f. runoff angiography
f. runoff arteriography
f. septum
f. shaft
f. shaft axis
f. shaft fracture
f. sheath
f. supracondylar fracture
f. torsion V angle
f. triangle
f. triangular content
f. tuberosity
f. vein
f. vein percutaneous insertion
f. venous approach
f. view

femorale
calcar f.

femoris
quadratus f.
quadriceps f.
rectus f.

femorocerebral catheter angiography
femorocrural graft
femorodistal popliteal bypass graft

femorofemoral
f. bypass graft
f. crossover
femorofemoropopliteal
femoropatellar joint
femoroperoneal in situ vein bypass graft
femoropopliteal
f. artery
f. atheromatous stenosis
f. bypass graft
f. Gore-Tex graft
f. system
f. thrombosis
f. vessel
femorotibial
f. angle (FTA)
f. bypass graft
FemoStop compression device
femtocurie
femtoliter
femtosecond laser system
femur, pl. **femora**
apex of f.
body of f.
distal f.
greater trochanter of f.
head of f.
isthmus of f.
f. length (FL)
f. length to abdominal
circumference
lesser trochanter of f.
neck of f.
NSA of f.
nutrient artery of f.
proximal f.
fencer's bone
fender fracture
fenestra, pl. **fenestrae**
fenestral otosclerosis
fenestrated
f. compression plate
f. sheath
f. tube
f. vessel
fenestration
aortopulmonary f.
apical f.
arterial f.
balloon catheter f.
f. of the basilar artery

F

NOTES

fenestration *(continued)*
    catheter-directed f.
    cusp f.
    f. of dissecting aneurysm
    falx f.
    interchordal space f.
    middle cerebral artery f.
    vertebral artery f.
fenoldopam mesylate
fentanyl citrate
Fe_3O_4
    magnetite
Ferguson
    F. angle
    F. method
    F. view
Fergusson method for measuring
  scoliosis
Feridex IV MRI contrast agent
fermium (Fm)
fermium-255 (^{255}Fm)
fern-like pattern
ferpentetate
    technetium-99m f.
Ferrein
    F. canal
    F. foramen
    F. ligament
ferric ammonium citrate-cellulose paste
ferrite
ferritin-labeled yttrium
ferrocalcinosis
    familial cerebral f.
ferrokinetic data
ferromagnetic
    f. artifact
    f. implant
    f. material
    f. microembolization
    f. microembolization treatment
    f. microsphere
    f. relaxation
    f. tamponade
ferrous citrate
ferruginous body
Fertinex
ferucarbotran MR imaging agent
feruglose contrast agent
ferumoxide imaging agent
ferumoxsil imaging agent
ferumoxtran-enhanced
    f.-e. echo-planar GRE T2*-weighted
      imaging
    f.-e. echo-planar SE T2-weighted
      and echo-planar GRE
    f.-e. echo-planar SE T2-weighted
      imaging

ferumoxtran imaging agent
FES
    fat embolism syndrome
    flame emission spectroscopy
    fluoroestradiol
fetal
    f. abdominal circumference
    f. abdominal cystic mass
    f. abdominal wall
    f. abdominal wall defect
    f. abnormality
    f. adenoma
    f. age
    f. alcohol syndrome
    f. amputation
    f. aortic flow volume
    f. ascites
    f. asphyxia
    f. attitude
    f. biometry
    f. biometry ulna
    f. biophysical profile score
    f. bowel obstruction
    f. BPS
    f. breathing movement (FBM)
    f. cardiac anomaly
    f. cardiosplenic syndrome
    f. cerebellum
    f. chest anomaly
    f. circulation
    f. CNS anomaly
    f. cranium
    f. cystic adenomatoid malformation
    f. cystic fibrosis
    f. death
    f. death in utero
    f. detail
    f. dystocia
    f. echocardiographic view
    f. echocardiography
    f. echocardiography in utero
    f. ectopia cordis
    f. epiphyseal bone center
    f. eye
    f. femoral length
    f. foot length measurement
    f. fracture
    f. gallbladder
    f. gastrointestinal anomaly
    f. goiter
    f. growth acceleration
    f. growth retardation
    f. hand malformation
    f. head circumference
    f. heart
    f. heart anomaly
    f. heart failure

fetal · ^{18}F-fluoro-2-deoxyglucose

f. hydrops
f. hypomineralization
f. incarceration
f. intraabdominal calcification
f. kidney lobation
f. lie
f. liver biopsy
f. lobe
f. lobulation
f. long bone measurement
f. lung hypoplasia
f. lymphoid tissue
f. mesenchymal tumor
f. mesenchymal tumor of kidney
f. midface
f. movement (FM)
f. musculoskeletal dysplasia
f. musculoskeletal system
f. neck anomaly
f. neck pseudomembrane
f. period
f. placenta
f. pleural effusion
f. pole
f. position
f. pyelectasis
f. renal function
f. renal hamartoma
f. renal obstruction
f. scalp edema
f. skin biopsy
f. small part
f. sonography
f. spine
f. stress test
f. swallowing
f. thoracic circumference
f. ultrasound
f. urinary tract anomaly
f. urogenital tract
f. uterus
f. ventricular heart disproportion
f. ventriculomegaly
f. weight

fetalis
chondrodystrophia f.
hydrops f.
nonimmune hydrops f.

fetal-pelvic
f.-p. disproportion
f.-p. index

feticide

fetogram
fetography
fetoliter
fetometry
fetus
amorphous f.
calcified f.
cephalic presentation of f.
demise of f.
disappearing f.
growth-retarded f.
impacted f.
intrauterine f.
malpositioned f.
maturity of f.
multiple f.'s
nonviable f.
paper-doll f.
f. papyraceus
parasitic f.
postterm f.
previable f.
retained dead f.
small for gestational age f.
small part of f.
stunted f.
syndactyly in f.
tissue of f.
trisomic f.
viable f.

Feuerstein-Mims syndrome
fever
San Joaquin Valley f.
FF
filtration fraction
FFA
free fatty acid
FFD
focal film distance
^{18}F-FDG, F-18 FDG
2-[fluorine-18]fluoro-2-deoxy-D-glucose
FFE
fast-field echo
FFF
fast Fourier flow
**F-1200, 2000, 4500 fluorescence
spectrophotometer**
**^{18}F-fluoro-6-thia-heptadecanoic acid
(FTHA)**
^{18}F-fluorocholine
radiation dosimetry of ^{18}F-f.
^{18}F-fluoro-2-deoxyglucose (FDG)

F

NOTES

^{18}F-fluorodeoxyglucose positron emission tomography (FDG-PET)

FFP

fast Fourier projection

FFT

fast Fourier transform

FG-36UX scanning echoendoscope

FHB

flexor hallucis brevis

FHC

familial hypertrophic cardiomyopathy

familial hypertrophy

FHF

fulminant hepatic failure

FHI

frontal horn index

FI

fusion inhibitor

FI method

FI projection

fiber

anular f.

asbestos f.

association f.

atrio-His f.

Bergman f.

bundle of Kent accessory bypass f.

cardiac muscle f.

cerebellar f.

climbing f.

differencing f.

gastric sling f.

Herxheimer f.

long f.

Mahaim and James f.

mossy f.

Müller f.

muscle f.

myocardial f.

nodoventricular bypass f.

notch from gastric sling f.

obliquely oriented f.

onionskin configuration of
  collagenous f.

parasympathetic f.

pontocerebellar f.

postganglionic gray f.

postganglionic sympathetic f.

precharred f.

Purkinje f.

radial glial f.

f. retraction

Sharpey f.

skeletal muscle f.

sling muscle f.

type I, II muscle f.

unmyelinated nerve f.

fiber-bundle striation

fibered

2 (x) 3, 4, 5, 6 f. Guglielmi
  detachable coil

fiberglass pneumoconiosis

Fiberlase laser

fiberoptic

f. bronchogram

f. bronchoscopy (FOB)

f. bundle

f. conductor

f. light source

f. probe

f. taper

f. video glasses

fiberscopic

fiber-shortening velocity

fiber-type disproportion

fibrillary

fibrillation

atrial f.

chondromalacia with f.

Fibrimage diagnostic imaging agent

fibrin

f. mass

f. platelet embolus

f. polymerization

f. sleeve stripping

fibrinogen

f. degradation

iodinated I-125 f.

labeled f.

radiolabeled f.

fibrinoid necrosis

fibrinolytic

f. therapy

f. treatment

fibrinopurulent pleurisy

fibrinous

f. degeneration

f. inflammation

f. pleurisy

f. pneumonia

f. polyp

fibrin-split product

fibroadenolipoma

breast f.

fibroadenoma

breast f.

calcified f.

cellular f.

degenerated f.

esophageal f.

giant breast f.

hyalinized breast f.

involuting f.

juvenile f.
noncalcified f.
fibroadenomatosis
breast f.
fibroadipose tissue
fibroareolar tissue
fibroblastic
f. meningioma
f. osteosarcoma
fibroblastoma
perineural f.
fibroblast radiosensitivity
fibrocalcific
f. cusp
f. residual
fibrocalcification
fibrocartilage
avascular f.
circumferential f.
f. complex
intraarticular plate of f.
labral f.
triangular f. (TFC)
fibrocartilaginous
f. disk
f. labrum
f. meniscus
f. nodule
f. overgrowth
f. pad
f. ridge
f. scar
f. tissue
f. volar plate
fibrocaseous
fibrocavitary infiltrate
fibrochondrogenesis
fibrocollagenous
f. connective tissue
f. stroma
fibrocongestive splenomegaly
fibrocystic
f. breast
f. breast disease
f. breast syndrome
f. change
f. lung disease
f. residual
fibroelastic
f. band
f. cartilage

fibroelastoma
f. of heart valve
papillary f.
fibroelastosis
endocardial f.
fibroepithelial
f. papilloma
f. urethral polyp
fibroepithelioma
urinary tract f.
fibrofatty
f. breast tissue
f. layer
f. plaque
fibrogenesis imperfecta ossium
fibrogenic pneumoconiosis
fibroglandular
f. density
f. element
f. tissue
fibrohistiocytic lesion
fibrohistiocytoma
fibrohistiocytosis
fibroid
f. adenoma
calcified f.
f. degeneration
f. embolization
exophytic f.
f. heart
intramural f.
f. lung
f. myocarditis
pedunculated uterine f.
f. polyp
submucosal f.
subserosal f.
f. tumor
uterine f.
f. uterus
fibrointimal hyperplasia
fibrolamellar
f. hepatocarcinoma
f. hepatocellular carcinoma
fibroleiomyoma
metastasizing f.
fibrolipoma
filum terminale f.
neural f.
fibrolipomatosis
pelvic f.
renal pelvic f.

F

NOTES

fibrolipomatous nerve hamartoma
fibroma
    ameloblastic f.
    aponeurotic f.
    benign pleural f.
    calcified f.
    cardiac f.
    cementifying f.
    cementoossifying f.
    central cementifying f.
    central ossifying f.
    chondromyxoid f. (CMF)
    concentric f.
    desmoplastic f.
    giant cell f.
    heart f.
    irritation f.
    juvenile aponeurotic f.
    juvenile ossifying f.
    f. of lung
    meningeal f.
    f. molle
    f. molle gravidarum
    f. molluscum
    musculoaponeurotic f.
    f. myxomatodes
    nonossifying f.
    nonosteogenic f.
    ossifying bone f.
    ossifying skull f.
    osteogenic bone f.
    ovarian f.
    periosteal f.
    peripheral ossifying f.
    periungual f.
    polypoid f.
    psammomatoid ossifying f.
    recurrent digital f.
    scrotal f.
    senile f.
    Shope f.
    sinonasal psammomatoid
      ossifying f.
    soft tissue f.
    subcutaneous f.
    subungual f.
    telangiectatic f.
    ungual f.
fibroma-thecoma tumor of ovary
fibromatogenic
fibromatoid
fibromatosis
    abdominal f.
    aggressive infantile f.
    f. colli
    congenital diffuse f.
    congenital generalized f.

    infantile digital f.
    juvenile f.
    mesenteric f.
    multicentric f.
    multiple congenital f.
    musculoaponeurotic f.
    palmar f.
    penile f.
    plantar f.
fibromatous
fibromuscular
    f. band
    f. dysplasia
    f. lesion
    f. pelvic floor
    f. ridge
    f. subaortic stenosis
    f. tissue
fibromyoma, pl. **fibromyomata**
fibromyositis
fibromyxoma
    kidney f.
    odontogenic f.
    pleural f.
fibronodular infiltrate
fibronuclear
fibroosseous
    f. attachment
    f. lesion
    f. pseudotumor of digit
    f. tunnel
fibroosteoma of the tooth
fibroplasia
    adventitial f.
    endomyocardial f.
    intimal f.
    medial f.
    perimedial f.
    retrolental f.
fibroplastic
    f. process
    f. proliferation
fibroproductive tuberculosis
fibroretractive
fibrosa
    hepatica f.
    osteitis f.
    osteodystrophia f.
    pseudoaneurysm of the mitral-
      aortic f.
fibrosarcoma
    ameloblastic f.
    bone f.
    cardiac f.
    central f.
    congenital kidney f.
    epididymal f.

infantile f.
inflammatory f.
nonmetastasizing f.
periosteal f.
f. variant
fibrosclerotic
fibrosed muscle
fibrosing
f. arachnoiditis
f. colonopathy
f. cryptogenic alveolitis
f. inflammation
f. inflammatory pseudotumor
f. mediastinitis
f. mesenteritis
f. mesothelioma
f. piecemeal necrosis
f. tissue
fibrosis
acute diffuse interstitial f.
alcoholic f.
anular f.
arachnoid f.
asbestos-induced pleural f.
basilar f.
benign meningeal f.
bone marrow f.
brachytelephalangic type of
cystic f.
breast f.
cirrhosis-related f.
confluent f.
congenital hepatic f. (CHF)
congenital liver f.
cystic f.
Davies endocardial f.
Davies endomyocardial f.
diffuse interstitial pulmonary f.
(DIPF)
endocardial f.
endomyocardial f. (EMF)
epidural anular f.
fetal cystic f.
focal f.
hepatic f.
horseshoe f.
hyalinized fibroadenoma with f.
idiopathic interstitial f.
idiopathic pulmonary f. (IPF)
inflammatory f.
interstitial diffuse pulmonary f.
interstitial prematurity f.

interstitial pulmonary f. (IPF)
intimal f.
intraalveolar f.
intralobular f.
leptomeningeal f.
f. of lung
massive f.
mediastinal f.
meningeal f.
mesenteric f.
mural endomyocardial f.
nodal f.
nodular subepidermal f.
noncirrhotic portal f. (NCPF)
nonnodular f.
pancreatic cystic f.
parietal lobe gray-matter cytosolic
choline pathogenetic mechanism
of myocardial f.
perialveolar f.
periaortic f.
peribronchial f.
pericentral f.
periductal f.
peridural f.
perihilar f.
perimuscular f.
perineural f.
periportal f.
periureteral f.
perivascular f.
perivenular f.
pipestem f.
portal f.
portal-to-portal f.
postinflammatory pulmonary f.
postradiation f.
posttraumatic f.
primary retroperitoneal f.
progressive interstitial pulmonary f.
progressive massive f. (PMF)
progressive nodular pulmonary f.
pulmonary idiopathic f.
pulmonary interstitial idiopathic f.
pulmonary vein f.
radiation-induced f. (RIF)
reactive f.
replacement f.
retroperitoneal f. (RPF)
secondary retroperitoneal f.
subadventitial f.
subintimal f.

F

NOTES

fibrosis *(continued)*
 subserosal f.
 Symmers f.
 transmural f.
fibrosum
 adenoma f.
 molluscum f.
 pericardium f.
fibrosus
 anulus f.
fibrothorax
fibrotic
 f. cavitating pattern
 f. change
 f. honeycombing
 f. island
 f. kidney
 f. plaque
 f. residual
 f. resolution
 f. scarring
 f. tissue
fibrous
 f. ankylosis
 f. attachment
 f. band
 f. bar
 f. bone lesion
 f. cap
 f. cartilage
 f. coalition
 f. connective tissue
 f. connective tissue tumor
 f. cord
 f. cortical defect
 f. GI tract polypoid lesion
 f. goiter
 f. hamartoma
 f. histiocytoma
 f. intima plaque
 f. mastopathy
 f. medullary defect
 f. meningioma
 f. metaphyseal-diaphyseal defect
 f. nodular pattern
 f. nodule
 f. nonunion
 f. obliterative cholangitis
 f. osteodystrophy
 f. osteoma
 f. pericardium
 f. plaque atherosclerosis
 f. pleural adhesion
 f. pneumonia
 f. renal capsule
 f. ring
 f. ring of disk

 f. scar tissue
 f. septum
 f. sheath
 f. skeleton
 f. temporal bone dysplasia
 f. tissue hyperplasia
 f. trigone
 f. tubercle
 f. tumor pleura
 f. union
 f. urinary tract polyp
 f. web
fibrovascular
 f. core
 f. polyp
 f. stalk
 f. tissue
fibroxanthoma
 malignant f.
 multiple f.'s
 pediatric f.
fibroxanthosarcoma
fibula, pl. **fibulae**
 apex of f.
 capitulum fibulae
 inferior tip of the f.
 malleolus fibulae
 nutrient artery of f.
 proximal f.
fibular
 f. articular surface
 f. collateral ligament
 f. fracture
 f. hallux sesamoid
 f. lymph node
 f. notch
 f. physis
 f. sesamoid bone
 f. vein
fibulotalar ligament
fibulotalocalcaneal (FTC)
 f. ligament
Ficat
 F. and Axlet staging system
 F. stage of avascular necrosis
 F. staging
Fick
 F. cardiac index
 F. equation
 F. first law of diffusion
 F. law
 F. method
 F. method for measuring cardiac
  output
 F. position
 F. principle
Ficoll gradient

FID
   flexion interspinous distance
   free-induction decay
FID-acquired echoes (FAcE)
fiducial
   f. alignment system
   f. movement
   f. skin marker
field
   f. alignment
   blocked vertex f.
   Brodmann cytoarchitectonic f.
   f. cancerization
   collapsed lung f.
   3D deformation f.
   f. defect
   dipole f.
   disk-to-magnetic f.
   f. drift
   f. echo (FE)
   electromagnetic f.
   electromagnetic focusing f. (EFF)
   electronic focusing f.
   f. emission tube
   f.-even echo rephasing (FEER)
   extremely low-frequency f.
   far f.
   fringe f.
   Gibbs random f.
   gonion gradient magnetic f.
   f. gradient
   gradient magnetic f.
   harmonic f.
   helmet f.
   high-powered f. (hpf)
   insonifying wave f.
   involved f.
   large hinge angle electron f.
   f. lock
   lower lung f.
   lung f.
   magnetic fringe f.
   mantle f.
   Markov random f.
   midlung f.
   near f.
   oscillating magnetic f.
   parietal eye f. (PEF)
   perturbing magnetic f.
   radiofrequency electromagnetic f.
   rotational f.
   skimming of magnetic f.

   spade f.
   static magnetic f.
   stationary f.
   stippling of lung f.
   stray neutron f.
   f. strength
   tangential breast f.
   tesla f.
   time-varying magnetic f.
   f. uniformity
   upper lung f.
   f. variation
   f. of view (FOV)
   Z axis f.
field-echo
   f.-e. difference
   f.-e. imaging
   f.-e. pulse sequence
   f.-e. sequence with even-echo
      rephasing (FEER)
   f.-e. sum
field-fitting
   f.-f. analysis
   f.-f. technique
Fielding-Magliato subtrochanteric
   fracture classification
field-of-view
   f.-o.-v. imaging
   f.-o.-v. information
field-profiling coil
Fiessinger-Leroy-Reiter syndrome
Fiessinger-Leroy syndrome
FIESTA imaging technique
fifth
   f. compartment
   f. cranial nerve
   f. intercostal space
   f. rib
   f. ventricle
fighter's fracture
FIGO
   F. stage carcinoma
   F. staging of adenocarcinoma of
      endometrium
figure-3 sign
figure-4 position
figure-8 appearance
filament
   f. emission
   f. transformer
filament-nonfilament count
filarial infection

F

NOTES

file
    Indian f.
filiform
    f. appendix
    f. polyp
    f. polyposis
filigree pattern
filipuncture
fill-and-spill of dye
filler block
filling
    augmented f.
    capillary f.
    compensatory capillary f.
    f. defect
    early venous f.
    f. factor
    late venous f.
    passive f.
    peak f.
    f. pressure
    rapid f. (RF)
    reduced f.
    retrograde f.
    subintimal f.
    ureteral f.
    ventricular f.
    vessel f.
    zero f.
film (*See* projection, radiograph, scan, view, x-ray)
    f. alternator
    anteroposterior f.
    f. badge
    biplane axial f.
    bitewing f.
    Bucky f.
    f. changer
    chest f.
    cine f.
    comparison f.
    corner f.
    crosstable lateral f.
    Curix Ultra UV-L f.
    cut and cine f.
    decubitus f.
    delayed f.
    f. density calibration
    f. diameter
    digital subtraction f.
    f. dispenser
    drain-out f.
    dual-emulsion mammography f.
    DuPont Cronex x-ray f.
    emulsion f.
    expiratory f.
    flat plate f.

f. fog
gamma f.
GLP7 f.
f. graininess
grid f.
f. hanger
high-contrast f.
horizontal beam f.
in-department f.
intraoperative f.
kidneys, ureter, and bladder f.
Knuttsen bending f.
Kodak Min-R f.
Kodak X-OMAT f.
late f.
lateral cervical spine f.
lateral decubitus f.
latitude f.
limited f.
low-contrast f.
low-dose f.
manual subtraction f.
mobility f.
nitrocellulose f.
normal chest f.
oblique f.
occlusal f.
overhead f.
overpenetrated f.
f. oxygenator
PA and lateral f.'s
panoramic x-ray f.
photo plotter f.
plain f.
Polaroid f.
port f.
portable chest f.
posteroanterior chest f.
postevacuation f.
postexercise f.
postreduction f.
postvoiding f.
preliminary f.
prone f.
radiochromic f.
right or left lateral decubitus f.
runoff f.
Scopix Laser f.
scout f.
f. screen cassette
f. screen contact test
screenless mammography f.
screen type f.
semierect f.
sequential f.'s
serial subtraction f.
shoot-through lateral x-ray f.

silver halide f.
simulation f.
skull f.
f. slippage
f. speed
spot f.
stress f.
suboptimal f.
subtraction f.
supine f.
survey f.
f. tube distance
UP7 f.
upright chest f.
upright compression spot f.
weightbearing f.
wide latitude f.
working f.
x-ray f.

film-based
f.-b. screening mammogram
f.-b. viewing
FilmFax teleradiology system
film hanger
filmless
f. imaging
f. radiography
film-screen
f.-s. magnification
f.-s. mammography
filter
bandpass f.
bird's nest f.
Butterworth f.
caval f.
compensating f.
density equalization f.
differencing f.
flattening f.
Greenfield vena cava f.
Günther Tulip vena cava MReye f.
Hann f.
helix f.
high-pass f.
inherent f.
Kalman f.
K-edge f.
Keeper vena cava f.
low-pass f.
Metz spatially varying f.
Mobin-Uddin vera cava f.
f. mold

nitinol inferior vena cava f.
10-pole Butterworth f.
ramp f.
rhodium f.
sigma f.
Simon Nitinol vena cava f.
software-controlled internal
  hardware f.
spatial f.
Tempofilter vena cava f.
temporal f.
Thoreau f.
translation-invariant f.
TrapEase inferior vena cava f.
TrapEase vena cava f.
vena caval f.
Vena Tech-LGM vena cava f.
wall f.
wedge f.
Weiner spatially varying f.
Wiener MRI f.
Wratten 6B f.
filtered
f. back-projection algorithm
f. back-projection method
filtering
3D low pass f.
3D post f.
dynamic f.
low-pass f.
morphologic f.
phase f.
filtration
beam f.
copper f.
dynamic beat f.
f. fraction (FF)
glomerular f.
postbeat f.
supplemental beam f.
filum
fatty f.
f. terminale
f. terminale fibrolipoma
fimbriated end
finding
angiographic f.
atypical f.
auscultatory f.
cardinal f.
characteristic f.
concomitant f.

F

NOTES

finding *(continued)*
    concordance of MR f.'s
    constellation of f.'s
    discordant f.
    equivocal f.
    focal lateralizing f.
    incidental f.
    lateralizing f.
    no discernible f.
    nonspecific f.
    pathognomonic f.
    roentgenographic f.
    secondary sonographic f.
    specious f.
    spurious f.
    ultrasonographic f.

fine
    f. calcification
    f. detail
    f. injection
    f. peripheral reticular pattern
    f. reticular pattern

fine-needle
    f.-n. aspiration
    f.-n. aspiration biopsy
    f.-n. puncture
    f.-n. transhepatic cholangiogram
    (FNTC)

fine-speckled appearance
finger
    base of f.
    baseball f.
    bolster f.
    bony tuft of f.
    clubbed f.
    Dawson f.
    drop f.
    football f.
    f. fracture
    hippocratic f.
    index f.
    jammed f.
    jersey f.
    little f.
    long f.
    f. lucent lesion
    mallet f.
    middle f.
    overlapping f.
    pedicle f.
    pulley of f.
    pulp of f.
    replantation of f.
    ring f.
    sausage f.
    spade f.
    speck f.
    spider f.
    stoved f.
    tapered f.
    trigger f.
    f. of tumor
    f. web
    webbed f.

finger-in-glove pattern
finger-like
    f.-l. mucous plug
    f.-l. projection
    f.-l. villus

fingerprint
    f. edema
    f. image compression
    f. mark artifact
    f. pattern

fingertip
    f. amputation
    f. calcification
    f. lesion

Finkelstein sign
firearm injury
FIRFT
    fast inversion-recovery Fourier transform

firing
    f. of ectopic atrial focus
    f. temperature

firm
    f. mass
    f. neoplasm

Firooznia
    threshold of F.

first
    f. branchial arch
    f. branchial cleft cyst
    f. carpal row
    f. cuneiform bone
    f. diagonal branch artery
    f. digital interosseous (FDI)
    f. duodenal sphincter
    f. major diagonal branch
    f. metatarsal angle
    f. metatarsal head (FMH)
    f. obtuse marginal artery
    f. parallel pelvic plane
    f. portion of duodenum
    f. ray instability
    f. rib
    f. septal perforator branch
    f. temporal gyrus
    f. ventricle of cerebrum
    f. visceral cleft

first-degree
    f.-d. AV block
    f.-d. heart block

first-fifth intermetatarsal angle

first-line therapy
first-order
 f.-o. chorda
 f.-o. reaction
first-pass
 f.-p. acquisition
 f.-p. cardiac perfusion
 f.-p. effect
 f.-p. examination
 f.-p. MUGA
 f.-p. myocardial perfusion imaging
 f.-p. myocardial perfusion MR
 f.-p. radionuclide angiography
  (FPRNA)
 f.-p. radionuclide exercise
  angiocardiography
 f.-p. radionuclide ventriculography
 f.-p. study
 f.-p. technique
 f.-p. thallium extraction
 f.-p. view
first-second intermetatarsal angle
first-trimester
 f.-t. bleeding
 f.-t. hemorrhage
 f.-t. nuchal translucency
 f.-t. placenta
Fischer sign
Fischgold
 F. bimastoid line
 F. biventer line
Fisher grade 1–4
fish flesh appearance
fishmeal worker's lung
fishmouth
 f. amputation
 f. configuration of mitral valve
 f. cusp
 f. fracture
 f. mitral stenosis
 f. mitral valve configuration
 f. vertebra
fishnet appearance
fish-scale gallbladder
fishtail
 f. tear
 f. vertebra
FISP
 fast imaging with steady-state precession
  mirrored FISP (mFISP)
  FISP pulse sequence

fission
 nuclear f.
 f. product
 f. track analysis
fissula
 ante fenestram f.
fissuration
fissure
 abdominal f.
 accessory f.
 anal f.
 f. in ano
 anterior interhemispheric f.
 anterior median f.
 antitragohelicine f.
 f. of anulus
 auricular f.
 azygos f.
 brain f.
 bulging lung f.
 calcarine f.
 callosomarginal f.
 central cerebellar f.
 cerebral f.
 choroidal f.
 chronic f.
 collateral f.
 cutaneous f.
 decidual f.
 dentate f.
 displacement of interhemispheric f.
 f. fracture
 glaserian f.
 hepatic f.
 hippocampal f.
 horizontal f.
 incomplete pulmonary f.
 inferior accessory f.
 inferior orbital f.
 interhemispheric f. (IHF)
 interlobar f.
 lateral f.
 ligamentum venosum f.
 liver f.
 longitudinal f.
 lung f.
 main f.
 major f.
 minor f.
 nasopalatal f.
 oblique f.
 occipital f.

F

NOTES

fissure *(continued)*
    oral f.
    orbital f.
    palpebral f.
    portal f.
    rolandic f.
    f. of Rolando
    f. sign
    studded f.
    superior orbital f.
    supraorbital f.
    sylvian f.
    transitional zone f.
    umbilical f.
    widened superior orbital f.
fissured atheromatous plaque
fisting
    rectal f.
fistula, pl. **fistulae, fistulas**
    abdominal f.
    aerodigestive f.
    anal f.
    f. in ano
    anorectal f.
    anovaginal f.
    aorta-left ventricular f.
    aorta-right ventricular f.
    aortic-enteric f.
    aortic sinus to right ventricle f.
    aortocaval f.
    aortoduodenal f.
    aortoenteric f.
    aortoesophageal f.
    aortojejunal f.
    aortopulmonary f.
    aortosigmoid f.
    arterial-arterial f.
    arterial-portal f.
    arteriobiliary f.
    arterioportobiliary f.
    arteriosinusoidal penile f.
    arteriovenous f. (AVF)
    biliary f.
    biliary-cutaneous f.
    biliary-duodenal f.
    biliary-enteric f.
    bilioenteric f.
    Blom-Singer tracheoesophageal f.
    BP f.
    branchial f.
    Brescia-Cimino f.
    bronchobiliary f.
    bronchocavitary f.
    bronchocutaneous f.
    bronchoesophageal f.
    bronchopleural f.
    bronchopulmonary f.

    cameral f.
    caroticocavernous f.
    carotid-cavernous f. (CCF)
    carotid-cavernous sinus f.
    carotid-dural f.
    carotid-jugular f.
    cavernous sinus f.
    cecocutaneous f.
    cerebral arteriovenous f.
    cerebrospinal fluid f.
    cholecystenteric f.
    cholecystocholedochal f.
    cholecystocolic f.
    cholecystocutaneous f.
    cholecystoduodenal f.
    cholecystoduodenocolic f.
    cholecystoenteric f.
    choledochal-colonic f.
    choledochoduodenal f.
    chylous f.
    coil closure of coronary artery f.
    colocolic f.
    colocutaneous f.
    colonic f.
    colovaginal f.
    colovesical f.
    communicating f.
    complex anorectal f.
    congenital pulmonary
      arteriovenous f.
    congenital tracheobiliary f.
    coronary arteriosystemic f.
    coronary arteriovenous f.
    coronary artery cameral f.
    coronary artery-pulmonary artery f.
    coronary artery to right
      ventricular f.
    cystic f.
    dialysis f.
    digestive-respiratory f.
    dorsal enteric f.
    duodenocolic f.
    duodenopancreatic f.
    dural arteriovenous f.
    dural carotid cavernous f. (DCCF)
    durocutaneous f.
    Eck f.
    enteric f.
    enterocolic f.
    enterocutaneous f.
    enteroenteral f.
    enterospinal f.
    enterourethral f.
    enterovaginal f.
    enterovesical f.
    esophagorespiratory f.
    esophagotracheal f.

external biliary f.
extrasphincteric anal f.
fecal f.
f. formation
gastric f.
gastrocolic f.
gastrocutaneous f.
gastroduodenal f.
gastrointestinal f.
gastrojejunocolic f.
genitourinary f.
graft-enteric f.
hepatic arteriovenous f.
hepatic artery-portal vein f.
hepatopleural f.
hepatoportal biliary f.
high-flow arteriovenous f.
horseshoe f.
H-type tracheoesophageal f.
hyperdynamic AV f.
iatrogenic iliocaval f.
ileosigmoid f.
infralevator f.
intersphincteric anal f.
intracranial arteriovenous f.
intradural retromedullary
　arteriovenous f.
intrahepatic arterial-portal f.
intrahepatic AV f.
intrapulmonary arteriovenous f.
jejunocolic f.
labyrinthine f.
Mann-Bollman f.
mediastinal f.
mesenteric f.
metroperitoneal f.
microvenoarteriolar f.
mucous f.
orofacial f.
f. ostium
pancreatic cutaneous f.
pancreaticopleural f.
paraprosthetic-enteric f.
parietal f.
periareolar f.
perineovaginal f.
persistent bronchopleural f.
pilonidal f.
pleural f.
pleurocutaneous f.
postbiopsy renal AV f.
premedullary arteriovenous f.

pulmonary arteriovenous f.
radial artery to cephalic vein f.
radiation f.
radiculomeningeal f.
rectal f.
rectovaginal f.
rectovesical f.
respiratory-esophageal f.
retroperitoneal f.
spinal dural arteriovenous f.
splanchnic AV f.
splenic AV f.
splenobronchial f.
supralevator f.
suprasphincteric f.
TE f.
thoracic duct-cutaneous f.
tracheobiliary f.
tracheobronchial f.
tracheobronchoesophageal f.
tracheoesophageal f. (TEF)
f. tract study
transdural f.
transsphincteric anal f.
trigeminal cavernous f.
type A carotid cavernous f.
ureteral f.
ureterocutaneous f.
ureterointestinal f.
ureteroperitoneal f.
ureterovaginal f.
urethrovaginal f.
urinary f.
vaginal f.
venobiliary f.
vertebrojugular f.
vertebrovertebral f.
vesical f.
vesicocolic f.
vesicovaginal f.
vitelline f.
fistulogram
cine f.
venous f.
fistulography
fistulous
f. gas communication
f. tract
fit
smoothed curve f.
fitting
peak f.

F

NOTES

Fitz-Hugh and Curtis syndrome
five-view chest x-ray
fixation
    f. articulation
    atlantoaxial rotary f.
    bowel loop f.
    catheter f.
    f. disk
    external f.
    external wire f.
    intramedullary f.
    intrapedicular f.
    metallic rod f.
    open reduction and internal f.
      (ORIF)
    plate and screw f.
    f. of scoliosis
    screw f.
    spinal f.
    suprasyndesmotic f.
    transsyndesmotic screw f.
    triangular external ankle f.
    wire f.
fixator
    dynamic axial f.
    f. muscle
fixed
    f. airway obstruction
    f. coronary obstruction
    f. flexion contracture
    f. gantry
    f. intracavitary filling defect
    f. mass
    f. perfusion defect
    f. pulmonary valvular resistance
    f. segment of bowel
    f. shaped coplanar or nonplanar
      radiation beam bouquet
    f. third-degree AV block
fixed-orifice aortic stenosis
fixer
fixing time
FL
    femur length
flabby heart
^{18}F-labeled
    fluorine-18-labeled
    ^{18}F-labeled fatty acid
    ^{18}F-labeled HFA-134a
    ^{18}F-labeled polyfluorinated ethyl
Flack sinoatrial node
flag
    Rudick red f.
flail
    f. air
    f. chest
    f. digit

    f. foot
    f. joint
    f. mitral valve
    f. shoulder
FLAIR
    fluid-attenuated inversion recovery
    FLAIR echo-planar imaging
    FLAIR image
FLAIR-FLASH imaging
FLAK
    flow artifact killer
    FLAK technique
flake
    f. fracture
    f. fracture of the hamate
flake-shaped injury
flaking of cartilage
flaky calcification
flame
    f. appearance
    f. emission spectroscopy (FES)
    f. ionization detector
Flamingo stent
flange
    shaft f.
flank
    f. bone
    f. stripe
flap
    bone f.
    bursal f.
    entry f.
    foramen ovale f.
    intimal f.
    Karapandzic f.
    liver f.
    localized intimal f.
    lytic area bone f.
    necrotic f.
    osteoplastic f.
    pedicle f.
    pericardial f.
    pleural f.
    f. positioning
    postangioplasty intimal f.
    rotary door f. (RDF)
    scapular f.
    scimitar-shaped f.
    subclavian f.
    f. tear
    f. valve ventricular septal defect
flap-like valve
flap-valve mechanism
flare
    condylar f.
    metaphyseal f.
    f. phenomenon

f. reaction
tibial f.
trochanteric f.
flared ilium
FLASH
fast low-angle shot
FLASH acquisition
diffusion/perfusion snapshot FLASH
(DPSF)
FLASH image
FLASH magnetic resonance
imaging
flashlamp-pulsed dye laser
flashlamp-pumped pulsed dye laser
flash photolysis
flask
Erlenmeyer f.
vascular f.
flask-shaped
f.-s. heart
f.-s. ulcer
flat
f. adenoma
f. bone
f. colorectal carcinoma
f. diastolic slope
f. electroencephalogram
f. facet
f. neck vein
f. pelvis
f. plate
f. plate of abdomen
f. plate film
f. suture
f. time-intensity profile
f. vertebral body
Flatau-Schilder disease
flat-field imaging
flatfoot
calcaneovalgus f.
f. deformity
Durham f.
flat-hand test
flat-panel megavoltage imager
flat-plate detector
flattened
f. arch
f. duodenal fold
f. E-to-F slope
f. longitudinal arch of foot
flattening
cortical f.

f. of diaphragm
f. filter
f. filter beam
f. of gyrus
f. of normal lordotic curvature
f. of normal lumbar curve
f. ratio (FR)
flat-top
f.-t. bladder
f.-t. talus
flava (*pl. of* flavum)
flaval ligament
flavone acetic acid (FAA)
flavum, pl. **flava**
ligamentum f.
pleating of ligamentum f.
flawed
f. image
f. imaging
flax-dresser disease
Flechsig bundle
Fleckinger view
fleck sign
fleecy mass
Fleet
F. Phospho-Soda bowel preparation
F. Prep Kit 1, 2, 3
fleeting lung infiltrate
Fleischmann bursa
Fleischner
F. line
F. position
F. sign
Fletcher
F. afterloader
F. factor
F. projection
F. rule of irradiation tolerance
Fletcher-Delclos dome cylinder
Fletcher-Suit-Delclos (FSD)
F.-S.-D. tandem
Fletcher-Suit system for radium therapy
fleur-de-lis pattern
flexa
coxa f.
flexible
f. biopsy needle
f. endofluoroscopy
f. nephroscope
f. over-wire system
f. radiofrequency coil
f. spastic equinovarus deformity

F

NOTES

351

flexible *(continued)*
  f. surface coil
  f. surface-coil-type resonator
    (FSCR)
flexible-tip guidewire
Flexiflo
Flexima biliary drainage catheter
flexion
  angle of greatest f. (AGF)
  f. contracture
  f. deformity
  f. and extension exercises
  f. and extension views
  external rotation in f. (ERF)
  internal rotation in f. (IRF)
  f. interspinous distance (FID)
  f. maneuver
  f. position
  f. teardrop fracture
flexion-adduction contracture
flexion-burst fracture
flexion-compression fracture
flexion-distraction
  f.-d. fracture
  f.-d. injury
flexion-extension
  f.-e. plane
  f.-e. projection
  f.-e. radiography
flexion-rotation injury
Flexi-Tip ureteral catheter
flexor
  f. bursa
  f. canal
  capital f.
  f. carpi radialis
  f. carpi radialis muscle
  f. carpi radialis tendon
  f. carpi ulnaris
  f. carpi ulnaris aponeurosis
  f. carpi ulnaris tendon
  f. digiti minimi
  f. digiti minimi brevis
  f. digiti quinti brevis
  f. digiti quinti brevis muscle
  f. digitorum brevis
  f. digitorum communis tendon
  f. digitorum longus
  f. digitorum longus muscle
  f. digitorum longus tendon
  f. digitorum profundus
  f. digitorum profundus muscle
  f. digitorum profundus tendon
  f. digitorum sublimis tendon
  f. digitorum superficialis
  f. digitorum superficialis muscle
  f. digitorum superficialis tendon

  f. hallucis brevis (FHB)
  f. hallucis brevis muscle
  f. hallucis brevis tendon
  f. hallucis longus
  f. hallucis longus tendon
  f. plate
  f. pollicis brevis
  f. pollicis brevis tendon
  f. pollicis longus
  f. pollicis longus tendon
  f. profundus tendon
  f. retinaculum
  f. sublimis tendon
  f. tendon sheath
  f. tenosynovitis
flexor-pronator muscle group
FlexStent
  Gianturco-Roubin F.
FlexStrand cable
flexure
  caudal f.
  cephalic f.
  cerebral f.
  cervical f.
  colonic f.
  cranial f.
  duodenojejunal f. (DJF)
  hepatic f.
  inferior duodenal f. (IDF)
  left colonic f.
  right colonic f.
  sigmoid f.
  splenic f.
flicker electroretinogram
Flint colon injury scale
flip
  f. angle
  spin f.
  tristimulus value f.
  value f.
flip-angle image
flip-flop
  f.-f. enhancement
  f.-f. pattern
flipped meniscus sign
floating
  f. arch fracture
  f. cartilage
  f. elbow
  f. endocardial centroid
  f. epicardial centroid
  f. gallbladder
  f. gallstone
  f. image
  f. kidney
  f. knee
  f. leaflet

f. ligament
f. liver
f. organ
f. osteophyte
f. patella
f. prostate
f. rib
f. spleen
f. teeth
f. thumb
f. villus
floccular fossa
flocculation of barium
flocculent
f. focus of calcification
flocculonodular
f. lobe
f. lobe of cerebellum
f. tumor
flocculus, pl. flocculi
Flocks and Kadesky system
flood
F. ligament
f. phantom
f. section
f. source
floor
bladder f.
fibromuscular pelvic f.
inguinal f.
f. of the orbit
pelvic f.
sellar f.
f. of ventricle
floppy
f. mitral valve
f. valve syndrome
floppy-thumb sign
Flo-Rester vessel occluder
florid
f. callus
f. cardiac tamponade
f. duct lesion
f. follicular hyperplasia
f. plaque
f. reactive periostitis
flow
absolute blood f.
f. acceleration
aliased f.
altered blood f.
anatomic shunt f.

antegrade bile f.
antegrade blood f.
antegrade diastolic f.
aortic f. (AF)
f. arrest
f. artifact killer (FLAK)
autoregulation of cerebral blood f.
azygos blood f.
backward f.
bile f.
blood f.
capillary blood f.
cephalization of blood f.
cerebral blood f. (CBF)
cerebral xenon-enhanced blood f.
(X-CBF)
chronic reserve f.
collateral blood f.
f. compensation (FC)
compromised f.
f. of contrast material
coronary blood f.
coronary reserve f. (CRF)
f. cytometric DNA measurement
f. cytometry
f. cytometry sample preparation
f. cytometry technique
dampened pulsatile f.
2D color-coded imaging of
blood f.
decreased cerebral blood f.
diastolic zero f.
Doppler study of blood f.
f. effect artifact
effective pulmonary blood f.
(EPBF)
effective renal plasma f. (ERFP,
ERPF)
electron f.
expiratory f.
fast Fourier f. (FFF)
fluid f.
flush f.
forward f.
Ganz formula for coronary sinus f.
global intracranial blood f.
great cardiac vein f. (GCVF)
hepatofugal f.
hepatopetal f.
high-velocity f.
hyperemic f.
f. imaging

F

NOTES

flow *(continued)*
    inspiratory f.
    intercoronary collateral f.
    internal carotid systolic peak f.
    (ICSPF)
    intrarenal arterial f.
    jet f.
    laminar f.
    left-to-right f.
    local bone blood f.
    low-velocity f.
    lung-volume loop f.
    maintenance of f.
    f. mapping technique
    maximum midexpiratory f. (MMEF)
    microcirculatory blood f.
    midexpiratory tidal f.
    mitral valve f.
    mixed petal-fugal f.
    f. mode ultrafast computed
    tomography
    myocardial blood f. (MBF)
    peak expiratory f. (PEF)
    peak flush f.
    peak velocity of blood f.
    peripheral blood f.
    petal-fugal f.
    f. phenomenon
    physiologic shunt f.
    plug f.
    Poiseuille f.
    portal f.
    f. portion of bone scan
    preferential f.
    protodiastolic reversal of blood f.
    pulmonary blood f. (PBF)
    pulmonic output f.
    pulmonic versus systemic f.
    f. quantification
    f. rate
    real-time phase-contrast f.
    f. redistribution
    regional cerebral blood f. (rCBF)
    regional myocardial blood f.
    regurgitant pandiastolic f.
    regurgitant systolic f.
    relative cerebral blood f.
    relative regional blood f. (rrBF)
    relative shunt f.
    resistance blood f.
    resting regional myocardial blood f.
    restoration of f.
    retrograde systolic f.
    reversed vertebral blood f.
    F. Rider microcatheter
    sluggish f.
    stasis of blood f.

    f. study
    supratentorial cerebral blood f.
    systemic blood f. (SBF)
    systemic output f.
    through-plane f.
    time-averaged f.
    tissue f.
    to-and-fro f.
    total cerebral blood f. (TCBF)
    f. tract
    transmitral f.
    tricuspid valve f.
    turbulent blood f.
    turbulent intraluminal f.
    unequal pulmonary blood f.
    uterine blood volume f.
    f. velocity
    f. velocity profile
    f. velocity signal
    f. velocity waveform
    f. void
    f. void effect
    f. volume
    zero net f.
flow-compensated
    f.-c. gradient-echo sequence
    f.-c. image
flow-compromising lesion
flow-controlled valve
flow-dependent obstruction
flow-encoding gradient
flow-function mismatch
flow-induced artifact
flowing
    f. anterior vertebra ossification
    f. spin
FloWire Doppler ultrasound
flow-limited expiration
flow-limiting
    f.-l. lesion
    f.-l. stenosis
flowmeter
    Doppler f.
    Gould electromagnetic f.
    Parks bidirectional Doppler f.
    pulsed Doppler f.
flowmetry
    blood f.
    Doppler f.
    laser Doppler f. (LDF)
    Narcomatic f.
    Parks 800 bidirectional Doppler f.
    Statham electromagnetic f.
flow-on gradient-echo image
flow-related
    f.-r. artifact
    f.-r. enhancement

f.-r. enhancement effect
f.-r. phase error
f.-r. phase shift
flow-sensitive MR imaging
flow-time curve
flow-volume loop
fluctuant mass
fluctuation
Poisson noise f.
fluence
energy f.
photon f.
f. profile
fluffy
f. infiltrate
f. margin
f. periosteal reaction
f. pulmonary nodule
f. rarefaction
fluid
abdominal collection of f.
f. accumulation
amnionic f. (AF)
anechoic f.
articular f.
ascitic f.
bloodless f.
bursal f.
cavitary f.
cerebrospinal f. (CSF)
f. collection
cystic f.
dammed-up cerebrospinal f.
f. density
edema f.
encapsulated f.
endometrial canal f.
f. expansion
extracellular f.
f. extravasation
extravascular f.
f. flow
free abdominal f.
free cul-de-sac f.
free peritoneal f.
high-signal intratendinous collection
of f.
increased interstitial f.
f. intake
f. interface
interstitial f.
intestinal f.

intraperitoneal f.
joint f.
f. level
loculated pleural f.
f. overload
pelvic f.
pericardial f.
pericerebral f.
pericholecystic f.
pericolonic f.
periesophageal f.
perigraft f.
peritoneal cavity f.
pleural f.
prostatic f.
f. resorption
retained fetal lung f.
f. retention
f. sequestration
serohemorrhagic f.
serosanguineous f.
f. signal
silicone f.
f. space
spinal f.
subgaleal cerebrospinal f.
subphrenic f.
subpulmonic f.
synovial f.
transudation of f.
transudative pericardial f.
f. volume
f. wave
fluid-attenuated
f.-a. inversion recovery (FLAIR)
f.-a. inversion recovery-fast low-
angle shot
fluid-blood layer
fluid-filled
f.-f. bronchogram
f.-f. catheter
f.-f. cyst
f.-f. kidney mass
f.-f. loop of bowel
f.-f. sac
fluid-flow artifact
fluid-fluid level
fluke
liver f.
lung f.
Oriental lung f.

F

NOTES

fluorescein
- f. angiogram
- f. angiography
- f. sodium
- f. uptake

fluorescence
- f. microscopy
- f. spectroscopy

fluorescence-activated cell sorter (FACScan)

fluorescent
- f. phosphor
- f. ray
- f. scan
- f. screen

Fluorescite injection

fluoride
- barium f.
- f. ion-positron emission tomography (F-18 PET)
- lithium f. (LiF)
- neodymium:yttrium-lithium f. (Nd:YLF)
- yttrium lithium f. (YLF)

fluorine (F)
- f. imaging agent

fluorine-18 (^{18}F, F-18)
- f.-18 fluorodeoxyglucose-positron emission tomography

fluorine-19 (^{19}F, F-19)
- f. spectroscopy

2-[fluorine-18]fluoro-2-deoxy-D-glucose (^{18}F-FDG)

fluorine-18-labeled (^{18}F-labeled)

Fluor-I-Strip

Fluor-I-Strip-AT

fluorocaptopril

fluorocarbon-based ultrasound contrast agent

fluorochloride
- barium f.

fluorochrome

fluorodeoxyglucose (FDG)
- ^{18}F f.
- f. F-18 injection
- f. imaging agent

2-fluoro 2-deoxyglucose (FDG)

fluorodeoxyglucose-6-phosphate

fluorodeoxyuridine

fluoro-DOPA

fluoroestradiol (FES)

fluorography
- digital f.
- spot film f.

fluorohalide
- europium-activated barium f.

fluorometer
- 96-well scanning f.

fluorometry
- image intensification f.
- two-plane f.

fluoromibolerone

fluoromisonidazole

fluoronephelometer

Fluoroplex

FluoroPlus
- F. angiography
- F. Cardiac digital fluoroscopy
- F. real-time digital imaging system

fluoropropylepidepride

fluoroptic thermometry system

fluoropyrimidine

fluororoentgenography

FluoroScan C-arm fluoroscopy

fluoroscope
- Edison f.

fluoroscopic
- f. assistance
- f. control
- f. guidance
- f. image
- f. imaging
- f. localization
- f. observation
- f. pushing technique
- f. road-mapping technique
- f. view

fluoroscopy
- airway f.
- biplane f.
- C-arm f.
- chest f.
- computed tomography f. (CTF)
- computerized f.
- digital f.
- electric joint f.
- FluoroPlus Cardiac digital f.
- FluoroScan C-arm f.
- high-resolution f.
- image-amplified f.
- mobile f.
- Orca C-arm f.
- orthogonal C-arm f.
- portable C-arm image intensifier f.
- real-time CT f.
- region of interest f.
- simultaneous f.

fluoroscopy-guided
- f.-g. condylar lift-off imaging
- f.-g. subarachnoid phenol block therapy

fluorosis
- osteophytosis in f.

fluorotamoxifen
Fluoro Tip cannula
FluoroTrak fluoroscopy-based surgical
  navigation system
fluorotropapride
fluorotyrosine
FluoroVision
flush
  f. angiogram
  f. aortogram imaging
  f. aortography
  cervical f.
  f. flow
flush-tank sign
flutter
  atrial fetal f.
flux, pl. **fluxes**
  electron f.
  improved photon f.
  magnetic f.
  photon f.
fluxionary hyperemia
flying
  f. focal spot
  f. spot excimer laser system
fly-through viewing
FM
  fetal movement
Fm
  fermium
²⁵⁵Fm
  fermium-255
FMAP
  feeding mean arterial pressure
FMH
  first metatarsal head
F-misonidazole
fMRA
  functional magnetic resonance
    angiography
fMRI
  functional magnetic resonance imaging
  cognitive fMRI
  integrated fMRI
  fMRI signal change
  VNS-synchronized BOLD fMRI
    vagus nerve stimulation-
      synchronized blood oxygen level-
      dependent functional MRI
fMR tube
FMS
  fatty meal sonogram

FNH
  focal nodular hyperplasia
  follicular nodular hyperplasia
FNTC
  fine-needle transhepatic cholangiogram
foam
  f. cushion
  f. embolus
  minimally attenuating medical-
    grade f.
  f. vacuum pillow
foam-padded Velcro restraint
foamy esophagus
FOB
  fiberoptic bronchoscopy
focal
  f. alimentary tract calcification
  f. alveolar infiltrate
  f. area of hemorrhage
  f. area of hypometabolism
  f. articular cartilage lesion
  f. asymmetric density
  f. asymmetry
  f. atrophy
  f. attenuation
  f. bacterial nephritis
  f. biliary cirrhosis
  f. bone sclerosis
  f. caliectasis
  f. cartilage erosion
  f. cecal apical thickening
  f. cerebellar dysplasia
  f. cerebral ischemia
  f. cold liver lesion
  f. colitis
  f. cortical dysplasia
  f. cortical hyperplasia
  f. damage
  f. decreased radiotracer uptake
  f. deficit
  f. degenerative change
  f. and diffuse lung texture analysis
  f. disk herniation
  f. distortion
  f. eccentric stenosis
  f. edema
  f. endocardial hemorrhage
  f. esophageal narrowing
  f. fat necrosis
  f. fatty infiltration of liver
  f. fibrocartilaginous dysplasia of
    tibia

F

NOTES

focal *(continued)*
- f. fibrosis
- f. film distance (FFD)
- f. gallbladder wall thickening
- f. gigantism
- f. hemispheric lesion
- f. hepatic necrosis
- f. high-intensity zone
- f. hot liver lesion
- f. hydronephrosis
- f. hyperinflation
- f. indentation
- f. inflammation
- f. interstitial infiltrate
- f. intimal thickening
- f. ischemic lesion
- f. lateralizing finding
- f. length
- f. limb abnormality
- f. liver hot spot
- f. liver scintigraphic defect
- f. lobular carcinoma
- f. lung disease
- f. malformation
- f. mass
- f. metabolic abnormality
- f. myometrial contraction
- f. neurologic sign
- f. nodular enhancement
- f. nodular hyperplasia (FNH)
- f. nuclear herniation
- f. organizing pneumonia
- f. osseous offset
- f. pancreatitis
- f. parenchymal brain lesion
- f. parenchymal cryptococcoma
- f. pattern
- f. perivascular infiltrate
- f. plane tomography
- f. plaque-like defect
- f. pleural plaque
- f. pool
- f. pooling of tracer
- f. pulmonary hemorrhage
- f. pulmonary uptake
- f. pyloric hypertrophy
- f. renal hypertrophy
- f. small-bowel disease
- f. splenic lesion
- f. spot (FS)
- f. spot blur
- f. spot-to-film angle
- f. spot-to-object distance
- f. spot tracking
- f. subluxation of vertebrae
- f. tumor
- f. ulcer
- f. wall motion abnormality
- f. white matter signal abnormality
- f. zone (FZ)

focal-dust emphysema
focally
- f. decreased renal neoplasm
- f. dilated duct
- f. increased renal echogenicity

focus, pl. foci
- Assmann f.
- atrial f.
- basal ganglia echogenic f.
- bright cystic f.
- brightly echogenic f.
- f. of calcification
- f. detection
- discrete hyperintense f.
- echogenic f.
- ectopic f.
- epileptic f.
- epileptogenic f.
- firing of ectopic atrial f.
- Ghon f.
- hemorrhagic f.
- hyperechoic f.
- hypermetabolic activity f.
- inflammatory f.
- junctional f.
- linear f.
- mesial frontal f.
- metastatic f.
- midline parasagittal f.
- multifocal residual f.
- multiple f.
- multizone transmit-receive f.
- nodular hyperintense f.
- f. object distance (FOD)
- occipital f.
- punctate hyperintense f.
- radiolucent f.
- residual f.
- satellite cartilaginous f.
- Simon f.
- stationary f.
- subependymal/subpial f.
- f. of tumor

focused
- f. abdominal sonography for trauma (FAST)
- f. appendix computed tomography (FACT)
- f. grid
- f. nuclear magnetic resonance
- f. segmented ultrasound machine
- f. ultrasound

focusing
- f. collimator

dynamic f.
zone f.
focus-skin distance (FSD)
FOD
focus object distance
fog
f. artifact
base f.
film f.
Fogarty
F. balloon embolectomy catheter
F. maneuver
fogging phenomenon
foil
scattering f.
Foix-Alajouanine syndrome
Foix-Chavany-Marie syndrome
fold
abnormal esophageal f.
abnormal small bowel f.
accordion f.
adipose f.
alar f.
amnionic f.
aryepiglottic f.
blunted mucosal f.
caval f.
cecal f.
cholecystoduodenocolic f.
circular f.
costocolic f.
crescentic submucosal f.
distorted mucosal f.
Douglas f.
duodenojejunal f.
duodenomesocolic f.
dural f.
effaced mucosal f.
epigastric f.
epiglottic f.
esophageal f.
falciform f.
flattened duodenal f.
fragmented mucosal f.
gastric f.
gastropancreatic f.
genital f.
giant gastric f.
glossoepiglottic f.
glossopalatine f.
gluteal f.
Guérin f.

haustral f.
Hensing f.
hepatopancreatic f.
hidebound small bowel f.
ileocecal f.
ileocolic f.
inferior transverse rectal f.
inframammary f.
inguinal f.
irregular mucosal f.
Kerckring f.
Kohlrausch f.
lateral umbilical f.
longitudinal esophageal f.
medical umbilical f.
mucosal f.
Nélaton f.
palatopharyngeal f.
paraduodenal f.
f. pattern
pericardial f.
peritoneal f.
pleuroperitoneal f.
prepyloric f.
rectal f.
rectouterine f.
rugal f.
sacrogenital f.
semilunar f.
sentinel f.
sickle-shaped f.
sigmoid f.
skin f.
smooth thickened mucosal f.
spiral f.
stack-of-coins mucosal f.
submucosal circular f.
superior duodenal f.
superior transverse rectal f.
tethered small bowel f.
thickened duodenal f.
thickened esophageal f.
thickened gastric f.
thickened nodular irregular small
bowel f.
thickened stomach f.
thickened straight small bowel f.
transverse esophageal f.
uteric f.
Vater f.
ventriculoinfundibular f.
vestigial f.

F

NOTES

folded
> f. fundus of gallbladder
> f. lung
> f. step ramp

folding potential analysis

foldover
> image f.

folia
> cerebellar f.
> shrunken f.

folial pattern

folium vermis

Folius muscle

follicle
> aggregated lymphatic f.
> anovular ovarian f.
> ascendant f.
> atretic ovarian f.
> dominant f.
> gastric lymphatic f.
> geographic f.
> graafian f.
> intestinal f.
> inverse f.
> luteinized unruptured f.
> lymphoid f.
> f. lysis
> malpighian f.
> nabothian f.
> primordial f.
> ruptured f.
> thyroid f.
> unruptured f.

follicular
> f. bronchiectasis
> f. bronchiolitis
> f. bronchitis
> f. center-cell lymphoma
> f. gastritis
> f. involution
> f. mixed small cleaved lymphoma
> f. nodular hyperplasia (FNH)
> f. ovarian cyst
> f. pattern
> f. phase
> f. predominantly large cell lymphoma
> f. predominantly small cell lymphoma
> f. salpingitis
> f. thyroid adenoma
> f. thyroid carcinoma

folliculare
> oophoroma f.

follicularis
> enteritis f.

follow-through
> small bowel f.-t. (SBFT)
> upper GI with small bowel f.-t.
> f.-t. view

follow-up duplex Doppler sonography

fomite

FONAR
> F.-360 MRI scanner
> F. Standing Ovation MRI system

Fong disease

Fontana canal

fontanelle, fontanel
> anterior f.
> anterolateral f.
> bregmatic f.
> bulging f.
> closed f.
> cranial f.
> frontal f.
> fused f.
> Gerdy f.
> mastoid f.
> occipital f.
> open f.
> overriding sutures of f.
> posterior f.
> posterolateral f.
> sagittal f.
> sphenoid f.
> tense f.
> triangular f.

Fontan operation

food
> f. bolus obstruction
> cholecystokinetic f.
> retention of f.

foot, pl. **feet**
> abnormal position of f.
> arch of f.
> f. architecture
> ball of f.
> calcaneocavus f.
> Charcot f.
> f. deformity
> digital artery of f.
> drop f.
> f. dysplasia
> flail f.
> flattened longitudinal arch of f.
> f. fracture
> Friedreich f.
> hollow f.
> large-vessel disease of diabetic f.
> lateral spring ligament of f.
> Madura f.
> march f.
> phalanges of f.

planovalgus f.
f. plate
f. revascularization
rocker-bottom f.
valgus f.
varus f.
foot-ankle complex
football
f. finger
f. sign
footling presentation
footprint analysis
foot-progression angle (FPA)
foramen, pl. **foramina**
alveolar f.
anterior condyloid f.
anterior palatine f.
anterior sacral f.
aortic f.
apical f.
arachnoidal f.
base of skull f.
Bichat f.
blind f.
Bochdalek f.
Botallo f.
brain mass in jugular f.
carotid f.
cecal f.
cervical neural f.
conjugate f.
costotransverse f.
cranial f.
Duverney f.
emissary sphenoidal f.
enlarged vertebral f.
enlargement of vertebral f.
epiploic f.
ethmoidal f.
external acoustic f.
Ferrein f.
Froesch f.
frontal f.
greater palatine f.
greater sciatic f.
great sacrosciatic f.
Huschke f.
Hyrtl f.
intertransverse f.
interventricular f.
intervertebral f.
jugular f.

f. lacerum
lesser sciatic f.
f. of Luschka
Magendie f.
f. magnum
f. magnum decompression
f. magnum herniation
mandibular f.
mastoid f.
f. of Monro
Morgagni f.
neural f.
nutrient f.
obturator f.
optic f.
f. ovale
f. ovale flap
ovale skull base of f.
f. ovale valve
palatine f.
parietal f.
petrosal f.
restrictive bulboventricular f.
Retzius f.
f. rotundum
sacral f.
sacrosciatic f.
skull-base f.
sphenopalatine f.
f. spinosum
spinous f.
Stensen f.
stylomastoid f.
sublabral f.
superior maxillary f.
supraorbital f.
thebesian f.
f. transversarium
f. venosum
vertebral f.
f. of Vesalius
Weitbrecht f.
f. of Winslow
zygomaticofacial f.
foraminal
f. encroachment
f. node
f. space
f. stenosis
force
coulomb f.
electromotive f. (emf)

F

NOTES

force *(continued)*
    magnetic lines of f.
    nuclear f.
    pascals of f.
    reserve f.
    rotational f.
    shearing f.
    stroke f.
    tensile f.
    torsion impaction f.
    transverse plane f.
forced
    f. expiratory volume
    f. flexion injury
force-frequency relation
forceful parasternal motion
force-length relation
force-velocity relation
forearm
    f. amputation
    f. fracture
forebrain
forefoot
    f. abduction deformity
    f. angulation
    narrowing of f.
foregut
    bronchopulmonary f.
    f. cyst
    f. duplication
foreign
    f. body (FB)
    f. body embolus
    f. body in esophagus
    f. body granuloma
    f. body upper airway obstruction
    f. debris
    f. material artifact
Forel
    H field of F.
foreshortened image data set
foreshortening
    anular f.
Forestier disease
forking
    aqueductal f.
    f. of sylvian aqueduct
form
    ring-shaped f.
Formad kidney
format
    cylindrical f.
    2D f.
    3D f.
    DICOM-3 compatible digital
      computer f.
    hemodynamic f.

    slice f.
    tag image file f. (TIFF)
formation
    abscess f.
    batwing f.
    beak-like osteophyte f.
    bone f.
    bony callus f.
    brainstem reticular f.
    bulla f.
    bunion f.
    callosal f.
    callus f.
    cellule f.
    Chiari f.
    cloacal f.
    degenerative microcystic f.
    eddy f.
    enchondral bone f.
    endogenous callus f.
    excessive callus f.
    exuberant atheroma f.
    fistula f.
    geode f.
    glomeruloid f.
    Gothic arch f.
    hematoma f.
    heterotopic bone f.
    hippocampal f. (HF)
    honeycomb f.
    hook-like osteophyte f.
    image f.
    intracavitary clot f.
    lateral reticular f.
    marginal osteophyte f.
    mesencephalic reticular f.
    microcystic f.
    midbrain reticular f. (MRF)
    mural thrombus f.
    mycetoma f.
    myelin ball f.
    neointima f.
    new bone f.
    nipple-like osteophyte f.
    osteoid f.
    osteophyte f.
    palisade f.
    pannus f.
    paramedian pontine reticular f.
      (PPRF)
    periosteal new bone f.
    pontine reticular f.
    pseudoaneurysm f.
    pseudogland f.
    pseudointimal f.
    pseudopod f.
    reticular f. (RF)

reticular activating f.
ruffled border f.
saccular f.
scar f.
semilunar bone f.
sparsity of bone f.
spur f.
thrombin f.
thrombus f.
tophus f.
vesical stone f.

formatter
former
low-risk single-stone f.
formic aldehyde
formula, pl. **formulas, formulae**
autotransformer f.
bayesian f.
Boyd f.
cigarroa f.
configurational f.
fan-beam f.
Poisson-Pearson f.
projection f.
rapid dissolution f.
Forney syndrome
fornicatus
gyrus isthmus f.
forniceal rupture
fornicis
corpora f.
fornix, pl. **fornices**
f. cerebri
vaginal f.
forward
f. flow
f. heart failure
f. positioning of head
f. stroke volume (FSV)
f. subluxation
f. transport
f. velocity
forward-angle light scattering
fossa, pl. **fossae**
acetabular f.
adipose f.
amygdaloid f.
anconal f.
antecubital f.
anterior recess of ischiorectal f.
articular f.
axillary f.

biloma in the gallbladder f.
bony f.
cardiac f.
condylar f.
coronoid f.
cranial f.
crural f.
cubital f.
digastric f.
digital f.
duodenal f.
duodenojejunal f.
epigastric f.
femoral f.
floccular f.
gallbladder f.
glenoid f.
Gruber f.
hepatorenal f.
hyaloid f.
hypoglossal f.
hypophyseal f.
iliac f.
infraspinous f.
infrasternal f.
infratemporal f.
intercondylar f.
intercondyloid f.
interpeduncular f.
intratemporal f.
ischiorectal f.
Jobert f.
Landzert f.
malleolar f.
mandibular f.
meningioma of posterior f.
mesentericoparietal f.
middle cranial f.
f. navicularis
olecranon f.
f. ovalis
f. ovalis cordis
ovarian f.
paraduodenal f.
pararectal f.
paravesical f.
patellar f.
pituitary f.
popliteal f.
posterior cranial f.
posterior pituitary f.
pterygoid f.

F

NOTES

363

fossa *(continued)*
- pterygopalatine f.
- radial f.
- rectouterine f.
- retroappendiceal f.
- rhomboid f.
- f. of Rosenmüller
- sphenoidal f.
- subscapular f.
- supraclavicular f.
- Sylvius f.
- temporal f.
- Treitz f.
- uterovesical f.
- valve of navicular f.
- Waldeyer f.

four-chamber
- f.-c. apical view
- f.-c. echocardiography
- f.-c. hypertrophy
- f.-c. plane

fourchette

four-dimensional
- f.-d. image
- f.-d. imaging

four element phased array coil

four-fiber therapy

four-field
- f.-f. technique
- f.-f. x-ray dosimetry

four-head camera

four-hour delayed thallium imaging

Fourier
- F. analysis
- F. coefficient
- F. direct transformation imaging
- F. discrete transformation
- F. domain
- F. imaging technique
- F. multislice modified KWE direct imaging
- F. optical theory
- F. pulsatility index
- F. transfer
- F. transform (FT)
- F. transformation reconstruction
- F. transformation zeugmatography
- F. transform imaging
- F. transform infrared spectroscopy
- F. transform NMR spectrometry
- F. transform Raman spectroscopy
- F. two-dimensional imaging
- F. two-dimensional projection reconstruction

Fourier-acquired
- F.-a. steady state (FAST)
- F.-a. steady state technique

Fourier-encoded

Fourmentin thoracic index

four-part fracture

four-phase bone scintigraphy

four-quadrant bar pattern

four-slice acquisition

fourth
- f. branchial arch
- f. branchial cleft pouch
- f. compartment
- f. cranial nerve
- f. intercostal space
- f. parallel pelvic plane
- f. turbinated bone
- f. ventricle (V4)
- f. ventricle diverticulum
- f. ventricle tumor

four-valve-tube rectification

four-vessel
- f.-v. arteriography
- f.-v. cerebral angiography
- f.-v. multiple projection biplane angiography

four-view
- f.-v. chest x-ray
- f.-v. wrist survey

FOV
- field of view
- FOV imaging

fovea
- f. capitis
- f. centralis
- f. inferior

foveal fat pad

foveated chest

foveola
- gastric f.

Fowler position

FP
- frontopolar
- FP artery

FPA
- foot-progression angle

F-18-PET
- fluoride ion-positron emission tomography

FPI
- femoral pulsatility index

FPRNA
- first-pass radionuclide angiography

FR
- flattening ratio
- frequency encode

fractal
- f. analysis
- f. dimension (FD)

fractal-based method

fraction
absorbed f.
active emptying f.
area-length method for ejection f.
blood flow extraction f.
blunted ejection f.
branching f.
cardiac scintigraphy ejection f.
computed ejection f.
depressed ejection f.
digital ejection f.
Dodge method for ejection f.
drug f.
ejection f. (EF)
filtration f. (FF)
gallbladder ejection f.
global ejection f.
globally depressed ejection f.
interval ejection f.
Kennedy method for calculating
  ejection f.
left atrial active-emptying f.
left ventricular ejection f. (LVEF)
Maddahi method of calculating
  right ventricular ejection f.
MB f.
myofibril volume f.
one-third ejection f.
oxygen extraction f. (OEF)
packing f.
penetration f.
photopeak f.
radionuclide ejection f.
regional ejection f.
regional oxygen extraction f.
  (rOEF)
regurgitant f.
resting left ventricular ejection f.
right ventricular ejection f. (RVEF)
scatter f.
shortening f.
shunt f.
S-phase f.
systolic ejection f.
Teichholz ejection f.
thermodilution ejection f.
thickening f.
unattached f.
ventricular ejection f.
well-preserved ejection f.
fractional
f. anisotropy (FA)

f. area
f. encephalography
f. moving blood volume
f. moving blood volume estimation
f. myocardial shortening
f. pneumoencephalography
f. shortening (FS)
f. shortening of left ventricle
f. vascular volume
f. volumetric analysis
fractionated
f. dose-survival curve
f. external beam radiation therapy
f. radiation
f. stereotactic radiation therapy
f. stereotactic radiotherapy (FSR)
fractionation
accelerated f.
fast f.
quasi-accelerated f.
S-phase f.
fracture (fx) (*See* fracture-dislocation)
abduction f.
abduction-external rotation f.
acetabular posterior wall f.
acetabular rim f.
acute avulsion f.
acute on chronic f.
adduction f.
adult-type III TIE f.
agenetic f.
Aitken classification of
  epiphyseal f.
alveolar bone f.
anatomic f.
Anderson-Hutchins tibial f.
angulated f.
ankle mortise f.
anterior column f.
anteroinferior corner f.
anterolateral compression f.
anular f.
AO classification of ankle f.
apophyseal f.
arch f.
articular mass separation f.
articular pillar f.
artificial f.
Ashhurst-Bromer classification of
  ankle f.
f. of astragalus
Atkin epiphyseal f.

F

NOTES

fracture *(continued)*

atlas f.
atrophic f.
avulsion chip f.
avulsion stress f.
axial compression f.
axial load teardrop f.
axial load three-part, two-plane f.
axis f.
backfire f.
banana f.
Bankart f.
Barton f.
Barton-Smith f.
basal neck f.
basal skull f.
baseball finger f.
basicervical f.
basilar femoral neck f.
basilar skull f.
bayonet f.
beak f.
bedroom f.
bending f.
Bennett comminuted f.
bicondylar T-shaped f.
bicondylar Y-shaped f.
bicycle spoke f.
bimalleolar ankle f.
bipartite f.
f. blister
blow-in f.
blowout f.
bone f.
boot-top f.
Bosworth f.
both-bone f.
both-column f.
bowing f.
boxer's f.
Boyd type II f.
f. bracing
bronchial f.
bucket-handle pattern of f.
bucket-handle pelvic f.
buckle f.
bumper f.
bunk-bed f.
Burkhalter-Reyes method of
  phalangeal f.
burst f.
bursting f.
butterfly f.
buttonhole f.
calcaneal avulsion f.
calcaneal displaced f.
calcaneal stress f.

f. callus
f. callus loading
calvarial f.
capitate f.
capitellar f.
capitulum radiale humeri f.
carpal bone stress f.
carpal navicular f.
carpal scaphoid bone f.
carpometacarpal joint f.
cartwheel f.
Cedell f.
cemental f.
central f.
cephalomedullary nail f.
cerebral palsy pathological f.
cervical spine f.
cervicotrochanteric f.
Chance spinal f.
Chaput f.
Charcot f.
chauffeur's f.
chevron f.
childhood f.
chip f.
chisel f.
chondral f.
Chopart f.
circumferential f.
f. classification
clavicular birth f.
clay shoveler's f.
cleavage f.
f. in close apposition
closed f.
closed-break f.
coccyx f.
Colles f.
collicular f.
combined flexion-distraction injury
  and burst f.
combined radial-ulnar-humeral f.
comminuted bursting f.
comminuted intraarticular f.
comminuted teardrop f.
complete f.
complex simple f.
complicated f.
composite f.
compound comminuted f.
compound complex f.
compound skull f.
compression f.
condylar split f.
congenital f.
Conrad-Bugg trapping of soft
  tissue in ankle f.

contrecoup f.
coracoid f.
corner f.
coronoid process f.
cortical f.
Cotton ankle f.
crack f.
craniofacial dysjunction f.
crush f.
crushed eggshell f.
cuboid f.
cuneiform f.
dancer's f.
Danis-Weber f.
Darrach-Hughston-Milch f.
dashboard f.
decompression of f.
f. deformity
Denis classification of spinal f.
dens f.
dentate f.
depressed skull f.
depression-type intraarticular f.
de Quervain f.
derby hat f.
Desault f.
f. deviation
diacondylar f.
diametric pelvic f.
diaphyseal f.
f. diastasis
diastatic f.
dicondylar f.
die-punch f.
direct f.
dishpan f.
f. dislocation
displaced f.
distal femoral epiphyseal f.
distal humoral f.
distal radial f.
distraction of f.
dome f.
dorsal rim distal radial f.
dorsal wing f.
double f.
Dupuytren f.
Duverney f.
dye punch f.
dyscrasic f.
El-Ahwany classification of humeral
  supracondylar f.

elbow f.
elementary f.
Ellis technique for Barton f.
f. en coin
f. en rave
epicondylar f.
epiphyseal plate f.
epiphyseal slip f.
epiphyseal tibial f.
Essex-Lopresti joint depression f.
explosion f.
extension teardrop f. (ETF)
extraarticular f.
extracapsular f.
extraoctave f.
facial f.
fatigue f.
femoral intertrochanteric f.
femoral neck f.
femoral shaft f.
femoral supracondylar f.
fender f.
fetal f.
fibular f.
fighter's f.
finger f.
fishmouth f.
fissure f.
flake f.
flexion-burst f.
flexion-compression f.
flexion-distraction f.
flexion teardrop f.
floating arch f.
foot f.
forearm f.
four-part f.
f. fragment
f. fragment separation
f. frame
Freiberg f.
frontal f.
Frykman classification of hand f.
Frykman radial f.
fulcrum f.
Gaenslen f.
Galeazzi f.
f. gap
Gartland classification of humeral
  supracondylar f.
glenoid rim f.
Gosselin f.

F

NOTES

fracture *(continued)*

greater trochanteric femoral f.
greater tuberosity f.
greenstick f.
grenade thrower's f.
gross f.
growth plate f.
Guérin f.
gunshot f.
Gustilo-Anderson open clavicular f.
gutter f.
hairline f.
hamate tail f.
hand f.
hangman's f.
Hawkins classification of talar f.
head-splitting humeral f.
healing f.
heat f.
hemicondylar f.
hemitransverse f.
Henderson f.
Herbert scaphoid bone f.
Hermodsson f.
hickory-stick f.
Hill-Sachs posterolateral
  compression f.
hip f.
hockey-stick f.
Hoffa f.
Holstein-Lewis f.
hook of the hamate f.
hoop stress f.
horizontal maxillary f.
humeral condylar f.
humeral head-splitting f.
humeral physeal f.
humeral supracondylar f.
Hutchinson f.
hyperextension teardrop f.
hyperflexion teardrop f.
ice skater's f.
idiopathic f.
ileofemoral wing f.
impacted subcapital f.
impacted valgus f.
implant f.
impression f.
incomplete f.
indented f.
indirect f.
inflammatory f.
infraction f.
insufficiency f.
intercondylar femoral f.
intercondylar humeral f.
intercondylar tibial f.

internally fixed f.
interperiosteal f.
intertrochanteric four-part f.
intraarticular calcaneal f.
intraarticular proximal tibial f.
intracapsular femoral neck f.
intraoperative f.
intraperiosteal f.
intrauterine f.
inverted-Y f.
ipsilateral femoral neck f.
ipsilateral femoral shaft f.
irreducible f.
ischioacetabular f.
isolated hook f.
Jefferson burst f.
Jefferson cervical f.
Jeffery classification of radial f.
joint depression f.
Jones classification of diaphyseal f.
juvenile Tillaux f.
juxtaarticular f.
juxtacortical f.
Kapandji radical f.
Key-Conwell classification of
  pelvic f.
Kilfoyle classification of
  condylar f.
knee f.
Kocher f.
labral and anterior inferior glenoid
  rim f.
LaGrange classification of humeral
  supracondylar f.
laryngeal f.
lateral column calcaneal f.
lateral condylar humeral f.
laterally displaced f.
lateral malleolar f.
lateral tibial plateau f.
lateral wedge f.
Laugier f.
lead pipe f.
Le Fort fibular f.
Le Fort I, II, III f.
Le Fort mandibular f.
Le Fort-Wagstaffe f.
lesser trochanteric f.
f. line
linear skull f.
f. line of consolidation
Lisfranc f.
local compression f.
local decompression f.
long bone f.
longitudinal tibial fatigue f.
long oblique f.

loose f.
lorry driver's f.
low-energy f.
low-T humerus f.
lumbar spine f.
lunate f.
Maisonneuve fibular f.
malar f.
Malgaigne pelvic f.
malleolar f.
mallet f.
malunited f.
mandibular f.
march f.
marginal f.
Mathews classification of
  olecranon f.
maxillary f.
maxillofacial f.
medial column calcaneal f.
medial epicondyle f.
medial malleolar f.
metacarpal f.
metaphyseal f.
metatarsal f.
midfacial f.
midfoot f.
midshaft f.
midwaist scaphoid f.
Milch classification of humeral f.
milkman's f.
minimally displaced f.
Moberg-Gedda f.
molar tooth f.
monomalleolar f.
Monteggia f.
Montercaux f.
Moore f.
Mouchet f.
multangular ridge f.
multipartite f.
multiple f.'s
multiray f.
nasal f.
nasomaxillary f.
nasoorbital f.
navicular body f.
navicular hand f.
naviculocapitate f.
f. of necessity
neck f.
Neer classification of shoulder f.

Neer-Horowitz classification of
  humeral f.
neoplastic f.
neural arch f.
neurogenic f.
neuropathic f.
neurotrophic f.
Newman classification of radial
  neck and head f.
nightstick f.
nonarticular radial head f.
noncontiguous f.
nondisplaced f.
nonphyseal f.
nonrotational burst f.
f. nonunion
nonunited f.
nutcracker f.
oblique spiral f.
O'Brien classification of radial f.
obturator avulsion f.
occipital condyle f.
occult osseous f.
odontoid condyle f.
Ogden classification of
  epiphyseal f.
olecranon tip f.
one-part f.
open f.
open-book f.
open-break f.
orbital blowout f.
orbital floor f.
osteochondral slice f.
osteoporotic compression f.
overlapping f.
Pais f.
panfacial f.
Papavasiliou classification of
  olecranon f.
paratrooper's f.
parry f.
pars interarticularis f.
patellar sleeve f.
pathologic f.
pedicle f.
pelvic insufficiency f.
pelvic rim f.
pelvic ring f.
pelvic straddle f.
penetrating f.
perforating f.

F

NOTES

fracture *(continued)*

periarticular f.
peripheral f.
periprosthetic f.
peritrochanteric f.
pertrochanteric f.
phalangeal diaphyseal f.
physeal plate f.
Piedmont f.
pillar f.
pillion f.
pillow f.
pilon ankle f.
ping-pong f.
pisiform f.
plafond f.
plaque f.
plastic bowing f.
plateau tibia f.
pond f.
Posada f.
posterior arch f.
posterior element f.
posterior ring f.
posterior wall f.
postirradiation f.
Pott ankle f.
pressure f.
pronation-abduction f.
pronation-eversion f.
proximal femoral f.
proximal humeral f.
proximal tibial metaphyseal f.
pseudo-Jefferson f.
puncture f.
pyramidal f.
Quinby classification of pelvic f.
radial head f.
radial neck f.
radial styloid f.
radiographically occult f.
f. reduction
resecting f.
retrodisplaced f.
reverse Barton f.
reverse Colles f.
reverse Monteggia f.
reverse Segond f.
rib f.
ring f.
ring-disrupting f.
Rolando f.
rotational burst f.
Ruedi-Allgower tibial plafond f.
f. running length of bone
sacral insufficiency f. (SIF)
sacroiliac f.

Sakellarides classification of
calcaneal f.
Salter-Harris classification of
epiphyseal f. 1–5
sandbagging f.
scaphoid hand f.
scottie dog f.
seatbelt f.
secondary f.
segmental bronchus f.
Segond f.
Seinsheimer classification of
femoral f.
senile subcapital f.
sentinel f.
SER-IV f.
shaft f.
shear f.
Shepherd f.
short oblique f.
sideswipe f.
silver fork f.
f. simple and depressed full-scale
deflection (FSD)
simple skull f.
f. site
skier's f.
Skillern f.
skull f.
sleeve f.
slice f.
Smith f.
snowboarder f.
sphenoid bone f.
spinal f.
spinous process f.
spiral oblique f.
splintered f.
split compression f.
split-heel f.
splitting f.
spontaneous f.
sprain f.
Springer f.
sprinter's f.
stability of f.
stable f.
stairstep f.
stellate skull f.
stellate undepressed f.
stepoff of f.
Stieda f.
straddle f.
strain f.
stress f.
strut f.
subcapital f.

subchondral f.
subcutaneous f.
subperiosteal f.
subtrochanteric f.
supination-adduction f.
supination-eversion f.
supination, external rotation type
  IV f.
supracondylar femoral f.
supracondylar humeral f.
supracondylar Y-shaped f.
surgical neck f.
T f.
talar avulsion f.
talar dome f.
talar neck f.
talar osteochondral f.
T condylar f.
teacup f.
teardrop burst f.
teardrop-shaped flexion-
  compression f.
temporal bone f.
tension f.
testis f.
thalamic f.
thoracic spine f.
thoracolumbar burst f.
thoracolumbar junction f.
three-part f.
f. threshold
through-and-through f.
thrower's f.
Thurston Holland f.
tibial bending f.
tibial condyle f.
tibial diaphyseal f.
tibial open f.
tibial pilon f.
tibial plafond f.
tibial plateau f.
tibial shaft f.
tibial triplane f.
tibial tuberosity f.
tibiofibular f.
Tillaux f.
Tillaux-Chaput f.
Tillaux-Kleiger f.
toddler's f.
tongue f.
tongue-type intraarticular f.
torsion f.

torus f.
total condylar depression f.
trabecular f.
tracheal f.
traction f.
trampoline f.
transcaphoid f.
transcapitate f.
transcervical femoral f.
transchondral talar f.
transcondylar f.
transepiphyseal f.
transhamate f.
transiliac f.
transsacral f.
transscaphoid dislocation f.
transtriquetral f.
transverse comminuted f.
transversely oriented endplate
  compression f.
transverse maxillary f.
transverse process f.
trapezium f.
traversing the f.
trimalleolar ankle f.
triplane f.
tripod f.
triquetral f.
trophic f.
T-shaped f.
tuft f.
two-part f.
ulnar f.
uncinate process f.
undepressed skull f.
undisplaced f.
unicondylar f.
unilateral f.
unimalleolar f.
unstable f.
ununited f.
upper thoracic spine f.
vertebral body f.
vertebral compression f.
vertebral plana f.
vertebral wedge compression f.
vertical shear f.
volar rim distal radial f.
Volkmann f.
V-shaped f.
Wagstaffe f.
Walther f.

F

NOTES

fracture *(continued)*
Weber C f.
wedge compression f.
wedge flexion-compression f.
western boot in open f.
willow f.
Wilson f.
Y f.
Y-T f.
ZMC f.
f. zone
zygomaticomaxillary f.

fractured
f. bronchus
f. kidney
f. vertebra

fracture-dislocation
Chopart f.-d.
cuneiform f.-d.
Galeazzi f.-d.
intermediate cuneiform f.-d.
Monteggia f.-d.
pedicolaminar f.-d.
perilunate f.-d.
posterior f.-d.

fragility
acquired f.

fragment
alignment of fracture f.
anteroinferior triangular f.
apoptic nuclear f.
articular f.
avulsed fracture f.
bayoneting of fracture f.
bone f.
butterfly fracture f.
calcified free f.
capital f.
chondral f.
cortical f.
f. depression
disk f.
displaced fracture f.
displaced osteochondral f.
extruded disk f.
fracture f.
free disk f.
free-floating cartilaginous f.
iodine-125-labeled f.
jagged bone f.
Klenow f.
loose osteochondral f.
LymphoScan Tc99m-labeled murine
 antibody f.
major fracture f.
malunion of fracture f.
metallic f.

nonunion of fracture f.
osteochondral fracture f.
overriding of fracture f.
retropulsed fracture f.
smear f.
Spengler f.
^{99m}Tc-labeled anti-E-selectin Fab f.
technetium-99m antimyosin Fab f.
torsion of fracture f.
union of fracture f.

fragmentation
f. of apophysis
f. of barium
collagen f.
electrohydraulic f.
meniscal f.
f. myocarditis
f. therapy
unilateral f.

fragmented
f. mucosal fold
f. pattern

fragmentocytosis

frame
adduction f.
adiabatic demagnetization in the
 rotating f. (ADRF)
Balkan fracture f.
Brown-Roberts-Wells f.
CT/MRI-compatible stereotactic
 head f.
fracture f.
imaging compatible stereotactic
 coordinate f.
ISAH stereotactic immobilization f.
Komai stereotactic head f.
Laitinen stereotactic head f.
Leksell D-shaped stereotactic f.
Leksell-Elekta stereotactic f.
Malcolm-Lynn C-RXF cervical
 retractor f.
pelvic fracture f.
radiolucent spine f.
Radionics CRW stereotactic head f.
Reichert-Mundinger-Fischer
 stereotactic f.
robotics-controlled stereotactic f.
stereotactic head f.
stereotactic localization f.
Stryker f.

frameless
f. stereotactic digital subtraction
 angiography
f. stereotactic guidance
f. stereotaxy

framing
exact f.

frank
>f. breech presentation
>f. cerebral gumma
>f. cirrhosis
>f. congestive heart failure
>f. disk herniation
>f. dislocation
>f. hemorrhage
>f. lesion
>f. necrosis
>f. pulmonary edema
>f. rupture
>F. vectorcardiography

Fränkel
>crossbar symptom of F.
>F. spinal cord injury classification
>F. typhus nodule
>F. white line

Frankfort
>F. horizontal plane
>F. line
>F. mandibular incisor angle
>F. mandibular notch

Franklin changer
Frank-Starling
>F.-S. curve
>F.-S. mechanism
>F.-S. relation

Franseen needle
fraternal twin
Fraunhofer zone
frayed
>f. disk
>f. metaphysis

frayed-string appearance
fraying
>chondromalacia with surface f.

Frederick-Miller tube
free
>f. abdominal fluid
>f. air passage
>f. air under diaphragm
>f. band of colon
>f. band of colon band
>f. body
>f. body calcification
>f. cul-de-sac fluid
>f. disk fragment
>f. electron
>f. fatty acid (FFA)
>f. fibered coil
>f. flap of cartilage

>f. gas bubble
>f. hepatic venography
>f. induction decay signal
>f. induction delay curve
>f. intraperitoneal air
>f. intraperitoneal gas
>f. knee joint
>f. pericardial space
>f. peritoneal air
>f. peritoneal fluid
>f. pleural effusion
>f. precession
>f. radical
>f. reflux
>f. subphrenic gas

FreeDop Doppler monitor
free-floating
>f.-f. cartilaginous fragment
>f.-f. loop of bowel
>f.-f. meniscus
>f.-f. retinaculum

FreeFlo stent-graft
free-fragment disk herniation
freehand
>f. interventional sonography
>f. interventional ultrasound
>f. probe

free-induction decay (FID)
freely movable mass
Freeman calcaneal fracture classification
free-radical dosimetry
freestanding workstation
Freiberg
>F. disease
>F. fracture
>F. infraction

French
>8-F. guiding catheter
>9-F. guiding catheter
>1.8-F. microcatheter
>2.1-F. microcatheter
>F. T-tube

frenulum of valve
frequency (f)
>f. analysis
>angular f.
>f. component
>disappearance f.
>f. domain
>f. domain image
>f. domain imaging (FDI)
>Doppler shift f.

F

NOTES

frequency *(continued)*
  f. encode (FE, FR)
  f. encoding
  energy f.
  f. estimation
  extremely low f. (ELF)
  false f.
  halftone f.
  f. intensification
  Larmor f.
  Nyquist f.
  offset f.
  pelvic mass f.
  precessional f.
  pulse repetition f.
  f. range
  raster f.
  resonance f.
  resonant f.
  respiratory f.
  rotational f.
  f. separation
  spatial f.
  f. spectrum
  f. synthesizer
  vibration f.
frequency-encoding gradient
frequency-related peak
frequency-selective
  f.-s. fat saturation
  f.-s. inversion
  f.-s. pulse
Fresnel
  F. zone
  F. zone plate
Freund anomaly
friability
friable
  f. anulus
  f. artery
  f. lesion
  f. mass
  f. mucosa
  f. thickened degenerated intima
  f. tumor
  f. vegetation
  f. wall
Fricke
  F. dosimetry
  F. gel
friction neuritis
Friedländer pneumonia
Friedman
  F. method
  F. position
Friedreich
  F. ataxic cardiomyopathy

  F. disease
  F. foot
  F. phenomenon
  F. sign
Fries score for rheumatoid arthritis classification
fringe
  f. field
  moiré f.
  f. of osteophyte
  f. skeleton extraction
  synovial f.
  f. thinning algorithm
FRODO technique
Froesch foramen
frogleg
  f. lateral projection
  f. lateral view
  f. position
  f. view of the hips
frog-like appearance
Frohse
  arcade of F.
  F. ligamentous arcade
Froment sign
frond
  villous f.
frond-like
  f.-l. appearance
  f.-l. filling defect
frondy lesion
frontal
  f. abscess
  f. arteriovenous malformation
  f. artery
  f. biauricular plane
  f. bone
  f. bossing
  f. bossing of Parrot
  f. cephalometric radiograph
  f. cortex
  f. crest
  f. defect
  f. eminence
  f. fontanelle
  f. foramen
  f. fracture
  f. gyrus
  f. horn
  f. horn asymmetry
  f. horn index (FHI)
  f. horn of lateral ventricle
  f. horn Mickey Mouse ear
  f. lobe
  f. lobe contusion
  f. lobe dysfunction
  f. lobe infarct

f. lobe lesion
f. lobe sign
f. lobe tumor
f. nerve
f. notch
f. plane loop
f. plane vectorcardiography
f. plate
f. pole
f. process
f. section
f. sinus
f. sinus mucocele
f. sulcus
f. suture
f. vein
f. view

frontalis
apertura sinus f.
f. sinus

frontier ulcer
frontocentral convexity
frontoethmoidal
f. encephalocele
f. giant cell reparative granuloma
f. mucocele
f. suture

frontolacrimal suture
frontomalar suture
frontomaxillary suture
frontomental diameter
frontonasal
f. duct
f. dysplasia
f. dysplasia malformation complex
f. process
f. suture

frontooccipital diameter
frontoorbital advancement
frontoparallel plane
frontoparietal
f. arteriovenous malformation
ascending f. (ASFP)
f. parasagittal cortex
f. suture

frontopolar (FP)
f. artery
f. point

frontopontine tract
frontosphenoidal
f. encephalocele
f. process

frontosphenoid suture
frontotemporal (FT)
f. atrophy
f. muscle
f. tract

frontozygomatic suture
Frostberg sign
frosted liver
frothy colonic mucosa
Frouin
quadrangulation of F.

frozen
f. hemithorax
f. joint
f. pelvis
f. shoulder

FRP
functional refractory period

Frykman
F. classification of hand fracture
F. distal radius fracture classification
F. radial fracture

FS
focal spot
fractional shortening
FS burst MR imaging

FS-069 sterile injectable sonography contrast agent
F-scan
FSCR
flexible surface-coil-type resonator

FSD
Fletcher-Suit-Delclos
focus-skin distance
fracture simple and depressed full-scale deflection

FSE
fast spin-echo

FSE-T2 with fat suppression
FSPGR
fast spoiled gradient-recalled echo
FSPGR technique

FSR
fractionated stereotactic radiotherapy

FSU
functional subunit

FSV
forward stroke volume

FT
Fourier transform
frontotemporal

F

NOTES

FTA
    femorotibial angle
FTC
    fibulotalocalcaneal
        FTC ligament
FTHA
    ^{18}F-fluoro-6-thia-heptadecanoic acid
Fuchs
    F. adenoma
    F. odontoid view
    F. position
    F. principle
fucose
Fuerbringer
fugax
    amaurosis f.
    coxitis f.
Fuji
    F. AC2 storage phosphor computed
    radiology system
    F. FCR9000 computed radiology
    system
    F. QA 771 workstation
Fukuyama
    F. congenital muscular disease
    (FCMD)
    F. congenital muscular dystrophy
    (FCMD)
fulcrum
    f. fracture
    joint f.
fulguration
    nephroscopic f.
full
    f. bladder ultrasound
    f. cervical spine series (FCS series,
    FCS series)
    f. cervical spine view
    f. column view
    f. lateral position
    f. length view
    f. ring scanner
    f. scan with interpolation
    f. scan with interpolation projection
    f. thickness
    f. three-dimensional mode
    f. width at half maximum
    (FWHM)
full-blown cardiac tamponade
full-body
    f.-b. CT scan
    f.-b. echo-planar system imager
full-column
    f.-c. barium enema
    f.-c. technique
full-energy peak efficiency
Fuller earth pneumoconiosis

full-field
    f.-f. digital mammography
    f.-f. digital mammography system
full-intensity needle
full-line scanning
full-scan
    f.-s. method
    f.-s. projection
full-thickness
    f.-t. button of aortic wall
    f.-t. Carrel button
    f.-t. chondral lesion
    f.-t. cleft
    f.-t. infarct
    f.-t. tear
full-to-empty VAD mode
full-volume loop spirometry
full-wave
    f.-w. rectification
    f.-w. rectifier
full-width
    f.-w. at half-maximum
    f.-w. at half-maximum of
    lorentzian curve
fully automated segmentation algorithm
fulminant
    f. cerebral lymphoma
    f. colitis
    f. fasciitis
    f. hepatic failure (FHF)
    f. hydrocephalus
    f. pulmonary edema
    f. tuberculosis
fulminating ulcerative colitis
function
    abnormal tubular f.
    atrial-phase volumetric f.
    autocorrelation f.
    brain f.
    bundle f.
    cerebrospinal fluid shunt f.
    commissural f.
    compromised ventricular f.
    contractile f.
    depressed right ventricular
        contractile f.
    edge response f. (ERF)
    excitation f.
    exercise LV f.
    fetal renal f.
    gaussian f.
    global ventricular f.
    gonadal f.
    harmonic f.
    impaired renal f.
    leaflet f.
    left atrial f.

left ventricular systolic/diastolic f.
left ventricular systolic pump f.
line spread f. (LSF)
midbrain f.
mitochondrial f.
modulation transfer f. (MTF)
myocardial contractile f.
nasal mucociliary clearance f.
pharyngoesophageal f.
point-spread f. (PSF)
rectosigmoid f.
regional left ventricular f.
regional myocardial f.
reserve cardiac f.
rest left ventricular f.
rest right ventricular f.
right and left atrial phasic
  volumetric f.
right ventricular systolic/diastolic f.
Shepp-Logan filter f.
sinusoid reference f.
stress perfusion and rest f.
swallowing f.
systolic f.
time correlation f. (TCF)
tubular f.
velocity distribution f. (F(v))
ventricular contractility f. (VCF)
volumetric f.
Zeeman hamiltonian f.

functional
  f. abnormality
  f. aerobic impairment
  f. anatomical mapping
  f. bladder capacity
  f. bowel syndrome
  f. brain imaging
  f. classification of congestive heart
    failure
  f. correlation
  f. data
  f. disorder
  f. diverticulum
  f. hyperlordosis
  f. hypertrophy
  f. ileus
  f. immaturity of bowel
  f. magnetic resonance angiography
    (fMRA)
  f. magnetic resonance imaging
    (fMRI)
  f. map

  f. marrow
  f. MRI
  f. MR tube
  f. neuroimaging
  f. ovarian cyst
  f. paraganglioma
  f. radioiodine scintigraphy
  f. reentry
  f. refractory period (FRP)
  f. residual capacity
  f. scoliosis
  f. sphincter
  f. spin-echo imaging
  f. subunit (FSU)
  f. units of spine
  f. ureteral obstruction
functioning
  f. neoplasm
  f. nodule
  f. pituitary adenoma
FuncTool software
fundal
  f. leiomyoma
  f. placenta
fundamental Doppler mode
fundi (*pl. of* fundus)
fundic-antral junction
fundic metaphysis
fundiform ligament
fundoplication
  Nissen f.
fundus, pl. **fundi**
  f. of aneurysm
  aneurysmal f.
  bald gastric f.
  bladder f.
  gallbladder f.
  gastric f.
  saddle-shaped uterine f.
  stomach f.
  urinary bladder f.
  f. uteri
  uterine f.
  vaginal f.
Funduscein injection
fungal
  f. hypha
  f. infection
  f. meningitis
  f. plaque
  f. pneumonia
fungating tumor

F

NOTES

fungoides
tumor d'emblee mycosis f.
funic souffle
funicular
f. inguinal hernia
funiculus
f. cuneatus
f. dorsalis
f. gracilis
funnel
f. chest
f. chest deformity
funnel-like cardiomegaly
funnel-shaped
f.-s. cavity
f.-s. pelvis
furifosmin
furosemide imaging agent
furrier's lung
fused
f. ankle
f. colliculi
f. commissure
f. fontanelle
f. image technology
f. kidney
f. papillary muscle
f. physis
f. rib
f. vertebrae
fusiform
f. aneurysm
f. bronchiectasis
f. defect
f. dilatation
f. enlargement of the optic nerve
f. gyrus
f. high signal intensity
f. malformation
f. narrowing of artery
f. shadow
f. swelling
f. syrinx
f. thickening
f. widening of duct
fusion
ankle f.
anterior cervical f. (ACF)
anterior spine f. (ASF)
atlantooccipital f.
bony f.
calcaneotibial f.
carpometacarpal f.
cervical interbody f.

cervical spine f.
cervicooccipital f.
chevron f.
f. of cusp
f. defect
diaphyseal-epiphyseal f.
extraarticular hip f.
facet f.
Hatcher-Smith cervical f.
image f.
f. inhibitor (FI)
interbody f.
interphalangeal f.
intersegmental laminar f.
interspinous process f.
intraarticular knee f.
joint f.
Kellogg-Speed lumbar spinal f.
metatarsocuneiform joint f.
metatarsophalangeal joint f.
multilevel f.
nuclear f.
occipitoatlantoaxial f.
occipitocervical f.
pantalar f.
f. plate
posterior lumbar interbody f.
(PLIF)
posterior spine f. (PSF)
sacroiliac joint f.
spinal f.
splenogonadal f.
talar body f.
talocrural f.
tibiocalcaneal f.
tibiotalocalcaneal f.
transfibular f.
two-stage f.
vertebral f.
fuzzy
f. clustering algorithm
f. echo
f. logic contrast correction
f. set theory
F(v)
velocity distribution function
FWHM
full width at half maximum
fx
fracture
FX-wire
Cragg FX-w.
FZ
focal zone

γ (*var. of* gamma)
G
  gauss
GA
  gestational age
Ga
  gallium
⁶⁷Ga
  gallium-67
    ⁶⁷Ga bone scan
    ⁶⁷Ga citrate scintigraphy
    ⁶⁷Ga examination
    ⁶⁷Ga excretion
    ⁶⁷Ga GABA uptake carrier
    ⁶⁷Ga higher dose
    ⁶⁷Ga SPECT
    ⁶⁷Ga uptake
⁶⁸Ga, Ga-68
  gallium-68
GABA
  gamma-aminobutyric acid
gadobenate dimeglumine (Gd-BOPTA)
gadobenic acid imaging agent
gadobutrol imaging agent
gadodiamide (Gd-DTPA-BMA)
  g. imaging agent
gadofosveset
  g. trisodium
  g. trisodium imaging agent
gadolinium (Gd)
  g. chelate
  g. chelate imaging agent
  g. complex
  g. diethylenetriamine pentaacetic acid (Gd-DTPA)
  g. diethylenetriamine pentaacetic acid bismethylamide (Gd-DTPA-BMA)
  g. enhancement
  g. Gd 159 hydroxycitrate
  intraarticular g.
  g. iron
  g. oxide imaging agent
  g. oxyorthosilicate
  g. scan
  g. sucralfate
  g. tetraazacyclododecanetetraacetic acid (Gd-DOTA)
  g. texaphyrin (Gd-Tex)
gadolinium-153
gadolinium-based contrast agent
gadolinium-DTPA
gadolinium-enhanced
  g.-e. elliptically reordered three-dimensional MR angiography
  g.-e. MR imaging
  g.-e. subtracted MR angiography, 3D
  g.-e. T1-weighted axial image
  g.-e. T1-weighted MRI image
  g.-e. venographic technique
Gadolite oral suspension contrast agent
gadopentate dimeglumine
gadopentetate
  g. contrast agent
  g. dimeglumine (Gd-DTPA)
  g. dimeglumine imaging agent
gadopentetic acid
gadopentolate-polylysine
gadoterate
  g. meglumine
  g. meglumine imaging agent
gadoterate-enhanced digital subtraction angiography
gadoteridol (Gd-DO3A, Gd-HP-DO3A)
  g. imaging agent
gadoversetamide imaging agent
gadoxetate
gadoxetic acid (Gd-EOB-DTPA)
Gaeltec catheter-tip pressure transducer
Gaenslen
  G. fracture
  G. sign
Gaertner (*var. of* Gärtner)
Gaffney joint
GAG
  glycosaminoglycan
gain
  accelerated phase g.
  brightness g.
  color g.
  Doppler g.
  phase g.
  power g.
  quadratic phase g.
  time-compensated g.
  time-varied g. (TVG)
Gaisböck syndrome
galactocele
galactogram
  mammary g.
galactography
galactophoritis
galactophorous
  g. canal
  g. duct
galactose-based suspension

G

galactose contrast medium
galactosyl human serum albumin (GSA)
Galassi arachnoidal cyst classification
galeal extension of tumor
Galeazzi
G. fracture
G. fracture-dislocation
G. sign
Galen
great cerebral vein of G.
G. Scan scanner
G. teleradiology system
G. vein aneurysm
G. ventricle
galenic venous malformation
Galileo intravascular radiotherapy
system
gallbladder
g. adenoma
g. agenesis
g. bed
bilobed g.
blunt trauma g.
body of g.
g. calculus
g. carcinoma
comet-tail artifact g.
contracted g.
Courvoisier g.
dilated g.
displaced g.
distended g.
g. diverticulum
double g.
g. duplication
ectopic g.
edematous g.
g. ejection fraction
g. empyema
enlarged g.
fetal g.
g. filling defect
fish-scale g.
floating g.
folded fundus of g.
g. fossa
g. function test
g. fundus
gangrene of the g.
g. gravel
hourglass constriction of g.
g. hydrops
g. hypoplasia
g. ileus
g. imaging
g. infundibulum
g. lift

mobile g.
multiseptated g.
neck of g.
nonfunctioning g.
nonvisualization of g.
pearl necklace g.
g. perforation
g. polyp
porcelain g.
porcine g.
g. septation
g. series (GBS)
shrunken g.
g. size
g. sludge
small g.
S-shaped g.
stasis g.
g. stone
strawberry g.
g. study
thick-walled g.
thin-walled g.
g. torsion
g. trauma
g. ultrasound
g. villus
g. wall
g. wall abscess
wandering g.
gallbladder-gastrointestinal series
gallbladder-vena cava line
gall duct
galli
ala cristae g.
crista g.
Gallie H-graft
gallium (Ga)
g. bone scintigraphy
g. Ga 57 citrate
g. imaging agent
g. lung imaging
g. lung scintigraphy
radioactive g.
g. scan
g. tumor scintigraphy
g. uptake
gallium-67 (^{67}Ga)
g. citrate
g. tumor imaging agent
gallium-68 (^{68}Ga, Ga-68)
gallium-67-avid lesion
gallium-67-labeled leukocyte
gallium-arsenide laser
gallium-avid thymic hyperplasia
gallium titrate Ga 67
gallium-transferrin complex

gallstone
> asymptomatic g.
> cholesterol g.
> dissolution of g.
> ectopic intraluminal g.
> faceted g.
> floating g.
> gas-containing g.
> g. ileus
> innocent g.
> intraluminal g.
> laminated g.
> layered g.
> layering of g.'s
> g. migration
> mulberry g.
> opacifying g.
> radiolucent g.
> retained g.
> silent g.
> solitary g.
> symptomatic g.

GALT
> gut-associated lymphoid tissue

galvanometer

gamekeeper's thumb

gamma, γ
> g. aminobutyrate
> g. camera
> g. cascade
> g. emission
> g. emitter
> g. encephalography
> g. factor
> g. film
> gamma tocopherol (gamma-T, γ-T)
> g. heating
> g. knife radiosurgery
> g. nail
> g. photon
> g. probe
> g. probe radiation detector
> g. radiation
> g. radiography
> g. ray
> g. ray attenuation
> g. ray capture
> g. ray counter
> g. ray level indicator
> g. ray scanner
> g. ray spectrometer
> g. ray spectrum

> g. ray therapy
> g. scan
> g. scanning
> g. signal
> g. spectrometric analysis
> g. transverse colon loop
> g. unit
> g. well counter

gamma-aminobutyric acid (GABA)

gamma-detection probe

gamma-emitting isotope

gammagram

gamma-irradiated plug

GammaPlan software

gamma-ribbon radiation therapy

gamma-T
> gamma tocopherol

Gammex
> G. RBA-5 radiation beam analyzer
> G. RMI DAP meter
> G. RMI scanner

gammography
> cerebral g.

gammopathy
> monoclonal g.

Gamna-Gandy
> G.-G. nodule

Gamna nodule

Gandy-Nanta disease

ganglia (*pl. of* ganglion)

gangliocytic paraganglioma

gangliocytoma
> dysplastic cerebellar g.

ganglioglioma
> cystic g.
> infantile g.
> intracerebral g.

gangliolysis
> radiofrequency g.

ganglioma
> intracerebral g.

ganglion, pl. ganglia
> aberrant g.
> acousticofacial g.
> Acrel g.
> aorticorenal g.
> auditory g.
> auricular g.
> basal g.
> calcification of basal g.
> cardiac g.
> carotid g.

NOTES

G

ganglion *(continued)*
    celiac g.
    g. cell tumor
    cervical g.
    cervicothoracic g.
    coccygeal g.
    g. cyst
    diffuse g.
    dorsal root g. (DRG)
    gasserian g.
    geniculate g.
    intraarticular g.
    intraosseous g.
    ipsilateral basal g.
    otic g.
    palmar g.
    paravertebral g.
    periosteal g.
    petrosal g.
    posterior root g.
    prevertebral g.
    pterygopalatine g.
    radiocapitellar joint g.
    g. ridge
    Scarpa g.
    sensory g.
    soft tissue g.
    sphenopalatine g.
    spinal g.
    submandibular g.
    superior cervical g.
    superior mesenteric g.
    sympathetic g.
    trigeminal g.
    uterine cervical g.
    vestibular g.
    Wrisberg cardiac g.
ganglioneuroblastoma (GNB)
ganglioneurofibromatosis
    mucosal g.
ganglioneuroma
    adrenal g.
ganglionic
    g. canal
    g. crest
gangrene
    bowel g.
    g. of the gallbladder
    g. of lung
gangrenous
    g. cholecystitis
    g. emphysema
    g. pneumonia
    g. tissue
Gans
    incisura dextra of G.
Ganser diverticulum

gantry
    g. angulation
    CT scan g.
    fixed g.
    g. rotation
    g. rotation time
    g. tilt
gantry-free gamma camera
Gantzer muscle
Ganz formula for coronary sinus flow
gap
    air g.
    artifactual g.
    Bochdalek g.
    g. calculation
    distraction g.
    fracture g.
    intersection g.
    interslice g.
Garden
    G. angle
    G. femoral neck fracture
        classification
garden spade deformity
GARD lesion
Gardner bone syndrome
Gardray dosimeter
Garland
    G. triad
    G. triangle
GARP
    globally optimized alternating phase
        rectangular pulse
Garré
    G. disease
    G. sclerosing osteomyelitis
Garren-Edwards gastric bubble
Garth view
Gartland classification of humeral
    supracondylar fracture
Gartner
    G. canal
    G. duct
    G. duct cyst
Gärtner, Gaertner
    G. phenomenon
gas, pl. **gases**
    abdominal g.
    accumulation of g.
    aneurysmal wall g.
    g. angiocardiography
    bile duct g.
    biliary tree g.
    bowel g.
    g. bubble
    g. collection
    coursing of g.

crescent of g.
g. CT cisternography
g. cupula
g. density line
displacement of bowel g.
g. entrapment
extraluminal g.
free intraperitoneal g.
free subphrenic g.
g. gangrene of uterus
genital tract g.
hyperpolarized ^{129}Xe g.
g. insufflation
intestinal g.
intrahepatic portal vein g.
intramural g.
intrauterine g. (IUG)
g. mediastinography
natural neon g.
noble g.
overlying bowel g.
g. pattern
paucity of bowel g.
portal venous g.
pulmonary g.
radioactive g.
radiopaque xenon g.
scrotal g.
small bowel g.
soft tissue g.
subcutaneous tissue g.
superimposed bowel g.
g. target
g. trapping
urinary tract g.
g. ventilation imaging
g. ventilation study
g. volume
gas-bloat syndrome
gas-containing
g.-c. gallstone
g.-c. stone
gaseous
g. cholecystitis
g. dilatation
g. distention
g. drainage
g. injection
g. mediastinography
g. oxygen artifact
gases (*pl. of* gas)
gas-filled detector

gas-fluid level
gasless abdomen
gasless laparoscopic system
gas-liquid phase chromatography (GLPC)
gasserian ganglion
Gasser syndrome
gastric
g. adenopapillomatosis
g. air bubble
g. antral erosion
g. antrum
g. artery
g. atony
g. atrophy
g. bypass surgery (GBS)
g. canal
g. capacity
g. cardia
g. channel
g. chloroma
g. content
g. decompression
g. diaphragm
g. dilatation
g. distention
g. diverticulum
g. duplication cyst
g. emphysema
g. emptying (GE)
g. emptying imaging
g. emptying scan
g. fistula
g. fold
g. fold enlargement
g. foveola
g. fundus
g. groove
g. hamartomatous polyposis
g. hemic calculus
g. hemorrhage
g. hernia
g. heterotopia
g. hypersecretion
g. impression
g. insufficiency
g. interposition
g. intramural-extramucosal lesion
g. leiomyoma
g. leiomyosarcoma
g. lumen
g. lymphatic follicle

G

NOTES

gastric *(continued)*
  g. lymph node
  g. lymphoma
  g. metastasis
  g. motor disorder
  g. mucosa imaging
  g. mucosal pattern
  g. narrowing
  g. omentum
  g. outlet obstruction
  g. outline
  g. parietography
  g. partition
  g. pit
  g. plexus
  g. pneumatosis
  g. polyp
  g. pool
  g. pouch
  g. pseudolymphoma
  g. pull-through procedure
  g. pull-up
  g. reflux of bile
  g. remnant
  g. remnant carcinoma
  g. remnant filling defect
  g. residual
  g. rugae
  g. sclerosis
  g. secretion
  g. sling fiber
  g. stump
  g. stump carcinoma
  g. surface
  g. thumbprinting
  g. transit time
  g. transposition
  g. ulcer (GU)
  g. varix
  g. vein
  g. volvulus
  g. wall deformity
  g. wall thickening
  g. window
  g. xanthoma
gastrica
  area g.
gastricae
gastrinoma
  duodenal g.
gastritis
  acute erosive g. (AEG)
  antral g.
  atrophic g.
  bile reflux g.
  chronic g.
  cirrhotic g.

  corrosive g.
  emphysematous g.
  erosive g.
  follicular g.
  giant hypertrophic g.
  hypertrophic g.
  necrotizing g.
  phlegmonous g.
  pseudomembranous radiation g.
  radiation g.
  reflux g.
  zonal g.
gastrocardiac syndrome
gastrocnemial ridge
gastrocnemius
  g. bursa
  g. muscle
  g. tendon
gastrocnemius-semimembranosus bursa
gastrocnemius-soleus
  g.-s. complex
  g.-s. contracture
  g.-s. junction
  g.-s. muscle group
  g.-s. tendon
gastrocolic
  g. fistula
  g. ligament
  g. omentum
gastrocutaneous fistula
gastrodiaphragmatic ligament
gastroduodenal
  g. artery
  g. artery complex
  g. fistula
  g. junction
  g. lumen
  g. lymph node
  g. mucosal prolapse
  g. orifice
gastroduodenitis
gastroduodenoscopy
gastroduodenostomy
  Billroth I, II g.
gastroenteritis
  cobblestone appearance
  eosinophilic g.
gastroenterocolitis
gastroenteroptosis
gastroenterostomy
  percutaneous g.
  g. stoma
gastroepiploic
  g. arcade
  g. artery
  g. lymph node

g. vein
g. vessel
gastroesophageal (GE)
g. angle
g. collateral
g. incompetence
g. junction
g. junction carcinoma
g. junction stricture
g. junction tumor
g. reflux (GER)
g. reflux disease (GERD)
g. variceal plexus
Gastrografin
G. enema
G. imaging agent
G. swallow
gastrohepatic
g. bare area
g. ligament
g. ligament node
g. omentum
gastrointestinal (GI)
g. adverse effect
g. bleeding
g. carcinoma
g. cyst
g. endoscopic ultrasound
g. endoscopy
g. fetal anomaly
g. fistula
g. lymphoma
g. malignancy
g. motility imaging
g. plaque
g. protein loss test
g. renal transplant hemorrhage
g. scintigraphy
g. series
g. stoma
g. stromal tumor (GIST)
g. tract
g. tract adenocarcinoma
g. tract obstruction
g. ulcer
upper g. (UGI)
gastrointestinal-associated lymphoid tissue
gastrojejunal mucosal prolapse
gastrojejunocolic fistula

gastrojejunostomy
Billroth I, II g.
g. catheter
gastrolienal ligament
GastroMARK oral imaging agent
gastroomental lymph node
gastropancreatic
g. fold
g. ligament
gastroparesis
diabetic g.
gastropathy
hyperplastic g.
gastropexy
gastrophrenic ligament
gastroplasty (GP)
Gastroport
gastroptosis
gastrorenal shunt
gastroschisis
gastroscope
Olympus XQ230 g.
Pentax ELLB 6000, 6500 ultrasound g.
gastroscopy
gastrosphincteric pressure gradient
gastrosplenic
g. ligament
g. omentum
gastrostomy
g. catheter
CT-guided percutaneous endoscopic g.
percutaneous endoscopic g. (PEG)
radiologic percutaneous g.
g. tube
gastrotomy
Gastroview imaging agent
Gastrovist imaging agent
gate array
gated
g. blood pool angiography
g. blood pool scan
g. blood pool scintigraphy
g. blood pool ventriculogram
g. cardiac blood pool imaging
g. CT scanner
g. 3D reconstruction
g. equilibrium blood pool scanning
g. equilibrium cardiac blood pool imaging

G

NOTES

385

gated *(continued)*
  g. equilibrium radionuclide angiography
  g. exercise examination
  g. image
  g. imaging study
  g. inflow magnetic resonance
  g. inflow technique
  g. magnetic resonance imaging
  g. nuclear angiography
  g. nuclear ventriculogram
  g. planar study
  g. radionuclide angiocardiography
  g. radionuclide ventriculogram
  g. RNA
  g. single-photon emission-computed tomography (GSPECT)
  g. SPECT myocardial perfusion imaging
  g. stress myocardial perfusion (GMP)
  g. stress myocardial perfusion slice
  g. system
  g. view

gating
  cardiac g.
  diastolic g.
  echocardiographic g.
  electrocardiographic g.
  heartbeat g.
  peripheral pulse g.
  respiratory g.
  retrospective respiratory g.
  spirometric g.
  systolic g.

Gaucher
  G. disease
  G. splenomegaly

gauge
  18-g. percutaneous access needle
  x-ray thickness g.

Ga-67 uptake
gauss (G)
gaussian
  g. curve
  g. distribution
  g. dose-volume histogram
  g. function
  g. line
  g. line saturation
  g. line shape
  g. mode profile laser beam
  g. noise
  g. radiofrequency
  g. smoothing

Gavard muscle

Gawkins talar neck fracture classification
Gaynor-Hart method
GB-GI series
GBM
  glioblastoma multiforme
  glomerular basement membrane
GBS
  gallbladder series
  gastric bypass surgery
GCH
  giant cavernous hemangioma
GCVF
  great cardiac vein flow
Gd
  gadolinium
Gd-153 imaging agent
Gd-BOPTA
  gadobenate dimeglumine
    Gd-BOPTA imaging agent
      gadobenate dimeglumine
Gd-BOPTA/Dimeg imaging agent
GDC
  Guglielmi detachable coil
    3/6-cm 3D GDC
    2/3-cm UltraSoft GDC
    2/6-cm UltraSoft GDC
    UltraSoft GDC
GDC-18
GDC-10 soft coil
Gd-DO3A
  gadoteridol
Gd-DOTA
  gadolinium tetraazacyclododecanetetraacetic acid
    Gd-DOTA contrast medium
Gd-DOTA-enhanced subtraction dynamic study
Gd-DTPA
  gadolinium diethylenetriamine pentaacetic acid
  gadopentetate dimeglumine
    Gd-DTPA PGTM imaging agent
    Gd-DTPA radioisotope
    Gd-DTPA with mannitol contrast agent
Gd-DTPA-BMA
  gadodiamide
  gadolinium diethylenetriamine pentaacetic acid bismethylamide
Gd-DTPA-enhanced turbo FLASH MRI
Gd-DTPA-labeled
    Gd-DTPA-l. albumin
    Gd-DTPA-l. dextran
Gd-enhanced imaging agent
Gd-EOB-DTPA
  gadoxetic acid

Gd-EOB-DTPA imaging agent
Gd-FMPSPGR imaging
Gd-HIDA chelate
Gd-HP-DO3A
  gadoteridol
  Gd-HP-DO3A imaging agent
Gd-Tex
  gadolinium texaphyrin
GE
  gastric emptying
  gastroesophageal
  General Electric
    GE 400AC/T;STAR II camera
    GE Advance PET scanner
    GE Advantage 1.5T imager
    GE CT Advantage scanner
    GE CT HiSpeed Advantage CT
     system
    GE CTI 9800 scanner
    GE CTI single detector scanner
    GE CT Max scanner
    GE CT Pace scanner
    GE CT/T 8800 scanner
    GE CT/T7 scanner
    GE 8800 CT/T scanner
    GE detector
    GE Echospeed 1.5T whole-body
     MR imager
    GE gamma camera
    GE Genesis CT scanner
    GE GN 500-MHz scanner
    GE GN300 7.05-T/89-mm bore
     multinuclear spectrometer
    GE 9800 high-resolution CT
     scanner
    GE HiSpeed Advantage helical CT
     scanner
    GE HiSpeed single detector
     scanner
    GE Lightspeed CT scanner
    GE MR Max scanner
    GE MR Signa scanner
    GE MR Vectra scanner
    GE Neurocam camera
    GE NMR spectrometer
    GE Omega 500-MHz scanner
    GE Pace CT scanner
    GE proton head coil probe
    GE QE 300-MHz scanner
    GE Senographe 2000D digital
     mammography system
    GE Signa 5.4 Genesis MR imager

    GE Signa 5.5 Horizon EchoSpeed
     MR imager
    GE Signa 4.7 MRI scanner
    GE Signa 1.5-T magnet
    GE Signa 1.5-T scanner
    GE Signa 5.2 with SR-230 three-
     axis EPI gradient upgrade scanner
    GE single-detector SPECT-capable
     camera
    GE SPECT
    GE Spiral CT scanner
    GE Starcam single-crystal
     tomographic scintillation camera
    GE Vectra MR scanner
    GE Viewer software
    GE Voluson 730 4D ultrasound
     system
Gee-Herter disease
Gee-Thaysen disease
GEG bubble
Gehan methodology
Geiger counter
Geiger-Müller
  G.-M. counter
  G.-M. detector
  G.-M. survey meter
  G.-M. tube
gel
  acoustic g.
  Fricke g.
  methylcellulose g.
  ultrasound g.
gelatin
  g. phantom
  g. sponge
  g. sponge particle
  g. sponge powder
gelatinous
  g. ascites
  g. brain pseudocyst
  g. carcinoma
  g. debris
  g. hematoma
  g. tissue
gemellary pregnancy
gemellus, pl. **gemelli**
gemistocytic astrocytoma
gemistocytoma
general
  g. pattern matching
General Electric (GE)

G

NOTES

generalisata
platyspondyly g.
generalized
g. angiofollicular lymph node hyperplasia
g. arteriosclerosis
g. breast hyperplasia
g. calcinosis
g. capillary leak
g. compensation for resonance offset and pulse length errors (GROPE)
g. cortical hyperostosis
g. cortical hyperstasis
g. emphysema
g. hamartomatosis
g. hazy opacity
g. increased liver echogenicity
g. interferography using spin echoes and stimulated echoes (GINSEST)
g. lymphadenopathy syndrome
g. lymphangiectasis
g. nephrographic (GNG)
g. osteoarthritis
g. pulmonary edema
g. seizure
generation
g. echo
g. 6 integrated radiotherapy system
generator
anterior current (AC) g.
carbon dioxide g.
g. characteristic
CO_2 g.
deuterium-tritium g.
direct current g.
^{166}Dy g.
dysprosium-holmium (^{166}Dy-166Ho) in vivo g.
electric g.
electrostatic g.
extraction g.
high-voltage g.
^{166}Ho in vivo g.
molybdenum-99 g.
molybdenum-technetium g.
nuclide g.
pizoelectric g.
polyphase g.
6-pulse, 3-phase g.
12-pulse, 3-phase g.
radiofrequency g.
radionuclide g.
resonance g.
spark gap g.
Super 50 CP high-voltage g.

supervoltage g.
g. system
technetium-99m g.
three-phase g.
Triphasix g.
Van de Graaf g.
video signal g.
VNUS radiofrequency g.
waveform g.
x-ray g.
generator-produced ^{188}Re
Genesis 2000 carbon dioxide laser
Genesys camera
gene therapy
genetically
g. homogeneous
g. significant dose
genial
g. tubercle
g. tubercle of mandible
geniculate
g. body
g. branch
g. ganglion
g. ganglion schwannoma
geniculocalcarine tract
geniculocalvarium
geniculum
genioglossus muscle
genital
g. blood pooling
g. canal
g. carcinoma
g. duct
g. eminence
g. fold
g. groove
g. ligament
g. ridge
g. tract
g. tract calcification
g. tract embryology
g. tract gas
g. visualization
genitalia
ambiguous g.
genitalis
genitoinguinal ligament
genitourinary (GU)
g. adverse effect
g. anomaly
g. carcinoma
g. fistula
g. injury
g. reflex
g. rhabdomyosarcoma
g. tract

g. tract trauma
g. tuberculosis
Gennari
G. band
line of G.
G. stripe
genome
mitochondrial g.
nuclear g.
genomic instability
GentleLASE Plus laser system
gentle lordosis
genu, pl. **genua**
g. of corpus callosum
g. recurvatum
g. valgum deformity
g. varum
g. varum deformity
geode formation
geographic
g. bone destruction
g. follicle
g. lesion
g. pattern
g. skull
geography
brain g.
geometric
g. blur
g. distortion
g. distribution
g. efficiency
g. optimization algorithm
g. unsharpness
geometrical efficiency
geometry
beam g.
coronary vessel g.
g. factor
Golay g.
scintillation camera g.
slice g.
geophagia artifact
GER
gastroesophageal reflux
GERD
gastroesophageal reflux disease
Gerdy
G. fontanelle
G. interatrial loop
G. interauricular loop

G. ligament
G. tubercle
Gerhardt
G. sign
G. triangle
geriatric
g. configuration
g. feature
germanate-68
bismuth g.
German horizontal plane
germanium
high-purity g. (HPGe)
germinal
g. bleed matrix
g. pole
germinolysis
subependymal g.
germinoma
intracranial g.
mediastinum g.
multicentric g.
pineal g.
suprasellar hemorrhagic g.
Gerota
G. capsule
G. fascia
G. method
Gerstmann-Straussler-Scheinker disease
Gerstmann syndrome
Gertzbein seatbelt injury classification
gestation
extrauterine g.
intrauterine g.
multiple g.
nonviable g.
normal g.
triplet g.
gestational
g. age (GA)
g. choriocarcinoma
g. sac (GS)
g. sac abnormality
g. sac diameter
g. sac measurement
g. trophoblastic disease (GTD)
g. trophoblastic neoplasm
g. trophoblastic tumor
g. week
geyser sign
GFR
glomerular filtration rate

G

NOTES

GGO
> ground-glass opacification

GHA
> glucoheptonate acid

GHCH
> giant hepatic cavernous hemangioma

Ghon
> G. complex
> G. focus
> G. node
> G. primary lesion
> G. tubercle

Ghon-Sachs complex

ghost
> g. image
> red cell g.
> g. reduction by equalized acquisition triplets (GREAT)
> separation of g.'s

ghosting artifact

GHz
> gigahertz

GI
> gastrointestinal
> GI bleed
> Imagent GI
> GI tract
> GI tract amyloidosis
> GI tract endometriosis
> GI tract lipoma
> GI tract lymphoid hyperplasia
> GI tract mastocytosis
> GI tract scintigraphy
> GI tract · trauma
> GI tract tuberculosis

Gianotti-Crosti syndrome

giant
> g. brain aneurysm
> g. breast fibroadenoma
> g. bullous emphysema
> g. cavernous hemangioma (GCH)
> g. cell adenocarcinoma
> g. cell astrocytoma
> g. cell carcinoma of thyroid gland
> g. cell fibroma
> g. cell interstitial pneumonia (GIP)
> g. cell lung carcinoma
> g. cell pneumonitis
> g. cell reparative granuloma
> g. cell sarcoma
> g. cell tumor
> g. cell tumor of the tendon sheath
> g. cell-type MFH
> g. colon
> g. duodenal ulcer
> g. follicle lymphoma
> g. follicular hyperplasia

> g. gastric fold
> g. hepatic cavernous hemangioma (GHCH)
> g. hyperplasia lymph node
> g. hypertrophic gastritis
> g. left atrium
> g. myofibroblastoma
> g. osteoid osteoma
> g. peptic ulcer
> g. saccular aneurysm
> g. serpentine aneurysm
> g. sigmoid diverticulum
> g. villous adenoma

Gianturco
> G. occlusion coil
> G. stent
> G. wool-tufted wire coil

Gianturco-Rosch biliary stent
Gianturco-Roubin FlexStent
Gianturco-Wallace-Anderson coil
Gianturco-Wallace-Chuang coil
gibbous deformity
Gibbs
> G. random field
> G. sampling

Gibbs-Donnan law
gibbus
> thoracic g.

Gierke respiratory bundle
gigahertz (GHz)
gigantiform cementoma
gigantism
> cerebral g.
> extremity g.
> focal g.

Gilchrist disease
gill
> g. arch skeleton
> g. cleft

Gillette
> G. joint
> G. suspensory ligament

Gillies suture
Gill lesion
Gimbernat ligament
gingival
> g. carcinoma
> g. crest
> g. curvature
> g. septum
> g. space

gingivitis
> erosive g.
> necrotizing ulcerative g. (NUG)

gingivobuccal groove
gingivodental ligament
gingivolabial groove

GINSEST
　　generalized interferography using spin
　　echoes and stimulated echoes
GIP
　　giant cell interstitial pneumonia
girdle
　　limb g.
　　pectoral g.
　　pelvic g.
　　shoulder g.
Girout method
girth
　　abdominal g.
Gissane
　　G. angle
　　crucial angle of G.
GIST
　　gastrointestinal stromal tumor
Given
　　G. diagnostic imaging system
　　G. imaging capsule/M2A capsule
GK-SRS boost
glabella
glabelloalveolar line
glabellomeatal line
glabrous cirrhosis
gladiolus
gladiomanubrial
GLAD lesion
gland
　　absorbent g.
　　accessory thyroid g.
　　admaxillary g.
　　adrenal g.
　　Albarran g.
　　alveolar g.
　　anteprostatic g.
　　aortic g.
　　apical g.
　　apocrine sweat g.
　　aporic g.
　　arterial g.
　　arteriococcygeal g.
　　axillary sweat g.
　　Bartholin g.
　　Bruch g.
　　Brunner g.
　　bulbocavernous g.
　　bulbourethral g.
　　calcified pineal g.
　　carotid g.
　　coccygeal g.

　　Duverney g.
　　ectopic g.
　　endocrine g.
　　enlarged thyroid g.
　　enlargement of lacrimal g.
　　enlargement of parotid g.
　　giant cell carcinoma of thyroid g.
　　globate g.
　　glomiform g.
　　haversian g.
　　hilar g.
　　interscapular g.
　　lacrimal g.
　　Littré g.
　　lymph g.
　　mammary g.
　　Montgomery g.
　　mucosal g.
　　ovary g.
　　pancreas g.
　　paramediastinal g.
　　paraurethral g.
　　parotid g.
　　periurethral g.
　　pineal g.
　　pituitary g.
　　prostate g.
　　salivary g.
　　Stensen g.
　　subaortic g.
　　sublingual g.
　　submandibular g.
　　submaxillary g.
　　substernal thyroid g.
　　supernumerary parathyroid g.
　　suprarenal g.
　　testicular g.
　　thymus g.
　　thyroid g.
　　urethral g.
　　Virchow g.
　　g. volume
　　Wharton g.
glandular
　　g. carcinoma
　　g. dose
　　g. proliferation
glandulography
glans
　　g. carcinoma
　　g. penis

NOTES

G

glare
  imaging chain veiling g.
  scatter and veiling g. (SVG)
  veiling g.
glaserian fissure
Glasgow
  G. outcome scale
  G. sign
glass
  g. blower's emphysema
  g. eye artifact
  fiberoptic video g.'s
  hepatic test of G.
  quartz g.
  g. ray
  g. tract detector
  vita g.
Glasscock-Jackson classification
glaze consistency
Glazunov tumor
Gleason grade
Glénard disease
Glenn
  G. anastomosis
  G. procedure
  G. shunt
glenohumeral
  g. dislocation
  g. instability
  g. joint
  g. ligament
glenoid
  g. articular rim disruption lesion
  g. cavity
  g. fossa
  g. labral ovoid body
  g. labrum
  g. labrum capsule
  g. labrum injury
  g. ligament
  g. ovoid mass
  g. point
  g. process
  g. rim
  g. rim fracture
  g. surface
glenolabral articular disruption lesion
Gliadel wafer
glial
  g. brain tumor
  g. limiting membrane
  g. nodule
  g. rest
  g. scarring
  g. stranding
  g. tumor calcification
GliaSite radiotherapy system

Glidecath
  RADIFOCUS G.
Glidecath
Glidecatheter
Glidewire
Glidewire
  angled G.
  0.035-inch G.
  long taper stiff shaft G.
  RADIFOCUS G.
gliding joint
glioblast
glioblastoma
  butterfly g.
  multicentric g.
  g. multiforme (GBM)
glioma
  anaplastic cerebral g.
  brainstem g.
  butterfly g.
  cerebral g.
  cystic g.
  high-grade g.
  hypothalamic g.
  intracranial g.
  low-grade g.
  malignant g.
  multicentric malignant g.
  nonanaplastic g.
  optic nerve g.
  pontine g.
  pontocerebellar g.
  recurrent high-grade malignant g.
  rolandoparietal g.
  spinal cord g.
  supratentorial g.
  tectal g.
  temporooccipital g.
  thalamic g.
gliomatosis
  arachnoidal g.
  g. cerebri
  g. peritonei
glioneural hamartoma
gliosarcoma
  cerebellar g.
gliosis
  astrocytic g.
  ischemic g.
  progressive subcortical g.
  reactive g.
  secondary g.
  g. of sylvian aqueduct
gliosis-induced microcystic degeneration
Glisson capsule
global
  g. cavus

g. cerebral hypoperfusion
g. cerebral ischemia
g. cortical defect
g. ejection fraction
g. hypokinesis
g. hypometabolism
g. intracranial blood flow
g. myocardial ischemia
g. phantogeusia
g. renal enlargement
g. tissue loss
g. ventricular function
g. wall motion abnormality
globally
g. depressed ejection fraction
g. optimized alternating phase
rectangular pulse (GARP)
globate gland
globe
optic g.
globe-orbit relationship
globoid heart
globular
g. cardiomegaly
g. chest
g. configuration
g. meningioma
g. tumor
g. valve
globulin
technetium-99m human immune g.
globulus, pl. **globuli**
Glofil-125 injection
glomangioma
glomera
choroid g.
glomerular
g. basement membrane (GBM)
g. filtration
g. filtration agent
g. filtration rate (GFR)
g. lesion
g. mesangial cell
g. nephritis
glomeruli (*pl. of* glomerulus)
glomerulocytoma
glomeruloid formation
glomerulonephritis
acute g.
chronic g.
crescent-shaped g.
membranous g.

necrotizing g.
proliferative g.
segmental necrotizing g.
glomerulopathy
glomerulosa
zona g.
glomerulosclerosis
glomerulus, pl. **glomeruli**
glomiform gland
glomus
body g.
g. body tumor
g. bone tumor
g. choroideum
g. of choroid plexus
g. jugulare
g. jugulare tumor
g. jugulotympanicum tumor
g. neck tumor
g. tympanicum
g. vagale
glomus-type arteriovenous malformation
glossoepiglottic
g. fold
g. ligament
glossopalatine fold
glossopharyngeal nerve
glottic
g. carcinoma
g. larynx
g. narrowing
glottis, pl. **glottides**
glove
optic g.
g. phenomenon
g. phenomenon artifact
radiation-attenuating surgical g.'s
gloved-finger
g.-f. shadow
g.-f. sign
glow
cathode g.
g. curve
g. modular tube
GLP7 film
GLPC
gas-liquid phase chromatography
glucagon imaging agent
glucagonoma
glucamoma
glucarate imaging agent
glucaric acid-labeled contrast medium

G

NOTES

gluceptate
    techneScan G.

glucoheptanoate
    ^{99m}Tc g.

glucoheptonate acid (GHA)

glucose
    g. water

glucosyl-galactosyl-pyridinoline
    urinary g.-g.-p.

glue
    Technovit 7210 VLC contact g.

glutamate spectroscopy

glutaric aciduria type I, II

gluteal
    g. bonnet
    g. fold
    g. line
    g. lymph node
    g. ridge

gluten-sensitive enteropathy

gluteus
    g. maximus
    g. medius
    g. minimus

glycerolphosphorylcholine (GPC)

glycogenic acanthosis

glycogen-rich pancreatic cystadenoma

glycol
    isoosmotic polyethylene g.
    polyethylene g. (PEG)

glycolysis
    enhanced g.

glycoprotein-secreting adenoma

glycosaminoglycan (GAG)

G-M counter

GMN
    gradient moment nulling

GMP
    gated stress myocardial perfusion

GMR
    gradient moment reduction
    gradient moment rephasing
    gradient motion rephasing

GM segmentation

gnathic osteosarcoma

GNB
    ganglioneuroblastoma

GNG
    generalized nephrographic
    GNG phase imaging

goblet-shaped pelvis

Godwin tumor

Goethe bone

goggles
    Avotec MR-compatible liquid
    crystal display g.

goiter
    adenomatous g.
    Basedow g.
    colloid g.
    congenital g.
    cystic g.
    diffuse toxic g.
    diving g.
    exophthalmic g.
    familial g.
    fetal g.
    fibrous g.
    intrathoracic g.
    iodide g.
    iodine-deficiency g.
    lingual g.
    multinodular g.
    nodular g.
    parenchymous g.
    retrotracheal g.
    retrovascular g.
    simple g.
    substernal g.
    suffocative g.
    thyroid g.
    toxic multinodular g.
    toxic nodular g.
    vascular g.
    wandering g.

goitrogen

Golay
    G. coil
    G. geometry

gold (Au)
    g. AU-198 imaging agent
    g. radioactive source
    g. seed

Goldblatt kidney

Golden
    motility of G.
    S sign of G.

Goldenhar syndrome

gold-195m
    g. radionuclide
    g. tracer

gold-marked stent

Goldsmith & Woodburne classification

Goldthwait sign

golfer's elbow

Golgi tendon

GoLYTELY bowel preparation

gonad
    indifferent g.

gonadal
    g. artery
    g. dose
    g. dysgenesis

g. function
g. neoplasm
g. shielding
g. stroma
g. stromal tumor
g. vein reflux
g. venography
g. venous ectasia
gonadoblastoma
gonadotroph cell adenoma
gonadotropin
chorionic g.
gonadotropin-secreting adenoma
gonecystic calculus
gonial angle
goniometer
Sceratti g.
gonion
g. gradient coil
g. gradient magnetic field
gonion-gnathion plane
Goodpasture syndrome
goose foot tendon
gooseneck
g. concept
g. outflow tract deformity
g. shape
Gordon-Brostrom single-contrast arthrography
Gordon sign
Gore 1.5T torso array MRI surface coil
Gorham disease
Gorlin
G. formula for aortic valve area
G. formula for mitral valve area
G. method for measuring cardiac output
G. syndrome
Gorlin-Goltz syndrome
Gosling pulsatility index
Gosselin fracture
Gosset
spiral band of G.
gossypiboma
Gothic arch formation
Gottron sign
gouge defect
Gould
G. electromagnetic flowmeter
G. Statham pressure transducer

gout
articular g.
tophaceous g.
gouty
g. arthritis
g. arthropathy
g. node
g. tophus
Gowers
G. bundle
G. bundle in cerebellum
G. column
G. fasciculus
G. sign
GP
gastroplasty
GPC
glycerolphosphorylcholine
g-probe localization
graafian
g. follicle
g. vesicle
Grace method of ratio of metatarsal length
gracile
g. bone
g. habitus
gracilis
funiculus g.
g. tendon
gradation
subtle g.
grade
Fisher g. 1–4
Gleason g.
histologic g.
Hunt and Hess aneurysm g. I–V
Hunt and Kosnik (grade 0–V) aneurysmal g.
g. 0, 2 insonation condition
osteoarthritis g.
placental g.
Scharff-Bloom-Richardson g.
g. 1–3 signal intensity
subarachnoid hemorrhage Fisher g. 1–4
thrombolysis in brain ischemia flow g.
graded
g. compression sonography
g. compression sonography technique

NOTES

G

graded *(continued)*
g. compression ultrasound
g. infusion
gradient
g. acquisition
g. across valve
g. amplifier
g. amplitude
aortic outflow g.
aortic valve g. (AVG)
aortic valve peak instantaneous g.
aortic valve pressure g.
arteriovenous pressure g.
atrioventricular g.
balanced g.
biliary-duodenal pressure g.
bipolar g.
brain-core g.
g. compensation
conjugate g.
coronary perfusion g.
dephasing g.
3D Fourier transform gradient-echo
  sequence with spoiler g.
diastolic g.
diffusion g.
diffusion-sensitizing g.
discontinuous density g.
g. drive current
duodenobiliary pressure g.
g. echo MR with magnetization
  transfer
echo-speed g.
electric field g. (EFG)
elevated g.
g. encoding
end-diastolic aortic-left ventricular
  pressure g.
fast PC cine MR sequence with
  echo-planar g.
Ficoll g.
field g.
flow-encoding g.
frequency-encoding g.
gastrosphincteric pressure g.
hepatic venous pressure g.
holosystolic g.
imaging g.
instantaneous g.
left ventricular outflow pressure g.
linear g.
g. linearity
magnetic field g. (MFG)
g. magnetic field
maximal estimated g.
mean mitral valve g.
mean systolic g.

mitral valve g.
g. moment nulling (GMN)
g. moment reduction (GMR)
g. moment rephasing (GMR)
motion-nulling g.
g. motion rephasing (GMR)
negligible pressure g.
nonisotropic g.
oscillating g.
osmotic g.
outflow tract g.
peak diastolic g.
peak instantaneous g.
peak pressure g.
peak right ventricular-right atrial
  systolic g.
peak systolic g.
peak-to-peak pressure g.
perfusion g.
phase-encoding g.
portosystemic g.
potential g.
Power Trak 6000 g.
pressure-flow g.
pre-TIPS g.
pullback pressure g.
pulmonary artery to right ventricle
  diastolic g.
pulmonary outflow g.
pulmonic valve g.
g. pulse
g. pump
readout g.
rephasing g.
residual g.
g. reversal
right ventricular to main pulmonary
  artery pressure g.
g. scheme
g. selection
sensitizing g.
g. sheet coil
g. slew rate
slice select g. (SS)
g.-spin echo
Stejskal-Tanner g.
stenotic g.
g. subsystem in MRI
subvalvular g.
g. switching noise
g. system
systolic g.
thoracoabdominal g.
g. timing
transaortic systolic g.
transjugular intrahepatic
  portosystemic shunt g.

translesional g.
transmitral g.
transpulmonic g.
transstenotic g.
transtricuspid valve diastolic g.
transvalvular pressure g.
tricuspid valve g.
twister g.
velocity g.
ventricular g.
voxel g.
washout g.
g. waveform
X g.
Z g.

gradient-echo
g.-e. axial image
g.-e. cine technique
g.-e. coronal image
g.-e. flow imaging
g.-e. imaging sequence
g.-e. method
g.-e. MR imaging
g.-e. phase imaging
g.-e. pulse sequence
g.-e. recall technique
g.-e. sequence imaging
spin lock g.-e. (SL-GRE)
g.-e. three-dimensional Fourier
transform volume imaging
g.-e. T2-weighted image

gradient-encoded image
gradient-induced phase dispersion
gradient-recalled
g.-r. acquisition in the steady state
(GRASS)
g.-r. echo
g.-r. echo image
spoiled g.-r.

gradient-refocused echo (GRE)
gradient-to-noise imaging
grading
gradually tapering border
Graf
G. alpha angle
G. hip dysplasia classification
G. method

graft
aorticorenal g.
aortic tube g.
aortofemoral bypass g. (AFBG)
aortoiliac bypass g.

aortoplasty with patch g.
arterial bypass g.
autogenous vein bypass g.
autologous patch g.
autologous vein g.
axillary-axillary bypass g.
axillary-brachial bypass g.
axillary-femoral bypass g.
axillary-femorofemoral bypass g.
axillobifemoral bypass g.
bifemoral g.
bifurcation g.
bilateral myocutaneous g.
bone g.
bone-tendon-bone g.
Brescia-Cimino g.
bypass g.
carotid-carotid venous bypass g.
Cloward bone g.
coronary artery bypass g. (CABG)
Corvita endoluminal g.
custom-fabricated g.
Dacron-covered stent g.
disk-shaped bone g.
donor g.
dowel-shaped bone g.
elephant trunk g.
endarterectomy g.
endoleak g.
endoscopic coronary artery
bypass g. (E-CABG)
endothelialized vascular g.
endovascular aortic g.
esophageal g.
expanded polytetrafluoroethylene g.
expanded polytetrafluoroethylene-
covered nitinol TIPS stent g.
extracavitary infected g.
extracavitary prosthetic arterial g.
g. failure
femorocrural g.
femorodistal popliteal bypass g.
femorofemoral bypass g.
femoroperoneal in situ vein
bypass g.
femoropopliteal bypass g.
femoropopliteal Gore-Tex g.
femorotibial bypass g.
H g.
hepatorenal saphenous vein
bypass g.
iliac-renal bypass g.

NOTES

G

graft *(continued)*
 ilioprofunda bypass g.
 infected thrombosed g.
 infrainguinal arterial bypass g.
 infrainguinal vein bypass g.
 inlay g.
 interbody bone g.
 internal thoracic artery g.
 interposition g.
 g. interstice
 intraabdominal arterial bypass g.
 ITA g.
 JOSTENT Peripheral Stent G.
 jump vein g.
 g. kinking
 limb of bifurcation g.
 loop g.
 modular stent g.
 occluded g.
 g. occlusion
 onlay g.
 osseous g.
 g. patency
 patency of vein g.
 pedicle bone g.
 polytetrafluoroethylene g.
 prosthetic femoral distal g.
 g. revascularization
 reversed vein g.
 g. roof impingement
 saphenous vein bypass g.
 Sauvage filamentous velour g.
 sequence bypass g.
 g. shrinkage
 in situ g.
 Smith-Robinson bone g.
 snake g.
 splenorenal arterial bypass g.
 g. stenosis
 straight interposition g.
 subcutaneous arterial bypass g.
 suprailiac aortic mesenteric g.
 synthetic vascular bypass g.
 Talent stent g.
 transluminally placed stented g.
 Varivas loop g.
 vascular bypass g.
 vein g.
 venous bypass g.
 venous interposition g.
 VIATORR transjugular intrahepatic
  portosystemic shunt stent g.
graft-enteric
 g.-e. erosion
 g.-e. fistula
graft-versus-host disease of the liver
graft-versus-tumor response

Graham-Burford-Mayer syndrome
Graham-Cole cholecystogram
grain handler's lung
graininess
 film g.
grand mal seizure
Granger
 G. line
 G. projection
 G. view
Grantham femur fracture classification
granular
 g. breast-cell myoblastoma
 g. calcification
 g. infiltrate
 g. kidney
 g. leukocyte
 g. lung-cell myoblastoma
 g. microcalcification
 g. opacity
 g. sella-cell myoblastoma
granularis
 ependymitis g.
granulation
 arachnoid g.
 Bayle g.
 pacchionian g.
 g. stenosis
 g. tissue
granule
 neurosecretory g.
granulocyte
 antibody-labeled circulating g.
 g. colony stimulating factor
granulocytic sarcoma
granuloma, pl. **granulomata**
 actinic g.
 apical g.
 aspergillotic g.
 beryllium g.
 bilharzial g.
 button sequestrum eosinophilic g.
 calcified cysticercus g.
 caseating g.
 ceroid gallbladder g.
 cholesterol ear g.
 coalescent g.
 cysticercus g.
 dental g.
 eosinophilic g.
 epithelioid g.
 extravascular g.
 foreign body g.
 frontoethmoidal giant cell
  reparative g.
 giant cell reparative g.
 Hodgkin g.

hyalinizing g.
inguinal g.
lethal midline g.
lung g.
malarial g.
mediastinal g.
midline g.
Mignon g.
miliary g.
noncaseating g.
paracoccidioidal g.
periapical g.
plasma cell g.
pseudopyogenic g.
pulmonary hyalinizing g.
reparative giant cell g.
reticulohistiocytic g.
rheumatic g.
root end g.
sarcoid g.
sea urchin g.
silicone g.
sperm g.
stellate g.
swimming pool g.
thorium dioxide g.
tracheal g.
tuberculous g.
umbilical g.
xanthomatous g.
zirconium g.

granulomatosis
allergic g.
bronchocentric g.
lipoid g.
lymphomatoid g.
mainline g.
Miescher g.
necrotizing respiratory g.
organic g.
pulmonary mainline g.
Wegener g.

granulomatous
g. brain abscess
g. enterocolitis
g. ileitis
g. inflammation of bronchus
g. lesion of sinus
g. lymphoma
g. myositis
g. pneumonia
g. pneumonitis

subacute g.
g. transmural colitis
g. uveitis

granulomonocyte
granulosa
g. cell carcinoma
pyoderma g.
g. theca neoplasm

granulosa-theca cell tumor
granulovacuolar degeneration
grape-like
g.-l. cluster
g.-l. vesicle

grape-skin lung cavity
graph
scatter g.
spin-phase g.
velocity-time g.

graphite fibrosis of lung
Graser diverticulum
Grashey
G. method
G. position
G. shoulder view

grasping technique
GRASS
gradient-recalled acquisition in the steady state
GRASS MR imaging
GRASS pulse sequence
spoiled GRASS (SPGR)
GRASS system

Gratiolet
G. convolution
radiation of G.

gravel
gallbladder g.

Graves disease
gravidarum
fibroma molle g.

gravid uterus
gravis
colitis ulcerosa g.

gravitational
g. edema
g. potential energy

Grawitz tumor
gray (Gy)
g. commissure
g. horns in spinal canal
g. lung
g. matter

G

NOTES

gray *(continued)*
  g. matter abnormality
  g. matter degeneration
  g. matter heterotopia
  g. matter-white matter differentiation
  periventricular g. (PVG)
  g. reticular
  g. scale
  g. unit
gray-level
  g.-l. histogram
  g.-l. spacing
  g.-l. thresholding
gray-scale
  g.-s. Doppler
  g.-s. endorectal ultrasound
  g.-s. ERU
  g.-s. examination
  g.-s. image
  g.-s. imaging
  g.-s. inversion
  g.-s. monitor
  g.-s. range
  g.-s. sonography
  g.-s. ultrasound
Grayson ligament
gray-to-white
  g.-t.-w. matter activity ratio
  g.-t.-w. matter contrast ratio
  g.-t.-w. matter interface
  g.-t.-w. matter utilization ratio
gray-white
  g.-w. differentiation
  g.-w. matter junction
GRE
  gradient-refocused echo
  GRE breath-hold hepatic imaging
  3D GRE
    3D gradient echo
  ferumoxtran-enhanced echo-planar
    SE T2-weighted and echo-planar GRE
  GRE gadolinium-chelate enhanced imaging
  GRE magnetic resonance imaging
  GRE technique
GREAT
  ghost reduction by equalized acquisition triplets
great
  g. cardiac plexus
  g. cardiac vein
  g. cardiac vein flow (GCVF)
  g. cerebral vein of Galen
  g. cistern
  g. sacrosciatic foramen

  g. terminal vertebra
  g. toe sesamoid bone
  g. vein of cerebrum
  g. vessel
  g. vessel transposition
  g. vessel view
greater
  g. arc injury
  g. circulation
  g. curvature of stomach
  g. curvature ulcer
  g. multangular bone
  g. omentum
  g. palatine canal
  g. palatine foramen
  g. pelvis
  g. peritoneal sac
  g. petrosal
  g. sac of peritoneal cavity
  g. saphenous system
  g. saphenous vein
  g. sciatic foramen
  g. sciatic notch
  g. sigmoid notch
  g. sphenoid wing
  g. superficial petrosal nerve
  g. trochanter
  g. trochanter of femur
  g. trochanteric femoral fracture
  g. tubercle
  g. tuberosity
  g. tuberosity fracture
green
  iodocyanine g. (ICG)
Greene
  G. biopsy set
  G. needle
Greenfield
  G. catheter
  G. vena cava filter
greenstick fracture
GRE-in
  G.-i. image
  G.-i. imaging
grenade thrower's fracture
grenz ray
GRE-out
  G.-o. image
  G.-o. imaging
Greulich
  G. and Pyle atlas
  G. and Pyle method
Grey Turner sign
grid
  antiscatter g.
  Bucky g.
  crosshatch g.

g. film
focused g.
localization g.
Lysholm g.
megavoltage g.
oscillating g.
Potter-Bucky g.
g. ratio
g. technique
g. therapy
Griesinger sign
griffe
simian g.
Griffith point
Grisel syndrome
Grocco sign
Grocott methenamine silver
groin
g. dissection
g. mass
Grollman pigtail catheter
groove
alveolingual g.
alveolobuccal g.
alveololabial g.
anal intersphincteric g.
anterior interventricular g.
anterolateral g.
anteromedian g.
arterial g.
atrioventricular g.
auriculoventricular g.
basilar g.
bicipital g.
bronchial g.
buccal g.
carotid g.
carpal g.
caudothalamic g.
cavernous g.
central g.
chiasmatic g.
coronary g.
costal g.
deltopectoral g.
dental g.
developmental g.
digastric g.
ectodermal g.
esophageal g.
ethmoidal g.
gastric g.

genital g.
gingivobuccal g.
gingivolabial g.
Harrison g.
infraorbital g.
interatrial g.
intercollicular g.
intercondylar g.
intertubercular g.
interventricular g.
labial g.
lacrimal g.
Liebermeister g.
meningeal artery g.
middle meningeal artery g.
neural g.
paravertebral g.
patellar g.
posterior coronary g.
posterior interventricular g.
proximal trochlear g.
radial neck g.
Ranvier g.
retromalleolar g.
sagittal g.
Sibson g.
spindle colonic g.
striatothalamic g.
supraorbital g. (SOG)
trochlear g.
trochleocapitellar g.
ulnar g.
urethral g.
vascular g.
venous g.
Verga lacrimal g.
vertebral g.
Waterston g.
grooved director
grooving of articular surface
GROPE
generalized compensation for resonance offset and pulse length errors
Groshong distal-valve catheter
gross
g. fracture
g. lesion
g. tumor
g. tumor volume (GTV)
Grossman
G. principle
G. scale for regurgitation

G

NOTES

ground

g. plate
g. state

ground-glass

g.-g. appearance
g.-g. attenuation
g.-g. definition
g.-g. density
g.-g. infiltrate
g.-g. lesion
g.-g. nodule
g.-g. opacification (GGO)
g.-g. opacity
g.-g. osteoporosis
g.-g. pattern
g.-g. texture

group

Dodd perforating vein g.
Eisenmenger g.
extensor-supinator g.
flexor-pronator muscle g.
gadolinium enhanced imaging g.
gastrocnemius-soleus muscle g.
interosseous muscle g.
iodinated tyrosine g.
thalamogeniculate g. (TGG)
g. viewing

growth

g. acceleration
g. arrest line
g. center of bone
g. center closure
g. disk
ectopic bone g.
epiphyseal chondroblastic g.
g. factor
g. hormone-producing adenoma
g. impairment
lepidic g.
morphologic g.
nutrient artery g.
papillomatous g.
g. parameter
g. plate
g. plate abscess
g. plate arrest
g. plate complex
g. plate fracture
g. plate injury
g. plate widening
g. retardation
spinal g.
targetoid g.
twin pregnancy discordant g.
Virchow law of skull g.

growth-retarded fetus

Gruber

G. fossa
petrosphenooccipital suture of G.
G. suture

grumous

g. debris
g. tissue

Grüntzig

G. balloon dilatation catheter
G. PTCA technique

Grynfeltt triangle
GS

gestational sac
GS diameter

GSA

galactosyl human serum albumin
GSA imaging agent

Gsell-Erdheim syndrome
GSPECT

gated single-photon emission-computed
tomography

GSW

gunshot wound

GTD

gestational trophoblastic disease

GTF-A

Olympus Gastrocamera G.-A.

GTV

gross tumor volume

GU

gastric ulcer
genitourinary
GU tract cholesteatoma
GU tract tuberculosis

gubernacular canal
Gubler

G. line
G. tumor

Guérin

G. fold
G. fracture
G. sinus

Guglielmi

G. detachable coil (GDC)
G. detachable coil embolization

guidance

active biplanar MR imaging g.
angioscopic g.
biplanar MR imaging g.
computerized tomography g.
fluoroscopic g.
frameless stereotactic g.
indirect ultrasound g.
mammographic g.
puncture g.
radiologic g.
sonographic g.

g. system selection
ultrasonic g.
Guidant ANCURE endograft procedure
guide
    Brown-Roberts-Wells CT
      stereotactic g.
    BRW CT stereotaxic g.
    CT stereotactic g.
    side-exiting g.
    Site Rite sonographic g.
guide-catheter
guided
    g. biopsy
    g. drainage
guideline
    Mallinckrodt Institute of
      Radiology g.
    MIR g.'s
    string g.
guidewire, guide wire
    Amplatz Super Stiff g.
    Athlete GT coronary g.
    Cope mandril g.
    g. entrapment
    exchange g.
    g. exchange technique
    extra stiff g.
    flexible-tip g.
    Hi-Torque Floppy g.
    Hi-Torque Modified J-GW g.
    Hi-Torque steerable g.
    0.010-inch g.
    0.016-inch Headliner g.
    0.016-inch hydrophilic g.
    0.035-inch hydrophilic angulated g.
    InQwire g.
    intracoronary Doppler flow g.
    J-tipped g.
    Katzen infusion g.
    Lunderquest-Ring g.
    Lunderquist exchange g.
    movable core g.
    Newton g.
    nitinol g.
    Platinum Plus g.
    RADIFOCUS hydrophilic coated g.
    Ring g.
    Roadrunner NaviGuide g.
    Rosen curved g.
    Silver Speed 0.010-inch g.
    Sniper Elite hydrophilic g.
    standard fixed core g.

    stiff g.
    straight g.
    super-stiff g.
    TAD steerable g.
    tapered core g.
    tapered-tip g.
    Teflon-coated g.
    torsion attenuating diameter g.
    variable stiffness g.
    WaveWire angioplasty g.
    x-shaped g.
guiding
    g. sheath
    g. shot
guillotine rib
guilt screen
Gumley seatbelt injury classification
gumma, pl. **gummas, gummata**
    frank cerebral g.
    g. of rib
gun
    automated biopsy g.
    Biopty biopsy g.
    electron g.
Gunn crossing sign
gunshot
    g. fracture
    g. wound (GSW)
gunstock deformity
Günther Tulip vena cava MReye filter
Günzberg ligament
Gustilo-Anderson
    G.-A. open clavicular fracture
    G.-A. tibial plafond fracture
      classification
gut
    aging g.
    blind g.
    g. edema
    large g.
    primitive g.
    g. signature
    small g.
gut-associated lymphoid tissue (GALT)
Guthrie muscle
gutter
    anterolateral g.
    g. fracture
    lateral g.
    left g.
    paracolic g.
    parapelvic g.

G

NOTES

gutter *(continued)*
    paravertebral g.
    peritoneal g.
    right g.
    sacral g.
    synovial g.
Guyon
    G. amputation
    G. canal
Gy
    gray
gymnast's wrist
gynecography
gynecoid pelvis
gynecologic endometriosis
gynecomastia
gynecophoric canal
gynogram
gynography
gyral
    g. abnormality
    g. brain enhancement
    g. crest
    g. infarct
gyration
Gyratome
gyri *(pl. of* gyrus)
    g. cerebri
gyriform
    g. calcification
    g. pattern
gyromagnetic ratio
Gyroscan
    G. ACS-NT
    G. ACS-NT MRI scanner
    G. ACS-NT MR unit
    G. ACS-NT 1.5 T MR scanner
    G. Interna scanner
    G. NT 10 magnet
    G. S15 scanner
    G. 1.5T superconducting magnet
gyrus, pl. **gyri**
    angular g. (AG)
    ascending parietal g.
    Broca g.
    callosal g.
    central g.
    g. cerebelli
    cingulate g.
    contiguous supramarginal g.

dentate g.
G. endourology system
fasciolar g.
first temporal g.
flattening of g.
frontal g.
fusiform g.
Heschl transverse g.
hippocampal g.
inferior frontal g.
inferior temporal g.
infracalcarine g.
insular g.
g. isthmus fornicatus
lamination of g.
lateral occipitotemporal g.
lingual g.
marginal g.
medial occipitotemporal g.
middle frontal g.
middle temporal g.
occipital g.
occipitotemporal g.
olfactory g.
orbital g.
paracentral g.
parahippocampal g.
paraterminal g.
parietal g.
postcentral g.
posterior central g.
precentral g.
preinsular g.
quadrate g.
g. recti
sensorimotor g.
short insular g.
subcallosal g.
subcollateral g.
superior frontal g.
superior parietal lobule g.
superior temporal g.
supracallosal g.
supramarginal g.
temporal g.
transverse temporal g.
Turner marginal g.
uncal g.
uncinate g.

H
    henry
    Holzknecht unit
    Hounsfield unit
    hydrogen
        H band
        H and D curve
        H disk
        H field of Forel
        H graft
        H ray

H1
    H1 catheter

H-1
    H-1 MR spectroscopic imaging
    H-1 MR spectroscopy

hν
    photon

Haas
    H. method
    H. position

habenula, pl. **habenulae**
habenular commissure calcification
habitus
    body h.
    gracile h.
    large h.
    twisted body h.

HADD
    hydroxyapatite deposition disease
hadron therapy
HAEC
    Hirschsprung-associated enterocolitis
Hageman factor (HF)
Hagie pin
HAGL
    humeral avulsion of the glenohumeral
      ligament
    HAGL lesion
Haglund
    H. deformity
    H. syndrome
Hahn
    H. cleft
    H. spin-echo sequence
Hahn-Steinthal capitellum fracture classification
HAI
    hepatic arterial infusion
Haifa camera
Haines-McDougall medial sesamoid ligament
hair artifact
hairbrush pattern

hairline
    h. crack
    h. fracture
hair-on-end
    h.-o.-e. appearance
    h.-o.-e. periosteal reaction
    h.-o.-e. of skull
hairpin vessel
hairy heart
Hajdu-Cheney syndrome
half-axial
    h.-a. anteroposterior projection
    h.-a. view
half-body radiation therapy
half-dose enhanced MRI with MT
half-Fourier
    h.-F. acquisition single-shot turbo
      spin-echo (HASTE)
    h.-F. imaging (HFI)
    h.-F. RARE image
    h.-F. three-dimensional technique
    h.-F. transformation technique
half-intensity needle
half-life (HL)
    antibody h.-l.
    biologic h.-l.
    effective h.-l.
    elimination h.-l.
    h.-l. layer
    positronium h.-l.
    radioactive h.-l.
    short h.-l.
half-maximum
    full-width at h.-m.
half-moon
    h.-m. artifact
    h.-m. patella
    h.-m. shape
    h.-m. sign
half-Nex imaging
half-scan (HS)
    h.-s. with extrapolation (HE)
    h.-s. with extrapolation projection
half-thickness
    narrow-beam h.-t.
half-time
    blood clearance h.-t.
    clearance h.-t.
    h.-t. of exchange
    pressure h.-t.
halftone
    h. banding
    h. frequency

H

halftoning
iterative h.
half-value layer (HVL)
half-wedged field technique
Hallermann-Streiff-François syndrome
hallmark
radiofrequency radiographic h.
hallucal pronation
hallucis
adductor h.
hyperdynamic abductor h.
hallux
h. abductovalgus
h. dorsiflexion angle (DFA)
h. elevatus
h. extensus
h. flexus deformity
h. interphalangeal joint
h. interphalangeus angle (HIA)
intrinsic minus h.
h. limitus (HL)
h. malleus deformity
h. migration
h. rigidus
h. rigidus deformity
h. saltans
h. sesamoid bone
h. sesamoid complex
h. valgus (HV)
h. valgus angle (HVA)
h. valgus deformity
h. valgus interphalangeus angle
h. valgus-metatarsus primus varus
complex
h. varus
h. varus deformity
halo
h. crown
h. device
h. effect
fatty h.
hypoechoic h.
lucent h.
nodule h.
pericardial h.
perinuclear h.
periventricular h.
radiolucent fat h.
h. ring
h. sign
h. sign of hydrops
sonolucent h.
subendometrial h.
h. vest
halogenated
h. phenolphthalein dye
h. pyrimidine

h. thymidine analog
h. thymidine analog radiosensitizer
hamartoma, pl. **hamartomata**
angiomatous lymphoid h.
astrocytic h.
benign fetal h.
bile duct multiple h.
brain h.
breast h.
cardiac h.
cartilaginous h.
chest wall h.
chondromatous h.
CNS cortical h.
cortical h.
duodenal wall h.
eccrine angiomatous h.
elevated retinal h.
endobronchial h.
extracerebral intracranial
glioneural h.
h. of the eye
fetal renal h.
fibrolipomatous nerve h.
fibrous h.
glioneural h.
hypothalamic h.
h. of the kidney
leiomyomatous kidney h.
lung h.
lymphoid h.
mesenchymal liver h.
multiple bile duct hamartomas
myoid h.
pancreatic h.
pigmented iris h.
pulmonary h.
renal h.
retrorectal cystic h.
h. spleen
splenic h.
subcortical CNS h.
subependymal h.
tuber cinereum h.
vascular h.
ventromedial hypothalamic h.
hamartomatosis
generalized h.
hamartomatous
h. gastric polyp
h. lesion
hamate
h. bone
h. facet
flake fracture of the h.
h. tail fracture
hamiltonian equation

Hamilton-Stewart formula for measuring cardiac output
Hamman-Rich syndrome
Hamman sign
hammered-brass appearance
hammered-silver
    h.-s. appearance
    h.-s. skull
hammer-marked skull
hammertoe deformity
hammocking of mitral valve leaflet
hammock ligament
Hampson unit
Hampton
    H. hump
    H. line
    H. maneuver
    H. technique
    H. view
hamstring tendon
hamulus
    pterygoideus h.
hand
    ape-like h.
    bear's paw h.
    bipenniform muscles of h.
    Breuerton view of h.
    calcium pyrophosphate dihydrate h.
    chiasm of digit of h.
    CPPD arthritis of the h.
    digital artery of h.
    h. fracture
    hypothenar muscle groups of h.
    h. injection
    h. injection of contrast medium
    h. motor deficit
    opera-glass h.
    h. osteoarthritis
    phalanges of h.
    spade-like h.
    tangential layer of h.
    trident h.
    ulnar h.
    h. vascularization
    windswept h.
hand-agitated imaging agent
hand-held
    h.-h. exploring electrode probe
    h.-h. mapping probe
    h.-h. 8-MHz Doppler probe
handle
    Amplatz radiolucent h.

hand-shaped bend
hands-up ergonomics
hand/wrist arthritis
hanging
    h. heart
    h. hip
hanging-block technique
hanging-fruit pattern
hangman's fracture
Hann filter
Hannover canal
Hanot cirrhosis
Hansen fracture classification
HAP
    hepatic arterial phase
Hapad metatarsal arch
HAPE
    high-altitude pulmonary edema
HARC-C wavelet compression technique
hard
    h. disk herniation
    h. palate carcinoma
    h. papilloma
    h. ray
hard-copy image
hardened
    h. lung
    h. pelvis
hardening
    h. artifact
    beam h.
    bone h.
Hardy-Clapham sesamoid classification
Hare syndrome
Harken valve
harlequin sign
harmonic
    h. field
    h. function
    h. imaging
Harms cage
harness-shaped distribution
Harrington
    H. rod
    H. rod insertion
Harris
    H. band
    H. flush enema
    H. line
    H. view
Harris-Beath axial hindfoot view

NOTES

H

Harrison
    H. curve
    H. groove
    H. sulcus
HART
    hyperfractionated accelerated radiation
      therapy
Hartmann
    H. closure of rectum
    H. point
    H. pouch
    H. solution
Harvard multidetector scanner
harvested vein
harvester's lung
Hashimoto thyroiditis
hashing
    image h.
HASTE
    half-Fourier acquisition single-shot turbo
      spin-echo
        magnetic resonance cholangiography
        with HASTE
Hatcher-Smith cervical fusion
hatchet
    h. defect
    h. sign
hatchet-head deformity
Hatle method to calculate mitral valve area
HAT-transformed imaging
Hausdorff
    H. error
    H. measurement
haustra (*pl. of* haustrum)
    h. coli
haustral
    h. blunting
    h. fold
    h. indentation
    h. marking
    h. pattern
    h. pouch
haustration
haustrum, pl. haustra
    colonic haustra
Haut-Einheits-Dosis
haversian
    h. canal
    h. canaliculus·
    h. channel
    h. fat pad
    h. gland
Hawkins
    H. accordion catheter drainage set
    H. accordion-type empyema
    H. breast lesion localization needle

    H. classification of talar fracture
    H. inside-out nephrostomy set
    H. line
    H. method
    H. one-stick needle
    H. sign
Hawkins-Akins needle
hay-fork sign
Haygarth node
hazard
    sandbag h.
haze
    hilar h.
haziness
    diffuse h.
    subtle h.
hazy
    h. density
    h. infiltrate
    h. opacity
hazy-opaque lung
HBCT
    helical biphasic contrast-enhanced CT
    HBCT imaging
HBE
    His bundle electrogram
HBI
HC
    head circumference
HC/AC ratio
    head circumference-to-abdominal
      circumference ratio
HCM
    hypertrophic cardiomyopathy
HCS
    hematocystic spot
HCTA
    helical computed tomographic
      angiography
HCTE
    helical CT-enteroclysis
H and D
    Hurter and Driffield
HD
    heart disease
    Hirschsprung disease
    Hodgkin disease
HDI
    high-definition imaging
      HDI 1000, 30000, 3500, 4000,
        5000 ultrasound imaging system
HDIC
    hepatodiaphragmatic interposition of
    colon
HDR
    high-dose rate

HE
    half-scan with extrapolation
³He
    helium-3
        ³He MRI
⁴He
    helium-4
head
    h. of barium column
    cartilaginous cap of phalangeal h.
    h. of the caudate nucleus
    h. circumference (HC)
    circumference of fetal h.
    h. circumference-to-abdominal
        circumference ratio (HC/AC ratio,
        HC/AC ratio)
    h. coil
    femoral h.
    h. of femur
    first metatarsal h. (FMH)
    forward positioning of h.
    h. of the humerus
    h. injury (HI)
    ischemic necrosis of femoral h.
        (INFH)
    large fetal h.
    long h.
    metatarsal h.
    h. and neck carcinoma
    h. of the pancreas
    pancreatic h.
    radial h.
    radial facing of metacarpal h.
    h. of rib
    h. shape
    short h.
    strawberry-shaped h.
    terminal h.
    transillumination of h.
    h. trauma
    ulnar h.
    ulnar facing of metacarpal h.
    ureter cobra h.
Headhunter catheter
Headisc
Headliner
    0.016-inch h. guidewire
headphones
    Avotec MR-compatible h.
head-splitting humeral fracture
Heaf test
healed gastric ulcer

healing
    bony h.
    h. flare response
    h. fracture
    h. infarct
    resorption phase of h.
    h. ulcer
heart
    abdominal h.
    air-driven artificial h.
    alcoholic h.
    h. amyloidosis
    angioreticuloendothelioma of h.
    angiosarcoma of h.
    h. anomaly
    anterior border of h.
    aortic opening of h.
    apex of the h.
    apical surface of h.
    armored h.
    artificial h.
    athlete's h.
    axis of h.
    balloon-shaped h.
    base of h.
    Baylor total artificial h.
    beer h.
    beriberi h.
    h. block
    boat-shaped h.
    bony h.
    booster h.
    boot-shaped h.
    h. border
    bread-and-butter h.
    h. bulb
    cardiogenic shock h.
    cervical h.
    chamber of h.
    chaotic h.
    cloudy swelling of h.
    conical h.
    coronary artery of h.
    h. count-to-mediastinum count ratio
        (H:M)
    crisscross h.
    H. CT scan
    h. decortication
    h. degeneration
    dextroversion of h.
    diaphragmatic surface of h.
    h. disease (HD)

NOTES

H

heart *(continued)*
dome-shaped h.
donor h.
double density h.
drop h.
dynamite h.
dysrhythmia of fetal h.
egg-on-its-side h.
electrocardiogram-gated multislice spiral CT of the h.
elongated h.
empty h.
encased h.
enlarged h.
h. failure (HF)
fatty h.
fetal h.
fibroid h.
h. fibroma
flabby h.
flask-shaped h.
globoid h.
h. and great vessels
hairy h.
hanging h.
Holmes h.
horizontal h.
hyperdynamic h.
hyperkinetic h.
hyperthyroid h.
hypertrophied h.
hypokinesis of h.
hypoplastic right h.
hypothermic h.
inferior border of h.
inflammation of h.
intermediate h.
irritable h.
ischemic h.
H. Laser
left border of h.
L-loop h.
malpositioned h.
massively enlarged h.
mesoversion of h.
mildly enlarged h.
movable h.
h. muscle necrosis
myxedema of h.
myxoma of h.
h. myxoma
one-ventricle h.
ovoid h.
ox h.
paracorporeal h.
parasternal view of h.
parchment h.

pear-shaped h.
pectoral h.
pendulous h.
h. position
posterior border of h.
h. pseudoaneurysm
pulmonary h.
Quain fatty degeneration of h.
h. rate reserve mechanism
h. remnant
resting h.
rhabdomyoma of h.
right border of h.
right ventricle of h.
round h.
sabot h.
h. sac
h. scintigraphy
semihorizontal h.
semivertical h.
h. shadow
shift of the h.
shoulder of h.
h. silhouette
single-outlet h.
snowman appearance of h.
soldier's h.
h. sound
spastic h.
squared-off h.
sternocostal surface of h.
stone h.
h. stroke volume
superior border of h.
superoinferior h.
suspended h.
swinging h.
systemic h.
h. tamponade
Taussig-Bing congenital malformation of h.
teardrop h.
three-chambered h.
thrush breast h.
thymoma of h.
tobacco h.
total artificial h.
h. transplant
transverse h.
Traube h.
triatrial h.
trilocular h.
h. tumor
univentricular h.
upstairs-downstairs h.
h. valve
h. valve calcification

h. valve leaflet
h. valve vegetation
venting of h.
vertical h.
wandering h.
water-bottle h.
heartbeat gating
heart-lung transplant
heart-shaped
h.-s. collimator
h.-s. pelvis
h.-s. uterus
heart-to-background ratio
heart-to-lung ratio (HLR)
heart-to-thorax volume
HeartView
H. cardiac reconstruction software
H. CT cardiac monitor
heat
h. fracture
h. shape
h. shaping
h. unit (HU)
heat-damaged ^{99m}**Tc-RBC**
heat-denatured autologous RBC SPECT imaging
heater
resistance wire h.
heat-generating source
heating
gamma h.
hot-source h.
interstitial conductive h.
nonablative h.
heave
h. and lift
sustained left ventricular h.
heavily penetrated view
heaving precordial motion
heavy
h. chain
h. charged particle
h. hydrogen
h. ion imaging
h. metal injection
h. particle therapy
h. water
heavy-chain disease
heavy-charged particle Bragg peak radiosurgery
heavy-duty standard exchange wire

Heberden
H. disease
H. node
Hecht pneumonia
Hector
tendon of H.
HEDP
hydroxyethylidene-1,1-diphosphonic acid
rhenium-186 HEDP
heel
black-dot h.
h. bone
h. effect
h. fat pad
h. pad thickening
Sorbol h.
h. spur
h. tendon
varus h.
Hegglin syndrome
Heidelberg
H. protocol
H. retina tomograph II (HRT II)
Heidenhain
H. pouch
H. variant
height
disk space h.
intervertebral disk space h.
knee joint space h.
radial h.
relative peak h.
vertebral body h.
Heim-Kreysig sign
Heineke-Mikulicz maneuver
Heinig view
Heister
valve of H.
helical
h. biphasic computed tomography
h. biphasic contrast-enhanced CT (HBCT)
h. computed tomographic angiography (HCTA)
h. CTA
h. CT angiography
h. CT-enteroclysis (HCTE)
h. CT holography
h. CT scanner
h. CT scanning protocol
h. hydro-CT
h. pattern

NOTES

H

helical *(continued)*
- h. technique
- h. thin-section CT
- h. thin-section CT scan

helices (*pl. of* helix)

helicine artery

helicoid

Helios
- H. diagnostic imaging
- H. laser system

Helioseal

helium
- hyperpolarized h.
- h. ion beam
- h. magnetic resonance imaging (He-MRI)

helium-3 (^{3}He)

helium-4 (^{4}He)

helium-cadmium laser

helium-filled balloon catheter

helium-neon (HeNe)
- h.-n. laser

helix, pl. **helices, helixes**
- H. camera
- h. filter

helmet
- collimator h.
- h. field

Helmholtz
- H. axis ligament
- H. coil
- H. configuration

helminthic infestation

helminthoma

heloma
- h. durum
- h. molle

hemal
- h. arch
- h. canal
- h. node

hemangioblastoma
- capillary h.
- cerebelloretinal h.
- craniospinal h.
- cystic h.
- retinal h.
- spinal capillary h.
- third ventricular h.

hemangioblastomatosis
- cerebelloretinal h.

hemangioendothelial
- h. bone sarcoma
- h. liver sarcoma

hemangioendothelioma
- capillary h.
- epithelioid h.

- infantile h.
- malignant h.
- osseous h.

hemangioepithelioma

hemangiofibroma

hemangiolymphangioma

hemangioma, pl. **hemangiomata**
- arteriovenous h.
- bone capillary h.
- brain calcification h.
- capillary h.
- cardiac h.
- cavernous brain h.
- choroidal h.
- epidural cavernous h.
- epithelioid h.
- extraaxial cavernous h.
- extramedullary h.
- extremity h.
- facial h.
- giant cavernous h. (GCH)
- giant hepatic cavernous h. (GHCH)
- hepatic h.
- infantile hepatic h.
- intraarticular h.
- intramuscular h.
- liver capillary h.
- lung h.
- orbital capillary h.
- osseous h.
- pediatric h.
- pulmonary sclerosing h.
- sclerosing h.
- small bowel h.
- soft tissue h.
- splenic h.
- subcutaneous h.
- subglottic h.
- synovial h.
- trigeminal h.
- umbilical cord h.
- urinary bladder h.
- vascular h.
- venous h.
- verrucous h.
- vertebral h.

hemangiomatosis
- pulmonary capillary h.

hemangiopericytoma
- meningeal h.
- primary pulmonary h.
- renal h.

hemangiosarcoma
- liver h.

hemarthrosis

hematobilia

hematocele
> scrotal h.

hematocrit effect

hematocystic spot (HCS)

hematogenous
> h. dissemination
> h. embolus
> h. osteomalacia
> h. route
> h. spread
> h. tuberculosis

hematologic parameter

hematoma
> acute intramural h.
> acute subdural h.
> adrenal h.
> aneurysmal h.
> aortic intramural h.
> axillary h.
> balancing subdural h.
> basal ganglia h.
> bladder flap h.
> bowel wall h.
> brain h.
> breast h.
> carotid plaque h.
> chronic subdural h. (CSDH)
> corpus luteum h.
> delayed traumatic intracerebral h. (DTICH)
> dissecting aortic h.
> dissecting intramural h.
> dural h.
> encapsulated subdural h.
> epidural h. (EDH)
> evolving h.
> extracerebral h.
> extradural brain h.
> h. formation
> gelatinous h.
> hemispheral h.
> infected pelvic h.
> interhemispheric subdural h.
> intermuscular h.
> interstitial loculated h.
> intracerebral h.
> intracranial h.
> intramural h.
> intraparenchymal h.
> intrarenal h.
> intraventricular h.
> isodense subdural h.

> mediastinal h.
> mural h.
> nasal septum h.
> nasopharyngeal h.
> organized h.
> parenchymal h.
> perianal h.
> periaortic mediastinal h.
> pericardial h.
> peridiaphragmatic h.
> perigraft h.
> perinephric h.
> perirenal h.
> posterior fossa h.
> postoperative breast h.
> primary intracerebral h.
> rectal sheath h.
> retromembranous h.
> retroperitoneal h.
> retropharyngeal h.
> retroplacental h.
> scalp h.
> spontaneous h.
> subacute subdural h.
> subcapsular renal h.
> subchorionic h.
> subdural interhemispheric h.
> subfascial h.
> subgaleal h.
> submembranous placental h.
> subperiosteal h.
> umbilical cord h.

hematomediastinum

hematometra

hematomyelia

hematopericardium

hematopoiesis
> extramedullary h.

hematopoietic
> h. bone marrow
> h. reticulum

hematopoietically active bone marrow

hematoporphyrin derivative photosensitizing agent (HpD)

hematosalpinx

hematoxylin and eosin stain

hemiagenesis

hemianopsia
> altitudinal h.

hemiarch

hemiatrophy
> cerebral h.

NOTES

H

hemiaxial view
hemiazygos vein
hemiballismus
hemiblock
    left anterosuperior h. (LASH)
    left bundle branch h.
hemibody radiotherapy
hemicardium
hemic calculus
hemicolon
hemicondylar fracture
hemicord
hemicranium
hemidecortication
    cerebral h.
hemidesmosome
hemidiaphragm
    accessory h.
    h. attenuation
    h. depression
    h. rupture
    tenting of h.
hemidiaphragmatic
hemifacial
    h. microsomia
    h. spasm
hemihypertrophy
hemimegalencephaly
    ipsilateral h.
hemimelia
hemimelica
    bilateral dysplasia epiphysealis h.
    dysplasia epiphysealis h.
hemimyelocele
hemiparkinsonism
hemipelvis
hemiplegia
    congenital h.
    infantile h.
    spinal h.
hemiscrotum
hemisection
    spinal cord h.
hemisensory syndrome
hemispheral
    h. hematoma
    h. mass effect
hemisphere
    h. atrophy
    cerebellar h.
    cerebral h.
    h. damage
    dominant h.
    left h.
    h. lesion
    mesial h.
    right h.

    h. stroke
    swollen brain h.
hemispheric
    h. demyelinating lesion
    h. infarct
    h. regional lateralization difference
    h. vein
hemithorax, pl. hemithoraces
    frozen h.
    h. opacification
hemitransverse fracture
hemitruncus
hemivertebra
    balanced h.
    unbalanced h.
hemivertebral
hemizygosity
Hemobahn
    H. PTFE-covered stent-graft
    H. stent
HemoCue photometer
hemodialysis catheter
hemodialysis-related venous stenosis
hemodynamic
    h. alteration
    h. assessment
    h. decompensation
    h. effect
    h. format
    h. impotence
    h. index
    h. pattern
    h. penumbra
    h. reserve impairment
    h. response
hemodynamically
    h. significant lesion
    h. significant stenosis
    h. weighted echo-planar MR
      imaging
hemolymph node
hemolytic splenomegaly
hemolyticuremic syndrome
hemomediastinum
hemoperfusion
hemopericardium
hemoperitoneum
hemophilic pseudotumor
hemopneumothorax
hemorrhage
    abdominal h.
    acute subarachnoid h.
    adrenal h.
    alveolar h.
    anastomotic h.
    aneurysmal h.
    antepartum h.

arterial h.
basilar intracerebral h.
bladder h.
brainstem h.
brain stenosis h.
bulbar intracerebral h.
capillary h.
carotid h.
catheter-induced pulmonary
  artery h.
cerebellar h.
cerebral h.
cerebromeningeal intracerebral h.
choroid plexus h.
chronic parenchymal h.
colonic diverticular h.
colorectal h.
concealed h.
h. consolidation
cortical intracerebral h.
delayed traumatic intracerebral h.
diffuse pulmonary alveolar h.
diffuse subarachnoid h.
Duret h.
eight-ball h.
epidural h.
exsanguinating h.
external h.
extradural h.
extraluminal h.
extramural h.
extrapleural h.
first-trimester h.
focal area of h.
focal endocardial h.
focal pulmonary h.
frank h.
gastric h.
gastrointestinal renal transplant h.
hypertensive brain h.
hypothalamic h.
infant gastrointestinal h.
internal capsule intracerebral h.
interstitial h.
intertrabecular h.
intraabdominal arterial h.
intracerebral h. (ICH)
intracranial subarachnoid h.
intradural h.
intraluminal h.
intramural arterial h.
intramural gastrointestinal tract h.

intraparenchymal h.
intraplaque h. (IPH)
intrapleural h.
intrapontine intracerebral h.
intrapulmonary h.
intrathecal h.
intratumoral h.
intraventricular h. (IVH)
intraventricular neonate h.
labyrinthine h.
life-threatening h.
lobar intracerebral h.
lower gastrointestinal h.
lung h.
massive exsanguinating h.
mediastinal h.
meningeal h.
neonatal choroid plexus h.
neonatal intracerebellar h.
neonatal intracranial h.
neonatal intraventricular h.
neonatal subdural h.
nonaneurysmal perimesencephalic
  subarachnoid h.
nondominant putaminal h.
nontraumatic epidural h.
old h.
periaqueductal h.
peribronchial h.
perigestational h.
perimesencephalic nonaneurysmal
  subarachnoid h.
perinephric space h.
perirenal h.
placental h.
plaque h.
pontine h.
postoperative mediastinal h.
posttraumatic h.
preplacental h.
pulmonary artery h.
putaminal h.
retrobulbar h.
retroperitoneal h.
retropharyngeal h.
retroplacental h.
salmon-patch h.
sentinel transoral h.
slit h.
small bowel h.
spinal epidural h. (SEH)
spinal subarachnoid h.

NOTES

hemorrhage (continued)
spinal subdural h. (SSH)
spontaneous renal h.
striate h.
subacute h.
subarachnoid h. (SAH)
subchorionic h.
subcortical intracerebral h.
subdural h. (SDH)
subependymal h.
subgaleal h.
submassive h.
submucosal h.
subperiosteal h.
subserosal h.
thalamic h.
traumatic meningeal h.
upper gastrointestinal h.
variceal h.
venous h.
ventricular intracerebral h.
vitreous h.

hemorrhagic
h. brain infarct
h. bronchopneumonia
h. consolidation of lung
h. corpus luteum cyst
h. duodenitis
h. focus
h. lesion
h. lung nodule
h. mediastinal adenopathy
h. metastasis
h. necrosis
h. ovarian cyst
h. pericarditis
h. pleural effusion
h. pleurisy
h. pneumonia
h. pulmonary edema
h. salpingitis
h. stroke
h. transformation

hemorrhagicum
corpus h.

hemorrhoidal plexus

hemosiderosis
idiopathic pulmonary h.

hemostatic puncture closure device

hemothorax, pl. **hemothoraces**

hemp seed calculus

He-MRI
helium magnetic resonance imaging
dynamic ventilation He-MRI

Henderson fracture

Henderson-Jones chondromatosis

HeNe
helium-neon
HeNe laser

Henke
H. triangle
H. trigone

Henle
H. canal
jejunal interposition of H.
jejunal loop interposition of H.
H. ligament
loop of H.
H. sheath
trapezoid bone of H.

Hennekam syndrome

Henry
master knot of H.
vertebral artery of H.

henry (H)

Henschke
H. afterloader
H. seed applicator

Hensen
H. canal
H. node
H. plane

Hensing
H. fold
H. ligament

hen worker's lung

hepar lobatum

hepatic
h. abscess
h. adenoma
h. anaplastic sarcoma
h. angiography
h. angiomyolipoma
h. angiosarcoma
h. angle
h. architecture
h. arterial dominant
h. arterial infusion (HAI)
h. arterial phase (HAP)
h. arteriography
h. arteriovenous fistula
h. artery
h. artery anatomy
h. artery aneurysm
h. artery-portal vein fistula
h. artery pseudoaneurysm
h. artery stenosis
h. artery system
h. artery thrombosis
h. bed
h. bleeding
h. calcification
h. calculus

h. capsular rupture
h. capsule
h. carcinoma
h. chemoembolization
h. cirrhosis
h. congestion
h. cord
h. cyst
h. degeneration
h. diverticulum
h. duct
h. ductal system
h. duct bifurcation
h. echo pattern
h. failure
h. fibrosis
h. fissure
h. flexure
h. fungal infection
h. hemangioma
h. hilum
h. hydrothorax
h. insufficiency
h. ligament
h. lipoma
h. lobe
h. lymph node
h. metabolism
h. metastasis
h. necrosis
h. neoplasm
h. nerve plexus
h. outflow tract
h. parenchyma
h. pattern echo
h. resistive artery index
h. sarcoidosis
h. sclerosis
h. sinusoid
h. steatosis
h. test of Glass
h. transplant
h. trauma
h. tumor
h. vein
h. vein disease
h. vein thrombosis
h. venography
h. veno-occlusive disease
h. venous outflow
h. venous outflow obstruction
h. venous pressure gradient

h. venous system
h. web
h. web dilatation
h. wedge pressure (HWP)
hepatica fibrosa
hepatis
parenchymal peliosis h.
phlebectatic peliosis h.
porta h.
sagittal porta h.
hepatitis, pl. **hepatitides**
acute h.
chronic h.
neonatal h.
radiation h.
recurrent pyogenic h.
hepatization
lung h.
hepatobiliary
h. carcinoma
h. contrast agent
h. disease
h. ductal system imaging
h. pathway
h. scan
h. scintigraphy
h. tree
hepatoblastoma
hepatocarcinogenesis
hepatocarcinoma
fibrolamellar h.
hepatocellular
h. adenoma
h. carcinoma
h. dysfunction
hepatocerebral
h. degeneration
h. disease
hepatocholescintigraphy
hepatoclavicular view
hepatocolic ligament
hepatocystocolic ligament
hepatocyte tracer uptake
hepatodiaphragmatic
h. interposition
h. interposition of colon (HDIC)
hepatoduodenal ligament
hepatoesophageal ligament
hepatofugal flow
hepatogastric ligament
hepatogastroduodenal ligament

NOTES

H

hepatogram
    emission h.
hepatography
hepatoid adenocarcinoma
hepatoiminodiacetic
    h. acid (HIDA)
    h. acid scan
hepatojejunal anastomosis
hepatojugular reflux
hepatolenticular degeneration
hepatolienography
Hepatolite
    H. imaging agent
    technetium-99m H.
hepatolithiasis
hepatoma
hepatomalacia
hepatomegaly
hepatopancreatic
    h. ampulla
    h. fold
hepatopancreatica
    ampulla h.
hepatopathy
hepatopetal flow
hepatophlebography
hepatophrenic ligament
hepatopleural fistula
hepatoportal
    h. biliary fistula
    h. sclerosis
hepatoportoenterostomy
hepatoptosis
hepatorenal
    h. angle
    h. fossa
    h. ligament
    h. pouch
    h. recess
    h. saphenous vein bypass graft
    h. syndrome (HRS)
hepatoscan
hepatosplenic
hepatosplenography
hepatosplenomegaly (HSM)
hepatoumbilical ligament
herald bleed
Herbert-Fisher fracture classification
Herbert scaphoid bone fracture
Hercules
    H. 7000 mobile x-ray unit
    H. power injector
hereditary
    h. amyloidosis
    h. flat adenoma syndrome
    h. multiple cartilaginous exostoses
    h. multiple exostoses (HME)

    h. nonpolyposis colorectal
      carcinoma (HNPCC)
    h. predisposition
Hering canal
Hermansky-Pudlak syndrome
hermaphroditism
    true h.
HERMES system
Hermodsson
    H. fracture
    H. tangential projection
hernia, pl. herniae
    abdominal wall h.
    axial hiatal h.
    Barth h.
    Beclard h.
    Bochdalek h.
    broad ligament h.
    h. canal
    cecal h.
    concentric h.
    congenital diaphragmatic h.
    h. defect
    diaphragmatic h.
    direct inguinal h.
    duodenal h.
    epigastric h.
    esophageal h.
    external h.
    femoral h.
    funicular inguinal h.
    gastric h.
    hiatal h.
    Holthouse h.
    incarcerated h.
    incisional h.
    incomplete h.
    indirect inguinal h.
    inguinal h.
    internal h.
    interstitial h.
    intrapericardial diaphragmatic h.
    Lesgaft h.
    lesser sac h.
    Littré h.
    lumbar h.
    mediastinal h.
    mixed h.
    Morgagni h.
    obturator h.
    ovarian h.
    pantaloon h.
    paraduodenal h.
    paraesophageal h.
    parahiatal h.
    paraileostomal h.
    h. paralysis

parastomal h.
peritoneal h.
peritoneopericardial diaphragmatic h.
h. pouch
properitoneal h.
Richter h.
Rieux h.
rolling hiatal h.
h. rupture
h. sac
scrotal h.
short esophagus-type hiatal h.
sliding hiatal h.
spigelian h.
strangulated inguinal h.
transient hiatal h.
traumatic diaphragmatic h.
Treitz h.
tubular hiatal h.
ultrasound-guided reduction of a
  spigelian h.
umbilical h.
ventral h.
hernial aneurysm
herniated
h. abdominal content
h. bowel
h. bowel loop
h. intervertebral disk (HID)
h. nucleus pulposus (HNP)
h. preperitoneal fat
herniation
brain tissue h.
central h.
cerebral h.
cervical disk h.
cingulate h.
cisternal h.
concentric h.
diencephalic h.
disk h.
fat lung h.
focal disk h.
focal nuclear h.
foramen magnum h.
frank disk h.
free-fragment disk h.
hard disk h.
hippocampal h.
impending h.
intercervical disk h.
internal disk h.

intradural disk h.
intraspongy nuclear disk h.
lateral disk h.
lumbosacral intervertebral disk h.
nuclear h.
nucleus pulposus h.
phalangeal h.
physiologic h.
h. pit
posterolateral disk h.
soft disk h.
subfalcine h.
subligamentous disk h.
supraligamentous disk h.
temporal lobe h.
tentorial notch h.
thoracic disk h.
tonsillar h.
transtentorial h.
uncal h.
herniography
heroin vapor leukoencephalopathy
herophili
torcular h.
herpes
h. esophagitis
h. simplex virus type 1
  encephalitis
h. thymidine kinase (HSV1-tk)
herpesvirus pneumonia
herpetic whitlow
herringbone pattern
Herring tube
hertz (Hz)
Herxheimer fiber
Heschl
H. convolution
H. transverse gyrus
Hesselbach
H. ligament
H. triangle
heterocladic anastomosis
heterocyclic free radical
heterogeneity
heterogeneous
h. appearance
h. breast mass
h. carotid plaque
h. color speckling
h. hyperattenuation
h. internal echo pattern
h. isodense enhancement

NOTES

H

heterogeneous *(continued)*
    h. microdistribution
    h. perfusion pattern
    h. radiation
    h. signal intensity
    h. uptake
heterogenicity
heterophilic leukocyte
heterotaxia, heterotaxy
    abdominal h.
    visceral h.
heterotopia
    band h.
    cerebellar h.
    gastric h.
    gray matter h.
    subependymal h.
heterotopic
    h. bone
    h. bone formation
    h. gray matter
    h. nodule
    h. pancreas
    h. pregnancy
    h. scar ossification
    h. white matter island
Heubner
    H. artery
    recurrent artery of H.
Hewlett-Packard (HP)
    H.-P. color flow imager
    H.-P. phased-array ultrasound
      imaging system
    H.-P. scanner
    H.-P. ultrasound
Hexabrix imaging agent
hexadactyly
hexafluoride
    sulfur h. (SF$_6$)
hexagonal configuration
hexametazime (HMPAO)
**hexamethylpropyleneamine oxime
(HMPAO)**
hexokinase reaction
Hey
    H. amputation
    H. ligament
HF
    Hageman factor
    heart failure
    hippocampal formation
    HF infrared laser
HFA-134a
    ^{18}F-labeled H.
HFD
    high-frequency Doppler

HFI
    half-Fourier imaging
H-graft
    Gallie H.-g.
HGSIL
    high-grade squamous intraepithelial
    lesion
HI
    head injury
HIA
    hallux interphalangeus angle
5-HIAA
    5-hydroxyindoleacetic acid
hiatal hernia
hiatus
    adductor h.
    aortic h.
    crus h.
    diaphragmatic esophageal h.
    esophageal h.
    patulous h.
    popliteal h.
    h. semilunaris
Hibbs metatarsocalcaneal angle
hibernating myocardium
hibernation
    myocardial h.
hibernoma
Hickey
    H. method
    H. position
Hickman
    H. line
    H. tunneled indwelling catheter
hickory-stick fracture
HID
    herniated intervertebral disk
HIDA
    hepatoiminodiacetic acid
    HIDA imaging
    HIDA scan
    TechneScan HIDA
hidebound small bowel fold
hierarchical
    h. information
    h. scanning pattern
Hieshima microcatheter
HIFU
    high-intensity focused ultrasound
high
    h. arch
    h. brachial artery catheterization
    h. cervical spinal cord lesion
    h. defect
    h. endothelial venule
    h. filling pressure
    h. frame rate

h. gradient field strength
h. hydrophylicity
h. interstitial pressure
h. jugular bulb (HJB)
h. lateral wall myocardial infarct
h. left main diagonal artery
h. linear energy transfer radiation
h. normal
h. pontine lesion
h. pulse repetition frequency
Doppler
h. reflectivity
h. right atrial electrogram (HRA)
h. right atrium (HRA)
h. signal intensity
h. small bowel obstruction
h. spatial frequency reconstruction
algorithm
h. spatial resolution algorithm
h. spatial resolution cine computed
tomography (HSRCCT)
h. spatial resolution cine CT
h. spatial resolution mode
h. spin
h. takeoff
h. temporal resolution
h. temporal resolution mode
h. tibial osteotomy
h. torque
h. velocity
h. wedge pressure
high-altitude pulmonary edema (HAPE)
high-amplitude
h.-a. echo
h.-a. impulse
high-attenuation stone
**high-caliber, low-velocity handgun
injury**
high-contrast film
high-definition
h.-d. imaging (HDI)
h.-d. three-dimensional analysis
high-density
h.-d. barium
h.-d. barium imaging agent
h.-d. lesion
h.-d. linear array
h.-d. rim
h.-d. structure
high-dose
h.-d. film dosimeter
h.-d. film dosimetry

h.-d. radiotherapy
h.-d. rate (HDR)
h.-d. therapy
high-dose-rate
h.-d.-r. intracavitary radiation
therapy
h.-d.-r. remote afterloading
high-energy
h.-e. bent-beam linear accelerator
h.-e. imaging
h.-e. laser
h.-e. proton
h.-e. trauma
high-field
h.-f. open MRI scanner
h.-f. system
high-field-strength
h.-f.-s. MR imaging
h.-f.-s. scanner
high-flow arteriovenous fistula
high-frame-rate run
high-frequency
h.-f. Doppler (HFD)
h.-f. Doppler ultrasound
h.-f. Doppler ultrasound imaging
h.-f. miniature probe
h.-f. therapeutic ultrasound
h.-f. transducer
high-grade
h.-g. AV block
h.-g. glioma
h.-g. infiltrative astrocytoma
h.-g. malignancy
h.-g. narrowing
h.-g. obstruction
h.-g. obstructive lesion
h.-g. partial tear
h.-g. proximal stenosis
h.-g. signal intensity
h.-g. squamous intraepithelial lesion
(HGSIL)
h.-g. surface osteogenic sarcoma
h.-g. surface osteosarcoma
h.-g. tumor
high-heat-capacity x-ray tube
high-impedance circulation
high-intensity
h.-i. focused ultrasound (HIFU)
h.-i. lesion
h.-i. signal
h.-i. transient signal (HITS)
h.-i. zone (HIZ)

NOTES

H

high-kV technique
highly
    h. mobile echo
    h. reflective echo
    h. vascular tumor
high-lying patella
high-minute ventilation
Highmore
    H. antrum
    antrum cardiacum of H.
high-osmolar contrast agent (HOCA)
high-osmolarity contrast medium
  (HOCM)
high-output
    h.-o. heart failure
    h.-o. state
high-pass filter
high-performance
    h.-p. liquid chromatography
    h.-p. size-exclusion chromatography
high-pitched signal
high-powered field (hpf)
high-pressure
    h.-p. Blue Max balloon
    h.-p. liquid chromatography
    h.-p. mercury arc lamp
high-probability lesion
high-pulse repetition frequency Doppler
  echocardiography
high-purity germanium (HPGe)
high-quality pitch
high-rate
    h.-r. detect interval
    h.-r. ventricular response
high-resolution
    h.-r. B-mode imaging
    h.-r. bone algorithm technique
    h.-r. collimator
    h.-r. computed tomography (HRCT)
    h.-r. coronal cut
    h.-r. CT imaging
    h.-r. CT mammography
    h.-r. 3DFT MR imaging
    h.-r. diffraction
    h.-r. 3D microcomputed tomography
    h.-r. 3D spoiled-GRASS image
    h.-r. fluoroscopy
    h.-r. infrared imaging (HRI)
    h.-r. linear array transducer
    h.-r. magnetic resonance (HR-MR)
    h.-r. magnification
    h.-r. MRI (HR-MRI)
    h.-r. multileaf collimator
    h.-r. multisweep (HRMS)
    h.-r. storage phosphor imaging
    h.-r. storage phosphor managing
    h.-r. transverse view image

    h.-r. ultrasound
    h.-r. ultrasound scanning
    h.-r. volumetric sequence
high-resolution,
    h.-r. fan-beam collimator
    h.-r. low-speed radiography
high-riding
    h.-r. patella
    h.-r. scapula
    h.-r. third ventricle
high-sensitivity measurement
high-signal
    h.-s. abnormality
    h.-s. intratendinous collection of
      fluid
    h.-s. lesion
    h.-s. mass
high-signal-intensity
    h.-s.-i. ischemic change
    h.-s.-i. yellow marrow
    h.-s.-i. zone
high-speech pitch
high-speed
    h.-s. gradient coil
    h.-s. imaging
high-temperature diffraction
high-temporal-resolution cine computed
  tomography (HTRCCT)
high-velocity
    h.-v. flow
    h.-v. gunshot wound
    h.-v. jet
    h.-v. signal loss
high-voltage
    h.-v. generator
    h.-v. pulsed galvanic stimulation
      (HVPGS)
    h.-v. radiotherapy
    h.-v. roentgen therapy
    h.-v. stimulation (HVS)
    h.-v. transformer
hila (*pl. of* hilum)
Hilal
    H. embolization apparatus
    H. microcoil
hilar
    h. adenopathy
    h. area
    h. artery
    h. cap
    h. cell tumor of ovary
    h. cholangiocarcinoma
    h. displacement
    h. extension
    h. gland
    h. haze
    h. height ratio

h. kidney lip
h. lipoma
h. lymph node
h. mass
h. obstruction
h. plate
h. prominence
h. reaction
h. shadow
h. sign
h. structure
h. tumor
h. vessel
Hildreth sign
Hilgenreiner
H. epiphyseal angle
H. line
HiLight Advantage System CT scanner
Hillock arch
Hill-Sachs
H.-S. defect (HSD)
H.-S. deformity
H.-S. dislocation
H.-S. posterolateral compression
  fracture
H.-S. shoulder lesion
Hill sign
Hilton
H. law
H. muscle
hilum, pl. **hila**
central fatty h.
hepatic h.
kidney h.
lip of h.
lung h.
hila measurement
pruned h.
pulmonary h.
renal h.
splenic h.
waterfall h.
hilus of tendon
Hinchey classification
hindbrain
h. deformity
h. dysgenesis
h. malformation
hindfoot
h. deformity
h. instability

h. joint complex
h. valgus
hindgut
h. duplication
primitive h.
Hine-Duley phantom
hinged implant
hinge joint
hip
h. bone
h. bump
h. capsule joint
congenital dislocation of h. (CDH)
congenital dysplasia of h.
developmental dysplasia of h.
  (DDH)
h. disarticulation
dislocated h.
h. dislocation
h. dysplasia
external snapping h.
h. flexion contracture
h. fracture
frogleg view of the h.'s
hanging h.
h. hump
h. joint space
h. muscle cross section
h. pinning
h. pointer
h. protrusion
h. replacement
snapping h.
transient osteoporosis of h.
transient synovitis of h.
hippocampal
h. atrophy
h. fissure
h. formation (HF)
h. gyrus
h. head, body, and tail
h. herniation
h. infarct
h. magnetic resonance volumetry
h. sclerosis
h. sulcus
h. volume
hippocampal-amygdaloid complex
hippocampus
electronic atlas of the h.
hippocratic finger

NOTES

H

423

hippuran
  I h.
  H. imaging agent
hip-to-ankle view
Hirschberg sign
Hirschfeld canal
Hirschsprung-associated enterocolitis (HAEC)
Hirschsprung disease (HD)
His
  H. angle
  atrioventricular node of H.
  atrioventricular opening of H.
  H. band
  H. bundle
  H. bundle electrogram (HBE)
  H. canal
  H. line
  H. spindle
His-Haas muscle transfer
HiSonic ultrasonic bone conduction hearing device
HiSpeed
  H. Advantage helical scanner
  H. Advantage System CT scanner
Hi-Star MRI system
histiocyte
  sinusoidal h.
histiocytic
  h. bone lymphoma
  h. bone tumor origin
  h. brain lymphoma
  h. chest lymphoma
histiocytoma
  angiomatoid malignant fibrous h.
  atypical benign fibrous h.
  benign fibrous h.
  fibrous h.
  malignant fibrous h. (MFH)
  malignant fibrous osseous h.
  myxoid malignant fibrous h.
  primary pulmonary malignant fibrous h.
  scrotal h.
  storiform-pleomorphic malignant fibrous h.
histiocytosis
  diffuse cerebral h.
  Langerhans lung cell h.
  sinus h.
  h. X
Histoacryl
  30–50% H.
  H. embolic agent
histogenesis
histogram
  average diffusivity h.

dose-surface h.
dose-volume h. (DVH)
h. equalization
h. equalization algorithm
gaussian dose-volume h.
gray-level h.
hose-volume h.
integrated optical density h.
multisectional dose-volume h.
volume h.
histogram-derived metrics
histograph
  Eppendorf pO$_2$ h.
histologic
  h. correlation
  h. grade
histology
  bone h.
histomorphometric
  h. image
  h. measurement
histomorphometry
  bone h.
histopathologic
  h. comparison
  h. CT correlation
histopathology
  ischemic h.
histoplasmoma
histoplasmosis
  disseminated CNS h.
  lung h.
  pulmonary h.
historadiography
Hitachi
  H. Altaire Open MRI system
  H. CT scanner
  H. EUB-555 diagnostic ultrasound system
  H. four-head system
  H. MR scanner
  H. Open MRI system scanner
  H. rotating detector array system
  H. SPECT 2000H-40 camera
  H. 0.3-T unit scanner
  H. ultrasound
Hi-Torque
  H.-T. Floppy guidewire
  H.-T. Modified J-GW guidewire
  H.-T. steerable guidewire
HITS
  high-intensity transient signal
HIV
  human immunodeficiency virus
  H. encephalitis
  H. encephalopathy

H. esophagitis
H. nephropathy
HIV-related TB
HIZ
high-intensity zone
HJB
high jugular bulb
HL
half-life
hallux limitus
HLA
horizontal long axial
HLA imaging
HLHS
hypoplastic left heart syndrome
HLR
heart-to-lung ratio
H:M
heart count-to-mediastinum count ratio
HMD
hyaline membrane disease
HME
hereditary multiple exostoses
H-mode echocardiography
HMPAO
hexametazime
hexamethylpropyleneamine oxime
^{99m}Tc HMPAO
1H-MRS
single voxel proton MR spectroscopy
HN
Huckman number
HNP
herniated nucleus pulposus
HNPCC
hereditary nonpolyposis colorectal
carcinoma
Hobb view
hobnail liver
HOC
hypertrophic obstructive cardiomyopathy
HOCA
high-osmolar contrast agent
hockey-stick
h.-s. appearance of catheter tip
h.-s. appearance of the ureter
h.-s. catheter
h.-s. deformity of tricuspid valve
h.-s. fracture
h.-s. tricuspid valve deformity

HOCM
high-osmolarity contrast medium
hypertrophic obstructive cardiomyopathy
Hodge plane
Hodgkin
H. disease (HD)
H. granuloma
H. lymphoma
H. tumor
Hodgson
H. aneurysmal dilatation of the
aorta
H. disease
Hodson-type kidney
Hoffa
H. disease
H. fat pad
H. fracture
Hoffmann
H. atrophy
H. sign
Hofmeister
H. anastomosis
H. procedure
**Hohl tibial condylar fracture
classification**
hold
single breath-h.
Holdaway ratio
Holdsworth spinal fracture classification
holdup in flow of barium
hole
black h.
h. pattern
hole-within-hole
h.-w.-h. appearance
h.-w.-h. bone lesion
holiday heart syndrome
Holl ligament
hollow
h. albumin microsphere
h. bone
h. chest
h. foot
h. organ
h. ribbon
h. structure
h. viscus
h. viscus injury
hollow-point bullet
holly leaf appearance

NOTES

H

Holmes
    H. cortical cerebellar degeneration
    H. heart
    H. syndrome
holmium
    h. imaging agent
    h. laser
    h. yttrium aluminum garnet laser
    (Ho:YAG laser)
holmium-166
holmium-YLF
holoacardia
holocord
    h. hydromyelia
    h. syringohydromyelia
Hologic
    H. 2000 densitometer
    H. QDR 1000W dual-energy x-ray
    absorptiometry scanner
    H. 2000 scanner
holography
    computerized tomographic h. (CTH)
    helical CT h.
    h. imaging
    medical h.
    multiple-exposure volumetric h.
    volumetric multiplexed transmission
      h.
    Voxgram multiple-exposure h.
holoprosencephaly
    alobar h.
    lobar h.
    microform of h.
    semilobar h.
holosystolic
    h. gradient
    h. mitral valve prolapse
holoventricle
Holstein-Lewis fracture
Holthouse hernia
Holt-Oram syndrome
Holzknecht
    H. space
    H. unit (H)
Holz phlegmon
homeostasis
    brain h.
Homer
    H. Mammalok needle
    H. needle/wire localizer
Homerlok needle
homing
    h. mechanism
    h. molecule
homogeneity
homogeneous
    h. appearance

    h. carotid plaque
    h. echo
    h. echo pattern
    h. enhancement
    genetically h.
    h. intrasellar mass
    h. lesion
    h. MR pattern
    h. opacity
    h. perfusion
    h. positive charge
    h. radiation
    h. signal intensity
    h. soft tissue density
    h. susceptibility distribution
    h. thallium distribution
homogeneously
homogenous echogenic uterine content
homograft
    aortic root h.
homology mapping
homonuclear spin system
homophilic Purkinje cell
homospoil
homovanillic acid (HVA)
homuncular
homunculus
Honda sign appearance
honeycomb
    h. appearance
    h. cyst
    h. degeneration
    h. formation
    h. lung
    h. pattern
    h. vertebra
honeycombing
    fibrotic h.
hood-shaped ureter
hooked
    h. acromion
    h. bone
    h. vertebra
hook of the hamate fracture
hook-like osteophyte formation
hookwire
    Kopans spring h.
hoop
    h. stress
    h. stress fracture
hoop-shaped loops of bowel
Hoover sign
Hopkins rod
Hopmann
    H. papilloma
    H. polyp

Horizon
H. LX scanner
H. LX 1.5-T superconducting
magnet
horizontal
h. beam film
h. beam study
h. boundary
h. dipole configuration
h. fissure
h. heart
h. lie
h. long axial (HLA)
h. long axis
h. long axis slice
h. long axis SPECT image
h. maxillary fracture
h. overframing
h. plane
h. plane loop
h. position
h. segment of middle cerebral
artery
h. striping
horizontal-beam radiography
hormesis
radiation h.
hormone
mediobasal hypothalamus luteinizing
hormone-releasing h.
hormone-receptor negative carcinoma
hormone-resistant prostate carcinoma
horn
Ammon h.
anterior h.
central h.
dorsal spinal cord h.
H. endootoprobe laser
enlarged frontal h.
frontal h.
iliac h.
lateral h.
meniscal h.
occipital h.
posterior gray h.
posterior spinal cord h.
projectile h.
spinal dorsal h.
splaying of frontal h.
temporal h.
uterine h.
h. of uterus

ventral h.
ventricular h.
Horner
H. muscle
H. sign
H. syndrome
horseshoe
h. abscess
h. appearance
h. configuration
h. configuration of brain
h. fibrosis
h. fistula
h. kidney
h. lung
h. osteophyte
h. placenta
h. shape
Horsley anastomosis
Horton disease
hose-pipe appearance of terminal ileum
hose-volume histogram
hot
h. area
h. cathode x-ray tube
h. caudate lobe
h. defect
h. laser
h. lesion
h. light
h. nose sign
h. quartz lamp
hot-cross
h.-c. bun appearance
h.-c. bun skull
hot-source heating
hot-spot
h.-s. artifact
h.-s. heart imaging
h.-s. myocardial imaging
hot-tipped laser probe
Hough
H. transform (HT)
H. transform mapping
Hounsfield
H. calcium density measurement
unit
H. number
H. unit (H, HU)
hourglass
h. bladder
h. chest

NOTES

H

hourglass *(continued)*
    h. configuration
    h. constriction
    h. constriction of gallbladder
    h. deformity
    h. membrane
    h. pattern
    h. phalanx
    h. shape
    h. stenosis
    h. stomach
    h. tumor
    h. ventricle
    h. vertebra
hourglass-shaped lesion
House grading system
housemaid's knee
housing
    x-ray tube h.
Houston
    H. muscle
    valve of H.
^{166}Ho in vivo generator
Howell-Evans syndrome
Howship-Romberg sign
Howtek Scanmaster DX scanner
Ho:YAG laser
HP
    Hewlett-Packard
    Profasi HP
    HP SONOS 5500 ultrasound
      echocardiography system
HPA
    hypothalamic-pituitary-adrenal
      HPA axis
HpD
    hematoporphyrin derivative
      photosensitizing agent
hpf
    high-powered field
HPGe
    high-purity germanium
      HPGe detector
HPS
    hypertrophic pyloric stenosis
HPV16-associated tumor
HPV18-associated tumor
H&R
    hysterectomy and radiation
HRA
    high right atrial electrogram
    high right atrium
HRARE
    hybrid rapid acquisition with relaxation
      enhancement
HRCT
    high-resolution computed tomography

    cystic airspace HRCT
    inhomogeneous lung attenuation
      HRCT
    interstitial nodule HRCT
HRI
    high-resolution infrared imaging
      HRI imaging
HR-MR
    high-resolution magnetic resonance
      sagittal HR-MR
HR-MRI
    high-resolution MRI
HRMS
    high-resolution multisweep
HRS
    hepatorenal syndrome
HRT II
    Heidelberg retina tomograph II
HS
    half-scan
    Hurler syndrome
H/S
    hysterosalpingogram
    hysterosalpingography
      H/S Elliptosphere balloon catheter
HSA
    human serum albumin
      ^{99m}Tc HSA
HSD
    Hill-Sachs defect
HSG
    hysterosalpingogram
    hysterosalpingography
    hysterosonography
      HSG catheter
H-shaped
    H.-s. vertebra
    H.-s. vertebral body
HSM
    hepatosplenomegaly
HSRCCT
    high spatial resolution cine computed
      tomography
HSSG
    hysterosalpingosonography
HSV1 encephalitis
HSV1-tk
    herpes thymidine kinase
HT
    Hough transform
HTRCCT
    high-temporal-resolution cine computed
      tomography
H-type tracheoesophageal fistula

HU
heat unit
Hounsfield unit
Huckman number (HN)
Hudson attachment
Hueck ligament
Hughes-Stovin syndrome
Hughston
H. Clinic injury classification
H. view
Huguier canal
Huisman percutaneous drainage set
Huldshinsky radiation
human
h. albumin microphere
h. aortic smooth muscle cell
h. immunodeficiency virus (HIV)
h. serum albumin (HSA)
h. serum albumin imaging agent
h. thrombin
h. visual sensitivity weighting
HumaSPECT imaging agent
humeral
h. avulsion of the glenohumeral
ligament (HAGL)
h. bone
h. capitellum
h. circumflex
h. condylar fracture
h. epicondyle
h. epiphysis
h. head-splitting fracture
h. length
h. line
h. mechanism
h. metaphysis
h. physeal fracture
h. ridge
h. supracondylar fracture
humeri (*pl. of* humerus)
humeroradial articulation
humeroulnar articulation
humerus, pl. **humeri**
capitulum humeri
epicondylar fracture of h.
head of the h.
surgical neck of h.
humidifier lung
hump
buffalo h.
diaphragmatic h.
dowager's h.

dromedary h.
Hampton h.
hip h.
Kumpe h.
humpback deformity
Humphry ligament
hunchback
Kokopelli h.
hundredth-normal solution
hunger
air h.
Hunner ulcer
Hunt
H. and Hess aneurysm grade I–V
H. and Hess aneurysm grading
system
H. and Hess subarachnoid
hemorrhage scale
H. and Kosnik (grade 0–V)
aneurysmal grade
Hunter
H. aneurysm ligation
H. canal
H. disease
H. ligament
hunterian ligation of aneurysm
Hunter-Schreger band
Hunter-Sessions
Hunt-Kosnik
H.-K. classification
H.-K. classification of aneurysm
Huppert disease
Hurler syndrome (HS)
Hurley-Schele syndrome
Hurst phenomenon
Hurter
H. and Driffield (H and D)
H. and Driffield curve
Hürthle cell adenoma
Huschke
H. canal
H. foramen
H. ligament
Hutch diverticulum
Hutchinson
H. fracture
H. plaque
H. syndrome
H. teeth
Hutchinson-Gilford syndrome
Hutchinson-type neuroblastoma
Hutinel-Pick syndrome

NOTES

H

Hutson loop
Huygens
    H. eyepiece
    H. principle
HV
    hallux valgus
HVA
    hallux valgus angle
    homovanillic acid
HVL
    half-value layer
HVPGS
    high-voltage pulsed galvanic stimulation
HVS
    high-voltage stimulation
HWP
    hepatic wedge pressure
hyaline
    h. arteriosclerosis
    h. articular cartilage
    h. cartilage endplate
    h. cartilage plate
    h. degeneration
    h. membrane disease (HMD)
    h. necrosis
hyalinized
    h. breast fibroadenoma
    h. fibroadenoma with fibrosis
    h. fibrocollagenous tissue
hyalinizing granuloma
hyalocapsular ligament
hyaloid
    h. artery
    h. canal
    h. canal of Cloquet
    h. fossa
hyaloserositis pleura
Hyams grading of esthesioneuroblastoma
  classification
hybrid
    h. detector configuration
    h. imaging
    h. magnet
    h. MRI imaging agent
    h. PET/SPECT camera
    h. probe
    h. rapid acquisition with relaxation
      enhancement (HRARE)
    h. subtraction technique
hybridization probe
hybridization-subtraction technique
hybrid-RARE imaging
hydatid
    alveolar h.
    h. heart cyst
    h. lung cyst
    h. mediastinum cyst

    Morgagni h.
    h. polyp
    h. pregnancy
    sessile h.
    Virchow h.
hydatidosis
    cardiac h.
    osseous h.
Hydradjust IV table
hydramnios, hydramnion
hydrated pyelogram
hydraulic
    h. chamber
    h. distention
    vascular h.'s
Hydra Vision Plus DR, ES, HP
  urological imaging system
hydrencephaly
hydrocalicosis
hydrocalyx
hydrocele
    congenital h.
    idiopathic h.
    infantile h.
    primary h.
    secondary h.
hydrocephalic obstruction
hydrocephalocele
hydrocephalus
    acquired h.
    acute h.
    asymptomatic h.
    bilateral h.
    chronic communicating h.
    communicating h.
    compensated h.
    congenital h.
    delayed h.
    extraventricular obstructive h.
    fulminant h.
    hyperdynamic h.
    idiopathic h.
    infantile h.
    intraventricular obstructive h.
    low-pressure h.
    mass-effect h.
    noncommunicating h.
    nonobstructive h.
    normal-pressure h.
    normotensive h.
    obstructive h.
    occult h.
    posthemorrhagic h.
    postinfectious h.
    posttraumatic h.
    primary h.
    progressive h.

secondary h.
shunted h.
symptomatic obstructive h.
unilateral h.
unshunted h.
hydrocolpocele
hydrocolpos
hydrocortisone enema
hydro-CT
helical h.-C.
hydrodynamic
h. potential of disk
h. thrombectomy system
hydroencephalocele
hydroencephalomeningocele
hydrogel plug
hydrogen (H)
heavy h.
hydrogen atom-# radioactive h.
h. peroxide enema
h. peroxide-enhanced anal
endosonography
h. peroxide imaging agent
h. proton imaging
h. spin density
hydrogen-1, -2, -3 MR spectroscopy
hydrography
MR h.
Hydrolyser hydrodynamic thrombectomy catheter
hydrolysis in vivo
hydrolyzed technetium
hydrometra
hydrometrocolpos
hydromyelia
holocord h.
hydromyoma
hydronephrosis
acute h.
chronic h.
congenital h.
focal h.
hydronephrotic
h. kidney
h. sac
hydropericardium
hydroperitoneum
hydrophilic
h.-coated guiding catheter
h. contrast agent
h. guidewire
0.035-inch h. angulated guidewire

0.016-inch h. guidewire
h. nonflocculating barium
hydrophilicity
hydrophone
needle h.
hydrophthalmos
hydrophylicity
high h.
hydropic
h. change
h. composition
h. degeneration
h. villus
hydropneumothorax
loculated h.
hydrops
h. canal
endolymphatic h.
fetal h.
h. fetalis
gallbladder h.
halo sign of h.
labyrinthine h.
nonimmune fetal h.
semicircular canal h.
transient gallbladder h.
hydropyonephrosis
hydrosalpinx
hydrosoluble contrast agent
hydrostatic
h. decompression
h. pressure of blood
hydrosyringomyelia
hydrothorax
hepatic h.
hydroureter
hydroureteronephrosis
hydroxide
iron h.
hydroxyapatite
air plasma spray h.
calcium h.
h. deposition disease (HADD)
h. implant
h. rheumatism
hydroxycitrate
gadolinium Gd 159 h.
hydroxyethylidene-1,1-diphosphonic acid (HEDP)
5-hydroxyindoleacetic acid (5-HIAA)
hygroma, pl. **hygromata**
cystic neck h.

NOTES

H

hygroma *(continued)*
    cystic orbital h.
    pseudocystic h.
    subdural h.
hyoepiglottic ligament
hyoglossus muscle
hyoid
    h. arch
    h. bar
    h. bone
hyopharyngeal carcinoma
hyoscine butylbromide imaging agent
Hypaque
    H. enema
    H. Meglumine imaging agent
    H. myelography
    H. Sodium imaging agent
    H. swallow
Hypaque-76 imaging agent
Hypaque-Cysto imaging agent
Hypaque-M imaging agent
hyparterial bronchus
hyperabduction
    h. maneuver
    h. syndrome
hyperactive peristalsis
hyperacute
    h. ischemic brain infarct
    h. myocardial infarct
    h. stroke
hyperaeration
hyperattenuated
    h. blood
    h. intrasellar mass
hyperattenuation
    heterogeneous h.
hypercalcemic supravalvular aortic stenosis
hypercellular reconverted bone marrow
hyperconcentration of contrast medium
hypercycloidal tomography
hyperdense
    h. brain lesion
    h. mass
    h. middle cerebral artery sign
    h. sinus secretion
    h. spleen
hyperdontia
hyperdynamic
    h. abductor hallucis
    h. AV fistula
    h. fourth ventricle
    h. heart
    h. hydrocephalus
    h. right ventricular impulse
hyperechogenicity

hyperechoic
    h. area
    h. breast mass
    h. focus
    h. region
    h. renal medulla
    h. renal nodule
    h. splenic spot
    h. structure with shadowing
    uniformly h.
hyperechoicity
hyperemia
    active h.
    arterial h.
    collateral h.
    diffuse h.
    fluxionary h.
    mucous membrane h.
    passive h.
    reactive h.
    subchondral marrow h.
    venous h.
hyperemic flow
hyperexpanded lobe
hyperexpansion
    compensatory lobe h.
hyperextensibility
    joint h.
hyperextension
    h. dislocation
    h. injury
    h. of neck
    h. teardrop fracture
hyperfine coupling
hyperfixation
    ^{99m}Tc HMPAO h.
hyperflexion
    spine h.
    h. teardrop fracture
hyperflexion/hyperextension cervical injury
hyperflexion/rotation injury
hyperfractionated
    h. accelerated radiation therapy (HART)
    h. radiation
    h. radiotherapy
hyperfractionation
hyperfunction
    adrenocortical h.
hypergastrinemia
hypergonadotropic hypogonadism
hyperinflation
    congenital lobar h.
    dynamic pulmonary h.
    focal h.
    pulmonary h.

hyperintense
- h. marrow space
- h. mass
- h. muscle
- h. periventricular brain lesion
- h. signal

hyperintensity
- cortical h.
- diffuse signal h.
- incidental punctate white matter h.
- localized h.
- multifocal area of h.
- muscle h.
- pulvinar h.
- punctate white matter h.
- sacral h.
- white matter signal h.

Hyperion LTK system
hyperkinesia
hyperkinesis
hyperkinetic
- h. heart
- h. segmental wall motion
- h. segmental wall motion abnormality

hyperlordosis
- functional h.

hyperlucency
hyperlucent
- h. lung
- h. rib

hypermaturation
hypermetabolic
- h. activity focus
- h. nodule
- h. region

hypermobile
- h. first ray
- h. joint
- h. kidney

hypermotility
hypermyelination
hypernephroid carcinoma
hypernephroma
hyperosmolar
hyperosmotic solution
hyperostosis
- ankylosing h.
- bony h.
- Caffey h.
- chronic infantile h.
- cortical h.

diffuse idiopathic skeletal h. (DISH)
- generalized cortical h.
- idiopathic cortical h. (ICH)
- infantile cortical h.
- h. of Morgagni
- senile ankylosing h.
- skeletal h.
- skull h.
- sternoclavicular h.
- vertebral h.

HyperPACS teleradiology system
hyperparathyroidism
- brown tumor of h.
- persistent h.
- primary h.
- recurrent h.
- secondary h.
- tertiary h. (tHPT)

hyperperfusion
- h. abnormality of liver
- ictal h.
- mesial h.
- septal h.

hyperperistalsis
hyperpermeability
- contrast medium-induced pulmonary vascular h.

hyperphenylalaninemia
hyperplasia
- adaptive h.
- adenomatous h.
- adrenal h.
- adrenocortical h.
- alveolar epithelial h.
- angiofibroblastic h.
- angiofollicular lymph node h.
- angiolymphoid h.
- antral G-cell h.
- atypical ductal h.
- atypical lobular h. (ALH)
- atypical lobular breast h.
- atypical regenerative h.
- benign prostatic h. (BPH)
- bone marrow lymphoid h.
- breast h.
- Brunner gland h.
- compensatory h.
- congenital adrenal h. (CAH)
- congenital adrenocortical h.
- cortical nodular h.
- cystic endometrial h.

NOTES

H

433

hyperplasia (*continued*)
    cystic glandular h.
    desquamated epithelial breast h.
    diffuse pulmonary neuroendocrine
      cell h.
    ductal epithelial h.
    endometrial h.
    epiphyseal h.
    epithelial h.
    explosive follicular h.
    fibrointimal h.
    fibrous tissue h.
    florid follicular h.
    focal cortical h.
    focal nodular h. (FNH)
    follicular nodular h. (FNH)
    gallium-avid thymic h.
    generalized angiofollicular lymph
      node h.
    generalized breast h.
    giant follicular h.
    GI tract lymphoid h.
    intimal h. (IH)
    intravascular papillary endothelial h.
    lipoid adrenal h.
    localized angiofollicular lymph
      node h.
    lung lymphoid h.
    lymphoid h.
    lymphonodular h.
    medial h.
    mucosal h.
    myointimal h.
    neointimal h.
    neoplastic h.
    nodular adrenal h.
    nodular lymphoid h.
    nodular regenerative h. (NRH)
    paracortical h.
    parathyroid h.
    physiologic h.
    pituitary h.
    plantar h.
    polypoid lymphoid h.
    prostatic h.
    pseudoangiomatous stromal h.
      (PASH)
    pseudointimal h.
    pulmonary neuroendocrine cell h.
    reactive follicular h.
    reactive lymphoid h.
    sclerosing duct h.
    sinus h.
    smooth h.
    splenic h.
    subadventitial h.
    tenocyte h.
    thymic h.
    thyroid h.
    torus h.
    unicentric angiofollicular lymph
      node h.

hyperplastic
    h. adenomatous polyp
    h. bone
    h. cholecystosis
    h. colon polyp
    h. gastric polyp
    h. gastropathy
    h. inflammation
    h. lesion
    h. stomach polyp
    h. synovium
    h. tissue

hyperpolarized
    h. ^{3}He imaging agent
    h. helium
    h. ^{129}Xe gas
    h. ^{129}Xe imaging agent

hyperpressure

hyperreactivity
    airway h. (AHR)

hyperreflexia
    detrusor h.

hyperreninemic hypertension

hyperrugosity

hypersecretion
    gastric h.
    mucous h.

hypersegmentation
    manubrium h.

hypersensitivity
    alveolar h.
    carotid sinus h.
    h. lung
    h. pneumonia
    h. pneumonitis
    h. reaction
    tracheobronchial h.

hypersplenism

hyperstasis
    generalized cortical h.

hyperstereoroentgenography

hyperstimulation of ovary

hypertelorism

hypertension
    acute thromboembolic pulmonary
      arterial h.
    arterial h.
    benign intracranial h.
    extrahepatic portal h.
    hyperreninemic h.
    hypoxic pulmonary h.
    idiopathic intracranial h.

idiopathic noncirrhotic portal h.
idiopathic portal h. (IPH)
h. injury
intracranial h.
obstructive pulmonary arterial h.
persistent pulmonary h.
portal h.
precapillary lung h.
primary pulmonary h. (PPH)
pulmonary arterial h.
pulmonary venous h.
refractory h.
renal artery h.
renal transplant h.
renal vascular h. (RVH)
renovascular h.
secondary intracranial h. (SIH)
segmental portal h.
sinistral portal h.
suprahepatic h.
systemic arterial h.
systemic venous h.
systolic h.
venous h.

hypertensive
h. arteriosclerosis
h. brain hemorrhage
h. cardiovascular disease
h. contrast concentration
h. diathesis
h. encephalopathy
h. ischemic ulcer
h. left ventricular hypertrophy
h. lower esophageal sphincter
h. renal disease
h. stroke
h. vascular degeneration
h. vascular disease

hyperthermia
anular phased-array h.
interstitial h.
locoregional h.
microwave h.
h. probe
radiofrequency h.
radiotherapy with h.
radiotherapy without h.
volumetric interstitial h.

hyperthyroid heart
hyperthyroidism
neonatal h.

hypertonic
h. airway
h. solution
hypertransradiancy
hypertrophic
h. asymmetry
h. bladder
h. cardiomyopathy (HCM)
h. cirrhosis
h. duct network
h. exostosis
h. gastritis
h. inflammation
h. infundibular subpulmonic stenosis
h. marginal spurring
h. nonunion
h. obstructive cardiomyopathy
  (HOC, HOCM)
h. olivary degeneration
h. pulmonary osteoarthropathy
h. pyloric stenosis (HPS)
h. pyloric string sign stenosis
h. pyloric target sign stenosis
h. pylorus
h. subaortic stenosis
h. tissue

hypertrophied
h. heart
h. intima
h. myocardium
h. trigone

hypertrophy
adaptive h.
asymmetric septal h. (ASH)
asymptomatic h.
benign prostatic h. (BPH)
biatrial h.
biventricular h.
bladder h.
bone h.
Brunner gland h.
cardiac h.
compensatory nodular kidney h.
complementary h.
concentric heart h.
contralateral h.
dilatation and h.
eccentric left ventricular h.
epiphyseal h.
familial h. (FHC)
focal pyloric h.
focal renal h.

NOTES

H

hypertrophy *(continued)*
    four-chamber h.
    functional h.
    hypertensive left ventricular h.
    interatrial septal h.
    left atrial h.
    left ventricular h. (LVH)
    ligamentous-muscular h.
    lipomatous h.
    muscular h.
    myocardial cellular h.
    olivary h.
    panchamber h.
    physiologic h.
    pyloric h.
    right atrial h.
    right ventricular h. (RVH)
    Romhilt-Estes score for left ventricular h.
    scalenus anticus muscle h.
    septal h.
    septate h.
    smooth muscle h.
    symmetric heart h.
    trigeminal trigonal h.
    trigonal h.
    type A–C right ventricular h.
    unilateral h.
    ventricular h.
    villous h.
    Wigle scale for ventricular h.
hypervariable
    h. region
    h. sequence
hypervascular
    h. arterialization
    h. granulation tissue
    h. hepatocellular carcinoma
    h. liver metastasis
    h. mediastinal mass
    h. pancreatic tumor
hypervascularity
hypervolemia of pregnancy
hypervolemic pulmonary edema
hypha
    fungal h.
hypoacousia
hypoaeration
hypoattenuating mass
hypoattenuation
hypocellular marrow
hypochordal arch
hypocycloidal tomography
hypodense
    h. area
    h. basal ganglion brain lesion
    h. mass

    h. mesencephalic low-density brain lesion
hypodensity
    periventricular h.
    white matter h.
hypodiploid tumor
hypodiploidy
hypodontia
hypoechogenic
    h. retroplacental myometrial zone
    h. tumor
hypoechogenicity
    false h.
hypoechoic
    h. area
    h. area of ultrasound
    h. band
    h. fluid collection
    h. halo
    h. layer
    h. liver
    h. mantle
    h. plaque
    h. renal sinus
    h. rim
    h. solid tumor
    h. structure
    h. testis
    h. tissue
    h. zone
hypofractionated radiation therapy
hypofrontality
hypoganglionosis of colon
hypogastric
    h. artery
    h. plexus
hypogastrium
hypogenetic lung
hypoglossal
    h. canal
    h. fossa
    h. nerve
    h. trigone
hypogonadism
    hypergonadotropic h.
hypoinflation of the lung
hypointense
    h. fibrous capsule
    h. nodule
    h. sella lesion
    h. signal
    h. signal inhomogeneity
    h. signal shadowing
hypointensity
    cortical h.
hypokinesis, hypokinesia
    apical h.

cardiac h.
diffuse ventricular h.
global h.
h. of heart
inferior wall h.
h. on echocardiography
regional h.
septal h.
wall h.
hypokinetic
h. left ventricle
h. myocardium
h. segment
h. segmental wall motion
h. segmental wall motion
abnormality
hypolordosis
hypolucency of lung
hypometabolic area
hypometabolism
bilateral superior parietal h.
biparietotemporal h.
focal area of h.
global h.
lesion h.
hypomineralization
fetal h.
hypoparathyroidism
idiopathic h.
secondary h.
hypoperfused state
hypoperfusion
acute alveolar h.
apical h.
cerebellar h.
cerebral h.
h. complex
global cerebral h.
peripheral h.
pulmonary h.
resting regional myocardial h.
septal h.
systemic h.
hypoperistalsis
hypopharyngeal
h. carcinoma
h. diverticulum
h. tumor
hypopharynx
hypophosphatemic osteomalacia
hypophyseal
h. fossa

h. pouch
h. Rathke duct
hypophysis
h. cerebri
infundibulum of h.
hypophysitis
lymphocytic h.
lymphoid h.
hypopituitarism
hypothalamic h.
hypoplasia
anular h.
aortic tract complex h.
ascending aorta h.
basiocciput h.
biliary h.
bone marrow h.
cartilage hair h.
cerebellar h.
cerebral white matter h.
condylar skull h.
congenital renal h.
conus h.
h. of the dens
endothelial h.
fetal lung h.
gallbladder h.
isolated cerebellar h.
left ventricular h.
lung h.
mandible h.
maxillary sinus h.
medullaris h.
occipital condyle h.
optic nerve h.
pontocerebellar h.
pulmonary h.
radius h.
seminal vesicle h.
sinus h.
skeletal h.
transverse h.
tubular aortic h.
uterine h.
vermian h.
vermian-cerebellar h.
vermis h.
hypoplastic
h. aortic arch
h. disk interval
h. emphysema
h. heart ventricle

NOTES

H

hypoplastic (*continued*)
- h. horizontal rib
- h. left heart syndrome (HLHS)
- h. left parietal syndrome
- h. left ventricle
- h. lung
- h. penis
- h. right heart
- h. right heart syndrome
- h. right ventricle
- h. subpulmonic outflow
- h. thumb
- h. tricuspid orifice
- h. valve

hypopnea
- obstructive h.

hyposensitization

hyposmia

hyposplenism

hypostatic
- h. bronchopneumonia
- h. congestion
- h. pneumonia
- h. pulmonary insufficiency

hypotelorism

hypotension
- arterial h.
- cerebral h.
- spontaneous intracranial h.

hypothalamic
- h. glioma
- h. hamartoma
- h. hemorrhage
- h. hypopituitarism
- h. hypothyroidism
- h. infundibulum
- h. lesion
- h. sulcus

hypothalamic-pituitary-adrenal (HPA)

hypothalamic-pituitary-adrenal axis

hypothalamic-pituitary axis

hypothalamic-pituitary-gonadal axis

hypothalamohypophysial tract

hypothalamoneurohypophyseal axis

hypothalamus
- anterior h.
- rostral h.
- h. tumor

hypothenar
- h. eminence
- h. muscle groups of hand

hypothermia
- scalp h.

hypothermic
- h. heart
- h. perfusion

hypothyroidism
- hypothalamic h.
- primary h.
- secondary h.
- tertiary h.

hypotonia

hypotonic
- h. bladder
- h. duodenography
- h. duodenography imaging

hypovascular zone

hypoventilation

hypovolemia trauma

hypovolemic
- h. complex
- h. shock

hypoxemia

hypoxia
- ischemic h.
- relative h.
- tumor h.

hypoxia-ischemia

hypoxic
- h. brain damage
- h. injury
- h. ischemic encephalopathy
- h. ischemic insult
- h. pulmonary hypertension
- h. pulmonary vasoconstriction

Hyrtl foramen

hysterectomy
- abdominal h.
- extrafascial h.
- h. and radiation (H&R)
- h. and radiation therapy
- supracervical h.
- Wertheim h.

hysteresis

Hysterocath hysterosalpingography device

hysterogram

hysterograph

hysterography
- conventional h.
- ultrasonic h.

hysterometry

hysteromyoma

hysterosalpingo-contrast sonography

hysterosalpingogram (H/S, HSG)

hysterosalpingography (H/S, HSG)
- h. catheter
- h. imaging
- ultrasonic h.

hysterosalpingosonography (HSSG)

hysteroscopy

hysterosonography (HSG)
- transvaginal h. (TVHS)

hysterotubogram
hysterotubography
Hz
    hertz

440-Hz   tone

NOTES

H

I
  iodine
  isoleucine
  I hippuran
^{123}I, I-123
  iodine-123
    ^{123}I BMIPP imaging
    ^{123}I brain imaging spectamine
    ^{123}I heptadecanoic acid
    ^{123}I iodoamphetamine
    ^{123}I isopropyl iodoamphetamine
    (IMP)
    ^{123}I metaiodobenzylguanidine
    ^{123}I metaiodobenzylguanidine
    scintigraphy
    ^{123}I OIH
^{125}I, I-125
  iodine-125
    ^{125}I fibrinogen scan
    ^{125}I interstitial radiation implant
^{127}I, I-127
  iodine-127
^{131}I, I-131
  iodine-131
    ^{131}I-mIB6
    ^{131}I radioactive iodine
    ^{131}I therapy
^{132}I, I-132
  iodine-132
    ^{132}I radioactive iodine
IA
  interbronchial angle
  intraarterial
IAB
  intraabdominal
IABP
  intraaortic balloon pump
IADSA
  intraarterial digital subtraction
    angiography
IAR
  instantaneous axis of rotation
IAS
  interatrial septum
iatrogenic
    i. avulsion
    i. cardiomegaly
    i. dural tear
    i. esophageal perforation
    i. iliocaval fistula
    i. pseudoaneurysm
    i. ureteral injury
IAVB
  incomplete atrioventricular block

**I-B1 radiolabeled antibody injection
  radiation therapy**
IBC
  inflammatory breast carcinoma
IBM
    IBM field-cycling research
      relaxometer
    IBM NMR spectrometer
IBTR
  ipsilateral breast tumor recurrence
ICA
  internal carotid artery
  intracranial aneurysm
    juxtasellar ICA
    petrous ICA
    supraclinoid ICA
ICE
  intracardiac echocardiography
ice
    i. cream cone shape
    i. skater's fracture
iceberg
    i. lesion
    i. radiotherapy
ice-pick view
ice-water swallow
ICG
  iodocyanine green
ICH
  idiopathic cortical hyperostosis
  intracerebral hemorrhage
ichorous pleurisy
ICIS
  integrated clinical information system
ICON
    Siemens I.
ICP
  intracranial pressure
ICP-AES
  inductively coupled plasma atomic
    emission spectrometry
    ICP-AES detection
ICRT
  intracoronary radiation therapy
ICRU
  International Commission on Radiation
    Units and Measurements
    ICRU reference point
ICS
  improved Chen-Smith
    ICS coder
ICSPF
  internal carotid systolic peak flow
ictal
    i. hyperperfusion

ictal *(continued)*
  i. PET scan
  i. phase study
  i. ^{99m}Tc HMPAO brain SPECT
ICUS
  intracoronary ultrasound
ICV
  internal cerebral vein
  intracerebroventricular
    ICV reservoir
ICW
  intracranial width
ID
  internal diameter
  interscan delay
IDA
  image display and analysis
    IDA scanning
IDC
  idiopathic dilated cardiomyopathy
  interlocking detachable coil
  intraductal carcinoma
IDD
  intraluminal duodenal diverticulum
identification
  particle i.
  peak i.
  phase i.
  topographic i.
IDF
  inferior duodenal flexure
idiopathic
  i. amyloidosis
  i. avascular necrosis
  i. cortical hyperostosis (ICH)
  i. diffuse cerebellar dysplasia
  i. dilated cardiomyopathy (IDC)
  i. dilated pulmonary artery
  i. edema
  i. epilepsy
  i. epiphyseolysis
  i. fibrous mediastinitis
  i. fracture
  i. gastric perforation
  i. hydrocele
  i. hydrocephalus
  i. hypertrophic subaortic sclerosis
    (IHSS)
  i. hypertrophic subaortic stenosis
  i. hypoparathyroidism
  i. interstitial fibrosis
  i. interstitial pneumonia
  i. interstitial pneumonitis
  i. intestinal pseudoobstruction
  i. intracranial hypertension
  i. megacolon
  i. multicentric osteolysis

  i. mural endomyocardial disease
  i. noncirrhotic portal hypertension
  i. obstruction
  i. osteolysis
  i. pleural calcification
  i. portal hypertension (IPH)
  i. pulmonary arteriosclerosis (IPA)
  i. pulmonary artery dilatation
  i. pulmonary fibrosis (IPF)
  i. pulmonary hemosiderosis
  i. restrictive cardiomyopathy
  i. right atrial dilatation
  i. scoliosis
  i. unilateral hyperlucent lung
  i. unilobar emphysema
  i. varicocele
idiosyncratic anaphylactoid reaction
idioventricular rhythm (IVR)
IDIS angiography system
IDK
  internal derangement of the knee
IDP
  imidodiphosphonate
IDSA
  intraoperative digital subtraction
  angiography
IDSI scanner
IDXrad radiology information system
I:E ratio
  inspiratory to expiratory ratio
IES
  inferior esophageal sphincter
IF
  screen-intensifying factor
IFT
  inverse Fourier transform
IgG
  immunoglobulin G
    ^{111}In IgG
    indium-111-labeled IgG
IGLLC
  inferior glenohumeral ligament labral
  complex
IH
  intimal hyperplasia
IHA
  intrahepatic atresia
IHF
  interhemispheric fissure
^{192}I high-dose-rate remote afterloader
IHSA
  iodinated human serum albumin
IHSS
  idiopathic hypertrophic subaortic
  sclerosis
IJV
  internal jugular vein

I-labeled
  [131]I.-l.
  I.-l. cholesterol
  [131]I.-l. human MoAb
  I.-l. macroaggregated albumin
  [131]I.-l. monoclonal Fab
  I.-l. rose bengal
[123]I-labeled Z-MIVE
ILBBB
  incomplete left bundle-branch block
ileal
  i. atresia
  i. conduit
  i. crypt
  i. inflow tract
  i. jejunization
  i. loop
  i. loopography
  i. motility
  i. neobladder
  i. obstruction
  i. pouch-anal anastomosis
  i. spill
  i. S pouch
  i. stenosis
ileitis
  backwash i.
  Crohn i.
  distal i.
  granulomatous i.
  obstructive dysfunctional i.
  prestomal i.
  reflux i.
  regional i.
  terminal i.
ileoanal pouch
ileocecal
  i. cystoplasty
  i. edema
  i. fat pad
  i. fold
  i. insufficiency
  i. junction
  i. orifice
  i. pouch
  i. recess
  i. syndrome
  i. valve
  i. valve abnormality
ileococcygeus muscle
ileocolic
  i. artery

  i. disease
  i. fold
  i. intussusception
  i. lymph node
  i. plexus
  i. vein
  i. vessel
ileocolitis
  Crohn i.
ileocolostomy
ileoentectropy
ileofemoral
  i. vein
  i. wing fracture
ileogram
ileoileal intussusception
ileorectal anastomosis (IRA)
ileosacral (IS)
ileosigmoid
  i. fistula
  i. knot
ileostogram
ileostomy
ileotransverse colon anastomosis
ileum
  antimesenteric border of distal i.
  cobblestone i.
  collapsed distal i.
  hose-pipe appearance of terminal i.
  jejunization of i.
  neoterminal i.
  terminal i.
ileus
  adhesive i.
  adynamic i.
  adynamic/paralytic i.
  cecal i.
  chronic duodenal i.
  colonic i.
  dynamic i.
  functional i.
  gallbladder i.
  gallstone i.
  localized i.
  mechanical i.
  meconium i.
  nonobstructive i.
  occlusive i.
  paralytic i.
  postoperative i.
  reflex i.
  spastic i.

NOTES

Ilfeld-Holder deformity
ilia (*pl. of* ilium)
iliac
    i. apophysitis
    i. artery
    i. artery aneurysm
    i. artery stenosis
    i. artery stenting
    i. bifurcation
    i. canal
    i. cancellous bone
    i. circumflex lymph node
    i. colon
    i. crest
    i. dowel
    i. fascia
    i. fossa
    i. fossa abscess
    i. horn
    i. index
    i. lesion
    i. plaque
    i. spine
    i. tubercle
    i. tuberosity
    i. vein
    i. vein obstruction
    i. venography
    i. vessel
    i. wing
iliac-renal bypass graft
iliacus
iliocaval
    i. junction
    i. thrombus
    i. tree
iliocostal muscle
iliofemoral
    i. artery
    i. crossover bypass
    i. ligament
    i. thrombosis
    i. triangle
    i. vein
    i. venous stenosis
ilioinguinal lymph node
ilioischial line
iliolumbar ligament
iliopectineal
    i. eminence
    i. ligament
    i. line
ilioprofunda bypass graft
iliopsoas
    i. abscess
    i. bursa
    i. bursitis

    i. compartment
    i. compartment enlargement
    i. muscle
    i. muscle shadow
    i. sign
    i. tendon
iliopubic
    i. eminence
    i. ligament
iliotibial (IT)
    i. band
    i. band friction syndrome
    i. ligament
    i. tract
iliotrochanteric ligament
ilium, pl. **ilia**
    flared i.
Ilizarov
    I. device
    I. ring
ill-defined
    i.-d. appearance
    i.-d. breast density
    i.-d. consolidation
    i.-d. margin
    i.-d. mass
    i.-d. multifocal lung density
illuminator
    Mammo Mask i.
ILUS
    intraluminal ultrasound
    ILUS catheter
IM
    intramedullary
    IM joint
    IM rod
    IM rodding
IMA
    inferior mesenteric artery
    intermetatarsal angle
    internal mammary artery
image (*See* imaging, film, projection, radiograph, radiography, scanning, scan, view, x-ray)
    acetazolamide dual-isotope i.
    i. acquisition
    i. acquisition-gated scan imaging
    Add-On Bucky radiographer detector i.
    i. aliasing
    alignment and registration of 3D i.
    i. amplifier
    amplitude i.
    i. analysis system
    anatomic i.
    arm-down i.
    arm-up i.

arterial flow-phase i.
artifact i.
attenuated i.
attenuation-corrected i.
axial fat-suppressed T2-weighted i.
axial gradient echo i.
axial proton-density-weighted i.
axial transabdominal i.
binarized i.
binary i.
bone phase i.
breath-hold fast spin-echo i.
bull's eye i.
calculated i.
cervicothoracic sagittal scout i.
i. chain
cine-encoded i.
cine magnetic resonance function i.
color-scale i.
column mode sinogram i.
i. compression
computer-generated i.
computerized transverse axial i.
cone-beam i.
confocal i.
contact i.
contiguous i.
i. contrast
contrast-enhanced MR i.
contrast-enhanced T1-weighted fat-
  suppressed i.
i. control
conventional transverse cross-
  sectional i.
i. converter
i. coregistration
coronal ECD brain SPECT i.
coronal GRE MR i.
coronal planar i.
coronal proton-density-weighted fast
  spin-echo i.
coronal SPIR i.
coronal T1-weighted i.
cross-sectional ultrasonographic i.
CTA i.
CT/MRI-defined tumor slice i.
CT/MRI-defined tumor volume i.
CT reconstruction i.
i. cytometry
3D-DSA i.
deformation-based surface-
  rendered i.

degradation of i.
delayed phase i.
2D gradient-encoded i.
diffusion-weighted i.
digitally fused CT and radiolabeled
  monoclonal antibody SPECT i.
digitized film i.
i. display
i. display and analysis (IDA)
i. distortion
Dixon quantitative chemical shift i.
2D portal i.
DSA i.
3D volume-rendering
  reconstruction i.
dynamic i.
ECG-triggered, flow-compensated
  gradient echo i.
echo-planar i.
endosonographic i.
excitation-spoiled fat-suppressed T1-
  weighted SE i.
exercise i.
expiratory i.
fast fluid-attenuation inversion
  recovery i.
fast Fourier transform i.
fast spin-echo T2-weighted i.
fat-saturated spin-echo proton
  density-weighted i.
fat-saturated T2-weighted fast spin-
  echo i.
fat-suppressed T1-weighted 3D
  spoiled gradient-echo i.
fat- and water-suppressed T2-
  weighted i.
FLAIR i.
FLASH i.
flawed i.
flip-angle i.
floating i.
flow-compensated i.
flow-on gradient-echo i.
fluoroscopic i.
i. foldover
i. formation
four-dimensional i.
frequency domain i.
i. fusion
gadolinium-enhanced T1-weighted
  axial i.

NOTES

image (continued)

gadolinium-enhanced T1-weighted MRI i.

gated i.

ghost i.

gradient-echo axial i.

gradient-echo coronal i.

gradient-echo T2-weighted i.

gradient-encoded i.

gradient-recalled echo i.

gray-scale i.

GRE-in i.

GRE-out i.

half-Fourier RARE i.

hard-copy i.

i. hashing

high-resolution 3D spoiled-GRASS i.

high-resolution transverse view i.

histomorphometric i.

horizontal long axis SPECT i.

imaginary i.

immediate postflow i.

inhomogeneous i.

in-phase T1-weighted i.

i. intensification

i. intensification fluorometry

i. intensifier

i. intensifier system

i. intensifier tube

intercondylar sagittal i.

intermediate i.

inversion recovery i.

inversion recovery-weighted i.

IR i.

large-field-of-view i.

late-phase i.

lateral sagittal i.

localizing i.

longitudinal i.

magnetic resonance multispectral color I.

magnetic susceptibility-weighted i.

magnetization transfer gradient-echo i.

magnitude i.

matrix i.

maximum intensity projection and source i.

midcoronal oblique i.

midplane sagittal i.

midsagittal MR i.

minimum intensity projection i.

MIP i.

mirror i.

misleading i.

i. modulation

modulus i.

motion-triggered cine kinematic MR i.

multiecho axial i.

multiecho coronal i.

multiplanar volume-reformatted i.

multiple planar gradient-recalled i.

native i.

negative i.

i. noise

nonattenuation-corrected i.

nonmagnetization transfer gradient-refocused echo i.

nonmagnified i.

nonsubtracted i.

nonsubtraction i.

nuclear magnetic resonance i.

opposed GRE i.

opposed-phase T1-weighted i.

overlapping i.

panoramic i.

parallel-tagged MR i.

parametric i.

parasagittal i.

parenchymal phase i.

phantom i.

phase i.

phase-corrected GRE i.

phase-velocity i.

pinhole i.

plain-paper i.

planar left anterior oblique i.

postexercise i.

post fire i.

postintraarticular paramagnetic contrast injection T1-weighted i.

i. postprocessing

i. postprocessing error artifact

poststress i.

prefire i.

i. processing workstation

projectional i.

proton-density axial i.

proton-density-weighted fast spin-echo i.

pulse-echo i.

PVP i.

i. quality

i. quality degradation

quasiradiographic i.

radiographic i.

rapid half-Fourier T2-weighted i.

real-time echo-planar i.

reconstructed i.

i. reconstruction

i. reconstruction algorithm

i. reconstruction computer

i. recording system
recovery time i.
reference i.
i. reformation
reformatted T1 magnetic
  resonance i.
i. registration
registration and alignment of 3D i.
renal i.
i. restoration algorithm
sagittal fat-suppressed T1-weighted
  3D spoiled gradient-echo i.
sagittal scout i.
sagittal T1-weighted MR i.
saturation recovery i.
scout i.
scrambled i.
second-echo i.
see-through i.
SE proton-density weighted i.
sequential postcontrast MR i.
i. set
i. shading
i. sharpness
short axis i.
short tau inversion recovery i.
single section 2D i.
single-slice gradient-echo i.
i. slice thickness
sliding thin-slab maximum intensity
  projection i.
smoked glass i.
spatial modulation of
  magnetization i.
i. spatial resolution
spectral-spatial i.
spin-echo pilot i.
spin-echo T1-weighted i.
spin-lock-induced T1-rho
  weighted i.
spot compression i.
spot-magnification i.
standard-dose enhanced conventional
  T1 weighted i.
static i.
stop-action i.
stress-and-rest i.
stress thallium i.
striation across i.
stroke count i.
stroke volume i.
subtracted i.

subtraction i.
T2 i.
tensor diffusion-weighted MR i.
T2-gradient refocused i.
thick slab 3D multiplanar
  reformatted i.
thin-collimation i.
thin-cut axial CT i.
thin-section axial i.
three-dimensional Fourier transform
  volume i.
transaxial fat-saturated 3D i.
transcoronal STIR i.
transient punctate cortical
  hyperintensities on T1-weighted i.
transverse ECD brain SPECT i.
transverse-plane PET i.
trauma register i.
TSE i.
turboSTIR i.
T1-weighted i. (T1WI)
T2-weighted i. (T2WI)
T1-weighted axial i.
T2-weighted axial i.
T1-weighted coronal i.
T1-weighted fat-suppressed i.
  (T1FS)
T1-weighted fat-suppressed
  gadolinium-enhanced SE i.
T1-weighted gadolinium-enhanced
  SE i.
T2-weighted sagittal oblique i.
T2-weighted spin-echo i.
T2-weighted turbo SE i.
ultrasonic tomographic i.
i. uniformity
unopposed i.
variance i.
velocity-encoded i.
ventilation i.
ventricular function equilibrium i.
i. volume
volume-rendered 3D i.
volumetric i.
x-ray i.
zebra stripe i.
image-acquisition
  i.-a. gated examination
  i.-a. time
image-amplified fluoroscopy
image-degrading scattering
image-forming system

NOTES

image-guided
    i.-g. radiofrequency tumor ablation
    i.-g. radiosurgery
    i.-g. surgery
    i.-g. therapy
image-intensifier node
ImageMASTER
Imagent
    I. BP
    I. GI
    I. GI, US imaging agent
    I. LN
image-processing software
imager
    Acuson 128EP i.
    Agfa LR 3300 laser i.
    DaTSCAN i.
    Digirad 2020tc i.
    Digital Fundus i.
    Drystar dry i.
    flat-panel megavoltage i.
    full-body echo-planar system i.
    GE Advantage 1.5T i.
    GE Echospeed 1.5T whole-body
      MR i.
    GE Signa 5.4 Genesis MR i.
    GE Signa 5.5 Horizon EchoSpeed
      MR i.
    Hewlett-Packard color flow i.
    I. II catheter
    Integris V3000 i.
    IRIS III i.
    Kodak Digital Science 1200, 3600
      distributed medical i.
    laser i.
    Magnetom SP MRI i.
    NeuroScan 3D i.
    Sonata i.
    Tesla magnetic resonance i.
    VOXAR Plug n View 3D i.
image-reconstruction time
imager/spectrometer
    1.5T Signa whole body i.
image-selected in vivo spectroscopy
imaginary
    i. image
    i. mode
    i. number
    i. signal
imaging (*See* image, MRI)
    3DFT gradient-echo MR i.
    3DFT volume i.
    3D magnetic source i.
    3D processed ultrafast
      computerized i.
    3D turbo SE i.
    3D ultrasound reconstruction i.

acetazolamide challenge brain
  SPECT i.
acoustic i.
acute cerebral infarct i.
adenosine stress i.
adrenal i.
A-FAIR i.
i. agent
agent detection i.
air-contrast i.
air enema fluoroscopic i.
Aloka i.
amplitude i.
AMT-25-enhanced MR i.
angiography i.
anisotropically rotational diffusion i.
anisotropic 3D i.
annotated i.
antegrade pyelography i.
anthropometric i.
antifibrin antibody i.
aortography i.
aperiodic functional MR i.
AquariusBLUE 3D i.
arteriovenous shunt i.
arthrography i.
Artoscan MRI i.
A-scan i.
ascending contrast phlebography i.
attenuation i.
axial breath-hold gradient-echo cine
  magnetic resonance i.
axial echo planar diffusion
  weighted i.
axial grade echo i.
axial plane i.
axial 0.2T T1-weighted spin-echo i.
balloon expulsion i.
balloon test occlusion i.
barium enema i.
barium swallow i.
bile duct i.
biliary tract CT scan i.
binary i.
bird-cage coil designed for wrist i.
black blood T2-weighted inversion-
  recovery MR i.
blipped echo planar i. (bEPI)
blood flow i.
blood oxygen level-dependent
  contrast i.
blood pool i.
BMIPP SPECT scan i.
B-mode i.
body coil i.
body section radiography i.
BOLD contrast i.

bolus challenge i.
bone age i.
bone density i.
bone length i.
bone marrow edema pattern on MR i.
bone mineral content i.
bone phase i.
bone scintiscan i.
brain scan i.
breath-hold segmented k-space gradient-echo i.
breath-hold T1-weighted gradient echo i.
breath-hold T1-weighted MP-GRE MR i.
breath-hold ungated i.
breath-hold velocity-encoded cine MR i.
bright-field i.
bronchial provocation i.
bronchogram i.
B-scan i.
bull's eye i.
Captopril-stimulated renal i.
cardiac blood pool i.
cardiac catheterization i.
cardiac positron emission tomography i.
cardiac radiography i.
cardiac wall motion i.
Cardiolite scan i.
cardiotocography i.
cardiovascular radioisotope scan and function i.
carotid duplex i.
carotid sinus i.
CAS i.
CEA-Scan diagnostic i.
cephalogram i.
cerebral perfusion SPECT i.
Ceretec brain i.
i. chain veiling glare
chemical-selective fat-saturation i.
chemical shift i. (CSI)
cholangiography i.
Chopper-Dixon fat suppression i.
cine CT i.
cine-gated i.
cine gradient-echo MR i.
cine gradient magnetic resonance i.

Cine Memory with color flow Doppler i.
cine phase contrast i.
cineradiography i.
cine view i.
cisternography i.
CKG i.
CMJ i.
coded-aperture i.
cognitive functional MR i.
coincidence i.
cold spot myocardial i.
collimation i.
color amplitude i.
color-coded Doppler flow i. (CDFI)
color-coded pulmonary blood flow i.
color Doppler i. (CDI)
color encoded brain MR i.
color-flow i. (CFI)
color-flow Doppler i.
color-flow Doppler real-time 2D blood flow i.
color-flow duplex i.
color velocity i.
column-mode sinogram i.
combined leukocyte-marrow i.
combined Myoscint/thallium i.
combined thallium-Tc-HMPAO i.
i. compatible stereotactic coordinate frame
Compuscan Hittman computerized i.
computed transmission tomography i.
computer fusion i.
continuous i. (CI)
continuous-wave Doppler i.
contrast-enhanced fundamental i.
contrast-enhanced magnetic resonance i.
contrast-enhanced T1-GRE i.
contrast-enhanced T1-weighted spin-echo high-field-strength MR i.
contrast enhancement of computed tomographic i.
contrast-enhancing parametric i.
conventional planar i. (CPI)
conventional spin-echo i.
convergent color Doppler i.
coronary artery scan i.
corpus cavernosonography i.
corrected gradient echo phase i.

NOTES

imaging *(continued)*

correlative diagnostic i.
correlative pertechnetate thyroid i.
cross-sectional i.
CSF-suppressed T2-weighted 3D MP-RAGE MR i.
CTAT i.
CT/SPECT fusion i.
cystography i.
cystourethroscopy i.
dacryocystography i.
darkfield i.
3D echo planar i.
delayed bone i.
DentaScan i.
DEXA bone density scan i.
dexamethasone suppression test i.
3D fast low-angle shot i.
3D fast spin-echo magnetic resonance i.
2D Fourier transformation i.
diagnostic i. (DI)
DIET fast SE i.
diffraction-enhanced i. (DEI)
diffusion magnetic resonance i.
diffusion tension i. (DTI)
diffusion tensor i. (DTI)
diffusion tensor MR i.
diffusion-weighted i. (DWI)
diffusion-weighted echo planar i.
diffusion-weighted MR i.
digital chest i.
digitally fused CT and radiolabeled i.
digital radiography i.
digital vascular i. (DVI, DVI mode)
dipyridamole echocardiography i.
dipyridamole handgrip i.
dipyridamole infusion i.
dipyridamole thallium-201 i.
dipyridamole thallium stress i.
direct Fourier transformation i.
discontinuous i.
displacement field-fitting MR i.
diuretic renal i.
2D KWE direct Fourier i.
3D KWE direct Fourier i.
2D modified KWE direct Fourier i.
Doppler color-flow i.
Doppler tissue i. (DTI)
Doppler ultrasonography i.
Doppler venous i.
double-dose gadolinium i.
double-helical CT i.

double-phase technetium-99m sestamibi i.
double pulse interlaced echo i. (DOPING)
3D projection reconstruction i.
dry laser i.
DSC MR i.
DT MR i.
3D T1-weighted gradient-echo i.
dual-coil i.
dual-echo DIET fast spin-echo i.
dual-echo and DT MR i.
dual-energy i.
dual isotope i.
dual-phase ^{99m}Tc-sestamibi i.
dual-tracer i.
duodenography i.
duplex carotid i.
duplex Doppler i.
dynamic contrast-enhanced magnetic resonance i. (DCE-MRI)
dynamic contrast-enhanced subtraction MR i.
dynamic magnetic resonance i.
dynamic renal i.
dynamic scintigraphy i.
dynamic susceptibility contrast magnetic resonance i.
dynamic volume i.
ECG-gated multislice MR i.
ECG-gated spin-echo MR i.
echo i.
echocardiogram planar i.
echocardiography i.
echo-planar i. (EPI)
echo-planar diffusion-weighted i.
echo-planar FLAIR i.
echo-planar GRE T2*-weighted i.
elastic i.
electric joint fluoroscopy i.
electrocardiogram-gated MRI i.
electrocardiography-gated echo-planar i.
electrodiagnostic i.
electromagnetic blood flow i.
electronic portal i.
electron paramagnetic resonance spatial i.
electron radiography i.
electrostatic i.
end-diastolic i.
endoanal MR i.
endocrine i.
endorectal surface-coil MR i.
enhanced i.
Ensemble contrast i. (ECI)
epicardial i.

epididymography i.
equilibrium MUGA i.
ERCP i.
esophageal function i.
esophagography i.
excretory urography i.
exercise thallium-201 stress i.
ex vivo magnetic resonance i.
fast cardiac phase contrast cine i.
fast Fourier i.
fast multiplanar inversion recovry i.
fast multiplanar spoiled gradient-
  recalled i.
fast scan magnetic resonance i.
fast spin-echo black blood i.
fast spin-echo and fast inversion
  recovery i.
fast spin-echo MR i.
fast spoiled gradient-recalled MR i.
fat-suppressed 3D spoiled gradient-
  recall echo i.
fat-suppressed gadolinium-
  enhanced i.
fat-suppressed three-dimensional
  spoiled gradient-echo FLASH
  MR i.
fat/water chemical shift i.
FDG-labeled positron i.
FDG myocardial i.
ferumoxtran-enhanced echo-planar
  GRE T2*-weighted i.
ferumoxtran-enhanced echo-planar
  SE T2-weighted i.
^{18}F FDG-negative i.
field-echo i.
field-of-view i.
filmless i.
first-pass myocardial perfusion i.
FLAIR echo-planar i.
FLAIR-FLASH i.
FLASH magnetic resonance i.
flat-field i.
flawed i.
flow i.
flow-sensitive MR i.
fluoroscopic i.
fluoroscopy-guided condylar lift-
  off i.
flush aortogram i.
four-dimensional i.
four-hour delayed thallium i.
Fourier direct transformation i.

Fourier multislice modified KWE
  direct i.
Fourier transform i.
Fourier two-dimensional i.
FOV i.
frequency domain i. (FDI)
FS burst MR i.
functional brain i.
functional magnetic resonance i.
  (fMRI)
functional spin-echo i.
gadolinium-enhanced MR i.
gallbladder i.
gallium lung i.
gastric emptying i.
gastric mucosa i.
gastrointestinal motility i.
gas ventilation i.
gated cardiac blood pool i.
gated equilibrium cardiac blood
  pool i.
gated magnetic resonance i.
gated SPECT myocardial
  perfusion i.
Gd-FMPSPGR i.
GNG phase i.
i. gradient
gradient-echo flow i.
gradient-echo MR i.
gradient-echo phase i.
gradient-echo sequence i.
gradient-echo three-dimensional
  Fourier transform volume i.
gradient-to-noise i.
GRASS MR i.
gray-scale i.
GRE breath-hold hepatic i.
GRE gadolinium-chelate enhanced i.
GRE-in i.
GRE magnetic resonance i.
GRE-out i.
i. guided catheter drainage
half-Fourier i. (HFI)
half-Nex i.
harmonic i.
HAT-transformed i.
HBCT i.
heat-denatured autologous RBC
  SPECT i.
heavy ion i.
Helios diagnostic i.

NOTES

imaging *(continued)*

helium magnetic resonance i. (He-MRI)

hemodynamically weighted echo-planar MR i.

hepatobiliary ductal system i.

HIDA i.

high-definition i. (HDI)

high-energy i.

high-field-strength MR i.

high-frequency Doppler ultrasound i.

high-resolution B-mode i.

high-resolution CT i.

high-resolution 3DFT MR i.

high-resolution infrared i. (HRI)

high-resolution storage phosphor i.

high-speed i.

HLA i.

H-1 MR spectroscopic i.

holography i.

hot-spot heart i.

hot-spot myocardial i.

HRI i.

hybrid i.

hybrid-RARE i.

hydrogen proton i.

hypotonic duodenography i.

hysterosalpingography i.

^{123}I BMIPP i.

image acquisition-gated scan i.

infarct-avid i.

infection i.

infrared i.

initial i.

in-phase GRE i.

integrated functional magnetic resonance i.

intermediate i.

interventional i.

interventional magnetic resonance i. (I-MRI)

intracoronary i.

intracranial i.

intraoperative i.

intraperitoneal technetium sulfur colloid i.

intrathecal i.

intravascular ultrasound i.

intravenous fluorescein angiography i.

inversion recovery echo planar i. (IR-EPI)

^{111}In white blood cell i.

iodine fluorescence i.

iodomethyl-norcholesterol scintigraphy i.

irreversible compression of MR i.

Isocam scintillation i.

isotope colloid i.

isotope hepatobiliary i.

isotope-labeled fibrinogen i.

isotope shunt i.

isotopic 3D i.

isotropic diffusion-weighted i.

IVFA i.

KCD i.

511-keV high-energy i.

kidney function i.

kidney radionuclide i.

kidneys, ureter, and bladder i.

kinematic magnetic resonance i.

kinestatic charge detector i.

KUB i.

laser-polarized helium MR i.

limitation of MR i.

limited i.

line i.

linear scan i.

lipid-polarized helium MR i.

lipid-sensitive MR i.

liver-spleen i.

localizing i.

longitudinal section i.

loopogram i.

lower extremity i.

lower limb venography i.

low-field-strength MR i.

low-flip-angle gradient-echo i.

low-resolution i.

lung i.

lymphangiography i.

lymphatic i.

lymph node i.

macromolecular contrast-enhanced MR i.

magic-angle spinning i.

Magnes 2500 whole-head i.

magnetic resonance i. (MRI)

magnetic resonance catheter i.

magnetic resonance diffusion i.

magnetic resonance perfusion i.

magnetic source i. (MSI)

magnetization and spin-lock transfer i.

magnetization transfer weighted i.

magnetoacoustic i.

malignant melanoma gallium i.

mammary ductogram i.

mammary galactogram i.

mangafodipir trisodium-enhanced MR i.

i. manifestation

marker transit i.

mass i.
material spin echocardiogram total
  volume i.
Matrix LR3300 laser i.
maxillofacial i.
maximum intensity projection i.
MCD i.
mediastinal cross-sectional i.
micro-CT i.
microscopic i.
microwave i.
middle-field-strength MR i.
midsagittal MR i.
miniature i.
minimum intensity projection i.
mirror i.
misleading i.
M-mode echocardiogram i.
morphologic i.
motion-free i.
moving tabletop MR i.
MRA i.
MR echo-planar i.
MR enteroclysis i.
MRI-guided laser-induced
  interstitial i.
MUGA cardiac blood pool i.
multiecho i.
multiformatted i.
multigated i.
multigated spectral Doppler i.
  (MSDI)
multimodality i.
multiorgan i.
multiplanar MR i.
multiplanar reformatted radiographic
  and digitally reconstructed
  radiographic i.
multiple-echo i.
multiple-gated blood pool i.
multiple line scan i. (MLSI)
multiple-plane i.
multiple slice i.
multisection diffuse-weighted
  magnetic resonance i.
multisection gradient-echo echo-
  planar i.
multishot echo-planar i. (MS-EPI)
multishot spin-echo echo-planar i.
multislice first-pass myocardial
  perfusion i.

multislice modified KWE direct
  Fourier i.
multitime point i.
multitracer i.
musculoskeletal i.
MUSTPAC ultrasound i.
myelography i.
myocardial I-123 MIBG i.
myocardial infarct i.
myocardial perfusion i. (MPI)
myocardial thallium i.
Myoscint i.
^{23}Na magnetic resonance i.
native tissue harmonic i. (NTHI)
navigated spin-echo diffusion-
  weighted MR i.
nephrostogram i.
nephrotomography i.
neurodiagnostic i.
neuroradiologic i.
neurotransmitter i.
NMR i.
nonavid infarct i.
noninvasive i.
nonsubtraction i.
nuclear bone i.
nuclear cardiovascular i.
nuclear gated blood pool i.
nuclear hepatobiliary i.
nuclear magnetic resonance i.
nuclear medicine i.
nuclear perfusion i.
oblique axial MR i.
oblique magnetic resonance i.
oblique sagittal EKG-gated spin-
  echo magnetic resonance i.
OCG i.
octreotide i.
off-resonance saturation pulse i.
one-dimensional chemical-shift i.
  (1D-CSI)
one-shot echo-planar i.
on-line portal i.
opposed-phase GRE, MR i.
optical surface i. (OSI)
optimum angle i.
oral cholecystogram i.
organ-specific scintigraphic i.
orthopantogram i.
orthoroentgenogram i.
out-of-phase GRE i.

NOTES

imaging *(continued)*

oxygenation-sensitive functional MR i.
oxygen-enhanced lung MR i.
PACS PathSpeed MR i.
pancreas ultrasonography i.
pancreatography i.
panoramic i.
parallel hole i.
paramagnetic enhancement accentuation by chemical shift i.
parathyroid ultrasonography i.
partial Fourier i.
PASTA i.
pediatric nuclear medicine i.
percutaneous intracoronary angioscopy i.
perfusion MR i.
perfusion and ventilation lung i.
perfusion-weighted i. (PWI)
perineogram i.
peripheral vascular i.
peritoneogram i.
Persantine thallium i.
PET lung i.
PET metabolic i.
PET myocardial fatty acid i.
PET perfusion metabolism i.
PETT i.
phased-array body coil MR i.
phased-array multicoil i.
phased-array surface coil MR i.
phase-dependent spectroscopic i.
phase-encode time-reduced acquisition sequence i.
phase-sensitive gradient-echo MR i.
phase velocity i.
photostimulable phosphor digital i.
physiologic i.
PIPIDA hepatobiliary i.
plain film i.
planar radionuclide i.
planar spin i.
planar thallium i.
i. plane
point i.
polarity-altered spectral-selective acquisition i.
POMP i.
portal venous phase i.
postcontrast MR i.
postdrainage i.
postexercise i.
postinjection i.
postmetrizamide CT i.
postoperative cholangiography i.
power Doppler i. (PDI)

precontrast i.
preoperative i.
pressure perfusion i.
pretherapy i.
projection reconstruction i.
projection tract i.
protodensity MR i.
proton chemical shift i.
proton-density-weighted i.
proton-electron double-resonance i. (PEDRI)
proton MR spectroscopic i.
pseudodynamic MR i.
pullback i.
pulmonary perfusion i.
pulmonary ventilation i.
pulsed electron paramagnetic i.
pulsed magnetization transfer MR i.
pulse-echo i.
pulse-inversion i.
pulse-inversion harmonic i. (PIHI)
pulse sequence echo-planar i.
pyelography i.
PYP i.
pyrophosphate i.
QCT i.
quantitative brain i.
quantitative chemical shift i. (QCSI)
quantitative fluorescence i.
quantitative lung perfusion i.
quantitative magnetic resonance i. (qMRI, QMRI)
quantitative spirometrically controlled CT i.
radioactive fibrinogen i.
radiographically normal i.
radioisotope cisternography i.
radioisotope gallium i.
radioisotope indium-labeled white blood cell i.
radioisotope technetium i.
radiolabeled antibody i.
radionuclide-gated blood pool i.
radionuclide milk i.
radionuclide renal i.
radionuclide renography i.
radionuclide thyroid i.
rapid axial MR i.
rapid-excitation MR i.
rapid-sequence i.
^{82}Rb-based cardiac i.
real-time color Doppler i.
real-time 2D blood flow i.
receptor i.
reconstructed radiographic i.

reconstruction from projections i.
reconstructive i.
rectilinear bone scan i.
redistribution thallium-201 i.
renal angiography i.
renal CT i.
renal cyst i.
renal duplex i.
renal ultrasonography i.
renogram i.
respiratory gated i.
resting MUGA i.
rest myocardial perfusion i.
rest redistribution i.
rest thallium-201 myocardial i.
reticuloendothelial i.
ring-type i.
rose bengal sodium I-131 biliary i.
rotating delivery of excitation off-
  resonance MR i.
rotating frame i.
rotationally invariant i.
row-mode sinogram i.
R-to-R i.
sagittal fast spin-echo T2-weighted
  MR i.
sagittal gradient-echo i.
sagittal oblique i.
sagittal transabdominal i.
saline-enhanced MR i.
scanogram i.
3-Scape real-time 3D i.
scintigraphic scan i.
scintillation i.
scout i.
second-harmonic i.
sector-scan echocardiography i.
segmental k-space turbo gradient-
  echo breath-hold sequence i.
segmented echo-planar i. (SEPI)
segmenting dual-echo MR i.
selective excitation projection
  reconstruction i.
selenium-labeled bile acid i.
sensitive plane projection
  reconstruction i.
sequence echo-planar i.
sequence quantitative MR i.
sequential first pass i.
sequential line i.
sequential plane i.
sequential point i.

sequential quantitative MR i.
serial contrast MR i.
serial duplex i.
serial dynamic i.
serialography i.
sestamibi stress scan i.
shaded surface display i.
short inversion recovery i.
short TI inversion recovery i.
shuntogram i.
sialography i.
silhouette i.
simultaneous volume i.
single-dose gadolinium i.
single-echo diffusion i.
single-shot gradient echo-planar i.
single voxel proton brain
  spectroscopy i.
sinus tract i.
slip-ring i.
small field-of-view MR i.
SmartScore CT i.
sodium i.
SonoCT real-time compound i.
source i.
spastic electron paramagnetic
  resonance i.
SPECT i.
spectamine brain i.
spectral Doppler i.
spike-related functional MR i.
spin-echo cardiac i.
spin-echo magnetic resonance i.
spin-echo T1-weighted transaxial
  MR i.
spin-lock and magnetization
  transfer i.
spin-warp i.
SPIO-enhanced MR i.
splanchnic vascular i.
spleen ultrasonography i.
splenoportography i.
split-brain i.
SSD i.
stacked-scan i.
static 3D FLASH i.
steady-state free precession i.
steady-state gradient-echo i.
STIR i.
stop-action i.
storage phosphor i.
strain-rate MR i.

NOTES

imaging *(continued)*
    stress-only perfusion i.
    stress-redistribution i.
    stress thallium-201 myocardial i.
    i. study
    subsecond FLASH i.
    subtraction i.
    superparamagnetic iron oxide
      MR i.
    i. surveillance
    susceptibility-weighted MR i.
    target-to-nontarget ratio for
      myocardial i.
    ^{99m}Tc-HMPAO cerebral perfusion
      SPECT i.
    ^{99m}Tc-labeled denatured autologous
      RBC i.
    ^{99m}Tc Myoview myocardial
      perfusion i.
    technetium-99m anti-CEA Fab
      murine monoclonal antibody i.
    technetium-99m Infecton i.
    technetium-99m tetrofosmin
      exercise-rest SPECT myocardial
      perfusion i.
    technetium stannous
      pyrophosphate i.
    technetium Tc 99m
      pyrophosphate i.
    technetium-thallium subtraction i.
    thallium-201 i.
    thallium myocardial perfusion i.
    thallium myocardial scan with
      SPECT i.
    thallium rest-redistribution i.
    thallium scintography i.
    thallium stress i.
    thick-slice i.
    thin-collimation i.
    thin-slice i.
    thoracic duct i.
    three-phase i.
    three-phase whole-body bone i.
      (TPWBBI)
    ThromboScan i.
    through-transfer i.
    thyroid ultrasonography i.
    i. time
    timed i.
    time-of-flight echo-planar i.
    TIPS i.
    tissue Doppler i.
    tissue harmonic i. (THI)
    TOF i.
    tomographic i.
    Toshiba Aspire continuous i.
    total body scan i.

transabdominal i.
transaxial i.
transcervical catheterization of
  fallopian tube i.
transcranial real-time color
  Doppler i.
transesophageal Doppler color
  flow i.
transfer i.
transform i.
transjugular intrahepatic
  portosystemic shunt i.
transthoracic i.
transverse breath-hold gradient-echo
  cine magnetic resonance i.
transverse section i.
triple-dose gadolinium i.
triple-phase bone scan i.
true dynamic joint i.
TSPP i.
tumor i.
turboFLAIR i.
turboFLASH i.
T1-weighted coronal i.
T1-weighted sagittal i.
two-frame gated i.
two-phase computed tomographic i.
two-phase CT i.
UBM i.
ultrafast CT i.
ultrasonic tomographic i.
ultrasound backscatter microscopy i.
ultrasound-based strain rate and
  strain i.
unenhanced MR i.
unsuppressed i.
urethrocystography i.
urography i.
vascular flow i.
vectorcardiography i.
velocity i.
velocity-density i.
velocity-encoded cine i. (VINNIE)
velocity-encoded cine MR i.
venography i.
venous i.
ventilation-perfusion i.
vesiculography i.
videofluoroscopic i.
virtual reality i.
Vitrea 3D i.
in vivo He-3 MR i.
volume i.
volumetric i.
V/Q i.
VScore with AutoGate cardiac i.
wall motion i.

water selective spin-echo i.
wavelet-encoded magnetic
resonance i.
wet laser i.
white blood cell i.
whole-body echo-planar MR i.
whole-body scan i.
whole-body thallium i.
i. workstation
xenon-133 SPECT i.
x-ray-sensitive vidicon i.

imaging-anatomic correlation
imaging-based stereotaxis
imaging-directed 3D volumetric
information
imaging-pathologic correlation
Imagopaque contrast medium
Imatron
I. C-100 EBT scanner
I. C-150L EBCT scanner
I. C-1000 UFCT scanner
I. C-100 Ultrafast CT scanner
I. C-150XL CT scanner
I. C-100XP CT scanner
I. Fastrac C-100 cine x-ray CT
scanner

imbalance
biomechanical i.
i. of gain artifact
i. of phase artifact
ventilatory capacity-demand i.

imbrication
capsular i.
facetal i.

IMED Gemini PC-2 volumetric
controller
IMI
inferior myocardial infarct

imidodiphosphonate (IDP)
immature
i. bone
i. lung
i. lung syndrome
i. ovarian teratoma
skeletally i.

immaturity
structural pulmonary i.

immediate
i. postflow image
i. postictal period

immediately detachable coil

immersion
i. B-scan ultrasound
i. technique

imminent
i. death
i. demise

immobilization
bone mineral i.

immobilizer
Angle-Iron skull i.
AP-PA skull i.
i. board
cross-table leg i.
dual leg i.
shoulder i.
tomographic skull i.

immovable joint
immune
i. electron microscopy
i. response

immunoblastic large-cell lymphoma
immunocytic amyloidosis
immunocytochemical staining
immunofluorimetric assay
immunoglobulin
i. G (IgG)
indium-111-labeled human
nonspecific i. G
^{111}In-labeled human nonspecific i.
G

immunologic injury
immunolymphoscintigraphy
immunomagnetic
i. bead
i. purging

Immuno-mini NJ-2300 microplate reader
immunoprecipitate
immunoproliferative small intestine
disease (IPSID)
immunoradioassay
immunoreactivity
immunoscintigraphy
immunoscintimetry
immunostained surface
ImmuRAID antibody imaging agent
IMN
intramammary node

imodoacetic acid imaging agent
IMP
^{123}I isopropyl iodoamphetamine
iodoamphetamine

NOTES

impacted
    i. calculus
    i. feces
    i. fetus
    i. subcapital fracture
    i. urethral stone
    i. valgus fracture
impaction
    anteromedial superior humeral
      head i.
    fecal i.
    lateral compartment i.
    i. lesion
    mucoid i.
    stone i.
impact velocity
impaired
    i. renal function
    i. renal perfusion
    i. tubular transit
    i. venous return
    i. ventilation-perfusion
impairment
    axonal transport i.
    circulatory i.
    functional aerobic i.
    growth i.
    hemodynamic reserve i.
    inspiratory muscle function i.
    motor i.
    posterior cingulate functional i.
    renal function i.
    sensory i.
IMPAX PACS system
impedance
    acoustic i.
    aortic i.
    diastolic notch i.
    i. matching
    i. MR phlebogram
    i. phlebography
    i. plethysmography (IPG)
    pulmonary arterial input i.
    pulmonary vascular bed i.
    respiratory modulation of
      vascular i.
    vascular i.
    i. venography
impeller basket catheter
impending
    i. herniation
    i. myocardial infarct
imperfecta
    amelogenesis i.
    dentinogenesis i.
    osteogenesis i. (OI)

    Sillence classification of
      osteogenesis i.
imperfect regeneration
imperforate anus
impingement
    anterolateral i.
    dural i.
    i. exostosis
    graft roof i.
    lateral i.
    ligamentous i.
    nerve root i.
    outlet i.
    posterior i.
    posterosuperior glenoid i.
    shoulder i.
    sidewall i.
    i. spur
    syndesmotic i.
    i. syndrome
    talar i.
    talofibular i.
    triquetral i.
    ulnolunate i.
impinging osteophyte
implant
    Baerveldt glaucoma drainage i.
    biodegradable i.
    bone i.
    bowel serosal endometrial i.
    carcinomatous i.
    cesium i.
    cobalt-chromium-molybdenum alloy
      metal i.
    cobalt-chromium-tungsten-nickel
      alloy metal i.
    cochlear i.
    Co-Cr-Mo alloy metal i.
    collapsed subpectoral i.
    i. collar
    double-lumen breast i.
    double-stem silicone lesser MP i.
    electrically activated i.
    endometrial i.
    endosseous i.
    epidural i.
    extraperitoneal i.
    ferromagnetic i.
    i. fracture
    hinged i.
    hydroxyapatite i.
    ^{125}I interstitial radiation i.
    interstitial low-dose-rate iridium-192
      needle i.
    intracavitary i.
    iridium-192 endobronchial i.
    iridium-192 wire i.

Joseph valve i.
Krupin-Denver eye valve-to-disc i.
malignant pleural i.
mammary i.
mechanically activated i.
metallic otologic i.
methyl methacrylate bead i.
ocular i.
open-cord tendon i.
otologic i.
palladium i.
^{103}Pd prostatic i.
penile i.
peritoneal metastatic i.
permanent interstitial i.
polymethyl methacrylate i.
prostate i.
prosthetic i.
retropectoral mammary i.
saline i.
serosal endometrial i.
silicone elastomer rubber ball i.
silicone wrist i.
single-lumen silicone breast i.
subpectoral i.
synthetic bone i.
temporary interstitial i.
total knee i.
transperineal i.
transvaginal i.
tumor i.
VDS i.

implantable
i. access catheter
i. drug delivery system
i. infusion port
i. infusion pump
i. vascular access device

implantation
i. cyst
epicardial i.
percutaneous transperineal seed i.
peroral i.
radon seed i.
i. site
subxiphoid i.
transluminal endograft i.
transvenous i.
two-staged stent i.

implanted
i. imaging opaque marker

i. NCP
i. pacemaker

impotence
arteriogenic i.
hemodynamic i.
vasogenic i.

impression
basilar i.
cardiac i.
colic i.
convolutional i.
digastric i.
duodenal i.
esophageal i.
extrinsic esophageal i.
extrinsic stomach i.
i. fracture
gastric i.
liver i.
renal i.
suprarenal i.

imprint
tissue i.

improved
i. Chen-Smith (ICS)
i. Chen-Smith coder
i. photon flux

improvement
interval i.

impulse
apical i.
bifid precordial i.
double systolic apical i.
downward displacement of apical i.
ectopic i.
high-amplitude i.
hyperdynamic right ventricular i.
jugular venous i.
nodal i.
prolonged left ventricular i.
sustained apical i.
systolic i.
undulant i.

I-MRI
interventional magnetic resonance
imaging

IMRT
intensity-modulated radiation therapy
intensity-modulated radiotherapy
treatment
SmartBeam IMRT

NOTES

459

IMT
   intimal-medial thickness
In
   indium
¹¹¹In, In-111
   indium-111
      ¹¹¹In antimyosin scintigraphy
      ¹¹¹In chloride
      ¹¹¹In DTPA
      ¹¹¹In imciromab pentetate
      ¹¹¹In labeling
      ¹¹¹In murine monoclonal antibody
      Fab to myosin
      ¹¹¹In octreotide
      ¹¹¹In-oxime-labeled leukocyte
      ¹¹¹In oxine
      ¹¹¹In oxine WBCs
      ¹¹¹In pentetreotide
      ¹¹¹In pentetreotide imaging agent
      ¹¹¹In satumomab pendetide
      ¹¹¹In WBCs
      ¹¹¹In white blood cell imaging
in
   in situ
   in situ graft
   in situ pinning
   in toto
   in utero
   in utero detection of cardiac
   anomaly
   in vitro evaluation of coil
   in vitro labeling
   in vivo
   in vivo balloon pressure
   in vivo correlation
   in vivo disposition study
   in vivo examination
   in vivo He-3 MR imaging
   in vivo labeling
   in vivo method
   in vivo microscopy
   in vivo optical spectroscopy
   (INVOS)
   in vivo proton MR spectroscopy
   in vivo stereologic assessment
   in vivo technique
inactivator
inactive
   i. endometrium
   i. mode
inadequate
   i. bowel preparation
   i. calvarial calcification
   i. cardiac output
   i. cranial calcification
   i. runoff
   i. visualization

inadvertent arterial injection
incarcerated
   i. hernia
   i. omentum
   i. placenta
incarceration
   fetal i.
incessant ovulation
incidence
incident
   i. angle
   i. ray
incidental
   i. finding
   i. lung uptake
   i. punctate white matter
   hyperintensity
incidentaloma
   adrenal i.
   brain i.
incision
   Brödel bloodless line of i.
incisional hernia
incisive
   i. bone
   i. canal
   i. suture
incisor
   fascial i.
   i. teeth
incisura, incisure, pl. **incisurae**
   i. angularis
   aortic i.
   cardiac i.
   i. defect
   i. dextra of Gans
   i. scapulae
   stomach defect i.
incisural
   i. epidermoidoma
   i. sclerosis
inciting
   i. event
   i. factor
inclination
   radial i.
   ulnar i.
   urethral i. (UI)
   i. verse
   volar i.
inclinometer
inclusion cyst
incoherence
   magnetic resonance spin i.
incoherent
   i. motion
   i. spin

incompetence
> aortic valvular i.
> chronotropic i.
> communicating vein i.
> deep venous i.
> gastroesophageal i.
> mitral valve i.
> myocardial i.
> postphlebitic valvular i.
> pulmonary i.
> saphenous vein i.
> sphincter i.
> traumatic tricuspid i.
> tricuspid i. (TI)
> valvular i.

incompetent
> i. blood-brain barrier
> i. cervix
> i. ileocecal valve
> i. perforator

incomplete
> i. atrioventricular block (IAVB)
> i. bladder emptying
> i. closure
> i. dislocation
> i. fracture
> i. fracture of bone
> i. heart block
> i. hernia
> i. left bundle-branch block
> (ILBBB)
> i. lower esophageal sphincter
> relaxation
> i. neurofibromatosis
> i. obstruction
> i. placenta previa
> i. pulmonary fissure
> i. resolution of pneumonia
> i. right bundle-branch block
> (IRBBB)
> i. stroke
> i. tumor
> i. ureteral duplication

incongruency
> patellofemoral i.

incongruity
> angle of i.
> facet joint i.
> joint i.

incontinence
> bladder i.
> bowel i.

> fecal i.
> motor urge i.
> stress i.

increased
> i. airway
> i. anteroposterior diameter
> i. attenuation
> i. basilar cistern
> i. bone density
> i. carrying angle
> i. central venous pressure
> i. cerebrovascular resistance
> i. density spleen
> i. echogenicity
> i. echo signal
> i. extracellular fluid volume
> i. interstitial fluid
> i. interstitial marking
> i. intracranial pressure
> i. intrapericardial pressure
> i. isotope uptake
> i. lateral joint space
> i. left ventricular ejection time
> i. marking of emphysema
> i. myocardial oxygen requirement
> i. outflow resistance
> i. peripheral resistance
> i. peristalsis
> i. prominence of pulmonary vessel
> i. pulmonary arterial pressure
> i. pulmonary obstruction
> i. pulmonary vascularity
> i. pulmonary vascular marking
> i. pulmonary vascular resistance
> i. pulmonary vasculature
> i. renal echogenicity cortex
> i. skull thickness
> i. splenic density
> i. thyroid uptake
> i. tracer activity
> i. tracer uptake
> i. uptake of radiotracer
> i. ventricular afterload

increase in intensity
increasingly dense nephrogram
increment
> i. in luminal diameter
> i. of perfusion

incremental
> i. dose
> i. risk factor

NOTES

patellofemoral i.
penile-brachial pressure i. (PBPI)
perfusion i.
pipe-stemming of ankle-brachial i.
Ponderal I.
portal vein congestion i.
positive cephalopelvic
  disproportion i.
postexercise i.
poststress ankle/arm Doppler i.
Pourcelot i.
predicted cardiac i.
profundal popliteal collateral i.
proliferative i.
pulmonary arterial resistance i.
pulmonary blood volume i. (PBVI)
pulmonary vascular resistance i.
  (PVRI)
pulmonic output i.
pulsatility indices
pyloric i.
qualitative i.
quantitative i.
quantum mottle i.
rectosigmoid i.
renal resistive i.
reproducibility i.
resistive i. (RI)
resting ankle pressure i. (RAPI)
right and left ankle i.
right ventricular stroke work i.
  (RVSWI)
Ritchie i.
runoff resistance i.
i. of runoff resistance
saturation i. (SI)
i. of sensitivity
short-increment sensitivity i.
Singh osteoporosis i.
stroke i. (SI)
stroke volume i. (SVI)
stroke-work i. (SWI)
superior-medial acetabular i.
  (SMAI)
systemic arteriolar resistance i.
systemic output i.
systemic vascular resistance i.
  (SvO$_2$, SVRI)
systolic pressure-time i.
systolic toe/brachial i.
talocalcaneal i.
tension-time i. (TTI)

therapeutic i.
thoracic i.
thymic i.
thymidine labeling i. (TLI)
tritiated thymidine labeling i.
truncated arch i.
tubular fertility i.
ulnar styloid process i. (USPI)
valgus i.
venous distensibility i. (VDI)
ventricular i. (VI)
vertebral body i.
wall motion score i.
water perfusable tissue i.
weighted-CT-dose i.
widened anterior meningeal i.
Wood unit i.
india ink artifact
Indian
  I. childhood cirrhosis
  I. file
Indiana pouch
indicator
  i. dilution curve
  i. dilution method of perfusion
    assessment
  i. dilution therapy
  i. fractionation principle
  gamma ray level i.
  xylol pulse i.
**indicator-dilution method for cardiac
  output measurement**
indices (*pl. of* index)
indicis
  extensor i.
Indiclor
indifferent gonad
indigo calculus
Indigo LaserOptic treatment system
indirect
  i. blood supply
  i. computed tomography
  i. CT
  i. fracture
  i. hernia sac
  i. inguinal hernia
  i. laryngoscopy
  i. MR arthrography
  i. MR arthrography of knee
  i. placentography
  i. ray
  i. ultrasound guidance

NOTES

indirect-contract transmission
indiscernible
indiscrete
indiscriminate lesion
indistinct
    i. endometrial margin
    i. interface
indium (In)
    cistern i.
    i. IgG
    i. imaging agent
    i. transferrin
indium-111 (^{111}In, In-111) *(See* ^{111}In)
indium-111-labeled
    i.-l. human nonspecific
      immunoglobulin G
    i.-l. IgG
    i.-l. leukocyte
    i.-l. white blood cell scan
indocyanine
    i. dilution curve
    i. green angiography
    i. green dye
    i. green imaging agent
indoleamine
indolent
    i. lesion
    i. myeloma
    i. radiation-induced rectal ulcer
Indomitable scanner
induced
    i. acoustic emission
    i. biopotential
    i. pneumothorax
    i. radioactivity
    i. thrombosis of aortic aneurysm
inducibility basal state
inducible
inductance
inductance-capacitance (LC)
induction
    dorsal i.
    electric i.
    electromagnetic i.
    magnetic i.
    neuromuscular system electric i.
    ovulation i.
    i. therapy
inductively coupled plasma atomic
   emission spectrometry (ICP-AES)
inductive reactance (XL)
indurated
    i. mass
    i. tissue
indurativa
    tuberculosis cutis i.

indurative
    i. necrosis
    i. pleurisy
    i. pneumonia
indwelling
    i. cannula
    i. Foley catheter
    i. nonvascular shunt
    i. stent
inelastic pericardium
inequality
    limb-length i.
    ventilation-perfusion i.
inert
    i. dust pneumoconiosis
    i. pneumoconiosis
inexorable progression
infant
    i. cranial Doppler ultrasonography
    i. gastrointestinal hemorrhage
infantile
    i. arteriosclerosis
    i. cardiomyopathy
    i. coarctation
    i. coarctation of aorta
    i. cortical hyperostosis
    i. digital fibromatosis
    i. embryonal carcinoma
    i. fibrosarcoma
    i. ganglioglioma
    i. hemangioendothelioma
    i. hemangioendothelioma of liver
    i. hemiplegia
    i. hepatic hemangioma
    i. hydrocele
    i. hydrocephalus
    i. lobar emphysema
    i. myofibromatosis
    i. pneumonia
    i. polycystic kidney disease
    i. pylorospasm
    i. thoracic dystrophy
    i. uterus
infantilism
    intestinal i.
infarct, infarction
    acute ischemic brain i.
    acute myocardial i.
    acute nonhemorrhagic i.
    acute renal i.
    age-indeterminate i.
    anemic i.
    anterior communicating artery
     distribution i.
    anterior myocardial i.
    anterior septal myocardial i.
    anterior wall myocardial i.

anteroinferior myocardial i.
anterolateral myocardial i.
anteroseptal myocardial i.
apical-lateral wall myocardial i.
apical myocardial i.
arrhythmic myocardial i.
atherothrombotic brain i.
atrial i.
basal ganglia i.
bicerebral i.
bilateral i.
bland i.
bone i.
bowel i.
brain i.
brainstem i.
capsular i.
capsulocaudate i.
capsuloputaminal i.
capsuloputaminocaudate i.
cardiac i.
cerebellar i.
cerebral artery i.
chronic ischemic brain i.
chronic renal i.
concomitant i.
cortical bone i.
diaphragmatic myocardial i. (DMI)
digital livedo reticularis i.
dominant hemisphere i.
dural sinus thrombosis i.
embolic cerebral i.
evolving myocardial i.
i. expansion
extensive anterior myocardial i.
frontal lobe i.
full-thickness i.
gyral i.
healing i.
hemispheric i.
hemorrhagic brain i.
high lateral wall myocardial i.
hippocampal i.
hyperacute ischemic brain i.
hyperacute myocardial i.
impending myocardial i.
inferior myocardial i. (IMI)
inferolateral wall myocardial i.
inferoposterior wall myocardial i.
inferoposterolateral myocardial i.
intestinal i.
ischemic brainstem i.

kidney i.
lacunar brain i.
lateral myocardial i.
lobar renal i.
marrow i.
medullary bone i.
mesencephalic i.
mesenteric i.
middle cerebral artery i.
multifocal i.
multiple cortical i.'s
muscle i.
myocardial i. (MI)
nonarrhythmic myocardial i.
nonembolic i.
nonhemorrhagic i.
nonseptic embolic brain i.
nontransmural myocardial i.
occipital lobe i.
occlusive mesenteric i.
old myocardial i.
omental i.
papillary muscle i.
paramedian i.
parenchymal i.
periventricular hemorrhagic i.
pituitary i.
placental i.
i. of pons
pontine i.
posterior cerebral territory i.
posterior wall myocardial i.
posterobasal wall myocardial i.
posteroinferior myocardial i.
posterolateral wall myocardial i.
postmyocardial i.
postmyocardiotomy i.
pulmonary i.
Q-wave myocardial i.
red i.
renal i.
right ventricular i.
rule out myocardial i. (ROMI)
i. scan
segmental bowel i.
segmental omental i.
septal myocardial i.
septic pulmonary i.
silent myocardial i.
sinoatrial node i.
i. size limitation
small bowel i.

NOTES

infarct (continued)
  small, deep, recent i. (SDRI)
  spinal cord i.
  splenic i.
  subacute ischemic brain i.
  subacute myocardial i.
  subcortical i.
  subendocardial i. (SEI)
  subendocardial myocardial i.
  temporal lobe i.
  testicular i.
  thalamic i.
  thromboembolic pontine i.
  thrombolysis in myocardial i.
    (TIMI)
  thrombotic i.
  transmural myocardial i.
  traumatic i.
  uncomplicated myocardial i.
  uninfected i.
  venous i.
  ventral pontine i.
  watershed brain i.
  wedge-shaped i.
  white matter i.
infarct-avid imaging
infarcted
  i. heart muscle
  i. lung segment
  i. myocardium
  i. scar
  i. testis
infarction (var. of infarct)
infarct-localized asynergy
infected
  i. aneurysm
  i. bone
  i. pelvic hematoma
  i. thrombosed graft
infection
  alveolar i.
  aortic graft i.
  buccal space i.
  diffuse i.
  diskovertebral i.
  disk space i.
  filarial i.
  fungal i.
  hepatic fungal i.
  i. imaging
  interstitial i.
  intraabdominal i.
  intracranial opportunistic i.
  masticator space i.
  mycotic lung i.
  opportunistic lung cavity i.
  orbital i.

  pelvic i.
  pneumocystic i.
  pulmonary parenchymal i.
  renal fungal i.
  respiratory tract i.
  retroperitoneal i.
  rickettsial lung i.
  sacroiliac i.
  salivary gland i.
  spinal i.
  subperiosteal i.
  superimposed fungal i.
  temporal space i.
  tendon sheath space i.
  vessel displacement brain i.
infectious
  i. aortitis
  i. bubbly bone lesion
  i. cardiomyopathy
  i. heart disease
  i. pulmonary disorder
  i. splenomegaly
infective
  i. embolus
  i. thrombosis
inferior
  i. accessory fissure
  apertura pelvis i.
  i. apical aspect of the myocardium
  i. aspect
  i. beaking
  i. border
  i. border of heart
  i. cardiac branch
  i. cerebellar peduncle
  i. colliculus
  i. dental canal
  i. displacement
  i. dorsal radioulnar ligament
  i. duodenal flexure (IDF)
  i. duodenal recess
  i. epigastric artery
  i. esophageal sphincter (IES)
  i. extensor retinaculum
  fovea i.
  i. frontal gyrus
  i. gemellus muscle
  i. glenohumeral ligament labral
    complex (IGLLC)
  i. jugular vein bulb
  i. lobe
  i. lobe bronchus
  i. lobe of lung
  i. longitudinal diameter
  i. margin of superior rib
  i. medial facet
  i. mediastinum

i. mesenteric artery (IMA)
i. mesenteric plexus
i. mesenteric vein
i. myocardial infarct (IMI)
i. olive
i. ophthalmic vein
i. orbital fissure
i. parietal lobule
i. peroneal retinaculum
i. pole
i. pubic ramus
i. pulmonary ligament
i. pulmonary vein
i. quadriceps retinaculum
i. rectal vein
i. sagittal sinus (ISS)
i. spur
i. syndrome of red nucleus
i. temporal gyrus
i. temporal lobule
i. thyroid vein
i. tip of the fibula
i. tip of scapula
i. transverse rectal fold
i. turbinated bone
i. vena cava (IVC)
i. vena cava diaphragm
i. vena cava duplication
i. vena cavagram
i. vena caval obstruction
i. vena cava orifice
i. vena cava syndrome
i. vena cava transposition
i. venacavography (IVCV)
i. wall
i. wall akinesis
i. wall branch
i. wall hypokinesis
i. wall MI
i. wall motion
zygapophysis i.
inferior-anterior count ratio
inferiormost
inferoapical
i. defect
i. segment
i. wall
inferobasal segment
inferolateral
i. displacement of apical beat
i. surface of prostate
i. wall myocardial infarct

inferolaterally
inferomedial
inferoposterior
i. segment
i. wall myocardial infarct
inferoposterolateral myocardial infarct
inferred presence
infestation
helminthic i.
INFH
ischemic necrosis of femoral head
infiltrate
active i.
acute alveolar i.
aggressive interstitial i.
aggressive perivascular i.
alveolar i.
apical i.
Assmann tuberculous i.
basilar zone i.
benign i.
bilateral interstitial pulmonary i.
bilateral upper lobe cavitary i.
bone marrow i.
brachial plexus i.
bronchocentric inflammatory i.
butterfly pattern of i.
calcareous i.
calcium i.
cavitary i.
chronic alveolar i.
circumscribed i.
confluent i.
consolidated i.
diffuse aggressive polymorphous i.
diffuse alveolar interstitial i.
diffuse bilateral alveolar i.
diffuse fatty liver i.
diffuse perivascular i.
diffuse reticulonodular i.
eosinophilic i.
epituberculous i.
fatty i.
fibrocavitary i.
fibronodular i.
fleeting lung i.
fluffy i.
focal alveolar i.
focal interstitial i.
focal perivascular i.
granular i.
ground-glass i.

NOTES

infiltrate *(continued)*
  hazy i.
  interstitial nonlobar i.
  invasive angiomatous interstitial i.
  linear i.
  lingular i.
  lung base i.
  lymphoplasmacytic i.
  marrow i.
  massive i.
  meningeal i.
  micronodular i.
  migratory patchy i.
  mottled i.
  multifocal aggressive i.
  mural i.
  parasitic i.
  patchy migratory i.
  peribronchial i.
  pericapsular fat i.
  perihilar batwing i.
  peripheral i.
  perivascular i.
  pneumonic i.
  pulmonary parenchymal i.
  pulmonic i.
  punctate i.
  recurrent fleeting i.
  reticular i.
  reticulonodular i.
  retrocardiac i.
  reverse peripheral bat-wing i.
  soft i.
  subcutaneous i.
  sulfasalazine-induced pulmonary i.
  transient symmetric pulmonary i.
  tuberculous i.
infiltrating
  i. adenocarcinoma
  i. breast epitheliosis
  i. ductal carcinoma
  i. esophageal carcinoma
  i. lesion
  i. lipoma
  i. lobular carcinoma
  i. plaque
infiltration
  dose i.
  marrow i.
  myocardial i.
  pathologic marrow i.
  i. pattern
  i. suture
infiltrative
  i. astrocytoma
  i. cardiomyopathy

  i. hemorrhagic element
  i. lymphoma
infinitesimal Z spectrum
inflamed
  i. bronchus
  i. pleura
inflammation
  abdominal i.
  acute phase of i.
  adhesive i.
  alveolar septal i.
  aortic i.
  atrophic i.
  i. of bone
  i. of brain
  bronchial i.
  bursal i.
  calcaneal bursa i.
  cardiac muscle i.
  chronic abdominal i.
  cirrhotic i.
  i. of colon
  diffuse i.
  disseminated i.
  i. of epididymis
  esophageal i.
  extrinsic intraabdominal i.
  fibrinous i.
  fibrosing i.
  focal i.
  i. of heart
  hyperplastic i.
  hypertrophic i.
  interstitial i.
  intrinsic intraabdominal i.
  lung i.
  meningeal i.
  mucosal i.
  myocardial i.
  necrotic i.
  obliterative i.
  parenchymatous i.
  pill-induced i.
  polyarticular symmetric tophaceous
    joint i.
  proliferative i.
  pseudomembranous i.
  radionuclide i.
  renal i.
  retrodiskal temporomandibular joint
    pad i.
  sclerosing i.
  spinal i.
  spleen i.
  subacute i.
  suppurative i.
  tendon i.

thyroid gland i.
transmural i.
tumor i.
vein i.
inflammatoria
dysphagia i.
inflammatory
i. adhesion
i. aortic aneurysm
i. bowel disease
i. bowel disease arthritis
i. breast carcinoma (IBC)
i. cholesteatoma
i. colonic polyp
i. edema
i. element
i. endometritis
i. esophagogastric polyp
i. fibroid polyp
i. fibrosarcoma
i. fibrosis
i. focus
i. fracture
i. heart block
i. idiopathic orbital pseudotumor
i. intestinal pseudotumor
i. joint effusion
i. lesion
i. MFH
i. myofibroblastic tumor
i. osteoarthritis
i. polypoid mass
i. reaction
i. spleen
i. stomach polyp
i. synovial process
inflation
air i.
balloon i.
delivered by balloon i.
sequential balloon i.
simultaneous balloon i.
inflow
aortic i.
blood i.
i. cuff
i. disease progression
third i.
i. tract of left ventricle
inflow/outflow method
influence
paramagnetic i.

information
field-of-view i.
hierarchical i.
imaging-directed 3D volumetric i.
infraapical
infraaxillary
infracalcaneal bursitis
infracalcarine gyrus
infracardiac-type total anomalous venous return
infraclavicular
i. area
i. node
i. pocket
infraclusion (*var. of* infraocclusion)
infracolic
i. compartment
i. midline
infracostal
infracristal ventricular septal defect
infraction
i. fracture
Freiberg i.
infradiaphragmatic
i. application
i. totally anomalous pulmonary venous drainage
i. vein
infragastric infragenicular popliteal artery
infragenicular
i. position
i. revascularization
infrageniculate popliteal artery
infraglenoid
i. recess
i. tuberosity
infraglottic
i. larynx
i. space
infragluteal crease
infrahepatic
i. arteriography
i. vena cava
infrahilar area
infra-His block
infrahyoid lymph node
infrainguinal
i. arterial bypass graft
i. bypass stenosis
i. percutaneous transluminal angioplasty

NOTES

infrainguinal *(continued)*
    i. revascularization
    i. vein bypass graft
infralevator fistula
inframammary
    i. crease
    i. fold
inframammillary
inframesocolic space
infranuclear lesion
infraocclusion, infraclusion
infraorbital
    i. canal
    i. groove
    i. line
    i. margin (IOM)
    i. suture
infraorbitomeatal line (IOML)
infrapatellar
    i. aspect
    i. bursa
    i. contracture syndrome (IPCS)
    i. ligament
    i. plica
    i. tendon
    i. view
infrapopliteal
    i. artery occlusion
    i. vessel
infrapulmonary position
infrared
    i. camera
    i. imaging
    i. light
    i. light-emitting diode
    i. navigational system
    near i. (NIR)
    i. radiation
    i. ray
    i. spectrum
    i. thermography
infrarenal
    i. abdominal aorta
    i. abdominal aortic aneurysm
    i. stenosis
infraroentgen ray
infrascapular
infraspinatus
    i. insertion erosion
    i. muscle
    i. tendon
infraspinous
    i. fascia
    i. fossa
infrasternal
    i. angle
    i. fossa

infratemporal fossa
infratentorial
    i. compartment
    i. gray matter
    i. Lindau tumor
infraumbilical
    i. mound
    i. omphalocele
infravesical obstruction
infundibula (*pl. of* infundibulum)
infundibular
    i. atresia
    i. chamber
    i. pulmonary stenosis
    i. septum
    i. stalk
    i. subpulmonic stenosis
    i. systolic/diastolic ratio
    i. tilt
    i. tumor
    i. ventricular septal defect
infundibular-to-bulb ratio
infundibuloovarian ligament
infundibulopelvic ligament
infundibuloventricular crest
infundibulum, pl. **infundibula**
    i. of bile duct
    bile duct i.
    cerebral i.
    ductus i.
    gallbladder i.
    i. of hypophysis
    hypothalamic i.
    junctional i.
    i. of kidney
    os i.
    pituitary i.
    right ventricular i.
    tumor of i.
    i. widening
Infuse-a-Port catheter
infuser
    IVAC P4000 i.
    Ohio i.
infusion
    arterial i.
    balloon-occluded arterial i.
    i. catheter
    circadian continuous i.
    continuous intravenous i. (CIVI)
    epidural i.
    graded i.
    hepatic arterial i. (HAI)
    intralymphatic i.
    intraportal i.
    isolated hepatic i.
    isoproterenol i.

local streptokinase i.
i. nephrotomography
pericardial i.
prostaglandin i.
protracted venous i. (PVI)
i. pyelogram
i. pyelography
retrograde coronary sinus i.
subcutaneous i.
superselective i.
i. transcatheter therapy
infusothorax
Ingenor silicone mixture
ingrowth
bone i.
peripheral perimeniscal capillary i.
porous i.
inguinal
i. bulge
i. canal
i. crease
i. floor
i. fold
i. granuloma
i. hernia
i. ligament
i. ligament syndrome
i. lymph node
i. lymph node metastasis
i. pseudoaneurysm
i. ring
i. triangle
i. trigone
inguinale
papilloma i.
inhalation
i. anthrax
i. bronchopneumonia
end i.
i. of krypton-77
i. pneumonia
radioactive xenon gas i.
i. study
i. technique
tin oxide i.
i. tuberculosis
inhaled
i. oxygen imaging agent
i. radionuclide
inherent
i. density
i. filter

inherited cavernous angioma-related posthemorrhage encephalomalacia
inhibited
atrial i. (AAI)
inhibition
competitive i.
inhibitor
fusion i. (FI)
inhibitory
i. neurotransmitter
i. syndrome
inhomogeneity
B_O field i.
contrast i.
i. correction
hypointense signal i.
metaphyseal-diaphyseal low-signal-intensity red marrow i.
off-axis dose i.
signal intensity i.
inhomogeneous
i. attenuation
i. contrast enhancement
i. echo
i. echo pattern
i. echo texture
i. image
i. lung attenuation HRCT
i. moderate enhancement
i. tracer distribution
iniencephaly
inion bump
initial
i. atelectasis
i. imaging
injectate
injection
accidental intradural i.
air i.
barium i.
bismuth i.
bolus intravenous i.
coarse i.
contrast i.
Definity suspension for IV i.
double i.
epidural steroid i.
ethanol i.
extraarachnoid i.
facet joint i.
fine i.
Fluorescite i.

NOTES

injection *(continued)*

fluorodeoxyglucose F-18 i.
Funduscein i.
gaseous i.
Glofil-125 i.
hand i.
heavy metal i.
inadvertent arterial i.
intraamniotic i.
intraarterial i.
intracavernosal i.
intradermal i.
intradiskal i.
intramuscular fetal i.
intraperitoneal fetal i.
intravascular i.
intravenous bolus i.
intravenous fetal i.
iobenguane I-123 i.
iodinated I-131 albumin
  aggregated i.
ipsilateral i.
kit for preparation of technetium
  Tc99m depreotide i.
machine i.
manual i.
i. mass
Miraluma i.
Omnipaque i.
opacifying i.
paratumoral i.
percutaneous ethanol i.
percutaneous ultrasound-guided
  thrombin i.
perinephric air i.
i. port
power i.
prostaglandin E_1 i.
radionuclide i.
rest i.
retrograde i.
i. scan interval (ISI)
sclerosing i.
selective arterial i.
serial i.
silicone i.
straight AP pelvic i.
subarachnoid i.
subdural contrast i.
test i.
transduodenal fiberscopic duct i.
ultrasonographically guided i.
venous i.

injector

Cordis i.
Hercules power i.
Mark V Plus automatic i.

Medrad automated power i.
Medrad contrast medium i.
Medrad power angiographic i.
MR-compatible power i.
Optistat power i.
power i.
pressure i.
Pulse-Spray i.
Renovist II i.
Spectris MR-compatible i.
Spectris power i.
Taveras i.

injury

acute radiation i.
acute stretch i.
acute traumatic aortic i. (ATAI)
ankle inversion i.
anterior cruciate ligament i.
anterior urethral i.
aortic-brachiocephalic i.
apophyseal i.
axial compression i.
axial loading i.
ballistic i.
barked i.
bilateral incomplete ureteral i.
blunt i.
bony trabecular i.
brachial plexus birth i.
burst i.
cervical spine i.
chronic ligamentous i.
closed head i. (CHI)
clothesline i.
cocking i.
compression flexion i.
compressive hyperextension i.
concomitant tracheal i.
contrecoup i.
crush i.
decelerative i.
diffuse axonal i. (DAI)
diffuse white matter i.
distraction hyperflexion i.
endothelial i.
epiphyseal plate i.
Erb i.
Erb-Duchenne-Klumpke i.
excitotoxic cord i.
extension i.
extensive head i.
firearm i.
flake-shaped i.
flexion-distraction i.
flexion-rotation i.
forced flexion i.
genitourinary i.

glenoid labrum i.
greater arc i.
growth plate i.
head i. (HI)
high-caliber, low-velocity
  handgun i.
hollow viscus i.
hyperextension i.
hyperflexion/hyperextension
  cervical i.
hyperflexion/rotation i.
hypertension i.
hypoxic i.
iatrogenic ureteral i.
immunologic i.
intercostal nerve i.
intraoperative gastrointestinal i.
intraperitoneal i.
inversion i.
irradiation i.
ischemic reperfusion i.
isolated airway i.
Klumpke brachial plexus i.
Kulkarni i.
labral i.
lateral bending i.
lateral compartment traumatic
  bony i.
lateral talar dome i.
lesser arc i.
lethal myocardial i.
Lisfranc i.
low back i.
Maisonneuve i.
matrix i.
mechanism of i.
medial talar dome i.
medial talar osteochondral i.
meniscal i.
metatarsal i.
midtarsal i.
mild head i.
mild traumatic brain i.
motor vehicle i.
multiple recurrent inversion i.'s
muscle crushing i.
myocardial reperfusion i.
nerve i.
nonlethal myocardial ischemic i.
occult osseous i.
osseous cervical spine i.
osteochondral i.

penetrating lung i.
pericarinal i.
perinatal i.
peripheral nerve i.
peroneal tendon i.
phrenic nerve i.
physeal i.
plexus i.
posterior cruciate ligament i.
posterior urethral i.
posterolateral corner i.
postnatal i.
prenatal i.
pronation-abduction i.
pronation-external rotation i.
proximity i.
pulmonary parenchymal i.
radial vascular thermal i.
radiation i.
radiation-induced skin i.
radiocontrast-induced i.
rapid deceleration i.
rectal radiation i.
renal i.
repetitive strain i. (RSI)
repetitive stress i. (RSI)
rotation-shearing i.
Sage-Salvatore classification of
  acromioclavicular joint i.
schemic i. (SE)
seatbelt i.
sesamoid i.
i. severity scale (ISS)
i. severity score (ISS)
shearing white matter i.
skier's i.
softball sliding i.
soft tissue i.
solid viscus i.
spinal cord i. (SCI)
straddle i.
stress i.
subendocardial i.
superior labral anterior-posterior i.
supination-adduction i.
supination-external rotation i.
supination-outward rotation i.
talar dome osteochondral i.
talofibular ligament i.
tensile i.
three-column i.
through-and-through i.

NOTES

injury *(continued)*
 throwing arm i.
 tracheobronchial i. (TBI)
 transcutaneous crush i.
 traumatic aortic i.
 traumatic brain i. (TBI)
 traumatic head i.
 two-column i.
 ultrasonic assessment of i.
 unilateral locked facet i.
 urethral straddle i.
 valgus-external rotation i.
 vesical i.
 wafer-shaped i.
 weightbearing rotational i.
 whiplash i.
 white matter shearing i.
 windup i.
inking the margin
In-labeled
 ^{111}In-labeled human nonspecific
 immunoglobulin G
 ^{111}In-labeled white blood cell
inlay graft
inlet
 esophageal i.
 pelvic i.
 i. position
 thoracic i.
 transaxial thoracic i.
inner
 i. adrenal cortex
 i. bright layer
 i. ear
 i. ear anatomy
 i. ear atresia
 i. ear mass
 i. ear vestibule
 i. stripe of Baillinger
 i. table
 i. table of frontal bone
 i. table of skull
 i. table thickening
innermost intercostal muscle
InnerVasc vascular access system
innervation
 sympathetic i.
Innervision MR scanner
innocent gallstone
innocuous
innominate
 i. absence of line
 i. aneurysm
 i. angiography
 i. artery
 i. artery buckling
 i. artery compression syndrome

 i. artery kinking
 i. artery stenosis
 i. artery stenting
 i. bone
 i. canaliculus
 i. vein
inoperable brain tumor
inorganic phosphorus
In-pentetreotide scintigraphy
in-phase
 i.-p. GRE imaging
 i.-p. sequence
 i.-p. T1-weighted image
in-plane
 i.-p. spatial resolution
 i.-p. vessel
InQwire guidewire
Insall ratio
Insall-Salvati
 I.-S. index
 I.-S. ratio
insertion
 anomalous i.
 Bosworth bone peg i.
 capsular i.
 catheter i.
 femoral vein percutaneous i.
 Harrington rod i.
 ligamentous i.
 percutaneous pin i.
 percutaneous tube i.
 sartorius i.
 tendinous i.
 velamentous i.
inside-out x-ray
inside-to-outside segmentation
InSightec
insoluble
insonation
 angle of i.
 i. condition
 Doppler i.
 transforaminal i.
 transtemporal i.
insonifying wave field
Inspec-100
inspection
 surgical i.
 visual i.
inspiration
 degree of i.
 i. and expiration views
 shallow i.
 suspended i.
inspiratory
 i. effort
 i. to expiratory

i. to expiratory ratio (I:E ratio, I:E ratio)
i. flow
i. flow rate
i. increase in venous pressure
i. muscle function impairment
i. phase
i. reserve volume (IRV)
i. retraction
i. spasm
i. view

inspired air

inspissated
i. feces
i. material
i. secretion

instability
alveolar i.
ankle i.
anterolateral rotary knee i.
articular i.
atlantoaxial i.
atraumatic, multidirectional, bilateral radial i. (AMBRI)
chronic functional i.
degenerative spinal i.
detrusor i.
dissociative i.
dorsal intercalated segmental i. (DISI)
first ray i.
genomic i.
glenohumeral i.
hindfoot i.
inversion i.
ischemic i.
joint i.
lateral rotatory ankle i.
ligamentous i.
microsatellite i.
midcarpal i.
nondissociative i.
osseous i.
perilunar i.
perilunate i.
phase i.
posterolateral rotatory i.
postlaminectomy i.
rotary ankle i.
rotational i.
rotatory i.
shoulder joint i.

sonographic measurement of subtalar joint i.
spinal i.
subtalar i.
sympathetic vascular i.
truncal i.
varus-valgus i.
ventricular electrical i.
volar-flexed intercalated segment i.
volar intercalated segment i. (VISI)

instantaneous
i. axis of rotation (IAR)
i. enhancement rate
i. gradient

InstaScan scanner

in-stent
i.-s. restenosis
i.-s. stenosis

instillation
contrast material i.
percutaneous ethanol i.
subarachnoid i.

instrument
ionization i.
Magnum biopsy i.
i. output
Sabouraud-Noiré i.
single-headed i.

instrumentation
advanced breast biopsy i. (ABBI)
interspinous segmental spinal i. (ISSI)

insufficiency
acute cerebrovascular i.
acute coronary i.
adrenal i.
aortic valvular i.
arterial i.
autonomic i.
basilar artery i.
brachial-basilar i.
cardiac i.
cardiopulmonary i.
cerebrovascular i.
chronic venous i.
congenital pulmonary valve i.
coronary i.
deep venous i. (DVI)
i. fracture
gastric i.
hepatic i.
hypostatic pulmonary i.

NOTES

insufficiency *(continued)*
    ileocecal i.
    mesenteric vascular i.
    mitral i. (MI)
    muscular i.
    myocardial i.
    nonocclusive mesenteric arterial i.
    nonrheumatic aortic i.
    pad sign of aortic i.
    parathyroid i.
    postirradiation vascular i.
    posttraumatic pulmonary i.
    primary adrenal i.
    pulmonary arterial flow i.
    pulmonary valve i.
    pulmonic i. (PI)
    pyloric i.
    renal i.
    respiratory i.
    rheumatic aortic i.
    secondary venous i.
    Sternberg myocardial i.
    thyroid i.
    transient ischemic carotid i.
    tricuspid i. (TI)
    uterine i.
    uteroplacental i.
    valvular aortic i.
    vascular i.
    velopharyngeal i.
    venous i.
    vertebrobasilar i. (VBI)
insufficient
    i. acoustic penetration
    i. cochlear turn
    i. venous opacification
insufflation
    air i.
    CO_2 i.
    gas i.
    mechanical i.
    perirenal i.
    retroperitoneal gas i.
    tubal i.
insula, pl. **insulae**
    roof of i.
    i. root
insular
    i. gyrus
    i. lobe
    i. region
    i. region of brain
    i. ribbon sign
    i. segment of middle cerebral
      artery
    i. triangle
insulinase

insulin-iodine
insulinoma
insult
    aortic i.
    bihemispheral i.
    cerebrovascular i.
    hypoxic ischemic i.
    mechanical i.
    myocardial i.
    notable cerebral i.
    occlusive cerebrovascular i.
    thermal i.
    vascular i.
Insyte Autoguard Shielded IV catheter
intact
    i. valve cusp
    i. ventricular septum
intake
    fluid i.
integral
    Choquet fuzzy i.
    i. dose
    systolic velocity-time i.
    time velocity i.
    i. uniformity scintillation camera
integrated
    i. clinical information system
      (ICIS)
    i. fMRI
    i. functional magnetic resonance
      imaging
    i. optical density (IOD)
    i. optical density histogram
    i. reference air kerma (IRAK)
Integrilin
Integris
    I. 3D RA
    I. III-V DSA system
    I. 3000 scanner
    I. V 3000 digital subtraction
      system
    I. V3000 imager
integrity
    spinal i.
Intelect Legend Combo stimulator and
    ultrasound unit
intense uptake
intensification
    i. factor
    frequency i.
    image i.
intensified radiographic imaging system
    (IRIS)
intensifier
    image i.
    portable C-arm i.

intensifying
    i. screen
    i. screen artifact
intensity
    absolute dose i. (ADI)
    amorphous high signal i.
    beam i.
    bright signal i.
    calcified sequestra of low signal i.
    central fat signal i.
    central intrasubstance signal i.
    dark signal i.
    decreased i.
    diminished marrow signal i.
    discrete hyperintense signal i.
    equal in i.
    fat signal i.
    fusiform high signal i.
    grade 1–3 signal i.
    heterogeneous signal i.
    high-grade signal i.
    high signal i.
    homogeneous signal i.
    increase in i.
    intermediate signal i.
    intrameniscal signal i.
    intravascular signal i.
    juxtaarticular low signal i.
    linear degenerative signal i.
    linear high signal i.
    low signal i.
    marrow fat signal i.
    maximal i.
    nuclear magnetic resonance
      signal i.
    ovoid high signal i.
    pedicle signal i.
    photostimulable luminescence i.
    radiation i.
    reduced signal i.
    reverse pattern of signal i.
    scene i.
    signal i. (SI)
    single photon/maximum i.
    site of maximal i.
    spatial average-pulse average i.
    spatial average-temporal average i.
    spatial peak-temporal average i.
    symmetric confluent high signal i.
    temporal average i.
    temporal peak i.
    time-to-peak i. (TTP)

    variable i.
    vertebral body marrow signal i.
    water-like signal i.
    i. windowing
intensity-modulated
    i.-m. arc therapy
    i.-m. photon beam
    i.-m. radiation therapy (IMRT)
    i.-m. radiotherapy treatment (IMRT)
intentional reversible thrombosis
interaction
    capacitive i.
    Compton i.
    dipolar i.
    dipole-dipole i.
    effector/target cell i.
    electric i.
    magnetic i.
    mind-body i.
    photoelectric i.
    proton dipole-dipole i.
interactive
    i. electronic scalpel
    i. gradient optimization
    i. MR-guided biopsy
interaorticobronchial diverticulum
interarch distance
interarticular
    i. cartilage
    i. disk
    i. ridge
interarticularis
    pars i.
interatrial
    i. baffle leak
    i. communication
    i. groove
    i. septal defect
    i. septal hypertrophy
    i. septum (IAS)
    i. transposition of venous return
interbody
    i. bone graft
    i. bone plug
    i. fusion
interbronchial
    i. angle (IA)
    i. diverticulum
    i. mass
intercalary defect
intercalated segment
intercalating agent

NOTES

intercalation
intercapital ligament
intercarpal
    i. angle
    i. articular
    i. articulation
    i. coalition
    i. joint
    i. ligament
intercartilaginous rim
intercaudate distance
intercaval band
intercavernous
    i. anastomosis
    i. sinus
intercellular
    i. edema
    i. space
Intercept
    I. esophagus microcoil
    I. prostate microcoil
    I. urethra microcoil
intercervical disk herniation
interchondral joint
interchordal space fenestration
interclavicular
    i. ligament
    i. notch
interclinoid ligament
intercollicular groove
intercomparison
    i. measurement
    i. measurement technique
intercondylar
    i. eminence
    i. femoral fracture
    i. fossa
    i. groove
    i. humeral fracture
    i. joint space
    i. notch
    i. process
    i. roof
    i. sagittal image
    i. tibial fracture
    i. tubercle
intercondyloid fossa
intercornual ligament
intercoronary collateral flow
intercostal
    i. artery
    i. artery angiography
    i. lymph node
    i. muscle
    i. nerve
    i. nerve injury
    i. neuromuscular bundle

    i. retraction
    i. space
    i. vein
    i. vessel
intercostobrachial nerve
intercristal diameter
intercuneiform ligament
interdigital
    i. clavus
    i. ligament
    i. neoplasm
    i. neuroma
interdigitation
    cerebral gyri i.
    i. of vastus lateralis
interecho spacing
interest
    region of i. (ROI)
    volume of i. (VOI)
interface
    acetabular-prosthetic i.
    acoustic i.
    air i.
    air–soft tissue i.
    bidirectional i.
    body i.
    bone-air i.
    bone-implant i.
    catheter-skin i.
    common gateway i. (CGI)
    dermal–subcutaneous fat i.
    Digital Imaging and
      Communications in Medicine i.
    disk-thecal sac i.
    fat-blood i. (FBI)
    fat-fluid density i.
    fat-water i.
    fluid i.
    gray-to-white matter i.
    indistinct i.
    joint i.
    lumen-intimal i.
    media-adventitia i.
    muscle-fat i.
    reactive i.
    shear i.
    i. sign
    socket-stump i.
    transducer-skin i.
interfacetal dislocation
interfacial canal
interference
    i. dissociation
    electromagnetic i. (EMI)
    i. phenomenon
    i. screw
    slice i.

interferential current therapy
interferometry
> phase-shifting i.

interfibrosis
interfollicular Hodgkin disease
interfoveolar ligament
interfraction interval
interfragmental compression
interfragmentary plate
intergluteal cleft
interhaustral septum
interhemispheric
> i. asymmetry
> i. cyst
> i. fissure (IHF)
> i. pathway
> i. subdural hematoma
> i. transfer

interictal
> i. brain SPECT
> i. normalization
> i. PET FDG study
> i. phase
> i. SPECT scan
> i. SPECT study
> i. spiking

interiliac
> i. lymph node
> i. plane

interinnominoabdominal cleft
interior surface of pancreas
interlacing
interlaminar distance
interleaved
> i. axial slab
> i. BOLD-fMRI scanning
> i. GRE sequence
> i. image acquisition
> i. imaging pass
> i. inversion-readout segment
> i. k-space coverage
> i. phase contrast technique

interligamentous bursa
interlobar
> i. artery
> i. empyema
> i. fissure
> i. pleurisy
> i. septal line
> i. septum
> i. space

interlobular
> i. bile duct
> i. emphysema
> i. lung septum
> i. septal thickening
> i. tissue
> i. vasculature
> i. vessel

interlocking detachable coil (IDC)
interloop abscess
intermaxillary
> i. bone
> i. spine
> i. suture

intermediate
> i. bronchus
> i. bursa
> i. callus
> i. coronary artery
> i. coronary syndrome
> i. CT slice
> i. cuneiform bone
> i. cuneiform fracture-dislocation
> i. fetal death
> i. heart
> i. image
> i. imaging
> i. nerve of Wrisberg
> i. ray
> i. signal intensity
> i. signal intensity layer
> i. signal intensity mass
> i. signal striation

intermediolateral
> i. gray column
> i. tract

intermedius
> bronchus i.
> nervus i.
> vastus i.

intermesenteric
> i. abscess
> i. plexus

intermetacarpal articulation
intermetatarsal
> i. angle (IMA)
> i. bursitis
> i. joint
> i. ligament
> i. space

NOTES

intermetatarsophalangeal
- i. bursa
- i. bursitis

intermittent
- i. diffuse esophageal spasm
- i. obstruction
- i. occlusion
- i. sinus arrest
- i. third-degree AV block

intermodality image registration

intermuscular
- i. hematoma
- i. septum

interna
- endometriosis i.
- theca i.

internal
- i. abdominal ring
- i. aberrant carotid artery
- i. architecture
- i. auditory canal
- i. auditory canal anatomy
- i. auditory canal enhancing lesion
- i. auditory meatus
- i. band
- i. biliary drainage
- i. biliary stent
- i. caliber
- i. capsule
- i. capsule intracerebral hemorrhage
- i. carotid
- i. carotid angiography
- i. carotid artery (ICA)
- i. carotid artery aneurysm
- i. carotid artery occlusion
- i. carotid balloon test
- i. carotid system
- i. carotid systolic peak flow (ICSPF)
- i. cerebral vein (ICV)
- i. cervical os
- i. clot
- i. collateral ligament
- i. conjugate diameter
- i. conversion
- i. conversion electron
- i. cyclotron target
- i. degeneration
- i. derangement
- i. derangement of the knee (IDK)
- i. diameter (ID)
- i. disk herniation
- i. echo
- i. echogenicity
- i. echotexture
- i. enhancement
- i. and external rotation views

- i. femoral rotation
- i. fixation device
- i. hernia
- i. iliac artery
- i. inguinal ring
- i. intercostal muscle
- i. intermuscular septum
- i. jugular bulb
- i. jugular triangle
- i. jugular vein (IJV)
- i. mammary artery (IMA)
- i. mammary artery pedicle
- i. mammary lymphatic chain
- i. mammary lymph node
- i. mammary lymphoscintigraphy
- i. oblique aponeurosis
- i. oblique radiograph
- i. pudendal artery
- i. pudendal vessel
- i. radiation therapy
- i. retention mechanism
- i. rotation deformity
- i. rotation in extension (IRE)
- i. rotation in flexion (IRF)
- i. table of calvaria
- i. thoracic artery (ITA)
- i. thoracic artery graft
- i. thoracic vein
- i. tibial torsion (ITT)
- i. tibiofibular torsion
- i. ureteral stent
- i. urethral orifice
- i. urethrotomy

internal/external catheter
internally fixed fracture
internasal suture
international
- i. reference preparation
- i. standard (IS)

internervous plane
internuclear distance
internus
- obturator i.

interobserver
- i. error
- i. variation

interopercular distance
interorbital distance
interossei
- dorsal i.
- palmar i.
- plantar i.

interosseous
- i. border
- i. cyst
- first digital i. (FDI)
- i. membrane (IOM)

i. muscle
i. muscle group
i. nerve
i. ridge
i. sacroiliac ligament
i. space
i. talocalcaneal ligament
i. tendon
interpalatine suture
interparietal
i. bone
i. suture
interpectoral lymph node
interpedicular
i. distance
i. distance widening
interpediculate
interpeduncular
i. cistern (IPC)
i. fossa
i. notch
i. space
interperiosteal fracture
interphalangeal
i. articulation
i. dislocation
distal i. (DIP)
i. fusion
i. joint
interpleural space
interpolation
i. algorithm
color space i.
cubic convolution i.
80-degree linear i.
full scan with i.
i. kernel
linear i.
object-based i.
prism i.
scene-based i.
sinc i.
trilinear i.
zero-fill i. (ZIP)
interpolator
color space i.
Interpore bone replacement material
interposed
i. colon segment
i. colon segment obstruction
interposition
colonic i.

gastric i.
i. graft
hepatodiaphragmatic i.
soft tissue i.
interpretation
mirror-image i.
radiographic i.
interpretive
i. criterion
i. variability
interpulse
i. interval
i. time
interpupillary line
interridge distance
interrogation
color duplex i.
deep Doppler velocity i.
Doppler i.
pulse Doppler i.
radiation i.
interrupted
i. duct sign
i. periosteal reaction
interruption
aortic arch i.
bony cortex i.
juxtahilar bronchus i.
pulmonary artery i.
surgical venous i.
intersacral canal
interscan delay (ID)
interscapular gland
interscapulothoracic amputation
intersection gap
intersegmental
i. aberration
i. laminar fusion
i. tract
intersesamoid ligament
intersex
i. female
true i.
intersigmoid recess
interslice
i. distance
i. gap
interspace
ballooning of vertebral i.
disk i.
vertebral disk i.
wedging of vertebral i.

NOTES

intersperse
interspersed lucency
intersphincteric
   i. abscess
   i. anal fistula
   i. plane
interspinal
   i. muscle
   i. plane
interspinous
   i. distance (ISD)
   i. ligament
   i. plane
   i. process
   i. process fusion
   i. segmental spinal instrumentation
    (ISSI)
   i. widening
interstice, pl. interstices
   bone i.
   graft i.
interstitial
   i. abnormality
   i. absorption
   i. afterloading nylon tube
   i. atrophy
   i. boost
   i. brachytherapy
   i. calcinosis
   i. change
   i. conductive heating
   i. congestion of epididymis
   i. cystitis
   i. diffuse pulmonary fibrosis
   i. ectopic pregnancy
   i. fibrotic lung disease
   i. fluid
   i. fluid hydrostatic pressure
   i. fluid space
   i. heat-generating source
   i. hemorrhage
   i. hernia
   i. hyperthermia
   i. hyperthermia treatment
   i. infection
   i. inflammation
   i. intestinal emphysema
   i. laser photocoagulation
   i. loculated hematoma
   i. low-dose-rate iridium-192 needle
    implant
   i. lung disease distribution
   i. lung disease with increased lung
    volume
   i. lung emphysema
   i. lung pattern
   i. marking

   i. meniscal tear
   i. nephritis
   i. nodule
   i. nodule HRCT
   i. nonlobar infiltrate
   i. organizing pneumonia
   i. plasma cell pneumonia
   i. pneumonia air leak
   i. pneumonitis
   i. prematurity fibrosis
   i. probe
   i. prominence
   i. pulmonary edema
   i. pulmonary fibrosis (IPF)
   i. radiation
   i. radiation therapy
   i. radioactive colloid therapy
   i. radioelement application
   i. radiosurgery
   i. radiotherapy
   i. radium therapy
   i. salpingitis
   i. scarring
   i. shadowing
   i. tear pattern
   i. thickening
   i. tissue
   i. water proton
interstitium
   lung i.
   pulmonary i.
intertarsal
interthalamic bridge
intertrabecular
   i. hemorrhage
   i. soft tissue
intertransverse
   i. foramen
   i. ligament
   i. muscle
intertrochanteric
   i. crest
   i. four-part fracture
   i. plate
   i. ridge
intertubercular
   i. bursitis
   i. diameter
   i. groove
   i. plane
intertwin membrane
interuncal distance (IUD)
interureteric ridge
interval
   acromiohumeral i. (AHI)
   i. articulation
   atlantoaxial i.

atlantodens i. (ADI)
basion axial i. (BAI)
basion dens i. (BDI)
i. change
confidence i. (CI)
i. development
i. ejection fraction
escape i.
high-rate detect i.
hypoplastic disk i.
i. improvement
injection scan i. (ISI)
interfraction i.
interpulse i.
i. intraatrial conduction
lucent i.
preejection i.
i. progression
prolonged i.
QRS i.
reconstruction i.
i. resolution
rotator i.
supracricoid i.
upper rate i.
ventriculoatrial i.

intervention
stage-matched i.
i. study
therapeutic i.

interventional
i. angiography
i. catheterization
i. imaging
i. magnetic resonance imaging (I-MRI)
i. neuroradiology
i. procedure
i. radiography
i. vascular angiogram

interventricular
i. block
i. foramen
i. groove
i. septal defect (IVSD)
i. septal rupture
i. septal thickness (IVST)
i. septum

intervertebral
i. cartilage calcification
i. disk
i. disk calcification

i. disk index
i. disk narrowing
i. diskogram
i. disk space
i. disk space height
i. disk space uniformity
i. foramen
i. joint
i. ligament
i. notch
i. osteochondrosis

intervillous
i. circulation
i. lacuna
i. placental thrombosis

interzone
intestinal
i. atony
i. Behçet syndrome
i. bypass procedure
i. calculus
i. canal
i. carcinoid tumor
i. conduit
i. congenital atresia
i. content
i. decompression
i. dilatation
i. distention
i. diverticulum
i. duplication
i. emphysema
i. fluid
i. follicle
i. gas
i. gas exchange
i. gas pattern
i. hypoperistalsis syndrome
i. infantilism
i. infarct
i. intussusception
i. kinking
i. lipodystrophy
i. loop
i. lumen
i. lymphangiectasis
i. mesentery
i. metaphysis
i. metaplasia
i. necrosis
i. obstruction
i. perforation

NOTES

intestinal *(continued)*
- i. polyposis
- i. prolapse
- i. tract
- i. tract malrotation
- i. tube
- i. ulcer
- i. ureter
- i. villous architecture
- i. villus
- i. wall
- i. web

intestinalis
- pneumatosis cystoides i.

intestine
- blind i.
- bullous emphysema of i.
- coils of i.
- congenital lymphangiectasia of i.
- kink in i.
- large i.
- malrotation of i.
- papillary adenoma of large i.
- small i.

intima
- arterial i.
- friable thickened degenerated i.
- hypertrophied i.
- pulmonary artery i.
- tunica i.

intimal
- i. arteriosclerosis
- i. atherosclerosis
- i. attachment of diseased vessel
- i. debris
- i. degeneration
- i. fibroplasia
- i. fibrosis
- i. flap
- i. hyperplasia (IH)
- i. irregularity
- i. proliferation
- i. remodeling
- i. tear
- i. thickening

intimal-medial
- i.-m. dissection
- i.-m. thickness (IMT)

intimate attachment

intraabdominal (IAB)
- i. abscess
- i. arterial bypass graft
- i. arterial hemorrhage
- i. calcification
- i. fat
- i. fetal calcification
- i. infection

- i. mass
- i. viscus

intraacetabular

intraacinar pulmonary artery

intraalveolar fibrosis

intraamniotic injection

intraaneurysmal
- i. flow circulation
- i. inflow pattern
- i. outflow pattern
- i. thrombus

intraaortic
- i. balloon assist
- i. balloon counterpulsation
- i. balloon pump (IABP)
- i. endovascular sonography

intraarterial (IA)
- i. chemotherapy catheter
- i. chemotherapy pump
- i. digital subtraction angiography (IADSA)
- i. filling defect
- i. injection
- i. stereotactic digital subtraction angiography
- i. superselective nimodipine
- i. thrombosis
- i. thrombus

intraarticular
- i. adhesion
- i. calcaneal fracture
- i. contrast
- i. debris
- i. gadolinium
- i. ganglion
- i. hemangioma
- i. knee fusion
- i. ligament
- i. localized nodular synovitis
- i. loose body
- i. plate of fibrocartilage
- i. proximal tibial fracture
- i. radiopharmaceutical therapy

intraatrial
- i. block
- i. electrogram
- i. filling defect
- i. reentry
- i. thrombus

intraauricular muscle

intraaxial
- i. brain lesion
- i. brain tumor
- i. varix

Intrabeam intraoperative radiotherapy system

intracanalicular

intracapsular
    i. ankylosis
    i. fat pad
    i. femoral neck fracture
    i. osteoid osteoma
intracardiac
    i. calcification
    i. calcium
    i. echocardiography (ICE)
    i. electrogram
    i. lead
    i. mass
    i. mixing
    i. pressure
    i. pressure waveform analysis
    i. thrombus
intracartilaginous
    i. bone
    i. ossification
Intracath catheter
intracaval
    i. endovascular ultrasonography
    i. fat mass
intracavernosal injection
intracavernous internal carotid artery
intracavitary
    i. afterloading applicator
    i. application brachytherapy
    i. clot formation
    i. delivery
    i. extension
    i. extension of tumor
    i. filling defect
    i. hyperthermia treatment
    i. implant
    i. radiation source
    i. radiation therapy
    i. radioactive colloid therapy
    i. radioelement application
    i. radiotherapy
    i. radium
intracavity mass
intracellular
    i. adhesion molecule
    i. water
intracerebral
    i. aneurysm
    i. arteriovenous malformation
    i. artery
    i. blood
    i. ganglioglioma
    i. ganglioma

    i. hematoma
    i. hemorrhage (ICH)
    i. lesion
    i. lymphoma
    i. thrombolysis
    i. tumor
    i. vascular malformation
intracerebroventricular (ICV)
intrachondral bone
IntraCoil
    I. endoprosthesis
    I. stent
intracompartmental
    i. edema
    i. ischemia
    i. tumor
intraconal
    i. lesion
    i. portion of the eye
intracondyloid
intracoronary
    i. artery radiation
    i. contrast echocardiography
    i. Doppler flow guidewire
    i. imaging
    i. radiation therapy (ICRT)
    i. stenting
    i. stent placement
    i. thrombolytic therapy
    i. ultrasound (ICUS)
intracorporeal liver
intracortical
    i. osteogenic sarcoma
    i. osteosarcoma
intracranial
    i. air
    i. aneurysm (ICA)
    i. arteriovenous fistula
    i. arteriovenous malformation
    i. berry aneurysm
    i. carotid artery atherosclerosis
    i. cavernous angioma
    i. circulation
    i. cryptococcosis
    i. dermoid cyst
    i. electroencephalography
    i. embolus
    i. empyema
    i. fat prolapse
    i. germinoma
    i. glioma
    i. hematoma

NOTES

intracranial *(continued)*
   i. hypertension
   i. imaging
   i. leptomeningeal vascular anomaly
   i. lipoma
   i. mass
   i. mass lesion
   i. metastasis
   i. MR angiography
   i. neoplasm
   i. neuroblastoma
   i. opportunistic infection
   i. physiologic calcification
   i. pneumatocele
   i. pneumocephalus
   i. pressure (ICP)
   i. pulse pressure
   i. saccular aneurysm
   i. seeding
   i. shift
   i. sinus thrombosis
   i. structure
   i. subarachnoid hemorrhage
   i. tuberculoma
   i. tumor
   i. vascular abnormality
   i. vascular lesion
   i. vascular occlusion
   i. vertebral artery
   i. vessel
   i. volume
   i. width (ICW)
intractable
   i. bleeding disorder
   i. heart failure
   i. ulcer
intracystic
   i. bleeding
   i. breast carcinoma
   i. breast papillary carcinoma in situ
   i. solid mass
intracytoplasmic
intradecidual sign
intradermal
   i. angioma
   i. injection
intradiaphragmatic aortic segment
intradiskal, intradiscal
   i. administration of gadolinium followed by MRI
   i. injection
intraductal
   i. breast filling defect
   i. breast papillomatosis
   i. bridge
   i. calcification

   i. carcinoma (IDC)
   i. mucin-producing tumor
   i. papillary carcinoma
   i. papillary mucinous tumor (IPMT)
   i. papillary mucinous tumor of the pancreas
   i. papilloma
   i. pressure
   i. solid mass
   i. ultrasonography
intraduodenal choledochal cyst
intradural
   i. abscess
   i. arachnoid cyst
   i. disk herniation
   i. epidermoidoma
   i. extramedullary lesion
   i. extramedullary mass
   i. extramedullary tumor
   i. hemorrhage
   i. intramedullary tumor
   i. lipoma
   i. nerve root
   i. retromedullary arteriovenous fistula
   i. rootlet
   i. spinal AVM
   i. vessel
intraforaminal vein
intragastric bubble
intragraft stenosis
intrahepatic
   i. abscess
   i. arterial-portal fistula
   i. atresia (IHA)
   i. AV fistula
   i. bile duct
   i. biliary atresia
   i. biliary calculus
   i. biliary carcinoma
   i. biliary cystic dilatation
   i. biliary ductal dilatation
   i. biliary neoplasm
   i. biliary stasis
   i. biliary tract
   i. biliary tract dilatation
   i. biliary tree
   i. biloma
   i. cholangiocarcinoma
   i. cholestasis
   i. portal vein branch
   i. portal vein gas
   i. sclerosing cholangitis
   i. stone
   i. umbilical vein
intra-His block

intrahisian block
intralabyrinthine
intralaminar thalamus
intraligamentary pregnancy
intraligamentous bursa
intralobar sequestration
intralobular
    i. connective tissue
    i. fibrosis
    i. interstitial thickening
    i. terminal duct
intraluminal
    i. adenocarcinoma
    i. air
    i. attenuation decrease
    i. brachytherapy
    i. debris
    i. dephasing
    i. detail
    i. dilatation
    i. dimension
    i. duodenal diverticulum (IDD)
    i. electrocoagulation
    i. embolus
    i. esophageal pressure
    i. filling defect
    i. foreign body
    i. gallstone
    i. hemorrhage
    i. intubation
    i. membrane
    i. plaque
    i. polyp
    i. stomach mass
    i. stone
    i. thrombus
    i. ultrasound (ILUS)
    i. ultrasound catheter
intralymphatic
    i. infusion
    i. radioactivity administration
intramammary
    i. lesion
    i. lymph node
    i. node (IMN)
intramedullary (IM)
    i. arteriovenous malformation
    i. canal
    i. compartment neoplasm
    i. cord lesion
    i. demyelination
    i. ependymoma

i. epidermoid cyst
i. fixation
i. fixation device
i. lipoma
i. marrow involvement
i. nail
i. osteosarcoma
i. rodding
i. skeletal kinetic distractor (ISKD)
i. skeletal kinetic distractor system
i. space-occupying lesion
i. spinal cord tumor
i. spinal lesion
i. tumor biopsy
intramembranous
    i. bone
    i. ossification
intrameniscal
    i. cyst
    i. mucoid degeneration
    i. signal intensity
intramesenteric abscess
intramural
    i. air in colon
    i. arterial hemorrhage
    i. clot
    i. colonic air
    i. coronary artery aneurysm
    i. diverticulum
    i. esophageal diverticulosis
    i. esophageal pseudodiverticulosis
    i. esophageal rupture
    i. fibroid
    i. filling defect
    i. gas
    i. gastric emphysema
    i. gastrointestinal tract hemorrhage
    i. hematoma
    i. hematoma of aorta
    i. leiomyosarcoma
    i. mapping
    i. mechanics
    i. myoma
    i. portion of distal ureter
    i. rupture of the esophagus
    i. thrombus
    i. tumor
    i. tunnel
intramural-extramucosal stomach lesion
intramuscular
    i. aortic segment
    i. fetal injection

NOTES

intramuscular *(continued)*
 i. fluid pressure
 i. hemangioma
 i. hemosiderin deposit
 i. venous malformation
intramyocardial
intranasal microbubble
intraneural ganglion cyst
intraneuronal neurofibrillary tangle
intranodal
 i. architecture
 i. block
 i. myofibroblastoma
in-transit metastasis
intranuclear
 i. cleft
 i. diskogram
intraobserver
 i. error
 i. variation
intraoccipital
 anterior synchondrosis i.
intraocular
 i. calcification
 i. foreign body
 i. lesion
 i. spread
Intra-Op autotransfusion system
intraoperative
 i. arteriography
 i. cardioplegic contrast echocardiography
 i. cholangiogram
 i. cholangiography
 i. device
 i. digital subtraction angiography (IDSA)
 i. Doppler
 i. electrocortical stimulation (IOECS)
 i. electrocortical stimulation mapping
 i. film
 i. fracture
 i. gamma probe
 i. gastrointestinal injury
 i. high dose rate (IOHDR)
 i. imaging
 i. laser photocoagulation
 i. lymphatic mapping
 i. pancreatography
 i. radiation therapy
 i. radiography
 i. radiolymphoscintigraphy
 i. radiotherapy
 i. red light therapy (IRLT)
 i. scanning technique

 i. sonography (IOS)
 i. ultrasound (IOUS)
 i. ventriculogram
 i. view
 i. x-ray visualization
intraoral
 i. periapical radiography
 i. projection
 i. radiograph
 i. radiology
 i. roentgentherapy
intraorbital air
intraosseous
 i. abscess
 i. arteriovenous malformation
 i. bone lesion
 i. desmoid tumor
 i. edema
 i. ganglion
 i. hemophilic pseudotumor
 i. keratin cyst
 i. lipoma
 i. low-grade osteosarcoma
 i. meningioma
 i. osteosarcoma
 i. vascular malformation
 i. venography
 i. wiring
intrapancreatic obstruction
intrapapillary terminus
intraparenchymal
 i. bleed
 i. blood
 i. cyst
 i. hematoma
 i. hemorrhage
 i. lung tumor
 i. lymph node
 i. meningioma
 i. metastasis
 i. microvessel
 i. tuberculoma
intrapatellar fat pad
intrapedicular fixation
intrapericardial
 i. bleeding
 i. diaphragmatic hernia
 i. patch lead placement
 i. portion
 i. pressure
intraperiosteal fracture
intraperitoneal
 i. abscess
 i. air
 i. cavity
 i. drug administration
 i. exposure

i. fetal injection
i. fluid
i. hyperthermic perfusion (IPHP)
i. injury
i. lesion
i. pregnancy
i. rupture
i. rupture of bladder
i. technetium sulfur colloid imaging
i. viscus
intrapixel sequential processing (IPSP)
intraplacental venous lake
intraplaque hemorrhage (IPH)
intrapleural
i. hemorrhage
i. pressure
intrapontine intracerebral hemorrhage
intraportal
i. endovascular ultrasonography
(IPEUS)
i. infusion
intrapulmonary
i. arteriovenous fistula
i. barotrauma
i. bronchogenic cyst
i. bronchus
i. hemorrhage
i. lymph node
i. pressure
intrarectal
i. coil
i. ultrasound
intrarenal
i. arterial flow
i. collecting system
i. hematoma
i. pelvis
i. reflux
i. stenosis
intrarun realignment
intrascapular ligament
intrascrotal abscess
intrasellar
i. brain mass
i. lesion
i. Rathke cleft cyst
i. tumor
intrasinus air-fluid level
Intrasound
Medtronic Pulsor I.
intraspinal
i. adenoma

i. dermoid cyst
i. enteric cyst
i. epidermoid cyst
i. lesion
i. neurenteric cyst
i. tumor
intraspongy nuclear disk herniation
intrastitial radiation source
intrasubstance cleavage tear
intrasynovial disease
intratemporal fossa
intratendinous
i. bursa
i. fluid collection
i. rupture
intratendon sheath
intratentorial lipoma
intratesticular
i. band
i. cyst
intrathecal (IT)
i. hemorrhage
i. imaging
i. root
i. space
intrathoracic
i. catheter drainage
i. cyst
i. dimension
i. dislocation of shoulder
i. fetal mass
i. goiter
i. Kaposi sarcoma
i. low-attenuation mass
i. pressure
i. stomach
i. thyroid
i. trachea
i. upper airway obstruction
intratracheal
intratumoral
i. accumulation
i. agent
i. calcification
i. cyst
i. hemorrhage
i. necrosis
i. structure
intrauterine
i. cardiac failure
i. demise
i. fetus

NOTES

intrauterine *(continued)*
- i. fracture
- i. gas (IUG)
- i. gestation
- i. growth restriction
- i. growth retardation (IUGR)
- i. heart failure
- i. membrane
- i. pregnancy (IUP)
- i. sac

intravaginal
- i. roentgentherapy
- i. torsion

intravasation
- venous i.

intravascular
- i. angiogenesis gene delivery
- i. clotting process
- i. coil
- i. congestion
- i. consumption coagulopathy
- i. content
- i. content extravasation
- i. contrast-enhanced computed tomography
- i. contrast-enhanced CT
- i. contrast medium
- i. filling defect
- i. foreign body
- i. injection
- i. leiomyosarcoma
- i. mass
- i. MRI catheter-based technique
- i. papillary endothelial hyperplasia
- i. radiopharmaceutical therapy
- i. sickling
- i. signal intensity
- i. space
- i. stent
- i. stent artifact
- i. stenting
- i. thrombosis
- i. tumor thrombus
- i. ultrasound (IVUS)
- i. ultrasound catheter
- i. ultrasound imaging
- i. volume depletion

intravenous (IV, I.V.)
- i. administration of contrast material
- i. angiocardiography
- i. aortography
- i. block
- i. bolus
- i. bolus injection
- i. cholangiogram (IVC)
- i. cholangiography
- i. cholecystography
- i. contrast medium
- i. digital subtraction angiography (IVDSA)
- i. fetal injection
- i. fluorescein angiography (IVFA)
- i. fluorescein angiography imaging
- i. infusion line
- i. injection of isotope
- i. microbubble contrast agent
- i. pyelography (IVP)
- i. renal angiography
- i. stereotactic digital subtraction angiography
- i. urography (IVU)

intravenously
- i. enhanced CT scan
- i. enhanced MRI

intraventricular
- i. aberration
- i. block (IVB)
- i. blood
- i. brain tumor
- i. conduction block
- i. conduction delay
- i. cryptococcal cyst
- i. heart block
- i. hematoma
- i. hemorrhage (IVH)
- i. mass
- i. meningioma
- i. neonate hemorrhage
- i. neuroblastoma
- i. neurocytoma
- i. obstructive hydrocephalus
- i. right ventricular obstruction
- i. septum
- i. systolic tension

intravertebral body vacuum cleft
intravesical
- i. obstruction
- i. stone
- i. ureter

intravital ultraviolet
intravoxel
- i. coherent motion
- i. dephasing
- i. incoherent motion (IVIM)
- i. phase dispersion

intrinsic
- i. cellular parameter
- i. compression
- i. deflection
- i. efficiency
- i. energy resolution
- i. factor
- i. field uniformity

i. field uniformity test
i. filling defect
i. foot muscle
i. intraabdominal inflammation
i. ligament
i. minus deformity
i. minus hallux
i. plus deformity
i. spatial linearity
i. stenotic lesion
i. stomach wall lesion
i. vein graft stenosis
introducer
  Desilets-Hoffman i.
  end-hole i.
  Tuohy-Borst i.
Intropaque
intubated small bowel series
intubation
  endotracheal i.
  esophagogastric i.
  intraluminal i.
  nasal i.
  nasogastric i.
  nasotracheal i.
  oral i.
  orotracheal i.
intussusception
  appendiceal i.
  bowel i.
  colocolic i.
  ileocolic i.
  ileoileal i.
  intestinal i.
  jejunoduodenogastric i.
  jejunogastric i.
  pneumatic reduction of i.
  rectal i.
  retrograde jejunoduodenogastric i.
  stomal i.
  transient i.
  vein i.
  venous i.
intussusceptum
intussuscipiens
Inutest
invagination
  basilar i.
  i. skull base
invasion
  arterial i.
  blood vessel i.

capillary lymphatic space i.
deep myometrial i.
early stromal i.
exogenous i.
mediastinal i.
neoplastic i.
occipital condyle i.
perineural i.
seminal vesicle i. (SVI)
transmural i.
tumoral i.
vascular i.
invasive
  i. angiomatous interstitial infiltrate
  i. assessment
  i. breast carcinoma
  i. lesion
  i. lobular carcinoma
  i. malignant sheath tumor
  i. papillomatosis
  i. pulmonary aspergillosis (IPA)
  i. radiological vascular procedure
  i. surgical staging (ISS)
  i. thermometry
inverse
  i. cerebellum
  i. comma appearance
  i. follicle
  i. follicle pattern
  i. Fourier transform (IFT)
  i. inspiratory-expiratory time ratio
  i. radiotherapy technique
  i. square law
  i. symmetry
inversion
  i. ankle stress view
  cardiac i.
  frequency-selective i.
  gray-scale i.
  i. injury
  i. injury of ankle
  i. instability
  isolated ventricular i.
  magnetic i.
  i. position
  i. pulse
  i. recovery (IR)
  i. recovery echo planar imaging (IR-EPI)
  i. recovery image
  i. recovery sequence
  i. recovery spin-echo (IRSE)

NOTES

inversion *(continued)*
    i. recovery spin-echo sequence
    i. recovery-weighted image
    selective population i. (SPI)
    i. sprain
    terminal i.
    i. time (TI)
    torcular-lambdoid i.
    i. transfer
    ventricular i.
inversion-eversion
inversion-prepared
    basis imaging with selective i.-p.
inversion-recovery
    selective partial i.-r. (SPIR)
    i.-r. technique
inversum
    duodenum i.
inversus
    abdominal situs i.
    complete situs i.
    situs i.
    situs viscerum i.
inverted
    i. Meckel diverticulum
    i. papilloma
    i. pelvis
    i. teardrop sign
    i. umbrella defect
    i. Y field radiotherapy
inverted-T
    i.-T appearance
    i.-T appearance mainstem bronchus
inverted-V sign
inverted-Y
    i.-Y block
    i.-Y complex
    i.-Y configuration
    i.-Y fracture
invertus
    cardiac situs i.
investing fascia
invisible
    i. light
    i. main pulmonary artery
    i. spectrum
involucrum, pl. involucra
involuting fibroadenoma
involution
    i. of duct
    follicular i.
    spontaneous i.
involutional breast calcification
involved
    i. field
involvement
    arcuate fiber i.

    axillary node i.
    contiguous organ i.
    cranial nerve i.
    extramedullary i.
    intramedullary marrow i.
    lymph node i.
    metastatic axillary i.
    pagetoid epidermal i.
    supraclavicular node i.
    thalamotegmental i.
INVOS
    in vivo optical spectroscopy
    INVOS 3100, 3100A cerebral
    oximeter monitoring system
    INVOS 2100 optical spectroscopy
inwardly displaced calcification
iobenguane I-123 injection
iobenzamic acid
iobitridol imaging agent
iocarmate meglumine
iocarmic acid
iocetamic
    i. acid
    i. acid imaging agent
IOCM
    isosmolar contrast medium
IOD
    integrated optical density
iodamine imaging agent
iodide
    i. contrast medium
    i. goiter
    potassium i.
    propidium i.
    silver i.
    sodium i. (NaI)
    thallium-activated sodium i.
    i. transport
iodinated
    i. CM-induced cardiac depression
    i. contrast material
    i. contrast material-induced cardiac
    depression
    i. human serum albumin (IHSA)
    i. I-131 aggregated albumin
    i. I-131 albumin aggregated
    injection
    i. I-125 fibrinogen
    i. imaging agent
    i. intravascular CM
    i. intravascular contrast medium
    i. I-125 serum albumin
    i. I-131 serum albumin
    i. nanoparticle
    i. radiologic contrast medium
    (IRCM)
    i. tyrosine group

iodination
iodine (I)
    i. allergy
    butanol-extractable i. (BEI)
    i. dose
    i. fluorescence imaging
    i. I-131 iodine PVP bond
    ^{132}I radioactive i.
    ^{131}I radioactive i.
    i. load
    protein-bound i. (PBI)
    radioactive i.
    i. radioactive source
    i. scintigraphy
    i. uptake
iodine-123 (^{123}I, I-123)
    i.-123 iodophenyl pentadecanoic
      acid (IPPA)
    i.-123 orthoiodohippurate (OIH)
    i.-123, -131 thyroid
iodine-125 (^{125}I, I-125)
iodine-127 (^{127}I, I-127)
iodine-131 (^{131}I, I-131)
    i.-131 antiferritin treatment
    i.-131 metaiodobenzylguanidine
    i.-131 OIH
    i.-131 orthoiodohippurate
    i.-131 outcome analysis
    sodium iodide i.-131
    i.-131 triolein
    i.-131 whole-body scan
    i.-131 whole-body scintigraphy
iodine-132 (^{132}I, I-132)
iodine-123-MIBG radioactive imaging
  agent
iodine-131-induced cellulitis
iodine-131-MIBG radioactive imaging
  agent
iodine-containing contrast medium
iodine-deficiency goiter
iodine-125-labeled
    i.-l. fragment
iodine-labeled product
iodine-to-particle ratio
iodipamide
    i. ethyl ester
    i. meglumine
    i. meglumine imaging agent
    i. methylglucamine
iodixanol contrast medium
iodized
    i. oil imaging agent

    i. oil study
    i. poppy seed oil
iodo
    5-i.-2-deoxyuridine imaging agent
iodoalphionic acid
iodoamphetamine (IMP)
    ^{123}I i.
    ^{123}I isopropyl i.
iodobenzamide
iodocholesterol
iodocyanine green (ICG)
iododeoxyuridine (IUdR)
    i. labeling
Iodo-gen imaging agent
iodohippurate
    i. sodium
    i. sodium imaging agent
iodomethamate
iodomethyl-norcholesterol-59 scintigraphy
iodomethyl-norcholesterol scintigraphy
  imaging
iodopanoic acid
iodophendylate contrast medium
iodophenyl pentadecanoic acid (IPPA)
Iodotope imaging agent
iodovinylestradiol
iodoxamate meglumine
IOECS
    intraoperative electrocortical stimulation
ioglunide contrast medium
ioglycamic acid contrast medium
ioglycamide
IOHDR
    intraoperative high dose rate
    IOHDR brachytherapy
iohexol
    i. CT ventriculogram
    i. imaging agent
IOM
    infraorbital margin
    interosseous membrane
iomeprol
Iomeron 150, 250, 300, 350 contrast
  medium
IOML
    infraorbitomeatal line
ion
    amphoteric dipolar i.
    calcium i.
    i. chamber
    i. pump

NOTES

ion-bound water
ion-exchange chromatography
ionic
    i. binding
    i. dimer contrast medium
    i. hexaiodinated dimer
    i. monomer
    i. monomeric contrast medium
    i. paramagnetic contrast medium
    i. paramagnetic imaging agent
    i. polar valence
    i. potassium
iON IntraOperative Navigation System
ionization
    i. chamber
    i. counter
    i. current
    i. density
    i. detector
    i. instrument
    i. potential
    i. radiation
    i. track
ionized atom
ionizing
    i. radiation
    i. radiation exposure
ionograph
ionography
iopamidol imaging agent
Iopamiron 310, 370 imaging agent
iopanoic
    i. acid
    i. acid imaging agent
iopentol nonionic imaging agent
iophendylate
    i. imaging agent
    i. oil
iopromide
    i. contrast medium
    i. nonionic imaging agent
iopydol
IOS
    intraoperative sonography
iosefamic acid imaging agent
iothalamate
    i. meglumine imaging agent
    i. sodium
    i. sodium imaging agent
iothalamic acid
iotrol, iotrolan
iotroxamide contrast medium
iotroxic acid imaging agent
IOUS
    intraoperative ultrasound
ioversol imaging agent

ioxaglate
    i. meglumine
    i. meglumine imaging agent
    i. sodium
    i. sodium imaging agent
ioxaglic
    i. acid
    i. acid contrast medium
ioxilan imaging agent
ioxithalamate contrast medium
ioxithalamic acid contrast agent
IPA
    idiopathic pulmonary arteriosclerosis
    invasive pulmonary aspergillosis
IPC
    interpeduncular cistern
IPCS
    infrapatellar contracture syndrome
IPEUS
    intraportal endovascular ultrasonography
IPF
    idiopathic pulmonary fibrosis
    interstitial pulmonary fibrosis
IPG
    impedance plethysmography
IPH
    idiopathic portal hypertension
    intraplaque hemorrhage
IPHP
    intraperitoneal hyperthermic perfusion
IP joint
I-Plant brachytherapy seeds
IPMT
    intraductal papillary mucinous tumor
ipodate
    i. calcium imaging agent
    i. sodium
    i. sodium imaging agent
ipodic acid contrast agent
ipomeanol
IPPA
    iodine-123 iodophenyl pentadecanoic
    acid
    iodophenyl pentadecanoic acid
IP-plus image processing software
IPSID
    immunoproliferative small intestine
    disease
ipsilateral
    i. antegrade arteriography
    i. antegrade site
    i. basal ganglion
    i. breast tumor recurrence (IBTR)
    i. bundle-branch block
    i. cortical diaschisis
    i. downstream artery
    i. femoral neck fracture

i. femoral shaft fracture
i. hemimegalencephaly
i. hemispheric carotid TIA
i. injection
i. jugular lymphatic bed
i. lateral ventricle
i. lung volume
i. margin
i. pleural effusion

IPSP
intrapixel sequential processing
IPSP neuron evaluation method

IR
inversion recovery
arrhythmia-insensitive flow-sensitive
alternating IR
IR image

Ir
iridium

^{192}Ir, Ir-192
iridium-192
^{192}Ir-loaded stent
^{192}Ir ribbon
^{192}Ir seed therapy
^{192}Ir wire

^{194}Ir, Ir-194
iridium-194

IRA
ileorectal anastomosis

IRA-400 resin

IRAK
integrated reference air kerma

IRBBB
incomplete right bundle-branch block

IRCM
iodinated radiologic contrast medium

IRE
internal rotation in extension

IR-EPI
inversion recovery echo planar imaging

Irex
I. Exemplar ultrasound
I. Exemplar ultrasound scanner

IRF
internal rotation in flexion

Iriditope

iridium (Ir)
i. imaging agent
i. needle
i. wire

iridium-192 (^{192}Ir, Ir-192)

i.-192 endobronchial implant
i.-192 wire implant

iridium-194 (^{194}Ir, Ir-194)

IRIS
intensified radiographic imaging system
IRIS III imager
IRIS scanner

iris-like stenosis

IRLT
intraoperative red light therapy

iron
i. accumulation in kidney
i. dextran
gadolinium i.
i. hydroxide
i. overload artifact
radioactive i.

iron-52 (^{52}Fe)

iron-55 (^{55}Fe)

iron-59 (^{59}Fe)

iron-ascorbate-DTPA
technetium-99m i.-a.-D.

iron-transporting protein mechanism

irradiating

irradiation
i. chamber
convergent beam i. (CBI)
i. injury
i. phenomenon
i. pneumonia
stereotactic external-beam i. (SEBI)
i. tolerance

irradiator
MDS-2000 microwave i.

irreducible
i. dorsal dislocation
i. fracture

irregular
i. block
i. bone
i. border
i. calcification
i. emphysema
i. enchondral ossification
i. extrinsic indentation
i. gallbladder wall thickening
i. hazy luminal contour
i. kidney
i. mass
i. mucosal fold

NOTES

irregular *(continued)*
    i. shape
    i. tapered appearance
irregularity
    avulsive cortical i.
    diffuse i.
    intimal i.
    luminal i.
    margin i.
    nodular i.
    sinus i. (SI)
    tendon i.
irregularly
    i. layered astrocytic component
    i. layered neuronal component
    i. shaped lesion
irreversible
    i. airway obstruction
    i. compression
    i. compression of MR imaging
    i. ischemia
    i. narrowing of bronchiole
    i. organ failure
irrigoradioscopy
irrigoscopy
irritability
    atrial i.
    cardiac i.
    muscle i.
    myocardial i.
    nerve root i.
    ventricular i.
irritable
    i. bowel syndrome
    i. colon
    i. heart
    i. stricture
irritant
    i. bronchitis
    primary i.
irritation
    chronic i.
    i. fibroma
IRSE
    inversion recovery spin-echo
IRSE sequence
IRV
    inspiratory reserve volume
IS
    ileosacral
    international standard
ISAH
    I. stereotactic immobilization frame
    I. stereotactic immobilizing mask
ischemia
    acute mesenteric i.
    anoxic i.

    balanced i.
    brachiocephalic i.
    brain i.
    brainstem i.
    cardiac i.
    carotid artery i.
    cerebral i.
    chronic cerebral i.
    chronic mesenteric i. (CMI)
    coronary i.
    cortical i.
    exercise-induced transient
      myocardial i.
    focal cerebral i.
    global cerebral i.
    global myocardial i.
    intracompartmental i.
    irreversible i.
    limb-threatening i.
    mesenteric i.
    myocardial i.
    neonatal intracranial i.
    nonhemorrhagic i.
    nonlocalized i.
    nonocclusive mesenteric i.
    organ i.
    periinfarction i.
    provocable i.
    radiation-induced i.
    radiation-related i.
    regional myocardial i.
    regional transmural i.
    remote i.
    reversible myocardial i.
    rostral brainstem i.
    segmental bronchus i.
    silent myocardial i.
    stress-induced i.
    subendocardial i.
    talar dome i.
    testicular i.
    transient cerebral i.
    transient myocardial i.
    vertebrobasilar i.
ischemic
    i. area
    i. bowel
    i. bowel disease
    i. brain damage
    i. brainstem infarct
    i. change
    i. colitis
    i. congestive cardiomyopathy
    i. contracture
    i. core
    i. decompensation
    i. defect

i. encephalopathy
i. episode
i. event
i. gliosis
i. heart
i. histopathology
i. hypoxia
i. index
i. instability
i. lesion
i. mesentery
i. necrosis
i. necrosis of femoral head (INFH)
i. penumbra
i. reperfused myocardium
i. reperfusion injury
i. segment
i. time
i. ulcer
i. viable myocardium
i. zone

ischemically mediated mitral regurgitation
ischial

i. bone
i. bursitis
i. spine
i. tuberosity

ischioacetabular fracture
ischiocapsular ligament
ischiocavernosus muscle
ischiofemoral ligament
ischiogluteal

i. bursa
i. bursitis

ischiopagus twin
ischiopubic ramus
ischiorectal

i. abscess
i. fat pad
i. fossa
i. fossa lesion
i. fossa plane

ischiospongiosus muscle of penis
ischium

ascending ramus of i.
ramus of i.
transverse diameter between i.'s

ISD

interspinous distance

ISG medical imaging workstation

ISI

injection scan interval

ISIS spectroscopy
ISKD

intramedullary skeletal kinetic distractor
ISKD system

island

bone i.
bony i.
cartilage i.
compact i.
endometrial i.
fat i.
fibrotic i.
heterotopic white matter i.
mucosal i.
Pander i.
i. of red marrow
Reil i.
sclerotic calvarium bone i.
tissue i.
i. of tissue

islet cell tumor
isoattenuating
isoattenuation
isobaric transition
isobar nuclide
isobutyl

dipyridamole technetium-99m-2-methoxy i.

Isocam

I. scintillation imaging
I. scintillation imaging system
I. SPECT imaging system

isocapnic hyperventilation-induced bronchoconstriction
isocenter

i. placement error
i. shift method
shoulder i.
single i.

isochromat
isoclosed curve
isocon camera
isodense

i. appearance
i. enhancement
i. mass
i. subdural hematoma

isodose

i. contour
i. curve

NOTES

isodose *(continued)*
    i. line
    i. plan
    i. shift method
    i. width
isoechoic
    i. breast mass
    i. clot
isoefamate contrast medium
isoeffect dose
isoeffective bronchial mucosa
isoelectric
    i. electroencephalogram
    i. line
    i. period
isoflurane
isoform
    CSF 14-3-3 i.
isoimmunization
    rhodium i.
isointense
    i. background fat
    i. lesion
    i. signal
    i. soft tissue
isointensity
Isolar rod
isolated
    i. airway injury
    i. cerebellar hypoplasia
    i. clustered calcifications
    i. dislocation
    i. focal cerebellar cortical dysplasia
    i. hepatic infusion
    i. hook fracture
    i. ventricular inversion
isolation perfusion
isoleucine (I)
isomer
    i. nuclide
    optical i.
isomeric
    i. decay
    i. transition
isomerism
    atrial i.
isonitrile
    dipyridamole technetium-99m-2-methoxy isobutyl i.
    methoxyisobutyl i.
isoosmotic polyethylene glycol
Isopaque contrast medium
isophil
isoporosis
isopotential line
isoproterenol infusion
isosceles triangular configuration

isosexual precocity
isosmolar contrast medium (IOCM)
isosmotic water solution
isotone nuclide
isotonicity
isotope
    beta-emitting i.
    i. bone scan
    i. calibrator
    carrier-free i.
    cistern i.
    i. clearance
    i. colloid imaging
    daughter i.
    i. decay
    i. dilution analysis
    i. effect
    gamma-emitting i.
    i. hepatobiliary imaging
    intravenous injection of i.
    isotope hepatobiliary imaging
      radioactive i.
    labeling of the i.
    i. meal
    i. nephrography
    neutron-deficient short-lived i.
    i. nuclide
    parent i.
    ^{103}Pd i.
    phosphorus i.
    poorly concentrated i.
    radioactive i.
    i. renogram
    rhenium i.
    i. scintigraphy
    short-range i.
    i. shunt imaging
    stable i.
    strontium i.
    i. uptake
    i. venography
    i. ventriculography
    i. voiding cystourethrography (IVCU)
isotope-labeled fibrinogen imaging
isotope-tagged marker
isotopic
    i. cisternography
    i. dilution
    i. 3D imaging
    i. 3D study
    i. lung scan
    i. ratio
    i. skeletal survey
    i. volume study
isotretinoin

isotropic
    i. diffusion-weighted imaging
    i. disk
    i. motion
    i. resolution
    i. tissue
    i. voxel
isotropy
isotype
isovolumetric
    i. contraction time
    i. period
    i. relaxation
isovolumic relaxation time (IVRT)
Isovue
    I. nonionic imaging agent
    I. prefilled syringe
Isovue-200, -250, -300, -370 imaging agent
Isovue-370 prefilled syringe
Isovue-M 200, 300 imaging agent
Israel camera
ISS
    inferior sagittal sinus
    injury severity scale
    injury severity score
    invasive surgical staging
ISSI
    interspinous segmental spinal
    instrumentation
isthmic
    i. coarctation
    i. organizer
    i. region
    i. spondylolisthesis
isthmus, pl. **isthmi, isthmuses**
    aortic i.
    i. of corpus callosum
    i. of femur
    pontine i.
    renal i.
    stenotic i.
    temporal i.
    thyroid i.
    uterine i.
    i. of uterus
    i. of Vieussens
IT
    iliotibial
    intrathecal
    IT band

ITA
    internal thoracic artery
ITA graft
iterative
    i. algorithm
    i. halftoning
    i. reconstruction
ITT
    internal tibial torsion
IUD
    interuncal distance
IUdR
    iododeoxyuridine
IUG
    intrauterine gas
IUGR
    intrauterine growth retardation
        asymmetric IUGR
        late flattening IUGR
        low-profile IUGR
        mixed IUGR
        symmetric IUGR
IUP
    intrauterine pregnancy
IV, I.V.
    intravenous
        supination-external rotation IV
        (SER-IV)
IVAC P4000 infuser
Ivalon
    I. particle
    I. plug
    I. sponge
IVB
    intraventricular block
IVC
    inferior vena cava
    intravenous cholangiogram
        solitary left IVC
IVCU
    isotope voiding cystourethrography
IVCV
    inferior venacavography
IVDSA
    intravenous digital subtraction
    angiography
Ivemark CHD syndrome
IVFA
    intravenous fluorescein angiography
        IVFA imaging
IVH
    intraventricular hemorrhage

NOTES

IVIM
  intravoxel incoherent motion
Ivor Lewis esophagectomy
ivory
  i. osteoma
  i. phalanx
  i. vertebra
IVP
  intravenous pyelography
    rapid-sequence IVP
IVR
  idioventricular rhythm
IVRT
  isovolumic relaxation time

IVSD
  interventricular septal defect
IVST
  interventricular septal thickness
IVU
  intravenous urography
IVUS
  intravascular ultrasound
    IVUS catheter
    2D IVUS
    3D IVUS

J

joule
J chain
J junction
J loop
J point
Jaboulay amputation
Jaccoud
J. arthropathy
J. sign
JACE-STIM electrotherapy unit
jackknife position
Jackson
J. sign
J. staging system
Jacobson canal
Jadassohn-Lewandowsky syndrome
Jaffe-Campanacci syndrome
Jaffe-Lichtenstein disease
jagged
j. bone fragment
j. osteophyte
Jahss dislocation classification
jail-bar
j.-b. appearance
j.-b. chest
j.-b. rib
James bundle
jammed finger
Janeway lesion
Jansen
J. disease
J. metaphyseal dysplasia
Jansen-type metaphyseal
chondrodysplasia
Jaquet apparatus
Jarcho-Levin syndrome
Jarjavay ligament
Jatene transposition
javelin thrower's elbow
jaw
ameloblastoma of the j.
j. bone
claudication of j.
independent j.
osteosarcoma of j.
Jefferson
J. burst fracture
J. cervical fracture
Jeffery classification of radial fracture
jejunal
j. diverticulosis
j. diverticulum
j. interposition of Henle
j. leiomyosarcoma

j. loop
j. loop interposition of Henle
j. motility
j. obstruction
j. pouch
j. ulcer
jejunitis
Crohn j.
ulcerative j.
jejunization
j. of colon
ileal j.
j. of ileum
vascular j.
jejunocolic fistula
jejunoduodenogastric intussusception
jejunogastric intussusception
jejunoileal (JI)
j. bypass (JIB)
j. diverticulum
j. shunt
jejunoileitis
ulcerative j.
jejunostomy catheter
jejunum
proximal j.
jelly-belly appearance
jeopardized myocardium
jersey finger
jet
aqueductal j.
j. flow
high-velocity j.
j. length (JL)
j. lesion
pressurized fluid j.
regurgitant j.
ureteral j.
ureteric j.
Jeune syndrome
Jewett nail
JGA
juxtaglomerular apparatus
J-hook
J.-h. deformity
J.-h. deformity of distal ureter
JI
jejunoileal
JI shunt
JIB
jejunoileal bypass
JL
jet length
J-modulation

J

JNPA
juvenile nasopharyngeal angiofibroma
Jobert fossa
Jod-Basedow phenomenon
Johnson-Jahss classification of posterior tibial tendon tear
Johnson position
joint
acromioclavicular j.
ankle j.
j. ankylosis
apophyseal j.
j. arthrography
j. articular surface
j. articulation
atlantoaxial j.
atlantooccipital j.
bail-lock knee j.
ball-and-socket j.
basal j.
Budin j.
calcaneocuboid j.
j. calculus
capitate hamate j.
capitolunate j.
j. capsule
j. capsule defect
j. capsule thickening
carpometacarpal j. (CMC)
carpophalangeal j.
j. cavity
Charcot j.
j. chondroma
Chopart j.
Clutton painful j.
computed tomography-guided
  percutaneous radiofrequency
  denervation of the sacroiliac j.
condyloid j.
j. contracture
coracoclavicular j.
costochondral j.
costotransverse j.
costovertebral j.
Cruveilhier j.
cubonavicular j.
cuneiform j.
j. cyst
j. debris
j. deformity
j. depression fracture
diarthrodial intervertebral j.
DIP j.
j. dislocation
distal interphalangeal j.
distal radioulnar j. (DRUJ)
j. distraction

j. effusion
elbow j.
ellipsoid j.
erythema of j.
facet j.
femoropatellar j.
flail j.
j. fluid
j. fluid extravasation
j. fluid extrusion
free knee j.
frozen j.
j. fulcrum
j. fusion
Gaffney j.
Gillette j.
glenohumeral j.
gliding j.
hallux interphalangeal j.
hinge j.
hip capsule j.
j. hyperextensibility
hypermobile j.
IM j.
immovable j.
j. incongruity
j. instability
intercarpal j.
interchondral j.
j. interface
intermetatarsal j.
interphalangeal j.
intervertebral j.
IP j.
j. kinematics
knee j.
j. laxity
lesser metatarsophalangeal j.
j. line
Lisfranc j.
loss of parallelism of facet j.
lunotriquetral j.
Luschka j.
manubriosternal j.
metacarpophalangeal j. (MCPJ)
metatarsal j.
metatarsocuneiform j.
metatarsophalangeal j.
midcarpal j.
middle facet of the subtalar j.
midtarsal j.
j. morphology
mortise j.
naviculocuneiform j.
near-anatomic position of j.
neuropathic tarsometatarsal j.
neurotrophic j.

occipitoaxial j.
osteolysis on both sides of j.
parallelism of facet j.
patellofemoral j.
perched facet j.
PIP j.
pisotriquetral j.
pivot j.
j. play
primary cartilage j.
proximal interphalangeal j. (PIP, PIPJ)
proximal radioulnar j.
pseudoneuropathic j.
pulvinar hip j.
radiocapitellar j.
radiocarpal j.
radioscaphoid j.
radioulnar j.
Regnauld degeneration of MTP j.
sacrococcygeal j.
sacroiliac j.
saddle j.
scaphocapitate j.
scapholunate j.
scaphotrapeziotrapezoid j.
scapulothoracic j.
seagull j.
secondary cartilaginous j.
j. segment
sesamoidometatarsal j.
shoulder j.
SI j.
signal j.
Silastic finger j.
SL j.
j. space
j. space narrowing
j. space pseudowidening
sternal j.
sternoclavicular j.
sternocostal j.
sternomanubrial j.
STT j.
subluxed facet j.
subtalar j.
j. survey
Swanson finger j.
j. swelling
symphysis cartilage j.
synovial diarthroidal j.
talocalcaneal j.

talocalcaneonavicular j.
talocrural j.
talofibular j.
talonavicular j.
tarsal j.
tarsometatarsal j.
temporomandibular j. (TMJ)
thoracic j.
tibiofibular j.
tibiotalar j.
j. tissue
transverse tarsal j.
trapeziometacarpal j.
trapezioscaphoid j.
trapeziotrapezoid j.
triquetrohamate j.
j.'s of trunk
uncovertebral j.
unstable j.
weightbearing j.
widened sacroiliac j.
j. widening
wrist j.
xiphisternal j.
zygapophyseal j.

Joliot method
Jomed peripheral stent-graft
Jones
    J. classification
    J. classification of diaphyseal fracture
    J. criterion
    J. view
Jones-Mote reaction
Joseph valve implant
JOSTENT Peripheral Stent Graft
Joubert
    J. focal cerebellar dysplasia
    J. malformation
    J. syndrome
joule (J)
    j. shock
JPA
    juvenile pilocytic astrocytoma
J-pouch
    small colonic J.-p.
JPS
    juvenile polyposis syndrome
JRA
    juvenile rheumatoid arthritis
J-sella deformity

NOTES

J-shaped
- J.-s. anastomosis
- J.-s. sella
- J.-s. stomach
- J.-s. tube
- J.-s. ureter

J-tipped guidewire

Jude
- J. pelvic view
- J. pelvic x-ray

Judet
- J. epiphyseal fracture classification
- J. view

Judkins
- J. coronary arteriography
- J. left coronary catheter
- J. right coronary catheter
- J. selective left coronary cinearteriography
- J. technique

jugal
- j. ligament
- j. suture

jugular
- j. bulb anomaly
- j. bulb tumor
- j. catheter
- j. compression maneuver
- j. foramen
- j. foramen schwannoma
- j. foramen syndrome
- j. foraminal mass
- j. lymph node
- j. megabulb
- j. node metastatic carcinoma
- j. process
- j. technique
- j. tubercle
- j. vein
- j. vein thrombosis
- j. venous access
- j. venous distention
- j. venous impulse
- j. venous oxygen saturation
- j. venous pressure
- j. venous pressure collapse

jugulare
- glomus j.

jugulodigastric
- j. chain
- j. node

juguloomohyoid lymph node

jumped facet

jumper's knee

jumping
- bite j.

jump vein graft

junction
- anomalous craniovertebral j.
- anorectal j. (ARJ)
- aortic sinotubular j.
- atlantooccipital j.
- atriocaval j.
- atrioventricular j.
- beaked cervicomedullary j.
- bird-beak taper at esophagogastric j.
- bulbous costochondral j.
- caniocervical j.
- cardioesophageal j.
- cardiophrenic j.
- cavoatrial j.
- CE j.
- cervicomedullary j.
- cervicothoracic j.
- choledochopancreatic ductal j.
- chondrosternal j.
- competence of ureterovesical j.
- corticomedullary j. (CMJ)
- costochondral j.
- craniocervical j.
- craniovertebral j.
- cystic-choledochal j.
- duodenojejunal j. (DJJ)
- esophagogastric j.
- fundic-antral j.
- gastrocnemius-soleus j.
- gastroduodenal j.
- gastroesophageal j.
- gray-white matter j.
- ileocecal j.
- iliocaval j.
- J j.
- lateral margin of the esophagogastric j.
- meniscocapsular j.
- meniscosynovial j.
- metaphyseal-diaphyseal j.
- midbrain-hindbrain j.
- mucocutaneous j.
- musculotendinous j.
- myoneural j.
- myotendinous j.
- neuromuscular j.
- occipitocervical j.
- pancreaticobiliary ductal j.
- pelviureteric j. (PUJ)
- phrenovertebral j.
- pontomedullary j.
- pontomesencephalic j.
- prostaticovesical j.
- pyloroduodenal j.
- rectosigmoid j.
- saphenofemoral j.

sinotubular j.
splenoportal j.
sternochondral j.
supraspinatus musculotendinous j.
sylvian-rolandic j.
temporooccipital j.
temporoparietooccipital j.
tracheoesophageal j.
ureteropelvic j. (UPJ)
ureterorenal j.
ureterovesical j.
uterovesical j.
venous j.
junctional
j. cortical defect
j. dilatation
j. epidermolysis bullosa
j. focus
j. infundibulum
j. nest
j. parenchymal kidney defect
j. zone
Junghans pseudospondylolisthesis
juvenile
j. ankylosing spondylitis
j. aponeurotic fibroma
j. autosomal recessive polycystic disease
j. breast papillomatosis
j. calcific diskitis
j. chronic polyarthritis
j. cirrhosis
j. embryonal carcinoma
j. epiphyseolysis
j. epiphysitis
j. fibroadenoma
j. fibromatosis
j. laryngeal papillomatosis
j. nasopharyngeal angiofibroma (JNPA)
j. nephronophthisis
j. orbital pilocytic astrocytoma
j. ossifying fibroma
j. osteoporosis
j. Paget disease
j. pelvis
j. pilocytic astrocytoma (JPA)
j. polyp
j. polyposis

j. polyposis syndrome (JPS)
j. rheumatoid arthritis (JRA)
j. spondyloarthropathy
j. Tillaux fracture
j. T-wave pattern
j. xanthogranuloma
juvenilis
kyphosis dorsalis j.
osteochondrosis deformans j.
juxtaanastomotic stenosis
juxtaarterial ventricular septal defect
juxtaarticular
j. fracture
j. low signal intensity
j. osteoid osteoma
juxtaarticulation
juxtacortical
j. bone lesion
j. chondroma
j. chondrosarcoma
j. fracture
j. osteogenic sarcoma
j. osteosarcoma
juxtacrural
juxtadiaphragmatic location
juxtaductal
j. aortic coarctation
j. coarctation of aorta
juxtaepiphyseal
juxtaglomerular
j. apparatus (JGA)
j. tumor
juxtahilar bronchus interruption
juxtaintestinal node
juxtapapillary diverticulum
juxtaphrenic peak
juxtaposition
atrial appendage j.
juxtapyloric ulcer
juxtarenal
j. aortic aneurysm
j. aortic atherosclerosis
j. cava
juxtarestiform body
juxtasellar ICA
juxtaspinal
juxtatricuspid ventricular septal defect
juxtavesical

J

NOTES

K
    potassium
      K capture
      K electron
      K radiation
      K shell
      K wire

^{38}**K**
    potassium-38
^{39}**K**
    potassium-39
^{40}**K**
    potassium-40
^{42}**K**
    potassium-42
^{43}**K**
    potassium-43

Kadish
    K. staging
    K. staging system
Kager triangle
Kahler disease
Kalamchi-Dawe congenital tibial deficiency classification
Kallmann syndrome
Kalman filter
Kanavel sign
Kantor string sign
kaolin pneumoconiosis
Kapandji radical fracture
Kaplan PenduLaser 115 laser system
Kaposi sarcoma (KS)
Karapandzic flap
Karplus
    K. relationship
    K. sign
    K. sign of pleural effusion
Kartagener
    K. syndrome
    K. triad
Kasabach-Merritt syndrome
Kasai procedure
Kast syndrome
Katayama syndrome
Katzen infusion guidewire
Katzman infusion of radionuclide cisternography
Katz-Wachtel phenomenon
Kawasaki disease
Kayser-Fleischer ring
Kazangia and Converse facial fracture classification
KBR
    kidney length to body height ratio
K-capture

KCC
    Kulchitsky cell carcinoma
KCD
    kinestatic charge detector
      KCD imaging
kCi
    kilocurie
Kearns-Sayre syndrome
K-edge filter
keel
    laryngeal k.
keeled chest
Keeper vena cava filter
Kehr sign
Keinböck disease
Keith
    K. node
    K. sinoatrial bundle
Keith-Flack sinoatrial node
Kellgren arthritis
Kellock
    K. sign
    K. sign of pleural effusion
Kellogg-Speed lumbar spinal fusion
Kelly-Goerss COMPASS stereotactic system
Kempe series
Kendall sequential compression device
Kennedy method for calculating ejection fraction
Kensey-Nash lithotrite
Kent
    bundle of Stanley K.
Kent-His bundle
keratectomy
    phototherapeutic k. (PTK)
keratin
    k. pearl
    k. plug
    k. testicular cyst
    k. urinary tract ball
keratinizing squamous metaplasia
keratocyst
    odontogenic k.
keratoma
Kerckring
    K. fold
    K. nodule
    K. ossicle
Kerley A, B, C line
kerma
    kinetic energy released per unit mass and
    kinetic energy released in medium
      air kerma

kerma *(continued)*
    integrated reference air kerma
      (IRAK)
    total reference air kerma (TRAK)
kerma-to-dose conversion factor
kernel
    dose k.
    interpolation k.
    large k.
    noise reconstruction k.
    k. size
    soft tissue k.
    spherical k.
kernel-of-corn appearance
Kernig sign
Kernohan brain tumor classification
Keshan disease
ketamine
ketanserin
ketene
ketone body
Kety equation
keV, kev
    kiloelectron volt
      keV gamma ray
      511-keV high-energy imaging
Key-Conwell
    K.-C. classification of pelvic
      fracture
    K.-C. pelvic fracture classification
keyhole deformity
keystone of calcar arch
kg
    kilogram
kHz
    kilohertz
kick
    atrial k.
Kidner lesion
kidney
    abdominal k.
    k. abscess
    absent k.
    k. adenocarcinoma
    k. adenoma
    k. amyloidosis
    k. anatomy
    k. aneurysm
    k. angiomyolipoma
    k. anomaly
    k. arteriosclerosis
    arteriosclerotic k.
    Ask-Upmark k.
    atrophic k.
    k. atrophy
    bilateral large k.
    bilateral small k.

blunt trauma k.
cake k.
k. calcification
k. calculus
k. carcinoma chromophobe
k. chloroma
cicatricial k.
congenital absence of k.
congested k.
contracted k.
contralateral k.
cortical scarring of k.
cross-ectopic k.
crush k.
cyanotic k.
k. cyst
cystic k.
discoid k.
k. disk
distended k.
double k.
doughnut k.
duplication of left k.
duplication of right k.
dysfunctional k.
dysgenetic k.
k. dyskeratosis
dysplastic k.
ectopic k.
edematous k.
enlarged k.
k. extraction efficiency
faceless k.
k. failure
fatty k.
fetal mesenchymal tumor of k.
k. fibromyxoma
fibrotic k.
floating k.
Formad k.
fractured k.
k. function imaging
k. function study
k. fungus ball
fused k.
Goldblatt k.
granular k.
hamartoma of the k.
k. hilum
Hodson-type k.
horseshoe k.
hydronephrotic k.
hypermobile k.
k. infarct
infundibulum of k.
iron accumulation in k.
irregular k.

k. leiomyoma
k. length to body height ratio
(KBR)
lobe of k.
lobulated k.
long axis of k.
lower pole of k.
lumbar k.
lump k.
k. lymphoma
k. malrotation
k. mass growth pattern
medullary sponge k.
mesonephric k.
k. metastasis
movable k.
multicystic k. (MCK)
multicystic dysgenetic k.
multicystic dysplastic k. (MCDK)
mural k.
k. mycetoma
native k.
k. neurofibromatosis
nonfunctioning k.
k. oxalosis
Page k.
pancake k.
k. papillary blush
partially polycystic k.
pelvis of k.
k. pole
pole-to-pole length of k.
polycystic k.
porous k.
Potter type IV k.
k. pseudotumor
ptotic k.
putty k.
k. radionuclide imaging
Rose-Bradford k.
sacciform k.
k. scan
scarred k.
sclerotic k.
k. shadow
shattered k.
shriveled k.
sigmoid k.
single functioning k.
k. sinus mass
k. size
sponge k.

k. stone
supernumerary k.
suspension of k.
thoracic k.
k. tomography
k. transplant
k. trauma
tree-barking k.
unicaliceal k.
unilateral large smooth k.
unilateral small k.
unipapillary k.
up-sloping curve of k.
k.'s, ureter, and bladder film
k.'s, ureter, and bladder imaging
k.'s, ureters, bladder (KUB)
k. vessel
wandering k.
k. washout
kidney-pancreas transplant
kidney-shaped
k.-s. distended cecum
k.-s. placenta
kidney-to-background ratio
**Kiel non-Hodgkin lymphoma
classification**
Kienböck
K. dislocation
K. unit (X)
Kienböck-Adamson point
Kikuchi disease
Kikuchi-Fujimoto disease
Kilfoyle
K. classification of condylar
fracture
K. condylar fracture classification
Kilian
K. line
K. pelvis
killer
flow artifact k. (FLAK)
Killian dehiscence
kilocurie (kCi)
kiloelectron volt (keV, kev)
kilogram (kg)
kilohertz (kHz)
kilomegacycle
kilovolt (kV)
kilovoltage (kV)
kilovolt peak (kVp)
Kimmelstiel-Wilson syndrome
Kimura classification

K

NOTES

Kimura-type choledochal cyst
kinase
    k. C antiglioma monoclonal
        antibody imaging agent
    herpes thymidine k. (HSV1-tk)
kindling phenomenon
kinematic
    joint k.'s
    k. magnetic resonance imaging
    k. MR cholangiopancreatography
    k. MRCP
    k. MRI study
    k. MR technique
    k. wrist device
kineradiography
kinesis
    color k.
kinestatic
    k. charge detector (KCD)
    k. charge detector imaging
kinetic
    k. cervical spine
    k. curve
    elimination k.'s
    k. energy
    k. energy released per unit mass
        and kinetic energy released in
        medium (kerma)
    exponential k.'s
    k. parameter analysis
    k. perfusion parameter
    sorption k.'s
    time-resolved imaging of
        contrast k.'s (TRICKS)
    washout k.'s
kinetocardiogram
kinetoscopy
Kinevac imaging agent
King classification of thoracic scoliosis
King-Moe
    K.-M. classification
    K.-M. scoliosis
kinin
kininogen
kininogenase
kink
    k. artifact
    cervicomedullary k.
    k. in intestine
    Lane k.
kinked
    k. aorta
    k. bowel
    k. ureter
kinking
    aortic k.
    arterial k.

blood vessel k.
bronchial k.
carotid artery k.
catheter k.
colon k.
graft k.
innominate artery k.
intestinal k.
patch k.
ureteric k.
Kinnier-Wilson disease
Kinsbourne syndrome
Kirchner diverticulum
Kirk distal thigh amputation
Kirklin meniscal complex
Kirner deformity
Kirsch laser
Kirschner wire (K-wire)
kissing
    k. artifact
    k. atherectomy technique
    k. balloon
    k. contraction
    k. lesion
    k. sequestrum
    k. spine
    k. stent
    k. ulcer
kissing-balloon technique
Kistler subarachnoid hemorrhage
    classification
Kistner tracheal button
kit
    Fleet Prep K. 1, 2, 3
    k. preparation
    k. for preparation of technetium
        Tc99m depreotide injection
    PYROLITE k.
    Ultra Tag k.
kite angle
Klatskin
    K. tumor
    K. tumor classification
kleeblatschädel deformity
kleeblattschadel
Kleffner-Landau syndrome
Klein
    K. muscle
    K. technique
Klemm sign
Klenow fragment
Klippel-Feil
    K.-F. deformity
    K.-F. sequence
    K.-F. syndrome
Klippel-Trenaunay syndrome
Klippel-Trenaunay-Weber syndrome

Klumpke
  K. brachial plexus injury
  K. paralysis
K-means
  K.-m. cluster
  K.-m. clustering algorithm
knee
  anterior cruciate deficit of k.
  k. arthrography bolster
  breaststroker's k.
  Brodie k.
  collateral ligament of k.
  corner of k.
  dislocated k.
  double camelback sign of k.
  k. flexion contracture
  floating k.
  k. fracture
  housemaid's k.
  indirect MR arthrography of k.
  internal derangement of the k.
    (IDK)
  k. joint
  k. joint effusion
  k. joint space height
  jumper's k.
  k. knob
  locked k.
  medial and lateral support
    structures of the k.
  motorcyclist's k.
  reefing of medial retinaculum
    of k.
  k. rest
  runner's k.
  spontaneous osteonecrosis of k.
    (SONK)
  tricompartmental chondromalacia of
    the k.
  k. view
  wrenched k.
kneecap
knee-like bend
Kniest dysplasia
knife, pl. **knives**
  Leksell 201-source cobalt-60
    Gamma k.
  roentgen k.
  UltraCision ultrasonic k.
knob
  absent aortic k.
  aortic k.

blurring of aortic k.
knee k.
notched aortic k.
knobby process
knocked-down shoulder
knock-knee deformity
knot
  false k.
  ileosigmoid k.
  lovers k.
  surfer's k.
  true umbilical cord k.
known primary carcinoma
knuckle
  aortic k.
  k. bone
  k. of colon
knuckle-shaped
Knuttsen bending film
Koch
  K. sinoatrial node
  K. triangle
  K. triangle apex
Kocher
  K. anastomosis
  K. dilatation ulcer
  K. fracture
  K. maneuver
**Kocher-Lorenz capitellum fracture
  classification**
Kodak
  K. Digital Science 1200, 3600
    distributed medical imager
  K. Min-R film
  K. Min-R screen
  K. RP X-OMAT processor
  K. software
  K. X-OMAT film
Koeppe nodule
Köhler
  K. disease
  K. line
Kohlrausch fold
Kokopelli hunchback
Köllicker nucleus
Komai stereotactic head frame
Kommerell
  K. diverticulum
  ductus of K.
Konica scanner
Konstram angle

K

NOTES

Kopans
    K. needle
    K. spring hookwire
Korányi-Grocco triangle
Kormed liver biopsy needle
Korotkoff test for collateral circulation
Kostuik-Errico spinal stability
   classification
Kovalevsky canal
Kr
   krypton
Kr 85
Krabbe
    K. diffuse sclerosis
    K. disease
K-radiation
Krause
    K. ligament
    transverse suture of K.
Krebs cycle
Kretztechnik ultrasound system
Krigel staging system
Kromayer lamp
Krönlein orbitotomy
Krukenberg tumor
Krupin-Denver eye valve-to-disc implant
Kruskal-Wallis test
krypton (Kr)
    k. laser
    k. laser photocoagulation
    k. scan
krypton-77
    inhalation of k.
krypton-81, 81m
KS
   Kaposi sarcoma
K-shell
k-space
    k-s. matrix
    k-s. trajectory
    k-s. velocity mapping
KTP
   potassium-titanyl-phosphate
   KTP laser
KUB
   kidneys, ureters, bladder
   KUB imaging
   KUB view
Kubelka-Munk theory
Kugel
    K. anastomosis
    K. artery

Kugelberg-Welander disease
Kulchitsky
    K. cell
    K. cell carcinoma (KCC)
Kulkarni injury
Kumar, Welti and Ernst method
Kumeral diverticulum
Kumpe
    K. catheter
    K. hump
Kupffer cell sarcoma
Kürner septum
Kussmaul-Maier disease
Kussmaul sign
kV
   kilovolt
   kilovoltage
kVp
   kilovolt peak
    kVp meter
kwashiorkor
KWE method
K-wire
   Kirschner wire
Ky
    sliding interleaved K. (SLINKY)
Kyle fracture classification
kyllosis
kymograph
kymography
   roentgen k.
kymoscopy
kyphoscoliosis
kyphoscoliotic
    k. heart disease
    k. pelvis
kyphosis
    Cobb method of measuring k.
    k. dorsalis juvenilis
    loss of thoracic k.
    lumbar k.
    lumbosacral k.
    postlaminectomy k.
    Scheuermann juvenile k.
    thoracic k.
    thoracolumbar k.
kyphotic
    k. angulation
    k. curvature
    k. pelvis
    k. view

Λ
Avogadro number
Ostwald solubility coefficient
radioactive constant
wavelength
L
lumbar vertebra
L electron
L shell
L5-S1 projection
LA
left atrium
L/A
liver-aorta
L/A peak ratio
LAA
left atrial appendage
left auricular appendage
LA:AR ratio
left atrium/aortic root ratio
LABA
laser-assisted balloon angioplasty
Labbé
L. triangle
L. vein
label
double l.
long wave-length photo l.
radioactive l.
radionuclide l.
single l.
triple l.
labeled
l. atom
l. fibrinogen
l. free fatty acid scintigraphy
l. leukocyte scan
l. phosphorus
l. positron
l. RBC
l. red blood cell sequestration
labeling
l. abnormality
antibody l.
^{111}In l.
iododeoxyuridine l.
l. of the isotope
microglobulin l.
pulse l.
pulsed arterial spin l.
radioactive l.
radioisotope l.
site-specific l.
technetium-99m antibody l.
technetium-tagged RBC l.

in vitro l.
in vivo l.
labial
l. groove
l. vein
labile blood pressure
labor dystocia
labral
l. and anterior inferior glenoid rim
fracture
l. capsular complex
l. fibrocartilage
l. injury
l. variant
labrum, pl. **labra**
acetabular l.
anterior glenoid l. (AGL)
articular l.
fibrocartilaginous l.
glenoid l.
labrum-ligament complex
labyrinth, labyrinthus
artery of l.
bony l.
cochlear l.
ethmoidal l.
membranous l.
osseous l.
renal l.
vestibular l.
labyrinthine
l. artery
l. fistula
l. hemorrhage
l. hydrops
l. structure
labyrinthitis ossificans
labyrinthus (*var. of* labyrinth)
LACD
left apex cardiogram, calibrated
displacement
lace-like
l.-l. appearance
l.-l. trabecular pattern
laceration
bladder l.
brain l.
liver l.
lung l.
parenchymal l.
spinal cord l.
spleen l.
tendon l.
lacerum
foramen l.

L

Lachman sign
laciniate
    l. ligament
    l. ligament of ankle
lack of acoustic penetration
lacrimal
    l. artery
    l. bone
    l. canal
    l. duct
    l. gland
    l. gland lesion
    l. groove
    l. mass
    l. nerve
    l. recess
    l. sac
    l. scan
    l. scintigraphy
lacrimoconchal suture
lacrimoethmoidal suture
lacrimomaxillary suture
lacrimoturbinal suture
lactate
    l. proton
    l. resonance
lactating adenoma
lacteal
    l. calculus
    l. vessel
lactiferous
    l. duct
    l. sinus
lactobezoar
lactoferrin production
lacuna, pl. lacunae, lacunas
    bone l.
    cartilage l.
    intervillous l.
    Morgagni l.
    osseous l.
    penis l.
    resorption l.
lacunaire
lacunar
    l. abscess
    l. brain infarct
    l. ligament
    l. node
    l. skull
    l. stroke
lacunas (*pl. of* lacuna)
lacune
LAD
    left anterior descending
    left axis deviation
LADARVision excimer laser

Ladd band
Ladder diagram
ladder-like pattern
Lady Windermere syndrome
LAE
    left atrial enlargement
LAFB
    left anterior fascicular block
LAG
    lymphangiogram
lag
    l. effect
    l. screw
Lagios classification system
LaGrange classification of humeral
    supracondylar fracture
LAID
    left anterior internal diameter
Laimer
    L. fascia
    triangle of L.
LAIS excimer laser
Laitinen
    L. CT guidance system
    L. stereotactic head frame
lake
    bile l.
    capillary l.
    intraplacental venous l.
    lipid l.
    maternal l.
    mucous l.
    venous intraplacental l.
    venous skull l.
lambda
    L. Plus PDL1, PDL2 laser
    white matter l.
lambdoid
    l. suture
    l. synostosis
lambdoidal cranial suture
Lambert
    L. canal
    L. channel
    L. projection
Lambert-Eaton myasthenic syndrome
lamella, pl. lamellae
    anular lamellae
    articular l.
    basal l.
    circumferential l.
    concentric l.
    enamel l.
lamellar
    l. body
    l. body density (LBD)

l. bone
l. periosteal reaction
lamina, pl. **laminae**
l. dura
external elastic l.
medullary l.
osseous spiral l.
l. papyracea
l. propria
vertebral l.
laminagram
laminagraph
laminagraphy (*var. of* laminography)
laminar
l. brain necrosis
l. flow
laminated
l. calcification
l. gallstone
l. intraluminal thrombus
lamination of gyrus
laminectomy
laminogram
laminography, laminagraphy
cardiac l.
laminoplasty
laminotomy
lamp
cold quartz lamp germicidal l.
high-pressure mercury arc l.
hot quartz l.
Kromayer l.
mercury arc l.
mercury vapor l.
quartz l.
sun l.
ultraviolet l.
Wood l.
xenon arc l.
lanceolate deformity
Lancisi
L. muscle
L. sign
Landau diamagnetism
Landau-Kleffner syndrome
landmark
anatomic l.
bony skull l.
l. registration
Landolfi sign
Landsmeer ligament
Landzert fossa

Lane
L. band
L. kink
Lanex medium screen
Langenbeck triangle
Langerhans lung cell histiocytosis
Langer line
Lannelongue ligament
lanthanide
l. metal
l. shift reagent (LSR)
lanthanide-induced shift
lanthanum
Lanz
L. line
L. point
LAO
left anterior oblique
LAO position
LAO projection
LAP
left atrial pressure
laparoscope
3D l.
laparoscopic
l. contact ultrasonography (LCU)
l. intracorporeal ultrasound (LICU)
l. laser
l. probe
l. ultrasound (LapUS, LUS)
l. ultrasound probe
laparoscopy
laparotomy
radioguided l.
Laplace
L. effect
L. mechanism
LapUS
laparoscopic ultrasound
large
l. airway
l. airway narrowing
l. bowel
l. bowel obstruction
l. cell neuroendocrine carcinoma (LCNEC)
l. cell undifferentiated carcinoma
l. cleaved cell lymphoma
l. clothing artifact
l. colloidal particle
l. duct papilloma
l. fetal head

L

NOTES

515

large *(continued)*
 l. field of view (LFV)
 l. field of view gamma camera
 l. for gestational age
 l. gut
 l. habitus
 l. hinge angle electron field
 l. intestine
 l. kernel
 l. loop excision
 l. obtuse marginal branch
 l. solid adrenal mass
 l. spleen
 l. susceptibility artifact
 l. thymus shadow
 l. utricle
 l. venous tributary
 l. vestibule
 l. volume joint effusion
large-bore
 l.-b. bile duct endoprosthesis
 l.-b. catheter
 l.-b. magnet
 l.-b. 0.6-T, 1.5-T imaging system scanner
large-caliber tube
large-core
 l.-c. technique
 l.-c. ultrasound-guided biopsy
large-droplet fatty liver
large-fiber demyelination
large-field
 l.-f. radiation therapy
 l.-f. radiotherapy
 l.-f. x-ray dosimetry
large-field-of-view image
large-for-dates uterus
large-vessel
 l.-v. disease of diabetic foot
 l.-v. thrombosis
Larkin position
Larmor
 L. equation
 L. frequency
 L. precession
Larsen syndrome
laryngeal
 l. atresia
 l. carcinoma
 l. cartilage
 l. edema
 l. fracture
 l. keel
 l. musculature fluorodeoxyglucose uptake
 l. nerve
 l. nodule

 l. papilloma
 l. papillomatosis
 l. part of pharynx
 l. polyp
 l. skeleton
 l. ventricle
 l. vestibule
 l. web
laryngectomy
 supraglottic l.
 vertical partial l.
larynges *(pl. of* larynx)
laryngitis
laryngocele
laryngogram
laryngography
 contrast l.
 double-contrast l.
laryngomalacia
laryngopharyngography
laryngopyocele
laryngoscope
 Olympus ENF-P2 l.
laryngoscopy
 indirect l.
larynx, pl. **larynges**
 appendix of ventricle of l.
 glottic l.
 infraglottic l.
 supraglottic l.
 ventricle of l.
 vestibule of l.
LASE
 laser-assisted spinal endoscopy
Lasègue sign
laser
 AccuLase excimer l.
 acupuncture l.
 alexandrite l.
 Apex Plus excimer l.
 ArF excimer l.
 argon l.
 argon/krypton l.
 argon-pumped dye l.
 Aura desktop l.
 Aurora diode soft-tissue l.
 l. beam
 l. biliary lithotripsy
 biocavity l.
 Candela 405-nm pulsed dye l.
 carbon dioxide l.
 CHRYS CO_2 l.
 ClearView CO_2 l.
 CO_2 l.
 Coherent CO2 surgical l.
 Coherent UltraPulse 5000C l.
 l. correlational spectroscopy (LCS)

coumarin pulsed dye l.
CTE:YAG l.
l. desiccation of thrombus
l. diffraction scanning
l. digitizer
diode l.
l. Doppler flowmetry (LDF)
l. Doppler velocimetry
dye l.
Eclipse TMR l.
endoscopic l.
l. energy
l. energy absorption
Epic ophthalmic 3-in-1 l.
EpiTouch l.
erbium:YAG infrared l.
ErCr:YAG l.
excimer l.
FeatherTouch CO_2 l.
Fiberlase l.
flashlamp-pulsed dye l.
flashlamp-pumped pulsed dye l.
gallium-arsenide l.
Genesis 2000 carbon dioxide l.
Heart l.
helium-cadmium l.
helium-neon l.
HeNe l.
HF infrared l.
high-energy l.
holmium l.
holmium yttrium aluminum
  garnet l. (Ho:YAG laser)
Horn endootoprobe l.
hot l.
Ho:YAG l.
    holmium yttrium aluminum garnet
    laser
l. imager
Kirsch l.
krypton l.
KTP l.
LADARVision excimer l.
LAIS excimer l.
Lambda Plus PDL1, PDL2 l.
L. Lancet laser device
laparoscopic l.
Lastec System angioplasty l.
LightSheer SC diode l.
Lightstic 180, 360 fiberoptic l.
low-energy l. (LEL)
LX 20 l.

Lyra l.
Mainster retina l.
Maloney endootoprobe l.
Microlase transpupillary diode l.
Microlight 830 l.
Microprobe l.
microsecond pulsed flashlamp
  pumped dye l.
midinfrared l.
Nd:YLF l.
NovaLine excimer l.
NovaPulse CO2 l.
Nuvolase 660 l.
OcuLight SL diode l.
OmniPulse-MAX holmium l.
Opmilas CO_2 multipurpose l.
OtoLAM l.
Pegasus PIV l.
Polaris 1.32 Nd:YAG l.
Prima l.
pulsed-dye l.
pulsed infrared l.
pulsed metal vapor l.
PulseMaster l.
Q-switched Nd:YAG l.
Q-switched ruby l.
l. sclerosis
Selecta 7000 l.
Sharplan SilkTouch Flashscan
  surgical l.
SLS l.
Spectranetics excimer l.
SPTL-1b vascular lesion l.
Surgilase 150 high-powered CO_2 l.
Surgilase Nd:YAG l.
l. system
TEC-2100 postioning l.
THC:YAG l.
Topaz CO_2 l.
UltraPulse CO_2 l.
Urolase fiber l.
l. uterosacral nerve ablation
  (LUNA)
VersaLight l.
VersaPulse holmium l.
Visulas Nd:YAG l.
Vitesse Cos l.
l. welding
Xanar 20 Ambulase CO_2 l.
YAG l.
yttrium-aluminum-garnet l.
Zeiss Visulas 690s l.

L

NOTES

laser-assisted
    l.-a. balloon angioplasty (LABA)
    l.-a. microvascular anastomosis
    l.-a. spinal endoscopy (LASE)
    l.-a. uvulopalatoplasty (LAUP)
laser-Doppler flowmetry probe
laser-induced
    l.-i. interstitial thermotherapy
    (LITT)
    l.-i. thermography (LITT)
    l.-i. thermotherapy (LITT)
laser-polarized
    l.-p. helium MRI
    l.-p. helium MR imaging
Laserprobe-PLR Plus
laserthermia
LASH
    left anterosuperior hemiblock
Lasix renography
Lastec System angioplasty laser
last normal vertebra (LNV)
lata
    fascia l.
    snapping fascia l.
latae
    tensor fasciae l.
Latarjet
    nerve of L.
LATC
    lateral talocalcaneal
late
    l. effect analysis
    l. effect of normal tissue (LENT)
    l. effect of normal tissues score
    l. effect toxicity score
    l. false aneurysm
    l. fetal death
    l. film
    l. flattening IUGR
    l. graft occlusion
    l. normal tissue sequela
    l. phase
    l. systolic bulge
    l. systolic retraction
    l. venous filling
latent
    l. coccidioidomycosis
    l. empyema
    l. pleurisy
late-onset dwarfism
late-phase
    l.-p. image
    l.-p. termination
lateral
    l. aneurysm
    l. anterior drawer stress view
    l. arcuate ligament

l. aspect
l. band
l. basal segmental bronchus
l. bending injury
l. bending view
l. border
l. cephalometric radiograph
l. cervical spine film
l. collateral ligament (LCL)
l. collateral ligament complex
l. column calcaneal fracture
l. compartment
l. compartment impaction
l. compartment traumatic bony
    injury
l. conal fascia
l. condylar humeral fracture
l. condyle
l. corticospinal tract
l. costotransverse ligament
l. crus
l. cystourethrogram
l. decubitus film
l. decubitus position
l. decubitus radiograph
l. decubitus view
l. disk herniation
l. divergence angle (LDA)
l. entrapment
l. epicondylar bursa
l. epicondylitis
exaggerated craniocaudal l. (XCCL)
l. extension view
l. facial cleft
l. femoral notch
l. femoral sulcus
l. fissure
l. flexion/extension radiograph
l. flexion view
l. geniculate body
l. gutter
l. horn
l. hypopharyngeal pouch (LHP)
l. impingement
l. joint line
l. joint space
l. left anterior oblique position
l. lemniscus tract
l. lobe of prostate
l. lumbar meningocele
l. lumbar support
l. malleolar fracture
l. malleolus
l. margin of the esophagogastric
    junction
l. mass
l. meniscal uncovering

l. myocardial infarct
l. oblique axial projection
l. oblique fascia
l. oblique jaw radiograph
l. oblique view
l. occipital sulcus
l. occipitotemporal gyrus
l. opposed beam
l. part of occipital bone
l. patellofemoral angle
l. placenta previa
l. plantar metatarsal angle
l. posterior choroidal (LPCh)
l. precordium
l. process of the talus
l. pterygoid muscle
l. pterygoid tendinous attachment
l. pyelography
l. ramus radiograph
l. recess
l. recess stenosis
l. recess syndrome
l. rectus muscle
l. reflection of colon
l. resolution
l. reticular formation
l. root
l. rotatory ankle instability
l. sagittal image
l. semicircular canal
l. sesamoid bone
l. shelf
l. sinus
l. skull radiograph
l. spinothalamic tract
l. spring ligament of foot
l. subluxation
l. talar dome
l. talar dome injury
l. talar process
l. talocalcaneal (LATC)
l. talocalcaneal angle
l. talocalcaneal ligament
l. talometatarsal angle
l. tarsometatarsal angle
l. temporal epileptogenic lesion
l. thoracic meningocele
l. tibial plateau fracture
l. tilt stress ankle view
l. tomography
l. transcranial projection
l. transfacial projection

l. ulnar collateral ligament (LUCL)
l. umbilical fold
l. ventricle
l. ventricle of cerebrum
l. ventricle trigone
l. wall refractive shadowing
l. web
l. wedge fracture
lateralis
interdigitation of vastus l.
meniscus l.
proboscis l.
sinus l.
vastus l.
laterality
lateralization deficit
lateralizing
l. finding
l. sign
laterally displaced fracture
laterocervical region
lateroconal fascia
lateromedial
l. oblique projection
l. oblique view
latex
Spli-Prest l.
LaTIS endovascular laser system
latissimus dorsi muscle
latitude film
lattice
l. index
l. relaxation time
l. vibration
l. work
Laubry-Pezzi syndrome
Laue pattern
Lauge-Hansen ankle fracture
classification
Laugier fracture
LAUP
laser-assisted uvulopalatoplasty
Laurin
L. angle
L. x-ray view
Lauth ligament
law
Angström l.
Avogadro l.
Beer l.
Bergonie-Tribondeau l.
Bragg l.

L

NOTES

519

law *(continued)*
    Coulomb l.
    Courvoisier l.
    Curie l.
    Doerner-Hoskins distribution l.
    Faraday l.
    Fick l.
    Gibbs-Donnan l.
    Hilton l.
    inverse square l.
    least square l.
    Le Borgne l.
    Lenz l.
    Ohm l.
    Poiseuille l.
    L. position
    Rayleigh scattering l.
    transformer l.
    L. view
    Wolff l.
Lawrence
    L. method
    L. position
lawrencium
laxative
    bulk l.
laxity
    chronic ligament complex l.
    joint l.
    ligamentous l.
    varus stress l.
layer
    basal l.
    Bekhterev l.
    boundary l.
    bright l.
    circumferential echo-dense l.
    echo-dense l.
    echo-free l.
    fibrofatty l.
    fluid-blood l.
    half-life l.
    half-value l. (HVL)
    hypoechoic l.
    inner bright l.
    intermediate signal intensity l.
    parietal l.
    seromuscular l.
    sonolucent l.
    subserosal l.
    tenth-value l.
    visceral l.
layered gallstone
layering
    l. calcification
    calcium l.
    l. of contrast material

    l. debris
    l. effusion
    l. of gallstones
Lazarus sign
Lazorthes
    posterior thalamic arteries of L.
LBBB
    left bundle-branch block
LBCD
    left border of cardiac dullness
LBD
    lamellar body density
L/B
    lesion-to-brain ratio
LC
    inductance-capacitance
L/C
    lesion-to-countersite ratio
LCA
    left coronary angiography
    left coronary artery
LC-DCP
    low-contact dynamic compression plate
LCDD
    light chain deposition disease
LCF
    left circumflex
LCIS
    lobular carcinoma in situ
LCL
    lateral collateral ligament
LCNEC
    large cell neuroendocrine carcinoma
LCP
    Legg-Calvé-Perthes disease
LCS
    laser correlational spectroscopy
LCT
    Leydig cell tumor
    liquid crystal thermography
LCU
    laparoscopic contact ultrasonography
LCX
    left circumflex
LDA
    lateral divergence angle
    left descending artery
LDD-gated SPECT with ^{201}Tl
LDF
    laser Doppler flowmetry
LE
    lower extremity
Le
    Lewis
        Le Borgne law
        Le Fort amputation
        Le Fort fibular fracture

Le Fort I, II, III fracture
Le Fort mandibular fracture
Le Fort-Wagstaffe fracture
lead (Pb)
l. apron shield
bipolar l.
chest l.
l. collimation
l. encephalopathy
l. eye shield
l. gonad shield
intracardiac l.
l. line
pacemaker l.
pacing l.
l. pellet marker
l. pin
l. pipe fracture
l. point
precordial l.
radioactive l.
leading edge
lead-pipe rigidity
lead-rubber apron
lead-time bias
leaf
l. of diaphragm
l. of mesentery
leafless tree appearance
leaflet
anterior motion of posterior mitral
valve l.
anterior tricuspid valve l.
apposition of l.
arching of mitral valve l.
bowing of mitral valve l.
coapted l.
commissural l.
doming of l.
floating l.
l. function
hammocking of mitral valve l.
heart valve l.
mitral l.
l. motion
myxomatous valve l.
noncalcified mitral l.
posterior mitral l. (pML)
posterior mitral valve l. (PMVL)
pseudomitral l.
redundant aortic valve l.
redundant mitral valve l.

l. retraction
l. separation
septal l.
spoon-like protrusion of l.
systolic prolapse of mitral valve l.
valve l.
leaf-like villus
leak
air l.
aortic paravalvular l.
ascites due to bile l.
baffle l.
blood l.
calibrated l.
capillary l.
cerebrospinal fluid l.
chyle l.
contained l.
current l.
femoral l.
generalized capillary l.
interatrial baffle l.
interstitial pneumonia air l.
light l.
Luschka duct l.
mitral l.
paraprosthetic l.
paravalvular l.
periprosthetic l.
perivalvular l.
transient chyle l.
leakage
anastomotic l.
bile l.
blood-tumor-barrier l.
chylous l.
contrast media l.
paraprosthetic l.
radiation l.
silicone implant l.
leaking
l. abdominal aortic aneurysm
l. vein
leaky
l. lung syndrome (LLS)
l. valve
lean mass
LEAP
Low Energy All Purpose
LEAP collimator
least
l. square (LS)

L

NOTES

least *(continued)*
  l. square algorithm
  l. square analysis
  l. square law
leather bottle stomach
leave-alone lesion
Leclercq test
ledge
  eccentric l.
left
  l. anterior chest wall wall
  l. anterior descending (LAD)
  l. anterior descending artery
  l. anterior fascicular block (LAFB)
  l. anterior hemiblock block
  l. anterior internal diameter (LAID)
  l. anterior oblique (LAO)
  l. anterior oblique position
  l. anterior oblique projection
  l. anterior oblique projection
    ventriculogram
  l. anterior oblique view
  l. anterosuperior hemiblock (LASH)
  l. apex cardiogram, calibrated
    displacement (LACD)
  l. atrial active-emptying fraction
  l. atrial appendage (LAA)
  l. atrial cannulation
  l. atrial chamber
  l. atrial end-diastolic pressure
  l. atrial enlargement (LAE)
  l. atrial function
  l. atrial hypertrophy
  l. atrial maximal volume
  l. atrial myxoma
  l. atrial pressure (LAP)
  l. atrioventricular groove artery
  l. atrium (LA)
  l. atrium/aortic root
  l. atrium/aortic root ratio (LA:AR
    ratio, LA:AR ratio)
  l. auricle
  l. auricular appendage (LAA)
  l. axillary artery catheterization
  l. axis deviation (LAD)
  l. border of cardiac dullness
    (LBCD)
  l. border of heart
  l. brain
  l. bundle branch
  l. bundle-branch block (LBBB)
  l. bundle branch hemiblock
  l. circumflex (LCF, LCX)
  l. circumflex coronary artery
  l. colon
  l. colonic flexure
  l. common carotid artery

  l. common femoral artery
  l. coronary angiography (LCA)
  l. coronary artery (LCA)
  l. coronary cusp
  l. coronary plexus
  l. coronary sinus
  l. crus
  l. descending artery (LDA)
  l. gastric artery
  l. gutter
  l. heart catheterization
  l. heart syndrome
  l. hemisphere
  l. hepatic vein (LHV)
  l. iliac system
  l. intercostal space (LICS)
  l. internal carotid artery (LICA)
  l. internal mammary artery (LIMA)
  l. internal mammary artery
    anastomosis
  l. lateral projection
  l. lobe of liver
  l. lower extremity (LLE)
  l. lower lobe (LLL)
  l. lower lobe lesion
  l. lower quadrant (LLQ)
  l. main coronary artery (LMCA)
  l. main stem bronchus
  l. mediastinum
  l. pleural apical hematoma cap
  l. posterior oblique (LPO)
  l. posterior oblique position
  l. posterior oblique projection
  l. primary bronchus
  l. pulmonary artery (LPA)
  l. pulmonary cusp
  l. pulmonary vein (LPV)
  l. respiratory nerve
  l. retroaortic renal vein
  l. sternal border (LSB)
  l. subclavian central venous
    pressure (LSCVP)
  l. upper lobe (LUL)
  l. upper lobe lesion
  l. upper quadrant (LUQ)
  l. ventricle
  l. ventricular afterload
  l. ventricular aneurysm
  l. ventricular angiography
  l. ventricular apex
  l. ventricular assist device (LVAD)
  l. ventricular asynergy
  l. ventricular cardiomyopathy
  l. ventricular cavity pressure
  l. ventricular chamber
  l. ventricular chamber volume
  l. ventricular configuration

l. ventricular contraction pattern
l. ventricular diastolic dimension (LVdd)
l. ventricular dilatation
l. ventricular dysfunction (LVD)
l. ventricular ejection fraction (LVEF)
l. ventricular ejection time (LVET)
l. ventricular end-diastolic dimension (LVEDD)
l. ventricular end-diastolic pressure (LVEDP)
l. ventricular end-diastolic volume
l. ventricular end-diastolic volume index (LVEDI)
l. ventricular end-systolic dimension (LVESD)
l. ventricular end-systolic volume index (LVESVI)
l. ventricular failure
l. ventricular fast filling time
l. ventricular filling pressure
l. ventricular fractional shortening index
l. ventricular free wall (LVFW)
l. ventricular functional shortening (LVFS)
l. ventricular function wall motion
l. ventricular gated blood pool scan
l. ventricular hypertrophy (LVH)
l. ventricular hypertrophy with strain
l. ventricular hypoplasia
l. ventricular inflow tract obstruction
l. ventricular inflow volume (LVIV)
l. ventricular internal diameter (LVID)
l. ventricular internal diastolic dimension (LVIDd, LVIDD)
l. ventricular internal dimension at end systole (LVIDs)
l. ventricular internal end systole
l. ventricular loading
l. ventricular mass (LVM)
l. ventricular mass index (LVMI)
l. ventricular maximal volume
l. ventricular muscle
l. ventricular noncompaction

l. ventricular outflow pressure gradient
l. ventricular outflow tract (LVOT)
l. ventricular outflow tract obstruction (LVOTO)
l. ventricular outflow volume (LVOV)
l. ventricular peak systolic pressure
l. ventricular posterior superior process
l. ventricular posterior wall (LVPW)
l. ventricular preload
l. ventricular pressure (LVP)
l. ventricular regional wall motion
l. ventricular regional wall motion abnormality
l. ventricular slow filling time
l. ventricular strain pattern
l. ventricular stroke volume
l. ventricular stroke work (LVSW)
l. ventricular stroke work index (LVSWI)
l. ventricular support system
l. ventricular systolic (LVs)
l. ventricular systolic/diastolic function
l. ventricular systolic functional reserve
l. ventricular systolic pressure
l. ventricular systolic pump function
l. ventricular systolic time interval ratio
l. ventricular wall (LVW)
l. ventriculogram (LVG)
left-dominant coronary anatomy
left-handedness
    ventricular l.-h.
left-right asymmetry
left-sided
    l.-s. empyema
    l.-s. heart failure
    l.-s. heart pressure
    l.-s. pleural effusion
left-sidedness
    bilateral l.-s.
left-side-down
    l.-s.-d. decubitus position
    l.-s.-d. decubitus scan
left-to-right
    l.-t.-r. flow

NOTES

L

left-to-right *(continued)*
    l.-t.-r. shift
    l.-t.-r. shunting of blood
leg
    l. axis
    baker's l.
    bayonet l.
    bowed l.'s
    champagne-bottle l.'s
    deep vein system of l.
    l. edema
    postphlebitic l.
    scissoring of l.'s
    l. shortening
    tennis l.
Legg-Calvé-Perthes disease (LCP)
Leggiero hydrophilic-coated microcatheter
leg-length discrepancy (LLD)
Leichtenstern sign
Leigh disease
leiomyoblastoma
leiomyoma, pl. **leiomyomata, leiomyomas**
    benign metastasizing l.
    degenerated uterine l.
    epithelioid l.
    esophageal l.
    fundal l.
    gastric l.
    kidney l.
    multiple vascular l.
    pedunculated l.
    renal l.
    small bowel l.
    stomach l.
    urinary bladder l.
    uterine l.
    vascular l.
leiomyomatosis
    esophageal l.
leiomyomatous kidney hamartoma
leiomyosarcoma
    duodenal l.
    esophageal l.
    gastric l.
    intramural l.
    intravascular l.
    jejunal l.
    retroperitoneal l.
    right atrial extension of uterine l.
    small bowel l.
    stomach l.
Leksell
    L. D-shaped stereotactic frame
    L. gamma unit

    L. 201-source cobalt-60 Gamma knife
    L. stereotactic system
Leksell-Elekta stereotactic frame
LEL
    low-energy laser
lemniscus, pl. **lemnisci**
    medial l.
lemon sign
Lenard ray tube
length
    basic cycle l. (BCL)
    basic drive cycle l. (BDCL)
    Beatson combined ankle l.
    cephalocaudad l.
    cervical l.
    crown-heel l.
    crown-rump l. (CR, CRL)
    CSF systole l.
    echo-train l. (ETL)
    effective path l. (EPL)
    femur l. (FL)
    fetal femoral l.
    focal l.
    Grace method of ratio of metatarsal l.
    humeral l.
    jet l. (JL)
    limb l.
    metacarpal l.
    metacarpophalangeal l.
    path l.
    pulse l.
    pyloric channel l.
    radial l.
    sinus cycle l. (SCL)
    track cone l.
    urethral l. (UL)
length-biased sampling
length-time bias
Lennox-Gastaut syndrome
Lenoir facet
lens
    acoustic l.
    right-angled telescopic l.
    Thorpe plastic l.
lens-sparing external beam radiation therapy (LSRT)
LENT
    late effect of normal tissue
    LENT score
    LENT scoring system
lenticular
    l. area
    l. bone
    l. carcinoma
    l. fasciculus

l. loop
l. nucleus
lenticulostriate
l. artery
l. supply
l. vasculopathy (LSV)
l. vessel
lentiform
l. bone
l. nucleus
Lenz law
leopard skin demyelination
lepidic growth
leptocyte
leptocytosis
leptomeningeal
l. anastomosis
l. angiomatosis
l. arachnoid cyst
l. artery
l. carcinoma
l. disease
l. fibrosis
l. ivy sign
l. metastasis
l. process
leptomeninges
leptomeningitis
leptomeningoencephalitis
leptomyelolipoma
lepton
Leri
melorheostosis of L.
L. pleonosteosis
L. sign
Leriche syndrome
Leri-Weill syndrome
LES
lower esophageal sphincter
Lesch-Nyhan syndrome
Lesgaft
L. hernia
L. triangle
lesion
acute cerebellar hemispheric l.
admixture l.
adrenal l.
afferent nerve l.
ALPSA l.
anechoic l.
angiocentric immunoproliferative l.
angiocentric lymphoproliferative l.

angulated l.
anterior labroligamentous periosteal
sleeve avulsion l.
anterior parietal l.
anterochiasmatic l.
Antopol-Goldman l.
anular constricting l.
aortic arch l.
aortic valve l.
apical l.
apophyseal l.
apple-core l.
Armanni-Ebstein l.
atheromatous l.
atherosclerotic l.
atrophic brain l.
Baehr-Lohlein l.
Bankart l.
barrel-shaped l.
basal hypodense ganglia l.
benign fibrous bone l.
benign lymphoepithelial l.
benign lymphoproliferative l.
benign vascular l.
Bennett l.
bifurcation l.
bilateral l.
bilobed polypoid l.
biparietal l.
bird's nest l.
black star breast l.
blastic l.
bleeding l.
blistering l.
blowout bone l.
Blumenthal l.
bone marrow l.
Bracht-Wachter l.
brain l.
brainstem l.
breast l.
Brown-Séquard l.
bubbling l.
bubbly bone l.
bulbourethral gland l.
bull's eye l.
butterfly l.
calcified l.
callosal l.
capsular drop l.
cardiac valvular l.
carinal l.

L

NOTES

lesion *(continued)*
    carpet l.
    cartilaginous l.
    cavernous sinus l.
    caviar l.
    cavitary lung l.
    cavitary pulmonary l.
    cavitary small bowel l.
    central medullary bone l.
    centrilobular l.
    cerebral l.
    cerebrospinal fluid-containing l.
    cervical cord l.
    chest wall l.
    Chiari I–IV l.
    chiasmal l.
    cholesterol-containing brain l.
    circular l.
    circumscribed l.
    cochlear l.
    coin l.
    cold l.
    collar-button chest l.
    colonic apple-core l.
    colonic carpet l.
    colonic saddle l.
    complete nerve l.
    complex sclerosing l.
    concentric l.
    congenital cystic neck l.
    constricting esophageal l.
    conus medullaris l.
    coordinates for target l.
    cord epidural extramedullary l.
    cord intramedullary l.
    coronary artery l.
    corpus callosum ring-enhancing l.
    cortical bone l.
    corticospinal pathway l.
    Cowper gland l.
    critical l.
    culprit l.
    cyclops l.
    cystic epididymis l.
    cystic intracranial fetal l.
    cystic liver l.
    cystic splenic l.
    deep-seated l.
    dendritic l.
    de novo l.
    dense enhancing brain l.
    dense lung l.
    desmoid l.
    destructive bone l.
    destructive diskovertebral l.
    l. detectability
    diaphyseal l.

Dieulafoy l.
differential diagnosis bone l.
difficult-to-treat vascular l.
diffuse ulcerative l.
discrete l.
disk l.
dominant hemisphere l.
dorsal root entry zone l.
doughnut l.
DREZ l.
dumbbell l.
Duret l.
Ebstein l.
eccentric medullary bone l.
eccentric restenosis l.
echogenic solid l.
ellipsoid l.
encapsulated fat-containing l.
encephaloclastic l.
endobronchial l.
enhancing brain l.
epicortical l.
epididymis l.
epidural extramedullary l.
epileptogenic l.
epiphyseal l.
esophageal apple-core l.
excitatory l.
expanding cavernous sinus brain l.
expansile lytic l.
expansile multilocular bone l.
expansile rib l.
expansile unilocular well-demarcated bone l.
extraaxial CNS l.
extraaxial low-attenuation l.
extracranial mass l.
extrahepatic l.
extramedullary compressive l.
extratemporal structural l.
extratesticular l.
extrathoracic l.
extrinsic l.
fast-flow l.
fat-containing breast l.
fibrohistiocytic l.
fibromuscular l.
fibroosseous l.
fibrous bone l.
fibrous GI tract polypoid l.
finger lucent l.
fingertip l.
florid duct l.
flow-compromising l.
flow-limiting l.
focal articular cartilage l.
focal cold liver l.

focal hemispheric l.
focal hot liver l.
focal ischemic l.
focal parenchymal brain l.
focal splenic l.
frank l.
friable l.
frondy l.
frontal lobe l.
full-thickness chondral l.
gallium-67-avid l.
GARD l.
gastric intramural-extramucosal l.
geographic l.
Ghon primary l.
Gill l.
GLAD l.
glenoid articular rim disruption l.
glenolabral articular disruption l.
glomerular l.
gross l.
ground-glass l.
HAGL l.
hamartomatous l.
hemisphere l.
hemispheric demyelinating l.
hemodynamically significant l.
hemorrhagic l.
high cervical spinal cord l.
high-density l.
high-grade obstructive l.
high-grade squamous
   intraepithelial l. (HGSIL)
high-intensity l.
high pontine l.
high-probability l.
high-signal l.
Hill-Sachs shoulder l.
hole-within-hole bone l.
homogeneous l.
hot l.
hourglass-shaped l.
hyperdense brain l.
hyperintense periventricular brain l.
hyperplastic l.
hypodense basal ganglion brain l.
hypodense mesencephalic low-
   density brain l.
hypointense sella l.
l. hypometabolism
hypothalamic l.
iceberg l.

iliac l.
impaction l.
indiscriminate l.
indolent l.
infectious bubbly bone l.
infiltrating l.
inflammatory l.
infranuclear l.
internal auditory canal enhancing l.
intraaxial brain l.
intracerebral l.
intraconal l.
intracranial mass l.
intracranial vascular l.
intradural extramedullary l.
intramammary l.
intramedullary cord l.
intramedullary space-occupying l.
intramedullary spinal l.
intramural-extramucosal stomach l.
intraocular l.
intraosseous bone l.
intraperitoneal l.
intrasellar l.
intraspinal l.
intrinsic stenotic l.
intrinsic stomach wall l.
invasive l.
irregularly shaped l.
ischemic l.
ischiorectal fossa l.
isointense l.
Janeway l.
jet l.
juxtacortical bone l.
Kidner l.
kissing l.
lacrimal gland l.
lateral temporal epileptogenic l.
leave-alone l.
left lower lobe l.
left upper lobe l.
lipomatous l.
liver l.
local l.
local glomerular l.
l. localization
localized l.
Löhlein-Baehr l.
low-attenuation l.
low-density mesencephalic l.
lower motor neuron l.

L

NOTES

lesion *(continued)*
    lucent finger l.
    lucent lung l.
    lumbar spine l.
    Lynch and Crues type 2 l.
    lytic bone l.
    macroscopic placental l.
    magnetic resonance-detected white
      matter l.
    malignant osseous l.
    Mallory-Weiss l.
    mammographically suspicious l.
    mass l.
    mass-like l.
    medial longitudinal fasciculus l.
    median nerve l.
    mediastinal l.
    mesencephalic low-density brain l.
    mesencephalodiencephalic l.
    mesenteric vascular l.
    mesial temporal epileptogenic l.
    metabolic l.
    metachronous l.
    metastatic l.
    micropapillary l.
    midbrain l.
    midline l.
    mixed fat-water density l.
    mixed sclerotic and lytic bone l.
    MLF l.
    mongolian spot-like l.
    monomelic bone l.
    Monteggia l.
    mucosal l.
    mulberry eye l.
    multicentric lytic l.
    multifocal enhancing brain l.
    multilocular cystic l.
    multiple lucent lung l.
    multiple lytic bone l.
    multiple osteosclerotic l.'s
    multiple parotid gland l.
    multiple stenotic l.'s
    muscular l.
    musculoskeletal l.
    nail bed l.
    napkin-ring anular l.
    necrotic l.
    needle localization of breast l.
    neoplastic l.
    neurogenic l.
    neurologic bladder l.
    neurovascular l.
    nidus of l.
    nodular l.
    nondominant hemisphere l.
    nonenhancing l.

    nonexpansile multilocular bone l.
    nonexpansile unilocular bone l.
    noninvasive l.
    nonmeningiomatous malignant l.
    nonproliferative l.
    nucleus ambiguus l.
    nucleus basalis l.
    obstructive l.
    occipital l.
    occlusive l.
    occult l.
    ocular l.
    onionskin l.
    optic nerve l.
    organic l.
    osseous l.
    osteoblastic l.
    osteocartilaginous l.
    osteochondral l.
    osteolytic l.
    osteosclerotic l.
    ostial l.
    outcropping of l.
    papillary l.
    papular l.
    papulonecrotic l.
    paradiskal l.
    paralabral l.
    paraorbital l.
    parasagittal l.
    parasellar l.
    parietal cortex l.
    parietal lobe l.
    parietooccipital l.
    parosteal bone l.
    partial l.
    patch l.
    pedunculated l.
    perforative l.
    periapical l.
    peripheral nerve l.
    perisellar vascular l.
    periventricular l.
    permeative l.
    Perthes l.
    Perthes-Bankart l.
    phosphaturic intraosseous l.
    photon-deficient bone l.
    plaque-like l.
    polyostotic bone l.
    polypoid l.
    pontine l.
    portal vein l.
    posterior column l.
    posterior compartment l.
    posterior fossa l.
    posterior fossa-foramen magnum l.

posterior language area l.
posterior vertebral element
  blowout l.
prechiasmal optic nerve l.
presacral cystic l.
pretectal l.
primary l.
proliferative l.
prostate hypoechoic l.
pulmonary l.
punched-out lytic bone l.
punctate l.
purulent l.
questionable l.
radial sclerosing l.
radiodense l.
radiofrequency l.
radiographic stability of l.
radiolucent l.
radiopaque l.
reactive fibrous l.
reactive lymphoid l.
rectal l.
rectosigmoid polypoid l.
recurrent l.
regurgitant l.
remote lower motor neuron l.
renal mass l.
resectable l.
retrochiasmal l.
retroglandular l.
reverse Hill-Sachs l.
rheumatic l.
rib l.
right lower lobe l.
right upper lobe l.
rim-enhancing l.
ring l.
ring-enhancing brain l.
ring-like l.
ring-wall l.
root entry-zone l.
rotator cuff l.
rounded l.
round lucent l.
saddle l.
satellite l.
scar l.
scirrhous l.
sclerosing l.
sclerotic l.
secondary l.

segmental bronchus l.
serial l.
sessile l.
sharply demarcated
  circumferential l.
sinonasal l.
sinusoidal l.
skeletal l.
skip l.
SLAP l.
slow-flow l.
slowly developing l.
small bowel cavitary l.
solid splenic l.
solid thymic l.
solitary cold l.
solitary osteosclerotic l.
solitary rib l.
solitary sternal l.
sonolucent cystic l.
space-occupying intracranial l.
spherical l.
spiculated scirrhous l.
spinal cord l.
spleen l.
splenic l.
spontaneous l.
stacked ovoid l.
stellate border breast l.
Stener l.
steno-obstructive l.
stenotic l.
sternal l.
Sterner l.
striatal l.
structural l.
subareolar l.
subchondral l.
subcortical intracranial l.
subcortical low-intensity l.
submucosal l.
subtentorial l.
subtotal l.
superficial l.
superior labral anterior-posterior l.
supraaortic l.
supranuclear l.
suprasellar low-density l.
supratentorial l.
suspicious l.
swan-neck tubular l.
synchronous l.

L

NOTES

lesion *(continued)*
>   systemic l.
>   tandem l.
>   target lung l.
>   teardrop-shaped l.
>   tectal l.
>   telangiectatic l.
>   temporal lobe l.
>   testicular cystic l.
>   thalamic l.
>   thoracic inlet l.
>   tight l.
>   total l.
>   trabeculated bone l.
>   transfer l.
>   transverse cord l.
>   trophic l.
>   true-negative l.
>   tuberculous l.
>   tubular l.
>   tumor-like l.
>   tumor-mimicking breast l.
>   ulcerative l.
>   ulnar nerve l.
>   umbilical cord l.
>   uncommitted metaphyseal l.
>   unilateral l.
>   unilocular cystic l.
>   unilocular well-demarcated bone
>   defect expansile l.
>   unresectable l.
>   unstable l.
>   upper motor neuron l.
>   valvular regurgitant l.
>   vascular l.
>   vasculitic l.
>   vegetative l.
>   vertebral expansile l.
>   visceral l.
>   Waldeyer ring l.
>   wedge-shaped l.
>   well-circumscribed l.
>   well-defined l.
>   white matter l.
>   white star breast l.
>   wide field l.
>   wire-loop l.
>   Wolin meniscoid l.
>   X, Y, and Z coordinates for
>   target l.

lesion-to-background ratio
**lesion-to-brain ratio (L:B ratio, L:B
ratio)**
lesion-to-cerebrospinal fluid noise
lesion-to-countersite ratio (L:C)
lesion-to-muscle ratio
lesion-to-nonlesion count ratio

lesion-to-normal tissue ratio
lesion-to-white matter noise
LESP
>   lower esophageal sphincter pressure
lesser
>   l. arc injury
>   l. atrophy
>   l. curvature of stomach
>   l. curvature ulcer
>   l. metatarsophalangeal joint
>   l. muscle
>   l. omentum (LO)
>   l. pancreas
>   l. pelvis
>   l. peritoneal sac
>   l. petrosal
>   l. sac hernia
>   l. sac of peritoneal cavity
>   l. saphenous system
>   l. saphenous vein
>   l. sciatic foramen
>   l. sciatic notch
>   l. trochanter
>   l. trochanter of femur
>   l. trochanteric fracture
>   l. tubercle
>   l. tuberosity
LET
>   linear energy transfer
lethal
>   l. bone dysplasia
>   l. dose
>   l. dwarfism
>   l. midline granuloma
>   l. musculoskeletal dysplasia
>   l. myocardial injury
>   l. neoplasm
lettering artifact
leucine radical
leucotomy
LEUHR
>   L. fan beam collimator
>   L. parallel-hole collimator
leukemia
>   acute lymphocytic l.
>   acute myeloid l.
>   chronic lymphocytic l.
>   chronic myeloid l.
>   Rieder cell l.
>   T-cell acute lymphoblastic l.
>   T-cell-type acute lymphoblastic l.
leukemic bone line
leukemid
leukemogenesis
leukemoid
leukocyte
>   agranular l.

autologous labeled l.
basophilic l.
endothelial l.
eosinophilic l.
gallium-67-labeled l.
granular l.
heterophilic l.
indium-111-labeled l.
^{111}In-oxime-labeled l.
mast l.
motile l.
neutrophilic l.
nongranular l.
nonmotile l.
polymorphonuclear l.
polynuclear neutrophilic l.
technetium-99m l.

leukodystrophy
congenital l.
leukoencephalitis
acute hemorrhagic l.
leukoencephalopathy
Cree l.
diffuse necrotizing l.
disseminated necrotizing l.
heroin vapor l.
multifocal l.
periventricular l.
postviral l.
progressive multifocal l. (PML)
radiation-induced l.
spongiform l.
toxic l.
leukomalacia
periventricular l. (PVL)
leukopenia
radiofrequency radiogenic l.
radiogenic l.
LeukoScan
L. imaging agent
technetium-99m HMPAO mixed leukocyte L.
Leur-par collimator
LeuTech radiolabeled imaging agent
levator
l. ani
l. muscle
l. palpebrae
l. scapulae
l. span
LeVeen plaque cracker

level
air-fluid l.
attenuation l.
contrast window l.
C-reactive protein l.
debris-fluid l.
energy l.
fat-fluid l.
fluid l.
fluid-fluid l.
gas-fluid l.
intrasinus air-fluid l.
l. I obstetric ultrasound
pontine-medullary l.
significance l.
stairstep air-fluid l.
supraventricular l.
window l.
zero reference l.
Zielke derotation l.
level-dependent
blood oxygenation l.-d. (BOLD)
Levenberg-Marquardt method
Levine tube
levoangiocardiogram
levocardiogram
levogram
levoposition
levorotary scoliosis
levorotatory
levoscoliosis
levotransposition (L-transposition)
levoversion
Levovist imaging agent
Lewis (Le)
L. angle
L. position
Leydig
L. cell adenoma
L. cell tumor (LCT)
Leyla arm
LFUS
low frequency ultrasound
LFV
large field of view
LGL
Lown-Ganong-Levine syndrome
LHBT tenosynovitis
Lhermitte-Duclos syndrome
LHP
lateral hypopharyngeal pouch

L

NOTES

LHV
    left hepatic vein
LI
    lumbar index
LICA
    left internal carotid artery
lichenoides
        tuberculosis l.
        tuberculosis cutis l.
Lichtenstein-Jaffe disease
licorice powder
LICS
    left intercostal space
LICU
    laparoscopic intracorporeal ultrasound
lidocaine-adrenaline solution
lidofenin
lie
        fetal l.
        horizontal l.
        longitudinal l.
        posterior l.
        transverse l.
        unusual fetal l.
Liebel-Flarsheim CT 9000 contrast delivery system
Lieberkühn crypt
Liebermeister groove
Liebow
        usual interstitial pneumonia of L. (UIP)
lienis
        sustentaculum l.
lienography
lienophrenic ligament
lienorenal ligament
Lieutaud trigone
LiF
    lithium fluoride
        LiF thermoluminescence dosimeter
        LiF thermoluminescence dosimetry
LifeJet catheter
Life-Pack 5 cardiac monitor
life-threatening
        l.-t. hemorrhage
        l.-t. pneumothorax
lift
        gallbladder l.
        heave and l.
        sternal l.
ligament
        accessory atlantoaxial l.
        acromioclavicular l.
        acromiocoracoid l.
        adipose l.
        alar l.
        anococcygeal l.

anterior cruciate l. (ACL)
anterior fibular l.
anterior inferior tibiofibular l.
anterior talofibular l. (ATF)
anterior tibiofibular l.
anterior tibiotalar l.
anular l.
apical l.
Arantius l.
arcuate l.
arterial l.
atlantal l.
attenuated l.
auricular l.
avulsed l.
axis l.
Bardinet l.
Barkow l.
beak l.
Bellini l.
Berry l.
Bertin l.
Bichat l.
bifurcated l.
Bigelow l.
Botallo l.
Bourgery l.
broad l.
Brodie l.
Burns l.
calcaneoclavicular l.
calcaneocuboid l.
calcaneofibular l. (CFL)
calcaneonavicular l.
calcaneotibial l.
Caldani l.
Campbell l.
Camper l.
capsular l.
Carcassonne l.
cardinal l.
caroticoclinoid l.
carpometacarpal l.
Casser l.
casserian l.
caudal l.
ceratocricoid l.
cervical mover l.
checkrein l.
cholecystoduodenal l.
chondroxiphoid l.
ciliary l.
Civinini l.
Clado l.
Cleland l.
clinoid l.
Cloquet l.

coccygeal l.
collateral l.
Colles l.
congenital laxity of l.
conjugate l.
conoid l.
conus l.
Cooper suspensory l.
coracoacromial l.
coracoclavicular l.
coracohumeral l.
corniculopharyngeal l.
coronary l.
costoclavicular l.
costocolic l.
costotransverse l.
costoxiphoid l.
cotyloid l.
Cowper l.
cricopharyngeal l.
cricothyroid l.
cricotracheal l.
cross l.
cruciate l.
cruciatum cruris l.
cruciform l.
Cruveilhier l.
cuboideonavicular l.
cuneocuboid l.
cuneonavicular l.
cystoduodenal l.
deep collateral l.
deltoid l.
Denonvilliers l.
dentate l.
denticulate l.
diaphragmatic l.
dorsal metacarpal l.
dorsal wrist l.
Douglas l.
duodenal l.
duodenorenal l.
epicondyloolecranon l.
l. of epididymis
epihyal l.
extracapsular l.
extrinsic l.
fabellofibular l.
falciform l.
fallopian l.
femoral l.
Ferrein l.

fibular collateral l.
fibulotalar l.
fibulotalocalcaneal l.
flaval l.
floating l.
Flood l.
FTC l.
fundiform l.
gastrocolic l.
gastrodiaphragmatic l.
gastrohepatic l.
gastrolienal l.
gastropancreatic l.
gastrophrenic l.
gastrosplenic l.
genital l.
genitoinguinal l.
Gerdy l.
Gillette suspensory l.
Gimbernat l.
gingivodental l.
glenohumeral l.
glenoid l.
glossoepiglottic l.
Grayson l.
Günzberg l.
Haines-McDougall medial
  sesamoid l.
hammock l.
Helmholtz axis l.
Henle l.
l.'s of Henry and Wrisberg
Hensing l.
hepatic l.
hepatocolic l.
hepatocystocolic l.
hepatoduodenal l.
hepatoesophageal l.
hepatogastric l.
hepatogastroduodenal l.
hepatophrenic l.
hepatorenal l.
hepatoumbilical l.
Hesselbach l.
Hey l.
Holl l.
Hueck l.
humeral avulsion of the
  glenohumeral l. (HAGL)
Humphry l.
Hunter l.
Huschke l.

L

NOTES

ligament *(continued)*

hyalocapsular l.
hyoepiglottic l.
iliofemoral l.
iliolumbar l.
iliopectineal l.
iliopubic l.
iliotibial l.
iliotrochanteric l.
inferior dorsal radioulnar l.
inferior pulmonary l.
infrapatellar l.
infundibuloovarian l.
infundibulopelvic l.
inguinal l.
intercapital l.
intercarpal l.
interclavicular l.
interclinoid l.
intercornual l.
intercuneiform l.
interdigital l.
interfoveolar l.
intermetatarsal l.
internal collateral l.
interosseous sacroiliac l.
interosseous talocalcaneal l.
intersesamoid l.
interspinous l.
intertransverse l.
intervertebral l.
intraarticular l.
intrascapular l.
intrinsic l.
ischiocapsular l.
ischiofemoral l.
Jarjavay l.
jugal l.
Krause l.
laciniate l.
lacunar l.
Landsmeer l.
Lannelongue l.
lateral arcuate l.
lateral collateral l. (LCL)
lateral costotransverse l.
lateral talocalcaneal l.
lateral ulnar collateral l. (LUCL)
Lauth l.
lienophrenic l.
lienorenal l.
limited proteoglycan matrix of l.
Lisfranc l.
Lockwood l.
longitudinal l.
lumbocostal l.
lunotriquetral interosseus l.

Luschka l.
Mackenrodt l.
macroscopic hemorrhage l.
Maissiat l.
Mauchart l.
Meckel l.
medial collateral l. (MCL)
median arcuate l.
median cruciate l.
median umbilical l.
meniscofemoral l.
meniscotibial l.
metacarpoglenoidal l.
metacarpophalangeal l.
microscopic hemorrhage of l.
mucosal suspensory l.
natatory l.
naviculocuneiform l.
nuchal l.
occipitoatlantoaxial l.
occipitoaxial l.
odontoid l.
opacification of posterior
   longitudinal l.
orbicular l.
Osborne l.
ossification of the longitudinal l.
ossification of the posterior
   longitudinal l. (OPLL)
ossified posterior longitudinal l.
ovarian suspensory l.
l. of ovary
palmar metacarpal l.
palmar radiocarpal l.
pectinate l.
pelvic ring l.
periodontal l.
peritoneal part of inguinal l.
Petit l.
Pétrequin l.
petroclinoid l.
phalangeal glenoidal l.
phrenicocolic l.
phrenicolienal l.
phrenicosplenic l.
phrenoesophageal l.
phrenogastric l.
phrenosplenic l.
pisohamate l.
pisometacarpal l.
pisounciform l.
pisouncinate l.
plantar l.
popliteal l.
posterior cruciate l. (PCL)
posterior inferior tibiofibular l.
posterior longitudinal l. (PLL)

posterior oblique l.
posterior talofibular l.
posterior tibiotalar l.
Poupart inguinal l.
pterygomandibular l.
pterygospinous l.
PTF l.
pubocapsular l.
pubocervical l.
pubofemoral l.
puboprostatic l.
pubovesical l.
pulmonary l.
quadrate l.
radial collateral l.
radial metacarpal l.
radiate sternocostal l.
radiocarpal l.
radiolunotriquetral l.
radioscaphocapitate l.
radioscaphoid l.
radioscapholunate l.
reflected edge of Poupart l.
reflected inguinal l.
l. reflecting edge
retinacular l.
Retzius l.
rhomboid l.
right triangular l.
ring l.
Robert l.
round l.
Rouviere l.
sacrodural l.
sacrospinous l.
sacrotuberous l.
Santorini l.
Sappey l.
scapholunate l. (LSS)
scaphotriquetral l.
l. of Scarpa
Schlemm l.
serous l.
sesamoid l.
sesamophalangeal l.
sheath l.
l. shelving edge
short radiolunate l.
Simonart l.
Soemmerring l.
sphenomandibular l.
spinoglenoid l.

spinous tarsus l.
spiral l.
splenocolic l.
splenorenal l.
spring l.
Stanley cervical l.
stellate l.
sternoclavicular l.
sternopericardial l.
stretched out l.
Struthers l.
stylohyoid l.
stylomandibular l.
stylomaxillary l.
superficial dorsal sacrococcygeal l.
superficial posterior
  sacrococcygeal l.
superficial transverse metacarpal l.
superficial transverse metatarsal l.
superior costotransverse l.
superior pubic l.
superior transverse scapular l.
suprascapular l.
supraspinous l.
suspensory l.
sutural l.
syndesmotic l.
synovial l.
talocalcaneal l.
talofibular l.
talonavicular l.
tarsal l.
tarsometatarsal l.
l. tear
tectoral l.
temporomandibular l.
Teutleben l.
Thompson l.
thyroepiglottic l.
thyrohyoid l.
tibial collateral l.
tibial sesamoid l.
tibiocalcaneal l.
tibiofibular l.
tibionavicular l.
torn meniscotibial l.
transverse atlantal l.
transverse carpal l.
transverse cervical l.
transverse crural l.
transverse genicular l.
transverse humeral l.

L

NOTES

ligament *(continued)*
transverse intertarsal l.
transverse metacarpal l.
transverse metatarsal l.
transverse perineal l.
transverse tibiofibular l.
trapezoid l.
l. of Treitz
triangular l.
triquetrohamate l.
triquetroscaphoid l.
Tuffier inferior l.
ulnar collateral l. (UCL)
ulnocarpal l.
ulnolunate l.
ulnotriquetral l.
umbilical l.
urachal l.
uterine l.
uterosacral l.
uterovesical l.
vaginal l.
venous l.
ventral sacrococcygeal l.
ventral sacroiliac l.
ventricular l.
vertebropelvic l.
vesicosacral l.
vesicoumbilical l.
vesicouterine l.
vestibular l.
vocal l.
volar carpal l.
Walther oblique l.
Weitbrecht l.
Winslow l.
Wrisberg l.
xiphicostal l.
xiphoid l.
Y-shaped l.
Zaglas l.
Zinn l.
ligamenta *(pl. of* ligamentum)
ligamentous
l. ankylosis
l. attachment
l. bouncing
l. box
l. calcification
l. complex
l. disruption
l. impingement
l. insertion
l. instability
l. laxity
l. luxation
l. strain

l. support
l. thickening
l. trauma
ligamentous-muscular hypertrophy
ligamentum, pl. **ligamenta**
l. arteriosum
l. flavum
l. flavum thickening
l. mucosum
l. nuchae
l. patellae
l. teres
l. teres notch
l. venosum fissure
ligand
l. agent
^{99m}Tc-labeled l.
ligation
Doppler-guided hemorrhoid artery l.
(DGHAL)
Hunter aneurysm l.
thoracic duct l.
light
l. bulb appearance
l. chain deposition disease (LCDD)
hot l.
infrared l.
invisible l.
l. leak
l. microscopy
l. pink lung
l. reflection rheography
l. scanning
structured l. (SL)
l. therapy
Wood l.
LightSheer SC diode laser
LightSpeed
L. multidetector CT scanner
L. QX/i scanner
L. Ultra CT system
Lightstic 180, 360 fiberoptic laser
Lightwood syndrome
Ligman-Sacks endocarditis disease
likelihood ratio (LR)
LILI
Lilienfeld position
Liliequist membrane
LILT
low-intensity laser therapy
LIMA
left internal mammary artery
LIMA anastomosis
limb
l. absence
l. of anterior capsule
l. of bifurcation graft

l. bone length ratio
l. bud
chronic lymphedematous l.
l. girdle
l. length
l. perfusion
l. reduction
l. reduction abnormality
l. reduction anomaly
Roux-en-Y l.
l. venography
vertebral, anal, cardiac, tracheal,
esophageal, renal, l. (VACTERL)
limb-body wall complex
limb-girdle muscular dystrophy
limbic
l. lobe
l. region
l. system
limb-length
l.-l. asymmetry
l.-l. discrepancy (LLD)
l.-l. inequality
limb-lengthening procedure
limb-threatening ischemia
limbus
l. suture
l. vertebra
l. of Vieussens
limit
eye exposure l.
Nyquist l.
quantum l.
tracking l.
limitation
beam l.
biophysical l.
infarct size l.
l. of joint motion
l. of MR imaging
l. of ultrasound
limited
l. examination
l. film
l. imaging
l. oxidative capacity
l. proteoglycan matrix of ligament
l. view
limited-cut plane
limited-slice computed tomography

limited-stage
l.-s. diffuse large-cell lymphoma
l.-s. DLCL
limiting membrane
limitus
hallux l. (HL)
LINAC
linear accelerator
LINAC radiosurgery
Varian LINAC
Linac
X-band L.
Lindblom position
Lindegaard ratio
line
absence of innominate l.
absorption l.
acanthiomeatal l.
acetabular l.
AC-PC l.
air-fluid l.
aneuploid cell l.
anorectal l.
anterior axillary l. (AAL)
anterior humeral l.
anterior junction l.
aortic vent suction l.
Arrow PICC l.
auricular l.
axillary l.
azygoesophageal l.
basilar l.
bimastoid l.
Blumensaat l.
Bolton-nasion l.
branching l.
Brödel avascular l.
calcification l.
Camper l.
canthomeatal l.
Cantlie l.
cement l.
central sacral l. (CSL)
central venous pressure l.
Chamberlain l.
Chaussier l.
clinoparietal l.
Conradi l.
Correra l.
costoclavicular l.
costophrenic septal l.
Crampton l.

NOTES

L

line *(continued)*
  crescent hip l.
  curved radiolucent l.
  curvilinear subpleural l.
  Cyma l.
  Daubenton l.
  demarcation l.
  dentate l.
  digastric l.
  displaced left paraspinal l.
  divisionary l.
  Ellis l.
  Ellis-Garland l.
  epiphyseal l.
  fat-density l.
  Feiss l.
  Fischgold bimastoid l.
  Fischgold biventer l.
  Fleischner l.
  l. focus principle
  fracture l.
  Fränkel white l.
  Frankfort l.
  F T l.
  gallbladder-vena cava l.
  gas density l.
  gaussian l.
  l. of Gennari
  glabelloalveolar l.
  glabellomeatal l.
  gluteal l.
  Granger l.
  growth arrest l.
  Gubler l.
  Hampton l.
  Harris l.
  Hawkins l.
  Hickman l.
  Hilgenreiner l.
  His l.
  humeral l.
  ilioischial l.
  iliopectineal l.
  l. imaging
  infraorbital l.
  infraorbitomeatal l. (IOML)
  innominate absence of l.
  l. integral concept
  interlobar septal l.
  interpupillary l.
  intravenous infusion l.
  isodose l.
  isoelectric l.
  isopotential l.
  joint l.
  Kerley A, B, C l.
  Kilian l.

  Köhler l.
  Langer l.
  Lanz l.
  lateral joint l.
  lead l.
  leukemic bone l.
  Linton l.
  Looser l.
  lorentzian l.
  lower lung l.
  low-intensity l.
  lucent l.
  Mach l.
  McGregor l.
  McKee l.
  McRae l.
  medial joint l.
  median l.
  Mees l.
  Merkel cell carcinoma cell l.
  Meyer l.
  midaxillary l.
  midclavicular l. (MCL)
  midhumeral l.
  midscapular l.
  midspinal l.
  midsternal l.
  Moyer l.
  Nélaton l.
  oblique prescription l.
  obturator l.
  Ogston l.
  Ohngren l.
  orbitomeatal l.
  orthogonal tag l.
  l. pair
  parallel M l.
  parallel pitch l.
  paramedian l.
  paraspinal l.
  pectinate l.
  peripheral intravenous infusion l.
  peripherally inserted central
    catheter l.
  Perkin l.
  photon therapy beam l.
  PICC l.
  l. placement
  pleural l.
  pleuroesophageal l.
  popliteal l.
  posterior axillary l.
  posterior cervical l.
  posterior junction l.
  posterior nipple l. (PNL)
  pronator quadratus l.
  properitoneal fat l.

psoas l.
pubococcygeal l. (PCL)
radiocapitellar l.
radiolucent crescent l.
raster l.
reference l.
Reid l.
resonance l.
l. of response (LOR)
l. of Retzius
Richter-Monroe l.
Rolando l.
sacrococcygeal inferior pubic
 point l.
Sappey l.
l. saturation
l. scanning (LS)
Schoemaker l.
scorbutic white l.
semilunar l.
septal l.
l. shadow
l. shape
Shenton l.
Simpson white l.
skin l.
Skinner l.
soleal l.
spectral l.
spinographic l.
spinolaminar l. (SLL)
l. spread function (LSF)
subchondral fracture l.
subclavian l.
subcutaneous fat l.
subpleural curvilinear l.
suture l.
transcondylar l.
transverse lucent metaphyseal l.
trough l.
Trümmerfeld l.
twining l.
Ullmann l.
ventral venous pressure l.
vertebral body l.
visualization of the Z l.
Wagner l.
water density l.
Wegner l.
white l.
l. width

Z l.
zero l.
linea, pl. **lineae**
l. alba
l. semilunaris
lineage
M4-M5 l.
linear
l. absorption coefficient
l. accelerator (LINAC)
l. accelerator isocenter motion
l. accelerator unit
l. actuator
l. amplifier
l. array echoendoscope
l. array-hydrophone assembly
l. array transducer
l. array transrectal ultrasound probe
l. artifact
l. attenuation
l. attenuation coefficient
l. band of maximal radiolucency
l. branching microcalcification
l. calcification
l. combination model software
l. compartmental system
l. defect
l. degenerative signal intensity
l. density
l. echo
l. electrode array
l. emphysema
l. energy transfer (LET)
l. erosion
l. focus
l. focus within cyst wall
l. gradient
l. high signal intensity
l. infiltrate
l. interpolation
l. interstitial disease pattern
l. low signal
l. lucency
l. margin
l. marking
l. measure
12- to 5-MHz l. array transducer
l. opacity
l. phased array
l. phosphate
l. photon
l. polarization

NOTES

linear *(continued)*
  l. prediction (LP)
  l. prediction with singular value
    decomposition
  l. radiopacity
  l. regression analysis
  l. scan imaging
  l. scanning
  l. sebaceous nevus syndrome
  l. shadow
  l. skull fracture
  l. stenosis
  l. structure
  l. tomography
  l. ulcer
linearity
  absolute l.
  gradient l.
  intrinsic spatial l.
  lung l.
  pulmonary l.
  scintillation camera l.
linearization
  perceptual l.
linearly polarized coil
linear-quadratic (LQ)
  l.-q. equation
linebacker's arm
line-pair measurement
line-shape sensitivity
lingual
  l. artery
  l. bone
  l. goiter
  l. gyrus
  l. nerve
  l. root
  l. thyroid
  l. tonsil
lingula, pl. lingulae
  l. pulmonis
  right middle lobe l.
lingular
  l. bronchus
  l. division of the left lung
  l. infiltrate
  l. mandibular bony defect (LMBD)
  l. nodule
  l. orifice
  l. pneumonia
lining
  mucosal l.
linitis
  l. plastica
  l. plastica carcinoma
link
  musculotendinous-osseous l.

Linsman water test
Linton line
Lintro-Scan
liothyronine sodium
LIP
  lymphocytic interstitial pneumonia
  lymphoid interstitial pneumonia
lip
  hilar kidney l.
  l. of hilum
  l. of lateral sulcus
  median cleft l.
  osteophytic bone l.
  posterior l.
  rhombic l.
  l. ring artifact
lipid
  l. cholecystitis
  l. content of storage fat
  l. cyst
  l. fraction relaxation rate
  l. lake
  l. signal
  l. zone
lipid-laden plaque
lipidosis
  cerebroside l.
  sphingomyelin l.
lipid-polarized helium MR imaging
lipid-rich material
lipid-sensitive
  l.-s. MR
  l.-s. MR imaging
Lipiodol
  L. embolization
  L. myelographic imaging agent
  70–50% L. Ultra-Fluid
  L. Ultra Fluid imaging agent
lip-like projection of cartilage
lipoblastic meningioma
lipoblastoma
lipocalcinogranulomatosis
lipodystrophy
  intestinal l.
  mesenteric l.
lipofibroadenoma
  breast l.
lipogenic tumor
lipogranuloma
  sclerosing l.
lipogranulomatosis
  disseminated l.
lipohemarthrosis
lipohyalinosis
lipoid
  l. adrenal hyperplasia
  l. dermatoarthritis

l. endogenous pneumonia
l. granulomatosis
l. pneumonitis
lipoleiomyoma
lipoma
l. arborescens
bone l.
brain l.
breast l.
cardiac l.
corpus callosum l.
diffuse synovial l.
epidural l.
GI tract l.
hepatic l.
hilar l.
infiltrating l.
intracranial l.
intradural l.
intramedullary l.
intraosseous l.
intratentorial l.
liver l.
l. macrodystrophia
mediastinum l.
pericallosal l.
soft tissue l.
spine l.
subpial l.
synovial diffuse l.
lipomatosa
macrodystrophia l.
lipomatosis
central sinus l.
epidural l.
esophageal l.
mediastinal l.
l. mediastinum
multiple symmetrical l.
pancreatic l.
pelvic l.
peripelvic l.
renal sinus l.
sinus l.
soft tissue l.
lipomatous
l. hypertrophy
l. hypertrophy of the interatrial
septum
l. lesion
l. polyp

l. tissue
l. tumor
lipomyelomeningocele
lipomyeloschisis
liponecrosis
l. macrocystica calcificans
l. microcystica calcificans
lipophilic
l. cationic diphosphine
l. compound
l. dye
l. imaging agent
l. oxine-indium
l. sequestration system
lipoplasty
ultrasound-assisted l. (UAL)
liposarcoma
metastatic pleomorphic l.
myxomatous l.
pleomorphic l.
retroperitoneal l.
liposarcomatous differentiation
liposclerotic mesenteritis
liposculpture
3D superficial l.
liposome
antibody-conjugated paramagnetic l.
(ACPL)
mannan-coated l.
Lipowitz metal
Lippes loop
lipping
osteophytic l.
Lippman-Cobb angle
LIQ
lower inner quadrant
liquefaction
l. degeneration
l. necrosis
liquefactive emphysema
liquid
l. barium suspension
l. calcium
l. crystal contact thermography
l. crystal display projector
l. crystal thermography (LCT)
l. embolic agent
l. food dysphagia
l. nylon
l. pleural effusion
l. scintillation analysis

L

NOTES

liquid *(continued)*
    l. scintillation spectrometer
    l. scintillation spectrometry
Lisch nodule
Lisfranc
    L. amputation
    L. dislocation
    L. fracture
    L. injury
    L. joint
    L. ligament
Lissauer
    L. column
    L. tract
lissencephaly, lissencephalia
    cobblestone l.
list
    l. mode data collection
    l. mode lithium
listeria encephalitis
Lister tubercle
lithiasis
    renal l.
lithium
    l. fluoride (LiF)
    list mode l.
lithium-7
lithoclast miniature pneumatic drill
lithogenic
    l. bile
    l. index
lithokelypedion
lithokelypedium
lithokelyphosis
litholysis
lithopedion
lithopedium
Lithostar nonimmersion lithotripter
lithotomy position
lithotripsy
    biliary l.
    candela l.
    electrohydraulic l. (EHL)
    electrohydraulic shockwave l.
    endoscopic l.
    extracorporeal shock wave l. (ESWL)
    laser biliary l.
    microexplosion l.
    pulsed-dye laser l.
    rotational contact l.
    ultrasonic l.
lithotripter, lithotriptor
    DoLi S extracorporeal shock wave l.
    Dornier compact l.
    Dornier HM3, HM4 l.

    Lithostar nonimmersion l.
    Modulith SL 20 l.
    Pulsolith laser l.
    Siemens Lithostar l.
    Sonolith Praktis l.
    Swiss lithoclast intracorporeal l.
    Wolf Piezolith 2200 l.
lithotrite
    Kensey-Nash l.
LithoTron
LITT
    laser-induced interstitial thermotherapy
    laser-induced thermography
    laser-induced thermotherapy
    LITT applicator
little
    l. finger
    L. Leaguer shoulder
Littré
    L. gland
    L. hernia
Litzmann obliquity
livedo reticularis
liver
    l. abscess
    l. agenesis
    alcoholic fatty l.
    amiodarone l.
    l. angiosarcoma
    l. bed
    biliary cirrhotic l.
    brimstone l.
    bronze l.
    l. calcification
    l. capillary hemangioma
    l. capsule
    cardiac impression on l.
    caudate lobe of l.
    l. cell adenoma
    centrilobular region of l.
    Chinese fluke l.
    l. cirrhosis
    cirrhotic l.
    l. coil
    l. cyst
    degenerative l.
    degraded l.
    diaphragmatic surface of l.
    l. dome
    l. echinococcosis
    echogenic l.
    l. edema
    l. edge
    enlarged l.
    extracorporeal l.
    l. failure
    fat-spared area in fatty l.

fatty l.
l. fissure
l. flap
floating l.
l. fluke
focal fatty infiltration of l.
frosted l.
graft-versus-host disease of the l.
l. hemangiosarcoma
hobnail l.
l. hydatid disease
hyperperfusion abnormality of l.
hypoechoic l.
l. impression
infantile hemangioendothelioma
  of l.
intracorporeal l.
l., kidneys, and spleen (LKS)
l. laceration
large-droplet fatty l.
left lobe of l.
l. lesion
l. lipoma
l. lymphoma
l. mass
l. metastasis
nodular l.
nodule-in-nodule l.
noncirrhotic l.
nutmeg appearance of l.
l. parenchyma
polycystic l.
polylobar l.
prominent l.
pyogenic l.
quadrate lobe of l.
right lobe of l.
l. scan
l. scintigraphy
l. scintiphotography
l. segment
shrunken l.
small-droplet fatty l.
l. span
l. spoked-wheel pattern
stasis l.
l. steatosis
tramline effect in the l.
l. transplant
l. trauma
undersurface of l.
visceral surface of l.

wandering l.
waxy l.
liver-aorta (L/A)
liver-like lung
liver-lung scan
Liverpool silicosis
liver-specific MRI contrast agent
liver-spleen
  l.-s. imaging
  l.-s. overlap
  l.-s. scan
liver-to-aorta peak ratio
liver-to-liver peak ratio
liver-to-muscle contrast ratio
Livierato sign
Livingston triangle
LKS
  liver, kidneys, and spleen
LL
  lower lobe
L-159, L-884
  ^{11}C L.
LLD
  leg-length discrepancy
  limb-length discrepancy
LLE
  left lower extremity
LLL
  left lower lobe
L-loop
  L.-l. heart
  L.-l. ventricular situs
L-looping
L/LP ratio
LLQ
  left lower quadrant
LLS
  leaky lung syndrome
L-malposition of aorta
LMBD
  lingular mandibular bony defect
LMCA
  left main coronary artery
L-methylmethionine
  ^{11}C L.-m.
LMR
  localized magnetic resonance
  Biosense-guided LMR
LN
  Imagent LN
LNV
  last normal vertebra

NOTES

L

LO
  lesser omentum
load
  combination flow and pressure l.
  exercise l.
  iodine l.
  osmotic l.
  predominant flow l.
  rotatory l.
loading
  axial weight l.
  coil l.
  contrast l.
  fracture callus l.
  left ventricular l.
  longitudinal l.
  peripheral l.
  spike l.
  l. technique
  uniform l.
lobar
  l. breast anatomy
  l. bronchus
  l. cavitation
  l. consolidation
  l. dysmorphism
  l. emphysema
  l. holoprosencephaly
  l. intracerebral hemorrhage
  l. lung atrophy
  l. nephronia
  l. pneumonia
  l. renal infarct
  l. resorption atelectasis
  l. sclerosis
lobation
  fetal kidney l.
  persistent cortical kidney l.
  persistent renal l.
lobatum
  hepar l.
lobatus
  ren l.
lobe
  accessory l.
  anterior tip of temporal l.
  association cortex of parietal l.
  l. of azygos vein
  calciform l.
  caudate l.
  collapsed l.
  cuneiform l.
  fetal l.
  flocculonodular l.
  frontal l.
  hepatic l.
  hot caudate l.

hyperexpanded l.
inferior l.
insular l.
l. of kidney
left lower l. (LLL)
left upper l. (LUL)
limbic l.
lower l. (LL)
medial temporal l.
middle l. (ML)
occipital l.
orbital aspect of frontal l.
parietal l.
polyalveolar l.
prominent pyramidal thyroid l.
pulmonary l.
pyramidal l.
ratio of caudate to right hepatic l.
Riedel l.
right lower l. (RLL)
right middle l. (RML)
right upper l. (RUL)
Rokitansky l.
sequestered l.
spigelian l.
succenturiate placental l.
superior l.
temporal l.
thyroid l.
uncus of temporal l.
upper l. (UL)
wedge-shaped l.
lobectomy
  sleeve l.
lobster-claw deformity
lobular
  l. alveolar pattern
  l. architecture
  l. atelectasis
  l. breast calcification
  l. breast microcalcification
  l. bronchiole
  l. carcinoma
  l. carcinoma in situ (LCIS)
  l. neoplasia
  l. pneumonia
lobulated
  l. border
  l. contour
  l. filling defect
  l. kidney
  l. mass
  l. paratracheal mediastinum
  l. saccular appearance
  l. shape
  l. tumor

lobulation
> fetal l.

lobule
> l. breast
> l. of epididymis
> fat l.
> inferior parietal l.
> inferior temporal l.
> lung l.
> paracentral l.
> primary pulmonary l.
> Reid l.
> secondary pulmonary l.
> splenic l.

LOCA
> low-osmolar contrast agent

local
> l. bone blood flow
> l. bulge of kidney contour
> l. bulge renal contour
> l. cavus
> l. coil
> l. compression fracture
> l. decompression fracture
> l. edema
> l. glomerular lesion
> l. gradient coil
> l. lesion
> l. metastasis
> l. misregistration
> l. nodal disease
> l. recurrence (LR)
> l. streptokinase infusion

LocaLisa cardiac navigation system

localization
> anatomic l.
> autologous white cell l.
> autoradiographic l.
> CT-directed hook-wire l.
> fluoroscopic l.
> g-probe l.
> l. grid
> lesion l.
> magnetic resonance imaging-guided wire l.
> MRI-guided wire l.
> needle l.
> needle-hookwire l.
> off-axis point l.
> pelvic film for IUD l.
> placental l.
> point l.

> preoperative l.
> radiopharmaceutical l.
> radiotherapy l.
> sagittal l.
> seizure l.
> stereotactic l.
> surface coil l.
> l. technique
> voxel l.
> l. window
> wire l.

localization-compression grid plate

localized
> l. angiofollicular lymph node hyperplasia
> l. caliectasis
> l. coarctation
> l. edema
> l. expansion
> l. fibrous mesothelioma
> l. fibrous tumor of pleura
> l. H1 spectroscopy
> l. hyperintensity
> l. ileus
> l. intimal flap
> l. lesion
> l. lucent lung
> l. lymphangioma
> l. magnetic resonance (LMR)
> l. mass effect
> l. myeloma
> l. necrosis
> l. obstructive emphysema
> l. osteopenia
> l. osteoporosis
> l. pleura tumor
> l. proton magnetic resonance spectroscopy
> l. pure ground-glass opacity
> l. shimming
> l. single-voxel proton spectrum
> l. uptake

localizer
> axial l.
> breast l.
> Homer needle/wire l.
> Picket Fence stereotactic l.
> T1-weighted axial l.

localizing
> l. image
> l. imaging

L

NOTES

localizing *(continued)*
  l. probe
  l. sign
locally invasive tumor
location
  juxtadiaphragmatic l.
loci (*pl. of* locus)
lock
  field l.
locked
  l. facet
  l. knee
  l. nuclear magnetization
locked-in syndrome
locking
  adiabatic off-resonance spin l.
  l. disk
lock-washer configuration
Lockwood ligament
LOCM
  low-osmolar contrast medium
locomotor pattern
locoregional
  l. breast carcinoma
  l. control
  l. disease
  l. field radiotherapy
  l. hyperthermia
locular
loculated
  l. empyema
  l. hydropneumothorax
  l. pleural effusion
  l. pleural fluid
  l. ventricle
loculation
locule
loculus, pl. **loculi**
locus, pl. **loci**
  scanning l.
Loehlein diameter
Löffler, Loeffler
  L. fibroplastic endocarditis
  L. pneumonia
  L. syndrome
Löfgren syndrome
log amplifier
Logic 700 MR transducer
log-rank test
Löhlein-Baehr lesion
Löhlein diameter
lollipop tree appearance
long
  l. axial oblique view
  l. axis
  l. axis acquisition
  l. axis of bone

  l. axis of kidney
  l. axis parasternal view
  l. axis ray
  l. axis of spleen
  l. bone
  l. bone fracture
  l. bone pseudoarthrosis
  l. bone survey
  l. dural tail
  l. fiber
  l. finger
  l. head
  l. head biceps tendon
  30-mm-l. Palmaz stent
  l. oblique fracture
  l. segmental diaphyseal uptake
    bone scintigraphy
  l. smooth esophageal narrowing
  l. smooth narrowing esophagus
  l. taper stiff shaft Glidewire
  l. TE MR spectroscopy
  l. tract
  l. tract sign
  l. TR/TE
  l. TR/TE sequence
  l. wave-length photo label
long-axis slice
long-bore collimator
long-chain fatty acid
long-echo-train fast spin-echo sequence
longitudinal
  l. acoustic wave
  l. arch
  l. arteriography
  l. axis
  l. band
  l. blood supply
  l. B-mode
  l. esophageal fold
  l. esophageal stricture
  l. fasciculus
  l. fissure
  l. image
  l. lie
  l. ligament
  l. loading
  l. magnetization
  l. muscle
  l. narrowing
  l. oval pelvis
  l. raphe
  l. recovery time
  l. relaxation
  l. relaxation time
  l. relaxivity (R1)
  l. renal ectopia
  l. ridge

l. scan
l. section imaging
l. section tomography
l. split biceps tendon
l. suture
l. taenia musculature
l. tear of the brevis tendon
l. tibial fatigue fracture
l. transarticular derangement
l. ultrasonic biometry
l. ultrasound view
longitudinalis medialis fasciculus
long-scale
l.-s. contrast
l.-s. imaging agent
long-term patency
longus
abductor pollicis l. (APL)
adductor l.
l. colli muscle
extensor carpi radialis l. (ECRL)
extensor digitorum l.
extensor hallucis l. (EHL)
extensor pollicis l. (EPL)
flexor digitorum l.
flexor hallucis l.
flexor pollicis l.
palmaris l.
peroneus l.
loop
access l.
afferent l.
air-filled l.
alpha sigmoid l.
bowel l.
capillary l.
cervical l.
cine l.
closed conducting l.
colonic l.
conductive l.
contiguous l.
Cope l.
Cordonnier ureteroileal l.
dextro l. (D-loop)
diathermic l.
dilated bowel l.
l. distribution
double reverse alpha sigmoid l.
duodenal l.
efferent l.
flow-volume l.

frontal plane l.
gamma transverse colon l.
Gerdy interatrial l.
Gerdy interauricular l.
l. graft
l. of Henle
herniated bowel l.
horizontal plane l.
Hutson l.
ileal l.
intestinal l.
J l.
jejunal l.
lenticular l.
Lippes l.
malrotation of bowel l.
matted bowel l.
matted small-bowel l.
Meyer l.
Meyer-Archambault l.
nonrotation of bowel l.
N-shaped sigmoid l.
l. ostomy bridge
P l.
peduncular l.
pressure-volume l.
puborectalis l.
reentrant l.
Roux l.
rubber vessel l.
sagittal plane l.
sentinel l.
separation of bowel l.
sigmoid l.
small bowel l.
Stoerck l.
subclavian l.
T l.
thickened bowel l.
transverse colon l.
unopacified bowel l.
vector l.
ventricular l.
vessel l.
Vieussens l.
Waltman l.
loopogram imaging
loopography
ileal l.
loose
l. fracture
l. intraarticular body

L

NOTES

loose *(continued)*
    l. mesenchymal tissue
    l. osteochondral fragment
    l. shoulder
Looser
    L. line
    L. transformation zone
lopamidol
LOQ
    lower outer quadrant
LOR
    line of response
LORAD
    L. full-field digital mammography
      system
    L. StereoGuide
Lorain-Lévi dwarfism
lordosis
    cervical l.
    gentle l.
    lumbar l.
    reversal of cervical l.
    spinal l.
    thoracic l.
lordotic
    l. aspect
    l. curve
    l. pelvis
    l. position
    l. view
lorentzian
    l. curve
    l. field mapping
    l. line
    l. line saturation
Lorenz position
lorry driver's fracture
LoSo Prep
loss
    l. of bone mass
    l. coincidence
    dead time l.
    l. of definition
    l. of distinction
    l. of elasticity of cartilage
    electron equilibrium l.
    global tissue l.
    high-velocity signal l.
    l. of parallelism of facet joint
    percentage signal intensity l.
    segmental bone l.
    l. of sigmoid curve
    signal l.
    single collision energy l.
    l. of thoracic kyphosis
    time-of-flight signal l.
    TOF signal l.

    transformer l.
    volume l.
lossless image data compression
lossy
    l. algorithm
    l. image data compression
lost
    l. intrauterine device
lotus position
Louis
    L. angle
    sternal angle of L.
Louis-Bar syndrome
lovers knot
low
    l. attenuation
    l. attenuation pulsation artifact
    l. back injury
    l. back syndrome
    l. cardiac output
    l. conus medullaris
    l. density
    L. Energy All Purpose (LEAP)
    l. frame rate
    l. frequency ultrasound (LFUS)
    l. interobserver variation
    l. lung volume
    l. metastatic potential
    l. normal
    l. osmolality
    l. right atrium (LRA)
    l. septal right atrium
    l. signal intensity
    l. signal intensity artifact
    l. signal intensity fibrous band
    l. signal intensity peripheral band
    l. signal intensity synchondrosis
    l. small bowel obstruction
    l. urethral pressure (LUP)
    l. yield
low-amplitude internal echo
low-angle
    l.-a. scattering
    l.-a. shot technique
low-attenuation
    l.-a. lesion
    l.-a. mediastinal mass
Low-Beers
    L.-B. position
    L.-B. projection
    L.-B. view
low-compliance, fixed diameter balloon
low-contact dynamic compression plate (LC-DCP)
low-contrast
    l.-c. film
    l.-c. structure

low-density
  l.-d. mesencephalic lesion
  l.-d. rim
  l.-d. ring
  l.-d. structure
low-dose
  l.-d. film
  l.-d. film mammographic technique
  l.-d. folic acid
  l.-d. mammography
  l.-d. screen-film technique
low-dose/high-dose protocol
Löwenberg canal
low-energy
  l.-e. collimator
  l.-e. fracture
  l.-e. laser (LEL)
  l.-e. photon attenuation
    measurement
  l.-e. radiofrequency conduction
    hyperthermia treatment
lower
  l. basilar aneurysm
  l. esophageal mucosal ring
  l. esophageal narrowing
  l. esophageal sphincter (LES)
  l. esophageal sphincter dysfunction
  l. esophageal sphincter pressure
    (LESP)
  l. extremity (LE)
  l. extremity arterial tree
  l. extremity imaging
  l. field visual sector
  l. gastrointestinal hemorrhage
  l. inner quadrant (LIQ)
  l. limb venography
  l. limb venography imaging
  l. lobe (LL)
  l. lobe lung mass
  l. lobe pneumonia
  l. lobe reticulation
  l. lung field
  l. lung line
  l. moiety ureter
  l. motor neuron
  l. motor neuron lesion
  l. outer quadrant (LOQ)
  l. pole
  l. pole collecting system
  l. pole of kidney
  l. pole of patella
  l. pole ureter

  l. pulmonary lobe atelectasis
  l. right quadrant (LRQ)
  l. sternal border (LSB)
  l. tract
  L. tubercle
low-field
  l.-f. magnetic resonance
  l.-f. MR angiography
  l.-f. MRI system
  l.-f. MR scanner
low-field-strength MR imaging
low-flip-angle gradient-echo imaging
low-flow syndrome
low-flux polysufone membrane
low-frame-rate run
low-frequency scatter
low-grade
  l.-g. astrocytoma
  l.-g. central osteogenic sarcoma
  l.-g. glioma
  l.-g. malignancy
  l.-g. neoplasm
low-intensity
  l.-i. laser therapy (LILT)
  l.-i. line
  l.-i. pulsed ultrasound
low-level echo
low-lying placenta
Lown-Ganong-Levine syndrome (LGL)
low-osmolar
  l.-o. contrast agent (LOCA)
  l.-o. contrast medium (LOCM)
low-output heart failure
low-pass
  l.-p. filter
  l.-p. filtering
  l.-p. three-dimensional postfiltering
low-photon energy
low-pressure
  l.-p. cardiac tamponade
  l.-p. hydrocephalus
  l.-p. mercury arc amp
low-profile
  l.-p. IUGR
  l.-p. mitral valve
low-resistance spectral waveform
low-resolution imaging
low-risk single-stone former
low-signal-intensity
  l.-s.-i. fibrous septum
  l.-s.-i. replacement
  l.-s.-i. tumor

L

NOTES

low-signal mass
Lowsley lobar anatomy
low-temperature diffraction
low-T humerus fracture
low-velocity flow
LP
    linear prediction
    lumbar puncture
    lymphomatous polyposis
LPA
    left pulmonary artery
LPAM
    L-phenylalanine mustard
LPCh
    lateral posterior choroidal
L-phenylalanine mustard (LPAM)
LPI laser system
LPO
    left posterior oblique
      LPO position
LPV
    left pulmonary vein
LQ
    linear-quadratic
      LQ ratio
LR
    likelihood ratio
    local recurrence
LRA
    low right atrium
L-radiation
LRQ
    lower right quadrant
LS
    least square
    line scanning
    lumbosacral
    lumbosacral spine
LSB
    left sternal border
    lower sternal border
LSCVP
    left subclavian central venous pressure
LSF
    line spread function
LSO
    cerium-doped lutetium oxyorthosilicate
LSR
    lanthanide shift reagent
LSRT
    lens-sparing external beam radiation
      therapy
LSS
    scapholunate ligament
LSV
    lenticulostriate vasculopathy

L-transposition
    levotransposition
LTX3000 lumbar rehabilitation system
L-tyrosine imaging agent
Lu
    lutetium
^{197}Lu
    lutetium-177
lucency
    area of l.
    interspersed l.
    linear l.
    sand-like l.
    slit-like residual l.
lucent
    l. band
    l. calculus
    l. center
    l. defect
    l. finger lesion
    l. halo
    l. hilar notch
    l. interval
    l. line
    l. lung lesion
lucite
    l. beam
    l. beam spoiler
LUCL
    lateral ulnar collateral ligament
Ludovici angle
Ludwig
    L. angle
    L. plane
luetic
    l. aortic aneurysm
    l. aortitis
    l. arteritis
    l. diaphysitis
luftsichel sign
LUL
    left upper lobe
lumazenil
    ^{11}C l.
lumbales
    vertebra l.
lumbar
    l. aortography
    l. arteriography
    l. artery
    l. curvature
    l. disk
    l. facet angle
    l. fascia
    l. flexion and extension study
    l. hernia
    l. index (LI)

l. kidney
l. kyphosis
l. lordosis
l. lordotic curve
l. lymph node
l. myelography
l. nerve root
l. part of diaphragm
l. plexus
l. pneumencephalography
l. puncture (LP)
l. rib
l. root avulsion
l. scoliosis
l. spinal canal
l. spinal stenosis
l. spine
l. spine dimension
l. spine fracture
l. spine lesion
l. spine view
l. synovial cyst
l. transverse process
l. vertebra (L)
l. vertebral body index
lumbarization
lumbarized spine
lumbocostal ligament
lumbocostoabdominal triangle
lumboperitoneal shunting
lumborum
    quadratus l.
lumbosacral (LS)
    l. agenesis
    l. canal
    l. dermal sinus
    l. disk
    l. intervertebral disk herniation
    l. joint angle
    l. kyphosis
    l. lateral recess
    l. myelography
    l. plexus
    l. projection
    l. series
    l. spine (LS)
    l. spine depth
    l. spine strain
    l. trunk
lumbrical tendon
lumen, pl. **lumina, lumens**
    aortic l.

arterial l.
l. assessment
attenuated l.
bile duct l.
bowel l.
bronchial l.
carotid l.
clot-filled l.
cloverleaf-shaped l.
crescentic l.
cystic duct l.
l. delineation
l. diameter
double l.
double-barrel l.
D-shaped vessel l.
duct l.
duodenal l.
eccentrically placed l.
elliptical l.
esophageal l.
false l.
gastric l.
gastroduodenal l.
intestinal l.
midgroove portion of l.
occluded l.
patent l.
scalloped bowel l.
slit-like l.
slit-shaped vessel l.
star-shaped vessel l.
tracheal l.
true l.
vascular l.
lumen-intimal interface
lumenogram (*var. of* luminogram)
luminal
    l. area
    l. caliber
    l. defect
    l. dimension
    l. distention
    l. encroachment
    l. irregularity
    l. narrowing
    l. plaque
    l. plug
    l. silhouette
    l. stenosis
    l. thrombosis
    l. wall

L

NOTES

luminance
    viewbox l.
Luminexx biliary stent
luminogram, lumenogram
    air l.
Lumiscan LS 85 scanner
Lumisys 20 digital x-ray scanner
lumpectomy bed
lump kidney
lumpy appearance of lung
LUNA
    laser uterosacral nerve ablation
Lunar
    L. DPX densitometer
    L. Expert densitometer
    L. scanner
lunate
    avascular necrosis l.
    l. bone
    l. dislocation
    l. facet
    l. fracture
    l. tilt
lunate-shaped trachea
lunate-triquetral coalition
lunatomalacia
Lunderquest-Ring guidewire
Lunderquist exchange guidewire
lung
    l. abscess
    acquired unilateral hyperlucent l.
    l. adenocarcinoma
    l. agenesis
    air conditioner l.
    air-filled l.
    airless l.
    amiodarone l.
    l. amyloidosis
    l. ankylosis spondylitis
    l. apex
    l. aplasia
    l. arch
    l. architecture
    arc welder's l.
    artificial l.
    atelectatic l.
    azygos lobe of l.
    l. base
    l. base infiltrate
    bauxite fibrosis of l.
    Bible printer's l.
    bilateral hyperlucent l.
    bird breeder's l.
    bird fancier's l.
    bird handler's l.
    black l.
    blunt border of l.

brown induration of l.
bubbly l.
budgerigar fancier's l.
l. calculus
l. capacity
l. carcinoma
l. cavity
cheese handler's l.
cheese washer's l.
chest fluke l.
cluster of grapes l.
coal miner's l.
coal worker's l.
l. coccidioidomycosis
coffee worker's l.
coin lesion of l.
collapsed l.
l. compliance
l. connectivity test
consolidated l.
contralateral l.
l. contusion
convexity of the l.
corundum smelter's l.
l. count curve
l. cylindroma
l. cyst
dark l.
l. decortication
l. density
dependent l.
drowned l.
dynamic l.
l. echinococcosis
eclipse effect l.
l. edema
l. emphysema
emphysematous l.
empty collapsed l.
expanded l.
l. expansion
farmer's l.
fibroid l.
fibroma of l.
fibrosis of l.
l. field
fishmeal worker's l.
l. fissure
l. fluke
folded l.
l. fungus ball
furrier's l.
gangrene of l.
grain handler's l.
l. granuloma
graphite fibrosis of l.
gray l.

l. hamartoma
hardened l.
harvester's l.
hazy-opaque l.
l. hemangioma
l. hemorrhage
hemorrhagic consolidation of l.
hen worker's l.
l. hepatization
l. hilum
l. histoplasmosis
honeycomb l.
horseshoe l.
humidifier l.
hyperlucent l.
hypersensitivity l.
hypogenetic l.
hypoinflation of the l.
hypolucency of l.
l. hypoplasia
hypoplastic l.
idiopathic unilateral hyperlucent l.
l. imaging
immature l.
inferior lobe of l.
l. infiltrate distribution
l. inflammation
l. interstitium
l. laceration
light pink l.
l. linearity
lingular division of the left l.
liver-like l.
l. lobule
localized lucent l.
lumpy appearance of l.
l. lymphangiectasis
l. lymphangioma
l. lymphoid hyperplasia
l. lymphoma
malt worker's l.
maple bark stripper's l.
l. marking
mason's l.
l. mass
meat wrapper's l.
l. metastasis
miller's l.
miner's l.
mottled gray l.
mushroom worker's l.
native l.

l. necrosis
l. nodularity
l. nodule
nondependent l.
l. opacity
l. overexpansion
l. overinflation
l. paragonimiasis
l. parenchyma
l. parenchyma consolidation
partial collapse of l.
l. perfusion
l. perfusion defect
l. perfusion radionuclide
l. periphery
physiologically immature l.
pigeon fancier's l.
polycystic l.
l. popcorn calcification
postperfusion l.
l. pseudocavitation
l. pseudolymphoma
pump l.
l. reexpansion
reperfusion injury of
  postischemic l.
right l.
l. root
rounded border of l.
rudimentary l.
l. sarcoid
l. scan
l. scintigraphy
l. segmentation
septic l.
sequestered lobe of l.
sharp border of l.
l. shock
shrunken l.
silicotic fibrosis of l.
silo-filler's l.
silver finisher's l.
silver polisher's l.
smoker's l.
solid edema of l.
l. starfish scar
static l.
l. stiffness
stiff noncompliant l.
l. stone
stretched l.
structurally immature l.

L

NOTES

lung *(continued)*
    subsegment of l.
    superior lobe of l.
    surface tension of l.
    l. talcosis
    l. torsion
    l. transplant
    l. tuberculoma
    l. tumor
    l. underinflation
    underventilated l.
    unilateral hyperlucent l.
    l. varix
    l. volume (V)
    l. washout
    welder's l.
    well-inflated l.
    wet l.
    white l.
    l. window
    l. zone
lung-airspace
lung/heart ratio of thallium 201 activity
lung-volume loop flow
lunocapitate bone
lunohamate arthritis
lunotriquetral
    l. interosseus ligament
    l. joint
lunula, pl. **lunulae**
LUP
    low urethral pressure
lupus
    drug-induced erythematous l.
    pernio l.
    systemic erythematosus l.
LUQ
    left upper quadrant
Luque rod
LUS
    laparoscopic ultrasound
Luschka
    L. bursa
    L. crypt
    L. duct leak
    foramen of L.
    L. joint
    L. ligament
    L. muscle
    sinuvertebral nerve of L.
lusoria
    arteria l.
    dysphagia l.
luteal
    l. cyst
    l. phase
    l. phase defect

luteinized
    l. unruptured follicle
    l. unruptured follicle syndrome
Lutembacher
    L. complex
    L. syndrome
lutetium (Lu)
    l. tantalate
lutetium-177 (^{197}Lu)
luxated bone
luxation
    ligamentous l.
Luxtec fiberoptic system
luxury
    l. perfusion
    l. perfusion syndrome
Luys body
LVAD
    left ventricular assist device
LVD
    left ventricular dysfunction
LVdd
    left ventricular diastolic dimension
LVEDD
    left ventricular end-diastolic dimension
LVEDI
    left ventricular end-diastolic volume
     index
LVEDP
    left ventricular end-diastolic pressure
LVEF
    left ventricular ejection fraction
       exercise first-pass LVEF
LVESD
    left ventricular end-systolic dimension
LVESVI
    left ventricular end-systolic volume index
LVET
    left ventricular ejection time
LVFS
    left ventricular functional shortening
LVFW
    left ventricular free wall
LVG
    left ventriculogram
LVH
    left ventricular hypertrophy
LVID
    left ventricular internal diameter
LVIDd, LVIDD
    left ventricular internal diastolic
     dimension
LVIDs
    left ventricular internal dimension at end
     systole
LVIV
    left ventricular inflow volume

LVM
left ventricular mass
LVMI
left ventricular mass index
LVOT
left ventricular outflow tract
LVOT flow rate
LVOTO
left ventricular outflow tract obstruction
LVOV
left ventricular outflow volume
LVP
left ventricular pressure
LVPW
left ventricular posterior wall
LVs
left ventricular systolic
LVs system
LVSW
left ventricular stroke work
LVSWI
left ventricular stroke work index
LVW
left ventricular wall
LX
LX EchoSpeed 1.5T CV/i, NVi
MR system
LX 20 laser
LX 8.3 software
Lyme carditis
lympangiomyomatosis
lymph
l. capillary
l. duct
l. gland
l. node
l. node eggshell calcification
l. node enlargement
l. node imaging
l. node involvement
l. node sinus
l. node syndrome
l. node tissue
l. plexus
l. vessel of prostate
lymphadenitis
regional granulomatous l.
lymphadenography
lymphadenopathy
angioblastic l.
angioimmunoblastic l.
axillary l.

benign l.
mesenteric l.
peripancreatic l.
persistent generalized l.
reactive l.
retrocrural l.
retroperitoneal l.
secondary axillary l.
superficial l.
l. syndrome
lymphangiectasis
acquired intestinal l.
congenital l.
generalized l.
intestinal l.
lung l.
primary pulmonary l.
pulmonary cystic l.
secondary l.
submucosal l.
subserosal l.
lymphangiogram (LAG)
lymphangiographic imaging agent
lymphangiography
bipedal l.
contrast l.
l. imaging
pedal l.
lymphangiohemangioma
lymphangioleiomyomatosis
lymphangioma
capillary l.
cardiac l.
cavernous l.
diffuse l.
localized l.
lung l.
l. mesentery
neck l.
orbital l.
pancreatic cystic l.
retroperitoneal l.
simple capillary l.
lymphangiomatosis
pulmonary l.
lymphangiomyomatosis
lymphangitic
l. carcinomatosis
l. metastasis
lymphangitis
lymphatic
l. canal

L

NOTES

lymphatic *(continued)*
- l. carcinomatosis
- l. channel
- l. cortex
- l. development
- dilated l.
- l. drainage pattern
- l. duct
- l. edema
- l. imaging
- l. malformation
- l. mapping
- l. medulla
- l. metastasis
- l. network
- l. obstruction
- paracervical l.
- prominent septal l.
- l. sac
- l. sarcoma
- subpleural l.
- l. tissue
- l. trunk
- l. tumor spread
- l. valve
- l. vessel

lymphatica
- pseudopolyposis l.

lymphaticovenous secondary edema

lymphatics

lymphaticum
- angioma l.

Lymphazurin imaging agent

lymphedema
- Meige l.
- Nonne-Milroy l.
- postmastectomy l.

lymphoblastic lymphoma

lymphoblastoma

lymphocapillary vessel

lymphocele
- renal transplant l.

lymphocyte-rich tumor

lymphocytic
- l. hypophysitis
- l. interstitial pneumonia (LIP)
- l. interstitial pneumonitis
- l. plasmacytoid lymphoma
- l. poorly-differentiated lymphoma
- l. well-differentiated lymphoma

lymphoepithelial parotid tumor

lymphoepithelioma
- salivary gland l.

lymphogenous
- l. dissemination
- l. embolus
- l. metastasis

lymphogranuloma venereum

lymphography
- MR l.
- time-lapse quantitative computed tomography l.

lymphoid
- l. follicle
- l. hamartoma
- l. hyperplasia
- l. hypophysitis
- l. interstitial pneumonia (LIP)
- l. interstitial pneumonitis
- l. polyp
- l. tissue
- l. tumor

lymphoma
- acute lymphoblastic l.
- adult T-cell l.
- African Burkitt l.
- anaplastic large cell l. (ALCL)
- angioimmunoblastic lymphadenopathy-like T-cell l.
- angiotropic large cell l.
- B-cell monocytoid l.
- bone l.
- brain l.
- breast l.
- Burkitt l.
- Burkitt-like l.
- butterfly l.
- B-zone small lymphocytic l.
- Castleman l.
- centroblastic l.
- centrocytic l.
- cerebral l.
- cleaved cell l.
- cobblestone appearance l.
- colorectal l.
- convoluted T-cell l.
- cutaneous B-cell l. (CBCL)
- cutaneous T-cell l.
- diffuse aggressive l.
- diffuse intermediate lymphocytic l.
- diffuse large-cell l. (DLCL)
- diffuse mixed small- and large-cell l.
- diffuse small-cell lymphocytic l.
- dural arachnoid l.
- enteropathy-associated T-cell l.
- epidural l.
- extranodal follicular l.
- follicular center-cell l.
- follicular mixed small cleaved l.
- follicular predominantly large cell l.
- follicular predominantly small cell l.

fulminant cerebral l.
l. gallium scintigraphy
gastric l.
gastrointestinal l.
giant follicle l.
granulomatous l.
histiocytic bone l.
histiocytic brain l.
histiocytic chest l.
Hodgkin l.
immunoblastic large-cell l.
infiltrative l.
intracerebral l.
kidney l.
large cleaved cell l.
limited-stage diffuse large-cell l.
liver l.
lung l.
lymphoblastic l.
lymphocytic plasmacytoid l.
lymphocytic poorly-differentiated l.
lymphocytic well-differentiated l.
macroglobulinemic l.
MALT l.
mantle cell l. (MCL)
marginal zone l. (MZL)
marginal zone B-cell l.
mediastinal l.
mesencephalic cerebral l.
mesenterial Castleman l.
mesenteric l.
metastatic testicular l.
mixed lymphocytic-histiocytic l.
mixed small and large cell l.
mucosa-associated lymphoid
  tissue l.
multifocal l.
noncleaved cell l.
orbital l.
osseous l.
pancreatic l.
peripheral l.
perirenal l.
plasmablastic l.
pleomorphic T-cell l.
polypoid l.
primary adrenal l.
primary bone l.
primary brain l.
primary CNS l.
primary cutaneous large B-cell l.
  (PCLBCL)

primary gastric non-Hodgkin l.
primary refractory Burkitt l.
pulmonary l.
pyothorax-associated pleural l.
recurrent l.
renal l.
retroperitoneal l.
Revised European American L.
  (REAL)
secondary brain l.
secondary cutaneous large B-cell l.
  (SCLBCL)
sinonasal l.
skeletal l.
small B-cell l.
small lymphocytic T-cell l.
spinal epidural l.
splenic B-cell l.
sporadic Burkitt l.
l. staging
systemic brain l.
T-cell lymphoblastic l.
thymic l.
thyroid l.
true histiocytic l.
T-zone l.
ulcerative l.
undefined l.
undifferentiated non-Hodgkin l.
urinary bladder l.
vitreous l.
Waldeyer ring l.
lymphomatoid granulomatosis
lymphomatosis
lymphomatosum
  cystadenoma l.
  papillary cystadenoma l.
lymphomatous
  l. lymph node
  l. mass
  l. polyposis (LP)
lymphonodular hyperplasia
lymphoplasmacytic infiltrate
lymphopneumatosis
  peritoneal l.
lymphoproliferative disorder
lymphoreticular tissue
LymphoScan
  L. imaging agent
  L. nuclear imaging system
  L. nuclear imaging system scanner

L

NOTES

LymphoScan *(continued)*
    L. Tc99m-labeled murine antibody
        fragment
lymphoscintigraphy
    cutaneous l.
    internal mammary l.
    radiocolloid l.
Lynch and Crues type 2 lesion
lyoluminescence
lyophilized
Lyra laser
lysate
Lyser
    trapezoid bone of L.
Lysholm
    L. grid
    L. method

lysis
    bony l.
    cystic l.
    follicle l.
lytic
    l. area
    l. area bone flap
    l. bone lesion
    l. change
    l. lesion of skull
    l. osteolysis
    l. osteosarcoma
    l. pattern

M
>M pattern
>3M scanner
>M shell

m
>meter

M1-M5 segment of middle cerebral artery

M1 segment aneurysm

M2A imaging capsule endoscopy

M4-M5 lineage

MAA
>macroaggregated albumin

maceration
>clot m.

Macewen sign

Mach
>M. band
>M. band effect
>M. line

machine
>Acoma portable x-ray m.
>Aestiva/5 MRI anesthesia m.
>cobalt megavoltage m.
>2D B-mode ultrasound m.
>Echospeed 1.5T MR m.
>focused segmented ultrasound m.
>m. injection
>neutron therapy m.
>panoramic rotating m.
>parallel virtual m. (PVM)

Mackenrodt ligament

Mackenzie point

Macklin effect

Macleod syndrome

Mac-Loc Ultrathane Cope nephroureterostomy stent

macrencephaly, macrencephalia

macroadenoma
>pituitary m.
>prolactin-secreting pituitary m.

macroaggregated
>m. albumin (MAA)
>m. albumin imaging agent

macroangiography

macrocalcification

macrocephalia, macrocephaly

macrocirculation

macrocolon

macrocyst
>adrenocortical m.

macrocystic
>m. adenoma
>m. cystadenoma
>m. encephalomalacia
>m. neoplasm
>m. pilocytic cerebellar astrocytoma

macrodacryocystography

macrodystrophia
>lipoma m.
>m. lipomatosa

macrofistulous arteriovenous communication

macroglobulinemic lymphoma

macrolobular cirrhosis

macromolecular
>m. content
>m. contrast-enhanced MR imaging
>m. contrast medium (MMCM)
>m. drug
>m. hydration effect
>m. imaging agent

macronodular pattern

macrophage inflammatory protein (MIP)

MACRO-P solution

macroradiography
>Buckland-Wright m.

macroreentrant circuit

macroscopic
>m. hemorrhage ligament
>m. magnetic moment
>m. magnetization vector
>m. placental lesion

Macrotec imaging agent

MacSpect real-time NMR workstation

macula, pl. **maculae**

macule
>coal m.

maculopathy bull's eye magnet

Maddahi method of calculating right ventricular ejection fraction

Madelung
>M. deformity
>M. neck

Madura foot

maduromycosis

Maffucci syndrome

MAG3
>mercaptoacetyltriglycine

magenblase

Magendie foramen

M

magenstrasse
Maggi biopsy needle
magic
> m. angle effect
> m. angle effect artifact
> m. angle phenomenon
> m. angle spinning NMR
> M. S/P Wallstent

magic-angle spinning imaging
Magilligan technique for measuring neutral anteversion
Maglinte catheter
magna
> abnormal cisterna m.
> arteria radicularis anterior m.
> chorda m.
> cisterna m.
> coxa m.
> mega cisterna m.

Magnascanner
> Picker M.

Magna-SL scanner
Magnes
> M. biomagnetometer
> M. biomagnetometer system
> M. 2500 whole-blood scanner
> M. 2500 whole-head imaging

magnesium
> m. chloride
> m. contrast medium

magnet
> air-core m.
> beam-bending m.
> cryostable m.
> doughnut m.
> Eindhoven m.
> Fe-Ex orogastric tube m.
> GE Signa 1.5-T m.
> Gyroscan NT 10 m.
> Gyroscan 1.5T superconducting m.
> Horizon LX 1.5-T superconducting m.
> hybrid m.
> large-bore m.
> maculopathy bull's eye m.
> Magnetom SP4000 m.
> Magnex m.
> m. mode
> nonenclosed m.
> open m.
> Oxford m.
> pancake MRI m.
> passively shimmed superconducting m.
> permanent m.
> Philips Gyroscan ACS NT superconducting m.

poor shimming of MRI m.
m. rate
resistive m.
m. response
shimmed m.
short-bore m.
m. stability
superconducting m.
superconductive m.
1.0T, 1.5T superconducting m.
tubular m.
Walker m.

magnetic
> m. anisotropy
> m. bolus tracking
> m. circuit
> m. dipole
> m. dipole-dipole coupling
> m. dipole moment
> m. disk
> m. domain
> m. field gradient (MFG)
> m. field perturbation
> m. field strength
> m. flux
> m. flux density
> m. focal plane
> m. fringe field
> m. induction
> m. induction device
> m. interaction
> m. inversion
> m. lines of force
> m. material
> m. nuclei
> m. particulate
> m. permeability
> m. pole
> m. radiation exposure
> m. resonance (MR)
> m. resonance angiography (MRA)
> m. resonance angiography-directed bypass procedure
> m. resonance arthrography
> m. resonance catheter imaging
> m. resonance cholangiogram (MRC)
> m. resonance cholangiography with HASTE
> m. resonance cholangiopancreatography (MRCP)
> m. resonance dacryocystography
> m. resonance depiction
> m. resonance-detected white matter lesion
> m. resonance detection
> m. resonance diffusion imaging

m. resonance digital subtraction
angiography (MRDSA)
m. resonance discriminator of
osseous metastasis
m. resonance elastography (MRE)
m. resonance enhancement pattern
m. resonance epidurography
m. resonance hydrographic
technique
m. resonance imaging (MRI)
m. resonance imaging-guided
focused ultrasound sector
transducer
m. resonance imaging-guided wire
localization
m. resonance mammography
(MRM)
m. resonance multispectral color
images
m. resonance myelography
m. resonance needle tracking
m. resonance neurography (MRN)
m. resonance pancreatography
(MRP)
m. resonance pelvimetry
m. resonance perfusion imaging
m. resonance phase velocity
mapping
m. resonance phlebography
m. resonance receptor agent
m. resonance sialography
m. resonance signal
m. resonance simulator
m. resonance spectroscopy (MRS)
m. resonance spin incoherence
m. resonance tomography (MRT)
m. resonance urography (MRU)
m. resonance user interface
software
m. resonance venogram (MRV)
m. resonance venography (MRV)
m. resonance volume estimation
m. retentivity
m. servomotor
m. shielding
m. source imaging (MSI)
m. stimulation
M. Surgery System
m. susceptibility
m. susceptibility artifact
m. susceptibility-weighted image
m. tape storage

magnetism
nuclear m.
magnetite (Fe_3O_4)
m. albumin imaging agent
magnetization
complementary spatial modulation
of m. (CSPAMM)
equilibrium m.
locked nuclear m.
longitudinal m.
net tissue m.
net transverse m.
m. precession angle
m. prepared (MP)
rephased transverse m.
residual m.
rest m.
spatial modulation of m.
m. and spin-lock transfer imaging
SSFP m.
steady-state free precession m.
m. transfer (MT)
m. transfer contrast (MTC)
m. transfer effect
m. transfer gradient-echo image
m. transfer ratio (MTR)
m. transfer technique
m. transfer weighted imaging
transverse m.
magnetization-prepared
m.-p. rapid acquisition gradient
echo
m.-p. rapid acquisition gradient-
echo sequence
m.-p. rapid gradient echo-water
excitation (MP-RAGE-WE)
magnetoacoustic
m. imaging
m. MRI
magnetoencephalogram
magnetoencephalography (MEG)
magnetogyric ratio
magnetohydrodynamic effect
Magnetom
M. Open system
M. Sonata 1.5T MR system
M. SP4000 magnet
M. SP MRI imager
M. SP63 scanner
M. Trio 3T unlimited MRI system
M. 1.5-T scanner
M. Vision MR unit

M

NOTES

Magnetom *(continued)*
 M. Vision scanner
 M. Vision 1.5T MR imaging
 system
magnetometer probe
magneton
 Bohr m.
magnetopharmaceutical
magnetoresistive sensor circuit
Magnevist
 M. gadopentate dimeglumine
 M. imaging agent
Magnex
 M. Alpha MR system
 M. magnet
 M. MR scanner
magnification (X)
 m. angiography
 electronic m.
 m. error
 m. factor (MF)
 film-screen m.
 m. hard copy
 high-resolution m.
 m. mammography
 m. radiography
 m. roentgenography
 signal m.
 spot m.
 m. and spot compression
 ultra-high m.
 m. view
magnitude
 m. calculation
 m. image
 m. of obliquity
 m. reconstruction
magnum
 M. biopsy instrument
 foramen m.
 vertebra m.
 visibility of the foramen m.
magnus
 adductor m.
Mahaim
 M. bundle
 M. and James fiber
main
 m. bundle
 m. energy substrate
 m. fissure
 m. glow peak
 m. magnetic field inhomogeneity
 artifact
 m. pancreatic duct (MPD)
 m. papillary duct (MPD)

 m. portal vein peak velocity
 (MPPv)
 m. pulmonary artery (MPA)
 m. timing event (MTE)
 m. tumor
mainline granulomatosis
mainstem
 m. bronchus
 m. carina
 m. coronary artery
Mainster retina laser
maintenance of flow
Maisonneuve
 M. fibular fracture
 M. injury
 M. sign
Maissiat
 M. band
 M. ligament
major
 m. aorticopulmonary collateral
 artery
 m. bronchus
 m. calix
 m. duodenal papilla
 m. fissure
 m. fracture fragment
 globus m.
 m. muscle
 psoas m.
 rhomboid m.
 teres m.
majus, pl. **majora**
 omentum m.
malabsorption
Malacarne antrum
maladie de Roger
malakoplakia, malacoplakia
 renal parenchymal m.
malaligned atrioventricular septal defect
malalignment
 patellar m.
 rotational m.
 subtle m.
malangulation
malar
 m. bone
 m. eminence
 m. fracture
 m. lymph node
malarial granuloma
Malcolm-Lynn C-RXF cervical retractor frame
maldescended testis
maldevelopment
 pubic bone m.

maldistribution of ventilation and perfusion
male
  m. genital tract calcification
  m. pelvis
  m. Turner syndrome
  m. urethra
Malecot nephrostomy catheter
malformation
  adenomatoid m.
  angiographically occult intracranial
    vascular m. (AOIVM)
  angiographically occult vascular m.
    (AOVM)
  angiographically visualized
    vascular m. (AVVM)
  anorectal m.
  aortic arch m.
  Arnold-Chiari m.
  arterial m. (AM)
  arteriovenous m. (AVM)
  arteriovenous brain m.
  arteriovenous colon m.
  arteriovenous cord m.
  arteriovenous kidney m.
  bronchopulmonary foregut m.
    (BPFM)
  capillary m.
  capillary-lymphatic m. (CLM)
  cardiovascular m.
  cavernous m.
  cerebral arteriovenous m.
  cerebral microarteriovenous m.
    (micro-AVM)
  cerebrovascular m.
  Chiari I–II m.
  cloacal m.
  computer-assisted resection of
    cerebral arteriovenous m.
  congenital cystic adenomatoid m.
    (CCAM)
  congenital heart m.
  congenital vascular m. (CVM)
  coronary artery m.
  cryptic vascular m. (CVM)
  cystic adenomatoid m.
  dancer's foot m.
  Dandy-Walker m.
  DeMyer system of cerebral m.
  Dieulafoy vascular m.
  diffuse m.
  dural arteriovenous m.

Ebstein m.
endocardial cushion m.
extremity m.
familial cavernous m.
fast-flow m.
fetal cystic adenomatoid m.
fetal hand m.
focal m.
frontal arteriovenous m.
frontoparietal arteriovenous m.
fusiform m.
galenic venous m.
glomus-type arteriovenous m.
hindbrain m.
intracerebral arteriovenous m.
intracerebral vascular m.
intracranial arteriovenous m.
intramedullary arteriovenous m.
intramuscular venous m.
intraosseous arteriovenous m.
intraosseous vascular m.
Joubert m.
lymphatic m.
Michel m.
mixed venous-lymphatic m.
molar tooth midbrain-hindbrain m.
Mondini m.
mural-type vein of Galen m.
neural axis vascular m.
occult cerebral vascular m.
  (OCVM)
occult vascular brain m.
pulmonary arterial m.
pulmonary arteriovenous m.
  (PAVM)
retromedullary arteriovenous m.
saccular m.
septal m.
sink-trap m.
slow-flow vascular m.
spinal cord m. (SCM)
spinal vascular m.
split spinal cord m. (SSCM)
subpial arteriovenous m.
telencephalic m.
valve m.
vascular m.
vein of Galen m.
venous vascular m.
Wyburn-Mason arteriovenous m.
malformed phlebectasia
Malgaigne pelvic fracture

M

NOTES

malignancy
    aggressive m.
    borderline m.
    epithelial m.
    extrapelvic m.
    gastrointestinal m.
    high-grade m.
    low-grade m.
    metastatic m.
    mimicker of m.
    myeloid m.
    pelvic m.
    primary pulmonary m.
    secondary m.
    m. threshold
    uroepithelial m.
    urogenital m.
    vulvar m.

malignant
    m. acetabular osteolysis
    m. adrenal mass
    m. airway obstruction
    m. bone aneurysm
    m. brain edema
    m. breast calcification
    m. chondrosarcoma
    m. degeneration
    m. duodenal tumor
    m. ependymoma
    m. external otitis
    m. fibrous histiocytoma (MFH)
    m. fibrous histiocytoma of bone (MFH-B)
    m. fibrous osseous histiocytoma
    m. fibrous xanthoma
    m. fibroxanthoma
    m. gastric ulcer
    m. glioma
    m. hemangioendothelioma
    m. mediastinum teratoid tumor
    m. melanoma gallium imaging
    m. melanoma staging
    m. meningioma
    m. myeloid sarcoma
    m. nephrosclerosis
    m. osseous lesion
    m. osteoid
    m. osteopetrosis
    m. ovarian germ cell tumor
    m. ovarian teratoma tumor
    m. pleomorphic adenoma
    m. pleural effusion
    m. pleural implant
    m. pleural mesothelioma
    m. pulmonary mesothelioma
    m. small bowel tumor
    m. teratoma

    m. thymoma
    m. transformation
    m. urethral neoplasm

malignum
    adenoma m.

Mallampati score

mallei (*pl. of* malleus)

malleolar
    m. fossa
    m. fracture

malleolus, pl. **malleoli**
    m. bone
    m. fibulae
    lateral m.
    medial m.
    m. tibiae

mallet
    m. finger
    m. fracture

mallet-finger deformity

malleus, pl. **mallei**

Mallinckrodt
    M. Institute of Radiology guideline
    M. scanner

Mallory-Weiss
    M.-W. esophageal tear
    M.-W. lesion
    M.-W. mucosal tear
    M.-W. syndrome

Malmo mammographic screening trial

malocclusion

malomaxillary suture

Maloney endootoprobe laser

malperfused

malperfusion

malpighian
    m. body
    m. body of the spleen
    m. follicle
    m. vesicle

malpositioned
    m. fetus
    m. heart
    m. testis

malrotation
    m. of bowel loop
    complete small bowel m.
    intestinal tract m.
    m. of intestine
    kidney m.
    midgut volvulus with m.
    partial small bowel m.
    renal m.
    small bowel m.

MALT
    mucosa-associated lymphoid tissue
    MALT lymphoma

malt worker's lung
malum perforans pedis
malunion of fracture fragment
malunited fracture
Malvern 2600 Sizer laser diffraction
  scanner
mamillary
  m. body
  m. suture
  m. system
mamillothalamic fasciculus
Mamm-Aire heart failure
Mammalock needle
mammaplasty (*var. of* mammoplasty)
mammary
  m. artery
  m. calculus
  m. cyst
  m. duct
  m. duct ectasia
  m. duct obstruction
  m. ductogram
  m. ductogram imaging
  m. dysplasia
  m. galactogram
  m. galactogram imaging
  m. gland
  m. implant
  m. parenchyma
  m. tissue
  m. tumorigenesis
MAMMEX TR computer-aided
  mammography diagnosis system
Mammo
  M. Mask dedicated viewer
  M. Mask illuminator
  M. Plus mammography system
  M. QC mammography
mammogram
  CAD-evaluated m.
  digitized contact m.
  false-negative m.
  film-based screening m.
  true-negative m.
mammographic
  m. evaluation of breast mass
  m. feature
  m. guidance
  m. measurement
  m. phantom
  m. technique
  m. view box

mammographically
  m. occult carcinoma
  m. suspicious lesion
mammographic-histopathologic
  correlation
mammography
  baseline m.
  computed tomography laser m.
    (CTLM)
  contoured tilting compression m.
  contrast-enhanced near-infrared
    laser m.
  contrast subtraction m.
  diagnostic m.
  digital m.
  digital subtraction m. (DSM)
  dual-energy m.
  Egan m.
  evaluation of mass m.
  film-screen m.
  full-field digital m.
  high-resolution CT m.
  low-dose m.
  magnetic resonance m. (MRM)
  magnification m.
  Mammomat B m.
  Mammo QC m.
  microfocal spot m.
  near-infrared optical m.
  NIR optical m.
  nonmagnified m.
  orthogonal projection m.
  positron emission m. (PEM)
  radionuclide m.
  screen-film m.
  screening m.
  Senographe 500T, 600T, 700T,
    800T m.
  single-view oblique m.
  spot compression magnification m.
  stage-matched intervention on
    repeat m.
  step-oblique m.
  stereo m.
  stereotactic m.
  m. technique
  two-view film-screen m.
  ultra-high magnification m.
    (UHMM)
  ultrasound augmented m.
  x-ray m.
Mammo-Lume

M

NOTES

Mammomat B mammography
mammoplasia
mammoplasty, mammaplasty
    augmentation m.
    postreduction m.
MammoReader
    M. computer-aided dectection
      system
    M. mammography system
Mammorex
MammoSite
    M. Radiation Therapy
    M. RTS
Mammospot
Mammotest
    M. breast biopsy system
    M. unit
Mammotome
    Biopsys M.
    M. ultrasound system
Mammotrax
Mammoviewer
man
    roentgen equivalent m. (REM)
management
    real-time position m. (RPM)
managing
    high-resolution storage phosphor m.
Manchester
    M. LDR implant system
    M. ovoid
mandible
    alveolar border of m.
    genial tubercle of m.
    m. hypoplasia
    m. osteolysis
    symphysis of the m.
mandibula, pl. **mandibulae**
    capitulum m.
    coronoid of m.
mandibular
    m. angle
    m. canal
    m. condyle
    m. disk
    m. division
    m. foramen
    m. fossa
    m. fracture
    m. lymph node
    m. nerve
    m. ramus
    m. triangle
mandibularis
    torus m.
mandibulofacial dysostosis
mandril, mandrin

maneuver
    Adson m.
    circumduction-adduction shoulder m.
    costoclavicular m.
    flexion m.
    Fogarty m.
    Hampton m.
    Heineke-Mikulicz m.
    hyperabduction m.
    jugular compression m.
    Kocher m.
    manual Matas m.
    Müller m.
    Osler m.
    Phalen m.
    pull m.
    push m.
    Rivero-Carvallo m.
    scalene m.
    squatting m.
    temporal artery tap m.
    transabdominal left lateral
      retroperitoneal m.
    Valsalva m.
mangafodipir
    m. trisodium
    m. trisodium agent
    m. trisodium-enhanced MR imaging
manganese (Mn)
    m. chloride
    m. chloride contrast medium
    m. citrate
    m. dipyridoxyl diphosphate
    m. imaging agent
    m. sulfate
    m. tetrasodium-meso-tetra (Mn-
      TPPS$_4$)
manganese-BOPTA
manganese-containing contrast agent
manifestation
    imaging m.
manifold
    three-stopcock m.
manipulation
    deformable m.
    rigid m.
Mankin method
man-made environmental radiation
mannan-coated liposome
Mann-Bollman fistula
mannitol and saline imaging agent
Mannkopf sign
manofluorography (MFG)
manometric
    m. measurement
    m. pattern

manometry
  anal m.
  aneroid m.
  anorectal m.
  biliary m.
  ERCP m.
  esophageal m.
  rectosigmoid m.
  sphincter of Oddi m.
mantle
  anechoic m.
  m. block
  brain m.
  m. cell lymphoma (MCL)
  cement m.
  cerebral m.
  m. complex
  m. field
  hypoechoic m.
  m. radiotherapy
manual
  m. compression
  m. injection
  m. Matas maneuver
  m. pressure over carotid sinus
  m. subtraction film
manubria (*pl. of* manubrium)
manubriosternalis
  symphysis m.
  synchondrosis m.
manubriosternal joint
manubrium, pl. **manubria**
  m. hypersegmentation
manus
  digiti m.
MAP
  mean arterial pressure
map (*See* mapping)
  acceleration m.
  ADC m.
  anisotropy m.
  bladder m.
  bull's eye polar m.
  cerebral blood volume m.
  cylindrical projection m.
  decimalized variance m.
  end-diastolic polar m.
  end-systolic polar m.
  functional m.
  sestamibi polar m.
  spherical m.
  trace m.

MAPCA
  multiple aortopulmonary collateral artery
map-guided partial endocardial ventriculotomy
maple
  m. bark disease
  m. bark stripper's lung
map-like skull
mapping
  activation-sequence m.
  advanced cardiac m.
  m. algorithm
  body surface Laplacian m. (BSLM)
  body surface potential m.
  brain electrical activity m. (BEAM)
  cardiac m.
  catheter m.
  m. of cerebral sulcus
  color-flow m.
  contour m.
  cortical m.
  2D m.
  m. of defect
  digital road m.
  direction-encoded color m. (DEC)
  Doppler color-flow m.
  2D pulsatility index m.
  2D resistance index m.
  eddy current m.
  electrophysiologic m.
  endocardial activation m.
  endocardial catheter m.
  epicardial m.
  functional anatomical m.
  homology m.
  Hough transform m.
  intramural m.
  intraoperative electrocortical
    stimulation m.
  intraoperative lymphatic m.
  k-space velocity m.
  lorentzian field m.
  lymphatic m.
  magnetic resonance phase
    velocity m.
  moving slice velocity m.
  MRI m.
  MR velocity m.
  pace m.
  parallel analog m.
  phase difference m.
  phase-shift velocity m.

M

NOTES

mapping *(continued)*
    precordial m.
    radiocolloid m.
    retrograde atrial activation m.
    road m.
    saphenous vein m.
    sinus rhythm m.
    spastic m.
    spatial m.
    susceptibility m.
    texture m.
    velocity m.
    volumetric magnetic resonance
     brain m.
marantic
    m. clot
    m. endocarditis
marble
    m. bone
    m. bone disease
marbling of pancreatic parenchyma
Marcacci muscle
march
    m. foot
    m. fracture
Marchiafava-Bignami disease
Marchiafava-Micheli syndrome
Marconi/Elscint MxTwin CT
Marcus Gunn syndrome
Marex MRI system
Marfan syndrome
margin
    anterior vertebral body m.
    m. of apposition
    band-like m.
    beveled m.
    blurring of disk m.
    cardiac m.
    circumscribed m.
    colon m.
    convex posterior m.
    cortical m.
    costal m.
    costodiaphragmatic m.
    depression of renal m.
    disk m.
    enhancing ventricular m.
    fluffy m.
    ill-defined m.
    indistinct endometrial m.
    infraorbital m. (IOM)
    inking the m.
    ipsilateral m.
    m. irregularity
    linear m.
    medial talar m.
    m. necrosis

    overhanging m.
    periarticular m.
    pleural m.
    posterior disk m.
    psoas m.
    m. of scapula
    scapular m.
    sclerotic m.
    sharp lateral m.
    spiculated m.
    stomach m.
    subcostal m.
    superomedial m.
    supraorbital m. (SOM)
    tumor m.
    vertebral body m.
marginal
    m. branch
    m. branch of left circumflex
     coronary artery
    m. branch of right coronary artery
    m. circumflex artery
    m. erosion
    m. exostosis
    m. fracture
    m. gyrus
    m. kidney depression
    obtuse m. (OM)
    m. osteophyte
    m. osteophyte formation
    m. placenta
    m. placenta previa
    m. ridge
    m. sclerosis
    m. serration
    m. sinus
    m. spur
    m. spurring
    m. syndesmophyte
    m. ulcer
    m. vein
    m. zone
    m. zone B-cell lymphoma
    m. zone lymphoma (MZL)
Marie-Bamberger disease
Marie-Strümpell disease
Marimastat
Marine-Lenhart syndrome
Mark
    M. II Kodros radiolucent awl
    M. V Plus automatic injector
marked
    m. hypoechogenicity shadowing
    m. sclerosis
    m. shunting of blood
markedly accentuated pulmonic
    component

marker
>   anatomic m.
>   external fiducial m.
>   fiducial skin m.
>   implanted imaging opaque m.
>   isotope-tagged m.
>   lead pellet m.
>   metallic m.
>   MicroMark tissue m.
>   myocardial-specific m.
>   needle m.
>   nipple m.
>   PINNACLE R/O II radiopaque m.
>   radioactive string m.
>   radiopaque gold m.
>   Sitzmarks radiopaque m.
>   m. transit imaging
>   m. transit study
>   tumor m.

marker-channel diagram

marking
>   absence of haustral m.
>   absence of vascular m.
>   accentuation of m.
>   bronchopulmonary m.
>   bronchovascular m.
>   bronchovesicular m.
>   coarse bronchovascular m.
>   confluence of vascular m.
>   convolutional m.
>   crowding of bronchovascular m.
>   digital m.
>   haustral m.
>   increased interstitial m.
>   increased pulmonary vascular m.
>   interstitial m.
>   linear m.
>   lung m.
>   peribronchial m.
>   perihilar m.
>   pullback arterial m.
>   pulmonary arterial m.
>   pulmonary vascular m.
>   sulcal m.
>   sutural m.
>   vascular m.

Markov
>   M. chain
>   M. chain Monte Carlo technique
>   M. random field

Marlex band

Maroteaux-Lamy syndrome

marrow
>   aberrant bone m.
>   m. agent bone scintigraphy
>   m. blush
>   bone m.
>   bright fatty m.
>   m. canal
>   cancellous hematopoietic m.
>   m. cavity
>   central nidus of high-intensity m.
>   m. dosimetry
>   m. edema pattern
>   epiphyseal hematopoietic m.
>   m. fat signal intensity
>   fatty m.
>   functional m.
>   hematopoietically active bone m.
>   hematopoietic bone m.
>   high-signal-intensity yellow m.
>   hypercellular reconverted bone m.
>   hypocellular m.
>   m. infarct
>   m. infiltrate
>   m. infiltration
>   island of red m.
>   peripheral hematopoietic
>   intermediate signal intensity m.
>   shunting of tracer to the bone m.
>   m. signal change
>   sternal m.
>   m. transplant
>   uptake in bone m.

Marshall vein

marshmallow bolus

Martin disease

Martorell
>   M. aortic arch syndrome
>   M. hypertensive ulcer
>   M. sign

masculine pelvis

masculinizing tumor

mask
>   convolution m.
>   m. data
>   ISAH stereotactic immobilizing m.
>   Orfit m.
>   particle m.
>   m. ventilation

mask-based approach

masking
>   unsharp m.
>   white m.

M

NOTES

Mason radial fracture classification
mason's lung
masquerading effect
mass
    abdominopelvic m.
    m. absorption coefficient
    adrenal cystic m.
    air-containing neck m.
    airless m.
    anechoic m.
    anterior mediastinal m.
    aortopulmonary window m.
    appendiceal m.
    apperceptive m.
    m. attenuation coefficient
    avascular brain m.
    avascular kidney m.
    avascular renal m.
    m. balance
    benign adrenal m.
    bilateral fetal chest m.
    bilateral renal m.
    bilobed m.
    brain m.
    calcified brain m.
    calcified intracranial m.
    calcified kidney m.
    calcified renal m.
    cardiophrenic right-angle m.
    carotid space m.
    cavitary m.
    cerebellar cystic m.
    circumscribed m.
    m. collision stopping power
    complex solid and cystic m.
    congenital nasal m.
    conglomerate m.
    conical m.
    cord intradural extramedullary m.
    cord-like m.
    critical m.
    cystic breast m.
    cystic teratomatous m.
    m. defect
    dense brain m.
    dense cerebral m.
    dirty m.
    discoid chest m.
    discrete m.
    doughy m.
    dumbbell brain m.
    dysplasia with associated lesion
      or m. (DALM)
    echogenic m.
    m. effect
    elongated m.
    encapsulated m.

    m. energy equivalence
    enhancing m.
    epidural m.
    expanding intracranial m.
    expansile m.
    external ear m.
    extracardiac m.
    extraosseous m.
    extraovarian m.
    extrapleural m.
    extrauterine pelvic m.
    extravascular m.
    fallopian tube m.
    fat-containing m.
    fat density m.
    fetal abdominal cystic m.
    fibrin m.
    firm m.
    fixed m.
    fleecy m.
    fluctuant m.
    fluid-filled kidney m.
    focal m.
    freely movable m.
    friable m.
    glenoid ovoid m.
    groin m.
    heterogeneous breast m.
    high-signal m.
    hilar m.
    homogeneous intrasellar m.
    hyperattenuated intrasellar m.
    hyperdense m.
    hyperechoic breast m.
    hyperintense m.
    hypervascular mediastinal m.
    hypoattenuating m.
    hypodense m.
    ill-defined m.
    m. imaging
    indurated m.
    inflammatory polypoid m.
    injection m.
    inner ear m.
    interbronchial m.
    intermediate signal intensity m.
    intraabdominal m.
    intracardiac m.
    intracaval fat m.
    intracavity m.
    intracranial m.
    intracystic solid m.
    intraductal solid m.
    intradural extramedullary m.
    intraluminal stomach m.
    intrasellar brain m.
    intrathoracic fetal m.

intrathoracic low-attenuation m.
intravascular m.
intraventricular m.
irregular m.
isodense m.
isoechoic breast m.
jugular foraminal m.
kidney sinus m.
lacrimal m.
large solid adrenal m.
lateral m.
lean m.
left ventricular m. (LVM)
m. lesion
liver m.
lobulated m.
loss of bone m.
low-attenuation mediastinal m.
lower lobe lung m.
low-signal m.
lung m.
lymphomatous m.
malignant adrenal m.
mammographic evaluation of
  breast m.
masticator space m.
mediastinal high-attenuation m.
mesenteric m.
middle ear m.
middle mediastinal m.
mixed attenuation m.
mixed density m.
mixed echogenic solid m.
mixed signal m.
mixed solid-cystic m.
mobile intraluminal gallbladder m.
molar m.
mulberry-like m.
multilobulated m.
multiloculated m.
mushroom-shaped m.
myocardial m.
nasal vault m.
nasopharyngeal m.
nodular m.
noncalcified nodular m.
nonhemorrhagic m.
nonhomogeneous hyperdense m.
nonopaque intraluminal m.
nonpulsatile abdominal m.
m. number
omental m.

orbital superolateral quadrant m.
ovarian m.
pancreatic m.
paraaortic m.
paracardiac m.
paranasal sinus m.
parasagittal intracranial m.
parasellar brain m.
paraspinal soft tissue m.
paravertebrally situated pelvic
  tumor m.
paravertebrally situated thoracic
  tumor m.
paucilocular cystic m.
pelvic cystic m.
periosseous soft tissue m.
perirenal m.
peritoneal m.
perivascular m.
petrous apex dumbbell m.
pharyngeal space m.
phlegmonous m.
phosphaturic m.
pineal m.
pleural m.
polypoid calcified irregular m.
porta hepatis low-density m.
posterior mediastinal m.
prepubertal testicular m.
presacral m.
prevertebral space m.
promontory m.
pulmonary m.
pulsating m.
red cell m. (RCM)
relativistic m.
renal sinus m.
reniform m.
retrobulbar m.
retrocardiac m.
retroperitoneal m.
retropharyngeal space m.
retrosternal m.
right cardiophrenic angle m.
right ventricular m. (RVM)
ring-enhancing m.
saccular m.
scrotal m.
soft tissue density m.
solid m.
solitary m.
sonolucent cystic m.

M

NOTES

mass *(continued)*
    space-occupying m.
    m. spectrometer
    spherical m.
    spiculated m.
    stellate m.
    stony m.
    subareolar m.
    subinsular m.
    suprasellar m.
    suspicious m.
    teratomatous m.
    thalamic-hypothalamic m.
    thymic m.
    m. thymus
    thyroid m.
    tissue m.
    torsed ovarian m.
    tubal m.
    tuboovarian m.
    tubular fluid-density adnexal m.
    tumor m.
    umbilical m.
    uncinate process m.
    unilateral adrenal m.
    unilateral fetal chest m.
    unilateral kidney m.
    urinary bladder extrinsic m.
    urinary bladder wall m.
    uterine m.
    ventricular m.
    wedge-shaped m.
    well-circumscribed breast m.
    well-defined m.
    woody m.
Massachusetts (General Hospital) Utility Multiprogramming System
mass-effect hydrocephalus
masseteric enlargement
masseter muscle
massive
    m. aortic regurgitation
    m. ascites
    m. embolus
    m. exsanguinating hemorrhage
    m. fibrosis
    m. hepatic necrosis
    m. herniated disk
    m. infiltrate
    m. osteolysis
    m. ovarian edema
    m. pleural effusion
    m. pneumonia
    m. pulmonary hemorrhagic edema
massively enlarged heart

mass-like
    m.-l. configuration
    m.-l. lesion
Masson body
MAST
    military antishock trousers
    motion artifact suppression technique
      MAST suit
mast
    m. cell-enhancing activity
    m. cell reticulosis
    m. leukocyte
mastectomy
    non-skin-sparing m. (non-SSM)
master knot of Henry
masticator
    m. muscle
    m. space
    m. space infection
    m. space mass
mastitis
    m. fibrosa cystica
    m. obliterans
mastocytosis
    bone m.
    GI tract m.
    systemic m.
mastoid
    m. antrum
    m. bone
    m. canal
    m. complex
    m. fontanelle
    m. foramen
    m. lymph node
    m. polytomography
    m. process
    m. sinus
    m. suture
mastopathy
    fibrous m.
mastoplasia
    cystic m.
match
    nontransmural m.
    transmural m.
    triple m.
matched peripheral dose (MPD)
matching
    atlas m.
    electron-photon field m.
    general pattern m.
    impedance m.
    m. network
matchline wedge
material *(See agent, contrast, medium)*
    anthracotic m.

atheromatous m.
ballistic m.
byproduct m.
coffee grounds m.
collection of contrast m.
columnization of contrast m.
contrast m.
dental contrast m.
embolic m.
extraneous m.
fecal m.
ferromagnetic m.
flow of contrast m.
inspissated m.
Interpore bone replacement m.
intravenous administration of
  contrast m.
iodinated contrast m.
layering of contrast m.
lipid-rich m.
magnetic m.
nonionic contrast m.
opaque m.
^{103}Pd radioactive m.
PET target m.
phosphaturic m.
radioactive m.
m. spin echocardiogram total
  volume imaging
superabsorbent polymer embolic m.
target m.
trophoblastic m.
uptake of radioactive m.
vessel cutoff of contrast m.

maternal
m. lake
m. placenta

**Mathews classification of olecranon
fracture**

matrix, pl. **matrices**
acquisition m.
bone tumor m.
calcific m.
m. calculus
cartilage m.
chondroid m.
decision m.
demineralized bone m. (DBM)
extracellular m.
germinal bleed m.
m. image
m. injury

k-space m.
M. LR3300 laser imaging
m. metalloprotease-3 (MMP-3)
m. mineralization
nuclear m.
osteoid m.
proteoglycan m.
quantization m. (QM)
reduced-acquisition m. (RAM)
m. size
solid m.
stromal m.
transformation m.
tumor m.

matted
m. bowel loop
m. small-bowel loop

matter
cortical gray m.
cortical white m.
cytotoxic edema of the gray m.
deep white ischemia m.
gray m.
heterotopic gray m.
infratentorial gray m.
particulate m.
periaqueductal gray m.
perilesional white m.
peritrigonal white m.
periventricular gray m.
periventricular white m.
pulverized plaque particulate m.
PVG m.
scalloped appearance of white m.
shearing of white m.
supratentorial gray m.
supratentorial white m.
white m.

maturation
bone m.
disk m.
m. index
pulmonary structural m.
skeletal m.

mature
m. bone
m. mediastinum teratoma
m. ovarian cystic teratoma
m. pancreatic pseudocyst
m. pseudocyst of pancreas
skeletally m.
m. vertebra

M

NOTES

maturity of fetus
Mauchart ligament
MAVIS
   mobile artery and vein imaging system
maxicamera
maxilla, pl. maxillae
maxillary
   m. antrum
   m. artery
   m. bone
   m. canal
   m. division
   m. fracture
   m. nerve anatomy
   m. process
   m. sinus
   m. sinus carcinoma
   m. sinus hypoplasia
   m. sinus opacification
   m. sinus puncture
   m. sinus radiograph
   m. spine
maxillofacial
   m. fracture
   m. imaging
Maxima II TENS unit
maximal
   m. estimated gradient
   m. intensity
   m. radiographic distention
   m. transaortic jet velocity
   m. volume of left atrium
   m. voluntary ventilation (MVV)
maximization
   ordered subset expectation m. (OSEM)
maximum
   m. amplitude constant
   m. anteroposterior diameter
   m. density (D_{max})
   m. diameter to minimum diameter ratio
   m. entropy processing
   full width at half m. (FWHM)
   m. inflation pressure
   m. inflation time
   m. intensity pixel (MIP)
   m. intensity projection (MIP)
   m. intensity projection algorithm
   m. intensity projection imaging
   m. intensity projection and source image
   m. likelihood algorithm
   m. midexpiratory flow (MMEF)
   m. midexpiratory flow rate (MMFR)
   m. permissible body burden

   m. permissible concentration
   m. predicted heart rate (MPHR)
   m. slew rate ramp
   time delay between excitation and echo m. (TE)
   m. venous outflow (MVO)
   m. ventricular elastance
maximum-intensity sliding thin slab projection
maximus
   gluteus m.
Max Plus MR scanner
Maxwell
   M. coil
   M. 3D field simulator
   M. pair
   M. theory of radiation
maxwellian distribution
Mayer
   M. position
   M. view
Mayer-Rokitansky-Küster-Hauser syndrome
May-Hegglin anomaly
Mayneord F factor
May-Thurner syndrome
Mazabraud syndrome
Mazur ankle evaluation classification
M-band myeloma
MBF
   myocardial blood flow
MB fraction
MBS-MRA
   minimum basis set magnetic resonance angiography
mC
   microcurie
MCA
   middle cerebral artery
   multichannel analyzer
   multiple congenital anomalies
MCAT
   myocardial contrast appearance time
McBurney point
McCabe-Fletcher classification
McCallum patch
McCune-Albright syndrome
MCD
   mean central dose
   molecular coincidence detection
   multicentric Castleman disease
     MCD imaging
MCDK
   multicystic dysplastic kidney
MCE
   myocardial contrast echocardiography

MCFSR
  mean circumferential fiber shortening
  rate
McGinn-White sign
McGregor line
Mci
  megacurie
mCi
  millicurie
mCi-hr
  millicurie-hour
McIlwain tissue chopper
MCK
  multicystic kidney
McKee line
McKusick-Kaufman syndrome
McKusick-type
  M.-t. metaphyseal chondrodysplasia
  M.-t. metaphyseal dysplasia
MCL
  mantle cell lymphoma
  medial collateral ligament
  midclavicular line
  MCL bursa
**McLain-Weinstein spinal tumor
  classification**
MCLC
  medial collateral ligament complex
MCLS
  mucocutaneous lymph node syndrome
McMurray test
McNamara coaxial catheter infusion set
MCP
  metacarpophalangeal
MCPJ
  metacarpophalangeal joint
MCPT
  Monte Carlo photon transport
  MCPT simulation
McRae line
MCS
  middle coronary sinus
MCT
  mean circulation time
MCTC
  metrizamide computed tomography
  cisternography
MCTD
  mixed connective-tissue disease
MCU
  micturating cystourethrogram

MDAC
  multiplying digital-to-analog converter
MDCT
  multidetector CT
  multidetector-row CT
MD-Gastroview imaging agent
MDP
  methylene diphosphonate
  TechneScan MDP
MDS-2000 microwave irradiator
MDT
  minimal deformation target
Meadows syndrome
meal
  barium m.
  Boyden test m.
  double-contrast barium m.
  Ewald test m.
  fatty m.
  isotope m.
  motor test m.
  opaque m.
  retention m.
  small bowel m.
  test m.
mean
  m. ankle-brachial systolic pressure
    index
  m. aortic flow velocity
  m. aortic pressure
  m. arterial pressure (MAP)
  m. blood pressure
  m. brachial artery pressure
  m. cardiac vector
  m. central dose (MCD)
  m. circulating time
  m. circulation time (MCT)
  m. circulatory filling pressure
  m. circumferential fiber shortening
    rate (MCFSR)
  m. corpuscular volume
  m. deviation
  m. diffusivity
  m. examination time
  m. free path
  m. gonad dose
  m. left atrial pressure
  m. mitral valve gradient
  m. perfusate temperature
  m. posterior wall velocity
  m. pulmonary artery pressure
    (MPAP)

M

NOTES

mean *(continued)*
    m. pulmonary artery wedge pressure
    m. pulmonary capillary pressure (MPCP)
    m. pulmonary flow velocity
    m. pulmonary transit time (MTT)
    m. right atrial pressure
    m. sac diameter (MSD)
    m. systolic gradient
    m. transit time (MTT)
    m. venous pulsation
    m. wall motion score
    m. wall motion score index
mean-diameter overframing
mean-square error
Meary metatarsotalar angle
measles pneumonia
measurable endpoint
measure
    linear m.
measurement
    ankle-brachial pressure m.
    antegrade perfusion pressure m. (APPM)
    appendicular bone mass m.
    attenuation m.
    automated cardiac flow m. (ACM)
    blood flow m.
    body composition m.
    bolus passage perfusion m.
    bone density m.
    breath pentane m.
    cardiac output m.
    cerebrospinal fluid flow m.
    Cerenkov m.
    Cobb m.
    densitometric m.
    diode m.
    Dixon fat-fraction m.
    end-diastolic velocity m.
    excitation function m.
    fat-fraction m.
    fetal foot length m.
    fetal long bone m.
    flow cytometric DNA m.
    gestational sac m.
    Hausdorff m.
    high-sensitivity m.
    hila m.
    histomorphometric m.
    indicator-dilution method for cardiac output m.
    intercomparison m.
    line-pair m.
    low-energy photon attenuation m.
    mammographic m.

    manometric m.
    microbubble concentration m.
    morphometric m.
    nondynamometric trunk strength m.
    nutation angle m.
    occlusion m.
    orbit m.
    phase-sensitive flow m.
    photon attenuation m.
    polarographic needle electrode m.
    pressure m.
    pulsatility m.
    pulse-echo distance m.
    quantitative regional myocardial flow m.
    regional washout m.
    renal length m.
    rocking curve m.
    root-mean-squared gradient m.
    segmental correction using x-ray m.
    segmental pressure m.
    semiquantitative m.
    signal intensity m.
    TCD m.
    temperature distribution m.
    thermodilution method of cardiac output m.
    thyroid uptake m.
    time-of-flight flow m.
    time-velocity m.
    topographic m.
    transcutaneous oxygen pressure m. ($tcPO_2$)
    true conjugate m.
    U1-NA cephalometric m.
    m. in vivo
    whole-brain magnetization transfer m.
    Wits m.
    xenon CT m.
    Z-score in bone mineral density m.
meatal segment
meatus, pl. **meati**
    acoustic m.
    external auditory m.
    internal auditory m.
    nasal m.
meat wrapper's lung
mebrofenin
mechanical
    m. augmentation
    m. axis
    m. biliary obstruction
    m. compound scan
    m. counterpulsation

m. duct obstruction
m. extrahepatic obstruction
m. genu varus
m. ileus
m. insufflation
m. insult
m. intestinal obstruction
m. potential energy
m. respiratory tract obstruction
m. sector scanner
m. small bowel obstruction
m. thrombectomy
m. thrombolysis
m. valve
m. ventilation
mechanically
m. activated implant
m. detachable platinum coil
m. sealed
mechanics
intramural m.
mechanism
blood-clotting m.
central extensor m. (CEM)
check-valve m.
compensatory m.
contrecoup m.
deglutition m.
excitotoxic m.
extensor m.
flap-valve m.
Frank-Starling m.
heart rate reserve m.
homing m.
humeral m.
m. of injury
internal retention m.
iron-transporting protein m.
Laplace m.
osseous pinch m.
pinchcock m.
propulsive m.
sinus m.
sodium-potassium ATPase dependent
   exchange m.
sphincteric m.
swallowing m.
Taylor-Blackwood m.
ventricular escape m.
watershed m.
Mecholyl test

Meckel
M. band
M. cavity
M. diverticulitis
M. diverticulum
M. ligament
M. plane
M. scan
M. syndrome
Meckel-Gruber syndrome
meclofenamic acid
meconium
m. aspiration
m. aspiration syndrome
m. ileus
m. ileus equivalent
m. peristalsis
m. peritonitis
m. plug
m. plug syndrome
m. pseudocyst
**MEDDARS cardiac catheterization
   analysis system**
media (*pl. of* medium)
media-adventitia interface
medial
m. angle
m. arch
m. arteriosclerosis
m. aspect
m. basal segmental bronchus
m. border
m. calcific sclerosis
m. carpal capsule
m. collateral ligament (MCL)
m. collateral ligament calcification
m. collateral ligament complex
   (MCLC)
m. column calcaneal fracture
m. compartment
m. condyle
m. crus
m. cuneiform bone
m. cystic necrosis
m. dissection
m. eminence
m. end of clavicle osteolysis
m. epicondylar bursa
m. epicondyle
m. epicondyle fracture
m. epicondylitis
m. extension

M

NOTES

medial (*continued*)
  m. femoral buttressing
  m. fibroplasia
  m. geniculate body
  m. geniculate fascia
  m. hyperplasia
  m. joint line
  m. joint space
  m. and lateral support structures of
    the knee
  m. lemniscus
  m. longitudinal fasciculus (MLF)
  m. longitudinal fasciculus lesion
  m. malleolar fracture
  m. malleolus
  m. malleolus periostitis
  m. oblique axial projection
  m. oblique view
  m. occipitotemporal gyrus
  m. papillary muscle
  m. physis
  m. plantar artery
  m. plica
  m. posterior choroidal (MPCh)
  m. pterygoid muscle
  m. rotation
  m. sagittal plane
  m. sesamoid bone
  m. shelf
  m. supraclavicular node
  m. talar dome injury
  m. talar margin
  m. talar osteochondral injury
  m. temporal lobe
  m. tibial stress syndrome
  m. traction spur
medialis
  meniscus m.
  vastus m.
medially
median
  m. antebrachial vein
  m. arcuate ligament
  m. arcuate ligament of diaphragm
  m. bar
  m. cleft lip
  m. cruciate ligament
  m. facial cleft
  m. lethal dose
  m. level echo
  m. line
  m. lip cleft
  m. lobe of prostate
  multiples of the m.
  m. nerve
  m. nerve entrapment
  m. nerve lesion

  m. palatine suture
  m. raphe
  m. raphe plane
  m. sacral artery
  m. sagittal plane
  m. septum
  m. umbilical ligament
mediastinal
  m. abscess
  m. adenoma
  m. adenopathy
  m. air
  m. angiolipoma
  m. arterial variant
  m. border
  m. bronchogenic cyst
  m. bulk
  m. collagenosis
  m. cross-sectional imaging
  m. crunch
  m. deviation
  m. dorsal enteric cyst
  m. duplication cyst
  m. emphysema
  m. fat
  m. fat edema
  m. fibrosis
  m. fistula
  m. granuloma
  m. hematoma
  m. hemorrhage
  m. hernia
  m. high-attenuation mass
  m. invasion
  m. lesion
  m. lipomatosis
  m. lung surface
  m. lymph node enlargement
  m. lymphoma
  m. node
  m. panniculitis
  m. pleura
  m. pleurisy
  m. prominence
  m. pseudomass
  m. retraction
  m. seminoma
  m. septum
  m. seroma
  m. shift
  m. structure
  m. teratoid tumor
  m. thickening
  m. thyroid tissue
  m. tube
  m. uptake
  m. vein

m. viscus
m. wedge
m. widening
m. window
mediastinitis
fibrosing m.
idiopathic fibrous m.
sclerosing m.
mediastinogram
mediastinography
gas m.
gaseous m.
opaque m.
mediastinoscopy
mediastinum
anterior m.
m. cerebelli
m. cerebri
m. dermoid
deviated m.
m. displacement
m. dysgerminoma
epidermoid m.
m. germinoma
inferior m.
left m.
m. lipoma
lipomatosis m.
lobulated paratracheal m.
middle m.
posterior m.
right m.
seminoma m.
superior m.
m. teratocarcinoma
teratoid m.
m. teratoma
m. testis
widened m.
medical
m. cyclotron
m. holography
m. internal radiation dosimetry
(MIRD)
M. Ultrasound Three-Dimensional
Portable Advanced
Communications (MUSTPAC)
m. umbilical fold
medicamentosa
thyrotoxicosis m.

medicine
Fellow of the American College of
Nuclear M.
nuclear m.
photonic m.
Medigraphics analyzer
**Medilase angioscope-laser delivery
system**
MedImage scanner
Medinvent
**mediobasal hypothalamus luteinizing
hormone-releasing hormone**
mediolateral
m. aspect
m. flow direction
m. oblique (MLO)
m. oblique projection
m. oblique view
m. radiocarpal angle
m. stress
m. view (MLO)
medionecrosis
cystic m.
medionodular cirrhosis
mediopatellar
MediPort catheter
Medison scanner
Medi-tech
M.-t. catheter
M.-t. ureteral stent system
medium, pl. **media** (*See* agent, contrast,
material)
barium sulfate contrast m.
benzoic acid contrast m.
bismuth contrast m.
brominized oil contrast m.
bullet kit culture m.
m. caliber
cerebral contrast m.
contrast m. (CM)
delayed excretion of contrast m.
diatrizoic acid contrast m.
endogenous adenosine contrast m.
Entero Vu contrast m.
EntroEase oral radiopaque
contrast m.
ethiodized oil contrast m.
ethyliodophenylundecyl contrast m.
extraluminal contrast m.
FDDNP PET scan contrast m.
galactose contrast m.
Gd-DOTA contrast m.

M

NOTES

medium *(continued)*
glucaric acid-labeled contrast m.
hand injection of contrast m.
high-osmolarity contrast m.
(HOCM)
hyperconcentration of contrast m.
Imagopaque contrast m.
intravascular contrast m.
intravenous contrast m.
iodide contrast m.
iodinated intravascular contrast m.
iodinated radiologic contrast m.
(IRCM)
iodine-containing contrast m.
iodixanol contrast m.
iodophendylate contrast m.
ioglunide contrast m.
ioglycamic acid contrast m.
Iomeron 150, 250, 300, 350
contrast m.
ionic dimer contrast m.
ionic monomeric contrast m.
ionic paramagnetic contrast m.
iopromide contrast m.
iotroxamide contrast m.
ioxaglic acid contrast m.
ioxithalamate contrast m.
isoefamate contrast m.
Isopaque contrast m.
isosmolar contrast m. (IOCM)
kinetic energy released per unit
mass and kinetic energy released
in m. (kerma)
low-osmolar contrast m. (LOCM)
macromolecular contrast m.
(MMCM)
magnesium contrast m.
manganese chloride contrast m.
meglumine salts contrast m.
methylglucamine contrast m.
Micropaque contrast m.
nephrotoxic contrast m.
Niopam contrast m.
nonionic dimer contrast m.
nonionic water-soluble contrast m.
oil-soluble contrast m. (OSCM)
opaque m.
potassium bromide contrast m.
radiochromic dosimetry m.
radiological contrast m.
radiolucent m.
radiopaque m.
rectal contrast m.
Resovist MR contrast m.
Solutrast 200, 250, 300, 370
contrast m.
sonicated saline contrast m.

tantalum-178 contrast m.
Telebrix contrast m.
tetraiodophenolphthalein contrast m.
topical water-soluble contrast m.
triiodobenzoic acid contrast m.
Triosil contrast m.
tunica m.
Uromiro contrast m.
water-soluble contrast m. (WSCM)
Xenetix 250, 300, 350 contrast m.
medium-detachment-pressure
medium-energy collimator
medium-sized bronchus
medius
digitus m.
gluteus m.
scalenus m.
Medos Hakim programmable valve
Medrad
M. automated power injector
M. contrast medium injector
M. Mrinnervu endorectal colon
probe coil
M. power angiographic injector
medronate
m. scan
Medsonic plethysmography
Medspec
M. MR imaging system
M. MR imaging system scanner
M. 30/80 tesla MR scanner
Med Tec Vac Loc immobilization
system
Medtronic
M. catheter
M. Minix
M. Pulsor Intrasound
M. radiofrequency receiver
medulla, pl. **medullae**
adrenal m.
hyperechoic renal m.
lymphatic m.
m. oblongata
ovarian m.
renal m.
rostral m.
spinal m.
medullare
corpus m.
osteoma m.
medullaris
artery of the conus m.
conus arteriosus m.
m. hypoplasia
low conus m.
medullary
m. artery

m. bone
m. bone infarct
m. breast carcinoma
m. calcification
m. canal
m. cavity
m. cone
m. cord
m. cystic disease
m. lamina
m. nephrocalcinosis
m. nephrogram
m. pyramid
m. rod
m. sinus
m. sponge
m. sponge kidney
m. tegmentum
m. thyroid carcinoma
m. vein
m. venous anatomy
medullary-type adenocarcinoma
medulloblastoma
m. metastasis
vermian m.
medusae
caput m.
Medusa hair-like opacity
Medweb clinical reporting system
Medx
M. camera
M. scanner
Mees line
mefenamic acid
MEG
magnetoencephalography
megabulb
jugular m.
megabulbus
duodenum m.
megacalicosis
mega cisterna magna
megacolon
acquired m.
aganglionic m.
congenital m.
m. dilatation
idiopathic m.
toxic m.
megacurie (Mci)
megacystic microcolon

megacystis-microcolon-intestinal hypoperistalsis syndrome
megaduodenum
megaesophagus of achalasia
megahertz (MHz)
megalencephaly
unilateral m.
MEGALINK stent
megalocornea
megalocystis
megaloencephaly
megalosplenia
megalothymus
megaloureter
megalourethra
megarectum
megaureter
primary m.
primary congenital m.
megavolt (MeV, MV)
m. therapy
megavoltage
m. grid
m. grid therapy
m. radiation
m. radiation therapy
m. radiotherapy
m. treatment beam
m. x-ray therapy
meglumine
m. acetrizoate
m. diatrizoate
gadoterate m.
iocarmate m.
iodipamide m.
m. iodipamide imaging agent
iodoxamate m.
m. iotroxate imaging agent
ioxaglate m.
m. salts contrast medium
megophthalmos
meibomian
m. cyst
m. gland carcinoma
Meiboom-Gill sequence
Meige lymphedema
Meigs
M. capillary
M. syndrome
Meigs-Cass syndrome
Meigs-Salmon syndrome
Meissner plexus

M

NOTES

melanosis coli
melanotic
    m. carcinoma
    m. neuroectodermal tumor
    m. whitlow
Melnick-Needles syndrome
Melone distal radius fracture
  classification
melorheostosis
    m. of Leri
    soft tissue pathoanatomy in m.
Melrose solution
melting sign
Meltzer sign
memberment
membranacea
    placenta m.
membranaceous tendon
membranaceum
membrane
    amnionic m.
    atlantooccipital m.
    Bichat m.
    m. of bone
    m. closure time
    cricothyroid m.
    glial limiting m.
    glomerular basement m. (GBM)
    hourglass m.
    interosseous m. (IOM)
    intertwin m.
    intraluminal m.
    intrauterine m.
    Liliequist m.
    limiting m.
    low-flux polysufone m.
    microporous m.
    mucous m.
    obturator m.
    m. oxygenator
    m. permeability
    m. phosphate
    rolling m.
    serous m.
    Shrapnell m.
    synovial m.
    Transwell m.
    vernix m.
membranous
    m. bronchiole
    m. glomerulonephritis
    m. labyrinth
    m. obstruction of inferior vena
      cava
    m. pregnancy
    m. septum
    m. subaortic stenosis

    m. subvalvular aortic stenosis
    m. urethra
    m. ventricular septal defect
    m. viscerocranium
memory
    Aloka color Doppler real-time 2D
      blood flow imaging with cine m.
    thermal shape m.
memory-intensive algorithm
Memotherm Nitinol self-expandable
  stent
MEMP
    multiecho multiplane
    contiguous slice MEMP (CSMEMP)
MEN
    multiple endocrine neoplasia
Mendelson syndrome
Ménétrier disease
Mengert index
Menghini
Mèniére
    M. disease
    M. syndrome
meningeal
    m. artery
    m. artery groove
    m. cell tumor
    m. enhancement
    m. fibroma
    m. fibrosis
    m. hemangiopericytoma
    m. hemorrhage
    m. infiltrate
    m. inflammation
    middle m.
    m. sarcoma
    m. tuberculosis
    m. vein
meninges (*pl. of* meninx)
meningioangiomatosis
meningioma
    angioplastic m.
    atypical m.
    cavernous sinus m.
    cerebellopontine angle m.
    clival m.
    convexity m.
    m. of cribriform plate
    cystic intraparenchymal m.
    ectopic m.
    endotheliomatous m.
    m. en plaque
    extracranial m.
    falcine m.
    falcotentorial m.
    fibroblastic m.
    fibrous m.

globular m.
intraosseous m.
intraparenchymal m.
intraventricular m.
lipoblastic m.
malignant m.
meningothelial m.
meningotheliomatous m.
multicentric m.
olfactory groove m.
optic nerve sheath m.
parasagittal m.
perioptic m.
posterior fossa m.
m. of posterior fossa
psammoma body m.
psammomatous m.
pulmonary m.
sphenoid ridge m.
sphenoid wing m.
sphenoorbital m.
spinal m.
subfrontal m.
suprasellar m.
temporal m.
tentorial m.
transitional m.
tuberculum sellae m.
meningiomatosis
meningitis, pl. **meningitides**
cryptococcal m.
fungal m.
meningocele
anterior sacral m.
anterior thoracic m.
cervical m.
cranial m.
dorsal m.
lateral lumbar m.
lateral thoracic m.
occipital m.
occult intrasacral m.
sacral m.
simple m.
traumatic m.
meningoencephalitis
meningoencephalocele
ethmoidal m.
sphenopharyngeal m.
meningofacial angiomatosis

meningohypophyseal
m. artery
m. trunk
meningomyelocele
meningothelial-like nodule
meningothelial meningioma
meningotheliomatous meningioma
meninx, pl. **meninges**
meninges of brain
meninges of spinal cord
meniscal
m. cleft
m. fragmentation
m. horn
m. injury
m. ossicle
menisci (*pl. of* meniscus)
meniscocapsular
m. attachment
m. junction
m. separation
meniscocondylar coordination
meniscofemoral
m. attachment
m. ligament
meniscosynovial junction
meniscotibial
m. attachment
m. ligament
m. separation
meniscus, pl. **menisci**
articular m.
m. articularis
discoid lateral m.
diverging m.
dysplastic m.
fibrocartilaginous m.
free-floating m.
m. lateralis
m. medialis
radiohumeral m.
m. sign
m. tear
meniscus-shaped calcification
Menkes syndrome
Mennell sign
mensuration algorithm
mental
m. canal
m. spine
mentoanterior
mentooccipital diameter

M

NOTES

mentoparietal diameter
Mentor prostatic biopsy needle
mentum
Menzel olivopontocerebellar degeneration
meralgia paresthetica
mercaptoacetyltriglycine (MAG-3)
    technetium-99m m.
mercaptoacetythiglycine
    ^{99m}Tc m.
Mercator
    M. atrial high-density array
      catheter
    M. projection
Merchant
    M. angle
    M. view
Mercuhydrin
mercurihydroxypropane
1-mercuri-2-hydroxypropane (MHP)
mercury
    m. arc lamp
    m. artifact
    millimeters of m. (mmHg, mm Hg)
    m. vapor lamp
Meridian echocardiography
Merkel
    M. cell carcinoma
    M. cell carcinoma cell line
Merland perimedullary arteriovenous
  fistula classification
mermaid
    m. deformity
    m. syndrome
meroacrania
merosin
merosin-deficient congenital muscular
  dystrophy
mertiatide
    technetium-99m m.
mesalamine enema
mesatipellic pelvis
mesencephalic
    m. artery
    m. cerebral lymphoma
    m. cistern
    m. cistern effacement
    m. infarct
    m. low-density brain lesion
    m. reticular formation
    m. tract
    m. vein
mesencephalitis
mesencephalodiencephalic lesion
mesencephalon aqueduct
mesenchymal
    m. abnormality
    m. chondrosarcoma

    m. liver hamartoma
    m. neoplasm
    m. tissue
    m. tumor
mesenchymoma
    atrial m.
    benign m.
    chest wall m.
mesenterial
    m. Castleman lymphoma
    m. sarcoma
mesenteric
    m. adenitis
    m. adenitis-ileitis complex
    m. adenopathy
    m. angiography
    m. apoplexy
    m. arterial thrombosis
    m. arteriography
    m. artery
    m. artery occlusion
    m. attachment
    m. border
    m. calcification
    m. cyst
    m. fat stranding
    m. fibromatosis
    m. fibrosis
    m. fistula
    m. infarct
    m. ischemia
    m. lipodystrophy
    m. lymphadenopathy
    m. lymph node pathology
    m. lymphoma
    m. mass
    m. metastasis
    m. node
    m. panniculitis (MP)
    m. phlegmon
    m. pregnancy
    m. rupture
    m. sclerosis
    superior m.
    m. tear
    m. thromboembolism (MTE)
    m. tissue
    m. triangle
    m. tuberculosis
    m. vascular insufficiency
    m. vascular lesion
    m. vascular occlusion
    m. vasculitis (MV)
    m. vein
    m. venous thrombosis
    m. vessel
    m. Weber-Christian disease

mesentericoparietal fossa
mesenteritis
    chronic fibrosing m.
    fibrosing m.
    liposclerotic m.
    retractile m.
    sclerosing m.
mesenterium commune
mesenteroaxial volvulus
mesentery
    fan-shaped m.
    fatty m.
    intestinal m.
    ischemic m.
    leaf of m.
    lymphangioma m.
    root of m.
    small intestine m.
    ventral m.
    Weber-Christian m.
mesh
    stent m.
    tantalum m.
    tubular wire m.
mesial
    m. aspect
    m. frontal focus
    m. hemisphere
    m. hyperperfusion
    m. temporal epileptogenic lesion
    m. temporal sclerosis
mesial-frontal cortex
mesiodens
mesiodistal plane
mesoappendix
mesoblastic nephroma
mesocardia
mesocaval shunt
mesocephalic head shape
mesocolic
    m. band
    m. shelf
mesocolon
    sigmoid m.
    transverse m.
mesocolonic
    m. fat
    m. vessel
mesocuneiform bone
mesoderm
    extraembryonic m.

mesodermal
    m. dysplasia
    m. sarcoma
mesomelia
mesomelic
    m. dwarfism
    m. dysplasia
mesometanephric carcinoma
mesonephric kidney
mesonephros, pl. **mesonephroi**
mesoporphyrine
    Bid-Gd m.
mesorectum
mesosigmoid colon
mesosternum
mesothelial cyst
mesothelioma
    asbestos-related m.
    atrioventricular nodal node m.
    benign m.
    cystic m.
    diffuse malignant peritoneal m.
    epithelioid malignant m.
    fibrosing m.
    localized fibrous m.
    malignant pleural m.
    malignant pulmonary m.
    peritoneal m.
    pleural m.
mesothorium
mesotympanum
mesoversion of heart
MESS
    multiple echo single shot
mesylate
    fenoldopam m.
metabolic
    m. alteration
    m. bone disease
    m. bone disorder
    m. bone series
    m. bone survey
    m. calculus
    m. cardiomyopathy
    m. cirrhosis
    m. lesion
    m. rate of oxygen
    m. response
    m. stone
    m. tracer uptake
metabolically inert area

M

NOTES

metabolism
    calcium m.
    carbon m.
    cerebral m.
    evaluation of glucose m.
    fat m.
    fatty acid m.
    hepatic m.
    myocardial m.
    oxidative m.
    phosphorus m.
metacarpal
    base of m.
    m. bone
    m. fracture
    m. index
    m. length
    m. sign
metacarpoglenoidal ligament
metacarpophalangeal (MCP)
    m. articulation
    m. bone marrow development
    m. joint (MCPJ)
    m. length
    m. ligament
metacarpus
metachronous
    m. lesion
    m. metastasis
    m. transitional cell carcinoma
metadiaphyseal
metadiaphysis
metaiodobenzylguanidine (MIBG)
    ^{123}I m.
    iodine-131 m.
metal
    m. chelate complex
    Co-Cr-W-Ni alloy implant m.
    lanthanide m.
    m. line-pair phantom
    Lipowitz m.
    radioactive m.
    m. technetium target
    transition m.
metallic
    m. artifact
    m. biliary endoprosthesis
    m. cage
    m. debris
    m. density
    m. distal end of tube
    m. echo
    m. foreign body (MFB)
    m. fragment
    m. marker
    m. needle
    m. otologic implant

    m. pointer
    m. rod fixation
    m. screw
    m. staple
    m. stent
    m. suture
    m. tip cannula
    m. track of bullet
metalloporphyrin
metalloprotease
    matrix m.-3 (MMP-3)
metanephric
    m. diverticulum
    m. vesicle
metanephros, pl. metanephroi
metaphyseal, metaphysial
    m. abscess
    m. chondrodysplasia
    m.-diaphyseal angle
    m. dysostosis
    m. dysplasia
    m. extension
    m. fibrous defect
    m. flare
    m. fracture
    m. lucent band
    m. metaphysis
metaphyseal-diaphyseal
    m.-d. junction
    m.-d. low-signal-intensity red
      marrow inhomogeneity
metaphyseal-epiphyseal angle
metaphysial (*var. of* metaphyseal)
metaphysis, pl. metaphyses
    agnogenic myeloid m.
    autoparenchymatous m.
    celomic m.
    columnar m.
    frayed m.
    fundic m.
    humeral m.
    intestinal m.
    metaphyseal m.
    myeloid m.
    primary myeloid m.
    secondary myeloid m.
    squamous m.
metaplasia
    agnogenic myeloid m.
    apocrine m.
    articular m.
    cartilaginous m.
    intestinal m.
    keratinizing squamous m.
    monarticular synovium-based
      cartilage m.
    osseous m.

osteocartilaginous m.
squamous m.
metaplastic
m. carcinoma
m. polyp
metapneumonic
m. empyema
m. pleurisy
metastable
m. radionuclide
m. state
m. trap
metastasis, pl. **metastases**
adnexal m.
adrenal m.
aortic node m.
axillary node m.
blastic m.
bone m.
brain m.
breast m.
calcareous m.
calcified ovarian metastases
calcifying m.
carcinomatous cavitary m.
cavitary m.
cavitating lung m.
celiac lymph node m.
cerebral m.
clivus m.
cystic m.
diffuse skeletal m.
distant m.
drop m.
echogenic liver m.
endobronchial m.
extracapsular m.
extrahepatic m. (EHM)
extrathoracic m.
gastric m.
hemorrhagic m.
hepatic m.
hypervascular liver m.
inguinal lymph node m.
intracranial m.
in-transit m.
intraparenchymal m.
kidney m.
leptomeningeal m.
liver m.
local m.
lung m.

lymphangitic m.
lymphatic m.
lymphogenous m.
magnetic resonance discriminator of osseous m.
medulloblastoma m.
mesenteric m.
metachronous m.
micronodular m.
MR discriminator of osseous m.
necrotic m.
neuroendocrine hepatic m.
nodal m.
occult bone m.
orbital m.
osseous m.
osteoblastic m.
osteolytic osseous m.
ovarian m.
m. to the pancreas
pancreatic m.
paracardiac m.
parasellar m.
parenchymal brain m.
peritoneal m.
placental m.
pleura m.
pulmonary m.
pulsating m.
renal m.
satellite m.
skeletal m.
skip m.
small bowel m.
solitary sternal m.
sphenoid sinus m.
spinal cord m.
splenic m.
testicular m.
uterine sarcoma m.
Virchow m.
white m.
widespread m.
metastasizing fibroleiomyoma
metastatic
m. adenocarcinoma
m. adenopathy
m. axillary involvement
m. bone survey
m. carcinoid syndrome
m. disease
m. focus

M

NOTES

metastatic *(continued)*
    m. lesion
    m. malignancy
    m. myocardial tumor
    m. osteosarcoma
    m. pleomorphic liposarcoma
    m. polyp
    m. renal neoplasm
    m. rhabdomyosarcoma
    m. seeding
    m. site
    m. soft tissue calcification
    m. testicular lymphoma
    m. urothelial carcinoma
metasynchronous tumor
metatarsal
    m. angle
    angle of declination of m.
    m. axis
    m. bone
    m. fracture
    m. head
    m. head width (MHW)
    m. injury
    m. joint
    m. length ratio
    m. parabola
    m. synostosis
metatarsocalcaneal angle
metatarsocuneiform
    m. joint
    m. joint fusion
metatarsophalangeal (MT, MTP)
    m. bone marrow development
    m. capsule
    m. joint
    m. joint arthritis
    m. joint fusion
metatarsotalar angle
metatarsus
    m. adductocavus deformity
    m. adductovarus deformity
    m. adductus
    m. adductus angle
    m. adductus deformity
    m. atavicus deformity
    m. latus deformity
    m. primus varus angle (MPVA)
    m. primus varus deformity
    m. valgus
    m. varus
    m. varus deformity
metatrophic
    m. dwarfism
    m. dysplasia
metencephalon
meter (m)

    analog rate m.
    counting rate m.
    dose-area product m.
    exposure m.
    Gammex RMI DAP m.
    Geiger-Müller survey m.
    kVp m.
    photovolt pH m.
    rate m. (R-meter)
    roentgen m.
    roentgen(s) (per) hour (at one) m. (rhm)
meters per second (mps)
methemoglobin effect
methiodal
methionine
    ^{11}C m.
method
    acoustic reflection m.
    Agatston calcium scoring m.
    Andren m.
    Arelin m.
    autoattenuation correction m.
    automated airway tree segmentation m.
    Ball m.
    Bayler-Pinneau m.
    Béclére m.
    Benassi m.
    Benedict-Talbot body surface area m.
    Bertel m.
    Bigliani and Morrison m.
    Blackett-Healy m.
    blood oxygen level-dependent fMRI m.
    border detection m. (BDM)
    Borell and Fernström m.
    Born m.
    Brasdor m.
    Bull m.
    Caldwell m.
    calibration m.
    Cameron m.
    CHESS m.
    Clauss m.
    Cleaves m.
    Cobb m.
    Colbert m.
    column extraction m.
    computer m.
    deconvolution m.
    2DFT m.
    double-echo m.
    downstream sampling m.
    dual-balloon m.
    echo-planar imaging m.

electrocardiographic trigger m.
ellipsoid m.
empirical m.
error diffusion m.
extraction m.
FBP m.
Ferguson m.
FI m.
Fick m.
filtered back-projection m.
fractal-based m.
Friedman m.
full-scan m.
Gaynor-Hart m.
Gerota m.
Girout m.
gradient-echo m.
Graf m.
Grashey m.
Greulich and Pyle m.
Haas m.
Hawkins m.
Hickey m.
inflow/outflow m.
in vivo m.
IPSP neuron evaluation m.
isocenter shift m.
isodose shift m.
Joliot m.
KWE m.
Lawrence m.
Levenberg-Marquardt m.
Lysholm m.
Mankin m.
Meyerding m.
Monte Carlo m.
multiple-line scanning m.
multiple-sensitive-point m.
multisection m.
paddle wheel m.
parallax m.
Pearson m.
m. of perpendiculars
Pfeiffer-Comberg m.
phase-inversion m.
phase-unwrapping m.
Pirie m.
pixel count m.
Porcher m.
Powell m.
pulse-echo m.
radioimmunoassay m.

radiotracer foil m.
ray-casting m.
receiver operating characteristic m.
ROC m.
rotational m.
Sansregret m.
m. of Scarpa
segmentation m.
selective excitation m.
selective saturation m.
SENSE m.
sensitivity encoding m.
Settegast m.
short-cannula coaxial m.
simulated annealing m.
spin-label m.
spin-warp m.
spiral imaging m.
Strickler m.
sum-peak m.
surface coil m.
Sweet m.
Thom m.
thresholding m.
time-of-flight m.
triangulation m.
two-dye m.
under-scan m.
Valdini m.
vertebral body ratio m.
volume-ratio m.
Wolf m.
Zimmer m.

methodology
Gehan m.

methoxyisobutyl
m. isonitrile
m. isonitrile SPECT

methoxystaurosporine
^{11}C m.

methyl
m. methacrylate bead
m. methacrylate bead implant
m. methacrylate imaging agent
m. proton

methyl-ABV

methylcellulose gel

methylene
m. blue enema
m. diphosphonate (MDP)
m. diphosphonate (MDP)
concentration

M

NOTES

methylglucamine
    m. contrast medium
    m. diatrizoate
    iodipamide m.
methylsulfate
    neostigmine m.
metopic suture
MET-PET
    ^{11}C-methionine positron emission
      tomography
    MET-PET scan
metrics
    histogram-derived m.
metrizamide
    m. computed tomography
      cisternography (MCTC)
    m. CT cisternogram
    m. imaging agent
    m. myelography
    m. ventriculogram
**metrizamide-assisted computed
tomography (CTMM)**
metrizoate
    m. imaging agent
metrizoic acid
metrography
metroperitoneal fistula
metroplasty
metrosalpingography
mets
    metastases
Metz spatially varying filter
MeV
    megavolt
    million electron volt
    million electron-volt
Mewissen infusion catheter
Meyer
    M. dysplasia
    M. line
    M. loop
    supratubercular ridge of M.
Meyer-Archambault loop
Meyerding method
**Meyer-McKeever tibial fracture
classification**
Meynet node
MF
    magnification factor
mf
    microfarad
MFB
    metallic foreign body
MFG
    magnetic field gradient
    manofluorography

MFH
    malignant fibrous histiocytoma
      giant cell-type MFH
      inflammatory MFH
      myxoid MFH
      postirradiation MFH
      storiform-pleomorphic MFH
MFH-B
    malignant fibrous histiocytoma of bone
mFISP
    mirrored FISP
MG
    Millenium MG
m/h
    midbrain-hindbrain
MHP
    1-mercuri-2-hydroxypropane
MH-908 slim ultrasonic probe
MHV
    middle hepatic vein
MHW
    metatarsal head width
MHz
    megahertz
      250 M. crossed-loop resonator
      7.5-M. linear transducer
MI
    mitral insufficiency
    myocardial infarct
      inferior wall MI
MIBG
    metaiodobenzylguanidine
      MIBG scintigraphy
      MIBG SPECT scan
      MIBG washout
MIC
    M. gastroenteric tube
    M. jejunal tube
micaceous
mica pneumoconiosis
Michaelis
    M. complex
    rhomboid of M.
Michaelis-Gutmann body
Michel
    M. anomaly
    M. aplasia
    M. deformity
    M. malformation
Michels classification
Mickey
    M. Mouse appearance
    M. Mouse ears pelvis
Mick seed applicator
Mi/Cr
    myoinositol-creatine ratio
micrencephaly, micrencephalia

microabscess
    m. of the spleen
    splenic m.
microadenoma
    adrenocorticotropin m.
    pituitary m.
microaggregated albumin
microaneurysm
    Charcot-Bouchard intracerebral m.
    retinal m.
microangioarchitecture
microangiogram
microangiography
microangiopathy
    mineralizing m.
    thrombotic m.
microangioscopy
microarchitecture
    bone m.
microarteriography
microatelectasis
micro-AVM
    cerebral microarteriovenous malformation
    single-shot embolization of micro-
        AVM
microballoon
    Rand m.
microbubble
    m. concentration measurement
    m. contrast enhancement
    intranasal m.
    sonicated albumin m.
microbubble-based contrast agent
microcalcification
    breast m.
    m. cluster
    coarse m.
    ductal breast m.
    granular m.
    linear branching m.
    lobular breast m.
    pleomorphic m.
    psammomatous m.
    sole cluster of m.
    subtle m.
microcalculus
microcardia
Micro-Cast collimator
microcatheter
    AngiOptic m.
    ball-tip m.

    Excel-14 m.
    Excelsior m.
    Flow Rider m.
    1.8-French m.
    2.1-French m.
    Hieshima m.
    Leggiero hydrophilic-coated m.
    20-mm Equinox balloon m.
    Rapid Transit m.
    Renegade m.
    Tracker 10 m.
microcavitation
microcinematography
microcirculation
    m. abnormality
    pulmonary m.
microcirculatory blood flow
microcluster
    biodegradable magnetic m.
microcoil
    Dacron-coated m.
    Hilal m.
    Intercept esophagus m.
    Intercept prostate m.
    Intercept urethra m.
    platinum m.
microcolon
    megacystic m.
microconidia
micro-CT imaging
microCT-20 scanner
microcurie (mC)
microcyst
    milk-of-calcium m.
microcystic
    m. adenoma
    m. degeneration
    m. encephalomalacia
    m. formation
    m. lumbar spine
    m. pancreatic tumor
    m. pilocytic cerebellar astrocytoma
microcystica
microcytosis
microdactylia
microdistribution
    heterogeneous m.
microdosimetry
microemboli (*pl. of* microembolus)
microembolism
    cerebral m.

M

NOTES

microembolization
> ferromagnetic m.

microembolus, pl. microemboli
> showers of microemboli

microendoscope
> ophthalmic laser m.

microenvironment
> bone marrow m.

microerosion

microexplosion lithotripsy

microextension

microfarad (mf)

microfixation plate

microfluidization

microfocal
> m. direct magnification in vitro x-ray tube
> m. spot mammography

microform of holoprosencephaly

microfracture
> subchondral m.
> trabecular m.

microgastria

microglandular adenosis

microglioma

microglobulin labeling

micrognathia

Micro-Guide

microhamartoma
> biliary m.

microimaging

microinfarct

microkymatotherapy

Microlase transpupillary diode laser

microlattice
> cerebral vascular m.

microlesion

Microlight 830 laser

microlith

microlithiasis
> alveolar m.
> pulmonary alveolar m.
> testicular m.

microlobular cirrhosis

microlobulation

micromanometer-tipped catheter

MicroMark tissue marker

micromelia
> bowed m.
> extreme m.

micromelic
> m. dwarfism
> m. dysplasia

micrometallic artifact

micrometastasis
> systemic m.

micrometer

MicroMewi multiple sidehole infusion catheter

micron

micronodular
> m. cirrhosis
> m. infiltrate
> m. metastasis
> m. pattern

micronodularity

micronodule
> centrilobular m.
> subpleural m.

micron-resolution retinal image in vivo

micropapillary
> m. carcinoma
> m. DCIS
> m. lesion
> m. tumor

Micropaque contrast medium

microperforation

micropipette

microplate reader

microporous membrane

Microprobe laser

microprolactinoma

micropuncture needle

microradiogram

microradiography

microreentrant circuit

microroentgen

microsatellite instability

microscintigraphy

microscope
> projection x-ray m.
> scanning acoustic m. (SAM)
> scanning electron m. (SEM)
> x-ray m.
> x-ray tomographic m. (XTM)

microscopic
> m. air bubble
> m. cortical dysplasia
> m. hemorrhage of ligament
> m. imaging
> m. polyangiitis

microscopy
> darkfield m.
> 3D magnetic resonance m.
> electron m.
> fluorescence m.
> immune electron m.
> light m.
> polarized light m.
> ultrasound backscatter m. (UBM)
> in vivo m.

microsecond pulsed flashlamp pumped dye laser

microSelectron-HDR

microSelectron rapid delivery system
microsnare
microsomia
   hemifacial m.
microsphere
   acrylic m.
   degradable starch m.
   EmboGold m.
   Embosphere m.
   ferromagnetic m.
   hollow albumin m.
   human albumin m.
   m. perfusion scintigraphy
   silicone m.
   stainless steel m.
   superparamagnetic m.
   technetium-99m albumin m.
   technetium-99m human albumin m.
   trisacryl gelatin m.
   ytterbium-90 m.
   yttrium-90 m.
microstructural architecture
micro tear
Microtek ScanMaker 9600XL scanner
microtomography
   view m.
Microtrast
microtrauma
   repetitive m.
Microtron accelerator
microvascular
   m. circulation
   m. decompression
   m. disease
   m. retrieval
microvasculature
   pulmonary m.
microvenoarteriolar fistula
microvesicular fat
microvessel
   intraparenchymal m.
microvolt
microwave
   m. ablation
   m. cardiac ablation system
   m. hyperthermia
   m. hyperthermia treatment
   m. imaging
   m. nonsurgical treatment
   m. therapy
   m. tumor coagulation
MI-Cr ratio

micturating
   m. cystourethrogram (MCU)
   m. cystourethrography
micturition cystourethrography
midabdominal wall
midaortic
   m. arch
   m. syndrome
midarterial phase
midaxillary line
midbody of vertebra
midbrain
   m. aqueduct
   m. function
   m. lesion
   m. reticular formation (MRF)
   m. tegmentum
midbrain-hindbrain (m/h)
   m.-h. junction
midcarpal
   m. compartment
   m. dislocation
   m. instability
   m. joint
   m. joint cavity
midcircumflex
midclavicular
   m. line (MCL)
   m. plane
midcolon
midcoronal
   m. oblique image
   m. plane
mid-diastole
mid-distal
middle
   m. aortic syndrome
   m. cardiac vein
   m. cerebral artery (MCA)
   m. cerebral artery bifurcation
   m. cerebral artery fenestration
   m. cerebral artery infarct
   m. cerebral artery occlusion
   m. coronary sinus (MCS)
   m. cranial fossa
   m. cuneiform bone
   m. ear
   m. ear choristoma
   m. ear mass
   m. ear neoplasm
   m. extrahepatic bile duct
   m. facet of the subtalar joint

M

NOTES

middle *(continued)*
    m. finger
    m. fossa syndrome
    m. frontal gyrus
    m. hepatic vein (MHV)
    m. lobe (ML)
    m. lobe bronchus
    m. lobe syndrome
    m. mediastinal mass
    m. mediastinum
    m. meningeal
    m. meningeal artery
    m. meningeal artery groove
    m. muscle
    m. palatine suture
    m. perforating collagen bundle
    m. pole
    m. pulmonary lobe atelectasis
    m. rectal vein
    m. temporal gyrus
    m. third shaft
    m. third of thoracic esophagus
    m. turbinate bone
middle-field-strength MR imaging
middorsal
midepigastrium
midesophageal diverticulum
midesophagus
midexpiratory tidal flow
midface
    fetal m.
    m. retrusion
midfacial fracture
midfemur
midfoot fracture
midfrontal
    m. plane
    m. plane coronal section
midget MRI scanner
midgraft stenosis
midgroove portion of lumen
midgut
    m. volvulus
    m. volvulus with malrotation
midhumeral line
midinfrared laser
midinguinal point
midlateral course
midleft sternal border
midline
    m. of brain cyst
    m. cerebellum
    m. cystic structure
    m. echoencephalograph
    m. granuloma
    m. herniation of disk
    m. incense presentation

    infracolic m.
    m. lesion
    m. longitudinal pontine cleft
    m. malignant reticulosis
    m. mucosa-sparing block
    m. parasagittal focus
    m. shift
midlung
    m. field
    m. zone
midmarginal branch
midpalmar
    m. abscess
    m. space
midpatellar tendon
midpelvis
midplane
    m. depth
    m. sagittal image
midpole
midportion
midsagittal
    m. diameter (MSD)
    m. MR image
    m. MR imaging
    m. plane
midscapular line
midshaft fracture
midshunt peak velocity (MSPv)
midsigmoid colon
midspinal line
midsternal
    m. area
    m. line
midsternum
midsystolic
    m. buckling of mitral valve
    m. notching of velocity spectrum
    m. retraction
midtarsal
    m. injury
    m. joint
midthalamic plane
midthigh amputation
midthoracic spine
midventricular short-axis slice
midwaist scaphoid fracture
midzonal necrosis
midzone
Miescher granulomatosis
Mignon granuloma
migrainous scintillation
migration
    m. abnormality
    m. of acetabular cup
    bowel m.
    catheter m.

coil m.
m. disorder
embolus m.
gallstone m.
hallux m.
m. index
neuronal m.
placenta m.
sesamoid m.
stent m.
tissue m.
migrational
m. anomaly
m. pattern
migratory
m. patchy infiltrate
m. pneumonia
Mikity-Wilson syndrome
Mikulicz
M. angle
M. disease
M. syndrome
Milch
M. classification of humeral
fracture
M. elbow fracture classification
mild
m. edema
m. head injury
m. recess
m. subcostal retraction
m. traumatic brain injury
mildly enlarged heart
Miles operation
miliary
m. aneurysm
m. embolus
m. granuloma
m. lung disease
m. nodule
m. parenchymal disease
m. pattern
m. pulmonary tuberculosis
military antishock trousers (MAST)
milk
m. of calcium
m. of calcium urinary tract cyst
m. leg syndrome
m. teeth
milk-alkali syndrome

milkmaid's
m. elbow
m. elbow dislocation
milkman
m. fracture
m. pseudofracture
M. syndrome
milk-of-calcium
m.-o.-c. calcification
m.-o.-c. microcyst
milky effusion
Millar catheter-tip transducer
Millenium MG
miller
M. double mushroom biliary stent
M. index
m. lung
M. position
Miller-Abbott tube
Miller-Dieker syndrome
millicurie (mCi)
millicurie-hour (mCi-hr)
millimeter (mm)
m.'s of mercury (mmHg, mm Hg)
millimole (mmol)
million electron-volt (MeV)
millirad (mrad)
millirem (mrem)
milliroentgen (mR, mr)
millisecond (ms, msec)
millivolt (mV)
Milroy disease
Milwaukee shoulder syndrome
MIMIC
multivane intensity modulation
compensator
mimic
mimicked
mimicker of malignancy
mimicking
mimosa pattern
Minaar classification of coalition
minced rib
mind-body interaction
mineralization
bone m.
matrix m.
stippled m.
mineralizing microangiopathy
mineralocorticoid secretion
mineral oil imaging agent
miner's lung

NOTES

M

miniature
- m. imaging
- m. stomach
- m. uterine cavity

miniaturized mitral valve
Mini-Balloon system
MINI 6000 C-arm
minicholecystostomy
minicoil
minification
minimal
- m. deformation target (MDT)
- m. intensity projection (minIP)
- m. interstitial thickening
- m. luminal diameter (MLD)
- m. port diameter (MPD)
- m. volume

minimally
- m. attenuating medical-grade foam
- m. displaced fracture
- m. invasive access set
- m. invasive endovascular stent placement

minimi
- flexor digiti m.
- opponens digiti m.

minimicroaggregated albumin colloid
minimizing bias
minimum
- m. basis set magnetic resonance angiography (MBS-MRA)
- m. blood pressure
- m. intensity projection image
- m. intensity projection imaging
- m. pixel density

minimum-intensity sliding thin slab projection
minimus
- digitus m.
- gluteus m.
- scalenus m.
- m. scalenus muscle

minIP
- minimal intensity projection

ministem shaft
Minix
- Medtronic M.

Mink-Deutsch classification
Minnesota tube
minor
- m. calix
- m. duodenal papilla
- m. fissure
- globus m.
- m. muscle
- rhomboid m.
- teres m.

minora (*pl. of* minus)
Minor sign
Minot-von Willebrand syndrome
minus, pl. **minora**
- omentum m.

minuscule
minus-density artifact
minute
- m. bleeding ulcer
- blood volume per m.
- cycle per m. (cpm)
- rotations per m. (rpm)
- m. ventilation
- m. vessel
- m. volume

minute-sequence study
MION
- monocrystalline iron oxide

MIP
- macrophage inflammatory protein
- maximum intensity pixel
- maximum intensity projection
- MIP algorithm
- MIP image
- MIP image processing
- MIP reconstruction

MIR
- M. guideline
- M. intrauterine tandem
- M. system

mirabile
- rete m.

Miraluma
- M. injection
- M. nuclear scan of breast

MIRD
- medical internal radiation dosimetry

Mirizzi syndrome
mirror
- beam-splitting m.
- m. image
- m. image aneurysm
- m. image reversal
- m. imaging
- polygon m.

mirrored FISP (mFISP)
mirror-image
- m.-i. artifact
- m.-i. brachiocephalic branching
- m.-i. interpretation

mirror-like echo
misalign
misalignment
- cytoskeletal m.
- neurofilamentous m.

miscommunication
- neural m.

misery perfusion
misinterpretation
misleading
    m. image
    m. imaging
mismapping
    phase m.
mismatch
    FDG-blood flow m.
    flow-function m.
    perfusion-metabolism m.
    ventilation-perfusion m.
    V/Q m.
misplaced thoracentesis
misregistration
    m. artifact
    local m.
    oblique flow m.
missed
    m. bronchogenic carcinoma
    m. testicular torsion
missile
    m. effect
    m. wound
missing pulse steady-state free
  precession sequence
Mitchell classification
Mitek bone anchor
mitochondrial
    m. ATP production
    m. encephalomyopathy
    m. function
    m. genome
    m. uncoupler
mitosis-karyorrhexis index (MKI)
mitral
    m. apparatus
    m. arcade
    m. component
    m. configuration of cardiac shadow
    m. deceleration slope
    m. flow velocity index
    m. inflow velocity
    m. insufficiency (MI)
    m. leaflet
    m. leak
    m. orifice (MO)
    posterior m. (PM)
    m. regurgitant signal area
    m. regurgitation (MR)
    m. regurgitation artifact
    m. ring calcification

    m. stenosis (MS)
    m. valve
    m. valve of anulus
    m. valve area (MVA)
    m. valve atresia
    m. valve calcification
    m. valve commissure
    m. valve cusp
    m. valve deformity
    m. valve echocardiography
    m. valve echogram
    m. valve flow
    m. valve gradient
    m. valve incompetence
    m. valve leaflet systolic prolapse
    m. valve leaflet tip
    m. valve myxomatous degeneration
    m. valve opening (MVO)
    m. valve orifice (MVO)
    m. valve prolapse (MVP)
    m. valve regurgitation
    m. valve replacement (MVR)
    m. valve ring
    m. valve septal separation
    m. valve stenosis (MVS)
    m. valve systolic anterior motion
mitralization
Mitsuyasu staging system
mixed
    m. aneurysm
    m. attenuation mass
    m. cell sarcoma
    m. connective-tissue disease
    (MCTD)
    m. density mass
    m. echogenic solid mass
    m. fat-water breast lesion density
    m. fat-water density lesion
    m. gonadal dysgenesis
    m. hernia
    m. IUGR
    m. lymphocytic-histiocytic
    lymphoma
    m. lytic and sclerotic pattern
    m. petal-fugal flow
    m. rheumatoid and degenerative
    arthritis
    m. sclerotic and lytic bone lesion
    m. sclerotic osteolysis
    m. signal mass
    m. small and large cell lymphoma
    m. solid-cystic mass

M

NOTES

mixed *(continued)*
m. venous blood
m. venous-lymphatic malformation
m. venous saturation
mixed-echo appearance
mixed-echoic
mixing
intracardiac m.
mixture
barium m.
Ingenor silicone m.
MKI
mitosis-karyorrhexis index
ML
middle lobe
ML 700 daylight processor
MLC
multileaf collimator
MLD
minimal luminal diameter
MLF
medial longitudinal fasciculus
MLF lesion
MLO
mediolateral oblique
mediolateral view
MLS
multiple line scan
MLSI
multiple line scan imaging
ML-Ultra balloon stent
mm
millimeter
3mm × 6 cm interlocking
detachable coil
4mm × 8 cm interlocking
detachable coil
MMCM
macromolecular contrast medium
MMEF
maximum midexpiratory flow
MMFR
maximum midexpiratory flow rate
mmHg, mm Hg
millimeters of mercury
M-mode
motion mode
M-mode cardiography
M-mode display
M-mode echocardiogram imaging
M-mode echocardiography
M-mode echophonocardiography
M-mode scanning
M-mode sector transducer
M-mode time motion scan
M-mode ultrasound

mmol
millimole
MMP-3
matrix metalloprotease-3
MMR
mobile mass x-ray
Mn
manganese
MnDPDP enhanced MRI
Mn-TPPS$_4$
manganese tetrasodium-meso-tetra
MO
mitral orifice
Mo
molybdenum
^{99}Mo
molybdenum-99
MoAb
^{131}I-labeled human MoAb
radiolabeled MoAb
Moberg-Gedda fracture
Mobetron
M. electron beam system
M. intraoperative radiation therapy
treatment system
mobile
m. artery and vein imaging system
(MAVIS)
cecum m.
cor m.
m. duodenum
m. fat ball
m. fluoroscopy
m. gallbladder
m. intraluminal gallbladder mass
m. magnetic resonance
m. mass x-ray (MMR)
m. radiography
m. spiral computed tomography
scanner
m. thrombus
m. without recapture
m. with recapture
mobility film
MobiTrak
M. automated table
M. moving table
modality
cross-sectional m.
diagnostic m.
multislice m.
neuroimaging m.
optimal m.
m. performed procedure step
(MPPS)
tomographic m.
modal velocity

mode

AAI rate-responsive m.
m. abandonment
active m.
asynchronous transfer m. (ATM)
blink m.
brightness m.
byte m.
cine m.
coincidence detection m.
continuous m.
decay m.
dispersion m.
dual-demand pacing m.
DVI m.
    digital vascular imaging
electron-capture decay m.
full three-dimensional m.
full-to-empty VAD m.
fundamental Doppler m.
high spatial resolution m.
high temporal resolution m.
imaginary m.
inactive m.
magnet m.
modified two-dimensional
    acquisition m.
motion m. (M-mode)
multiplanar m.
multislice m.
noncommitted m.
pulsed m.
road-mapping m.
semicommitted m.
sequential m.
step-and-shoot m.
stimulated echo acquisition m.
    (STEAM)
stimulation m.
triggered-flow m.
triggered pacing m.
underdrive m.
unipolar pacing m.
volume m.

model

modeling

compartmental m.
3D m.
electromagnetic m.
Monte Carlo m.
thermal m.

ultrasonographic m.
vascular and airway m.
moderately dilated ureter
moderate-sized volume joint effusion
moderator band
modest caliber
Modic disk abnormality classification
modification
thiol m.
modified
m. Bernoulli equation
m. bird-cage coil
m. Blalock-Taussig shunt patency
m. electron-beam CT scanner
m. linear accelerator
m. linear accelerator radiosurgery
m. projection
m. Simpson rule
m. stage exercise
m. two-dimensional acquisition
    mode
m. vessel image processor software
modiolus, pl. **modioli**
modular stent graft
modulation
amplitude m. (A-mod)
brightness m.
image m.
object m.
off-center m.
print reflectance m.
specific m.
m. transfer function (MTF)
module
detecting m.
E-TOF detecting m.
tube geometry m.
Modulith SL 20 lithotripter
modulus image
mogul
cardiac m.
third cardiac m.
Mohn-Wriedt brachydactyly
Mohr syndrome
moiety, pl. **moieties**
upper pole m.
moiré
m. fringe
m. fringes artifact
m. pattern
M. photography
molal solution

M

NOTES

molar
- m. mass
- m. pregnancy
- m. teeth
- m. tooth appearance
- m. tooth configuration
- m. tooth fracture
- m. tooth midbrain-hindbrain malformation
- m. volume

mold
- filter m.

molding
- atheroma m.
- m. of skull

molecular
- m. coincidence detection (MCD)
- m. diffusion
- m. recognition unit (MRU)
- m. vibration
- m. weight dependence of relaxation

molecule
- accessory adhesion m.
- homing m.
- intracellular adhesion m.
- signaling m.

molecule-1
- vascular cell adhesion m.-1 (VCAM-1)

molle
- fibroma m.
- heloma m.
- papilloma m.

molluscum, pl. **mollusca**
- fibroma m.
- m. fibrosum

Molnar disk

Molteno
- M. double plate drainage device
- M. single plate drainage device

molybdenum (Mo)
- m. anode
- m. target
- m. target tube

molybdenum-99 (^{99}Mo)
- m. breakthrough test
- m. generator

molybdenum-molybdenum target filter combination (Mo-Mo)

molybdenum-rhodium target filter combination (Mo-Rh)

molybdenum-technetium generator

moment
- macroscopic magnetic m.
- magnetic dipole m.
- nuclear magnetic m.
- quadrupole m.
- zeroth m.

momentum
- angular m.

Mo-Mo
- molybdenum-molybdenum target filter combination

monarticular
- m. process
- m. synovium-based cartilage metaplasia

Mönckeberg
- M. arteriosclerosis
- M. calcification
- M. degeneration

Mondini
- M. anomaly
- M. dysplasia
- M. malformation

Mondor disease

mongolian spot-like lesion

mongoloid feature

moniliasis

moniliform ectasia

monitor
- air m.
- beam m.
- blood perfusion m. (BPM)
- Brilliance 109 MP PC m.
- cardiac m.
- Doppler blood flow m.
- Doppler ultrasonic fetal heart m.
- FreeDop Doppler m.
- gray-scale m.
- HeartView CT cardiac m.
- Life-Pack 5 cardiac m.
- N-Cat N-500 tonometric blood pressure m.
- Nicolet Elite Doppler m.
- radiation beam m.
- tonometric blood pressure m.
- m. unit

monitoring
- electrode m.
- photoplethysmographic m.
- ultrasound m.
- video electroencephalography m.
- whole-body dose m.

monoamine oxidase

monoarticular

monochorionic
- m. diamniotic twin pregnancy
- m. monoamniotic twin pregnancy

monochorionic-monoamniotic twin

monochromatic
- m. synchrotron
- m. synchrotron radiation

m. x-ray
m. x-ray beam
monochromatization
monoclonal
    m. antibody imaging agent
    m. gammopathy
monocrystalline iron oxide (MION)
monocuspid tilting disk valve
monocusp valve
monocyte
monodactylism
monodermal dermoid
monodisk
monodisperse iodinated macromolecular
  blood pool agent
monoenergetic radiation
Monoject hypodermic needle
monomalleolar fracture
monomelic bone lesion
monomer
    ionic m.
    nonionic triiodinated m.
monophasic
monophosphate
    cyclic adenosine m.
    cyclic guanosine m.
monopolar
    m. electrode
    m. radiofrequency electrocautery
Monopty
    M. core biopsy
    M. needle
monoradicular filling defect
monorchia
monosomy X
monostotic
    m. fibrous dysplasia
    m. Paget disease
monoventricle
monoxide
    ^{11}C carbon m.
monozygotic twin
Monro
    M. aqueduct
    M. bursa
    foramen of M.
Monroe-Kellie doctrine
mons pubis
Monte
    M. Carlo calculation
    M. Carlo method
    M. Carlo modeling

M. Carlo photon transport (MCPT)
M. Carlo photon transport
  simulation
M. Carlo technique
Monteggia
    M. dislocation
    M. fracture
    M. fracture-dislocation
    M. lesion
Montercaux fracture
Montgomery gland
Moore fracture
morcellation
morcellized bone
Morgagni
    M. appendix
    column of M.
    M. crypt
    M. foramen
    M. hernia
    M. hydatid
    hyperostosis of M.
    M. lacuna
    M. nodule
    sinus of M.
    M. syndrome
    tubercle of M.
    M. ventricle
Morgagni-Adams-Stokes syndrome
morgagnian cyst
Mo-Rh
    molybdenum-rhodium target filter
    combination
Morison pouch
morphine-augmented study
morphine sulfate scintigraphy
morphologic
    m. criterion
    m. filtering
    m. growth
    m. imaging
    m. left ventricle
morphological
    m. correlation
    m. and physiological image
    coregistration
morphologically normal
morphology
    disk m.
    enhancement m.
    joint m.
    ovarian m.

M

NOTES

morphology · motion

morphology *(continued)*
    residuum m.
    spine m.
morphometric
    m. measurement
    m. x-ray absorptiometry
morphometry
    MRI m.
    pelvic m.
Morquio
    M. sign
    M. syndrome
Morquio-Brailsford syndrome
Morris point
mortise
    ankle m.
    ball-and-socket ankle m.
    m. of bone
    cuneiform m.
    diaphyseal cortical m.
    m. joint
    m. projection
    m. radiograph
    m. view
Morton
    M. neuroma
    M. plane
    M. toe
morula
morula-like epithelial cell
mosaic
    m. artifact
    m. attenuation pattern
    m. detector configuration
    m. duodenal mucosal pattern
    m. jet signal
    m. oligemia
    m. perfusion
MOS capacitator
Moschcowitz test
Mossbauer spectrometer
Mosse syndrome
Moss gastrostomy tube
mossy fiber
Motarjeme catheter
moth-eaten
    m.-e. appearance
    m.-e. bone destruction
    m.-e. pattern
motile leukocyte
motility
    antroduodenal m.
    colonic m.
    m. disorder
    esophageal m.
    m. of Golden
    ileal m.

    jejunal m.
    small bowel m.
    m. study
motion
    akinetic segmental wall m.
    anterior wall m.
    apical wall m.
    m. artifact
    m. artifact suppression technique
      (MAST)
    m. averaging
    m. blur
    bowel m.
    brisk wall m.
    brownian water m.
    cardiac wall m.
    catheter tip m.
    chest wall paradoxical m.
    m. compensation gradient pulse
    CSF oscillatory m.
    cusp m.
    m. degradation
    discernible venous m.
    dyskinetic segmental wall m.
    forceful parasternal m.
    heaving precordial m.
    hyperkinetic segmental wall m.
    hypokinetic segmental wall m.
    incoherent m.
    inferior wall m.
    intravoxel coherent m.
    intravoxel incoherent m. (IVIM)
    isotropic m.
    leaflet m.
    left ventricular function wall m.
    left ventricular regional wall m.
    limitation of joint m.
    linear accelerator isocenter m.
    mitral valve systolic anterior m.
    m. mode (M-mode)
    nonoscillatory m.
    paradoxical leaflet m.
    paradoxical septal m.
    parasternal m.
    patient m.
    phantom simulating cardiac m.
    photoreceptor m.
    posterior wall m.
    posterolateral wall m.
    precessional m.
    random m.
    rapid oscillatory m.
    regional hypokinetic wall m.
    respiratory m.
    rocking precordial m.
    rotational m.
    scapulothoracic m.

segmental wall m.
septal wall m.
stationary zero-order m.
sustained anterior parasternal m.
swirling m.
systolic anterior m. (SAM)
time m. (TM)
translational m.
trifid precordial m.
m. unsharpness
venous m.
ventricular wall m.
vibratory m.
visible anterior m.
wall m.
within-view m.
motional narrowing
motion-compensating format converter
motion-free
m.-f. imaging
m.-f. positioning
motion-induced phase shift
motion-nulling gradient
motion-triggered cine kinematic MR image
motoneuron
motor
m. area
m. branch
m. cortex
m. impairment
m. meal barium GI series
m. nucleus
programmable stepper m.
m. reinnervation
m. root
m. test meal
m. tract
m. urge incontinence
m. vehicle injury
versive m.
motorcyclist's knee
MOTSA
multiple overlapping thin-slab acquisition
Mott body
mottle
photon m.
quantum m.
radiographic m.
mottled
m. appearance
m. calcification

m. density
m. distribution
m. echotexture
m. gas collection
m. gray lung
m. hepatic uptake
m. infiltrate
m. liver uptake
m. pattern
m. thickening
mottling
diffuse m.
m. of renal parenchyma
Mouchet fracture
mound
infraumbilical m.
Mounier-Kuhn syndrome
Mountain View transducer
mouse
m. ear erosion
peritoneal m.
mouth (os)
tapir's m.
movable
m. core guidewire
m. heart
m. kidney
m. vertebra
movement
arcuate m.
m. artifact
bowel m.
fetal m. (FM)
fetal breathing m. (FBM)
fiducial m.
m. pattern
pendulum m.
propulsive m.
spontaneous fetal m.
systolic anterior m.
table m.
moving
m. slice velocity mapping
m. slot radiography
m. table technique
m. tabletop MR imaging
moving-bed infusion tracking MRA
moyamoya
m. disease
m. syndrome
m. vascularity
Moyer line

M

NOTES

Moynahan syndrome
MP
> magnetization prepared
> mesenteric panniculitis
>> MP inversion pulse

MPA
> main pulmonary artery

MPAP
> mean pulmonary artery pressure
> multipurpose access port

MPCh
> medial posterior choroidal

MPCP
> mean pulmonary capillary pressure

MPD
> main pancreatic duct
> main papillary duct
> matched peripheral dose
> minimal port diameter
> multiplanar display

MPGR
> multiplanar gradient recall
>> MPGR technique

MPHR
> maximum predicted heart rate

MPI
> myocardial perfusion imaging

mPower PET scanner
MPPS
> modality performed procedure step

MPPv
> main portal vein peak velocity

MPR
> multiplanar reconstruction
> multiplanar reformation
> myocardial perfusion reserve
>> MPR view

MP-RAGE
>> MP-RAGE protocol
>> MP-RAGE technique

MP-RAGE-WE
> magnetization-prepared rapid gradient
> echo-water excitation

mps
> meters per second

MPS types I–IV
MPVA
> metatarsus primus varus angle

MPVR
> multiplanar volume reformation

MR
> magnetic resonance
> mitral regurgitation
>> BP MR
>>> biphasic magnetic resonance
>> MR catheter imaging and
>> spectroscopy system scanner

chemical-selective fat-saturation MR
MR colonography
combined multisection diffuse-
weighted and hemodynamically
weighted echo-planar MR
contrast-enhanced MR
MR discriminator of osseous
metastasis
echo FLASH MR
MR echo-planar imaging
MR enteroclysis imaging
first-pass myocardial perfusion MR
MR flow quantification study
MR hydrography
lipid-sensitive MR
MR lymphography
oxygenation-sensitive functional MR
MR proton spectroscopy
renal artery stenosis screening MR
MR velocity mapping

mR, mr
> milliroentgen

MRA
> magnetic resonance angiography
>> body-coil-based contrast-enchanced
>> MRA
>> bolus-chase stepping-table 3D MRA
>> contrast-enhanced MRA
>> 3D MRA
>>> three-dimensional magnetic
>>> resonance angiography
>> MRA imaging
>> moving-bed infusion tracking MRA
>> multiphase MRA
>> stepping-table MRA
>> ultrafast contrast-enhanced MRA
>> MRA using 3D k-space reordering

MRC
> magnetic resonance cholangiogram

MR-compatible power injector
MRCP
> magnetic resonance
> cholangiopancreatography
>> kinematic MRCP
>> secretin-enhanced dynamic MRCP
>> MRCP using HASTE with a
>> phased array coil

MRDSA
> magnetic resonance digital subtraction
> angiography
>> 2D MRDSA
>>> two-dimensional magnetic
>>> resonance digital subtraction
>>> angiography

MRE
> magnetic resonance elastography

mrem
millirem
MRF
midbrain reticular formation
MR-guided
M.-g. laser-induced thermotherapy
M.-g. lumbar sympathicolysis
MRI
magnetic resonance imaging (*See*
imaging)
body-coil MRI
BOLD contrast functional MRI
breath-hold contrast-enhanced MRI
cardiac MRI
chondroitin sulfate iron colloid-
enhanced MRI
cine MRI
coregistered MRI
coronal FLAIR MRI
MRI CSF flow study
digital reformatting knee MRI
double-dose delayed-contrast MRI
dynamic-contrast MRI
dynamic contrast-enhanced MRI
electrocardiogram-gated MRI
endoluminal MRI
Excelart short-bore MRI
extremity MRI (E-MRI)
functional MRI
Gd-DTPA-enhanced turbo FLASH
MRI
gradient subsystem in MRI
^{3}He MRI
high-resolution MRI (HR-MRI)
intradiskal administration of
gadolinium followed by MRI
intravenously enhanced MRI
laser-polarized helium MRI
magnetoacoustic MRI
MRI mapping
MnDPDP enhanced MRI
MRI morphometry
multinuclear MRI
multiplanar MRI
nonproton MRI
OPART MRI
open MRI
opposed-phase MRI
perfusion-weighted MRI
phase-contrast cine MRI
phased-array MRI
MRI prescan

MRI probehead
proton-density-weighted MRI
MRI segmentation
Subtraction ictal SPECT
coregistered to MRI (SISCOM)
susceptibility contrast-weighted MRI
3T MRI
T2 quantitative MRI
ultrafast MRI
vagus nerve stimulated functional
MRI (VNS-fMRI)
vagus nerve stimulation-
synchronized blood oxygen level-
dependent functional MRI (VNS-
synchronized BOLD fMRI)
MRI-compatible electrode
MRI-guided
M.-g. breast biopsy
M.-g. focused ultrasound transducer
M.-g. laser-induced interstitial
imaging
M.-g. laser-induced interstitial
thermotherapy
M.-g. periradicular nerve root
infiltration therapy
M.-g. wire localization
MRM
magnetic resonance mammography
MRN
magnetic resonance neurography
MRP
magnetic resonance pancreatography
MRS
magnetic resonance spectroscopy
slice-point MRS
MRT
magnetic resonance tomography
MRU
magnetic resonance urography
molecular recognition unit
ThromboScan MRU
MRUI software
MRV
magnetic resonance venogram
magnetic resonance venography
MS
mitral stenosis
ms
millisecond
MS-325 contrast agent
MSAD
MSA syndrome

M

NOTES

MSCT technique
MSCV
    multislice cardiovolume
MSD
    mean sac diameter
    midsagittal diameter
MSDI
    multigated spectral Doppler imaging
        simultaneous MSDI
msec
    millisecond
MS-EPI
    multishot echo-planar imaging
M-shaped
    M.-s. mitral valve pattern
    M.-s. pattern of mitral valve
MSI
    magnetic source imaging
MSPv
    midshunt peak velocity
MT
    magnetization transfer
    metatarsophalangeal
        half-dose enhanced MRI with MT
        MT saturation
        triple-dose gadolinium-enhanced MR
            imaging without MT
MTC
    magnetization transfer contrast
MTE
    main timing event
    mesenteric thromboembolism
MTF
    modulation transfer function
MTP
    metatarsophalangeal
        semiflexed MTP
MTR
    magnetization transfer ratio
MTSA
    multiple thin slab acquisition
MTT
    mean pulmonary transit time
    mean transit time
m-tyrosine
mucicarmine stain
mucin-hypersecreting carcinoma
mucinous
    m. adenocarcinoma
    m. adenoma
    m. breast carcinoma
    m. bronchogram
    m. cyst
    m. cystadenoma
    m. degeneration
    m. ductal ectasia of pancreas
    m. ductectatic tumor of pancreas

    m. ovarian cystadenocarcinoma
    m. ovarian tumor
    m. pancreatic cystic neoplasm
mucin-producing
    m.-p. adenocarcinoma
    m.-p. carcinoma
mucocele
    appendix m.
    breast m.
    bronchial m.
    frontal sinus m.
    frontoethmoidal m.
    orbital m.
    paranasal sinus m.
mucocutaneous
    m. junction
    m. lymph node syndrome (MCLS)
mucoepidermoid
    m. carcinoma
    m. carcinoma parotitis
mucoid
    m. degeneration of umbilical cord
    m. impaction
    m. impaction of bronchus
    m. plugging of airway
    m. umbilical cord degeneration
mucopolysaccharidosis types I–IV
mucopyocele
mucosa, pl. mucosae
    bowel m.
    bronchial m.
    buccal m.
    burned-out m.
    cobblestone m.
    colorectal m.
    endocervical m.
    friable m.
    frothy colonic m.
    isoeffective bronchial m.
    muscularis m.
    m. muscularis
    outpocketings of m.
    polypoid m.
    prolapsed antral m.
    prolapsed gastric m.
    sloughed m.
mucosa-associated
    m.-a. lymphoid tissue (MALT)
    m.-a. lymphoid tissue lymphoma
mucosal
    m. abnormality
    m. bridge
    m. crinkling
    m. destruction
    m. esophageal nodule
    m. esophageal tumor
    m. fold

m. fold pattern
m. ganglioneurofibromatosis
m. gland
m. hyperplasia
m. inflammation
m. island
m. lesion
m. lining
m. mass collecting system
m. necrosis
m. prolapse syndrome
m. relief radiography
m. relief roentgenography
m. ring
m. suspensory ligament
m. thickening
m. ulcer
mucosa-sparing block
mucosum
ligamentum m.
mucous
m. bronchogram
m. carcinoma
m. degeneration
m. fistula
m. hypersecretion
m. lake
m. lake of stomach
m. membrane
m. membrane hyperemia
m. plug
m. plugging
m. polyp
m. pseudomass
m. retention cyst
mucus-filled small airway
mud
biliary m.
Mueller (*var. of* Müller)
MUGA
multiple gated acquisition
MUGA cardiac blood pool imaging
first-pass MUGA
MUGA scan
Muir-Torre syndrome
Mukherjee-Sivaya view
mulberry
m. calculus
m. eye lesion
m. gallstone
m. ovary
mulberry-like mass

mulberry-type
m.-t. calcification
m.-t. classification
Mulder sign
Müller, Mueller
M. canal
M. fiber
M. humerus fracture classification
M. maneuver
M. muscle
M. sign
M. test
M. tray
müllerian
m. duct
m. duct anomaly
m. duct cyst
m. mucinous borderline tumor
multangular
m. bone
m. ridge fracture
multangulum
multiaccess catheter
multiarc LINAC radiosurgery
multiaxial classification
multibreath washout study
multicentric
m. angiofollicular lymph node
m. basal cell carcinoma
m. carcinoid tumor
m. Castleman disease (MCD)
m. fibromatosis
m. germinoma
m. glioblastoma
m. invasive lobular carcinoma
m. lytic lesion
m. malignant glioma
m. meningioma
m. osteogenic sarcoma
m. osteosarcoma
m. reticulohistiocytosis
multicentricity
multichannel analyzer (MCA)
multicoil
phased-array m.
multicolor flow cytometry
multicompartment clearance
multicoupled loop-gap resonator
multicrystal
m. BGO ring system
m. gamma camera

M

NOTES

multicystic
- m. acoustic neuroma
- m. dysgenetic kidney
- m. dysplasia
- m. dysplastic kidney (MCDK)
- m. encephalomalacia
- m. kidney (MCK)

multidetector
- m. computed tomography
- m. CT (MDCT)
- m. CTA
- m. CT scanner
- m. helical CT
- m. helical scanner
- m. system

multidetector-row CT (MDCT)
multi-detector row CT scan
MultiDop P, T, X transcranial Doppler device
multidose vial
multidrug-resistant tuberculosis
multiecho
- m. axial
- m. axial image
- m. coronal image
- m. imaging
- m. multiplane (MEMP)
- m. sequence
- standard m.

multielectrode catheter
multielemental neutron activation analysis
multiexponential relaxation
multifactorial etiologies
multifield beam
multifocal
- m. aggressive infiltrate
- m. anaplastic astrocytoma
- m. area of hyperintensity
- m. autonomic adenoma
- m. brain tumor
- m. breast carcinoma
- m. enhancing brain lesion
- m. glioblastoma multiforme
- m. infarct
- m. invasive lobular carcinoma
- m. leukoencephalopathy
- m. lymphoma
- m. nephroblastomatosis
- m. osteosarcoma
- m. residual focus
- m. short stenosis
- m. subperitoneal sclerosis

multifollicular ovary
multiformat camera
multiformatted imaging

multiforme
- glioblastoma m. (GBM)
- multifocal glioblastoma m.

multiform ventricular complex
multigated
- m. angiography
- m. imaging
- m. pulsed Doppler flow system
- m. spectral Doppler analysis software
- m. spectral Doppler imaging (MSDI)

multigate Doppler
MultiHance imaging agent
multihole collimator
multiilluminant color correction
multiinfarct dementia
multiinterval
multilamellar periosteal reaction
multilaminar body
multileaf
- m. collimating system
- m. collimator (MLC)

multilevel fusion
multiline scanning technique
multilobular
- m. cirrhosis
- m. configuration

multilobulated mass
multilocular
- m. cystic lesion
- m. cystic nephroma
- m. renal cyst

multiloculated mass
multilog effect
multimodal image fusion technique
multimodality
- m. imaging
- m. therapy

multinodular
- m. goiter
- m. thyroid

multinuclear MRI
multiorgan imaging
multiparametric color composite display
multiparticle cyclotron
multipartite
- m. fracture
- m. patella

multipennate muscle
multiphase MRA
multiphasic
- m. helical CT
- m. multislice MRI technique
- m. multislice spin-echo imaging technique
- m. renal computerized tomography

multiplanar
 m. compression
 m. display (MPD)
 m. endorectal ultrasound
 m. gradient-echo software
 m. gradient recall (MPGR)
 m. gradient-recalled echo
 m. gradient refocus
 m. gradient refocused sequence
 m. mode
 m. MRI
 m. MR imaging
 phase-offset m. (POMP)
 phase-ordered m. (POMP)
 m. reconstruction (MPR)
 m. reformation (MPR)
 m. reformatted radiographic and digitally reconstructed radiographic imaging
 m. reformatting
 m. reformatting view
 m. scanning
 m. transducer
 m. transesophageal echocardiography
 m. volume reformation (MPVR)
 m. volume-reformatted image

multiplane
 m. dosage calculation
 multiecho m. (MEMP)

multiple
 m. accessory spleen
 m. aortopulmonary collateral artery (MAPCA)
 m. bile duct hamartomas
 m. block
 m. bone myeloma
 m. bull's eye lesions bowel wall
 m. cartilaginous exostoses
 m. chords
 m. coil array
 m. colon filling defect
 m. concentric GI rings
 m. congenital anomalies (MCA)
 m. congenital fibromatosis
 m. cortical infarcts
 m. echo single shot (MESS)
 m. emboli
 m. enchondromatosis
 m. endocrine neoplasia (MEN)
 m. endocrine neoplasia syndrome
 m. epiphyseal dysplasia
 m. fetuses

 m. fibroxanthomata
 m. focal lesions of spinal cord
 m. focus
 m. fractures
 m. gated acquisition (MUGA)
 m. gated acquisition scan
 m. gated blood pool scan
 m. gestation
 m. gland disease
 m. hereditary exostoses
 m. idiopathic hemorrhagic sarcoma
 m. jointed digitizer
 m. jointed digitizer scanner
 m. kidney myeloma
 m. line scan (MLS)
 m. line scan imaging (MLSI)
 m. loops of small bowel
 m. lucent lung lesion
 m. lung nodules
 m. lytic bone lesion
 m.'s of the median
 m. mucosal neuroma syndrome
 m. mural dilatation
 m. organ failure
 m. osteochondromatosis
 m. osteolysis
 m. osteosclerotic lesions
 m. overlapping thin-slab acquisition (MOTSA)
 m. parotid gland lesion
 m. peripheral papilloma
 m. planar gradient-recalled image
 m. pleural density
 m. polyposis
 m. polyps
 m. pregnancy
 m. projection biplane angiography
 m. pterygium syndrome
 m. pulmonary calcifications
 m. pulmonary cysts
 m. pulmonary necrobiotic nodule
 m. quantum coherence
 m. recurrent inversion injuries
 m. sclerosis
 m. sclerosis plaque
 m. sclerotic osteosarcoma
 m. sensitive points
 m. slice acquisition
 m. slice imaging
 m. small bowel filling defect
 m. small bowel stenosis
 m. small bowel ulcers

M

NOTES

multiple *(continued)*
    m. spin echo
    m. stenotic lesions
    m. stenotic lesions of small bowel
    m. stones
    m. symmetrical lipomatosis
    m. system atrophy
    m. system atrophy syndrome
    m. thin slab acquisition (MTSA)
    m. thin-walled lung cavity
    m. thyroid cysts
    m. trauma
    m. vascular leiomyoma
multiple-beam interface spacing
multiple-echo imaging
multiple-exposure volumetric holography
multiple-gated blood pool imaging
multiple-headed gamma camera
multiple-lesion osteosclerosis
multiple-line scanning method
multiple-plane imaging
multiple-sample clearance
multiple-sensitive-point method
multiple-side-hole infusion system
multiple-suture synostosis
multiplex
    dysostosis m.
    dysplasia epiphysealis m.
multiplexing
multiplying digital-to-analog converter (MDAC)
multiply tuned coil
Multi-Pro biopsy needle
multipurpose
    m. access port (MPAP)
    m. catheter
multiray fracture
multirod collimator
multiscalar
multiscale image detail contrast amplification (Musica)
multisection
    m. diffuse-weighted magnetic resonance imaging
    m. gradient-echo echo-planar imaging
    m. method
    m. multirepetition acquisition
multisectional dose-volume histogram
multisensor
    m. structured light range digitizer
    m. structured light-range digitizer scanner
multiseptate appearance
multiseptated gallbladder

multishot
    m. echo-planar imaging (MS-EPI)
    m. spin-echo echo-planar imaging
multi-sideport infusion catheter
multislab magnetic resonance angiography
multislice
    m. acquisition
    m. cardiovolume (MSCV)
    m. computed tomography
    m. CT
    m. CT scanner
    2D m.
    ECG-gated m.
    m. first-pass myocardial perfusion imaging
    m. FLASH 2D
    m. flow-related enhancement
    m. full line scan
    m. modality
    m. mode
    m. modified KWE direct Fourier imaging
    m. spin-echo sequence
    m. spin-echo technique
    m. spiral weighting
multispectral diffuse transillumination
multispin relaxation
Multistar
    M. angiographic unit
    M. Top Plus DSA system
multisweep
    high-resolution m. (HRMS)
multitime point imaging
multitracer
    m. imaging
    m. study
multivane intensity modulation compensator (MIMIC)
multivariant regressional analysis
multiwire proportional chamber
multizone transmit-receive focus
mural
    m. aneurysm
    m. arch
    m. architecture
    m. change
    m. clot
    m. CNS nodule
    m. defect
    m. degeneration
    m. dilatation
    m. endomyocardial fibrosis
    m. fibrosing alveolitis
    m. hematoma
    m. infiltrate
    m. kidney

m. leaflet of mitral valve
m. nodulation
m. pregnancy
m. stratification
m. thickening
m. thrombus
m. thrombus formation
mural-type vein of Galen malformation
mu rhythm
muscarinic receptor
muscle
abductor digiti quinti m.
abductor hallucis m.
abductor pollicis brevis m.
accessory m.
adductor magnus m.
Aeby m.
Albinus m.
anconeus m.
anomalous m.
anterior papillary m. (APM)
antigravity m.
m. artifact
auricular m.
axillary m.
BBC m.
belly of m.
biceps femoris m.
bipennate m.
Bochdalek m.
Bovero m.
Bowman m.
brachioradialis m.
Braune m.
Brücke m.
bulbi m.
bulbocavernosus m.
m. bulk
cardiac m.
Casser m.
casserian m.
cervical m.
Chassaignac m.
circular m.
Coiter m.
conal papillary m.
cone of extraocular m.
m. contracture
Crampton m.
cricopharyngeus m.
m. crushing injury
dartos m.

deep m.
m. of deglutition
detrusor m.
digastric m.
dorsal m.
Dupré m.
Duverney m.
ECRB m.
ECRL m.
ECU m.
EDB m.
EDC m.
EDL m.
EDQ m.
EIP m.
EPB m.
EPL m.
extensor carpi radialis brevis m.
extensor carpi radialis longus m.
extensor carpi ulnaris m.
extensor digiti quinti m.
extensor digitorum brevis m.
extensor digitorum communis m.
extensor digitorum longus m.
extensor hallucis longus m.
extensor indicis proprius m.
extensor pollicis brevis m.
extensor pollicis longus m.
external oblique m.
extraocular m.
extrinsic foot m.
fast-twitch m.
FDL m.
FDQB m.
FDS m.
m. fiber
m. fiber wasting
fibrosed m.
fixator m.
flexor carpi radialis m.
flexor digiti quinti brevis m.
flexor digitorum longus m.
flexor digitorum profundus m.
flexor digitorum superficialis m.
flexor hallucis brevis m.
Folius m.
frontotemporal m.
fused papillary m.
Gantzer m.
gastrocnemius m.
Gavard m.
genioglossus m.

M

NOTES

611

muscle *(continued)*

Guthrie m.
Hilton m.
Horner m.
Houston m.
hyoglossus m.
hyperintense m.
m. hyperintensity
ileococcygeus m.
iliocostal m.
iliopsoas m.
m. infarct
infarcted heart m.
inferior gemellus m.
infraspinatus m.
innermost intercostal m.
intercostal m.
internal intercostal m.
interosseous m.
interspinal m.
intertransverse m.
intraauricular m.
intrinsic foot m.
m. irritability
ischiocavernosus m.
Klein m.
Lancisi m.
lateral pterygoid m.
lateral rectus m.
latissimus dorsi m.
left ventricular m.
lesser m.
levator m.
longitudinal m.
longus colli m.
Luschka m.
major m.
Marcacci m.
masseter m.
masticator m.
medial papillary m.
medial pterygoid m.
middle m.
minimus scalenus m.
minor m.
Müller m.
multipennate m.
mylohyoid m.
myocardial m.
nonstriated m.
oblique m.
obturator internus m.
occipitofrontalis m.
Ochsner m.
Oddi m.
ODQ m.
Oehl m.

omohyoid m.
opponens digiti quinti m.
opposing m.
organic m.
m. ossification
palatal m.
papillary m.
paralaryngeal m.
paraspinal m.
Passavant m.
pectineus m.
pectoralis major m.
pectoralis minor m.
peroneal m.
peroneus quartus m.
pharyngeal m.
Phillips m.
piriform m.
piriformis m.
plantaris m.
platysma m.
posterior papillary m. (PPM)
Pozzi m.
psoas m.
pterygoid m.
pubococcygeus m.
pupillary constrictor m.
pyloric m.
quadrate m.
quadriceps m.
reactive disease of smooth m.
m. recruitment pattern
rectus m.
Reisseisen m.
retronuchal m.
rhomboideus major m.
ribbon m.
rider's m.
Riolan m.
rotator cuff m.
Rouget m.
round m.
Ruysch m.
sacrospinalis m.
Santorini m.
sartorius m.
scalenus anterior m.
Sebileau m.
semimembranous m.
semispinal m.
semitendinous m.
septal papillary m.
serratus anterior m.
m. sheath
short m.
shoulder m.
Sibson m.

skeletal m.
slow-twitch m.
smooth m.
Soemmerring m.
soleus m.
somatic m.
m. spasm
sphenomandibularis m.
m. spindle
spindle-shaped m.
sternocleidomastoid m.
sternohyoid m.
sternothyroid m.
m. strain
strap m.
striated m.
styloglossus m.
stylohyoid m.
subaortic m.
subscapularis m.
sucking m.
superficial m.
supraspinatus m.
synergic m.
tailor's m.
temporalis m.
tendinous part of epicranius m.
tensor veli palatini m.
Theile m.
thenar m.
thigh m.
m. tissue
Tod m.
Toynbee m.
transversus abdominis m.
trapezius m.
Treitz m.
triangular m.
trigonal m.
true back m.
two-bellied m.
unipennate m.
m. uptake
Valsalva m.
vascular smooth m.
vastus medialis m.
ventral m.
vertical m.
visceral m.
vocal m.
vocalis m.
voluntary m.

Wilson m.
wrinkler m.
muscle-eye-brain disease
muscle-fat interface
muscular
    m. atrioventricular septum
    m. branch
    m. bridge
    m. crus
    m. crus of diaphragm
    m. degeneration
    m. dystrophy
    m. hypertrophy
    m. insufficiency
    m. lesion
    m. ring esophagus
    m. slip
    m. subaortic stenosis
    m. tube
    m. twig
    m. ventricular septal defect
muscularis
    mucosa m.
    m. mucosa
    m. propria
musculature
    axial m.
    cervical m.
    longitudinal taenia m.
    paraspinous m.
    paravertebral m.
    scalene m.
musculi (*pl. of* musculus)
musculoaponeurotic
    m. fibroma
    m. fibromatosis
musculocutaneous sarcoidosis
musculofascial pedicle
musculophrenic
    m. artery
    m. branch
    m. vessel
musculoskeletal
    m. imaging
    m. imaging study
    m. lesion
    m. radiography
    m. system
    m. tumor
musculotendinous
    m. cuff
    m. junction

M

NOTES

musculotendinous *(continued)*
    m. retraction
    m. unit
musculotendinous-osseous link
musculotubal canal
musculus, pl. **musculi**
    m. uvula
mushroom
    m. appearance
    m. picker's disease
    m. shape
    m. worker's lung
mushroom-shaped mass
Musica
    multiscale image detail contrast
    amplification
Musset sign
mustard
    L-phenylalanine m. (LPAM)
MUSTPAC
    Medical Ultrasound Three-Dimensional
    Portable Advanced Communications
    MUSTPAC ultrasound imaging
mutant
mutation
    point m.
    reelin m.
mutational dysostosis
mutilans
    arthritis m.
muzzle velocity
MV
    megavolt
    mesenteric vasculitis
MVA
    mitral valve area
MVO
    maximum venous outflow
    mitral valve opening
    mitral valve orifice
MVP
    mitral valve prolapse
MVR
    mitral valve replacement
MVS
    mitral valve stenosis
MVV
    maximal voluntary ventilation
mycalamide A
mycetoma
    m. formation
    kidney m.
mycoplasmal pneumonitis
mycosis, pl. **mycoses**
mycotic
    m. aortic aneurysm
    m. brain aneurysm

    m. intracranial aneurysm
    m. lung infection
    m. plaque
    m. pneumonia
    m. sinusitis
myelencephalon
myelin
    m. ball
    m. ball formation
    m. sheath
myelination
    delayed m.
    nerve fiber m.
    optic pathway m.
myelinolysis
    central pontine m.
    extrapontine m.
    pontine m.
myelitis
    acute transverse m.
    radiation m.
    subacute necrotizing m.
    transverse m.
myeloblastoma
myelocele
myelocisternoencephalography
myelo-CT
myelocystocele
myelocystography
myelodysplasia
myelofibrosis
    acute m.
    m. osteosclerosis
myelogenesis
myelogram
myelographic imaging agent
myelography
    air m.
    cervical m.
    complete m.
    computed m.
    computer-assisted m. (CAM)
    CT m.
    extraarachnoid m.
    Hypaque m.
    m. imaging
    lumbar m.
    lumbosacral m.
    magnetic resonance m.
    metrizamide m.
    oil m.
    opaque m.
    oxygen m.
    Pantopaque m.
    positive contrast m.
    thoracic m.
    water-soluble m.

myeloid
> m. malignancy
> m. metaphysis

myelolipoma
> adrenal m.

myeloma
> amyloidosis of multiple m.
> endothelial m.
> indolent m.
> localized m.
> M-band m.
> multiple bone m.
> multiple kidney m.
> plasmablastic m.
> sclerosing m.
> solitary bone m.
> spinal plasma cell m.

myelomalacia
> cystic m.

myelomatosis

myelopathy
> acute posttraumatic m.
> carcinomatous m.
> cervical spondylotic m. (CSM)
> cystic m.
> delayed posttraumatic m.
> necrotizing m.
> paracarcinomatous m.
> posttraumatic ascending m.
> posttraumatic cystic m.
> progressive posttraumatic m.
> radiation m.
> spondylotic m.
> subacute necrotizing m.

myelophthisic splenomegaly

myeloproliferative disorder

myeloschisis

myelosclerosis

myelotomography

myenteric
> m. plexus
> m. plexus of Auerbach

Myerson sign

mylohyoid
> m. muscle
> m. ridge

myoblastoma
> granular breast-cell m.
> granular lung-cell m.
> granular sella-cell m.

myocardial
> m. blood flow (MBF)

m. blush
m. bridge
m. calcification
m. cellular degeneration
m. cellular hypertrophy
m. centroid
m. contractile function
m. contractility
m. contracture
m. contrast appearance time (MCAT)
m. contrast echocardiography (MCE)
m. contusion
m. depression
m. dilatation
m. disarray
m. fiber
m. fibrous degeneration
m. function assessment
m. hibernation
m. I-123 MIBG imaging
m. incompetence
m. infarct (MI)
m. infarct imaging
m. infarction recovery index
m. infiltration
m. inflammation
m. insufficiency
m. insult
m. irritability
m. ischemia
m. jeopardy index
m. mass
m. metabolism
m. muscle
m. necrosis
m. O_2 demand index
m. oxygen consumption
m. perfusion
m. perfusion echocardiography
m. perfusion imaging (MPI)
m. perfusion imaging Q-complex
m. perfusion reserve (MPR)
m. perfusion scan
m. perfusion scintigraphy
m. perfusion tomography
m. preservation
m. protection
m. recovery
m. reperfusion injury
m. revascularization

M

NOTES

myocardial *(continued)*
  m. rupture
  m. scar
  m. stunning
  m. tagging
  m. texture analysis
  m. thallium imaging
  m. thickening
  m. tissue viability
  m. twist
  m. uptake
  m. wall
  m. work
myocardial-specific marker
myocardiopathy
myocarditis
  fibroid m.
  fragmentation m.
myocardium
  asynergic m.
  calcification of m.
  dilated m.
  hibernating m.
  hypertrophied m.
  hypokinetic m.
  infarcted m.
  inferior apical aspect of the m.
  ischemic reperfused m.
  ischemic viable m.
  jeopardized m.
  necrotic m.
  noninfarcted m.
  nonperfused m.
  perfused m.
  recovery period of m.
  refractory period of m.
  reperfused m.
  rupture of m.
  salvage of m.
  senile m.
  sparkling appearance of m.
  stunned m.
  thinned m.
  ventricular m.
  viable m.
myocardium-to-abdomen count ratio
myocyte
  cardiac m.
  m. membrane purinoceptor
myoepithelial sialadenitis
myoepithelioma
myofascial
  m. disruption
  m. pain-dysfunction syndrome
myofibrillar disintegration
myofibril volume fraction

myofibroblastoma
  giant m.
  intranodal m.
myofibrohistiocytic proliferation
myofibromatosis
  infantile m.
myogenesis
myoid hamartoma
myoinositol-creatine ratio (Mi/Cr)
myointimal
  m. hyperplasia
  m. proliferation
myoma
  complicated m.
  intramural m.
  pedunculated subserous m.
  serosal m.
  submucous m.
  uncomplicated m.
  uterine m.
myometrial
  m. contraction
  m. septum
myometrium
  uterine m.
myonecrosis
  calcific m.
myoneural junction
myopathy
  carcinomatous m.
myosarcoma
Myoscint
  M. imaging
  M. imaging agent
myosin
  [111]In murine monoclonal antibody
    Fab to m.
myosis
  endolymphatic stromal m.
myositis
  brucellar m.
  eye m.
  granulomatous m.
  m. ossificans circumscripta
myostatic contracture
myotendinous
  m. junction
  m. junction rupture
  m. strain
myotube
Myoview imaging agent
myxadenoma
myxedema
  m. of heart
  pretibial m.
myxoglobulosis

myxoid
    m. cyst
    m. degenerative change
    m. extraskeletal chondrosarcoma
    m. malignant fibrous histiocytoma
    m. MFH
myxoma, pl. **myxomata, myxomas**
    atrial m.
    biatrial m.
    cardiac m.
    complex m.
    familial m.
    heart m.
    m. of heart
    left atrial m.
    odontogenic m.
    pedunculated uterine m.
    vascular m.
    ventricular m.
myxomatodes
    fibroma m.
myxomatous
    m. degeneration
    m. liposarcoma
    m. proliferation
    m. valve leaflet
myxomembranous colitis
myxopapillary ependymoma
MZL
    marginal zone lymphoma

NOTES

M

N

nitrogen

¹³**N**

^{13}N ammonia radioactive tracer
^{13}N ammonia uptake

¹⁴**N**

nitrogen-14

¹⁵**N**

nitrogen-15

²³**Na**

sodium-23
^{23}Na magnetic resonance imaging

²⁴**Na**

sodium-24

nabothian

n. cyst
n. follicle

Naclerio

V-sign of N.

nadir

untransformed n.

Naegele obliquity
Naffziger sign
Nägele pelvis
NaI

sodium iodide
NaI detector

nail

n. bed lesion
body of n.
gamma n.
intramedullary n.
Jewett n.
orthopedic n.
n. plate
n. plate avulsion
Smith-Petersen n.
spoon-shaped n.
triflanged n.
Zickel supercondylar n.

nailing

elastic stable intramedullary n.
(ESIN)

nail-patella syndrome
nail-plate device
Nakata index
naked-facet sign
naloxone imaging agent
Namaqualand hip dysplasia
nanocolloid

technetium-99m n.

nanocurie (nCi)
nanogram (ng)
nanoparticle

iodinated n.

nanoparticulate imaging agent
napkin-ring

n.-r. anular lesion
n.-r. anular stenosis
n.-r. anular tumor
n.-r. trachea

Napoleon hat sign
Narcomatic flowmetry
naris, pl. **nares**
narrow

n. anteroposterior diameter
n. beam
n. caliber
n. chest
n. collimation
n. gating tolerance

narrow-band spectral-selective
radiofrequency pulse
narrow-beam half-thickness
narrowed

n. orifice
n. valve

narrowing

airway n.
antral stomach n.
arterial n.
arteriolar n.
n. of artery
artificial lumen n.
n. asymmetry
atherosclerotic n.
beak-like n.
bile duct n.
bird-beak configuration or n.
bronchiolar n.
n. of bronchiolar passage
carinal angle n.
circumferential n.
colonic n.
concentric n.
degenerative n.
diffuse n.
discrete n.
disk space n.
duodenal n.
eccentric n.
esophageal n.
n. exchange
focal esophageal n.
n. of forefoot
gastric n.
glottic n.
high-grade n.
intervertebral disk n.
joint space n.

N

narrowing *(continued)*
    large airway n.
    longitudinal n.
    long smooth esophageal n.
    lower esophageal n.
    luminal n.
    motional n.
    nasopharyngeal n.
    neural foraminal n.
    oropharyngeal n.
    pancompartmental joint space n.
    rectal n.
    residual luminal n.
    retropharyngeal n.
    segmental bronchus n.
    smooth esophageal n.
    n. of spinal canal
    stomach n.
    subcritical n.
    subglottic n.
    supraglottic n.
    symmetric n.
    n. of thecal sac
    tracheal n.
    vallecular n.
nasal
    n. airway resistance
    n. bone
    n. bridge
    n. canal
    n. cavity
    n. cavity wall
    n. concha
    n. fracture
    n. intubation
    n. meatus
    n. mucociliary clearance function
    n. part of pharynx
    n. polyp
    n. septum
    n. septum hematoma
    n. sinus
    n. spine
    n. suture
    n. tip deformity
    n. turbinate
    n. vault mass
nasal-to-plasma radioactivity ratio
nasi
    agger n.
nasion recession
nasobregmatic arc
nasociliary nerve
nasofrontal
    n. duct
    n. suture

nasogastric
    n. intubation
    n. (NG) tube
nasojejunal feeding tube
nasolabial
    n. cyst
    n. lymph node
nasolacrimal
    n. canal
    n. duct
nasomaxillary
    n. fracture
    n. suture
nasooccipital arc
nasoorbital fracture
nasopalatal fissure
nasopalatine canal
nasopharyngeal
    n. atresia
    n. carcinoma (NPC)
    n. craniopharyngioma
    n. hematoma
    n. mass
    n. mucous retention cyst
    n. narrowing
    n. reflux
    n. squamous cell carcinoma
nasopharyngography
nasopharynx
nasotracheal
    n. intubation
    n. tube
natatory ligament
natiform skull
native
    n. aorta
    n. aortic valve
    n. aortic valve closure
    n. atherosclerosis
    n. coronary artery
    n. image
    n. kidney
    n. kidney renal artery stenosis
    n. kidney renal vein thrombosis
    n. lung
    n. tissue harmonic imaging (NTHI)
    n. ventricle
    n. vessel
natural
    n. neon gas
    n. radiation
    n. radioactivity
Naumoff syndrome
Navarre catheter
navel
    n. ring artifact
    n. string

Navi Ball guidance system
navicular
> n. body
> n. body fracture
> n. bone
> carpal n.
> n. to first metatarsal angle
> n. hand fracture
> ossific nucleus of n.
> n. projection
> protrusion of n.
> target n.
> tarsal n.
> n. tuberosity
> n. view

naviculare
> os n.

navicularis
> fossa n.

naviculocapitate fracture
naviculocuneiform
> n. joint
> n. ligament

navigable echo signal
navigated spin-echo diffusion-weighted MR imaging
navigation
> computer-assisted intracranial n.

navigator
> N. computer workstation
> n. echo
> n. echo-based real-time respiratory gating and triggering
> n. echo motion correction technique
> n. pulse
> n. shift

Navigus cranial electrode system
Navi-Star ablation catheter
Navitrack computer-assisted surgery system
NB
> neuroblastoma

N-butyl-2-cyanoacrylate embolization
N-Cat N-500 tonometric blood pressure monitor
NCCT
> noncontrast head CT

nCi
> nanocurie

NCP
> noncontrast phase
> implanted NCP

NCPF
> noncirrhotic portal fibrosis

Nd:YAG
> neodymium:yttrium-aluminum-garnet
> Nd:YAG CTLC
> Nd:YAG laser catheter

Nd:YLF
> neodymium:yttrium-lithium fluoride
> Nd:YLF laser

near
> n. field
> n. infrared (NIR)
> n. infrared spectroscopy (NIRS)

near-anatomic
> n.-a. position
> n.-a. position of joint

near-infrared optical mammography
near-normal radiotracer uptake
near-resonance spin-lock contrast
near-water
> n.-w. attenuation
> n.-w. density

NEC
> noise effective count

necessity
> fracture of n.

neck
> anatomic n.
> n. of aneurysm
> aneurysmal n.
> aneurysm remnant n.
> n. of bladder
> bone n.
> n. coil
> dental n.
> n. emphysema
> femoral n.
> n. of femur
> n. fracture
> n. of gallbladder
> n. germ-cell tumor
> hyperextension of n.
> n. lymphangioma
> Madelung n.
> n. of pancreas
> pancreatic n.
> n. phantom
> posterior triangle of the n.
> potato tumor of n.

NOTES

N

neck (*continued*)
    n. of rib
    selective occlusion of
      aneurysmal n.
    n. shaft angle
    surgical n.
    n. of talus
    n. teratoma
    uterine wry n.
    vesical n.
    webbed n.
neck-space anatomy
necleotherapy
necrobiotic nodule
necrolytic
necrosis, pl. **necroses**
    acute cortical n.
    acute native kidney tubular n.
    acute renal transplant tubular n.
    acute sclerosing hyaline n. (ASHN)
    acute tubular n. (ATN)
    alveolar septal n.
    aortic idiopathic n.
    arteriolar n.
    aseptic n.
    asphyxia-related renal n.
    avascular n. (AVN)
    avascular bone n.
    avascular cortical infarction n.
    avascular femoral head n.
    avascular tarsal scaphoid n.
    avascular vertebral body n.
    bilateral cortical n.
    biliary piecemeal n.
    bloodless zone of n.
    bony n.
    bowel n.
    breast fat n.
    bridging n.
    caseous n.
    central n.
    centrilobular n.
    coagulation n.
    colliquative n.
    colonic n.
    comedo n.
    contraction band n.
    cortical kidney n.
    cystic medial n.
    diffuse n.
    dirty n.
    embolic n.
    epiphyseal ischemic n.
    Erdheim cystic medial n.
    fascial margin n.
    fat n.
    fatty n.

fibrinoid n.
fibrosing piecemeal n.
Ficat stage of avascular n.
focal fat n.
focal hepatic n.
frank n.
heart muscle n.
hemorrhagic n.
hepatic n.
hyaline n.
idiopathic avascular n.
indurative n.
intestinal n.
intratumoral n.
ischemic n.
laminar brain n.
liquefaction n.
localized n.
lung n.
margin n.
massive hepatic n.
medial cystic n.
midzonal n.
mucosal n.
myocardial n.
Paget quiet n.
pancreatic n.
papillary n.
peripheral n.
piecemeal n.
postbiopsy fat n.
postpartum pituitary n.
postsurgical fat n.
posttraumatic aseptic n.
posttraumatic fat n.
pressure n.
progressive emphysematous n.
punctate n.
radiation n.
radiation-induced n. (RIN)
radium n.
renal allograft n.
renal cortical n.
renal papillary n.
renal tubular n.
septal n.
septic n.
soft tissue n.
strangulation n.
stromal n.
subacute hepatic n.
subcapsular hepatic n.
subcutaneous fat n.
subendocardial n.
submassive hepatic n.
superficial n.
total n.

tracheobronchial mucosal n.
transmural n.
traumatic fat n.
tubular n.
tumor n.
vascular n.
ventricular muscle n.
Zenker n.

necrotic
n. bone
n. bone pseudocyst
n. debris
n. flap
n. inflammation
n. lesion
n. metastasis
n. myocardium
n. renal cell carcinoma
n. sequestrum
n. tissue
n. tumor
n. ulcer

necrotizing
n. aspergillosis
n. emphysema
n. enterocolitis
n. external otitis
n. fasciitis
n. gastritis
n. glomerulonephritis
n. myelopathy
n. pancreatitis
n. pneumonia
n. respiratory granulomatosis
n. thrombosis
n. ulcerative gingivitis (NUG)

NECT
nonenhanced computed tomography

NED
no evidence of disease

needle
Abrams biopsy n.
abscission n.
Accucore II biopsy n.
Amplatz angiography n.
Arrow Fischell Evan N.
aspiration biopsy n.
Bauer Temno biopsy n.
B-D bone marrow biopsy n.
beveled n.
Bierman n.
BioPince n.

biopsy n.
n. biopsy
Biopty cut n.
blood-containment n.
blunt-end sialogram n.
BV2 n.
cesium n.
Chiba n.
coaxial sheath cut-biopsy n.
Colapinto n.
Conrad-Crosby bone marrow
  biopsy n.
Cope biopsy n.
core biopsy n.
Cournand arteriography n.
Cournand-Grino angiography n.
n. deviation
Dos Santos aortography n.
dumbbell n.
Echo-Coat ultrasound biopsy n.
E-Z-EM cut biopsy n.
flexible biopsy n.
Franseen n.
full-intensity n.
18-gauge percutaneous access n.
Greene n.
half-intensity n.
Hawkins-Akins n.
Hawkins breast lesion
  localization n.
Hawkins one-stick n.
Homerlok n.
Homer Mammalok n.
n. hydrophone
iridium n.
Kopans n.
Kormed liver biopsy n.
n. localization
n. localization of breast lesion
n.-localized breast biopsy (NLBB)
Maggi biopsy n.
Mammalock n.
n. marker
Mentor prostatic biopsy n.
metallic n.
micropuncture n.
2.1-mm automated biopsy n.
Monoject hypodermic n.
Monopty n.
Multi-Pro biopsy n.
nonferromagnetic n.
OSTYCUT bone biopsy n.

N

NOTES

needle *(continued)*
PercuCut cut-biopsy n.
n. pyelography
Quick-Core biopsy n.
Quincke spinal n.
^{226}Ra n.
Rosch-Uchida n.
scalp vein n.
Seldinger n.
self-aspirating cut-biopsy n.
sheath n.
sialography n.
single-wall n.
skinny n.
Sos Pulse-Vu Bloodless Entry N.
spinal n.
spring-loaded biopsy n.
Temno II cutting n.
T-fastener delivery n.
TLA n.
translumbar aortography n.
Tuohy aortography n.
n. visualization
Westcott n.
Whitacre spinal n.
Yeuh centesis n.
needle-guided excisional biopsy
needle-hookwire localization
needle-shaped breast calcification
needle-tip bioimpedance
Neel temperature
Neer
N. classification of shoulder
fracture
N. impingement sign
N. lateral view
N. transscapular view
Neer-Horowitz
N.-H. classification of humeral
fracture
N.-H. humerus fracture
classification
NEFA
nonesterified fatty acid
N. scintigraphy
Neff percutaneous access set
negative
n. contrast imaging agent
n. contrast left atriography
n. EMA result
n. image
n. image pulmonary edema
n. Mach band
n. mucin result
n. predictive value
pulmonary edema photographic n.
true n. (TN)

negative-ion cyclotron
negatron emission
negligible pressure gradient
Nélaton
N. dislocation
N. fold
N. line
Nelson syndrome
NEMD
nonspecific esophageal motility disorder
neoadjuvant
n. hormonal therapy
n. radiotherapy
neoangiogenesis
neoaorta
neoaortic valve
neobladder
ileal n.
neocerebellum
neocholangiole
neocortex
neodensity
neodymium:YAG laser therapy
neodymium:yttrium-aluminum-garnet
(Nd:YAG)
n. laser
n. laser catheter
neodymium:yttrium-lithium fluoride
(Nd:YLF)
neofissure
neogalactosyl albumin
neointima formation
neointimal
n. hyperplasia
n. proliferation
Neo-Iopax
neonatal
n. adrenal ultrasound
n. ascites
n. cardiac failure
n. choroid plexus hemorrhage
n. cystic pulmonary emphysema
n. heart failure
n. hepatitis
n. hyperthyroidism
n. intracerebellar hemorrhage
n. intracranial hemorrhage
n. intracranial ischemia
n. intraventricular hemorrhage
n. omphalitis
n. osteomyelitis
n. pneumonia
n. radiography
n. subdural hemorrhage
n. transfontanellar brain ultrasound
n. wet lung disease

neonate
    n. encephalomalacia
    n. mediastinal shift
neonatorum
    edema n.
neon particle protocol
neopallium
neoplasia
    exophytic n.
    extrinsic n.
    lobular n.
neoplasm, pl. neoplasia
    adrenocortical n.
    benign n.
    bone n.
    breast n.
    bronchopulmonary n.
    cavitating n.
    cervical intraepithelial n.
    choroid plexus n.
    colonic n.
    connective tissue n.
    cranial nerve n.
    cystic splenic n.
    ductectatic mucinous cystic n.
    encapsulated n.
    epithelial n.
    esophageal n.
    external ear n.
    firm n.
    focally decreased renal n.
    functioning n.
    gestational trophoblastic n.
    gonadal n.
    granulosa theca n.
    hepatic n.
    interdigital n.
    intracranial n.
    intrahepatic biliary n.
    intramedullary compartment n.
    lethal n.
    low-grade n.
    macrocystic n.
    malignant urethral n.
    mesenchymal n.
    metastatic renal n.
    middle ear n.
    mucinous pancreatic cystic n.
    multiple endocrine n. (MEN)
    neuroepithelial n.
    NK-cell n.
    osteocartilaginous parasellar n.

    ovarian n.
    pancreatic n.
    papillary epithelial n.
    papillary pancreatic cystic n.
    pearly n.
    pineal gland n.
    primary n.
    second malignant n. (SMN)
    skeletal n.
    soft tissue n.
    spherical n.
    supratentorial n.
    T-cell n.
    thoracic spinal n.
    thymic n.
    transitional cell n.
    trochlear nerve n.
    vaginal intraepithelial n.
    vulvar intraepithelial n.
    well-circumscribed n.
neoplastic
    n. aneurysm
    n. calcification
    n. cyst
    n. destruction of spinal element
    n. fracture
    n. hyperplasia
    n. invasion
    n. lesion
    n. process
    n. stenosis
    n. tissue
Neoprobe
    N. 1000, 1500 portable
       radioisotope detector
    N. radioactivity detector
neopterin
neorectum
Neoscan
NeoSpect diagnostic imaging agent
neosphincter
neostigmine methylsulfate
NeoTect imaging agent
neoterminal ileum
neovagina
neovascularity
    tumor n.
neovascularization
    choroidal neovascularization (CNV)
neovasculature
    tumor n.
nepheline pneumoconiosis

NOTES

nephritic calculus
nephritis, pl. **nephritides**
    acute diffuse bacterial n.
    acute focal bacterial n.
    acute interstitial n. (AIN)
    bacterial n.
    Balkan n.
    chronic hereditary n.
    diffuse bacterial n.
    focal bacterial n.
    glomerular n.
    interstitial n.
    nephrocalcinosis n.
    radiation n.
    salt-losing n.
    tubulointerstitial n.
nephroblastoma
    classical n.
    cystic partially differentiated n.
    polycystic n.
nephroblastomatosis
    multifocal n.
    superficial diffuse n.
nephrocalcinosis
    cortical n.
    medullary n.
    n. nephritis
    renal cortical n.
nephrogenic, nephrogenetic
    n. bladder adenoma
    n. diabetes insipidus
    n. phase
nephroglastomatosis
    panlobar n.
nephrogram
    cortical rim n.
    delayed unilateral n.
    increasingly dense n.
    medullary n.
    obstructive n.
    persistent increasing n.
    rim n.
    n. rim
    segmental n.
    shell n.
    n. shock
    soap-bubble n.
    spotted n.
    striated angiographic n.
    sunburst n.
    Swiss cheese n.
    tubular n.
nephrographic
    generalized n. (GNG)
    n. phase (NP)
nephrography
    isotope n.

nephrolithiasis
nephrolithotomy
    percutaneous n. (PCNL)
nephroma
    congenital mesoblastic n.
    cystic n.
    mesoblastic n.
    multilocular cystic n.
NephroMax balloon catheter
nephronia
    lobar n.
nephronophthisis
    juvenile n.
nephropathic cystinosis
nephropathy
    analgesic n.
    Balkan n.
    contrast media-induced n.
    diabetic n.
    HIV n.
    obstructive n.
    radiation n.
    radiocontrast-induced n.
    radiographic contrast media-
      induced n.
    reflux n.
    urate n.
    uric acid n.
nephroptosis
nephropyelography
nephrosclerosis
    arterial n.
    benign n.
    malignant n.
    senile n.
nephroscope
    Alken-Marberger n.
    flexible n.
    percutaneous n.
    Wickham-Miller n.
nephroscopic fulguration
nephroscopy
nephrosis, pl. **nephroses**
    congenital Finnish n.
nephrosonography
nephrostogram
    n. imaging
    postprocedure n.
nephrostolithotomy
    caliceal n.
    percutaneous n. (PCNL)
nephrostomy
    n. catheter
    circle wire n.
    Cope loop n.
    percutaneous n.

n. puncture
n. track
nephrotic
n. edema
n. syndrome
nephrotomogram
nephrotomography
n. imaging
infusion n.
nephrotoxic contrast medium
nephrotoxicity
contrast media n.
cyclosporin n.
drug-induced n.
nephroureteral
n. stent
n. stent system
nephroureterectomy
nephroureterostomy stent
nephrourography
nephrouroradiology
Neptune trident appearance
neptunium
NER
no evidence of recurrence
NERD
no evidence of recurrent disease
Nernst equation
nerve
accessory n.
acoustic n.
afferent digital n.
cluneal n.
cochlear n.
cranial n.
dorsal ramus of spinal n.
efferent digital n.
n. entrapment
excrescentic thickening of the
optic n.
facial n.
femoral n.
n. fiber myelination
fifth cranial n.
fourth cranial n.
frontal n.
fusiform enlargement of the
optic n.
glossopharyngeal n.
greater superficial petrosal n.
hypoglossal n.
n. injury

intercostal n.
intercostobrachial n.
interosseous n.
lacrimal n.
laryngeal n.
n. of Latarjet
left respiratory n.
lingual n.
mandibular n.
median n.
nasociliary n.
oculomotor n.
ophthalmic n.
optic n.
peripheral n.
periradicular n.
peroneal n.
petrosal n.
pinched n.
n. plexus
posterior interosseous n. (PIN)
recurrent laryngeal n.
recurrent meningeal n.
n. root
n. root axillary pouch
n. root compression
n. root edema
n. root embarrassment
n. root impingement
n. root irritability
n. roots of the cauda equina
n. root sheath
n. root sheath effacement
n. root sleeve
n. root tumor
rostral cervical n.
sacral n.
saphenous n.
second cranial n.
n. sheath tumor
spinal accessory n.
subcostal n.
supraspinatus n.
sural n.
trochlear n.
n. trunk
vagus n.
vein, artery, n.
vestibular division of eighth
cranial n.
vestibulocochlear n.
vidian n.

N

NOTES

VIII nerve complex
nervus intermedius
nesidioblastoma
nesidioblastosis
nest
    junctional n.
net
    n. magnetization factor
    n. magnetization vector
    n. shunt
    n. tissue magnetization
    n. transverse magnetization
network
    articular n.
    artificial neural n.
    hypertrophic duct n.
    lymphatic n.
    matching n.
    neural n.
    vascular n.
    venous n.
neural
    n. arch cleft
    n. arch fracture
    n. axis vascular malformation
    n. canal
    n. crest origin
    n. crest tissue
    n. evaluation algorithm
    n. fibrolipoma
    n. foramen
    n. foramen remodeling
    n. foraminal narrowing
    n. groove
    n. miscommunication
    n. network
    n. origin bone tumor
    n. pathway
    n. placode
    n. sheath
    n. tube
    n. tube defect (NTD)
    n. tuberculosis
    n. vertebral arch
neuralgia
    sphenopalatine n.
neuraxis
    n. radiation therapy
    n. staging
neuraxonal dystrophy
neurenteric canal
neurilemoma, neurilemmoma
neurinoma (*var. of* neuroma)
neuritic
    n. plaquing
    n. senile plaque
neuritis, pl. **neuritides**

    axial n.
    brachial plexus n.
    friction n.
    optic n.
Neuro
    N. Lobe software
    N. SPGR software
neuroangiography
neuroarthropathy
neuroaugmentation
neuroblastoma (NB)
    adrenal n.
    cerebral n.
    chest wall n.
    dumbbell-type n.
    Hutchinson-type n.
    intracranial n.
    intraventricular n.
    olfactory n.
    stage 4S n.
    n. staging
neuroblockage
neurocentral synchondrosis
neurocutaneous syndrome
neurocysticercosis
neurocytoma
    central n.
    intraventricular n.
neurodegenerative disease
neurodiagnostic
    n. imaging
    n. scanner
NeuroEcho software
neuroectodermal
    n. dysplasia
    n. origin
    n. tumor
neuroendocrine
    n. hepatic metastasis
    n. small-cell carcinoma
    n. tumor
neuroendovascular interventional
    procedure
neuroenteric cyst
neuroepithelial neoplasm
neurofibrillary tangle
neurofibroma
    aryepiglottic fold n.
    craniofacial plexiform n.
    dumbbell n.
    extraspinal n.
    paraspinal n.
    plexiform n.
neurofibromatosis
    abortive n.
    central n.
    incomplete n.

kidney n.
peripheral n.
segmental n.
type 1, 2 n.
n. with bilateral acoustic neuroma
neurofibrosarcoma
neurofilamentous misalignment
NeuroFOCUS scanner
neurogenic
n. disorder
n. fracture
n. intestinal obstruction
n. lesion
n. pulmonary edema
n. sarcoma
n. tumor
neuroglial tumor
neurography
magnetic resonance n. (MRN)
neuroimaging
3D n.
functional n.
n. modality
neurointerventional radiology
NeuroLink II data acquisition system
Neurolite imaging agent
neurologic
n. bladder lesion
n. sequelae
neuroma, neurinoma
acoustic n.
digital n.
interdigital n.
Morton n.
multicystic acoustic n.
neurofibromatosis with bilateral
acoustic n.
postamputation n.
posttraumatic n.
neuromatosa
elephantiasis n.
neuromeningeal trunk
neuromorphometry
neuromuscular
n. junction
n. system electric induction
neuromyelitis optica
neuromyopathy
carcinomatous n.
neuron
lower motor n.
nigrostriatal dopaminergic n.

pyramidal n.
upper motor n.
neuronal
n. cell origin tumor
n. cytotoxic edema
n. migration
n. plasticity
n. proliferation
neuronavigation
neurootologist
Neuropac
neuropathic
n. ankle
n. arthropathy
n. fracture
n. midfoot deformity
n. osteoarthropathy
n. tarsometatarsal joint
neuropathicum
papilloma n.
neuropathy
compression n.
entrapment n.
radiation-related optic n. (RON)
neuropore
neuroradiologic
n. examination
n. imaging
neuroradiology
interventional n.
pediatric n.
neuroreceptor
neuroroentgenography
neurosarcoidosis
neurosarcoma
NeuroScan 3D imager
neurosecretory granule
NeuroSector
N. ultrasound
N. ultrasound system
neurosonogram
neurosonography
neurosonology
neurospectroscopy
neuroticum
papilloma n., papilloma
neuropathicum
neurotomography
neurotoxic effect
neurotransmitter
excitatory n.
n. imaging

N

NOTES

neurotransmitter (continued)
    inhibitory n.
    n. precursor
neurotrophic
    n. fracture
    n. imaging agent
    n. joint
neurovascular
    n. bundle
    n. compression
    n. lesion
neurSector scanner
neurulation
neutral
    adduction to n.
    n. amyloid probe
    n. hip position
neutralization plate
neutrino
    electron n.
neutron
    n. absorption process
    n. activation analysis
    n. beam
    n. bombardment
    epithermal n.
    fast n.
    n. number
    n. radiation
    n. radiography
    slow n.
    n. therapy
    n. therapy machine
    thermal n.
neutron-deficient
    n.-d. nucleus
    n.-d. short-lived isotope
neutron/gamma
    n. transmission
    n. transmission method
    n. transmission therapy
neutron-rich biomedical tracer
neutropenic enterocolitis
neutrophilic leukocyte
Neviaser frozen shoulder classification
nevoid
    n. basal cell carcinoma
    n. basal cell carcinoma syndrome
nevus verrucosus
new bone formation
Newman
    N. classification of radial neck and
        head fracture
    N. radial fracture classification
NewTom CT scanner
Newton guidewire

Newvicon camera tube
NEX
    number of excitation
ng
    nanogram
Nicoladoni-Branham sign
Nicolet
    N. Elite Doppler monitor
    N. NMR spectrometer
Nicoll bone
nicotinamide
    n. imaging agent
    n. radiosensitizer
Nidek EC-5000 excimer laser system
nidus
    n. angle
    arteriovenous malformation n.
    n. demarcation
    n. of lesion
    n. patency
    thrombus n.
    tumor n.
Niemann-Pick disease
Niemeier gallbladder perforation
Nievergelt
    N. disease
    N. syndrome
Niewenglowski ray
nightstick fracture
nigra
    substantia n.
nigricans
    acanthosis n.
nigrostriatal dopaminergic neuron
Nihon Kohden Neurofax
    Electroencephalograph
nimodipine
    n. imaging agent
    intraarterial superselective n.
niobium/titanium superconductor
Niopam
    N. contrast medium
    N. imaging agent
NIP
    nonspecific interstitial pneumonia
nipple
    adenoma of n.
    aortic n.
    deep to the n.
    n. marker
    out-of-profile n.
    n. retraction
    n. ring artifact
    n. sector
    n. shadow
nipple-areolar complex

nipple-like
> n.-l. common bile duct
> n.-l. osteophyte formation

NIPS
> noninvasive programmed stimulation

NIR
> near infrared
> NIR contrast agent
> NIR optical mammography

NIRS
> near infrared spectroscopy

Nishimoto Sangyo scanner

Nissen
> N. antireflux operation
> N. fundoplication
> N. fundoplication procedure

Ni-Ti alloy stent

nitinol
> n. guidewire
> n. inferior vena cava filter
> n. U-clips
> n. wire core

Nitinol Symphony stent

niton

nitric oxide

nitrocellulose film

nitrogen (N)
> n. washout

nitrogen-13
> nitrogen-13 ammonia imaging agent

nitrogen-14 (^{14}N)

nitrogen-15 (^{15}N)

nitroxide-stable free radical

NK-cell neoplasm

NLBB
> needle-localized breast biopsy

N-methylspiperone

N-methylspiroperidol (NMS)
> ^{11}C N.-m.

NMR
> nuclear magnetic resonance
> continuous-wave NMR
> 2D NMR
> NMR imaging
> NMR LipoProfile test
> magic angle spinning NMR
> NMR magnetometer probe
> pulse NMR
> pulsed-electron paramagnetic NMR
> NMR quadrature detection array
> NMR scan
> NMR signal

> NMR spectrometer
> surface coil NMR

NMS
> N-methylspiroperidol

no
> no discernible finding
> no evidence of disease (NED)
> no evidence of recurrence (NER)
> no evidence of recurrent disease (NERD)
> no frequency wrap

noble
> n. gas
> n. gas in magnetic resonance study
> N. position

***Nocardia* brain abscess**

nocardial osteomyelitis

no-carrier-added
> n.-c.-a. ^{18}F imaging agent
> n.-c.-a. radionuclide

nocturnal polysomnography

nodal
> n. conduction
> n. disease
> n. fibrosis
> n. impulse
> n. metastasis
> n. point
> n. premature contraction
> n. rhythm
> n. rupture
> n. staging
> n. tissue

node
> abdominal lymph n.
> accessory lymph n.
> anorectal lymph n.
> aortic lymph n.
> aortic window n.
> apical lymph n.
> appendicular lymph n.
> Aschoff n.
> Aschoff-Tawara n.
> atrioventricular n.
> auricular lymph n.
> AV n.
> axillary lymph n. (ALN)
> azygos lymph n.
> benign n.
> bifurcation lymph n.
> Bouchard n.
> brachial lymph n.

NOTES

node *(continued)*
brachiocephalic lymph n.
bronchopulmonary lymph n.
buccinator lymph n.
n. calcification
calcified lymph n.
cardiac n.
cartilaginous n.
caval lymph n.
celiac lymph n.
central lymph n.
cervical paratracheal lymph n.
Cloquet inguinal lymph n.
common iliac lymph n.
companion lymph n.
coronary n.
cubital lymph n.
cystic lymph n.
Delphian lymph n.
deltopectoral lymph n.
diaphragmatic lymph n.
Dürck n.
eggshell calcification of lymph n.
epicolic lymph n.
epigastric lymph n.
epitrochlear lymph n.
Ewald n.
external iliac lymph n.
fibular lymph n.
Flack sinoatrial n.
foraminal n.
gastric lymph n.
gastroduodenal lymph n.
gastroepiploic lymph n.
gastrohepatic ligament n.
gastroomental lymph n.
Ghon n.
giant hyperplasia lymph n.
gluteal lymph n.
gouty n.
Haygarth n.
Heberden n.
hemal n.
hemolymph n.
Hensen n.
hepatic lymph n.
hilar lymph n.
ileocolic lymph n.
iliac circumflex lymph n.
ilioinguinal lymph n.
image-intensifier n.
infraclavicular n.
infrahyoid lymph n.
inguinal lymph n.
intercostal lymph n.
interiliac lymph n.
internal mammary lymph n.

interpectoral lymph n.
intramammary n. (IMN)
intramammary lymph n.
intraparenchymal lymph n.
intrapulmonary lymph n.
jugular lymph n.
jugulodigastric n.
juguloomohyoid lymph n.
juxtaintestinal n.
Keith n.
Keith-Flack sinoatrial n.
Koch sinoatrial n.
lacunar n.
lumbar lymph n.
lymph n.
lymphomatous lymph n.
malar lymph n.
mandibular lymph n.
mastoid lymph n.
medial supraclavicular n.
mediastinal n.
mesenteric n.
Meynet n.
multicentric angiofollicular lymph n.
nasolabial lymph n.
obturator lymph n.
occipital lymph n.
Osler n.
pancreatic lymph n.
pancreaticoduodenal lymph n.
pancreaticolienal lymph n.
pancreaticosplenic n.
paraaortic lymph n.
paracardial lymph n.
paracolic lymph n.
paramammary lymph n.
pararectal lymph n.
parasternal lymph n.
paratracheal lymph n.
parauterine lymph n.
paravaginal lymph n.
paravesicular lymph n.
parietal lymph n.
parotid lymph n.
Parrot n.
pectoral lymph n.
pelvic lymph n.
periaortic lymph n.
peribronchial lymph n.
pericardial lymph n.
pericholedochal n.
perisplenic n.
phrenic lymph n.
popliteal n.
porta hepatis n.
postaortic lymph n.
postcaval lymph n.

posterior mediastinal n.
postvesicular lymph n.
potato n.
preaortic lymph n.
precaval lymph n.
prececal lymph n.
prelaryngeal n.
prepericardial lymph n.
pretracheal lymph n.
prevertebral lymph n.
prevesicular lymph n.
pulmonary juxtaesophageal
  lymph n.
pyloric lymph n.
Ranvier n.
rectal lymph n.
regional lymph n.
retroaortic lymph n.
retroauricular lymph n.
retrocecal lymph n.
retrocrural n.
retroperitoneal n.
retropharyngeal lymph n.
retropyloric n.
retrorectal lymph n.
right hilar lymph n.
Rosenmüller n.
Rotter n.
Rouviere n.
SA n.
sacral lymph n.
satellite n.
scalene n.
Schmorl n.
sentinel lymph n. (SLN)
sick sinus n.
sigmoid lymph n.
signal n.
singer's n.
sinoatrial n. (SAN)
sinoauricular n.
sinus node
Sister Mary Joseph n.
solitary lymph n.
spinal accessory lymph n.
splenic lymph n.
subcarinal lymph n.
subcentimeter n.
submandibular lymph n.
submental lymph n.
subpyloric n.
subscapular lymph n.

superficial inguinal lymph n.
supraclavicular lymph n.
suprapyloric n.
supratrochlear n.
syphilitic n.
Tawara atrioventricular n.
thyroid lymph n.
tibial n.
tracheal lymph n.
tracheobronchial lymph n.
Troisier n.
vesicular lymph n.
vestigial left sinoatrial n.
Virchow sentinel n.
Virchow-Troisier n.
visceral lymph n.
node-negative carcinoma
node-positive carcinoma
nodosa
  periarteritis n.
  polyarteritis n. (PAN)
  salpingitis isthmica n.
nodosum
nodoventricular
  n. bypass fiber
  n. pathway
  n. tachycardia
nodular
  n. adrenal hyperplasia
  n. aneurysm
  n. appearance
  n. density
  n. enhancement
  n. goiter
  n. hyperintense focus
  n. induration of temporal artery
  n. irregularity
  n. lesion
  n. liver
  n. liver regeneration
  n. lung disease
  n. lymphoid hyperplasia
  n. mass
  n. obstruction
  n. proliferation
  n. pulmonary parenchymal opacity
  n. regenerative hyperplasia (NRH)
  n. sclerosis Hodgkin disease
  n. subepidermal fibrosis
  n. synovitis
  n. thyroid disease

N

NOTES

nodularity
  calcified n.
  coarse n.
  lung n.
  noncalcified n.
  pulmonary n.
  surface n.
  tendon n.
  vein n.
nodulated
nodulation
  mural n.
nodule
  acinar n.
  airspace n.
  Albini n.
  aortic valve n.
  Arantius n.
  Aschoff n.
  autonomous thyroid n. (ATN)
  Bianchi n.
  calcified lung n.
  Caplan n.
  cartilaginous n.
  cavitating lung n.
  cerebral n.
  circumscribed n.
  cirrhotic n.
  cold thyroid n.
  conglomerate pulmonary n.
  cortical n.
  Cruveilhier n.
  cutaneous n.
  Dalen-Fuchs n.
  discordant thyroid n.
  discrete pulmonary n.
  dysplastic liver n.
  eccentric enhancing n.
  echogenic n.
  enhancing n.
  esophageal mucosal n.
  fibrocartilaginous n.
  fibrous n.
  fluffy pulmonary n.
  Fränkel typhus n.
  functioning n.
  Gamna n.
  Gamna-Gandy n.
  glial n.
  ground-glass n.
  n. halo
  hemorrhagic lung n.
  heterotopic n.
  hyperechoic renal n.
  hypermetabolic n.
  hypointense n.
  interstitial n.

  Kerckring n.
  Koeppe n.
  laryngeal n.
  lingular n.
  Lisch n.
  lung n.
  meningothelial-like n.
  miliary n.
  Morgagni n.
  mucosal esophageal n.
  multiple lung n.'s
  multiple pulmonary necrobiotic n.
  mural CNS n.
  necrobiotic n.
  noncavitary n.
  nondelineated n.
  nonenhancing n.
  nonfunctioning thyroid n.
  ossific n.
  peripheral n.
  pleura-based lung n.
  pleural n.
  prostatic hyperplastic n.
  pulmonary n.
  regenerative liver n.
  rheumatoid n.
  Rokitansky n.
  satellite n.
  Scheuermann n.
  Schmorl n.
  semiautonomous n.
  shaggy lung n.
  silicotic n.
  singer's n.
  Sister Mary Joseph n.
  solitary metastatic lung n.
  solitary pulmonary n. (SPN)
  solitary pulmonary necrobiotic n.
  subcutaneous n.
  surfer's n.
  tendon n.
  thyroid adenoma n.
  thyroid colloid n.
  tobacco n.
  toxic n.
  tuberculous n.
  typhoid n.
  typhus n.
  warm n.
nodule-in-a-nodule appearance
nodule-in-nodule liver
nodulus Arantius
nodus arcus venae azygos
nofetumomab diagnostic imaging agent
noire
  atrophie n.

noise
> digitalization n.
> echogenic n.
> n. effective count (NEC)
> gaussian n.
> gradient switching n.
> image n.
> lesion-to-cerebrospinal fluid n.
> lesion-to-white matter n.
> pixel n.
> quantum n.
> radiographic n.
> Rayleigh n.
> n. reconstruction kernel
> n. spike artifact
> statistical n.
> structured n.
> subtractive n.
> systematic n.
> thermal n.
> total image n.

Nölke position
nomifensine
nominal
nomogram
nonablative heating
nonanaplastic glioma
nonaneurysmal perimesencephalic subarachnoid hemorrhage
nonarrhythmic myocardial infarct
nonarticular radial head fracture
nonatherosclerotic disease
nonattenuation-corrected
> n.-c. image
> n.-c. slice

nonavid infarct imaging
nonaxial beam technique
nonbony union
noncalcareous renal calculus
noncalcified
> n. carcinoma
> n. coronary stenosis
> n. fibroadenoma
> n. mitral leaflet
> n. nodularity
> n. nodular mass
> n. ocular process

noncardiac
> n. angiography
> n. pulmonary edema

noncardiogenic pulmonary edema

noncaseating
> n. granuloma
> n. tubercle

noncavitary nodule
nonchromaffin paraganglioma
noncircularity degree
noncirrhotic
> n. liver
> n. portal fibrosis (NCPF)

nonclassifiable interstitial pneumonia
noncleaved cell lymphoma
non-CNS PNET
noncoaxial catheter tip position
noncoiled umbilical cord
noncollagenous pneumonoconiosis
noncollinear directions
noncolonic structure
noncommitted mode
noncommunicating
> n. cyst
> n. hydrocephalus

noncompaction
> left ventricular n.

noncompliant plaque
noncontact imaging technology
noncontiguous fracture
noncontractile scar tissue
noncontrast
> n. CT scan
> n. head CT (NCCT)
> n. phase (NCP)

noncoplanar
> n. arch technique
> n. arc technique
> n. beam technique
> n. therapy beam

noncoronary
> n. cusp
> n. sinus

noncritical
> n. soft tissue
> n. stenosis

nondeciduate placenta
nondecremental
nondelineated nodule
nondependent lung
nondetachable
> n. balloon
> n. balloon catheter

nondilated system
nondisplaced fracture
nondissociative instability

N

NOTES

nondominant
- n. hemisphere lesion
- n. putaminal hemorrhage
- n. vessel

nondynamometric trunk strength measurement

non-ECG-assisted multidetector row CT

nonechogenic tumor

nonembolic infarct

nonenclosed magnet

nonenhanced
- n. computed tomography (NECT)
- n. CT
- n. CT scan

nonenhancing
- n. lesion
- n. nodule

nonesterified
- n. fatty acid (NEFA)
- n. fatty acid scintigraphy

nonexpansile
- n. multilocular bone lesion
- n. osteolysis
- n. unilocular bone lesion
- n. well-demarcated multilocular bone defect
- n. well-demarcated unilocular bone defect

nonfamilial intestinal pseudoobstruction

nonferromagnetic
- n. needle
- n. positioning device

nonfetal
- n. complication
- n. uterine condition

nonfilarial chylocele

nonfilling venous segment

nonforeshortened angiographic view

nonfunctioning
- n. gallbladder
- n. heart valve
- n. islet cell tumor
- n. kidney
- n. pituitary adenoma
- n. thyroid nodule

nonfusion of cranial suture

nongated CT scan

nongranular leukocyte

nonhemorrhagic
- n. infarct
- n. ischemia
- n. mass

nonhomogeneous
- n. consolidation
- n. enhancement
- n. hyperdense mass

nonhyperfunctioning adrenal adenoma

non-idiosyncratic anaphylactoid reaction

nonimmune
- n. fetal hydrops
- n. hydrops fetalis

noninducible tachycardia

noninfarcted
- n. myocardium
- n. segment

noninflammatory joint effusion

noninvasive
- n. aspergillosis
- n. assessment
- n. imaging
- n. imaging study
- n. lesion
- n. programmed stimulation (NIPS)
- n. technique
- n. thermometry
- n. thymoma
- n. ultrasound

nonionic
- n. contrast material
- n. dimer contrast medium
- n. iodinated contrast agent
- n. paramagnetic contrast imaging agent
- n. triiodinated monomer
- n. water-soluble contrast medium

nonionizing radiation

nonischemic congestive cardiomyopathy

nonisotropic gradient

nonlethal
- n. dwarfism
- n. dysplasia
- n. myocardial ischemic injury

nonlinear
- n. excitation profile
- n. sampling

nonlinearity

nonlingular
- n. branch
- n. branch of upper lobe bronchus

nonlocalized ischemia

nonmagnetization transfer gradient-refocused echo image

nonmagnified
- n. image
- n. mammography

nonmeningiomatous malignant lesion

nonmetastasizing fibrosarcoma

nonmotile leukocyte

nonmucinous adenocarcinoma

Nonne-Milroy lymphedema

nonneoplastic
- n. cyst
- n. tumor

nonnephrotoxic contrast agent

nonnipple sector
nonnodular
  n. fibrosis
  n. silicosis
nonobstructive
  n. atelectasis
  n. cardiomyopathy
  n. hydrocephalus
  n. ileus
nonocclusive
  n. mesenteric arterial insufficiency
  n. mesenteric ischemia
nonodontogenic
nonolfactory cortex
nononcogenic
nonopaque
  n. calculus
  n. intraluminal mass
  n. stone
nonorthogonal plane
nonoscillatory motion
nonossifying fibroma
nonosteogenic fibroma
nonperfused myocardium
nonphyseal fracture
nonplanar slice
nonpolar crevice
nonpregnant horn of bicornuate uterus
nonproliferative lesion
nonproton MRI
nonpulsatile abdominal mass
nonradiopaque
  n. foreign body
  n. stone
nonreplantable amputation
nonresonance Raman spectroscopy
nonrheumatic
  n. aortic insufficiency
  n. valvular aortic stenosis
non-rib-bearing vertebra
nonrotational burst fracture
nonrotation of bowel loop
nonsecretor
nonsegmental areas of opacification
nonselective
  n. angiography
  n. pulse
nonseminomatous germ cell tumor
nonseptate
nonseptic embolic brain infarct
non-skin-sparing mastectomy (non-SSM)
non-small cell lung carcinoma (NSCLC)

nonspecific
  n. accumulation
  n. bowel gas pattern
  n. change
  n. conglomerate
  n. esophageal motility disorder
    (NEMD)
  n. finding
  n. interstitial pneumonia (NIP,
    NSIP)
non-SSM
  non-skin-sparing mastectomy
nonstanding lateral oblique view
nonstress
  n. fetal test
  n. test (NST)
nonstriated muscle
nonsubperiosteal cortical defect
nonsubtracted image
nonsubtraction
  n. image
  n. imaging
nonsuppurative
  n. ascending cholangitis
  n. destructive cholangitis
nonsurgical ablative therapy
nonsyndromic
  n. bicoronal synostosis
  n. focal cerebellar dysplasia
  n. unicoronal synostosis
nontarget embolization
nonthromboembolic condition
nontrabeculated atrium
nontransmural
  n. match
  n. myocardial infarct
nontraumatic epidural hemorrhage
nontriggered phase-contrast MR
  angiography
non-tuberculosis mycobacteria
nonuniform
  n. attenuation
  n. excitation
  n. rotational defect (NURD)
nonunion
  atrophic n.
  bony n.
  fibrous n.
  fracture n.
  n. of fracture fragment
  hypertrophic n.
  torsion wedge n.

N

NOTES

nonunited fracture
nonvalved conduit
nonviable
    n. fetus
    n. gestation
    n. scar
    n. tissue
nonviral vector
nonvisualization
    n. of fetal stomach
    n. of gallbladder
    n. of spleen
nonweightbearing view
Noonan syndrome
no-reflow phenomenon
Norland
    N. bone densitometry
    N. pQCT XCT2000 scanner
    N. XR26 bone densitometer
normal
    n. anatomic position
    n. anatomic variation
    n. anteroposterior view
    n. axis
    n. bladder caliber
    borderline n.
    n. calcification
    n. caliber bowel
    n. caliber duct
    n. chest film
    n. echogenicity
    n. fold urethrogram
    n. gestation
    n. hemodynamic liver parameter
    high n.
    n. lordotic curve
    low n.
    n. lower esophageal sphincter
      resting pressure
    morphologically n.
    n. ossification
    n. ovarian surface epithelium
      (NOSE)
    n. perfusion pressure breakthrough
    n. planar MR anatomy
    n. range
    n. renal parenchyma
    n. sinus rhythm
    n. spleen weight
    upper limits of n.
    n. variant
    n. variant fluorodeoxyglucose
      uptake distribution
    n. variant of Ga-67 uptake
    n. whole body fluorodeoxyglucose
      distribution
normal-appearing bronchus

normalization
    interictal n.
    spatial n.
normalized
    n. cross-section
    n. to plasma activity
    n. plateau slope
normal-pressure hydrocephalus
normal-region pixel
normochromasia
normochromia
normotensive hydrocephalus
normoxia
Norrie disease
NOS
    not otherwise specified
NOSE
    normal ovarian surface epithelium
nose
    anteater n.
    beak-shaped n.
    n. ring artifact
nose-chin position
nose-forehead position
notable cerebral insult
notch
    anacrotic n.
    angular n.
    antegonial n.
    aortic n.
    apical n.
    auricular n.
    cardiac n.
    cerebellar n.
    clavicular n.
    coracoid n.
    costal n.
    craniofacial n.
    dicrotic n.
    digastric n.
    ethmoidal n.
    fibular n.
    Frankfort mandibular n.
    n. from gastric sling fiber
    frontal n.
    greater sciatic n.
    greater sigmoid n.
    interclavicular n.
    intercondylar n.
    interpeduncular n.
    intervertebral n.
    lateral femoral n.
    lesser sciatic n.
    ligamentum teres n.
    lucent hilar n.
    n. projection
    radial sigmoid n.

sacrosciatic n.
scapular n.
sciatic n.
semilunar n.
septal n.
sigmoid n.
spinoglenoid n.
splenic n.
sternal n.
suprasternal n.
trochlear n.
ulnar n.
n. view

notched
n. aortic knob
n. vertebra

notching
cortical n.
pelvic n.
n. of pulmonic valve
rib n.
n. ureter
ureteral n.

Nothnagel syndrome
no-threshold
n.-t. body
n.-t. concept

notochordal
n. canal
n. process

notochord remnant
not otherwise specified (NOS)
Novacor left ventricular assist system
NovaLine excimer laser
Novalis radiosurgery system
NovaPulse CO2 laser
novel agent
Novopaque
Novus Medical Image Card
NOX
number of excitation

nozzle effect
NP
nephrographic phase

NPC
nasopharyngeal carcinoma

⁵⁹NP scintigraphy
NRC
NRH
nodular regenerative hyperplasia

NSA
number of signal average
NSA of femur

NSCLC
non-small cell lung carcinoma

N-shaped sigmoid loop
NSIP
nonspecific interstitial pneumonia

NST
nonstress test

NTD
neural tube defect

NTHI
native tissue harmonic imaging

NTP
nucleoside triphosphate

nuchae
ligamentum n.

nuchal
n. cord
n. cyst
n. ligament
n. plane
n. skin thickening
n. translucency

nuchofrontal projection
Nuck
N. canal
N. diverticulum

nuclear
n. aggregation
n. angiography
n. anular differentiation
n. atom
n. bone imaging
n. cardiovascular imaging
n. chemistry
n. decay
n. disintegration
n. electric quadripole relaxation
n. emulsion
n. enema
n. energy
n. fission
n. force
n. fusion
n. gated blood pool imaging
n. gated blood pool testing
n. genome
n. hepatobiliary imaging
n. herniation

NOTES

nuclear *(continued)*
    N. Magnetic Device Lypoo Profile device
    n. magnetic moment
    n. magnetic resonance (NMR)
    n. magnetic resonance Fourier transformation
    n. magnetic resonance image
    n. magnetic resonance imaging
    n. magnetic resonance phantom
    n. magnetic resonance relaxation rate enhancement
    n. magnetic resonance scan
    n. magnetic resonance scanning sequence
    n. magnetic resonance signal intensity
    n. magnetic resonance spectography
    n. magnetic resonance spectral parameter
    n. magnetic resonance spectrometer
    n. magnetic resonance spectroscopy
    n. magnetic resonance spectrum
    n. magnetic resonance tomography
    n. magnetism
    n. matrix
    n. medicine
    n. medicine camera
    n. medicine imaging
    n. medicine information system
    n. Overhauser effect
    n. particle
    n. perfusion imaging
    n. pleomorphism
    n. polarization
    n. probe
    n. pulse amplifier
    n. radiationoccupational radiation
    n. reaction
    n. reactornuclear relaxation
    n. renal scintigraphy
    n. scanner
    n. scanning
    n. signal
    n. spin
    n. spin quantum number
    n. structure
nuclei (*pl. of* nucleus)
nucleide
nucleiform
nucleography
nucleoid
nucleon number
nucleoside
    n. phosphonate
    n. triphosphate (NTP)
nucleotide scan

Nucletron
    N. applicator
    N. MicroSelectron/LDR remote afterloader
nucleus, pl. **nuclei**
    n. ambiguus lesion
    arcuate n.
    basal n.
    n. basalis lesion
    n. of Cajal
    caudate n.
    cranial n.
    n. of Darkschewitsch
    dentate nuclei
    dorsomedial n.
    head of the caudate n.
    inferior syndrome of red n.
    Köllicker n.
    lentiform n., lenticular nucleus
    magnetic nuclei
    motor n.
    neutron-deficient n.
    oculomotor-trochlear n.
    ossific n.
    parafascicular n.
    pretectal n.
    n. pulposus herniation
    quadripolar n.
    residual n.
    sensory n.
    sixth n.
    n. of the solitary tract
    ventral cochlear n.
nuclide
    n. analysis
    daughter n.
    n. generator
    isobar n.
    isomer n.
    isotone n.
    isotope n.
    parent n.
    radioactive n.
NUG
    necrotizing ulcerative gingivitis
nulled
nulling
    gradient moment n. (GMN)
null point
NuLytely bowel preparation
number
    average gradient n.
    Avogadro n. (Λ)
    body atomic n.
    clonogen n.
    CT n.
    effective atomic n.

Euler n.
n. of excitation (NEX, NOX)
Hounsfield n.
Huckman n. (HN)
imaginary n.
mass n.
neutron n.
nuclear spin quantum n.
nucleon n.
n. profile
quantum n.
Reynolds n.
S n.
n. of signal average (NSA)
spin quantum n.
numerary renal anomaly
nummular pneumonia
NURD
nonuniform rotational defect
Nurick
N. classification of spondylosis
N. spondylosis classification
nursemaid's elbow
nutation
n. angle
n. angle measurement

nutcracker
n. esophagus
n. fracture
n. phenomenon
n. syndrome
nutmeg appearance of liver
nutrient
n. artery of femur
n. artery of fibula
n. artery growth
n. foramen
nutritional cirrhosis
Nuvolase 660 laser
NYHA
NYHA congestive heart failure classification
nylon
n. catheter
liquid n.
Nyquist
N. criterion
N. frequency
N. limit
N. sampling theorem

NOTES

N

O
  O shell
O₂
  oxygen
  O_2 consumption index
¹⁵O
  oxygen-15
¹⁶O
  oxygen-16
¹⁷O
  oxygen-17
¹⁸O
  oxygen-18
OA
  osteoarthritis
OAF
  off-axis factor
OAR
  off-axis ratio
  OAR malleolar rule
Oasis
  O. thrombectomy catheter
  O. triple-lumen catheter
oat cell carcinoma
OAV
  oculoauriculovertebral
object
  o. coordinate system
  o. modulation
  side-by-side o.
  unidentified bright o. (UBO)
object-based
  o.-b. interpolation
  o.-b. visualization
object-film distance (OFD)
object-plane blur
oblique
  o. annihilation photon pair
  o. axial MR imaging
  o. coronal plane
  o. diameter
  o. film
  o. fissure
  o. flow misregistration
  o. lateral projection
  left anterior o. (LAO)
  left posterior o. (LPO)
  o. magnetic resonance imaging
  mediolateral o. (MLO)
  o. muscle
  o. pericardial sinus
  o. position
  o. prescription line
  o. radiograph
  o. ridge

  right anterior o. (RAO)
  right posterior o. (RPO)
  o. sagittal EKG-gated spin-echo
    magnetic resonance imaging
  o. sagittal sequence
  o. slice
  o. spiral fracture
  superior o.
  trauma o.
  T2-weighted fast spin-echo
    coronal o.
  o. vein
  o. vein of left atrium
  o. view
oblique-angle reconstruction
obliquely
  o. oriented axon
  o. oriented fiber
obliquity
  degree of neck o.
  Litzmann o.
  magnitude of o.
  Naegele o.
  pelvic o.
  Roederer o.
  varying degrees of o.
obliterans
  arteriosclerosis o. (ASO)
  atherosclerosis o. (ASO)
  bronchiolitis fibrosa o.
  endarteritis o.
  mastitis o.
  postinfectious bronchiolitis o.
  thromboangiitis o.
obliterated costophrenic angle
obliteration
  balloon-occluded transvenous o.
  subdeltoid fat plane o.
obliterative
  o. arteriosclerosis
  o. bronchiolitis
  o. cardiomyopathy
  o. inflammation
oblongata
  medulla o.
O'Brien
  O. classification of radial fracture
  O. radial fracture classification
OBS
  organic brain syndrome
obscuration arteriosclerosis
observation
  fluoroscopic o.
observed maximal uptake
observer variation

O

obstetric, obstetrical
    o. sonography
    o. ultrasound
obstipation
obstructed shunt tube
obstructing embolus arteriosclerosis
obstruction
    acute abdominal o.
    adynamic intestinal o.
    airway o.
    aortic arch o.
    aortic outflow o.
    aortic valve o.
    aortoiliac o.
    aqueductal o.
    arachnoid villi o.
    arterial o.
    ball-valve o.
    benign biliary o. (BBS)
    bilateral o.
    bile flow o.
    biliary tract o.
    biliary tree o.
    bladder outlet o.
    bowel o.
    bronchial o.
    bronchiolar o.
    cardiac o.
    catheter o.
    central venous o.
    cerebrospinal fluid o.
    chronic airway o.
    closed-loop intestinal o.
    colonic o.
    common bile duct o.
    complete bowel o.
    congenital duodenal o.
    congenital left-sided outflow o.
    congenital pelviureteric junction o.
    congenital subpulmonic o.
    congenital ureteric o.
    distal common bile duct o.
    duct o.
    duodenal-gastric outlet o.
    efferent loop o.
    embolic o.
    endobronchial o.
    esophageal o.
    extrahepatic binary o.
    extrathoracic o.
    extrinsic malignant o.
    false colonic o.
    fecal o.
    fetal bowel o.
    fetal renal o.
    fixed airway o.
    fixed coronary o.

    flow-dependent o.
    food bolus o.
    foreign body upper airway o.
    functional ureteral o.
    gastric outlet o.
    gastrointestinal tract o.
    hepatic venous outflow o.
    high-grade o.
    high small bowel o.
    hilar o.
    hydrocephalic o.
    idiopathic o.
    ileal o.
    iliac vein o.
    incomplete o.
    increased pulmonary o.
    inferior vena caval o.
    infravesical o.
    intermittent o.
    interposed colon segment o.
    intestinal o.
    intrapancreatic o.
    intrathoracic upper airway o.
    intraventricular right ventricular o.
    intravesical o.
    irreversible airway o.
    jejunal o.
    large bowel o.
    left ventricular inflow tract o.
    left ventricular outflow tract o.
      (LVOTO)
    low small bowel o.
    lymphatic o.
    malignant airway o.
    mammary duct o.
    mechanical biliary o.
    mechanical duct o.
    mechanical extrahepatic o.
    mechanical intestinal o.
    mechanical respiratory tract o.
    mechanical small bowel o.
    neurogenic intestinal o.
    nodular o.
    otic o.
    outflow o.
    outlet o.
    pancreatic duct o.
    paralytic colonic o.
    partial small bowel o.
    pelvic venous o.
    porta hepatis o.
    post transplantation ureteric o.
    posttuberculous o.
    postural ureteric o.
    preocclusive o.
    primary acquired nasolacrimal
      duct o. (PANDO)

prostatic o.
pulmonary artery o.
pulmonary outflow o.
pulmonary vascular o.
pulmonary venous o.
pyloric outlet o.
pyloroduodenal o.
rectal o.
renal o.
respiratory tract o.
right ventricular outflow o.
Rigler triad of small bowel o.
secondary o.
segmental biliary o.
sequence o.
simple mechanical o.
small bowel o. (SBO)
strangulated o.
strangulating o.
subclavian artery o.
subpulmonic o.
subrectus o.
subvalvular aortic o.
subvalvular diffuse muscular o.
superior vena cava o. (SVCO)
suprapancreatic o.
supravesical o.
thrombotic o.
transient shunt o.
tubal o.
upper airway o.
ureteral renal transplant o.
ureteropelvic junction o.
ureterovesical junction o.
urethral o.
urinary o.
vascular o.
venous o.
ventricular o.
vesical outlet o.

obstructive
o. abnormality
o. airway disease
o. atelectasis
o. biliary cirrhosis
o. calculus
o. component
o. dysfunctional ileitis
o. emphysema
o. hydrocephalus
o. hypertrophic cardiomyopathy
o. hypopnea

o. lesion
o. lung disease
o. nephrogram
o. nephropathy
o. pancreatitis
o. plaque
o. pneumonia
o. pulmonary arterial hypertension
o. pulmonary disease (OPD)
o. pulmonary overinflation
o. renal dysplasia
o. thrombus
o. uropathy
o. ventilatory defect

obturating embolus
obturator
o. avulsion fracture
o. externus
o. foramen
o. hernia
o. internus
o. internus fascia
o. internus muscle
o. internus tendon
o. line
o. lymph node
o. membrane
o. nodal chain
o. sign

obtuse
o. marginal (OM)
o. marginal branch (OMB)
o. marginal coronary artery

occipital
o. artery
o. bone
o. bossing
o. cephalocele
o. condyle
o. condyle fracture
o. condyle hypoplasia
o. condyle invasion
o. eminence
o. encephalocele
o. fissure
o. focus
o. fontanelle
o. gyrus
o. horn
o. lesion
o. lobe
o. lobe infarct

NOTES

O

occipital *(continued)*
    o. lymph node
    o. meningocele
    o. plane
    o. pole
    o. protuberance
    o. sinus
    o. suture
    o. tip
    o. vessel
    o. view
    o. view of skull
occipitalization
    atlas o.
occipitoanterior
occipitoatlantoaxial
    o. anomaly
    o. fusion
    o. ligament
occipitoaxial
    o. joint
    o. ligament
occipitocervical
    o. angle
    o. articulation
    o. fusion
    o. junction
    o. plate
occipitofrontal
    o. diameter (OFD)
    o. fasciculus
occipitofrontalis muscle
occipitomastoid suture
occipitomental
    o. diameter
    o. projection
occipitoparietal suture
occipitopontine tract
occipitoposterior
occipitosphenoid suture
occipitotemporal
    o. convolution
    o. gyrus
    o. sulcus
occiput
occluded
    o. graft
    o. lumen
occluder
    ameroid o.
    CardioSEAL o.
    clamshell double umbrella o.
    Flo-Rester vessel o.
    radiolucent plastic o.
    Rashkind o.

occluding
    o. agent
    o. spring embolus
occlusal
    o. facet
    o. film
    o. plane
    o. radiograph
    o. segment
    o. surface
occlusion
    angiographic o.
    o. angiography
    o. aorta
    aqueductal o.
    arterial o.
    o. of artery
    atrial septal defect o.
    balloon test o.
    basilar o.
    bilateral o.
    carotid artery o.
    carotid-cavernous fistula o.
    celiac axis o.
    cerebral sinovenous o.
    complete o.
    coronary o.
    deep venous o.
    diathermic vascular o.
    ductus arteriosus o.
    dural sinus o.
    embolic o.
    fallopian tube o.
    graft o.
    infrapopliteal artery o.
    intermittent o.
    internal carotid artery o.
    intracranial vascular o.
    late graft o.
    o. measurement
    mesenteric artery o.
    mesenteric vascular o.
    middle cerebral artery o.
    parent artery o.
    parent vessel o.
    percutaneous thermal o.
    pulmonary arterial o.
    selective test o.
    side-branch o.
    snowplow o.
    subclavian artery o.
    subclavian vein o.
    subtotal o.
    superficial femoral artery o.
    tandem ICA/MCA o.
    tapering o.
    test balloon o.

thermal o.
thrombotic o.
top of carotid T o.
total o.
transrenal ureteric o.
transvenous o.
traumatogenic o.
tubal o.
unilateral o.
ureteral o.
vascular brain o.
vein graft o.
venous o.
vertebral artery o.
vertebrobasilar o.
vertebrobasilar artery o.
vessel o.
occlusive
   o. arterial thrombus
   o. cerebrovascular disease
   o. cerebrovascular insult
   o. ileus
   o. impedance phlebography
   o. lesion
   o. mesenteric infarct
occult
   o. blood
   o. bone metastasis
   o. cerebral vascular malformation
    (OCVM)
   o. detection
   o. hydrocephalus
   o. intrasacral meningocele
   o. lesion
   o. osseous fracture
   o. osseous injury
   o. papillary carcinoma
   o. pericardial constriction
   o. phosphaturic mesenchymal tumor
   o. primary tumor of testis
   o. residual herniated disk
   roentgenographically o.
   o. spinal dysraphism
   o. subluxation
   o. thyroid carcinoma
   o. vascular brain malformation
occulta
   spina bifida o. (SBO)
occupational lung disease
OCD
   osteochondral defect

OCG
   oral cholecystogram
   OCG imaging
ochronosis
Ochsner muscle
OCL bowel preparation
O'Connor finger dexterity test
OCR
   off-center ratio
OCT
   optical coherence tomography
octagonal configuration
Octane postprocessing workstation
OctreoScan
   O. 111 radioactive imaging agent
   O. system
octreotide
   o. imaging
   O. imaging agent
   ^{111}In o.
   o. paraganglioma scintigraphy
   ^{99m}Tc-labeled o.
   o. tumor localization scan
ocular
   o. adnexa
   o. globe topography
   o. implant
   o. lesion
   o. magnification system
   o. pneumoplethysmography (OPG)
   o. radiation therapy (ORT)
   o. rhabdomyosarcoma
   o. trauma
OcuLight SL diode laser
oculoauriculovertebral (OAV)
oculomotor
   o. apparatus
   o. nerve
oculomotor-trochlear nucleus
oculopharyngeal dystrophy
oculoplethysmography (OPG)
oculoplethysmography/carotid
  phonoangiography (OPG/CPA)
oculopneumoplethysmography
oculosubcutaneous syndrome of Yuge
OCVM
   occult cerebral vascular malformation
OD
   optical density
odd-echo dephasing

NOTES

O

Oddi
    O. muscle
    sphincter of O.
Odelca camera unit
O'Donoghue unhappy triad
odontogenic
    o. cyst
    o. fibromyxoma
    o. keratocyst
    o. myxoma
    o. tumor
odontoid
    o. bone
    o. condyle fracture
    o. dysplasia
    o. erosion
    o. fracture types I–III
    o. ligament
    pannus deformity of o.
    o. process
    o. vertebra
    o. view
odontoma
odontoradiograph
ODQ
    ODQ muscle
odynophagia
OEC Series 9600 cardiac system
OEF
    oxygen extraction fraction
Oehl muscle
OER
    oxygen extraction rate
OFD
    object-film distance
    occipitofrontal diameter
off-axis
    o.-a. dose inhomogeneity
    o.-a. factor (OAF)
    o.-a. point localization
    o.-a. ratio (OAR)
    o.-a. rotational acquisition
off-center
    o.-c. cut
    o.-c. modulation
    o.-c. ratio (OCR)
off-lateral projection
off-resonance
    3D rotating delivery of
      excitation o.-r.
    rotating delivery of excitation o.-r.
      (RODEO)
    o.-r. saturation
    o.-r. saturation pulse imaging
    o.-r. spin-locking
offset
    chemical shift spatial o.

E-zero o.
focal osseous o.
o. frequency
quarter-detector o.
o. radiofrequency spin echo
    resonance o.
Ogden
    O. classification of epiphyseal
      fracture
    O. epiphyseal fracture classification
Ogilvie syndrome
Ogston line
Ohio
    O. infuser
    O. Nuclear Delta 50 FS, 2000
      scanner
Ohm law
Ohngren line
OHP
    orthogonal-hole test pattern
OI
    osteogenesis imperfecta
OIH
    iodine-123 orthoiodohippurate
    orthoiodohippurate
    ^{123}I OIH
    iodine-131 OIH
oil
    brominated o.
    chloriodized o.
    o. cyst
    o. embolus
    o. emulsion imaging agent
    ethiodized o.
    iodized poppy seed o.
    iophendylate o.
    o. myelography
    silicone o.
oil-aspiration pneumonia
oil-soluble contrast medium (OSCM)
oil-water phantom
okadaic acid
Okuda transhepatic obliteration of
   varix
old
    o. hemorrhage
    o. myocardial infarct
olecranon
    o. bursa
    o. bursitis
    o. fossa
    o. process
    o. tip fracture
oleoperitoneography
oleothorax
Olerud and Molander fracture
   classification

olfactory
> o. area
> o. bulb
> o. canal
> o. groove meningioma
> o. gyrus
> o. neuroblastoma
> o. sulcus
> o. tract

oligemia
> mosaic o.

oligemia-related cyanotic CHD
oligoastrocytoma
> anaplastic mixed o.
> recurrent vermian o.

oligodactylia
oligodendroglia
oligodendroglioma
> bifrontal o.
> subependymal o.

oligohydramnios
oligomeganephronia
oligonucleotide
> antisense o.
> o. probe
> radiolabeled antisense o.

olisthesis
olivary
> o. degeneration
> o. hypertrophy

olive
> amiculum of o.
> inferior o.
> posterior o.

Oliver-Cardarelli sign
olivopontocerebellar
> o. atrophy
> o. degeneration (OPCD)

Ollier disease
Olshevsky tube
Olympus
> O. CF-1T100L colonoscope
> O. CF-200Z colonoscope
> O. CHF-BP30 transduodenal choledochofiberscope
> O. endoscopic ultrasound
> O. endoscopic ultrasound scanner
> O. ENF-P2 laryngoscope
> O. EU-M30 system
> O. EVIS Q-200V endoscope
> O. Gastrocamera GTF-A

> O. GF-UM2, GF-UM3 echoendoscope
> O. GIF-1T10 echoendoscope
> O. JF1T10 duodenoscope
> O. JF-UM20 echoendoscope
> O. MH-908 slim ultrasonic probe
> O. SIF-100 video enteroscope
> O. S20-20R transendoscopic ultrasound probe
> O. TJF-100 endoscope
> O. VU-M2 echoendoscope
> O. XIF-UM3 echoendoscope
> O. XQ230 gastroscope

OM
> obtuse marginal
> orbitomeatal
> OM artery

OMB
> obtuse marginal branch

omega-sella
Omenn syndrome
omenta (*pl. of* omentum)
omental
> o. band
> o. bursa
> o. cake
> o. cyst
> o. infarct
> o. mass
> o. tuberosity

omentoportography
omentum, pl. **omenta**
> colic o.
> gastric o.
> gastrocolic o.
> gastrohepatic o.
> gastrosplenic o.
> greater o.
> incarcerated o.
> lesser o. (LO)
> o. majus
> o. minus
> pancreaticosplenic o.
> sigmoid o.
> splenogastric o.

Omni
> O. Flush 3F, 4F, 5F catheter
> O. Selective 0-3 catheter

Omnipaque
> O. 140, 180, 240, 300, 350 imaging agent
> O. injection

NOTES

O

OmniPulse-MAX holmium laser
Omniscan imaging agent
Omniscience valve
Omnisense 7000S bone sonometer
omohyoid muscle
omovertebral bone
omphalic
omphalitis
    neonatal o.
omphalocele
    infraumbilical o.
omphaloma
omphalomesenteric
    o. artery
    o. duct
    o. duct cyst
    o. remnant
omphalopagus twin
onchocerciasis
oncocalyx
oncocytic thyroid adenoma
oncocytoma
    pituitary o.
oncogenesis
    radiation o.
oncogenic osteomalacia
on-column preparation
OncoRad OV103
OncoScint
    O. CR103
    O. CR/OV breast imaging agent
    O. OV103
    O. PR
oncosis
OncoTrac
oncotropic
one-dimensional
    o.-d. chemical-shift imaging (1D-CSI)
    o.-d. phase encoding
one-part fracture
one-shot echo-planar imaging
one-sided image reconstruction
one-stage amputation
OneStep paracentesis drainage catheter
one-step production
one-stick system
one-third ejection fraction
one-ventricle heart
onion peel appearance
onion-shaped dilatation of duodenum
onionskin
    o. appearance
    o. configuration of collagenous fiber
    o. lesion
    o. periosteal reaction

onlay graft
on-line portal imaging
Onodi cell
on-off phenomenon
onset
on-the-fly random correction
onychoosteodysplasia
    familial o.
oocyte retrieval
oophoroma folliculare
opacification
    arterial o.
    collecting system o.
    contrast o.
    early segmental o.
    extravesical o.
    ground-glass o. (GGO)
    hemithorax o.
    insufficient venous o.
    maxillary sinus o.
    nonsegmental areas of o.
    pedal artery o.
    o. of posterior longitudinal ligament
opacified
opacifying
    o. gallstone
    o. injection
opacity
    abnormal lung o.
    airspace o.
    asymmetric lung o.
    basilar reticular o.
    branching centrilobar o.
    bubbly o.
    centrilobar o.
    chronic diffuse confluent lung o.
    chronic multifocal ill-defined lung o.
    coarse linear o.
    coarse reticular o.
    conglomerate o.
    dependent o.
    diffuse airspace o.
    generalized hazy o.
    granular o.
    ground-glass o.
    hazy o.
    homogeneous o.
    linear o.
    localized pure ground-glass o.
    lung o.
    Medusa hair-like o.
    nodular pulmonary parenchymal o.
    parenchymal o.
    patchy alveolar o.
    pleura-based area of increased o.

o. profusion
reticular o.
rounded o.
tree-in-bud o.
tubular o.
uterine o.
whole-lung o.
opaque
o. arthrography
o. branching structure
o. calculus
o. enema
o. foreign body
o. material
o. meal
o. mediastinography
o. medium
o. myelography
o. powder
o. stone
o. synovium
o. wire suture
OPART MRI
OPCD
olivopontocerebellar degeneration
OPD
obstructive pulmonary disease
Opdima digital mammography system
**OPD-Scan optical path difference
scanning system**
open
o. beam
o. bronchus sign
o. dislocation
o. fontanelle
o. fracture
o. magnet
o. magnetic resonance defecography
o. MRI
o. MRI system
o. neural tube defect
o. pneumothorax
o. reduction
o. reduction and internal fixation
(ORIF)
o. tuberculosis
open-architecture system
open-book fracture
open-break fracture
**open-configuration magnetic resonance
system**
open-cord tendon implant

open-ended guidewire
opening
aortic o. (AO)
aortic valve o.
buttonhole o.
caval o.
esophageal o.
mitral valve o. (MVO)
o. slope
tubal fimbrial o.
valvular o.
open-mouth
o.-m. odontoid view
o.-m. projection
OpenPACS system
opera-glass hand
operating voltage
operation
3D connect o.
Fontan o.
Miles o.
Nissen antireflux o.
pulsed-mode o.
Senning o.
Whipple o.
operative
o. arteriography
o. cholangiogram
operator-dependent positioning
operator exposure
opercula (*pl. of* operculum)
opercular
o. cortex
o. segment of middle cerebral
artery
operculofrontal artery
operculum, pl. **opercula**
cerebral o.
parietal o. (PO)
sylvian o.
OPES
oropharyngoesophageal scintigraphy
OPG
ocular pneumoplethysmography
oculoplethysmography
ophthalmoplethysmography
OPG/CPA
oculoplethysmography/carotid
phonoangiography
ophenoxic acid
ophthalmic
o. artery

NOTES

O

ophthalmic *(continued)*
    o. biometry by ultrasound echography
    o. laser microendoscope
    o. nerve
    o. vein
ophthalmoplegia
ophthalmoplethysmography (OPG)
ophthalmoscope
    Panoramic 200 nonmydriatic o.
ophthalmoscopy
    scanning laser o.
opisthion
opisthotonic position
Opitz thrombophlebitic splenomegaly
OPLL
    ossification of the posterior longitudinal ligament
        thoracic OPLL
Opmilas
    O. CO_2 multipurpose laser
    O. 144 Plus laser system
Oppenheim sign
opponens
    o. digiti minimi
    o. digiti quinti muscle
    o. pollicis
opportunistic lung cavity infection
opposed
    o. GRE image
    o. loop-pair quadrature NMR coil
opposed-phase
    o.-p. GRE, MR imaging
    o.-p. MRI
    o.-p. sequence
    o.-p. T1-weighted image
opposing
    o. articular surfaces
    o. muscle
    o. pleural surfaces
opsonized
OPTA balloon stent-graft
optic
    o. canal
    o. chiasm
    o. chiasm disease
    o. complex tumor
    o. excrescentic thickening
    o. foramen
    o. glioma pathway
    o. globe
    o. glove
    o. nerve
    o. nerve atrophy
    o. nerve compression
    o. nerve Drusen
    o. nerve enlargement

    o. nerve fusiform thickening
    o. nerve glioma
    o. nerve hypoplasia
    o. nerve lesion
    o. nerve sheath meningioma
    o. neuritis
    o. papilla
    o. pathway myelination
    o. radiation
    o. recess
    o. strut
optica
    neuromyelitis o.
optical
    o. coherence tomography (OCT)
    o. density (OD)
    o. isomer
    O. Path Difference-Scan optical device
    o. surface imaging (OSI)
Opticath catheter
opticochiasmatic cistern
Opti-Flow dialysis catheter
optimal
    o. imaging plane
    o. modality
    o. visualization
optimally positioned view
OptiMARK
optimization
    acquisition o.
    interactive gradient o.
    o. parameter
optimum angle imaging
option
    post reconstruction filtering o.
optional target-to-background ratio
Optiplanimat automated unit
OptiQue catheter
Optiray 10, 240, 300, 320, 350 imaging agent
Optison sterile injectable sonography contrast agent
Optispike dispensing pin
Optistar MR contrast delivery system
Optistat power injector
OR1 electronic system
ora (*pl. of* os)
Orabilex
Oracle
    O. MegaSonics catheter
    O. Micro Plus catheter
    O. PTCA catheter
Oragrafin
    O. calcium imaging agent
    O. sodium imaging agent

oral
> o. cavity tumor
> o. cephalocele
> o. cholecystogram (OCG)
> o. cholecystogram imaging
> o. cholecystography
> o. contrast imaging agent
> o. fissure
> o. intubation
> o. magnetic particle
> o. part of pharynx
> o. radiology
> o. urography

oral-enhanced CT scan

orange
> acridine o.

orbicular
> o. bone
> o. ligament

orbicularis
> zona o.

orbit
> angular process of o.
> o. artifact
> body contour o.
> bony o.
> egg-shaped o.
> electron o.
> floor of the o.
> o. measurement
> Rhese view of o.

orbital
> o. abscess
> o. amyloidosis
> o. aneurysm
> o. angiography
> o. apex
> o. apex syndrome
> o. aspect of frontal lobe
> o. base
> o. blood cyst
> o. blowout fracture
> o. bone
> o. canal
> o. capillary hemangioma
> o. cavity
> o. cellulitis
> o. childhood tumor
> o. chocolate cyst
> o. dermoid cyst
> o. edema
> o. electron

> o. emphysema
> o. fissure
> o. floor fracture
> o. granulocytic sarcoma
> o. gyrus
> o. infection
> o. juvenile pilocytic astrocytoma
> o. lymphangioma
> o. lymphoma
> o. mass compression
> o. metastasis
> o. mucocele
> o. plane
> o. plate
> o. pseudotumor
> o. rhabdomyosarcoma
> o. rim
> o. rim stepoff
> o. sarcoidosis
> o. schwannoma
> o. space
> o. superolateral quadrant mass
> o. teratoma
> o. varix
> o. varix ophthalmic vein
> o. wall

orbitofrontal
> o. cortex
> o. dominance

orbitography

orbitomeatal (OM)
> o. line

orbitopathy
> thyroid o.

orbitosphenoidal bone

orbitotomy
> Krönlein o.

Orbix x-ray unit

Orca C-arm fluoroscopy

order
> phase-encoding o.

ordered
> o. phase encoding
> o. subset expectation maximization (OSEM)

Orfit mask

organ
> accessory o.
> adjacent o.
> anulospiral o.
> o. capsule
> circumventricular o.

NOTES

O

organ *(continued)*
Corti o.
critical o.
extraperitoneal o.
floating o.
hollow o.
o. ischemia
o. piping
pole of o.
retroperitoneal o.
rudimentary o.
sanctuary o.
secondary retroperitoneal o.
target o.
o. transplant
Zuckerkandl o.
organelle
sphere o.
organic
o. anion transporter polypeptide
o. brain syndrome (OBS)
o. free radical
o. granulomatosis
o. lesion
o. muscle
organification defect
organization
World Health O. (WHO)
organized hematoma
organizer
embryonic o.
isthmic o.
organizing
o. focal pneumonia
o. interstitial pneumonia
organoaxial
o. rotation
o. volvulus
organogenesis
organoid structure
organomegaly
organ-sparing treatment approach
organ-specific concentration
organ-specific scintigraphic imaging
Oriental
O. cholangiohepatitis
O. lung fluke
orientation
angle of o.
axial o.
coronal o.
cruciate o.
disk-to-magnetic field o.
disturbed o.
sagittal o.
scan o.

slice o.
spatial o.
temporal o.
transverse o.
ORIF
open reduction and internal fixation
orifice
anal o.
aortic o.
atrioventricular nodal o.
cardiac o.
coronary o.
double coronary o.
esophagogastric o.
external urethral o.
gastroduodenal o.
hypoplastic tricuspid o.
ileocecal o.
inferior vena cava o.
internal urethral o.
lingular o.
mitral o. (MO)
mitral valve o. (MVO)
narrowed o.
pharyngeal o.
pulmonary o.
pyloric o.
rectal o.
regurgitant o.
segmental bronchus o.
slit-like o.
tricuspid o.
ureteral o.
urethral o.
vaginal o.
valvular o.
orifice-to-anulus ratio
origin
anomalous o.
o. of artery
brown fat o.
histiocytic bone tumor o.
neural crest o.
neuroectodermal o.
spatial o.
o. of vessel
Ormond disease
orodigitofacial syndrome
oroendotracheal tube
orofacial fistula
orogastric tube
oropharyngeal
o. airway
o. dysfunction
o. dysphagia

o. emptying
o. narrowing
oropharyngoesophageal scintigraphy (OPES)
oropharynx
orotracheal intubation
ORT
ocular radiation therapy
Orthicon
O. camera
O. tube
orthocephalic
orthodeoxia
orthodiagram
orthodiagraph
orthodiagraphy
orthodiascopy
orthogonal
o. angiographic projection
o. C-arm fluoroscopy
o. plane
o. projection mammography
o. radiofrequency coil
o. tag line
o. view
o. view on angiography
orthogonal-hole test pattern (OHP)
orthogonally
orthoiodohippurate (OIH)
iodine-123 o. (OIH)
iodine-131 o.
orthonormal diameter
orthopantogram imaging
orthopantograph
orthopantomograph
Orthopantomograph-panoramic digital radiography unit
orthopantomography
orthopedic
o. nail
o. pin
o. plate
o. rod
o. screw
o. staple
orthoroentgenogram imaging
orthoroentgenography
orthostereoscope
orthotic plate
orthotopic
o. total heart replacement

o. ureter
o. ureterocele
orthovoltage
o. radiation therapy
o. radiotherapy
Ortner syndrome
Ortolani
O. sign
O. test
os, pl. **ora, ossa**
bone
mouth
o. acetabulum
o. acromiale
o. calcis
o. calcis bone
coronary sinus o.
o. coxae
external o.
o. fabella
o. infundibulum
internal cervical o.
o. naviculare
o. peroneum
o. peroneum syndrome
o. pubis
o. styloidium
o. supranaviculare
o. sustentaculi
o. terminale
o. tibiale externum
o. trigonum
o. trigonum syndrome
Osborne ligament
OSCAR ultrasonic bone cement removal system
oscillating
o. Bucky
o. electron
o. gradient
o. grid
o. magnetic field
oscillation
resonant frequency of o.
oscillatory shear rate
oscillography
oscilloscope tuning station
OSCM
oil-soluble contrast medium
OSEM
ordered subset expectation maximization
Osgood-Schlatter disease

O

NOTES

OSI
optical surface imaging
Osler
O. disease
O. maneuver
O. node
O. sign
O. triad
Osler-Libman-Sacks syndrome
Osler-Weber-Rendu
O.-W.-R. syndrome
O.-W.-R. telangiectasia
Osm
osmole
osmium-194
osmolality
low o.
osmole (Osm)
osmotic
o. edema
o. effect
o. gradient
o. load
ossa (*pl. of* os)
osseocartilaginous
o. arch
o. thoracic cage
osseoligamentous arch
osseous, osteal
o. abnormality
o. activity
o. bone contusion
o. bridge
o. cervical spine injury
o. coalition
o. defect
o. destructive process
o. dysplasia
o. graft
o. hemangioendothelioma
o. hemangioma
o. hydatidosis
o. instability
o. labyrinth
o. lacuna
o. lesion
o. lymphoma
o. metaplasia
o. metastasis
o. metastatic disease
o. patellar outgrowth
o. pinch mechanism
o. polyp
o. rarefaction
o. remodeling
o. spiral lamina
o. structure

o. survey
o. trauma
o. tumor of soft tissue
o. union
ossicle
accessory o.
benign Bergman o.
Kerckring o.
meniscal o.
Riolan o.
ossiferous
ossific
o. nodule
o. nucleus
o. nucleus of navicular
ossificans
fasciitis o.
labyrinthitis o.
panniculitis o.
pseudomalignant myositis o.
subacute myositis o.
ossification
abnormal o.
o. of cartilaginous structure
o. center
diaphyseal o.
disk o.
dural o.
ectopic o.
enchondral o.
extraarticular posterior o.
flowing anterior vertebra o.
heterotopic scar o.
intracartilaginous o.
intramembranous o.
irregular enchondral o.
o. of the longitudinal ligament
muscle o.
normal o.
paravertebral o.
periarticular heterotopic o. (PHO)
peripheral o.
o. of the posterior longitudinal
  ligament (OPLL)
primary center of o.
scar o.
secondary center of o.
soft tissue o.
spine o.
unilateral o.
o. variant
vertebral arch ligament o.
ossified
o. body
o. cartilage
o. posterior longitudinal ligament
o. scar

ossiform
ossifying
o. bone fibroma
o. cochleitis
o. epiphysis
o. skull fibroma
ossium
fibrogenesis imperfecta o.
osteal (*var. of* osseous)
osteite
osteitic lesion of the sternum
osteitis
o. deformans
diffuse periapical sclerosing o.
o. fibrosa
o. fibrosa cystica
o. pubis
radiation o.
synovitis, acne, pustolosis, hyperostosis, o. (SAPHO)
ostemia
ostempyesis
OsteoAnalyzer bone densitometry device
osteoarthritic
o. cartilage
o. change
o. spur
osteoarthritis (OA)
degenerative o.
early o.
erosive o.
generalized o.
o. grade
o. grading classification
hand o.
inflammatory o.
posttraumatic o.
premature o.
traumatic o.
osteoarthropathy
hypertrophic pulmonary o.
neuropathic o.
primary hypertrophic o.
pulmonary o.
osteoarticular
osteoblastic
o. activity
o. bone regeneration
o. lesion
o. metastasis
o. osteosarcoma

o. presentation
o. tumor
osteoblastoma
benign o.
expansile o.
osteocartilaginous
o. defect
o. exostosis
o. lesion
o. metaplasia
o. parasellar neoplasm
o. tissue
o. tumor
osteochondral
o. defect (OCD)
o. fracture fragment
o. injury
o. lesion
o. loose body
o. slice fracture
osteochondritis dissecans
osteochondrodysplasia
osteochondrodystrophia deformans
osteochondrodystrophy
osteochondrofibroma
osteochondrolysis
osteochondroma
benign o.
coat hanger o.
epiphyseal o.
soft tissue o.
osteochondromatosis
bursal o.
multiple o.
synovial o.
tenosynovial o.
osteochondromyxoma
osteochondrophyte
osteochondrosarcoma
osteochondrosis
o. deformans juvenilis
o. dissecans
intervertebral o.
spinal o.
vertebral o.
osteochondrotic
o. loose body
o. separation of epiphysis
osteoclasis
osteoclastic
o. erosion
o. resorption

O

NOTES

osteoclast-mediated bone resorption
osteoclastoma
osteoconductive polymer
osteocyte
osteocytoma
osteodentin
osteodermia
osteodiastasis
osteodystrophia fibrosa
osteodystrophy
>   Albright hereditary o.
>   azotemic o.
>   congenital renal o.
>   fibrous o.
>   renal o.

osteoenchondroma
osteofibroma
osteofibromatosis
>   cystic o.

osteofibrous dysplasia
osteogenesis
>   distraction o.
>   o. imperfecta (OI)
>   o. imperfecta tarda

osteogenic
>   o. bone fibroma
>   o. sarcoma

Osteo-Gram bone density test
osteoid
>   o. carcinoma
>   o. formation
>   malignant o.
>   o. matrix
>   o. osteoma
>   o. seam
>   tumor o.

osteoid-origin tumor
osteolipochondroma
osteolipoma
osteolucency
osteolysis
>   blade-of-grass o.
>   candle-flame o.
>   carpotarsal o.
>   essential o.
>   expansile o.
>   idiopathic o.
>   idiopathic multicentric o.
>   lytic o.
>   malignant acetabular o.
>   mandible o.
>   massive o.
>   medial end of clavicle o.
>   mixed sclerotic o.
>   multiple o.
>   nonexpansile o.
>   o. on both sides of joint

periprosthetic o.
sacral o.
scalloping o.
skull o.
temporomandibular joint o.
trabeculated o.
o. tuft
unilocular o.

osteolytic
>   o. lesion
>   o. osseous metastasis

osteoma, pl. **osteomas**
>   cancellous osteoid o.
>   choroidal o.
>   compact o.
>   cortical osteoid o.
>   costal o.
>   o. cutis
>   o. durum
>   o. eburneum
>   fibrous o.
>   giant osteoid o.
>   intracapsular osteoid o.
>   ivory o.
>   juxtaarticular osteoid o.
>   o. medullare
>   osteoid o.
>   parosteal o.
>   soft tissue o.
>   o. spongiosum
>   spongy o.
>   subperiosteal osteoid o.
>   trabecular o.
>   tropical ulcer o.
>   ulcer o.

osteomalacia
>   axial o.
>   hematogenous o.
>   hypophosphatemic o.
>   oncogenic o.
>   renal tubular o.
>   senile o.

osteomalacic pelvis
osteomas, osteomata (pl. of osteoma)
osteomatoid
osteomatosis
osteomesopyknosis
osteomyelitic sinus
osteomyelitis
>   Ackerman criteria for o.
>   active o.
>   acute hematogenous o. (AHO)
>   bacterial o.
>   brucellar o.
>   central vertebral o.
>   childhood o.
>   chronic recurrent multifocal o.

chronic sclerosing o.
cystic tuberculous o.
diskovertebral o.
early o.
Garré sclerosing o.
neonatal o.
nocardial o.
puncture wound o.
pyogenic o.
recurrent multifocal o.
sacral o.
o. scintigraphy
sclerosing nonsuppurative o.
sneaker o.
spinal o.
subligamentous vertebral o.
tuberculous o.
vertebral o.
osteomyelofibrosis
osteomyelography
osteonal bone
osteonecrosis
radiation o.
spontaneous o.
osteopathia
osteopenia
localized o.
osteopenic bone
osteopetrosis
autosomal-dominant benign form
of o.
cranial o.
malignant o.
osteophyte
anterior o.
bony o.
bridging o.
cervical o.
discogenic o.'s
floating o.
o. formation
fringe of o.
horseshoe o.
impinging o.
jagged o.
marginal o.
posterior o.
spinal o.
osteophytic
o. bone lip
o. bridge
o. defect

o. lipping
o. proliferation
o. spurring
osteophytosis in fluorosis
osteoplastic flap
osteopoikilosis
osteoporosis
o. of bone
o. circumscripta
corticosteroid-induced o.
disuse o.
ground-glass o.
juvenile o.
localized o.
partial transient o.
periarticular o.
picture-framing o.
postmenopausal o.
posttraumatic o.
regional migratory o.
regional transient o.
senile o.
transient regional o.
osteoporotic
o. bone
o. compression fracture
osteoradiology
osteoradionecrosis
osteosarcoma
cardiac o.
central o.
chondroblastic o.
classical o.
conventional o.
epithelioid o.
extraosseous o.
extraskeletal o.
extremity o.
fibroblastic o.
gnathic o.
high-grade surface o.
intracortical o.
intramedullary o.
intraosseous o.
intraosseous low-grade o.
o. of jaw
juxtacortical o.
lytic o.
metastatic o.
multicentric o.
multifocal o.
multiple sclerotic o.

O

NOTES

osteosarcoma *(continued)*
  osteoblastic o.
  parosteal o.
  periosteal o.
  sacral o.
  sclerosing o.
  secondary o.
  small-cell o.
  surface o.
  telangiectatic o.
osteosarcomatosis
osteosarcomatous
osteosclerosis
  constitutional o.
  diffuse o.
  multiple-lesion o.
  myelofibrosis o.
  solitary o.
  subchondral o.
  o. tuft
  o. vertebral sarcoidosis
osteosclerotic lesion
osteosis
osteospongioma
osteosynthesis
  biological o.
osteothrombosis
osteotomy
  high tibial o.
OsteoView
  O. desktop hand x-ray system
  O. digital bone densitometer
  O. 2000 digital imaging system
ostia *(pl. of* ostium)
ostial
  o. cannulation
  o. lesion
  o. renal artery stenosis
ostiomeatal
  o. complex
  o. unit
ostitis deformans
ostium, pl. ostia
  aneurysmal o.
  aortic o.
  artery o.
  atrioventricular nodal o.
  conus branch ostia
  coronary artery o.
  coronary sinus o.
  fistula o.
  o. primum
  o. primum atrial septal defect
  o. secundum
  o. secundum atrial septal defect
Ostreg spinal marker system
Ostwald solubility coefficient (Λ)

OSTYCUT bone biopsy needle
2.OT
  SPECTRO-20000 2.OT
OTD
otic
  o. capsule
  o. ganglion
  o. obstruction
otitis
  malignant external o.
  necrotizing external o.
OtoLAM laser
otologic implant
otosclerosis
  cochlear o.
  fenestral o.
  retrofenestral o.
  stapedial o.
otospongiosis
Ottawa ankle rule
Otto
  O. disease
  O. pelvis
Otto-Krobak pelvis
OURQ
  outer upper right quadrant
out
  rule o. (R/O)
  silhouetted o.
outcropping of lesion
outer
  o. anular/posterior longitudinal
    ligament complex
  o. border of uterus
  o. canthus
  o. table of skull
  o. table thickening
  o. upper right quadrant (OURQ)
outer-air
  o.-a. region
  o.-a. segmentation
outflow
  double o.
  o. effect
  hepatic venous o.
  hypoplastic subpulmonic o.
  maximum venous o. (MVO)
  o. obstruction
  subpulmonic o.
  swan-neck shape of ventricular o.
  o. tract
  o. tract gradient
  o. of ventricle
outgrowth
  osseous patellar o.
outlet
  cervical o.

o. impingement
o. obstruction
pelvic o.
pyloric o.
thoracic o.
ventricular o.
o. view
o. view radiograph
widened thoracic o.

outline

absent kidney o.
double o.
gastric o.
renal o.
trabeculated o.

out-of-field count
out-of-phase

o.-o.-p. gradient echo
o.-o.-p. GRE imaging

out-of-profile nipple
out-of-slice artifact
outpocketings of mucosa
outpouching

aneurysmal o.
saccular o.

output

adequate cardiac o.
o. amplitude
augmented cardiac o.
cardiac o. (CO, Q)
Dow method for measuring cardiac o.
Fick method for measuring cardiac o.
Gorlin method for measuring cardiac o.
Hamilton-Stewart formula for measuring cardiac o.
inadequate cardiac o.
instrument o.
low cardiac o.
o. point
pulmonic o.
reduced systemic cardiac o.
stroke o.
systemic o.
thermodilution cardiac o.
ventricular o.

outrigger arm
outside-to-inside segmentation
OV

ovarian

OV103

OncoRad O.
OncoScint O.

ova (*pl. of* ovum)
Ovadia-Beals tibial plafond fracture classification
oval

o. aneurysm
o. aneurysm with bleb
o. shape
o. window

ovalbumin
ovale

centrum o.
foramen o.
patent foramen o. (PFO)
o. skull base of foramen

ovalis

anulus o.
fossa o.

ovarian (OV)

o. abscess
o. anatomy
o. artery
o. carcinoma
o. choriocarcinoma
o. cortex
o. cystadenofibroma
o. cystadenoma
o. dermoid
o. dermoid cyst
o. Doppler signal
o. dysgenesis
o. dysgerminoma
o. edema
o. fibroma
o. fishnet weave pattern
o. follicular cyst
o. fossa
o. hernia
o. hyperstimulation syndrome
o. image signature cyst
o. mass
o. medulla
o. mesonephroid tumor
o. metastasis
o. morphology
o. neoplasm
o. pregnancy
o. remnant syndrome
o. retention cyst
o. serous cystadenocarcinoma

NOTES

O

ovarian *(continued)*
    o. size
    o. suspensory ligament
    o. systic teratoma
    o. torsion
    o. vein
    o. vein embolization
    o. vein syndrome
    o. vein thrombosis
    o. venography
    o. volume
ovarioabdominal pregnancy
ovary
    atrophied o.
    clear cell neoplasm of o.
    cystic o.
    embryonic o.
    fibroma-thecoma tumor of o.
    o. germ cell tumor
    o. gland
    hilar cell tumor of o.
    hyperstimulation of o.
    ligament of o.
    mulberry o.
    multifollicular o.
    palpable postmenopausal o.
    pearly white o.
    polycystic o.
    postmenopausal o.
    sclerocystic o.
    stromal carcinoid tumor of o.
    suspensory ligament of o.
    teratoblastoma of o.
    teratocarcinoma of o.
    thecoma of o.
    transposition of o.
Ovation falloposcopy system
overaeration
overcirculation
    pulmonary vessel o.
    o. vascularity
overcouch
    o. exposure
    o. tube
    o. view
overdamping
overdevelopment
    bone o.
overdiagnostic bias
overdistention
    alveolar o.
    o. of alveolar populations
    pulmonary o.
overdrainage
overdrive suppression

overexpansion
    lung o.
    pulmonary o.
overexposure
overframing
    horizontal o.
    mean-diameter o.
    subtotal o.
overgrowth
    bony o.
    cuticular o.
    epiphyseal o.
    fibrocartilaginous o.
    vertebral body o.
overhanging
    o. border
    o. margin
Overhauser effect
overhead
    o. film
    o. oblique view
overinflation
    lung o.
    obstructive pulmonary o.
    pulmonary o.
    unilateral o.
overlap
    liver-spleen o.
    o. shadow
overlapping
    o. finger
    o. fracture
    o. image
    o. rib
    o. suture
overlay
    anatomic o.
    o. plate
    venous o.
overlie
overload
    acute hemodynamic o.
    cardiac o.
    chronic hemodynamic o.
    diastolic o.
    fluid o.
    pressure o.
    right ventricular o.
    systolic ventricular o.
    transfusional iron o.
    volume o.
overlying
    o. attenuation artifact
    o. bowel content
    o. bowel gas
    o. bowel shadows
    o. branching pattern

overpenetrated film
overread
overrelaxation factor
override
    aortic o.
overriding
    o. aorta
    o. of fracture fragment
    o. great artery
    o. sutures of fontanelle
    o. toe
over-the-wire design
overventilation
    alveolar o.
overview angiogram
overvoltage
oviductal pregnancy
ovoid
    afterloading tandem and o.
    o. heart
    o. high signal intensity
    Manchester o.
    o. ossification center
    o. shape
    tandem and o.
ovulation
    incessant o.
    o. induction
ovulatory
    o. failure
    o. phase
ovum, pl. ova
    aspiration of ova
Owen view
owl's eye appearance
oxalosis
    bone o.
    kidney o.
    primary o.
Oxford
    O. magnet
    O. 2-T large-bore imaging system
      scanner
ox heart
oxidase
    cytochrome o. (COX)
    monoamine o.
oxidation
    Baeyer-Villiger o.
    o. state
oxidative metabolism

oxide
    monocrystalline iron o. (MION)
    nitric o.
    superparamagnetic agent iron o.
    superparamagnetic iron o. (SPIO)
    ultrasmall superparamagnetic iron o.
      (USPIO)
oxidized complex
oxidronate
Oxilan imaging agent
oxime
    hexamethylpropyleneamine o.
      (HMPAO)
    ^{99m}Tc hexamethylpropylene
      amine o.
    technetium-99m hexamethylpropylene
      amine o.
oxine
    ^{111}In o.
oxine-indium
    lipophilic o.-i.
oxycephaly
oxygen (O_2)
    activation-induced uncoupling of
      cerebral o.
    cerebral metabolic rate of o.
      ($CMRO_2$)
    cistern o.
    o. cisternography
    o. consumption (QO_2)
    o. effect
    o. extraction fraction (OEF)
    o. extraction rate (OER)
    o. imaging agent
    metabolic rate of o.
    o. myelography
    regional cerebral metabolic rate
      for o. ($rCMRO_2$)
    o. saturation
oxygen-15 (^{15}O)
oxygen-16 (^{16}O)
oxygen-17 (^{17}O)
    o. NMR spectroscopy
oxygen-18 (^{18}O)
oxygenated perfluorocarbon blood
substitute
oxygenation
    extracorporeal membrane o.
    tissue o.
oxygenation-sensitive
    o.-s. functional MR
    o.-s. functional MR imaging

O

NOTES

oxygenator
 bubble o.
 disk o.
 extracorporeal membrane o.
 film o.
 membrane o.
 rotating disk o.
 screen o.

oxygen-dependent emphysema
oxygen-enhanced lung MR imaging
oxyorthosilicate
 cerium-doped lutetium o. (LSO)
 gadolinium o.
oxyphilic adenoma
oyster-pearl breast calcification

P

phosphorus
posterior
    P loop
    P pulmonale pattern
P-32 (*var. of* ³²P)
    sodium phosphate
P792
P1-P4 segment of posterior cerebral artery
P2 segment aneurysm
³²P, P-32
    phosphorus-32
        sodium phosphate ³²P
PA

parathyroid adenoma
pathology
posteroanterior
pulmonary artery
    PA and lateral films
    PA position
    PA projection
P/A

perimeter-area ratio
Pa

protactinium
Paas disease
PABP

pulmonary artery balloon pump
pacchionian

p. body
p. depression
p. granulation
pace

p. mapping
P. Plus System scanner
pacemaker

p. artifact
bipolar p.
p. effect
implanted p.
p. lead
p. wire
pachydermoperiostosis
pachygyria
pachymeningitis
pachymeninx, pl. **pachymeninges**
pachypleuritis
pacing

p. artifact
p. lead
Packard Merlin life-monitoring system
packed bead
packing

edge p.

endosaccular p.
p., extraction, and calculation technique
p. fraction
PACS

picture archiving and communication system
    P. PathSpeed MR imaging
    P. workstation
pad

antimesenteric fat p.
decubitus p.
p. effect
epicardial fat p.
esophagogastric fat p.
fat p.
fibrocartilaginous p.
foveal fat p.
haversian fat p.
heel fat p.
Hoffa fat p.
ileocecal fat p.
intracapsular fat p.
intrapatellar fat p.
ischiorectal fat p.
patellar fat p.
pericardial fat p.
pre-Achilles fat p.
Sat P.
scalene fat p.
p. sign of aortic insufficiency
thickened heel p.
UltraEase ultrasound p.
ultrasound p.
padding

antral p.
zero p.
paddle

compression p.
spot compression p.
p. wheel method
PADP-PAWP

pulmonary artery diastolic pressure and pulmonary artery wedge pressure
PAEDP

pulmonary artery end-diastolic pressure
Page kidney
Paget

P. abscess
P. carcinoma
P. disease of bone
P. jaw disease
P. osteitis deformans
P. quiet necrosis
pagetic

P

pagetoid
    p. bone
    p. epidermal involvement
Paget-von Schroetter syndrome
PAH
    paraaminohippurate
pain
    periumbilical p.
painful
    p. disk derangement
    p. osmotic demyelination syndrome
painless thyroiditis
pain provocation response
paint brush striation
pair
    electron-positron p.
    line p.
    Maxwell p.
    oblique annihilation photon p.
    p. production
    transaxial annihilation photon p.
paired
    p. inferior vena cava
    p. parietal branch
    p. visceral branch
Pais fracture
palatal muscle
palate
palatina
    uvula p.
palatine
    p. bone
    p. canal
    p. foramen
    p. ridge
    p. root
    p. shelf
    p. suture
palatoethmoidal suture
palatoglossus
palatograph
palatography
palatomaxillary
    p. canal
    p. suture
palatomyograph
palatopharyngeal fold
palatopharyngeus
palatovaginal canal
paleopathologic and radiologic study
palisade formation
palladium (Pd)
    p. imaging agent
    p. implant
palladium-103 (^{103}Pd, Pd-103)

palliative
    p. esophagostomy
    p. radiation therapy
pallidotomy
pallidum
pallidus
    globus p.
palmar
    p. angulation
    p. aponeurosis
    p. arterial arch
    p. cutaneous vein
    p. displacement
    p. fascia
    p. fasciitis
    p. fibromatosis
    p. ganglion
    p. interossei
    p. metacarpal ligament
    p. plate
    p. radiocarpal ligament
    p. slope
    p. surface
    p. tilt
    p. wrist
palmaris
    p. brevis
    p. longus
    p. longus tendon
Palmaz
    P. PS 424 stent
    P. P 394 stainless steel balloon-expandable stent
palmitate
    ^{11}C p.
palmitic acid
palmoplantar
palpable
    p. aortic ejection sound
    p. postmenopausal ovary
    p. presystolic bulge
    p. pulmonic ejection sound
Palpagraph breast mapping device
palpatory T-stage prostate carcinoma
palpebra, pl. **palpebrae**
    levator palpebrae
palpebral
    p. fissure
    p. raphe
palsy
    dyskinetic cerebral p.
    progressive supranuclear p.
    waiter's tip p.
PAM
    pulmonary artery mean pressure
    PAM pressure

pamidronate
  p. disodium
  p. therapy
pampiniform plexus
PAN
  polyarteritis nodosa
panacinar emphysema
panagraphy
panaortic
panbronchiolitis
  diffuse p.
pancake
  p. appearance
  p. compression
  p. kidney
  p. MRI magnet
pancarpal destructive arthritis
panchamber
  p. enlargement
  p. hypertrophy
Pancoast
  P. syndrome
  P. tumor
pancolitis
pancompartmental joint space
  narrowing
pancreas, pl. **pancreata**
  aberrant p.
  accessory p.
  anterior surface of p.
  anular p.
  Aselli p.
  body of the p.
  p. cystadenoma
  degeneration of p.
  p. divisum
  dorsal p.
  ectopic p.
  fat-spared area in p.
  p. gland
  head of the p.
  heterotopic p.
  interior surface of p.
  intraductal papillary mucinous
    tumor of the p.
  lesser p.
  mature pseudocyst of p.
  metastasis to the p.
  mucinous ductal ectasia of p.
  mucinous ductectatic tumor of p.
  neck of p.
  posterior surface of p.

  tail of p.
  p. transplant
  p. ultrasonography imaging
  uncinate process of p.
  ventral p.
pancreatic
  p. abscess
  p. angiography
  p. arteriography
  p. ascites
  p. atrophy
  p. calcification
  p. calculus
  p. carcinoma
  p. cholera syndrome
  p. cutaneous fistula
  p. cyst
  p. cystadenocarcinoma
  p. cystic fibrosis
  p. cystic lymphangioma
  p. degeneration
  p. disease
  p. divisum
  p. dorsal anlage
  p. duct
  p. ductal adenocarcinoma
  p. duct branch
  p. duct dilatation
  p. duct obstruction
  p. duct sphincter
  p. duct stent
  p. fluid collection
  p. hamartoma
  p. head
  p. islet cell tumor
  p. lipomatosis
  p. lymph node
  p. lymphoma
  p. macrocystic adenoma
  p. mass
  p. metastasis
  p. microcystic adenoma
  p. neck
  p. necrosis
  p. neoplasm
  p. phlegmon
  p. pseudocyst
  p. pseudocyst drainage
  p. scan
  p. trauma
  p. vein
pancreatic-enteric continuity

NOTES

P

pancreaticobiliary
  p. common channel
  p. disease
  p. ductal junction
  p. function variant
  p. sphincter
  p. tract
  p. ultrasound
pancreaticoblastoma
pancreaticoduodenal
  p. artery
  p. lymph node
pancreaticoduodenectomy
pancreaticohepatic syndrome
pancreaticolienal lymph node
pancreaticopleural fistula
pancreaticosplenic
  p. node
  p. omentum
pancreatitis
  acute p.
  chronic calcifying p.
  chronic obstructive p.
  diffuse p.
  edematous p.
  focal p.
  necrotizing p.
  obstructive p.
  phlegmonous p.
  p. pseudoaneurysm
  Santiani-Stone classification of p.
  suppurative p.
  tropical p.
pancreatocholangiogram
  retrograde p.
pancreatogram
pancreatography
  endoscopic retrograde p.
  p. imaging
  intraoperative p.
  magnetic resonance p. (MRP)
  percutaneous p.
  retrograde p.
pancreatolithiasis
pancytopenia-dysmelia syndrome
panda appearance
Pander island
PANDO
  primary acquired nasolacrimal duct
    obstruction
panduriform placenta
panencephalitis
  progressive rubella p.
  sclerosing p.
  subacute sclerosing p. (SSPE)
panfacial fracture
panhypopituitarism

panlobar nephroglastomatosis
panlobular emphysema
panmyelopathy
panmyelosis
Panner disease
panniculitis
  mediastinal p.
  mesenteric p. (MP)
  p. ossificans
  systemic nodular p.
pannus, pl. **panni**
  p. deformity
  p. deformity of odontoid
  p. formation
  synovial p.
  p. of synovium
pan-oral radiography
panoramic
  p. CT scan
  p. image
  p. imaging
  P. 200 nonmydriatic
    ophthalmoscope
  p. radiograph
  p. radiography
  p. rotating machine
  p. surface projection
  p. tomography
  p. view
  p. x-ray film
Panorex view
pansinusitis
pan synovitis
pansystolic mitral regurgitation
pantalar fusion
pantaloon
  p. embolus
  p. hernia
pantomogram
pantomographic view
pantomography
  concentric p.
  eccentric p.
Pantopaque
  P. cisternography
  P. imaging agent
  P. myelography
PAOD
  peripheral arterial occlusive disease
PAP
  pulmonary alveolar proteinosis
  pulmonary artery pressure
**Papavasiliou classification of olecranon
  fracture**
paper-doll fetus
Papile classification
papilla, pl. **papillae**

aberrant p.
acoustic p.
bile p.
circumvallate p.
p. of columnar epithelium
duodenal p.
major duodenal p.
minor duodenal p.
optic p.
renal p.
Santorini p.
sloughed p.
smudged p.
urethral p.
p. of Vater
p. of Vater enlargement
p. of Vater stenosis

papillary
p. adenoma of large intestine
p. apocrine change
p. bile duct stenosis
p. breast carcinoma
p. cystadenoma lymphomatosum
p. cystic adenoma
p. DCIS
p. duct of Bellini
p. epididymal cystadenoma
p. epithelial neoplasm
p. excrescence
p. fibroelastoma
p. lesion
p. muscle
p. muscle infarct
p. muscle rupture
p. necrosis
p. pancreatic cystic neoplasm
p. projection
p. proliferation
p. renal cell carcinoma
p. serous adenocarcinoma
p. serous carcinoma
p. thyroid carcinoma
p. tumor

papilledema
papillocarcinoma
papillogram
papilloma, pl. **papillomas, papillomata**
p. acuminata
basal cell p.
benign intraductal p.
p. of bladder
breast p.

choroid plexus p.
cockscomb p.
p. diffusum
ductal p.
p. durum
fibroepithelial p.
p. of the fourth ventricle
hard p.
Hopmann p.
p. inguinale
intraductal p.
inverted p.
large duct p.
laryngeal p.
p. molle
multiple peripheral p.
p. neuropathicum
p. neuroticum
penile squamous p.
schneiderian p.
soft p.
transitional urethral cell p.
villous p.

papillomatosis
intraductal breast p.
invasive p.
juvenile breast p.
juvenile laryngeal p.
laryngeal p.
pulmonary p.
recurrent respiratory p.
tracheobronchial p.

papillomatous growth
Papillon-Léfevré syndrome
Papillon technique
papillotomy
papular lesion
papulonecrotic lesion
PAPVR
partial anomalous pulmonary venous
return
papyracea
lamina p.
papyraceus
fetus p.
PAR
plain abdominal radiography
paraaminobenzoic acid
paraaminohippurate (PAH)
paraaminohippuric acid
paraaminosalicylic acid (PAS)
paraanastomotic aneurysmal repair

NOTES

P

paraaortic
p. lymph node
p. mass
paraarticular
p. bone remodeling
p. calcification
parabola
digital p.
metatarsal p.
parabolic velocity profile
paracarcinomatous myelopathy
paracardiac
p. mass
p. metastasis
p. tumor
**paracardiac-type total anomalous venous
return**
paracardial lymph node
paracecal appendix
paracentesis
abdominal p.
paracentral
p. artery
p. gyrus
p. lobule
paracervical lymphatic
parachute
p. deformity of mitral valve
p. mitral valve deformity
paracicatricial emphysema
paracoccidioidal granuloma
paracolic
p. abscess
p. gutter
p. lymph node
paracorporeal heart
paracortical hyperplasia
paracostal
paracystic pouch
paradigm
block p.
coregistration p.
event-related p.
paradiskal lesion
paradoxical
p. bronchospasm
p. cerebral embolus
p. colon dilatation
p. embolization
p. enhancement
p. leaflet motion
p. middle turbinate
p. septal motion
p. suppression
paradoxicum
paradoxus
pulsus p.

paraduodenal
p. fold
p. fossa
p. hernia
p. recess
paraesophageal
p. hernia
p. varix
paraesophagogastric devascularization
parafascicular
p. nucleus
p. thalamotomy
paraffin-embedded tissue
paraffinoma
paraganglioma
adrenal p.
chromaffin p.
extraadrenal p.
functional p.
gangliocytic p.
nonchromaffin p.
thoracic p.
paragangliomatosis
paraglenoid cyst
paragonimiasis
brain p.
lung p.
paragranuloma
parahiatal hernia
parahilar
parahippocampal gyrus
paraileostomal hernia
**para-isopropyl-iminodiacetic acid
(PIPIDA)**
**para-isopropyl-iminodiacetic acid
technetium-99m hepatobiliary scan**
paralabral
p. cyst
p. lesion
paralaryngeal
p. muscle
p. space
parallax
p. method
p. view
parallel
p. analog mapping
p. array
p. cine
p. data acquisition coil
p. hole imaging
p. mean translation
p. M line
p. opposed unmodified port
p. pitch line
p. ray
p. and spiral flow pattern

p. tag plane
p. virtual machine (PVM)
parallel-hole
p.-h. medium sensitivity collimator
p.-h. scintigram
parallelism
p. of articular surface
p. of facet joint
parallel-line
p.-l.-equal-space bar
p.-l. equal spacing (PLES)
parallel-opposed beams
parallel-tagged MR image
paralysis, pl. **paralyses**
p. of diaphragm
diaphragmatic p.
hernia p.
Klumpke p.
phrenic nerve p.
vocal cord p.
paralytic
p. chest
p. colonic obstruction
p. ileus
paralytica
dysphagia p.
paramagnetic
p. artifact
p. cation
p. contrast agent
p. contrast-enhanced MR study
p. contrast enhancement
p. effect
p. enhancement accentuation
p. enhancement accentuation by
chemical shift imaging
p. influence
p. shift
p. shift relaxation
paramagnetism
apparent p.
collective p.
paramalleolar artery
paramammary lymph node
paramedian
p. infarct
p. line
p. pontine reticular formation
(PPRF)
p. position
p. sagittal plane

p. section
p. thalamic artery
p. thalamopeduncular artery
p. triangle
paramediastinal gland
parameningeal rhabdomyosarcoma
parameniscal cyst
paramesonephric
p. duct
p. duct cyst
parameter
clinical p.
extrinsic cellular p.
growth p.
hematologic p.
intrinsic cellular p.
kinetic perfusion p.
normal hemodynamic liver p.
nuclear magnetic resonance
spectral p.
optimization p.
physiologic p.
rendering p.
scan p.
sonographic p.
thermal treatment p.
timing p.
ventricular function p.
parametrectomy
radical p.
parametria (*pl. of* parametrium)
parametrial fat
parametric image
parametrium, pl. **parametria**
paranasal
p. sinus
p. sinus carcinoma
p. sinusitis
p. sinus mass
p. sinus mucocele
paraneoplastic
p. cerebellar degeneration
p. process
p. syndrome
p. thromboembolism
paraorbital lesion
paraosteoarthropathy
paraovarian
p. cyst
p. varicosity
parapatellar plica

NOTES

P

parapelvic
>   p. cyst
>   p. gutter

parapharyngeal
>   p. abscess
>   p. space
>   p. space cyst

parapneumonic effusion

paraprosthetic
>   p. leak
>   p. leakage

paraprosthetic-enteric fistula

pararectal
>   p. abscess
>   p. fossa
>   p. lymph node
>   p. pouch

pararenal
>   p. abscess
>   p. aortic aneurysm
>   p. aortic atherosclerosis
>   p. space

parasagittal
>   p. depression
>   p. image
>   p. intracranial mass
>   p. lesion
>   p. meningioma
>   p. plane

parasellar
>   p. brain mass
>   p. cistern
>   p. dermoid tumor
>   p. lesion
>   p. metastasis

paraseptal
>   p. emphysema
>   p. position

parasinoidal

parasitic
>   p. fetus
>   p. infiltrate

paraspinal
>   p. abnormality
>   p. abscess
>   p. calcification
>   p. line
>   p. muscle
>   p. neurofibroma
>   p. pleural stripe
>   p. soft tissue mass
>   p. soft tissue shadowing

paraspinous musculature

parasternal
>   p. bulge
>   p. long-axis view

>   p. long-axis view echocardiography
>   p. lymph node
>   p. motion
>   p. scanning
>   p. short-axis view
>   p. short-axis view echocardiography
>   p. view of heart
>   p. window

parastomal hernia

parastriate cortex

parasympathetic
>   p. fiber
>   p. ganglia tumor
>   p. nervous system

paraterminal gyrus

paratesticular
>   p. rhabdomyosarcoma
>   p. tumor

parathyroid
>   p. adenoma (PA)
>   p. carcinoma
>   p. cyst
>   ectopic p.
>   p. hyperplasia
>   p. insufficiency
>   p. scintigraphy
>   technetium-99m sestamibi p.
>   p. tumor
>   p. ultrasonography imaging
>   p. vein

parathyroidectomy
>   radioguided p.

P:A ratio

paratracheal
>   p. adenopathy
>   p. convexity
>   p. lymph node
>   p. region
>   p. soft tissue
>   p. tissue stripe

paratrooper's fracture

paratubal serous cyst

paratumoral injection

paraumbilical
>   p. anterior abdominal wall
>   p. vein

paraureteral diverticulum

paraurethral
>   p. canal
>   p. cyst
>   p. duct
>   p. gland

parauterine lymph node

paravaginal
>   p. lymph node
>   p. soft tissue

paravalvular
  p. leak
  p. regurgitation
paravertebral
  p. ganglion
  p. groove
  p. gutter
  p. musculature
  p. nerve plexus
  p. ossification
  p. scanning
  p. venous plexus
paravertebrally
  p. situated pelvic tumor mass
  p. situated thoracic tumor mass
paravesical
  p. fossa
  p. pouch
paravesicular lymph node
parcellation of structure
parchment
  p. heart
  p. right ventricle
parenchyma
  bleeding into brain p.
  brain p.
  breast p.
  cerebral p.
  computerized texture analysis of
    lung nodules and lung p.
  hepatic p.
  liver p.
  lung p.
  mammary p.
  marbling of pancreatic p.
  mottling of renal p.
  normal renal p.
  pulmonary p.
  renal p.
  spinal cord p.
  testicular p.
parenchymal
  p. blastoma
  p. blood
  p. brain metastasis
  p. breast pattern
  p. change
  p. cone
  p. consolidation
  p. echogenicity
  p. enhancement
  p. extension

  p. fibrous band
  p. hematoma
  p. infarct
  p. laceration
  p. lung band
  p. opacity
  p. peliosis hepatis
  p. phase image
  p. scarring
  p. tissue
  p. tracer accumulation
  p. transit
parenchymatous
  p. atrophy
  p. cerebellar degeneration
  p. inflammation
  p. phase
  p. pneumonia
parenchymography
  endoscopic retrograde p. (ERP)
parenchymous goiter
parent
  p. artery occlusion
  p. element
  p. isotope
  p. nuclide
  p. radionuclide
  p. vein
  p. vessel
  p. vessel occlusion
parentheses-like calcification
Parenti-Fraccaro disease
paresthetica
  meralgia p.
Parham-Martin band
parietal
  p. association area
  p. band
  p. bone
  p. bone thinning
  p. boss
  p. cephalohematoma
  p. convexity
  p. cortex
  p. cortex lesion
  p. diameter
  p. eminence
  p. encephalocele
  p. extension
  p. extension of infundibular septum
  p. eye field (PEF)
  p. fistula

NOTES

parietal *(continued)*
   p. foramen
   p. gyrus
   p. layer
   p. lobe
   p. lobe gray-matter cytosolic
     choline pathogenetic mechanism
     of myocardial fibrosis
   p. lobe lesion
   p. lymph node
   p. middle cerebral artery
   p. operculum (PO)
   p. pelvic fascia
   p. pericardial calcification
   p. pericardium
   p. peritoneum
   p. pleura
   p. pleural scarring
   p. pregnancy
   p. presentation
   p. suture
parietography
   gastric p.
parietomastoid suture
parietooccipital
   p. area
   p. branch of posterior cerebellar
     artery
   p. lesion
   p. region
   p. sulcus
   p. suture
parietoorbital projection
parietotemporal
   p. area
   p. suture
Parinaud syndrome
Paris ultrasound system
park
   p. bench position
   P.'s bidirectional Doppler flowmeter
   P.'s 800 bidirectional Doppler
     flowmetry
   P. Medical Systems scanner
Parkes-Weber syndrome
paroöphoron
parosteal
   p. bone lesion
   p. chondrosarcoma
   p. osteogenic sarcoma
   p. osteoma
   p. osteosarcoma
   p. soft tissue angiosarcoma
parotid
   p. abscess
   p. duct
   p. gland

   p. gland sialography
   p. lymph node
   p. pleomorphic adenoma
   p. pneumatocele
   p. tumor
parotitis
   adenoid cystic carcinoma p.
   benign mixed tumor p.
   cylindroma p.
   mucoepidermoid carcinoma p.
   pleomorphic adenoma p.
parovarian cyst
paroxysmal
   p. auricular tachycardia
   p. AV block
   p. change
   p. pulmonary edema
parrot
   frontal bossing of P.
   P. node
parrot-beak
   p.-b. labral tear
   p.-b. meniscus tear
   p.-b. pattern
parry fracture
pars, *pl.* **partes**
   p. flaccida cholesteatoma
   p. interarticularis
   p. interarticularis defect
   p. interarticularis fracture
   pedicles and p.
   p. tensa cholesteatoma
Parsons
   third intercondylar tubercle of P.
   P. tubercle
part
   fetal small p.
   presenting p.
partes (*pl. of* pars)
partial
   p. anomalous pulmonary venous
     connection
   p. anomalous pulmonary venous
     return (PAPVR)
   p. atrioventricular canal defect
   p. bursal surface tear
   p. collapse of lung
   p. complex seizure
   p. corpus callosum agenesis
   p. dislocation
   p. dislodgement
   p. flip-angle fast-scan technique
   p. Fourier imaging
   p. Fourier technique
   p. heart block
   p. k-space sampling
   p. lesion

p. liquid ventilation
p. liquid ventilation with perflubron
p. obliteration of lateral ventricle
p. pericardial abscess
p. pericardial absence
p. placenta previa
p. pulmonary venous connection
p. saturation (PS)
p. saturation pulse sequence
p. saturation spin echo
p. saturation technique
p. small bowel malrotation
p. small bowel obstruction
p. thickening
p. thickness split tear
p. transient osteoporosis
p. transposition of great artery
p. tubular appearance
p. ureter duplication
p. volume averaging
p. volume effect artifact

partial-brain radiation therapy
partially
p. polycystic kidney
p. relaxed Fourier transform
(PRFT)
partial-ring bismuth germanate-crystal
scanner
particle
accelerated p.
p. accelerator
alpha p.
p. approach
beta p.
bone p.
calcium/oxyanion-containing p.
charged-p.
embosphere p.
gelatin sponge p.
heavy charged p.
p. identification
Ivalon p.
large colloidal p.
p. mask
nuclear p.
oral magnetic p.
polyvinyl alcohol p.
PVA p.
p. size determination
submicron magnetic p.'s
superparamagnetic iron oxide p.

viral p.
Zimmermann elementary p.
particle-beam radiation therapy
particulate
p. arterial embolization
p. debris
p. echo
p. embolic agent
magnetic p.
p. matter
partition
atrial p.
p. coefficient
gastric p.
partitioning
recursive p.
parturient canal
parturition
PAS
paraaminosalicylic acid
pulmonary artery systolic pressure
pascals of force
PASH
pseudoangiomatous stromal hyperplasia
PASP-SASP ratio
pass
p. coaxially
interleaved imaging p.
PASSA
proximal articular set angle
passage
adiabatic fast p. (AFP)
adiabatic rapid p. (ARP)
biliary p.
free air p.
narrowing of bronchiolar p.
p. pressure
Passager Nitinol self-expandable stent
Passavant
P. bar
P. muscle
P. ridge
passive
p. atelectasis
p. chest expansion
p. clot
p. edema
p. filling
p. hepatic congestion
p. hyperemia
p. pneumonia
p. shielding

NOTES

P

passive · patency

passive *(continued)*
    p. shimming
    p. track detector
    p. vascular congestion
    p. venous distention
passively
    p. congested lung tissue
    p. shimmed superconducting magnet
PASTA imaging
paste
    ferric ammonium citrate-cellulose p.
pastille, pastil
    p. radiometer
    Sabouraud p.
PASV
    pressure-activated safety valve
    PASV catheter
Patau syndrome
patch
    ash leaf p.
    blood p.
    p. crinkling
    p. electrode
    epidural blood p.
    p. graft reconstruction
    p. kinking
    p. lesion
    McCallum p.
    Peyer p.
    pigskin p.
    sclerotic calvarial p.
    subcutaneous p.
patch-graft aortoplasty
patchy
    p. alveolar opacity
    p. area of consolidation
    p. area of density
    p. area of pneumonia
    p. atelectasis
    p. atrophy of renal cortex
    p. colonic ulcer
    p. distribution of tracer
    p. edema
    p. migratory infiltrate
    p. zone
patella, pl. **patellae**
    p. alta
    apex of head of p.
    p. baja
    bipartite p.
    chondromalacia p.
    dislocation of p.
    floating p.
    half-moon p.
    high-lying p.
    high-riding p.
    ligamentum patellae

    lower pole of p.
    multipartite p.
    pebble-shaped p.
    skyline view of p.
    squared p.
    subluxation of p. (SLP)
    subluxing p.
    undersurface of p.
patellar
    p. bursa
    p. bursitis
    p. button
    p. cartilage thickness
    p. chondromalacia
    p. contour
    p. dislocation
    p. edge
    p. entrapment
    p. fat pad
    p. fossa
    p. groove
    p. ligament-patellar ratio
    p. malalignment
    p. pole
    p. retinaculum
    p. shaving
    p. shelf
    p. skyline view
    p. sleeve fracture
    p. subluxation
    p. tendinopathy
    p. tendinosis
    p. tendon
    p. tilt
patellectomy
patelliform
patellofemoral
    p. angle
    p. articular cartilage
    p. articulation
    p. compartment
    p. congruence
    p. disorder
    p. incongruency
    p. index
    p. joint
    p. joint space
    p. realignment
patelloquadriceps tendon
patency
    arterial p.
    p. of artery
    coronary artery bypass graft p.
    ductus arteriosus p.
    ductus venosus p.
    graft p.
    long-term p.

modified Blalock-Taussig shunt p.
nidus p.
p. rate
short-term p.
shunt p.
p. trifurcation
p. and valvular reflux of deep
  vein
vascular p.
vein p.
p. of vein graft
p. of vessel

patent

p. bifurcation
p. ductus arteriosus (PDA)
p. foramen ovale (PFO)
p. lumen
p. stent
p. urachus
p. vessel
widely p.

Paterson-Parker system

path

p. length
mean free p.
puncture p.
water p.

pathognomonic

p. finding
p. imaging characteristic

pathologic, pathological

p. correlation
p. dislocation
p. fracture
p. intracranial calcification
p. marrow infiltration

pathology (PA)

acute aortic p.
mesenteric lymph node p.
radiographic p.

pathophysiologic change

pathway

amygdalofugal p.
anomalous p.
antegrade fast p.
anterior internodal p.
atrio-His p.
cerebellar p.
cerebropontocerebellar p.
cerebrospinal fluid p.
corticospinal motor p.
dentatoolivary p.

dual atrioventricular node p.
Embden-Meyerhof glycolytic p.
hepatobiliary p.
interhemispheric p.
neural p.
nodoventricular p.
optic glioma p.
reticulocortical p.
retrovestibular neural p.
septal accessory p.
striatal output p.
synaptic p.
Thorel p.

patient

p. motion
p. motion artifact
p. volume

pattern

abnormal lung p.
acinar p.
activation p.
airway p.
alveolar p.
anhaustral colonic gas p.
anular tear p.
arborization p.
architectural p.
arterial deficiency p.
atypical vessel colposcopic p.
ballerina-foot p.
basket-weave p.
beam p.
benign-appearing p.
bigeminal p.
blood flow p.
bony trabecular p.
bowel gas p.
branching p.
broken bough p.
bronchiectatic p.
bronchopneumonia p.
bronchovascular p.
bubbly p.
butterfly p.
cavitating p.
centrum semiovale p.
cerebral cortical gyral p.
circadian p.
coarse p.
cobblestone p.
cobweb p.
coiled spring p.

NOTES

P

pattern *(continued)*

collimator plugging p.
colonic urticaria p.
comedo p.
concertina p.
contractile p.
contrast enhancement p.
convolutional p.
corduroy cloth p.
corkscrew p.
crazy paving p.
cribriform p.
cross-sectional p.
cystic p.
degenerative nuclear p.
p. of destruction
diffraction p.
diffuse contrast agent
  distribution p.
dissemination p.
divergent spiculated p.
dot-and-dash p.
3D physiologic flow p.
ductal p.
early repolarization p.
echo p.
echo-dense p.
echolucent p.
edema p.
enhancement p.
esophageal achalasia p.
extended p.
feathery p.
fern-like p.
fibrotic cavitating p.
fibrous nodular p.
filigree p.
fine peripheral reticular p.
fine reticular p.
finger-in-glove p.
fingerprint p.
fleur-de-lis p.
flip-flop p.
focal p.
fold p.
folial p.
follicular p.
four-quadrant bar p.
fragmented p.
gas p.
gastric mucosal p.
geographic p.
ground-glass p.
gyriform p.
hairbrush p.
hanging-fruit p.
haustral p.

helical p.
hemodynamic p.
hepatic echo p.
herringbone p.
heterogeneous internal echo p.
heterogeneous perfusion p.
hierarchical scanning p.
hole p.
homogeneous echo p.
homogeneous MR p.
honeycomb p.
hourglass p.
infiltration p.
inhomogeneous echo p.
interstitial lung p.
interstitial tear p.
intestinal gas p.
intraaneurysmal inflow p.
intraaneurysmal outflow p.
inverse follicle p.
juvenile T-wave p.
kidney mass growth p.
lace-like trabecular p.
ladder-like p.
Laue p.
left ventricular contraction p.
left ventricular strain p.
linear interstitial disease p.
liver spoked-wheel p.
lobular alveolar p.
locomotor p.
lymphatic drainage p.
lytic p.
M p.
macronodular p.
magnetic resonance enhancement p.
manometric p.
marrow edema p.
micronodular p.
migrational p.
miliary p.
mimosa p.
mixed lytic and sclerotic p.
moiré p.
mosaic attenuation p.
mosaic duodenal mucosal p.
moth-eaten p.
mottled p.
movement p.
M-shaped mitral valve p.
mucosal fold p.
muscle recruitment p.
nonspecific bowel gas p.
orthogonal-hole test p. (OHP)
ovarian fishnet weave p.
overlying branching p.
parallel and spiral flow p.

parenchymal breast p.
parrot-beak p.
permeative p.
phlebographic p.
pin p.
PLES bar p.
pneumoencephalographic p.
postembolization angiographic p.
P pulmonale p.
proliferative p.
prominent ductal p.
pseudohomogeneous edema p.
pseudoinfarct p.
pseudomantle zone p.
pulmonary flow p.
pulmonary vascular p.
pulsation p.
QR p.
quantum mottling p.
railroad track p.
ray p.
recurrence p.
relief p.
restrictive p.
reticular interstitial disease p.
reticular lung p.
reticulogranular p.
reticulonodular p.
reverberating flow p.
rheologic p.
right ventricular strain p.
ring-like p.
rosary bead p.
rugal p.
salt-and-pepper chromatin p.
sawtooth excretory p.
sclerotic p.
segmental alveolar p.
seizure p.
sheet-like growth p.
shish kabob p.
sigmoid hair p.
signet ring p.
sinus p.
slice-of-sausage breast p.
small bowel mucosal p.
snowflake p.
snowstorm breast p.
solid p.
speckled p.
SPECT perfusion p.
spectral p.

spiral flow p.
spoiler gradient p.
spoked wheel p.
p. of spread
star p.
star test p.
start test p.
stellate p.
storiform p.
storiform-pleomorphic p.
strain p.
sulcal p.
sunburst gyral p.
surface convexity p.
Tabar p.
tagging p.
task-rest p.
temporal sawtooth p.
thermal convection p.
tigroid p.
trabecular p.
tram-track p.
transducer beam p.
tree-in-bud p.
trigeminal p.
tubular gas p.
typical cobblestone p.
V p.
variegated p.
ventricular contraction p.
vesicular p.
white branching linear p.
Wolfe DY, NI, P1, P2 p.
Wolfe mammographic
  parenchymal p.
zebra-striped p.

patulous
  p. cardia
  p. esophagogastric region
  p. hiatus
pauciarticular
paucilocular
  p. cystic mass
  p. tumor
pauciostotic
paucity
  alveolar p.
  p. of bowel gas
Pauli exclusion principle
Pauly point
pause
  asystolic p.

NOTES

P

pause *(continued)*
    compensatory p.
    postextrasystolic p.
    sinus p.
Pauwel
    P. angle
    P. femoral neck fracture
      classification
paving-stone degeneration
PAVM
    pulmonary arteriovenous malformation
Pawlik
    P. triangle
    P. trigone
Pawlow
    P. position
    P. projection
PAWP
    pulmonary artery wedge pressure
Payr sign
Pb
    lead
PBD
    percutaneous biliary drainage
PBF
    pulmonary blood flow
PBI
    protein-bound iodine
PBPI
    penile-brachial pressure index
PBVI
    pulmonary blood volume index
PC
    phase contrast
    posterior commissure
      PC MR angiography
PCA
    posterior cerebral artery
    posterior communicating artery
PCAVC
PCC
    peripheral cholangiocarcinoma
PCD
    percutaneous catheter drainage
    posterior capsular distance
pCi
    picocurie
PCIS
    postcardiac injury syndrome
PCL
    posterior cruciate ligament
    pubococcygeal line
PCLBCL
    primary cutaneous large B-cell
      lymphoma

PCNL
    percutaneous nephrolithotomy
    percutaneous nephrostolithotomy
PCoA
    posterior communicating artery
PCOD
    polycystic ovarian disease
PCOS
    polycystic ovary syndrome
PCP
    pulmonary capillary pressure
PCRA
    percutaneous coronary rotational
      atherectomy
PCS
    proximal coronary
PCWP
    pulmonary capillary wedge pressure
Pd
    palladium
^{103}Pd, Pd-103
    palladium-103
      ^{103}Pd isotope
      ^{103}Pd prostatic implant
      ^{103}Pd radioactive material
PDA
    patent ductus arteriosus
    poorly differentiated adenocarcinoma
    posterior descending artery
PDD
    percentage depth dose
    progressive diaphyseal dysplasia
pDEXA
    peripheral dual energy x-ray
      pDEXA x-ray peripheral bone
        densitometer
PDI
    power Doppler imaging
PDR
    pulsed dose rate
PDS
    power Doppler sonography
PDT
    photodynamic therapy
PE
    pericardial effusion
    phase encoding
    photographic effect
    polyethylene
    pulmonary edema
    pulmonary embolus
      PE catheter
Peacock system
peak
    p. airway pressure
    p. amplitude
    p. aortic flow velocity

p. area
backscatter p.
Bragg ionization p.
carotid pulse p.
p. count density
p. diastolic gradient
diffraction p.
p. dP/dt
p. early diastolic filling velocity
early systolic p.
p. expiratory flow (PEF)
p. filling
p. filling rate (PFR)
p. fitting
p. flow variability
p. flush flow
frequency-related p.
p. identification
p. inflation pressure
p. instantaneous gradient
juxtaphrenic p.
kilovolt p. (kVp)
p. late diastolic filling velocity
main glow p.
p. of maximum enhancement
   (PME)
p. parenchymal activity
photon p.
pressure p.
p. pressure gradient
p. profile
p. pulmonary flow velocity
recirculation p.
p. regurgitant flow velocity
p. regurgitant wave pressure
p. right ventricular-right atrial
   systolic gradient
p. scatter factor
p. shape
single p.
spread Bragg p.
p. systolic aortic pressure
p. systolic and diastolic ratio
p. systolic gradient
p. systolic velocity
temporal p. (TP)
time-to-p.
p. transmitted velocity
p. velocity of blood flow
peak-to-peak pressure gradient
pearl
   keratin p.

p. necklace gallbladder
scrotal p.
pearl-like breast calcification
pearly
   p. body
   p. CNS tumor
   p. neoplasm
   p. white ovary
pear-shaped
   p.-s. defect
   p.-s. heart
   p.-s. urinary bladder
   p.-s. uterus
Pearson
   P. attachment
   P. correlation coefficient
   P. method
   P. position
   P. syndrome
pea-size
pebble-shaped patella
Pecquet
   cistern of P.
pecten pubis
pectinate
   p. ligament
   p. line
pectineal
pectineus muscle
pectoral
   p. girdle
   p. heart
   p. lymph node
   p. ridge
pectoralis
   p. major muscle
   p. major syndrome
   p. minor muscle
pectus
   p. carinatum deformity
   p. excavatum
   p. excavatum deformity
   p. recurvatum
pedal
   p. artery opacification
   p. bone
   p. lymphangiography
pedes (*pl. of* pes)
pediatric
   p. biplane TEE probe
   p. bronchiolitis
   p. fibroxanthoma

NOTES

P

pediatric (*continued*)
   p. hemangioma
   P. IngestaScan metal detector
   p. neuroradiology
   p. nuclear medicine imaging
   p. primary brain tumor
   p. radiology
   p. scintigraphy
   p. solid tumor
pedicle
   p. bone graft
   p. erosion
   p. finger
   p. flap
   p. fracture
   musculofascial p.
   p.'s and pars
   phrenic p.
   p. plate
   pulmonary p.
   p. sclerosis
   p. signal intensity
   spinal p.
   splaying of p.'s
   vascular p.
   p. of vertebra
pedicolaminar fracture-dislocation
pedis
   malum perforans p.
   calcar p.
   digitus p.
   dorsalis p.
   dorsum p.
   pollex p.
pedobarography
   dynamic p.
PEDRI
  proton-electron double-resonance
  imaging
peduncle
   cerebellar p.
   cerebral p.
   inferior cerebellar p.
peduncular
   p. loop
   p. segment of superior cerebellar
   artery
pedunculated
   p. leiomyoma
   p. lesion
   p. polyp
   p. subserous myoma
   p. thrombus
   p. uterine fibroid
   p. uterine myxoma
   p. vesical tumor
pedunculation

peel
   pleura p.
peel-away sheath
PEF
   parietal eye field
   peak expiratory flow
PEG
   percutaneous endoscopic gastrostomy
   pneumoencephalogram
   pneumoencephalography
   polyethylene glycol
peg
   cerebellar p.
   rete p.
Pegasus PIV laser
Pegasys workstation
peizoelectric
PELA
   peripheral excimer laser angioplasty
peliosis
   spleen p.
Pelizaeus-Merzbacher disease
Pellegrini-Stieda
   P.-S. calcification
   P.-S. disease
pellet
   alanine-silicone p.
   p. artifact
   radiopaque p.
pellucidum
   cavum septum p.
   septum p.
pelves (*pl. of* pelvis)
pelvic
   p. abscess
   p. aneurysm
   p. arteriography
   p. artery
   p. bone
   p. brim
   p. canal
   p. chocolate cyst
   p. collateral vessel
   p. colon
   p. congestion syndrome
   p. cystic mass
   p. diameter
   p. diaphragm
   p. exenteration
   p. exostosis
   p. fascia
   p. femoral angle
   p. fibrolipomatosis
   p. film for IUD localization
   p. floor
   p. fluid
   p. fracture frame

p. girdle
p. infection
p. inflammatory disease
p. inlet
p. insufficiency fracture
p. lipomatosis
p. lymph node
p. malignancy
p. mass complex
p. mass frequency
p. morphometry
p. notching
p. obliquity
p. outlet
p. peritoneal surface
p. peritoneum
p. phased-array coil
p. plane
p. plexus
p. rim fracture
p. ring
p. ring fracture
p. ring ligament
p. sidewall
p. sonography
p. space
p. spot
p. steal
p. steal test
p. straddle fracture
p. ultrasound
p. ultrasound CT scan
p. unleveling
p. vascular trauma
p. vein thrombosis
p. venous obstruction
p. venous stenosis
p. view
p. viscus
p. wall
pelvicaliceal
p. change
p. dilatation
p. distention
pelvicaliectasis
pelvicephalography
pelvicephalometry
pelviectasis
pelvimetry
magnetic resonance p.
radiographic p.
pelviography

pelvioradiography
pelvioscopy
pelviradiography
pelviroentgenography
pelvis, pl. **pelves**
aditus p.
android p.
anthropoid p.
assimilation p.
beaked p.
bifid p.
bony p.
brachypellic p.
brim of the p.
champagne glass p.
contracted p.
cordate p.
cordiform p.
Deventer p.
diameter obliqua p.
diameter transversa p.
dolichopellic p.
dwarf p.
elephant ears p.
extrarenal renal p.
false p.
female p.
flat p.
frozen p.
funnel-shaped p.
goblet-shaped p.
greater p.
gynecoid p.
hardened p.
heart-shaped p.
intrarenal p.
inverted p.
juvenile p.
p. of kidney
Kilian p.
kyphoscoliotic p.
kyphotic p.
lesser p.
longitudinal oval p.
lordotic p.
male p.
masculine p.
mesatipellic p.
Mickey Mouse ears p.
Nägele p.
osteomalacic p.
Otto p.

NOTES

P

pelvis *(continued)*
    Otto-Krobak p.
    platypelloid p.
    postmenarchal female p.
    pseudoosteomalacic p.
    rachitic p.
    renal p.
    reniform p.
    Rokitansky p.
    scoliotic p.
    small p.
    spider p.
    spondylolisthetic p.
    tombstone p.
    transverse oval p.
    trident p.
    true p.
    wine glass p.
pelviureteric junction (PUJ)
pelviureterography
pelvocaliceal
    p. effacement
    p. system
pelvocephalography
PEM
    positron emission mammography
Pena Shokeir syndrome
pencil
    p. dosimeter
    p. electron beam
pencil-beam
    p.-b. approach
    p.-b. navigator echo
pencil-in-cup deformity
penciling
    p. deformity
    p. of the distal clavicle
    p. of rib
    p. of terminal tuft
pencil-like deformity
pencil-point metatarsal deformity
pendent positioning
pendetide
    [111]In satumomab p.
Pendred syndrome
pendulous
    p. heart
    p. pouch
    p. reference axis (PRA)
    p. urethra
pendulum
    cor p.
    p. movement
penes (*pl. of* penis)
penetrability
penetrating
    p. aortic ulcer

    p. atherosclerotic ulcer
    p. fracture
    p. lung injury
    p. trauma
    p. TRD
    p. wound
penetration
    acoustic p.
    bowel wall p.
    p. fraction
    insufficient acoustic p.
    lack of acoustic p.
    radiographic p.
    rectal p.
penetrometer
    Benoist p.
penile
    p. artery
    p. fibromatosis
    p. implant
    p. plaque
    p. raphe
    p. sonography
    p. squamous papilloma
    p. urethra
    p. vein
    p. vessel
penile-brachial pressure index (PBPI)
penis, pl. **penes**
    bulb of p.
    bulbospongiosus muscle of p.
    clubbed p.
    concealed p.
    corpora cavernosa p.
    corpus spongiosum p.
    crus of p.
    deep fascia of p.
    dorsal artery of p.
    dorsal nerve of p.
    dorsum of p.
    double p.
    glans p.
    hypoplastic p.
    ischiospongiosus muscle of p.
    p. lacuna
    root of p.
    suspensory ligament of p.
    webbed p.
peniscopy
penoscrotal
PenRad mammography clinical reporting system
pentacene
pentagastrin imaging agent
pentalogy
    p. of Cantrell
    p. of Fallot

pentavalent DMSA imaging agent
Pentax ELLB 6000, 6500 ultrasound
   gastroscope
Pentax-Hitachi FG32UA endosonographic
   system
pentetate
   ^{111}In imciromab p.
pentetic acid imaging agent
pentetide
   satumomab p.
pentetreotide
   p. imaging agent
   ^{111}In p.
   p. tumor localization scan
pentose cycle
penultimate section
penumbra, pl. **penumbrae**
   dosimetric p.
   hemodynamic p.
   ischemic p.
   p. zone
PEP
   preejection period
Pepper
   P. syndrome
   P. tumor
peppermint oil imaging agent
pepper-pot pitting
peptic
   p. esophagitis
   p. stricture
   p. ulcer
   p. ulcer disease (PUD)
peptide imaging agent
percentage
   p. classification
   p. depth dose (PDD)
   p. signal intensity loss
Perception scanner
perceptual linearization
perched facet joint
Percheron
   artery of P.
perchlorate
   potassium p.
   p. washout test
Perclose
   P. arterial closure device
   P. PVS suture system
percreta
   placenta p.
PercuCut cut-biopsy needle

Percuflex stent
percussion sensitivity
percutaneous
   p. abscess drainage
   p. antegrade biliary drainage
   p. antegrade pyelography
   p. antegrade urography
   p. arterial closure device
   p. atherectomy
   p. automated diskectomy
   p. biliary drainage (PBD)
   p. catheter drainage (PCD)
   p. cavity drainage catheter
   p. cecostomy
   p. cholecystotomy catheter
   p. choledochoscopy
   p. coronary rotational atherectomy
   (PCRA)
   p. dilatation of biliary duct
   p. dissolution of thrombus
   p. electrical nerve stimulation
   p. embolectomy
   p. embolotherapy
   p. endofluoroscopy
   p. endoluminal placement
   p. endometrial drug delivery
   p. endopyelotomy
   p. endoscopic gastrostomy (PEG)
   p. endoscopy
   p. ethanol injection
   p. ethanol injection therapy
   p. ethanol instillation
   p. ethanol sclerotherapy
   p. femoral arteriography
   p. gastroenterostomy
   p. hepatobiliary cholangiography
   p. interventional radiology
   p. intraaortic balloon
   p. intracoronary angioscopy imaging
   p. microwave coagulation therapy
   p. nephrolithotomy (PCNL)
   p. nephroscope
   p. nephrostolithotomy (PCNL)
   p. nephrostomy
   p. pancreatography
   p. pericardioscopy
   p. peritoneovenous shunt creation
   p. pin insertion
   p. radiofrequency catheter ablation
   p. retrograde transfemoral technique
   p. splenoportography
   p. stent

NOTES

P

percutaneous *(continued)*
    p. thermal occlusion
    p. transcatheter therapy
    p. transhepatic biliary drainage
      (PTBD)
    p. transhepatic cholangial drainage
      (PTCD)
    p. transhepatic cholangiogram (PTC,
      PTCA, PTHC)
    p. transhepatic cholangiography
      (PTHC)
    p. transhepatic cholecystostomy
    p. transhepatic decompression
    p. transhepatic endoluminal biliary
      biopsy
    p. transhepatic liver biopsy
    p. transhepatic portography
    p. transluminal angioplasty (PTA)
    p. transluminal balloon dilatation
    p. transluminal coronary angioplasty
      (PTCA)
    p. transluminal coronary
      recanalization technique
    p. transluminal renal angioplasty
      (PTRA)
    p. transperineal seed implantation
    p. transtracheal bronchography
    p. tube insertion
    p. tumor treatment
    p. ultrasound-guided thrombin
      injection
    p. vascular surgical device
    p. vertebroplasty
    7 (x) 40 mm p. transluminal
      angioplasty balloon
percutaneously cannulated
Perez sign
Perflex stainless steel balloon-expandable
  stent
perflubron
    p. imaging agent
    partial liquid ventilation with p.
perfluorocarbon-exposed sonicated
  dextrose albumin (PESDA)
perfluorocarbon imaging agent
perfluorochemical
perfluorooctyl bromide (PFOB)
perflutren lipid microsphere injectable
  suspension
perforans
perforated
    p. aortic cusp
    p. cholecystitis
    p. diverticulum
    p. gangrenous appendix
    p. hollow viscus
    p. ulcer

perforating
    p. aneurysm
    p. artery
    p. branch
    p. colorectal carcinoma
    p. fracture
    p. vein
    p. wound
perforation
    bladder p.
    bowel p.
    cardiac p.
    colonic p.
    common bile duct spontaneous p.
    duodenal ulcer p.
    esophageal p.
    gallbladder p.
    iatrogenic esophageal p.
    idiopathic gastric p.
    intestinal p.
    Niemeier gallbladder p.
    renal transplant GI tract p.
    septal p.
    spontaneous p.
    transseptal p.
    ulcer p.
    ureteral p.
    vascular p.
    ventricular p.
perforative lesion
perforator
    incompetent p.
    septal p.
    p. vessel
Performa mammography system
perfusate vessel
perfused
    p. myocardium
    p. twin
perfusion
    p. abnormality
    adequate coronary p.
    p. agent
    antegrade p.
    blood p.
    brain p.
    capillary p.
    continuous hyperthermic
      peritoneal p.
    p. CT
    decreased distal p.
    diminished airway p.
    diminished systemic p.
    first-pass cardiac p.
    gated stress myocardial p. (GMP)
    p. gradient
    homogeneous p.

hypothermic p.
impaired renal p.
increment of p.
p. index
intraperitoneal hyperthermic p. (IPHP)
isolation p.
limb p.
lung p.
p. lung scan
luxury p.
maldistribution of ventilation and p.
p. measurement technique
misery p.
mosaic p.
p. MR imaging
myocardial p.
peripheral p.
poor p.
p. pressure
pulsatile p.
quantitative cardiac p.
regional cerebral p.
regional pulmonary p.
regional vascular p.
renal p.
resting p.
retrograde cardiac p.
p. scintigraphy
p. study
p. time
tissue p.
unilateral lung p.
p. and ventilation lung imaging
perfusion-metabolism mismatch
perfusion-weighted
p.-w. imaging (PWI)
p.-w. MRI
perialveolar fibrosis
periampullary
p. carcinoma
p. diverticulum
p. duodenal tumor
perianal
p. abscess
p. hematoma
periaortic
p. area
p. fibrosis
p. lymph node
p. mediastinal hematoma

periaortitis
chronic p.
periapical
p. cemental dysplasia
p. granuloma
p. lesion
p. radiograph
periappendiceal
p. abscess
p. structure
periaqueductal
p. gray matter
p. hemorrhage
periareolar fistula
periarteriolar lymphoid sheath
periarteritis nodosa
periarticular
p. calcification
p. fluid collection
p. fracture
p. heterotopic ossification (PHO)
p. margin
p. osteoporosis
p. tissue
periauricular region
peribiliary cyst
peribronchial
p. alveolar space
p. connective tissue
p. cuffing
p. distribution
p. fibrosis
p. hemorrhage
p. infiltrate
p. lymph node
p. marking
p. thickening
peribronchovascular interstitial compartment
peribursal fat
pericaliceal cyst
pericallosal
p. artery
p. lipoma
p. vein
p. vessel
pericapsular fat infiltrate
pericardia (*pl. of* pericardium)
pericardiacophrenic vein
pericardiac pleura
pericardial
p. aorta

NOTES

P

pericardial *(continued)*
  p. calcification
  p. cavity
  p. chyle with tamponade
  p. defect
  p. diaphragmatic adhesion
  p. disease
  p. duplication cyst
  p. effusion (PE)
  p. empyema
  p. fat pad
  p. flap
  p. fluid
  p. fold
  p. halo
  p. hematoma
  p. infusion
  p. knock sound
  p. lymph node
  p. reserve volume
  p. sac
  p. silhouette
  p. sinus
  p. space
  p. vein
  p. window
pericardiectomy
pericardioperitoneal canal
pericardioscopy
  percutaneous p.
pericarditis
  bread-and-butter p.
  constrictive p.
  diffuse p.
  hemorrhagic p.
  postmeningococcal p.
  radiation-induced p.
pericardium, pl. **pericardia**
  adherent p.
  autologous p.
  p. calcareous deposit
  calcified p.
  congenitally absent p.
  crus p.
  diaphragmatic p.
  p. fibrosum
  fibrous p.
  inelastic p.
  parietal p.
  rheumatic adherent p.
  roughened state of p.
  serous p.
  shaggy p.
  soldier's patches of p.
  visceral p.
pericarinal injury
pericatheter thrombus

pericaval
pericavernous
pericecal abscess
pericentral fibrosis
pericerebral fluid
pericholecystic
  p. abscess
  p. edema
  p. fluid
  p. fluid collection
pericholedochal
  p. node
  p. varix
perichondral
  p. bone
  p. cell seeding
  p. ring
perichondrium
pericicatricial emphysema
pericolic abscess
pericolonic
  p. abscess
  p. fat
  p. fluid
pericranii
  sinus p.
pericyst
pericystic edema
peridental space
peridiaphragmatic hematoma
peridiploid
peridiverticulitis
periductal
  p. calcification
  p. fibrosis
peridural fibrosis
periesophageal fluid
perifascial fluid-like collection
perifocal emphysema
perigastric
  p. deformity
  p. fat
perigestational hemorrhage
perigraft
  p. fluid
  p. hematoma
  p. seroma
perihepatic
  p. abscess
  p. space
perihepatitis
perihilar
  p. area
  p. batwing infiltrate
  p. density
  p. edema
  p. fat

p. fibrosis
p. lung disease
p. marking
p. region
periileal
periinfarction
p. block
p. ischemia
perilabral sulcus
perilesional white matter
perilobular
p. connective tissue
p. duct
perilunar
p. dislocation
p. instability
perilunate
p. dislocation
p. fracture-dislocation
p. instability
perimedial
p. dysplasia
p. fibroplasia
p. renal fibroplasia artery
perimedullary
perimembranous ventricular septal defect
perimeniscal capsular plexus
perimesencephalic
p. cistern
p. nonaneurysmal subarachnoid hemorrhage
perimeter-area ratio (P/A)
perimetry testing
perimuscular
p. fibrosis
p. plexus
perimylolysis
perinatal
p. anoxia
p. asphyxia
p. injury
perinea (*pl. of* perineum)
perineal
p. descent
p. fascia
p. sinus
p. space
perineogram imaging
perineoplastic edema
perineovaginal fistula

perinephric
p. abscess
p. air injection
p. fat
p. fluid collection
p. hematoma
p. space
p. space hemorrhage
perinephritic abscess
perineum, pl. **perinea**
perineural
p. arachnoid cyst
p. fat
p. fibroblastoma
p. fibroblastoma tumor
p. fibrosis
p. glial proliferation
p. invasion
p. sacral cyst
p. tumor spread
perinuclear halo
period
antegrade refractory p.
diastasis heart p.
diastolic filling p.
effective refractory p. (ERP)
embryonic p.
fetal p.
functional refractory p. (FRP)
immediate postictal p.
isoelectric p.
isovolumetric p.
phase-encoding p.
postbiopsy p.
preejection p. (PEP)
radiofrequency p.
rapid filling p.
raster p.
reduced ventricular filling p.
relative refractory p. (RRP)
retrograde refractory p.
systolic ejection p. (SEP)
total atrial refractory p. (TARP)
ventricular effective refractory p. (VERP)
window p.
periodicity
circadian p.
periodic synchronous discharge (PSD)
periodontal
p. disease
p. ligament

NOTES

P

689

perioptic meningioma
periorbital
    p. bidirectional Doppler
    p. directional Doppler
      ultrasonography
    p. edema
periosseous soft tissue mass
periosteal
    p. artery
    p. bone
    p. bone collar
    p. creep
    p. desmoid
    p. dysplasia
    p. elevation
    p. fibroma
    p. fibrosarcoma
    p. ganglion
    p. new bone formation
    p. osteosarcoma
    p. reaction
    p. resorption
    p. sarcoma
periosteum, pl. periostea
    p. of rib
periostitis
    florid reactive p.
    medial malleolus p.
periotic bone
peripancreatic
    p. artery
    p. fluid collection
    p. lymphadenopathy
peripartum dilated cardiomyopathy
peripelvic
    p. collateral vessel
    p. cyst
    p. fat proliferation
    p. lipomatosis
peripheral
    p. airspace disease
    p. arterial disease
    p. arterial occlusive disease
    (PAOD)
    p. arteriography
    p. arteriosclerosis
    p. blood
    p. blood flow
    p. bolus chase
    p. border
    p. cholangiocarcinoma (PCC)
    p. chondrosarcoma
    p. circulation
    p. circulatory vasoconstriction
    p. consolidation
    p. cutaneous vasoconstriction
    p. directional atherectomy

    p. dual energy x-ray (pDEXA)
    p. embolus
    p. excimer laser angioplasty
    (PELA)
    p. expansion
    p. fracture
    p. hematopoietic intermediate signal
      intensity marrow
    p. hypoperfusion
    p. infiltrate
    p. intravenous infusion line
    p. laser angioplasty
    p. lesion enhancement
    p. loading
    p. lung disease
    p. lymphoma
    p. meniscocapsular tear
    p. MR angiography
    p. necrosis
    p. nerve
    p. nerve decompression
    p. nerve injury
    p. nerve lesion
    p. nervous system
    p. neuroectodermal tumor
    p. neurofibromatosis
    p. nodule
    p. ossification
    p. ossifying fibroma
    p. parenchymal atelectasis
    p. perfusion
    p. perimeniscal capillary ingrowth
    p. pneumonia
    p. pseudoaneurysm
    p. puddling
    p. pulmonary artery stenosis
    (PPAS)
    p. pulse gating
    p. quantitative computed
      tomography (pQCT)
    p. runoff
    p. skeleton
    p. small airway study
    p. synovitis
    p. vascular disease (PVD)
    p. vascular imaging
    p. vascular occlusive disease
    p. vascular resistance (PVR)
    p. vasculature
    p. vasogenic edema
    p. venography
    p. vessel
peripherally
    p. inserted central catheter (PICC)
    p. inserted central catheter line
periphery
    p. of the anulus

echogenic p.
lung p.

periportal
p. area
p. cirrhosis
p. collar
p. fibrosis
p. sinusoidal dilatation
p. tracking
p. tracking of blood

periprosthetic
p. bone resorption
p. fracture
p. leak
p. osteolysis

periradicular
p. nerve
p. sheath

perirectal
p. abscess
p. fat

perirenal
p. abscess
p. air study
p. bleeding
p. compartment
p. fat
p. hematoma
p. hemorrhage
p. insufflation
p. lymphoma
p. mass
p. septum
p. space

perirolandic parietal cortex
perisellar vascular lesion
perisigmoid colon
perisinusoidal space
perisplenic node
peristalsis
abnormal esophageal p.
absence of primary p.
absent p.
accelerated p.
anterograde p.
bowel p.
decreased p.
esophageal p.
hyperactive p.
increased p.
meconium p.
primary esophageal p.

retrograde p.
reversed p.
secondary p.
small bowel p.
ureteral seesaw p.
visible p.
yo-yo esophageal p.
yo-yo ureteral p.

peristaltic
p. activity
p. contraction
p. rush
p. sequence
p. wave

peristriate cortex
perisylvian cortex
peritendinitis
peritendinous
p. adhesion
p. calcification

perithyroid vein
peritoneal
p. abscess
p. attachment
p. band
p. carcinomatosis
p. cavity
p. cavity fluid
p. dialysis catheter
p. effusion
p. enhancement
p. fold
p. gutter
p. hernia
p. inclusion cyst
p. lymphopneumatosis
p. mass
p. mesothelioma
p. metastasis
p. metastatic implant
p. mouse
p. part of inguinal ligament
p. recess
p. sac
p. scintigraphy
p. seeding
p. shunting
p. sign
p. space

peritoneal-venous shunt patency test
peritonei
carcinomatosis p.

NOTES

P

peritonei *(continued)*
  gliomatosis p.
  pseudomyxoma p.
peritoneocele
peritoneogram imaging
peritoneography
  CT, MR p.
peritoneopericardial diaphragmatic
  hernia
peritoneopleural communication
peritoneoscintigraphy
peritoneovenous shunt (PVS)
peritoneum
  p. desmoid tumor
  parietal p.
  pelvic p.
  visceral p.
peritonitis
  chemical p.
  meconium p.
  tuberculous p.
peritrigonal white matter
peritrochanteric fracture
peritubular
  p. vascular bed
peritumoral
  p. cyst
  p. edema
  p. tissue
periumbilical
  p. pain
  p. swelling
periungual fibroma
periureteral fibrosis
periurethral gland
perivalvular
  p. leak
  p. pseudoaneurysm
perivascular
  p. cloaking
  p. cuffing
  p. distribution
  p. edema
  p. fibrosis
  p. infiltrate
  p. mass
  p. pseudorosette
  p. space
periventricular
  p. bright signal
  p. calcification
  p. echogenicity (PVE)
  p. gray (PVG)
  p. gray matter
  p. halo
  p. hemorrhagic infarct
  p. hypodensity

  p. lesion
  p. leukoencephalopathy
  p. leukomalacia (PVL)
  p. plaque
  p. white matter
perivenular fibrosis
perivesical
Perkin line
permanent
  p. brachytherapy
  p. callus
  p. interstitial implant
  p. magnet
  p. stoma
PermCath
  Quinton P.
permeability
  capillary p.
  p. constant
  constant p.
  Crone-Renkin index of p.
  magnetic p.
  membrane p.
  pulmonary capillary p.
  p. pulmonary edema
  tumor capillary p.
permeation
permeative
  p. bone destruction
  p. lesion
  p. pattern
permutation
pernio lupus
peroneal
  p. artery
  p. bone
  p. brevis tendon
  p. longus tendon
  p. muscle
  p. nerve
  p. retinaculum
  p. sign
  p. tendon injury
  p. tendon subluxation
  p. tenosynovitis
  p. thrombus
  p.-to-anterior compartment ratio
  p. trochlea
  p. tubercle
  p. vein
  p. vessel
peroneum
  os p.
peroneus
  p. brevis tendon
  p. longus
  p. longus muscle avulsion

p. longus tendon
p. quartus muscle
p. tertius tendon
peroral
    p. cone radiation therapy
    p. implantation
    p. retrograde pancreaticobiliary
     ductography
perosteal cloaking
peroxidase
    tracer horseradish p.
peroxyl
perpendicular mean translation
perpendiculars
    method of p.
Persantine
    P. imaging agent
    P. thallium imaging
persistent
    p. bronchopleural fistula
    p. common atrioventricular canal
    p. cortical kidney lobation
    p. ductus arteriosus
    p. fetal circulation
    p. generalized lymphadenopathy
    p. hyperparathyroidism
    p. increasing nephrogram
    p. left inferior vena cava
    p. left superior vena cava
    p. metopic suture
    p. ossiculum terminale
    p. ostium atrioventriculare commune
    p. primitive trigeminal artery
    p. pulmonary hypertension
    p. pylorospasm
    p. renal lobation
    p. sciatic artery
    p. splenomegaly
    p. truncus arteriosus (PTA)
personal ionization chamber
perspective volume rendering (PVR)
Pertechnegas
pertechnetate
    p. scintigraphy
    sodium p.
Perthes
    P. disease
    P. epiphysis
    P. lesion
Perthes-Bankart lesion
pertrochanteric fracture

perturbation
    cytoskeletal p.
    magnetic field p.
    radiation dose p.
perturbing magnetic field
pertussoid eosinophilic pneumonia
perversus
    situs p.
pes, pl. **pedes**
    p. abductus
    p. adductus
    p. anserine bursa
    p. anserinus
    p. anserinus bursitis
    p. arcuatus
    p. arcuatus clawfoot deformity
    p. calcaneocavus
    p. calcaneovalgus
    p. calcaneus
    p. calvaneovalgus
    p. cavovalgus
    p. cavovarus
    p. cavus
    p. cavus clawfoot deformity
    p. equinovalgus
    p. equinovarus
    p. equinus
    p. malleus valgus
    p. planovalgus
    p. planovalgus deformity
    p. plantigrade planus
    p. planus deformity
    p. pronation
    p. pronatus
    p. varus
PESDA
    perfluorocarbon-exposed sonicated
    dextrose albumin
PET
    positron emission tomography
    PET balloon
    cardiac PET
    PET compound
    PET full-ring scanner
    PET lung imaging
    PET measurement of dopamine
     receptor availability
    PET metabolic imaging
    PET myocardial fatty acid imaging
    PET perfusion metabolism imaging
    PET radioligand
    PET radiopharmaceutical

NOTES

P

PET *(continued)*
  PET scan
  PET target material
  tyrphostin radiotracer for PET
petal-fugal flow
PET/CT scanner
petiole
petit
  P. ligament
  p. mal seizure
  P. sinus
PETite scanner
Pétrequin ligament
petrobasilar suture
petroclinoid ligament
petromastoid
petrosal
  p. bone
  p. cerebellum
  p. foramen
  p. ganglion
  greater p.
  lesser p.
  p. nerve
  p. sinus
  p. vein
petrositis
  apical p.
petrosphenobasilar suture
petrosphenoid
petrosphenooccipital
  p. suture
  p. suture of Gruber
petrosquamosal suture
petrosquamous suture
petrous
  p. apex
  p. apex dumbbell mass
  p. carotid canal
  p. carotid canal stenosis
  p. ICA
  p. pyramid
  p. pyramid scalloping
  p. ridge
  p. segment of internal carotid
  artery
  p. temporal bone
  p. tip
PETT
  positron emission transaxial tomography
  positron emission transverse tomography
  PETT imaging
  PETT VI PET scanner
Peutz-Jeghers
  P.-J. gastrointestinal polyposis
  P.-J. polyp
  P.-J. syndrome

Peyer patch
Peyronie disease
PFA
  platelet function analyzer
PFA-100 system
Pfaundler-Hurler disease
Pfeiffer
  P. acrocephalosyndactyly
  P. disease
  P. syndrome
Pfeiffer-Comberg method
PFFD
  proximal focal femoral deficiency
Pfizer
  P. 200 FS, 400 scanner
PFO
  patent foramen ovale
PFOB
  perfluorooctyl bromide
Pfoundler-Hurler syndrome
PFR
  peak filling rate
PGSE
  pulsed-gradient spin echo
PHA
  proper hepatic artery
  pulse-height analyzer
phagedenic ulcer
phakomatosis, pl. **phakomatoses**
phalangeal
  p. bone
  p. branch
  p. diaphyseal fracture
  p. glenoidal ligament
  p. herniation
  p. preponderance
  p. shortening
phalanx, pl. **phalanges**
  base of p.
  drumstick p.
  phalanges of foot
  phalanges of hand
  hourglass p.
  ivory p.
  rectangular p.
Phalen
  P. maneuver
  P. position
phantogeusia
  global p.
phantom
  Alderson anthropomorphic p.
  p. bone
  p. breast tumor
  p. dosimetry
  flood p.
  gelatin p.

Hine-Duley p.
p. image
p. limb syndrome
p. lung tumor
mammographic p.
metal line-pair p.
neck p.
nuclear magnetic resonance p.
oil-water p.
p. pregnancy
p. radiograph
reference p.
p. simulating cardiac motion
p. study
velocity-evaluation p.
wax p.

phantosmia
birhinal p.
unirhinal p.

pharmacoangiography
pharmacologic
p. dilatation
p. stress
p. stress dual-isotope myocardial
  perfusion SPECT
p. stress echocardiography

**pharmacoradiologic disimpaction of
esophageal foreign body**
pharmacoradiology
PharmaSeed palladium-103 seeds
pharyngeal
p. abscess
p. area
p. artery
p. canal
p. muscle
p. orifice
p. plexus
p. pouch
p. recess
p. space mass
p. tonsil
p. wall carcinoma

pharynges (*pl. of* pharynx)
pharyngobasilar fascia
pharyngoesophageal
p. diverticulum
p. function
p. sphincter

pharyngoesophagogram
pharyngoesophagography
pharyngography

pharyngotonsillitis
pharyngotympanic tube
pharynx, pl. **pharynges**
p. cross-section
laryngeal part of p.
nasal part of p.
oral part of p.
postcricoid p.

phase
accelerated p.
accumulation p.
p. analysis
p. angle
arterial p.
blastic p.
blood pool p.
p. cancellation
cardiac p.
chronic p.
p. coherence
p. contrast (PC)
p. correction
corticomedullary p.
p. cycling
p. delay
delayed p.
diastolic depolarization p.
p. difference mapping
p. discontinuity artifact
p. effect
p. encoding (PE)
equilibrium p.
excretory p. (EP)
expiratory p.
fat-water out of p.
p. filtering
follicular p.
p. gain
hepatic arterial p. (HAP)
p. identification
p. image
inspiratory p.
p. instability
interictal p.
late p.
luteal p.
midarterial p.
p. mismapping
nephrogenic p.
nephrographic p. (NP)
noncontrast p. (NCP)
ovulatory p.

NOTES

P

phase *(continued)*
  parenchymatous p.
  plateau p.
  portal venous p. (PVP)
  portal venous-dominant p. (PVP)
  prolonged expiratory p.
  prolonged inspiratory p.
  rapid early repolarization p.
  rapid ventricular filling p.
  p. relation
  p. sampling ratio (PSR)
  p. shift
  spent p.
  static bone p.
  thallium redistribution p.
  vascular p.
  p. velocity imaging
  ventilation scintigraphy
    equilibrium p.
  wash-in p.
  washout p.
  zero p.
phase-angle display redundancy
phase-contrast
  p.-c. angiography
  p.-c. cine MRI
phase-corrected GRE image
phased-array
  p.-a. body coil MR imaging
  2.0-MHz p.-a. probe
  p.-a. MRI
  p.-a. multicoil imaging
  p.-a. multicoils
  p.-a. scanner
  p.-a. surface coil
  p.-a. surface coil MR imaging
  p.-a. torso coil
  p.-a. transducer
phase-dependent spectroscopic imaging
phase-encode
  p.-e. pulse
  p.-e. time-reduced acquisition
    sequence
  p.-e. time-reduced acquisition
    sequence imaging
phase-encoding
  p.-e. direction
  p.-e. gradient
  p.-e. motion artifact
  p.-e. order
  p.-e. period
  p.-e. step
phase-inversion method
phase-offset multiplanar (POMP)
phase-ordered multiplanar (POMP)
phase-preserving reconstruction

phase-sensitive
  p.-s. detector
  p.-s. flow measurement
  p.-s. gradient-echo MR imaging
phase-shift
  p.-s. artifact
  p.-s. effect
  p.-s. velocity mapping
phase-shifting interferometry
phase-specific action
phase-unwrapping method
phase-velocity image
phasic
  p. contraction
  p. pressure
phasicity
phasing-in time
Phemister triad
phenazopyridine
phenobarbital
  p. biliary atresia
  p. imaging agent
phenoltetrachlorophthalein
**phenomenological effective surface
  potential**
phenomenon, pl. **phenomena** *(See* disease,
  syndrome)
  Ashman p.
  Austin Flint p.
  autoimmune p.
  Bancaud p.
  Bell p.
  common cavity p.
  crankshaft p.
  Cushing p.
  dip p.
  embolic p.
  extinction p.
  flare p.
  flow p.
  fogging p.
  Friedreich p.
  Gärtner p.
  glove p.
  Hurst p.
  interference p.
  irradiation p.
  Jod-Basedow p.
  Katz-Wachtel p.
  kindling p.
  magic angle p.
  no-reflow p.
  nutcracker p.
  on-off p.
  pivot shift p.
  Raynaud p.
  resonance p.

R-on-T p.
Schiff-Sherrington p.
seizure p.
spin-phase p.
staircase p.
steal p.
treppe p.
truncation p.
unilateral Raynaud p.
vacuum disk p.
vertebral steal p.
Wenckebach p.

phenoxyacetic acid
phentetiothalein
phenyloxazolyl
pheochromocytoma
adrenal p.
bladder p.
p. rule of 10

Philips
P. DVI 1 system
P. Gyroscan ACS, NT, NT5,
NT15, S5, T5 scanner
P. Gyroscan ACS NT
superconducting magnet
P. Integris 5000 digital subtraction
angiography system
P. linear accelerator
P. 1.5-T NT MR scanner
P. Tomoscan 350, SR 6000 CT
scanner
P. 4.7-T small-bore system scanner

Phillips muscle
phlebectasia
malformed p.

phlebectatic peliosis hepatis
phlebitis
postvenography p.

phlebogram
ascending contrast MR p.
direct puncture MR p.
impedance MR p.

phlebograph
phlebographic pattern
phlebography
ascending contrast p.
cervical magnetic resonance p.
(CMRP)
direct puncture p.
impedance p.
magnetic resonance p.
occlusive impedance p.

phlebolith
phlebolith-like calcification
phleborheography (PRG)
phlebosclerosis
phlebostasis
phlebostenosis
phlebothrombosis
phlegmon
Holz p.
mesenteric p.
pancreatic p.

phlegmonous
p. abscess
p. gastritis
p. mass
p. pancreatitis

PHO
periarticular heterotopic ossification

phocomely, phocomelia
phonation study
phonoangiography
carotid p.
oculoplethysmography/carotid p.
(OPG/CPA)

phonocardiography
phonophotography
**PhorMax CR desktop workstation
system**
phosphate
chromium p.
p. enema
linear p.
membrane p.
phosphorus-32 sodium p.
sodium p. (P-32)
^{99m}Tc p.

phosphaturic
p. intraosseous lesion
p. mass
p. material
p. tumor

phosphaturic-inducing tumor
phosphomonoester (PME)
phosphonate
nucleoside p.

phosphor
cesium iodide input p.
fluorescent p.
photostimulable p. (PSP)
p. plate

phosphorated
phosphorescence

NOTES

P

phosphoric acid imaging agent
phosphorus (P)
  colloidal chromic p.
  p. imaging agent
  inorganic p.
  p. isotope
  labeled p.
  p. magnetic resonance spectroscopy
    (P-MRS)
  p. metabolism
  radioactive p.
phosphorus-31
  p.-31 magnetic resonance
    spectroscopy
phosphorus-32 (^{32}P, P-32)
  p. sodium phosphate
phosphorylase
  thymidine p. (TP)
Phospho-Soda
phosphosoda enema
Phosphotope oral solution
photic
photo
  analog p.
  p. plotter film
  p. transformation
photoacoustic ultrasound
photoactinic
photoaffinity
photoaging
photoangioplasty
photocathode
photocell plethysmography
photochemotherapy
  extracorporeal p.
photochromogen
photocoagulation
  interstitial laser p.
  intraoperative laser p.
  krypton laser p.
photocoagulator
  xenon arch p.
photodeficient region
photodensitometry
photodetector
  CCD p.
photodiode
photodisintegration
photodisplay unit
photodisruption
photodynamic therapy (PDT)
photoechoic effect
photoelasticity
photoelectric
  p. absorption
  p. effect

  p. emission
  p. interaction
  p. system
photoelectron
photoexcitation
photoflow
photofluorogram
photofluorographic
photofluorography
photofluoroscope
photographic
  p. effect (PE)
  p. radiometer
photography
  CT bone window p.
  Moiré p.
photolysis
  flash p.
photometer
  HemoCue p.
photomicrograph
  cystic hyperplasia p.
photomultiplier (PM)
  p. tube (PMT)
photon (hν)
  annihilation p.
  p. attenuation
  p. attenuation measurement
  P. cataract removal system
  Compton scattering p.
  p. correlation spectroscopy
  p. deficiency
  degraded p.
  p. densitometry
  p. density
  dual p.
  p. energy
  p. fluence
  p. flux
  gamma p.
  p. interaction depth
  linear p.
  p. mottle
  p. peak
  P. Radiosurgery System (PRS)
  soft p.
  p. theory of radiation
  p. therapy beam line
photon-deficient
  p.-d. area
  p.-d. bone lesion
  p.-d. lesion bone scintigraphy
photoneutron
photonic medicine
**photon-neutron mixed-beam radiation
  therapy**

photonuclear
  p. effect
  p. reaction
photooptical detection
photopeak
  p. breadth
  p. fraction
photopenia
photopenic
  p. area
  p. defect
  p. region
Photopic Imaging ultrasound system
photoplethysmographic
  p. digit
  p. monitoring
photoplethysmography (PPG)
PhotoPoint photodynamic therapy
photoprotein
photoradiation
photoradiometer
photoreceptor
  p. fractional velocity error
  p. motion
photorecording
photoroentgenography
photoscan
photoscanner
photostimulable
  p. luminescence intensity
  p. phosphor (PSP)
  p. phosphor computed radiography
  p. phosphor dental radiography
  p. phosphor digital imaging
  p. phosphor plate
phototherapeutic keratectomy (PTK)
photothermal sclerosis
phototimer
phototoxic
phototoxicity
phototube output circuit
photovolt pH meter
PHP
  pseudohypoparathyroidism
phrenic
  p. ampulla
  p. artery
  p. lymph node
  p. nerve injury
  p. nerve paralysis
  p. pedicle
phrenicocolic ligament

phrenicoesophageal (*var. of*
  phrenoesophageal)
phrenicolienal ligament
phrenicosplenic ligament
phrenoesophageal, phrenicoesophageal
  p. ligament
phrenogastric ligament
phrenopericardial angle
phrenosplenic ligament
phrenovertebral junction
phrygian
  p. cap
  p. cap deformity
phrynoderma
phthalocyanine
phthinoid chest
phthisis
  p. bulbi
phyllode
  cystosarcoma p.
  p. tumor
physeal
  p. bar
  p. bony bridging
  p. cartilage
  p. closure
  p. damage
  p. distraction
  p. injury
  p. plate fracture
physes (*pl. of* physis)
physician
  Fellow of the American College of
    Nuclear P.'s
physics
  radiation p.
physiologic
  p. atrophy
  p. herniation
  p. high activity
  p. hyperplasia
  p. hypertrophy
  p. imaging
  p. ovarian cyst
  p. parameter
  p. regurgitation
  p. shunt flow
  p. sphincter
  p. uterine blush
physiologically immature lung
physis, pl. **physes**
  distal tibial p.

NOTES

physis *(continued)*
    fibular p.
    fused p.
    medial p.
    unfused p.
phytobezoar
PI
    pulmonic insufficiency
pia arachnoid
pial
    p. AVM
    p. vessel
piano key sign
PICA
    posterior-inferior cerebellar artery
pica artifact
PICC
    peripherally inserted central catheter
    PICC line
PICD
Pick
    P. body
    P. bundle
    P. disease
    P. tubular adenoma
Picker
    P. camera
    P. Magnascanner
    P. MR scanner
    P. PQ 5000 helical CT scanner
    P. PQ 2000 spiral CT scanner
    P. PRISM 3000 PET scanner
    P. SPECT attenuation correction
    P. Synerview 600 scanner
    P. system
picket
    p. fence appearance
    P. Fence stereotactic localizer
pick-off artifact
pickup tube
picocurie (pCi)
picometer (pm)
picomole (pmol)
picosecond pulse
picture
    p. archiving and communication
        system (PACS)
    p. element
    p. frame appearance
    p. frame pattern of vertebral body
    p. frame vertebra
picture-frame-like
picture-framing osteoporosis
PIE
    postinfectious encephalomyelitis
    pulmonary interstitial emphysema

piece
    chin-occiput p.
    pole p.
piecemeal necrosis
Piedmont fracture
Pierre Robin syndrome
piezoelectric
    p. effect
    p. transducer
pigeon
    p. chest
    p. fancier's lung
pigeon-breast deformity
Pigg-O-Stat pediatric positioning device
pigmented
    p. basal cell carcinoma
    p. iris hamartoma
    p. villonodular synovitis
pigment stone
pigskin patch
pigtail
    p. catheter
    p. stent
PIHI
    pulse-inversion harmonic imaging
pilar
    p. sheath
    p. tumor
pilaris
pile
    sentinel p.
pill
    barium p.
    p. esophagitis
pillar
    faucial p.
    p. fracture
    p. projection
    tonsillar p.
    P. view
pill-induced inflammation
pillion fracture
pillow
    cervical skull p.
    foam vacuum p.
    p. fracture
pilocytic
    p. astrocytoma
    p. tumor
piloid astrocytoma
pilomatricoma
pilon ankle fracture
pilonidal
    p. cyst
    p. fistula
    p. sinus
    p. tract

pilorum
    vortices p.
pilosebaceous unit
pilosity
PIN
    positive-intrinsic-negative
    posterior interosseous nerve
        PIN diode
pin
        Hagie p.
        lead p.
        Optispike dispensing p.
        orthopedic p.
        p. pattern
        resorbable p.
        revolving Ge-68 p.
        track of p.
pinchcock
        p. effect
        p. mechanism
pinched nerve
pinch-off syndrome
pincushion distortion
Pindborg tumor
pineal
        p. apoplexy
        p. body
        p. cyst
        p. dysgerminoma
        p. germ-cell tumor
        p. germinoma
        p. gland
        p. gland calcification
        p. gland neoplasm
        p. gland shift
        p. gland teratocarcinoma
        p. gland tumor
        p. gland tumor classification
        p. mass
        p. parenchymal tumor
        p. region
        p. region tumor
        p. teratoma
        p. ventricle
pinealcytoma
pinealoblastoma, pineoblastoma
pinealoma
    ectopic p.
pineocytoma
ping-pong
        p.-p. ball deformity

        p.-p. fracture
        p.-p. heart volume
pinhole
        bone p.
        p. camera
        p. collimator
        p. image
        p. scintigram
        p. technique
pink tetralogy
Pinnacle[3] radiotherapy planning system
PINNACLE R/O II radiopaque marker
pinning
        hip p.
        in situ p.
Pinpoint stereotactic arm
Pins sign
pion
        p. beam
        p. dosimetry
PIOPED
    prospective investigation of pulmonary
    embolus diagnosis
        PIOPED criteria
Piotrowski sign
PIP
    proximal interphalangeal joint
        PIP articulation
        PIP joint
pipe
    endoscopic washing p.
pipestem
        p. artery
        p. cirrhosis
        p. fibrosis
        p. ureter
pipe-stemming of ankle-brachial index
PIPIDA
    para-isopropyl-iminodiacetic acid
        PIPIDA hepatobiliary imaging
        PIPIDA scan
        technetium-99m PIPIDA
piping
    organ p.
PIPJ
    proximal interphalangeal joint
Pipkin femoral fracture classification
Pirie
        P. bone
        P. method
        P. transoral projection

NOTES

P

piriform, pyriform
- p. muscle
- p. recess
- p. sinus
- p. sinus carcinoma

piriformis, pyriformis
- apertura p.
- p. muscle

Pirogoff
- P. amputation
- P. angle

PISA
- proximal isovelocity surface area

pisiform
- p. bone
- p. fracture

pisohamate ligament
pisometacarpal ligament
pisoscaphoid distance
pisotriquetral
- p. articulation
- p. joint

pisounciform ligament
pisouncinate ligament
pistol-grip femur deformity
pistoning
piston-like reflux
pit
- anal p.
- articular p.
- auditory p.
- central p.
- colonic p.
- costal p.
- cutaneous p.
- gastric p.
- herniation p.
- pitch ratio p.
- postanal p.
- primitive p.
- scan pitch p.
- spiral CT pitch p.
- p. of stomach
- synovial herniation p.

pitch
- calcaneal p.
- high-quality p.
- high-speech p.
- p. ratio
- p. ratio pit
- recon p.
- scan p.
- spiral CT p.

pitchblende
pitted cartilage
pitting
- pepper-pot p.

Pittsburgh pneumonia
pituicytoma
pituilith
pituitary
- p. adenoma
- p. adenoma chromophobe
- p. apoplexy
- p. bright spot
- p. cyst
- p. dwarfism
- p. failure
- p. fossa
- p. gland
- p. gland anatomy
- p. gland enlargement
- p. hyperplasia
- p. infarct
- p. infundibulum
- p. macroadenoma
- p. microadenoma
- p. oncocytoma
- p. stalk
- p. stone
- p. tumor

pivot
- p. of calcar
- p. joint
- p. shift
- p. shift phenomenon

pivoting table
pivot-shift sign
pixel
- p. block
- p. count method
- edge-region p.
- maximum intensity p. (MIP)
- p. noise
- normal-region p.
- p. shift program
- p. value

pixel-oriented algorithm
pixel shift program
Pixsys FlashPoint camera
pizoelectric generator
PLA
- polylactic acid

placement
- anular p.
- catheter p.
- intracoronary stent p.
- intrapericardial patch lead p.
- line p.
- minimally invasive endovascular stent p.
- percutaneous endoluminal p.
- radiotherapy field p.
- shim p.

shunt p.
subanular p.
subject p.
superselective microcatheter p.
transcatheter filter p.
transjugular portosystemic stent
  shunt p.
transluminal endovascular stent-
  graft p.
transpapillary p.
placenta, pl. **placentae**
abnormal adherence of p.
abruptio placentae
accessory p.
p. accreta
adherent p.
anterofundal p.
anular p.
battledore p.
bilobate p.
p. biopsy
chorioallantoic p.
circummarginate p.
cirsoid p.
deciduate p.
Duncan p.
p. enlargement
extrachorial p.
fetal p.
first-trimester p.
fundal p.
horseshoe p.
incarcerated p.
p. increta
kidney-shaped p.
low-lying p.
marginal p.
maternal p.
p. membranacea
p. migration
nondeciduate p.
panduriform p.
p. percreta
premature senescence p.
p. previa
retained p.
p. rotation
Schultze p.
second-trimester p.
third-trimester p.
p. tumor
vascular space of the p.

velamentous p.
villous p.
placental
p. abruption
p. circulation
p. disk
p. edema
p. grade
p. hemorrhage
p. infarct
p. localization
p. metastasis
p. polyp
p. septal cyst
p. septum
p. souffle
p. villus
placentation
placentogram
displacement p. (DPG)
placentography
indirect p.
placode
neural p.
unneurulated neural p.
plafond
p. fracture
tibial p.
plagiocephaly
deformation posterior p.
posterior p.
synostotic posterior p.
plain
p. abdominal radiography (PAR)
p. film
p. film imaging
p. radiograph
p. tomogram
p. view
plain-paper image
plan
isodose p.
posterior transaxial scan p.
plana
coxa p.
vertebra p.
planar
p. circular coil
p. detector
p. diagnostic 1231 scintigraphy
p. exercise thallium-201
  scintigraphy

NOTES

P

planar *(continued)*
  p. left anterior oblique image
  p. plate
  p. radionuclide imaging
  p. spin imaging
  p. thallium imaging
  p. thallium scan
  p. thallium with quantitative
    analysis
  p. view
Planck
  P. constant
  P. quantum theory
plane
  AC-PC p.
  Aeby p.
  anatomic p.
  areolar p.
  axial p.
  axiolabiolingual p.
  axiomesiodistal p.
  Baer p.
  biparietal p.
  bite p.
  Blumenbach p.
  Bolton p.
  Bolton-nasion p.
  Broadbent-Bolton p.
  buccolingual p.
  Calvé vertebra p.
  capsular p.
  circular p.
  p. of cleavage
  clip-editing p.
  coronal p.
  count per p.
  cross-sectional p.
  Daubenton p.
  E p.
  eye-ear p.
  facial p.
  fascial p.
  fat p.
  first parallel pelvic p.
  flexion-extension p.
  four-chamber p.
  fourth parallel pelvic p.
  Frankfort horizontal p.
  frontal biauricular p.
  frontoparallel p.
  German horizontal p.
  gonion-gnathion p.
  Hensen p.
  Hodge p.
  horizontal p.
  imaging p.
  interiliac p.

internervous p.
intersphincteric p.
interspinal p.
interspinous p.
intertubercular p.
ischiorectal fossa p.
limited-cut p.
Ludwig p.
magnetic focal p.
Meckel p.
medial sagittal p.
median raphe p.
median sagittal p.
mesiodistal p.
midclavicular p.
midcoronal p.
midfrontal p.
midsagittal p.
midthalamic p.
Morton p.
nonorthogonal p.
nuchal p.
oblique coronal p.
occipital p.
occlusal p.
optimal imaging p.
orbital p.
orthogonal p.
parallel tag p.
paramedian sagittal p.
parasagittal p.
pelvic p.
Poschl p.
principal p.
radial p.
p. of reference
reverse Waters p.
sagittal p.
scan p.
sella-nasion p.
semicoronal p.
sensitive p.
p. sensitivity
short axis p.
slicing p.
spinous p.
sternoxiphoid p.
subadventitial p.
subcostal p.
subintimal cleavage p.
supracristal p. (SCP)
suprasternal notch p.
p. suture
tag p.
temporal p.
thalamic p.
thoracic p.

transaxial scan p.
transmedial p.
transpyloric p.
transtubercular p. (TTP)
transumbilical p. (TUP)
transverse p.
tumor cleavage p.
umbilical p.
valve p.
varus-valgus p.
vertical p.
Virchow p.
XY p.
ZY p.
planigram
planigraphic principle
planigraphy
planimeter
planimetry
planing
planithorax
planning
3D radiation treatment p.
radiation therapy p. (RTP)
radiation treatment p. (RTP)
p. target volume (PTV)
planogram
planography
planovalgus
p. foot
p. foot deformity
pes p.
plantar
p. aponeurosis
p. arterial arch
p. aspect
p. axial view
p. bursa
p. calcaneal enthesophyte
p. calcaneal spur
p. capsule
p. compartment
p. compartmental anatomy
p. fasciitis
p. fibromatosis
p. flexion-inversion deformity
p. flexion stress view
p. hyperplasia
p. interossei
p. ligament
p. metatarsal angle
p. metatarsal artery

p. plate
p. shift
p. surface
p. vault
plantarward
plantodorsal projection
planum sphenoidale
planus
pes plantigrade p.
plaque
arterial p.
arteriosclerotic p.
asbestos pleural p.
atheromatous p.
atherosclerotic p.
b-amyloid senile p.
calcified p.
carotid artery p.
p. cleaving
p. compression
concentric atherosclerotic p.
p. constituent
p. cracker
discrete p.
disrupted p.
eccentric atherosclerotic p.
echogenic p.
echolucent p.
endocardial p.
p. erosion
esophageal p.
fatty p.
fibrofatty p.
fibrotic p.
fibrous intima p.
fissured atheromatous p.
florid p.
focal pleural p.
p. fracture
fungal p.
gastrointestinal p.
p. hemorrhage
heterogeneous carotid p.
homogeneous carotid p.
Hutchinson p.
hypoechoic p.
iliac p.
infiltrating p.
intraluminal p.
lipid-laden p.
luminal p.
meningioma en p.

NOTES

P

705

plaque *(continued)*
  multiple sclerosis p.
  mycotic p.
  neuritic senile p.
  noncompliant p.
  obstructive p.
  penile p.
  periventricular p.
  pleural p.
  pleuroparenchymal p.
  pulverized p.
  Randall p.
  p. regression
  p. remodeling
  residual p.
  p. rupture
  sclerotic p.
  senile p.
  sequential paired opposed p.
  (SPOP)
  sessile p.
  p. splitting
  stenotic p.
  talc p.
  p. tearing
  ulcerated atheromatous p.
  ulcerated carotid artery p.
  uncalcified pleural p.
  p. vaporization
plaque-containing artery
plaque-like
  p.-l. lesion
  p.-l. linear defect
plaquing
  p. calcification
  neuritic p.
plasma
  p. cell granuloma
  p. cell pneumonia
  p. emission spectroscopy
  P. 1000 ICP-AES unit
  p. iron turnover
  p. radioiron disappearance rate
  p. radioiron turnover rate
  p. volume
plasmablast
plasmablastic
  p. lymphoma
  p. myeloma
plasmacytoma
  anaplastic p.
  extramedullary p. (EMP)
  primary pulmonary p.
  solitary p.
  solitary bone p. (SBP)
plasmodium embolus

plaster
  x-ray in p. (XIP)
  x-ray out of p. (XOP)
plastic
  p. bowing fracture
  carbon fiber-reinforced p.
  p. clot
  p. pleurisy
plastica
  linitis p.
plasticity
  brain p.
  neuronal p.
plate
  acetabular reconstruction p.
  alar p.
  amorphous selenium p.
  anal p.
  anchor p.
  auditory p.
  axial p.
  basal p.
  blade p.
  bone fixation p.
  bony p.
  buttress p.
  cap p.
  cardiogenic p.
  cartilaginous growth p.
  cloacal p.
  cloverleaf p.
  compression p.
  condylar p.
  connecting p.
  cortical p.
  cranial fixation p.
  cribriform p.
  3D p.
  dorsal p.
  dual p.
  end p.
  epiphyseal cartilage p.
  epiphyseal growth p.
  ethmovomerine p.
  femoral p.
  fenestrated compression p.
  fibrocartilaginous volar p.
  flat p.
  flexor p.
  foot p.
  Fresnel zone p.
  frontal p.
  fusion p.
  ground p.
  growth p.
  hilar p.
  hyaline cartilage p.

interfragmentary p.
intertrochanteric p.
localization-compression grid p.
low-contact dynamic compression p. (LC-DCP)
meningioma of cribriform p.
microfixation p.
nail p.
neutralization p.
occipitocervical p.
orbital p.
orthopedic p.
orthotic p.
overlay p.
palmar p.
pedicle p.
phosphor p.
photostimulable phosphor p.
planar p.
plantar p.
Plexiglas p.
prochordal p.
PSP imaging p.
pterygoid p.
quadrigeminal p.
quadrilateral p.
p. reader
resorbable p.
p. and screw fixation
selenium p.
septal cartilage p.
sinodural p.
skull p.
Spli-Prest p.
stabilization p.
stainless steel p.
stem base p.
subchondral bone p.
supracondylar p.
tarsal p.
tectal p.
tendon p.
tissue p.
titanium p.
vertebral body p.
volar p.
xeroradiographic selenium p.
Y bone p.
plateau
    p. phase
    p. tibia fracture
    tibial p.

platelet-fibrin embolus
platelet function analyzer (PFA)
platelet-rich thrombus
plate-like atelectasis
platform
    positioning p.
platinocyanoide
    barium p.
platinum (Pt)
    p. coil
    p. coil embolization
    0.0015-inch p. wire
    0.00175-inch p. wire
    p. microcoil
    P. Plus guidewire
platinum-marked stent
platinum-resistant ovarian carcinoma
platybasia
platycephaly
platypelloid, platypellic
    p. pelvis
platypodia
platysma muscle
platyspondylia
platyspondylosis
platyspondyly generalisata
play
    joint p.
pleat
    accordion-shaped p.
pleating
    p. of ligamentum flavum
    p. of small bowel
pleomorphic
    p. adenoma parotitis
    p. calcification
    p. liposarcoma
    p. lung adenoma
    p. microcalcification
    p. rhabdomyosarcoma
    p. sarcoma
    p. T-cell lymphoma
    p. type
    p. xanthoastrocytoma (PXA)
pleomorphism
    nuclear p.
pleonosteosis
    Leri p.
PLES
    parallel-line equal spacing
    PLES bar
    PLES bar pattern

NOTES

P

plesiocurie therapy
plesiography
plesiosectional tomography
plesiotherapy
plethora-related cyanotic CHD
plethysmograph
plethysmography
    air p.
    body box p.
    computer strain-gauge p. (CSGP)
    digital p.
    Doppler ultrasonic velocity detector
      segmental p.
    exercise strain gauge venous p.
    impedance p. (IPG)
    Medsonic p.
    photocell p.
    segmental bronchus p.
    strain-gauge p.
    thermistor p.
    venous p.
pleura, pl. pleurae
    cervical p.
    congested p.
    costal p.
    costodiaphragmatic recess of p.
    crus p.
    diaphragmatic p.
    edematous p.
    fibrous tumor p.
    hyaloserositis p.
    inflamed p.
    localized fibrous tumor of p.
    mediastinal p.
    p. metastasis
    parietal p.
    p. peel
    pericardiac p.
    p. pseudotumor
    pulmonary p.
    scarification of p.
    silicotic visceral p.
    solitary fibrous tumor of the p.
      (SFTP)
    visceral p.
    wrinkled p.
pleura-based
    p.-b. area of increased opacity
    p.-b. lung nodule
pleural
    p. apical hematoma cap
    p. calcification
    p. canal
    p. cavity
    p. change
    p. cupula
    p. cyst

p. density
p. disease
p. effusion
p. empyema
p. fibromyxoma
p. fistula
p. flap
p. fluid
p. fluid aspiration
p. fluid collection
p. line
p. margin
p. mass
p. mesothelioma
p. nodule
p. plaque
p. reaction
p. recess
p. rind
p. sac
p. scarring
p. shunting
p. space
p. stripe
p. thickening
p. tube
pleurisy
    acute p.
    Bends asbestos p.
    blocked p.
    chronic p.
    circumscribed p.
    costal p.
    diaphragmatic p.
    diffuse p.
    double p.
    dry p.
    encysted p.
    exudative p.
    fibrinopurulent p.
    fibrinous p.
    hemorrhagic p.
    ichorous p.
    indurative p.
    interlobar p.
    latent p.
    mediastinal p.
    metapneumonic p.
    plastic p.
    primary p.
    proliferation p.
    pulmonary p.
    pulsating p.
    purulent p.
    sacculated p.
    secondary p.
    septic p.

serofibrous p.
serous p.
single p.
suppurative p.
typhoid p.
visceral p.
wet p.
pleuritic pneumonia
pleuritis
viral p.
pleurocutaneous fistula
pleurodesis
chemical p.
pleuroesophageal
p. line
p. stripe
pleurography
pleuroparenchymal
p. plaque
p. reflection
pleuropericardial
p. adhesion
p. canal
p. cyst
p. effusion
pleuroperitoneal
p. canal
p. communication
p. fold
pleuropulmonary
p. adhesion
p. blastoma
pleuroscopy
plexiform neurofibroma
Plexiglas plate
plexogenic pulmonary arteriopathy
plexus, pl. **plexus, plexuses**
abdominal aortic p.
anterior coronary p.
anterior pulmonary p.
aortic p.
autonomic p.
axillary p.
basilar p.
Batson p.
biliary p.
brachial p.
cardiac p.
carotid p.
cavernous p.
celiac p.
cervical p.

choroid p.
ciliary ganglionic p.
coccygeal p.
colic p.
colonic myenteric p.
common carotid p.
coronary p.
cystic p.
dangling choroid p.
deep cardiac p.
deferential p.
enteric p.
epidural venous p.
esophageal p.
Exner p.
extradural vertebral p.
facial p.
femoral p.
gastric p.
gastroesophageal variceal p.
glomus of choroid p.
great cardiac p.
hemorrhoidal p.
hepatic nerve p.
hypogastric p.
ileocolic p.
inferior mesenteric p.
p. injury
intermesenteric p.
left coronary p.
lumbar p.
lumbosacral p.
lymph p.
Meissner p.
myenteric p.
nerve p.
pampiniform p.
paravertebral nerve p.
paravertebral venous p.
pelvic p.
perimeniscal capsular p.
perimuscular p.
pharyngeal p.
posterior coronary p.
posterior pulmonary p.
presacral p.
prostatic venous p.
pterygoid p.
pulmonary p.
rectal p.
retrovertebral p.
right coronary p.

NOTES

P

plexus *(continued)*
    sacral p.
    sciatic p.
    solar p.
    spinal nerve p.
    subareolar p.
    submucosal venous p.
    superficial p.
    superior hypogastric p.
    superior mesenteric p.
    tympanic p.
    uterovaginal p.
    vaginal p.
    vascular p.
    venous p.
    vertebral venous p.
    vesical venous p.
plica, pl. **plicae**
    infrapatellar p.
    medial p.
    parapatellar p.
    suprapatellar p.
    symptomatic lateral synovial p.
    p. syndrome
    synovial p.
plicated dural sheath
plication
    p. defect
    disk p.
    transmesenteric p.
PLIF
    posterior lumbar interbody fusion
P-LINK software
PLL
    posterior longitudinal ligament
plot
    box-and-whisker p.
plug
    bile p.
    bone p.
    collagen p.
    dermoid p.
    echogenic p.
    finger-like mucous p.
    p. flow
    gamma-irradiated p.
    hydrogel p.
    interbody bone p.
    Ivalon p.
    keratin p.
    luminal p.
    meconium p.
    mucous p.
    P. n View 3D medical imaging software
    Porstmann Ivalon p.

plugging
    mucous p.
plug-like appearance
Plumbicon
plumbline view
Plummer
    P. disease
    P. sign
Plummer-Vinson syndrome
plump vessel
plurality of slices
plural pregnancy
pluripotential bronchial epithelial stem cell
plus-density artifact
4096 Plus PET scanner
plutonism
plutonium
    environmental p.
PM
    photomultiplier
    posterior mitral
Pm
    promethium
pm
    picometer
PMC
    primary motor cortex
PMC activation
PME
    peak of maximum enhancement
    phosphomonoester
        time to PME (tPME)
PMF
    progressive massive fibrosis
PML
    progressive multifocal leukoencephalopathy
pML
    posterior mitral leaflet
pmol
    picomole
PMRA
    pulmonary magnetic resonance angiography
P-MRS
    phosphorus magnetic resonance spectroscopy
PMT
    photomultiplier tube
        PMT imaging agent
        PMT robotic fulcrumless tomographic system
PMV
    prolapsed mitral valve
PMVL
    posterior mitral valve leaflet

PNC
premature nodal contraction
PNET
primitive neuroectodermal tumor
non-CNS PNET
pneumarthrogram
pneumarthrography
pneumatic
p. bone
p. reduction of intussusception
pneumatization
pneumatocele
p. cranii
extracranial p.
intracranial p.
parotid p.
postinfectious p.
traumatic p.
pneumatocyst
pneumatogram
pneumatograph
pneumatosis
p. coli
cystic p.
p. cystoides intestinalis
epidural p.
gastric p.
p. sphenoidale
stomach p.
pneumencephalography
lumbar p.
pneumoalveolography
pneumoangiogram
pneumoangiography
pneumoarthrogram
pneumoarthrography
pneumobilia
pneumocardiograph
pneumocardiography
pneumocele
pneumocephalus
intracranial p.
pneumocolon
pneumoconiosis, pl. **pneumoconioses**
aluminum p.
barium p.
bauxite p.
p. classification
coal worker's p. (CWP)
complicated p.
fiberglass p.
fibrogenic p.

Fuller earth p.
inert p.
inert dust p.
kaolin p.
mica p.
nepheline p.
rheumatoid p.
sericite p.
silicate p.
sillimanite p.
talc p.
tungsten carbide p.
zeolite p.
pneumoconstriction
pneumocystic infection
pneumocystography
breast p.
pneumocystosis
cutaneous p.
pneumocystotomography
pneumoencephalogram (PEG)
pneumoencephalographic pattern
pneumoencephalography (PEG)
cerebral p.
fractional p.
pneumoencephalomyelogram
pneumoencephalomyelography
pneumoenteric
p. canal
p. defect
pneumofasciogram
pneumogastrography
pneumogram
pneumography
cerebral p.
retroperitoneal p.
pneumogynogram
pneumohemothorax
pneumohydrothorax
pneumointestinalis
pneumolith
pneumomediastinogram
pneumomediastinography
pneumomediastinum
postoperative p.
radiolucent p.
spontaneous p.
traumatic p.
pneumomyelography
pneumonectomy chest
pneumonia
acute eosinophilic p.

NOTES

pneumonia *(continued)*

acute interstitial p. (AIP)
adenovirus p.
alcoholic p.
allergic p.
alveolar p.
anthrax p.
apical p.
aspiration p.
asthmatic p.
atypical bronchial p.
atypical interstitial p.
atypical measles p.
atypical primary p.
bilateral lower lobe p.
bilious bronchial p.
bronchiolitis obliterans with
  organizing p. (BOOP)
Buhl desquamative p.
capillary p.
caseous p.
catarrhal p.
cavitating p.
central p.
cerebral p.
cheesy p.
chelonian p.
chemical p.
chronic interstitial p.
community-acquired p.
concomitant p.
consolidative p.
contusion p.
cryptogenic organizing p.
deglutition p.
delayed resolution of p.
desquamative interstitial p. (DIP)
diffuse p.
double p.
Eaton agent p.
embolic p.
endogenous lipid p.
eosinophilic p.
ephemeral p.
exogenous lipoid p.
extensive bilateral p.
fibrinous p.
fibrous p.
focal organizing p.
Friedländer p.
fungal p.
gangrenous p.
giant cell interstitial p. (GIP)
granulomatous p.
Hecht p.
hemorrhagic p.
herpesvirus p.

hypersensitivity p.
hypostatic p.
idiopathic interstitial p.
incomplete resolution of p.
indurative p.
infantile p.
inhalation p.
interstitial organizing p.
interstitial plasma cell p.
irradiation p.
lingular p.
lipoid endogenous p.
lobar p.
lobular p.
Löffler p.
lower lobe p.
lymphocytic interstitial p. (LIP)
lymphoid interstitial p. (LIP)
massive p.
measles p.
migratory p.
mycotic p.
necrotizing p.
neonatal p.
nonclassifiable interstitial p.
nonspecific interstitial p. (NIP,
  NSIP)
nummular p.
obstructive p.
oil-aspiration p.
organizing focal p.
organizing interstitial p.
parenchymatous p.
passive p.
patchy area of p.
peripheral p.
pertussoid eosinophilic p.
Pittsburgh p.
plasma cell p.
pleuritic p.
postobstructive p.
posttraumatic p.
purulent p.
pyogenic p.
radiation p.
recurrent p.
resolving p.
right-sided p.
round p.
secondary p.
segmental p.
septic p.
superficial p.
suppurative p.
terminal p.
toxic p.
traumatic p.

tuberculous p.
tularemic p.
unresolved p.
usual interstitial p. (UIP)
walking p.
white p.
pneumonic infiltrate
pneumonitis
acute interstitial p.
acute radiation p.
aspiration p.
bacterial p.
basilar p.
chemical p.
chronic p.
diffuse p.
drug-induced p.
early p.
giant cell p.
granulomatous p.
hypersensitivity p.
idiopathic interstitial p.
interstitial p.
lipoid p.
lymphocytic interstitial p.
lymphoid interstitial p.
mycoplasmal p.
radiation p.
unusual interstitial p.
usual interstitial p.
ventilation p.
pneumonocirrhosis
pneumonoconiosis
noncollagenous p.
pneumonograph
pneumonography
pneumoorbitography
pneumopathy
cobalt p.
pneumopericardium
pneumoperitoneal
pneumoperitoneum
balanced p.
diagnostic p.
drop test for p.
transabdominal p.
pneumoplethysmography
ocular p. (OPG)
pneumopreperitoneum
pneumopyelogram
pneumopyelography
pneumorachicentesis

pneumorachis
pneumoradiography
retroperitoneal p.
pneumoretroperitoneum
pneumoroentgenogram
pneumoroentgenography
pneumoscrotum
pneumothorax, pl. **pneumothoraces** (**PT**)
artificial p.
basilar p.
blowing p.
catamenial p.
closed p.
congenital p.
diagnostic p.
extrapleural p.
induced p.
life-threatening p.
open p.
positive-pressure p.
pressure p.
recurrent p.
simultaneous bilateral
spontaneous p. (SBSP)
spontaneous tension p.
sucking p.
tension p.
therapeutic p.
traumatic p.
tuberculous p.
uncomplicated p.
valvular p.
pneumotomography
pneumoventriculogram
pneumoventriculography
PNL
posterior nipple line
pnuemoperitoneography
PO
parietal operculum
Po
polonium
pocket
air p.
p. chamber
p. Doppler
p. dosimeter
infraclavicular p.
rectus sheath p.
regurgitant p.
p. shot
subcutaneous p.

NOTES

P

713

pocket *(continued)*
    subpectoral p.
    valve p.
    p. of Zahn
pocketed calculus
pocketing of barium
POEMS
    polyneuropathy, organomegaly,
    endocrinopathy, monoclonal
    gammapathy, skin changes
    POEMS syndrome
point
    A p.
    Addison p.
    alveolar p.
    apophyseal p.
    auricular p.
    p. Ba
    bleeding p.
    Bolton p.
    branch p.
    breast trigger p.
    Cannon p.
    Cannon-Boehm p.
    cardinal p.
    Chauffard p.
    choroid p.
    Clado p.
    coaptation p.
    commissural p.
    congruent p.
    Cope p.
    coplanar contour p.
    craniometric p.
    Crowe pilot p.
    D p.
    dorsal p.
    end p.
    entry p.
    equilibrium p.
    Erb p.
    frontopolar p.
    glenoid p.
    Griffith p.
    Hartmann p.
    ICRU reference p.
    p. imaging
    J p.
    Kienböck-Adamson p.
    Lanz p.
    lead p.
    p. localization
    Mackenzie p.
    McBurney p.
    midinguinal p.
    Morris p.
    multiple sensitive p.'s

    p. mutation
    nodal p.
    null p.
    output p.
    Pauly p.
    preauricular p.
    pressure p.
    random p.
    reentry p.
    Rolando p.
    sacrococcygeal inferior pubic p.
    (SCIPP)
    saddle p.
    scanned focal p. (SFP)
    p. scanning
    seed p.
    sensitive p.
    p. sensitivity
    Sudeck p.
    sylvian p.
    target p.
    time p.
    white p.
pointer
    hip p.
    metallic p.
    shoulder p.
point-in-space stereotactic biopsy
point-resolved
    p.-r. spectroscopy localization
    technique
    p.-r. spectroscopy sequence
    (PRESS)
point-spread function (PSF)
point-to-point protocol (PPP)
Poiseuille
    P. flow
    P. law
poisoning
    radiation p.
Poisson
    P. distributed activity concentration
    P. distribution
    P. noise fluctuation
    P. ratio
Poisson-Pearson formula
poker spine
Poland
    P. epiphyseal fracture classification
    P. syndrome
polar-bound water
polar coordinate system
Polaris 1.32 Nd:YAG laser
polarity-altered
    p.-a. spectral-selective acquisition
    p.-a. spectral-selective acquisition
    imaging

polarization
  cell p.
  chemically-induced dynamic
    nuclear p.
  cross p. (CP)
  dynamic nuclear p. (DNP)
  linear p.
  nuclear p.
polarized light microscopy
polarographic
  p. needle electrode
  p. needle electrode measurement
Polaroid film
pole
  abapical p.
  10-p. Butterworth filter
  cephalic p.
  fetal p.
  p. figure texture analysis
  frontal p.
  germinal p.
  inferior p.
  kidney p.
  lower p.
  magnetic p.
  middle p.
  occipital p.
  p. of organ
  patellar p.
  p. piece
  scaphoid p.
  p. of scaphoid bone
  superior p.
  temporal p.
  p. tip
  upper p.
  p. of vessel
pole-to-pole length of kidney
Polhemus
  P. 3D digitizer
polidocanol sclerosing agent
polka-dot appearance
pollex pedis
pollicis
  adductor p.
  p. longus tendon
  opponens p.
pollicization
  Riordan finger p.
pollicized ray
polonium (Po)

polyadenopathy
  angiofollicular and plasmacytic p.
polyalveolar lobe
polyangiitis
  microscopic p.
Pólya procedure
polyarcuate diaphragm
polyarteritis nodosa (PAN)
polyarthritis
  juvenile chronic p.
polyarthropathy
polyarticular symmetric tophaceous joint inflammation
polychondritis
  relapsing p.
polychromatic radiation
polycycloidal tomography
polycystic
  p. kidney
  p. kidney disease
  p. liver
  p. liver disease
  p. lung
  p. nephroblastoma
  p. ovarian disease (PCOD)
  p. ovary
  p. ovary syndrome (PCOS)
polydactyly
  Wassel classification of thumb p.
polydirectional tomography
polyethylene (PE)
  p. catheter
  p. glycol (PEG)
  p. stent
  p. tube
Polyflex stent
polyglycolide
  self-reinforced p.
polygonal elongate cell
polygon mirror
polygyria
polyhydramnios
polylactic acid (PLA)
polylobar liver
polymastia
polymer
  p. dosimetry
  osteoconductive p.
polymerization
  fibrin p.
polymerizing agent
polymethyl methacrylate implant

NOTES

P

polymicrogyria
polymorphonuclear leukocyte
polymyalgia rheumatica
polynesian bronchiectasis
polyneuropathy, organomegaly,
    endocrinopathy, monoclonal
    gammapathy, skin changes (POEMS)
polynomial stepwise multilinear
    regression
polynuclear neutrophilic leukocyte
polyostotic
    p. bone lesion
    p. fibrous dysplasia
polyp
    adenomatous p. (AP)
    angiomatous nasal p.
    antral p.
    antrochoanal p.
    bleeding p.
    broad-based p.
    bronchial p.
    cardiac p.
    carpet p.
    cervical p.
    choanal p.
    cholesterol gallbladder p.
    colonic adenomatous p.
    colonic hamartomatous p.
    colorectal p.
    cyst or p.
    cystic p.
    dental p.
    duodenal p.
    endometrial p.
    epithelial colonic p.
    fibrinous p.
    fibroepithelial urethral p.
    fibroid p.
    fibrous urinary tract p.
    fibrovascular p.
    filiform p.
    gallbladder p.
    gastric p.
    hamartomatous gastric p.
    Hopmann p.
    hydatid p.
    hyperplastic adenomatous p.
    hyperplastic colon p.
    hyperplastic gastric p.
    hyperplastic stomach p.
    inflammatory colonic p.
    inflammatory esophagogastric p.
    inflammatory fibroid p.
    inflammatory stomach p.
    intraluminal p.
    juvenile p.
    laryngeal p.

    lipomatous p.
    lymphoid p.
    metaplastic p.
    metastatic p.
    mucous p.
    multiple p.'s
    nasal p.
    osseous p.
    pedunculated p.
    Peutz-Jeghers p.
    placental p.
    postinflammatory p.
    rectal p.
    regenerative gastric p.
    retention colon p.
    retention stomach p.
    sessile p.
    sigmoid p.
    single p.
    p. stalk
    tubular p.
    tubulovillous p.
    uterine fibroid p.
    vascular fibrous p.
    villoglandular p.
    villous stomach p.
polypeptide
    organic anion transporter p.
polyphase generator
polyphebus
polyphosphate
polyphosphonate
    technetium p.
polypoid
    p. adenoma
    p. calcified irregular mass
    p. carcinoma
    p. dysplasia
    p. fibroma
    p. fibroma collecting system
    p. filling defect
    p. lesion
    p. lesion of the lower esophagus
    p. lymphoid hyperplasia
    p. lymphoma
    p. mucosa
polyposa
    colitis p.
polyposis
    diffuse mucosal p.
    familial adenomatous p. (FAP)
    familial colorectal p.
    familial gastrointestinal p.
    familial intestinal p.
    familial juvenile p.
    familial multiple p.
    filiform p.

gastric hamartomatous p.
intestinal p.
juvenile p.
lymphomatous p. (LP)
multiple p.
Peutz-Jeghers gastrointestinal p.
postinflammatory p.
sinonasal p.
polypropylene catheter
polyradiculomyelitis
polyradiculoneuropathy
polyradiculopathy
polysomnogram
polysomnography
nocturnal p.
polysplenia syndrome
polystotic
polytetrafluoroethylene (PTFE)
p. graft
polythelia
polytomogram
polytomographic radiology
polytomography
mastoid p.
polytrauma
polyurethane
p. foam embolus
p. stent
polyvinyl
p. alcohol (PVA)
p. alcohol particle
p. alcohol particle embolization
p. butyral (PVB)
p. chloride (PVC)
polyvinylpyrrolidone (PVP)
POMP
phase-offset multiplanar
phase-ordered multiplanar
POMP imaging
Pompe disease
Ponderal Index
pond fracture
pons
bifid p.
caudal p.
infarct of p.
rostral p.
tegmentum of p.
pontine, pontile
p. angle
p. angle tumor
p. artery

central p.
p. cistern
p. contusion
p. glioma
p. hemorrhage
p. hydatid cyst
p. infarct
p. isthmus
p. lesion
p. myelinolysis
p. reticular formation
p. tegmentum
pontine-medullary level
pontis
basis p.
brachium p.
pontocerebellar
p. fiber
p. glioma
p. hypoplasia
pontomedullary
p. junction
p. sulcus
pontomesencephalic
p. junction
p. vein
pool
blood p.
focal p.
gastric p.
vascular blood p.
pooling
genital blood p.
venous p.
poor
p. perfusion
p. screen/film contact
p. sensitivity
p. shimming of MRI magnet
p. vascular reserve
p. visualization
poorly
p. circumscribed tumor
p. concentrated isotope
p. differentiated adenocarcinoma (PDA)
p. differentiated tumor
popcorn calcification
popcorn-like appearance
popliteal
p. artery
p. artery aneurysm

NOTES

P

popliteal *(continued)*
> p. artery entrapment syndrome
> p. artery occlusive disease
> p. artery pulsation artifact
> p. artery trifurcation
> p. cavity
> p. cyst
> p. fossa
> p. hiatus
> p. ligament
> p. line
> p. node
> p. recess
> p. space
> p. tendon
> p. tendonitis
> p. vein

popliteus
> p. bursa
> p. tendon

poppet
> barium-impregnated p.
> disk p.

poppy seed-like calcification
population
> overdistention of alveolar p.
> uneven recruitment of alveolar p.

porcelain
> p. aorta
> p. gallbladder

Porcher method
porcine
> p. gallbladder
> p. heart xenograft

porencephalic cyst
porencephaly
> acquired p.
> agenetic p.
> encephaloclastic p.
> true p.

porosis
> cerebral p.

porous
> p. bone
> p. ingrowth
> p. kidney
> p. metallic stent

Porstmann Ivalon plug
PORT
> postoperative radiotherapy
> PORT radiofrequency electrode
> design

port
> Cordis multipurpose access p.
> p. film
> implantable infusion p.
> injection p.

multipurpose access p. (MPAP)
parallel opposed unmodified p.
radiation p.
radiotherapy p.
simulation of converging p.
single p.
subcutaneous implanted injection p.
tangential p.
treatment p.

porta
> p. cirrhosis
> p. hepatis
> p. hepatis defect
> p. hepatis low-density mass
> p. hepatis node
> p. hepatis obstruction

portable
> p. C-arm image intensifier
> fluoroscopy
> p. C-arm intensifier
> p. chest film
> p. radiography
> p. view
> p. x-ray

portacamera
Port-A-Cath
portacaval
> p. shunt
> p. space

portal
> p. canal
> p. decompression
> p. fibrosis
> p. fissure
> p. flow
> p. hypertension
> p. portography
> radiation p.
> radiocarpal p.
> simulation of tangential p.
> p. space
> superomedial p.
> p. triad
> p. vascular bed
> p. vein
> p. vein aneurysm
> p. vein cavernoma
> p. vein congestion index
> p. vein enhancement
> p. vein lesion
> p. vein system
> p. vein thrombosis
> p. vein velocity
> p. venography
> p. venous dominant
> p. venous-dominant phase (PVP)
> p. venous gas

p. venous phase (PVP)
p. venous phase imaging
p. venous pressure (PVP)
portal-phased spiral CT scan
portal-to-portal
p.-t.-p. bridge
p.-t.-p. fibrosis
PortalVision radiation oncology system
port-catheter system
portion
cavernous p.
intrapericardial p.
supraclinoid p.
portio vaginalis
portogram
portography
arterial p.
computed tomography during
arterial p. (CTAP)
double-spiral CT arterial p.
percutaneous transhepatic p.
portal p.
splenic p.
transhepatic p.
transjugular p.
umbilical p.
portohepatic
portomesenteric venous thrombosis
portophlebography
portopulmonary shunt
portosplenic thrombosis
portosplenography
portosystemic
p. anastomosis
p. collateral
p. collateral circulation
p. collateral vessel
p. gradient
p. shunt
portovenography
portovenous
Posada fracture
Posadas-Wernicke coccidioidomycosis
Poschl plane
Posicam HZ PET scanner
position
abduction p.
adduction p.
Albers-Schönberg p.
Albert p.
anatomic p.
anterior oblique p.

anteroposterior p.
barber chair p.
bayonet fracture p.
beach chair p.
Béclére p.
Benassi p.
Bertel p.
bladder neck p.
Broden p.
brow-down p.
brow-up p.
Caldwell p.
cardiac p.
catheter tip p.
central venous line p.
Chassard-Lapiné p.
Cleaves p.
Clements-Nakayama p.
cock-robin p.
conus medullaris p.
cross-table lateral p.
decubitus p.
dorsal decubitus p.
dorsal recumbent p.
dorsosacral p.
dwell p.
p. encoding
erect p.
eversion p.
extension p.
Feist-Mankin p.
fetal p.
Fick p.
figure-4 p.
Fleischner p.
flexion p.
Fowler p.
Friedman p.
frogleg p.
Fuchs p.
full lateral p.
Grashey p.
Haas p.
heart p.
Hickey p.
horizontal p.
infragenicular p.
infrapulmonary p.
inlet p.
inversion p.
jackknife p.
Johnson p.

NOTES

position *(continued)*
LAO p.
Larkin p.
lateral decubitus p.
lateral left anterior oblique p.
Law p.
Lawrence p.
left anterior oblique p.
left posterior oblique p.
left-side-down decubitus p.
Lewis p.
Lilienfeld p.
Lindblom p.
lithotomy p.
lordotic p.
Lorenz p.
lotus p.
Low-Beers p.
LPO p.
Mayer p.
Miller p.
near-anatomic p.
neutral hip p.
Noble p.
Nölke p.
noncoaxial catheter tip p.
normal anatomic p.
nose-chin p.
nose-forehead p.
oblique p.
opisthotonic p.
PA p.
paramedian p.
paraseptal p.
park bench p.
Pawlow p.
Pearson p.
Phalen p.
prone p.
pulmonary capillary wedge p.
reclining p.
rectus p.
recumbent p.
reverse Trendelenburg p.
reverse Waters p.
right anterior oblique p.
right posterior oblique p.
right-side-down decubitus p.
Schüller p.
semiaxial p.
semierect p.
semi-Fowler p.
semilateral p.
semirecumbent p.
semisupine p.
semiupright p.
Settegast p.

side-lying p.
Sims p.
spatial p.
squatting p.
Staunig p.
Stecher p.
steep Trendelenburg p.
Stenver p.
stepping-source p.
submentovertex p.
supine p.
swimmer's p.
Tarrant p.
Taylor p.
three-quarters prone p.
tibial sesamoid p.
Titterington p.
Towne p.
Trendelenburg p.
tripod p.
Twining p.
upright p.
ventral decubitus p.
verticosubmental p.
Walcher p.
Waters p.
Wigby-Taylor p.
Zanelli p.

positional
p. dysfunction
p. variation

positioner
basilar block skull p.
dual lateral hand p.
dual oblique hand p.
Waters p.

positioning
arms-up p.
automatic endoscopic system for
optimal p. (AESOP)
p. error
flap p.
motion-free p.
operator-dependent p.
pendent p.
p. platform

positive
p. cephalopelvic disproportion index
p. contrast encephalography
p. contrast myelography
p. electron
p. end-expiratory pressure
ER p.
estrogen-receptor p.
p. node basin
p. predictive value (PPV)
p. ray

true p. (TP)
p. washout test
positive-intrinsic-negative (PIN)
positive-intrinsic-negative diode
positive-ion cyclotron
positive-pressure pneumothorax
positrocephalogram
positron (*See* PET, PETT)
p. decay
p. emission mammography (PEM)
p. emission tomography (PET)
p. emission transaxial tomography (PETT)
p. emission transverse tomography (PETT)
p. emitting radionucleotide
energetic p.
labeled p.
p. matter-antimatter annihilation reaction
p. range
p. scanning
p. scintillation camera
positron-coincidence
positronium half-life
post
p. Diamox state
p. ECT sequelae
p. fatty meal cholecystography
p. fire image
p. PTCA residual stenosis
p. reconstruction filtering option
p. transplantation ureteric obstruction
postablation
postamputation neuroma
postanal pit
postangioplasty
p. angiography
p. aortography
p. intimal flap
p. mural thrombosis
p. restenosis
p. stenosis
postaortic lymph node
postaugmentation
postbeat filtration
postbiopsy
p. change
p. eggshell calcification
p. fat necrosis
p. period

p. renal AV fistula
p. scarring
postbulbar
p. duodenum
p. ulcer
postbypass spasm
postcapillary venule
postcaptopril radioisotope study
postcardiac injury syndrome (PCIS)
postcardiotomy lymphocytic splenomegaly
postcatheterization pseudoaneurysm
postcaval
p. lymph node
p. ureter
postcentral
p. gyrus
p. sulcus
postchemoembolization liver abscess
postcontrast
p. echocardiography
p. MR imaging
postcricoid
p. area
p. carcinoma
p. defect
p. pharynx
p. soft tissue
p. web
postcubital
postdilatation arteriography
postdrainage
p. cystogram
p. imaging
p. projection
postductal
p. aortic coarctation
p. coarctation of aorta
Postel destructive coxarthrosis
postembolization
p. angiographic pattern
p. angiography
p. syndrome
postenhancement sequence
posterior (P)
p. abdominal wall
p. acoustic enhancement
p. acoustic shadowing
ampulla ossea p.
p. anulus
p. aorta transposition of great artery

NOTES

P

posterior *(continued)*
p. apical segment
p. arch fracture
p. aspect
p. auricular vein
p. axillary line
p. basal segmental bronchus
p. border
p. border of heart
p. calcaneal bursitis
p. capsular distance (PCD)
p. cardinal vein
p. central gyrus
p. central indentation
p. cerebral artery (PCA)
p. cerebral territory infarct
p. cervical line
p. cervical space
p. cervical triangle
p. choroidal artery
p. cingulate functional impairment
p. circulation territory
p. circumflex humeral artery
p. cistern
p. colliculus
p. column deficit
p. column demyelination
p. column lesion
p. column of spine
p. column syndrome
p. commissure (PC)
p. communicating artery (PCA, PCoA)
p. communicating artery aneurysm
p. compartment
p. compartment lesion
p. concavity
p. coronary groove
p. coronary plexus
p. cranial fossa
p. cruciate ligament (PCL)
p. cruciate ligament injury
p. cusp
p. descending artery (PDA)
p. descending branch
p. disk margin
p. element fracture
p. embryotoxon
p. epidural fat
p. fascicular block
p. fontanelle
p. fossa circulation
p. fossa cyst
p. fossa-foramen magnum lesion
p. fossa hematoma
p. fossa lesion
p. fossa meningioma

p. fossa tumor
p. fracture-dislocation
p. free wall
p. gray column of cord
p. gray horn
p. iliac crest
p. impingement
p. impingement syndrome
p. inferior iliac spine
p. inferior spine
p. inferior tibiofibular ligament
p. intercostal artery
p. intercostal branch
p. interosseous nerve (PIN)
p. interosseous nerve entrapment
p. interventricular groove
p. interventricular sulcus
p. interventricular vein
p. intraoccipital synchondrosis
p. joint syndrome
p. junction line
p. language area lesion
p. lateral talar process
p. leaflet prolapse
p. lie
p. lip
p. longitudinal ligament (PLL)
p. longitudinal ligament tear
p. lumbar interbody fusion (PLIF)
p. lumbar vessel
p. median septum
p. mediastinal mass
p. mediastinal node
p. mediastinum
p. membrane articulation
p. metatarsal arch
p. midbody of corpus callosum
p. mitral (PM)
p. mitral leaflet (pML)
p. mitral valve leaflet (PMVL)
p. neck surface coil
p. neural arch
p. nipple line (PNL)
p. oblique ligament
p. olive
p. osteophyte
p. palatine suture
p. papillary muscle (PPM)
p. parietal artery
p. patch aortoplasty
p. pharyngeal wall carcinoma
p. pituitary fossa
p. pituitary gland ectopia
p. plagiocephaly
p. pleural recess
p. predominance
p. probability

p. projection
p. pulmonary plexus
p. rectus sheath
p. retrocrural approach
p. reversible encephalopathy
 syndrome (PRES)
p. ring fracture
p. root entry zone
p. root ganglion
p. scalloping of vertebra
p. semicircular canal
p. septal space
p. skull view
p. spinal artery
p. spinal cord horn
p. spine fusion (PSF)
p. spinocerebellar tract
p. spur
p. subluxation
superior labral anterior to p.
 (SLAP)
superior labral anterior p.
p. surface
p. surface of pancreas
p. surface of prostate
p. talofibular (PTF)
p. talofibular ligament
p. temporal artery
p. temporal vertical (PTV)
p. thalamic arteries of Lazorthes
p. tibial artery
tibialis p.
p. tibial tendon (PTT)
p. tibiotalar ligament
p. tracheal band
p. transaxial scan plan
p. transcaval approach
p. triangle of the neck
p. turn of the aortic arch
p. urethra
p. urethral injury
p. urethral valve (PUV)
p. urethrovesical angle (PUVA)
p. vagal trunk
p. ventricular branch
p. vertebral element blowout lesion
p. vertebral scalloping
p. wall (PW)
p. wall fracture
p. wall motion
p. wall myocardial infarct
p. wall thickness (PWT)

posterior-inferior
 p.-i. cerebellar artery (PICA)
posteroanterior (PA)
 p. chest film
 p. lordotic projection
 p. view
posteroapical defect
posterobasal
 p. segment
 p. wall myocardial infarct
posteroexternal
posteroinferior myocardial infarct
posterointernal
posterolateral
 p. aspect
 p. capsule
 p. compartment
 p. corner injury
 p. disk herniation
 p. fontanelle
 p. rotatory instability
 p. rotatory subluxation
 p. sclerosis
 p. segment
 p. spinal artery
 p. wall
 p. wall motion
 p. wall myocardial infarct
posteromedial
 p. compartment
 p. tibia
posteromedian
posterooblique view
posteroparietal
posterosuperior glenoid impingement
posterotransverse diameter
postevacuation
 p. film
 p. view
postexercise
 p. echocardiography
 p. film
 p. image
 p. imaging
 p. index
 p. stunning
postextrasystolic
 p. pause
 p. potentiation
postfiltering
 low-pass three-dimensional p.
postgadolinium scan

NOTES

P

postganglionic
- p. gray fiber
- p. sympathetic fiber

postglomerular arteriolar constriction

postglucose loading examination

posthemorrhagic hydrocephalus

posthepatic cirrhosis

postictal cerebral blood flow scan

postimplant radiation survey

postinfarction
- p. ventricular aneurysm
- p. ventriculoseptal defect

postinfectious
- p. bronchiectasis
- p. bronchiolitis obliterans
- p. demyelination
- p. encephalitis
- p. encephalomyelitis (PIE)
- p. hydrocephalus
- p. pneumatocele

postinflammatory
- p. adenopathy
- p. polyp
- p. polyposis
- p. pulmonary fibrosis
- p. renal atrophy
- p. scarring

postinjection
- p. attenuation scan
- p. echocardiography
- p. imaging
- p. scan delay

postintraarticular paramagnetic contrast injection T1-weighted image

postirradiation
- p. fracture
- p. MFH
- p. osteogenic sarcoma
- p. vascular insufficiency

postischemic
- p. atrophy
- p. recovery

postlaminectomy
- p. instability
- p. kyphosis

postlumpectomy skin thickening

postlymphangiography

postmastectomy lymphedema

postmaturity syndrome

postmediastinal

postmediastinum

postmenarchal female pelvis

postmeningococcal pericarditis

postmenopausal
- p. adnexal cyst
- p. endometrial thickness
- p. endometrium
- p. estrogen therapy
- p. osteoporosis
- p. ovary
- p. uterine atrophy

postmetrizamide
- p. CT imaging
- p. CT scan

postmyelography CT

postmyocardial
- p. infarct
- p. infarction echocardiography
- p. infarction syndrome

postmyocardiotomy infarct

postmyocarditis dilated cardiomyopathy

postnatal injury

postnecrotic
- p. cirrhosis
- p. scarring

postobstructive
- p. atelectasis
- p. pneumonia
- p. renal atrophy

postoperative
- p. angiography
- p. breast hematoma
- p. cholangiography
- p. cholangiography imaging
- p. chylothorax
- p. emphysema
- p. ileus
- p. mediastinal hemorrhage
- p. pneumomediastinum
- p. radiotherapy (PORT)
- p. resorption atelectasis
- p. scar tissue
- p. seroma
- p. skull defect
- p. stenosis
- p. thoracic deformity
- p. view

postorchiectomy paraaortic radiation therapy

postpartum
- p. cardiomyopathy
- p. pituitary apoplexy
- p. pituitary necrosis

postperfusion lung

postpericardiotomy syndrome

postpharyngeal soft tissue

postphlebitic
- p. leg
- p. valvular incompetence

postpolio syndrome

postprimary pulmonary tuberculosis

postprocedure nephrostogram

postprocessing
- image p.

p. procedure
p. workstation
postprocessor
postpyelonephritis cortical scarring
postradiation
p. calcification
p. fibrosis
postradiotherapy implant survey reading
postreduction
p. film
p. mammoplasty
p. view
p. x-ray
postrelease radiography
postrheumatic cusp retraction
postrolandic parietal cortex
postsphenoid bone
poststenotic dilatation
poststress
p. ankle/arm Doppler index
p. image
p. stunning
postsurgical
p. change
p. emphysema
p. fat necrosis
p. pseudoaneurysm
p. recurrent ulcer
posttemporal middle cerebral artery
postterm
p. fetus
p. pregnancy
posttherapy change
postthoracotomy change
postthrombolytic coronary reocclusion
posttourniquet occlusion angiography
posttransplant
p. acute renal failure
p. coronary artery disease
p. lymphoproliferative disorder
posttraumatic
p. angulation
p. ascending myelopathy
p. aseptic necrosis
p. atrophy of bone
p. cavus
p. central spinal cord syrinx
p. chondrolysis
p. cystic myelopathy
p. fat necrosis
p. fibrosis
p. hemorrhage

p. hydrocephalus
p. intradiploic pseudomeningocele
p. neuroma
p. oil cyst
p. osteoarthritis
p. osteoporosis
p. pneumonia
p. pulmonary insufficiency
p. spinal cord cyst
p. subcapsular hepatic fluid
  collection
p. syringomyelia
posttuberculous obstruction
postulate
Avogadro p.
postulnar bone
postural
p. reduction
p. ureteric obstruction
posture
benediction p.
postvagotomy
p. dysphagia
p. effect
p. small-bowel distention
postvasectomy change in epididymis
postvenography phlebitis
postvesicular lymph node
postviral leukoencephalopathy
postvoid
p. radiography
p. residual urine
p. residual urine volume
p. view
postvoiding film
Potain sign
potassium (K)
p. bromide contrast medium
p. imaging agent
p. iodide
ionic p.
p. perchlorate
total exchangeable p. (TEK)
potassium-38 (^{38}K)
potassium-39 (^{39}K)
potassium-40 (^{40}K)
potassium-42 (^{42}K)
potassium-43 (^{43}K)
potassium-titanyl-phosphate (KTP)
potato
p. node
p. tumor of neck

NOTES

P

725

potential
 p. difference
 electrostatic p.
 p. energy
 p. gradient
 ionization p.
 low metastatic p.
 phenomenological effective
  surface p.
 recruitment p.
 resting phase of cardiac action p.
 sorption p.
 upstroke phase of cardiac action p.
 variable tube p.
potentiation
 postextrasystolic p.
potentiator
potentiometer
Pott
 P. abscess
 P. aneurysm
 P. ankle fracture
 P. disease
 P. puffy tumor
Potter
 P. classification
 P. dysplasia
 P. sequence
 P. syndrome
 P. type IV kidney
Potter-Bucky
 P.-B. diaphragm
 P.-B. grid
Potts shunt
pouce flottant
pouch
 antral p.
 apophyseal p.
 arachnoid retrocerebellar p.
 axillary p.
 Blake p.
 blind upper esophageal p.
 branchial p.
 Broca pudendal p.
 celomic p.
 collecting venous p.
 deep perineal p.
 Douglas rectouterine p.
 dural root p.
 endodermal p.
 endorectal ileal p.
 fourth branchial cleft p.
 gastric p.
 Hartmann p.
 haustral p.
 Heidenhain p.
 hepatorenal p.

 hernia p.
 hypophyseal p.
 ileal S p.
 ileoanal p.
 ileocecal p.
 Indiana p.
 jejunal p.
 lateral hypopharyngeal p. (LHP)
 Morison p.
 nerve root axillary p.
 paracystic p.
 pararectal p.
 paravesical p.
 pendulous p.
 pharyngeal p.
 Prussak p.
 Rathke p.
 rectal p.
 rectouterine p.
 rectovaginal p.
 rectovaginouterine p.
 rectovesical p.
 renal p.
 Seessel p.
 S-shaped p.
 superficial inguinal p.
 superficial perineal p.
 suprapatellar p.
 two-loop ileal J p.
 ultimobranchial p.
 uterovesical p.
 venous p.
 vesicouterine p.
 Willis p.
 W-shaped ileal p.
 Zenker p.
pouchogram
pouchography
 evacuation p.
poudrage
 thoracoscopic p.
Poupart inguinal ligament
Pourcelot index
powder
 barium p.
 bone p.
 gelatin sponge p.
 licorice p.
 opaque p.
 p. pseudocalcification
 tantalum p.
Powell method
power
 p. Doppler
 p. Doppler imaging (PDI)
 p. Doppler signal
 p. Doppler sonography (PDS)

p. Doppler ultrasound
p. gain
p. injection
p. injector
mass collision stopping p.
p. ratio
resolving p.
scanning p.
p. spectral analysis (PSA)
stopping p.
stroke p.
POWERstation LNX workstation
Power Trak 6000 gradient
PowerVision ultrasound
Pozzi muscle
PPAS
peripheral pulmonary artery stenosis
PPG
photoplethysmography
PPH
primary pulmonary hypertension
PPM
posterior papillary muscle
PPP
point-to-point protocol
PPRF
paramedian pontine reticular formation
PPV
positive predictive value
pQCT
peripheral quantitative computed
tomography
PQCT scanner
PQ 5000 CT scanner
P:QRS ratio
P wave to QRS wave ratio
PR
pulmonic regurgitation
OncoScint PR
Pr
praseodymium
PRA
pendulous reference axis
practicable
as low as readily p. (ALARP)
praecox
Praestholm
praseodymium (Pr)
PRE
proton relaxation enhancement
T2 PRE
T2 proton relaxation enhancement

preablation
pre-Achilles fat pad
preacinar arterial wall thickness
preamplifier
preampullary portion of bile duct
preangioplasty stenosis
preaortic lymph node
preauricular point
precancer
precancerous change
precapillary lung hypertension
precaptopril radioisotope study
precarcinomatous
precatheterization
precaval lymph node
prececal lymph node
precentral
p. artery
p. cerebellar vein
p. gyrus
p. sulcus
precentroblast
precessing proton
precession
p. angle
fast imaging with steady-state p.
(FISP)
free p.
Larmor p.
reverse fast imaging with steady-
state free p. (PSIF)
steady-state free p. (SSFP)
true fast imaging with steady-
state p. (TrueFISP)
precessional
p. frequency
p. motion
precharred fiber
prechiasmal optic nerve lesion
precipitate evacuation
precipitating event
precipitation
contrast p.
precision
test-retest p.
precocity
isosexual p.
precommunicating
p. segment of anterior cerebral
artery
p. segment of posterior cerebral
artery

NOTES

P

precontrast
    p. echocardiography
    p. imaging
    p. scan
precordial
    p. bulge
    p. lead
    p. mapping
precordium, pl. **precordia**
    active p.
    anterior p.
    bulging p.
    lateral p.
precoronal sagittal sinus
precuneus
precursor
    BH4 p.
    bone marrow myeloid p.
    neurotransmitter p.
    p. sign to rupture of aneurysm
predental space
predetector
predicted
    p. cardiac index
    p. maximal uptake
    p. target heart rate
prediction
    linear p. (LP)
predictor
predisposition
    hereditary p.
prediverticular
    p. change
    p. disease
predominance
    anterior p.
    basilar p.
    posterior p.
    temporal p.
predominant flow load
preductal aortic coarctation
preejection
    p. interval
    p. period (PEP)
preembolization aortography
preemphasis
preenhancement sequence
preepiglottic
    p. soft tissue
    p. space
preesophageal dysphagia
preexcitation
    ventricular p.
preexposure prophylaxis
preferential flow
pre-filtering
    3D p.-f.

prefire image
preformed clot
prefragmentation
prefrontal
    p. artery
    p. bone of von Bardeleben
pregnancy
    abdominal ectopic p.
    ampullar p.
    anembryonic p.
    bigeminal p.
    broad ligament p.
    cervical p.
    combined p.
    compound p.
    compromised p.
    cornual ectopic p.
    diamniotic p.
    dichorionic diamniotic twin p.
    ectopic p. (EP)
    extrauterine p.
    failed p.
    fallopian p.
    false p.
    gemellary p.
    heterotopic p.
    hydatid p.
    hypervolemia of p.
    interstitial ectopic p.
    intraligamentary p.
    intraperitoneal p.
    intrauterine p. (IUP)
    membranous p.
    mesenteric p.
    molar p.
    monochorionic diamniotic twin p.
    monochorionic monoamniotic
     twin p.
    multiple p.
    mural p.
    ovarian p.
    ovarioabdominal p.
    oviductal p.
    parietal p.
    phantom p.
    plural p.
    postterm p.
    prevalence ectopic p.
    prolonged p.
    pseudointraligamentary p.
    ruptured ectopic p.
    sarcofetal p.
    sarcohysteric p.
    selective reduction of p.
    sextuplet p.
    spurious p.
    stump p.

tubal p.
tuboabdominal p.
tuboligamentary p.
tuboovarian p.
tubouterine p.
p. tumor
twin ectopic p.
uteroabdominal p.
uterotubal p.
p. wastage
pregnancy-induced uterine blush
pregnant
    p. uterus
    p. uterus rupture
preinjection echocardiography
preinsular gyrus
preintegration complex
preinterparietal bone
preinvasive
    p. carcinoma
    p. disease of cervix, vagina, and vulva
Preiser disease
prelaryngeal node
preliminary
    p. film
    p. view
preload
    left ventricular p.
    p. reserve
preloading radiation survey
premalleolar bursa
premamillary branch
premammillary artery
premasseteric
    p. space
    p. space abscess
premature
    p. atherosclerosis
    p. calcification
    p. closure of ductus arteriosus
    p. mid diastolic closure of mitral valve
    p. nodal contraction (PNC)
    p. osteoarthritis
    p. placental senescence
    p. senescence placenta
    p. suture synostosis
    p. uterine membrane rupture
    p. valve closure
    p. ventricular contraction (PVC)
prematurely closed suture

premaxillary
    p. bone
    p. suture
premedication
premedullary arteriovenous fistula
premolar teeth
premonitory sign
premotor
    p. area
    p. coret activation
    p. cortex
premyocardial infarction echocardiography
prenatal
    p. injury
    p. radiation
preocclusive obstruction
preoperative
    p. angiography
    p. imaging
    p. localization
    p. radiotherapy
    p. resting MUGA scan
    p. view
preosteonecrosis marrow edema
prep
    preparation
    LoSo Prep
prepapillary bile duct
preparation (prep)
    bowel p.
    Colyte bowel p.
    crush p.
    dry bowel p.
    Dulcolax bowel p.
    Emulsoil bowel p.
    p. error
    Evac-Q-Kwik bowel p.
    Fleet Phospho-Soda bowel p.
    flow cytometry sample p.
    GoLYTELY bowel p.
    inadequate bowel p.
    international reference p.
    kit p.
    NuLytely bowel p.
    OCL bowel p.
    on-column p.
    Tridrate bowel p.
    wet bowel p.
    X-Prep bowel p.
prepared
    magnetization p. (MP)

NOTES

P

prepatellar
p. bursa
p. bursitis
prepectoral fascia
prepectorally
prepericardial lymph node
preperitoneal fat
preplacental hemorrhage
preponderance
phalangeal p.
prepontine
p. cistern
p. white epidermoidoma
prepubertal
p. female breast
p. testicular mass
prepulse
spin-lock p.
prepyloric
p. antrum
p. atresia
p. fold
p. sphincter
p. ulcer
p. vein
prereduction
p. view
p. x-ray
prerenal
p. aortic aneurysm
p. failure
p. fat
prerupture of aneurysm
PRES
posterior reversible encephalopathy
syndrome
presacral
p. anomaly
p. cystic lesion
p. mass
p. plexus
p. space
presaturation
p. bolus tracking
fat-selective p.
p. projection
p. pulse
spatial p.
p. technique
presbyesophagus
presbyophrenia
prescan
MRI p.
prescapula
presence
inferred p.
presenile arteriosclerosis

presentation
breech p.
brow p.
cephalic p.
compound p.
cord p.
face p.
footling p.
frank breech p.
midline incense p.
osteoblastic p.
parietal p.
shoulder p.
transverse p.
vertex p.
presenting part
preservation
myocardial p.
p. of native aortic valve
sphincter p.
zone of partial p. (ZPP)
presinusoidal
preslip
p. change
p. staging
presphenoid bone
PRESS
point-resolved spectroscopy sequence
pressor unit
pressure
acoustic p.
airway p.
alveolar p.
p. amplitude
ankle-arm p.
ankle systolic p.
aortic root p.
arterial peak systolic p.
atmospheric p.
atrial p.
A-wave p.
bile duct p.
blood p.
bone marrow p. (BMP)
brachial artery cuff p.
brachial artery end-diastolic p.
brachial artery peak systolic p.
brachial artery pulse p.
bursting p.
capillary hydrostatic p.
capillary wedge p.
cardiac filling p.
cardiovascular p.
catheter bursting p.
central aortic p.
central venous p. (CVP)
cerebral perfusion p. (CPP)

colloid oncotic p. (COP)
coronary perfusion p.
coronary wedge p.
p. cuff
C-wave p.
damping of catheter tip p.
diastolic filling p. (DFP)
diastolic perfusion p.
distal coronary perfusion p.
Doppler ankle systolic p.
Doppler blood p.
draining with venous p.
drifting wedge p.
elevated lower esophageal sphincter
  resting p.
endocardial p.
end-systolic p. (ESP)
p. epiphysis
p. equalization
equalized diastolic p.
esophageal peristaltic p.
extravascular p.
feeding mean arterial p. (FMAP)
filling p.
p. fracture
p. half-time
p. half-time technique
hepatic wedge p. (HWP)
high filling p.
high interstitial p.
high wedge p.
increased central venous p.
increased intracranial p.
increased intrapericardial p.
increased pulmonary arterial p.
p. injector
inspiratory increase in venous p.
interstitial fluid hydrostatic p.
intracardiac p.
intracranial p. (ICP)
intracranial pulse p.
intraductal p.
intraluminal esophageal p.
intramuscular fluid p.
intrapericardial p.
intrapleural p.
intrapulmonary p.
intrathoracic p.
jugular venous p.
labile blood p.
left atrial p. (LAP)

left atrial end-diastolic p.
left-sided heart p.
left subclavian central venous p.
  (LSCVP)
left ventricular p. (LVP)
left ventricular cavity p.
left ventricular end-diastolic p.
  (LVEDP)
left ventricular filling p.
left ventricular peak systolic p.
left ventricular systolic p.
lower esophageal sphincter p.
  (LESP)
low urethral p. (LUP)
maximum inflation p.
mean aortic p.
mean arterial p. (MAP)
mean blood p.
mean brachial artery p.
mean circulatory filling p.
mean left atrial p.
mean pulmonary artery p. (MPAP)
mean pulmonary artery wedge p.
mean pulmonary capillary p.
  (MPCP)
mean right atrial p.
p. measurement
minimum blood p.
p. necrosis
normal lower esophageal sphincter
  resting p.
p. overload
PAM p.
passage p.
p. peak
peak airway p.
peak inflation p.
peak regurgitant wave p.
peak systolic aortic p.
perfusion p.
p. perfusion imaging
p. perfusion study
phasic p.
p. pneumothorax
p. point
portal venous p. (PVP)
positive end-expiratory p.
pulmonary arterial systolic pressure
  to systemic arterial systolic p.
pulmonary arterial wedge p.
pulmonary artery p. (PAP)

NOTES

P

731

pressure *(continued)*
    pulmonary artery diastolic pressure and pulmonary artery wedge p. (PADP-PAWP)
    pulmonary artery end-diastolic p. (PAEDP)
    pulmonary artery mean p. (PAM)
    pulmonary artery peak systolic p.
    pulmonary artery systolic p. (PAS)
    pulmonary artery wedge p. (PAWP)
    pulmonary capillary p. (PCP)
    pulmonary capillary wedge p. (PCWP)
    pulmonary venous wedge p.
    pulmonary wedge p. (PWP)
    pulse p.
    p. reading
    recoil p.
    regional cerebral perfusion p. (rCPP)
    right atrial p. (RAP)
    right-sided heart p.
    right ventricular p. (RVP)
    right ventricular diastolic p.
    right ventricular end-diastolic p.
    right ventricular peak systolic p.
    right ventricular volume p.
    segmental bronchus lower extremity Doppler p.
    shockwave p.
    stump p.
    subatmospheric p.
    superior vena cava p.
    supersystemic pulmonary artery p.
    systemic diastolic blood p.
    systemic mean arterial p. (SMAP)
    systolic-diastolic blood p.
    torr p.
    transmyocardial perfusion p.
    transpulmonary p. (Ptp)
    venous p.
    ventricular p.
    ventricularization of p.
    in vivo balloon p.
    V-wave p.
    p. wave
    p. waveform
    wedge p.
    wedge hepatic venous p. (WHVP)
    withdrawal p.
    X-wave p.
    Y-wave p.
    Z-point p.
pressure-activated safety valve (PASV)
pressure-controlled intermittent coronary occlusion technique

pressure-detachable silicone balloon
pressure-flow gradient
pressure-gradient wire system
pressure-volume loop
PressureWire sensor
pressurized fluid jet
prestenotic dilatation
prestomal ileitis
prestyloid recess
pretectal
    p. lesion
    p. nucleus
pretendinous
    p. band
    p. cord
pretherapy imaging
pretibial
    p. dimple
    p. myxedema
pre-TIPS gradient
pretracheal lymph node
prevalence ectopic pregnancy
prevertebral
    p. fascia
    p. ganglion
    p. lymph node
    p. soft tissue
    p. soft tissue swelling
    p. space
    p. space mass
    p. width
prevesicular lymph node
previa
    central placenta p.
    complete placenta p.
    incomplete placenta p.
    lateral placenta p.
    marginal placenta p.
    partial placenta p.
    placenta p.
    total placenta p.
    vasa p.
previable fetus
PRFT
    partially relaxed Fourier transform
PRG
    phleborheography
prickle cell carcinoma
Prima laser
primary
    p. achalasia
    p. acquired cholesteatoma
    p. acquired nasolacrimal duct obstruction (PANDO)
    p. adrenal insufficiency
    p. adrenal lymphoma
    p. amyloidosis

p. aspergillosis
p. atelectasis
p. auditory cortex
p. beam
p. benign liver tumor
p. biliary cirrhosis
p. bone lymphoma
p. brain lymphoma
cancer of unknown p. (CUP)
p. cartilage joint
p. center of ossification
p. CNS cholesteatoma
p. CNS lymphoma
p. CNS tumor classification
p. coccidioidomycosis
p. complex
p. congenital megaureter
p. cutaneous large B-cell
 lymphoma (PCLBCL)
p. cyst of spleen
p. digital acquisition
p. esophageal peristalsis
p. familial xanthomatosis
p. gastric non-Hodgkin lymphoma
p. hepatocellular carcinoma
p. HIV encephalitis
p. hydrocele
p. hydrocephalus
p. hyperparathyroidism
p. hypertrophic osteoarthropathy
p. hypothyroidism
p. implanted tumor
p. intracerebral hematoma
p. intracranial germ cell tumor
p. intraosseous carcinoma
p. irritant
p. left bronchus
p. lesion
p. malignant liver tumor
p. megaureter
p. motor cortex (PMC)
p. motor strip
p. myeloid metaphysis
p. neoplasm
p. neuroendocrine small-cell
 carcinoma
p. optic atrophy
p. ovarian choriocarcinoma
p. oxalosis
p. peristaltic wave
p. pigmented nodular adrenocortical
 disease

p. pleurisy
p. progressive cerebellar
 degeneration
p. pulmonary hemangiopericytoma
p. pulmonary hypertension (PPH)
p. pulmonary lobule
p. pulmonary lymphangiectasis
p. pulmonary malignancy
p. pulmonary malignant fibrous
 histiocytoma
p. pulmonary plasmacytoma
p. pulmonary tuberculosis
p. radiation
p. ray
p. refractory Burkitt lymphoma
p. renal tumor
p. retroperitoneal fibrosis
p. rhabdomyosarcoma
p. right bronchus
p. sarcoma
p. sclerosing cholangitis
p. sequestrum
p. teeth
p. temporal bone cholesteatoma
p. thrombus
p. tumor bed
unknown p.
p. vasospasm
p. vesical calculus
p. visual cortex
p. vitreous
p. yolk sac
PRIME
priming effect
primitive
p. acoustic artery
p. bone
p. dislocation
p. gut
p. hindgut
p. hypoglossal artery
p. neuroectodermal tumor (PNET)
p. neuroepithelial tumor
p. pit
p. streak
p. trigeminal artery (PTA)
p. ventricle
p. vertebra
p. yolk sac
primordial
p. follicle
p. tooth cyst

NOTES

P

primum
    ostium p.
    septum p.
primus
    digitus p.
PrinceStar electrophysiologic imaging study system
principal
    p. artery of pterygoid canal
    p. bronchus
    p. eigenvector
    p. plane
principle
    Dodge p.
    Doppler shift p.
    Fick p.
    Fuchs p.
    Grossman p.
    Huygens p.
    indicator fractionation p.
    line focus p.
    Pauli exclusion p.
    planigraphic p.
    tracer p.
    uncertainty p.
print reflectance modulation
prion protein (PrP)
prior probability
prism
    p. interpolation
    p. method for ventricular volume
PRISM three-head system
PROACT
    Prolyse in acute cerebral
    thromboembolism
    P. I, II trial
proactinium
probability
    absolute emission p.
    emission p.
    posterior p.
    prior p.
PROBE
    proton brain examination
probe
    AngeLase combined mapping-laser p.
    P. balloon dilatation system
    biplane sector p.
    Cardiac View p.
    p. dilatation
    Doppler flow echocardiographic p.
    electrohydraulic p.
    electromagnetic flow p.
    fiberoptic p.
    freehand p.
    gamma p.

gamma-detection p.
GE proton head coil p.
hand-held exploring electrode p.
hand-held mapping p.
hand-held 8-MHz Doppler p.
high-frequency miniature p.
hot-tipped laser p.
hybrid p.
hybridization p.
hyperthermia p.
interstitial p.
intraoperative gamma p.
laparoscopic p.
laparoscopic ultrasound p.
laser-Doppler flowmetry p.
linear array transrectal
    ultrasound p.
localizing p.
magnetometer p.
MH-908 slim ultrasonic p.
2.0-MHz phased-array p.
neutral amyloid p.
NMR magnetometer p.
nuclear p.
oligonucleotide p.
Olympus MH-908 slim
    ultrasonic p.
Olympus S20-20R transendoscopic
    ultrasound p.
pediatric biplane TEE p.
relaxation p.
scintillation p.
shift p.
side-firing p.
side-hole cannulated p.
Teflon p.
transesophageal echocardiography p.
Transonics flow p.
truncated NMR p.
ultrasonic p.
ultrasound p.
USCI p.
Versadopp ultrasonic Doppler p.
probehead
    MRI p.
probe-surface distance
PROBE-SV
    single-voxel proton brain examination
    PROBE-SV spectrometry
problematic abdominal activity
proboscis lateralis
Probst callosal bundle
procedure
    artificial pleural effusion p.
    button p.
    Cabrol composite graft p.
    catheter-directed interventional p.

Chamberlain p.
Damus-Kaye-Stansel p.
diagnostic p.
DKS p.
edge-detection p.
Eloesser p.
endoscopic p.
gastric pull-through p.
Glenn p.
Guidant ANCURE endograft p.
Hofmeister p.
interventional p.
intestinal bypass p.
invasive radiological vascular p.
Kasai p.
limb-lengthening p.
magnetic resonance angiography-
    directed bypass p.
neuroendovascular interventional p.
Nissen fundoplication p.
Pólya p.
postprocessing p.
provocative p.
psoas hitch p.
revascularization p.
Roux-en-Y p.
segmentation p.
Senning p.
spatial localization p.
stereotactic p.
Swenson pull-through p.
two-step p.
Whipple p.

process

accessory p.
acromion p.
alar p.
alveolar consolidative p.
apical p.
articular p.
ascending p.
auditory p.
basilar p.
bony p.
bremsstrahlung p.
calcaneal p.
capitular p.
carrier-free separation p.
caudate p.
clinoid p.
cochleariform p.
condyloid p.

conoid p.
consolidative p.
coracoacromial p.
coracoid p.
coronoid p.
costal p.
cribriform p.
cystic p.
destructive p.
2D filtering p.
energy transfer p.
ensiform p.
ethmoidal p.
falciform p.
fanning of the spinous p.
fibroplastic p.
frontal p.
frontonasal p.
frontosphenoidal p.
glenoid p.
inflammatory synovial p.
intercondylar p.
interspinous p.
intravascular clotting p.
jugular p.
knobby p.
lateral talar p.
left ventricular posterior superior p.
leptomeningeal p.
lumbar transverse p.
mastoid p.
maxillary p.
monarticular p.
neoplastic p.
neutron absorption p.
noncalcified ocular p.
notochordal p.
odontoid p.
olecranon p.
osseous destructive p.
paraneoplastic p.
posterior lateral talar p.
prominent xiphoid p.
pterygoid p.
radial styloid p.
radiostyloid p.
sacral p.
sacralized transverse p.
Sand p.
space-occupying p.
spinous p.
SSFP p.

NOTES

P

process (continued)
 Stieda p.
 styloid p.
 superior articulating p.
 supracondylar p.
 supracondyloid p.
 temporal p.
 p. tomography (PT)
 transverse p.
 trigonal p.
 trochlear p.
 ulnar styloid p.
 uncinate p.
 vermiform p.
 vertebral p.
 vertebrospinous p.
 within-slice filtering p.
 xiphoid p.
 zygomatic p.
processing
 digital imaging p. (DIP)
 enterocytic p.
 intrapixel sequential p. (IPSP)
 maximum entropy p.
 MIP image p.
 signal p.
processor
 array p.
 conventional p.
 daylight p.
 fast-array p.
 Kodak RP X-OMAT p.
 ML 700 daylight p.
 RP X-OMAT p.
 p. sensitometry
 sequence p.
processus vaginalis
prochordal plate
procoagulant
ProCol vascular bioprosthesis
proctogram
 balloon p.
 video p.
proctographic feature
proctography
 evacuation p.
proctopathy
 radiation p.
proctostat
procurvature deformity
product
 brightness area p. (BAP)
 decay p.
 dose area p. (DAP)
 fibrin-split p.
 fission p.
 iodine-labeled p.

 respiratory burst p.
 spallation p.
production
 Cerenkov radiation p.
 fast routine p.
 lactoferrin p.
 mitochondrial ATP p.
 one-step p.
 pair p.
 radionuclide p.
 radiopharmaceutical p.
 remote-controlled p.
 secondary electron p.
Profasi HP
profile
 CH20 Kernal and slim 2 p.
 3D dose p.
 excitation p.
 flat time-intensity p.
 flow velocity p.
 fluence p.
 P. mammography system
 nonlinear excitation p.
 number p.
 parabolic velocity p.
 peak p.
 projection p.
 p. ray view
 rectangular section p.
 section-sensitivity p.
 slice sensitivity p. (SSP)
 ultra-low p. (ULP)
 velocity p.
profilogram
profluens
Proforma catheter
profundal popliteal collateral index
profundus
 flexor digitorum p.
 p. tendon
profusion
 opacity p.
progeny
 radon p.
progeria
 adult p.
prognathic dilatation
prognathism
programmable
 p. stepper motor
 p. ventricular shunt valve
programmer
 pulse p.
 p. wand
progression
 inexorable p.

inflow disease p.
interval p.

progressive

p. coccidioidomycosis
p. degeneration
p. diaphyseal dysplasia (PDD)
p. dysphagia
p. emphysematous necrosis
p. familial cirrhosis
p. hydrocephalus
p. interstitial pulmonary fibrosis
p. massive fibrosis (PMF)
p. multifocal leukoencephalopathy
  (PML)
p. nodular pulmonary fibrosis
p. posttraumatic myelopathy
p. primary tuberculosis
p. rubella panencephalitis
p. spin saturation
p. stroke
p. subcortical gliosis
p. suppurative cholangitis
p. supranuclear palsy
p. systemic sclerosis
p. uptake

ProHance imaging agent
projectile horn
projection

p. angiogram
anterior p.
anteroposterior lordotic p.
AP p.
apical lordotic p.
average pixel p. (APP)
axial p.
axillary p.
back p.
ball-catcher p.
base p.
basilar p.
basovertical p.
p. binning
biplane p.
blowout view p.
bony vertebra p.
brow-down p.
brow-up p.
Caldwell p.
carpal tunnel p.
cartographic p.
caudad p., caudal p.
caudocranial p.

centroid-based maximum
  intensity p.
Chassard-Lapiné p.
Chausse III p.
Chaussier p.
coronal maximum-intensity p.
craniocaudal p.
cross-sectional transverse p.
cross-table lateral p.
cylindrical map p.
divergent ray p.
dorsoplantar p.
3D stereotactic surface p.
erect fluoro spot p.
fan-beam p.
fast Fourier p. (FFP)
FI p.
p. fiber damage
finger-like p.
Fletcher p.
flexion-extension p.
p. formula
frogleg lateral p.
full-scan p.
full scan with interpolation p.
Granger p.
half-axial anteroposterior p.
half-scan with extrapolation p.
Hermodsson tangential p.
intraoral p.
Lambert p.
LAO p.
lateral oblique axial p.
lateral transcranial p.
lateral transfacial p.
lateromedial oblique p.
left anterior oblique p.
left lateral p.
left posterior oblique p.
Low-Beers p.
L5-S1 p.
lumbosacral p.
maximum intensity p. (MIP)
maximum-intensity sliding thin
  slab p.
medial oblique axial p.
mediolateral oblique p.
Mercator p.
minimal intensity p. (minIP)
minimum-intensity sliding thin
  slab p.
modified p.

NOTES

P

projection *(continued)*
mortise p.
navicular p.
notch p.
nuchofrontal p.
oblique lateral p.
occipitomental p.
off-lateral p.
open-mouth p.
orthogonal angiographic p.
PA p.
panoramic surface p.
papillary p.
parietoorbital p.
Pawlow p.
pillar p.
Pirie transoral p.
plantodorsal p.
postdrainage p.
posterior p.
posteroanterior lordotic p.
presaturation p.
p. profile
radiographic p.
ramp-filtered back p.
ray-sum p.
p. reconstruction imaging
recumbent lateral p.
reversed Stenvers p.
Rhese p.
right anterior oblique p.
right posterior oblique p.
rotating tomographic p.
Runström p.
saturation inversion p. (SIP)
scaphoid p.
Schüller p.
semiaxial anteroposterior p.
semiaxial transcranial p.
Settegast p.
simulated annealing method p.
skyline p.
sliding thin-slab maximum
    intensity p. (STS-MIP)
steep left anterior oblique p.
steep Towne p.
Stenver p.
stereographic p.
stereo right lateral p.
stereotactic surface p. (SSP)
straight lateral p.
stress p.
Stryker notch p.
submentovertex p.
sunrise p.
superoinferior p.
surface p.

swimmer's p.
tangential p.
thin-slab minimum intensity p.
Towne p.
p. tract imaging
transaxial maximum-intensity p.
transthoracic p.
tunnel p.
under-filled submentovertical p.
under-scan method p.
variable p. (VARPRO)
verticosubmental p.
Vogt bone-free p.
Waters p.
p. x-ray microscope
projectional image
projection-reconstruction technique
projector
cine p.
liquid crystal display p.
white light pattern p.
prolactin-secreting pituitary
    macroadenoma
prolapse
anterior leaflet p.
p. of aortic valve
billowing mitral valve p.
cord p.
gastroduodenal mucosal p.
gastrojejunal mucosal p.
holosystolic mitral valve p.
intestinal p.
intracranial fat p.
mitral valve p. (MVP)
mitral valve leaflet systolic p.
posterior leaflet p.
rectal p.
p. of right aortic valve cusp
p. of spleen
systolic p.
tricuspid valve p.
p. of umbilical cord
valve p.
prolapsed
p. antral mucosa
p. gastric mucosa
p. mitral valve (PMV)
p. stoma
p. tumor
proliferation
angiofibroblastic p.
p. area
astrocytic p.
benign sclerosing ductal p.
bile duct p.
bizarre parosteal
    osteochondromatous p.

bizarre subparosteal
  osteochondromatous p.
p. of bone
bony p.
collagen tissue p.
connective tissue p.
extranodal p.
fibroplastic p.
p. of fibrous tissue
glandular p.
intimal p.
myofibrohistiocytic p.
myointimal p.
myxomatous p.
neointimal p.
neuronal p.
nodular p.
osteophytic p.
papillary p.
perineural glial p.
peripelvic fat p.
p. pleurisy
p. rate
reactive fibrovascular arachnoid p.
synovial p.
villous p.
proliferative
  p. bronchiolitis
  p. change
  p. glomerulonephritis
  p. index
  p. inflammation
  p. lesion
  p. pattern
  p. phase endometrium
prolonged
  p. ejection time
  p. expiratory phase
  p. inspiratory phase
  p. interval
  p. left ventricular impulse
  p. pregnancy
**Prolyse in acute cerebral
  thromboembolism (PROACT)**
promethium (Pm)
prominence
  aortic p.
  p. of bone
  bony p.
  hilar p.
  interstitial p.
  mediastinal p.

styloid p.
tibial tubercle p.
upper lobe vein p.
prominent
  p. ductal pattern
  p. ductal vascular structure
  p. liver
  p. pyramidal thyroid lobe
  p. rim of radiolucency
  p. septal lymphatic
  p. spur
  p. tubercle
  p. uptake
  p. vertebra
  p. xiphoid process
promontory
  p. mass
  sacral p.
pronate
pronation
  hallucal p.
  pes p.
pronation-abduction
  p.-a. fracture
  p.-a. injury
pronation-eversion fracture
pronation-external
  p.-e. rotation
  p.-e. rotation injury
pronator
  p. quadratus
  p. quadratus line
  round p.
  p. teres (PT)
  p. teres tendon
pronatus
  pes p.
prone
  p. film
  p. lateral view
  p. position
pronephron
  rudimentary p.
pronephros, pl. **pronephroi**
pronunciation
  artifact p.
propagation speed artifact
proper
  p. digital nerve branch
  p. hepatic artery (PHA)
properitoneal
  p. fat

NOTES

P

properitoneal *(continued)*
  p. fat line
  p. flank stripe
  p. hernia
prophylaxis
  preexposure p.
propidium iodide
proportion
  aneurysmal p.
proportional
  p. counter
  p. ratio
proportionality
  cephalofacial p.
propria
  lamina p.
  muscularis p.
  substantia p.
  tunica p.
propulsive
  p. mechanism
  p. movement
propyliodone imaging agent
prosencephalon
ProSound SSD-5500 ultrasound
prospective
  p. analysis
  p. investigation of pulmonary
    embolus diagnosis (PIOPED)
  p. synchronization
ProSpeed CT scanner
prostaglandin
  p. E_1
  p. E_1 injection
  p. infusion
Prostalase laser system
**Prostar XL 8, 10 suture mediated
  closure device**
ProstaScint
  P. monoclonal antibody imaging
    agent
  P. scan
prostate
  p. abscess
  p. anatomy
  apex of p.
  p. capsule
  p. carcinoma
  floating p.
  p. gland
  p. hypoechoic lesion
  p. implant
  inferolateral surface of p.
  lateral lobe of p.
  lymph vessel of p.
  median lobe of p.
  posterior surface of p.

  p. seeding
  transrectal ultrasound-guided biopsy
    of the p.
  transurethral incision of p.
  transurethral resection of p.
    (TURP)
  visual laser ablation of p. (VLAP)
prostatectomy
  transurethral ultrasound-guided laser-
    induced p. (TULIP)
prostatic
  p. adenoma
  p. bed
  p. calculus
  p. carcinoma
  p. cyst
  p. duct
  p. fluid
  p. hyperplasia
  p. hyperplastic nodule
  p. obstruction
  p. sinus
  p. stent
  p. transition zone
  p. urethra
  p. urethroplasty
  p. uterus
  p. venous plexus
prostaticovesical junction
prostatitis
  cavitary p.
  diverticular p.
prostatography
prosthetic
  p. cup
  p. femoral distal graft
  p. heart valve
  p. implant
  p. mitral valve
  p. replacement
  p. valve embolus
prostrema
  area p.
protactinium (Pa)
protection
  p. factor
  myocardial p.
  radiation p.
  region of p.
protein
  carrier p.
  CSF 14-3-3 p.
  macrophage inflammatory p. (MIP)
  prion p. (PrP)
proteinase
protein-bound iodine (PBI)
protein-losing enteropathy

protein-nucleic acid synthesis in tumor cell
proteinosis
    alveolar p.
    pulmonary alveolar p. (PAP)
proteoglycan matrix
Proteus syndrome
protium
protocol
    axial BMD center with agreed joint p.
    axial T1-SE p.
    biphasic injection p.
    Cornell p.
    CT scan with renal stone p.
    default display p.
    2D GRE dynamic p.
    Ellestad p.
    Heidelberg p.
    helical CT scanning p.
    low-dose/high-dose p.
    MP-RAGE p.
    neon particle p.
    point-to-point p. (PPP)
    proton relaxometric p.
    telomere repeat amplification p.
    transmission control protocol/Internet p. (TCP/IP)
    UCLA imaging p.
protodensity MR imaging
protodiastolic reversal of blood flow
proton
    p. beam
    p. brain examination (PROBE)
    p. chemical shift imaging
    p. dipole-dipole interaction
    p. electron dipole-dipole
    high-energy p.
    interstitial water p.
    lactate p.
    p. magnetic resonance
    methyl p.
    p. MR spectroscopic imaging
    p. nuclear magnetic resonance spectroscopy
    p. nuclear magnetic resonance spectrum
    precessing p.
    p. relaxation
    p. relaxation enhancement (PRE)
    p. relaxometric protocol
    p. spin-lattice relaxation time

proton-density
    p.-d. axial image
    p.-d. axial MR scan
proton-density-weighted
    p.-d.-w. fast spin-echo image
    p.-d.-w. imaging
    p.-d.-w. MRI
proton-electron double-resonance imaging (PEDRI)
proton-proton magnetization exchange
protoplasmic astrocytoma
protopulmonary bilharziasis
protracted
    p. exposure sensitization
    p. radiation
    p. venous infusion (PVI)
protruded disk
protruding
    p. atheroma
    p. fat
protrusio acetabuli
protrusion
    acetabular p.
    anal p.
    broad-based disk p.
    coil p.
    p. of cystocele
    disk p.
    hip p.
    p. of navicular
    spicular p.
    spoon-like p.
    vascular p.
protuberance
    bony p.
    occipital p.
protuberans
    dermatofibrosarcoma p.
provisional callus
provocable ischemia
provocative procedure
proximal
    p. acinar emphysema
    p. anterior descending artery
    p. anterior tibial artery
    p. aorta
    p. articular set angle (PASSA)
    p. aspect
    p. brain shift
    p. carpal row
    p. circumflex artery
    p. coil

NOTES

P

proximal *(continued)*
- p. colon
- p. convoluted tubule
- p. coronary (PCS)
- p. digital artery
- p. dilation
- p. and distal portion of vessel
- p. esophagitis dilatation
- p. femoral fracture
- p. femur
- p. fibula
- p. focal femoral deficiency (PFFD)
- p. humeral fracture
- p. interphalangeal joint (PIP, PIPJ)
- p. interphalangeal joint articulation
- p. isovelocity surface area (PISA)
- p. jejunum
- p. left anterior descending artery
- p. loop syndrome
- p. part of dorsal duct
- p. popliteal artery
- p. radioulnar joint
- p. segment
- p. small bowel
- p. third shaft
- p. tibia
- p. tibial metaphyseal fracture
- p. trochlear groove
- p. tubular adenoma

proximally

proximity
- p. arteriography
- p. injury
- stent p.

PrP
- prion protein

PRS
- Photon Radiosurgery System

prune belly syndrome

pruned
- p. appearance of pulmonary vasculature
- p. hilum

pruned-tree appearance

pruned-tree-appearance bile duct

pruning
- p. of pancreatic duct branch
- pulmonary artery p.

Prussak
- P. pouch
- P. space

PS
- partial saturation
- pulmonary sequestration

PSA
- power spectral analysis

psammoma
- p. body
- p. body meningioma
- Virchow p.

psammomatoid ossifying fibroma

psammomatous
- p. calcification
- p. meningioma
- p. microcalcification

psathyrosis

PSD
- periodic synchronous discharge

pseudarthrosis *(var. of pseudoarthrosis)*

pseudoacardia

pseudoachondroplasia

pseudoaneurysm
- anastomotic p.
- aortic p.
- arterial p.
- chronic posttraumatic aortic p.
- p. formation
- heart p.
- hepatic artery p.
- iatrogenic p.
- inguinal p.
- p. of the mitral-aortic fibrosa
- pancreatitis p.
- peripheral p.
- perivalvular p.
- postcatheterization p.
- postsurgical p.
- renal transplant p.
- saccular p.
- splenic artery p.
- traumatic aortic p.
- uterine artery p.

pseudoangiomatous stromal hyperplasia (PASH)

pseudoangiosarcoma

pseudoarthritis

pseudoarthrosis, pseudarthrosis
- long bone p.
- tibial p.

pseudoarticulation

pseudoascites

pseudo-AV block

pseudobulbar affect

pseudocalcification
- powder p.

pseudocalculus bile duct

pseudocapsule
- radiopaque p.

pseudocarcinoma

pseudocarcinomatous

pseudocavitation
- lung p.

pseudochylous effusion

pseudocirrhosis
    cholangiodysplastic p.
pseudocoarctation of aorta
pseudocolor B-mode
pseudocryptorchidism
pseudocyst
    adrenal p.
    gelatinous brain p.
    mature pancreatic p.
    meconium p.
    necrotic bone p.
    pancreatic p.
    pulmonary p.
    splenic p.
    subarticular p.
    umbilical cord p.
pseudocystic hygroma
pseudo-Dandy-Walker malformation
pseudodefect
pseudodextrocardia
pseudodiffusion
pseudodisease
pseudodislocation
pseudodissection
pseudodiverticula
    small bowel p.
pseudodiverticulosis
    intramural esophageal p.
pseudodiverticulum
    retrograde ureteral p.
pseudodynamic MR imaging
pseudoepiphysis
pseudoexstrophy
pseudofollicle
pseudofollicular salpingitis
pseudofracture
    p. artifact
    milkman's p.
pseudogating
    diastolic p.
pseudogestational sac
pseudogland formation
pseudoglioma
pseudogout
pseudogynecomastia
pseudohaustration
pseudohermaphroditism
    female p.
pseudohomogeneous edema pattern
pseudo-Hurler deformity
pseudohypertrophy
pseudohypoparathyroidism (PHP)

pseudoinfarct pattern
pseudointimal
    p. formation
    p. hyperplasia
pseudointraligamentary pregnancy
pseudointussusception
pseudo-Jefferson fracture
pseudojoint
pseudolesion
pseudoluxation
pseudolymphoma
    breast p.
    gastric p.
    lung p.
pseudomalignant
    p. myositis ossificans
    p. tumor
pseudomantle zone pattern
pseudomass
    mediastinal p.
    mucous p.
pseudomembrane
    fetal neck p.
pseudomembranous
    p. colitis
    p. inflammation
    p. radiation gastritis
pseudomeningocele
    posttraumatic intradiploic p.
pseudomitral leaflet
pseudomucinous cystadenocarcinoma
pseudomyxoma peritonei
pseudoneoplasm
pseudonephritis
    athlete's p.
pseudoneuroma
pseudoneuropathic joint
pseudoobstruction
    bowel p.
    chronic idiopathic intestinal p.
    (CIIP)
    colonic p.
    familial intestinal p.
    idiopathic intestinal p.
    nonfamilial intestinal p.
pseudoomphalocele
pseudoorbital tumor
pseudoosteomalacic pelvis
pseudopancreatitis
pseudoperiostitis
pseudoplaque
pseudopneumoperitoneum

NOTES

P

pseudopod formation
pseudopodia
pseudopolyp definition
pseudopolyposis lymphatica
pseudoporencephaly
pseudopost Billroth I appearance
pseudopregnancy
pseudopseudohypoparathyroidism
pseudo-pseudotumor
pseudopyogenic granuloma
pseudorosette
    perivascular p.
pseudosac
pseudosacculation
pseudosarcoma
    esophageal p.
pseudosarcomatous fasciitis
pseudosclerosis
    spastic p.
pseudosheath
pseudospondylolisthesis
    Junghans p.
pseudostenosis
    sigmoid p.
pseudostone
pseudostricture
    colon p.
pseudosubluxation
    C-spine p.
pseudotear
pseudothickening
pseudothrombophlebitis syndrome
pseudothrombosis
pseudotrabecula
pseudotrochanteric bursitis
pseudotruncus arteriosus
pseudotumor
    abdominal p.
    p. appearance
    atelectatic asbestos p.
    p. cerebri (PTC)
    fibrosing inflammatory p.
    hemophilic p.
    inflammatory idiopathic orbital p.
    inflammatory intestinal p.
    intraosseous hemophilic p.
    kidney p.
    orbital p.
    pleura p.
    renal p.
    small bowel p.
    vermian p.
    xanthomatous p.
pseudo-Turner syndrome
pseudoulceration
pseudoureterocele
pseudovagina

pseudo-Whipple disease
pseudowidening
    joint space p.
pseudoxanthoma elasticum
pseudo-Zollinger-Ellison syndrome
PSF
    point-spread function
    posterior spine fusion
PSH-25GT transcranial imaging
    transducer
PSIF
    reverse fast imaging with steady-state
    free precession
psoas
    p. abscess
    p. fascia
    p. hitch procedure
    p. line
    p. major
    p. margin
    p. muscle
    p. shadow
    p. shadow angle
    p. sign
    p. stripe
psoralen and ultraviolet A (PUVA)
PSP
    photostimulable phosphor
      PSP imaging plate
^{31}P spectroscopy
PSR
    phase sampling ratio
PSSE
PT
    pneumothorax
    process tomography
    pronator teres
Pt
    platinum
PTA
    percutaneous transluminal angioplasty
    persistent truncus arteriosus
    primitive trigeminal artery
PTBD
    percutaneous transhepatic biliary drainage
PTC
    percutaneous transhepatic cholangiogram
    pseudotumor cerebri
PTCA
    percutaneous transhepatic cholangiogram
    percutaneous transluminal coronary
      angioplasty
PTCD
    percutaneous transhepatic cholangial
      drainage
pterion
pterional transsylvian approach

p-terphenyl
pterygium colli
pterygoid
> p. artery
> p. bone
> p. canal
> p. chest
> p. fossa
> p. muscle
> p. plate
> p. plexus
> p. process

pterygoideus hamulus
pterygomandibular
> p. ligament
> p. raphe

pterygopalatine
> p. canal
> p. fossa
> p. ganglion

pterygospinous ligament
PTF
> posterior talofibular

PTFE
> polytetrafluoroethylene

PTFE stent
PTF ligament
PTHC
> percutaneous transhepatic cholangiogram
> percutaneous transhepatic
>   cholangiography

PTK
> phototherapeutic keratectomy

pTL
ptosis, pl. **ptoses**
ptotic kidney
Ptp
> transpulmonary pressure

PTRA
> percutaneous transluminal renal
>   angioplasty

PTT
> posterior tibial tendon
> pulse transit time

PTV
> planning target volume
> posterior temporal vertical

ptyalography
pubescent uterus
pubic
> p. arch
> p. bone

> p. bone maldevelopment
> p. crest
> p. ramus
> p. symphysis
> p. tubercle

pubica
> symphysis p.

pubis
> mons p.
> os p.
> osteitis p.
> pecten p.
> symphysis ossium p.
> widened symphysis p.

pubocapsular ligament
pubocervical ligament
pubococcygeal line (PCL)
pubococcygeus muscle
pubofemoral ligament
puboischial area
puboprostatic ligament
puborectalis loop
pubovesical ligament
PU catheter
Puck film changer
PUD
> peptic ulcer disease

puddle sign
puddling
> p. of contrast
> peripheral p.

pudenda
> ulcerating granuloma of p.

pudendal
> p. blood supply
> p. branch
> p. canal
> p. cleft
> p. vein
> p. vein reflux

PUJ
> pelviureteric junction

pullback
> p. across aortic valve
> aortic p.
> p. arterial marking
> p. esophagram
> p. imaging
> p. pressure gradient
> p. pressure recording
> p. study

NOTES

P

pulley
>   bone p.
>   p. of finger

pull maneuver

pull-type gastrostomy tube

pull-up
>   gastric p.-u.

pulmoaortic canal

pulmogram

pulmolith

pulmolithiasis

pulmonale
>   atrium p.
>   cor p.

pulmonary
>   p. abscess
>   p. adenopathy
>   p. alveolar microlithiasis
>   p. alveolar proteinosis (PAP)
>   p. alveolus
>   p. amyloidosis
>   p. angioma
>   p. aplasia
>   p. arborization
>   p. arc
>   p. arterial circulation
>   p. arterial flow insufficiency
>   p. arterial hypertension
>   p. arterial input impedance
>   p. arterial malformation
>   p. arterial marking
>   p. arterial occlusion
>   p. arterial resistance index
>   p. arterial systolic pressure to
>   systemic arterial systolic pressure
>   p. arterial vent
>   p. arterial wedge pressure
>   p. arteriography
>   p. arteriolar resistance
>   p. arteriolar vasoconstriction
>   p. arteriosclerosis
>   p. arteriovenous aneurysm
>   p. arteriovenous fistula
>   p. arteriovenous malformation
>   (PAVM)
>   p. artery (PA)
>   p. artery agenesis
>   p. artery apoplexy
>   p. artery atresia
>   p. artery balloon pump (PABP)
>   p. artery bifurcation
>   p. artery blockage
>   p. artery-bronchus ratio
>   p. artery compression ascending
>   aortic aneurysm

>   p. artery diastolic pressure and
>   pulmonary artery wedge pressure
>   (PADP-PAWP)
>   p. artery dilatation
>   p. artery embolization
>   p. artery end-diastolic pressure
>   (PAEDP)
>   p. artery hemorrhage
>   p. artery interruption
>   p. artery intima
>   p. artery mean pressure (PAM)
>   p. artery obstruction
>   p. artery peak systolic pressure
>   p. artery pressure (PAP)
>   p. artery pruning
>   p. artery to right ventricle diastolic
>   gradient
>   p. artery sarcoma
>   p. artery stenosis
>   p. artery stenting
>   p. artery systolic pressure (PAS)
>   p. artery wedge angiography
>   p. artery wedge pressure (PAWP)
>   p. asbestosis
>   p. aspergillosis
>   p. aspiration
>   p. atrium
>   p. barotrauma
>   p. blood flow (PBF)
>   p. blood flow redistribution
>   p. blood flow study
>   p. blood volume
>   p. blood volume index (PBVI)
>   p. calcification
>   p. capillary endothelium
>   p. capillary hemangiomatosis
>   p. capillary permeability
>   p. capillary pressure (PCP)
>   p. capillary wedge position
>   p. capillary wedge pressure
>   (PCWP)
>   p. capillary wedge tracing
>   p. and cardiac sclerosis
>   p. cartilage
>   p. cavitation
>   p. cavity
>   p. cirrhosis
>   p. confluence
>   p. consolidation
>   p. contusion
>   p. cyst
>   p. cystic lymphangiectasis
>   p. density
>   p. dysmaturity
>   p. edema (PE)
>   p. edema photographic negative
>   p. embolic septic disease

p. embolus (PE)
p. failure
p. flow pattern
p. function test
p. gas
p. gas exchange
p. hamartoma
p. heart
p. hilum
p. histoplasmosis
p. hyalinizing granuloma
p. hyperinflation
p. hypoperfusion
p. hypoplasia
p. idiopathic fibrosis
p. incompetence
p. infarct
p. interstitial abnormality
p. interstitial disease
p. interstitial emphysema (PIE)
p. interstitial idiopathic fibrosis
p. interstitial thinning
p. interstitium
p. juxtaesophageal lymph node
p. Kaposi sarcoma
p. lesion
p. ligament
p. linearity
p. lobe
p. lymphangiomatosis
p. lymphoid disorder
p. lymphoma
p. magnetic resonance angiography
 (PMRA)
p. mainline granulomatosis
p. mass
p. meningioma
p. metastasis
p. microcirculation
p. microvasculature
p. neuroendocrine cell hyperplasia
p. nodularity
p. nodule
p. nodule enhancement
p. orifice
p. osteoarthropathy
p. outflow gradient
p. outflow obstruction
p. overdistention
p. overexpansion
p. overinflation
p. papillomatosis

p. parenchyma
p. parenchymal change
p. parenchymal infection
p. parenchymal infiltrate
p. parenchymal injury
p. parenchymal window
p. pedicle
p. perfusion imaging
p. perfusion MRI contrast agent
p. perfusion and ventilation
p. pleura
p. pleurisy
p. plexus
p. pseudocyst
p. quantitative differential function
 study
p. resection
p. sarcoidosis
p. scar
p. scintigraphy
p. sclerosing hemangioma
p. segment
p. sequestration (PS)
p. sequestration spectrum
p. sinus
p. sling
p. sling complex
p. squamous cell carcinoma
p. stable echo-enhancer
p. stenosis
p. structural maturation
p. subcutaneous encephalitis
 emphysema
p. sulcus
p. talcosis
p. telangiectasia
p. thromboembolic disease
p. thromboembolism
p. thromboembolization
p. thrombosis
p. time activity curve
p. trunk
p. trunk bifurcation
p. trunk idiopathic dilatation
p. tuberculosis
p. tumor
p. valve
p. valve anulus
p. valve area
p. valve atresia
p. valve cusp
p. valve deformity

NOTES

P

pulmonary *(continued)*
    p. valve dysplasia
    p. valve insufficiency
    p. valve stenosis
    p. valve stenosis dilatation
    p. varix
    p. vascular bed
    p. vascular bed impedance
    p. vascular congestion
    p. vascularity
    p. vascular marking
    p. vascular obstruction
    p. vascular pattern
    p. vascular redistribution
    p. vascular reserve
    p. vascular resistance (PVR)
    p. vascular resistance index (PVRI)
    p. vasculature
    p. vasoreactivity
    p. vein
    p. vein apoplexy
    p. vein atresia
    p. vein fibrosis
    p. vein stenosis
    p. vein wedge angiography
    p. venous congestion (PVC)
    p. venous drainage
    p. venous hypertension
    p. venous obstruction
    p. venous return
    p. venous system
    p. venous-systemic air embolus
    p. venous wedge pressure
    p. ventilation imaging
    p. vesicle
    p. vessel
    p. vessel overcirculation
    p. wedge pressure (PWP)
pulmonic
    p. area
    p. atresia
    p. infiltrate
    p. insufficiency (PI)
    p. output
    p. output flow
    p. output index
    p. regurgitation (PR)
    p. stenosis
    p. valve (PV)
    p. valve gradient
    p. valve regurgitation
    p. valvular stenosis
    p. versus systemic flow
pulmonic-systemic flow ratio
pulmonis
    crista p.
    lingula p.

pulp
    p. abscess
    p. canal
    p. of finger
    p. space
    p. stone
pulpal abscess
pulposus
    herniated nucleus p. (HNP)
pulsatile perfusion
pulsatility
    arterial p.
    p. indices
    p. measurement
pulsating
    p. current
    p. empyema
    p. mass
    p. metastasis
    p. pleurisy
    p. vein
pulsation
    p. artifact
    capillary p.
    mean venous p.
    p. pattern
pulse
    adiabatic slice-selective
      radiofrequency p.
    p. amplifier
    balanced fast-field-echo p.
    compensated composite spin-lock p.
    composite p.
    dampened obstructive p.
    DANTE-selective p.
    depth p.
    p. design
    diastolic depolarization p.
    Doppler p.
    p. Doppler interrogation
    2D spatially selective
      radiofrequency p.
    p.-echo image
    p.-echo imaging
    p.-echo technique
    E point of cardiac apex p.
    p. fashion pulse spray
    fat suppression p.
    p. flip angle
    frequency-selective p.
    globally optimized alternating phase
      rectangular p. (GARP)
    gradient p.
    p. height spectral analysis
    inversion p.
    p. labeling
    p. length

motion compensation gradient p.
MP inversion p.
narrow-band spectral-selective
  radiofrequency p.
navigator p.
p. NMR
nonselective p.
phase-encode p.
6-p., 3-phase generator
12-p., 3-phase generator
picosecond p.
presaturation p.
p. pressure
p. programmer
radiofrequency p.
radiofrequency excitation p.
p. reappearance time
p. repetition frequency
p. repetition time
resting p.
RF p.
saturation p.
section-select p.
selective p.
p. sequence
p. sequence echo-planar imaging
p. shape
small water-hammer p.
spatially selective inversion p.
synchronous carotid arterial p.
tailored p.
tidal wave of carotid arterial p.
time following inversion p. (TI)
p. transit time (PTT)
trough of venous p.
twin-peaked p.
velocity-compensating gradient p.
vertical synchronization p.
p. voltage
p. volume recording (PVR)
p. volume waveform
V peak of jugular venous p.
p. width (PW)
p. width variation
pulsed
  p. arterial spin labeling
  p. arterial spin labeling sequence
  p. Doppler flowmeter
  p. Doppler transesophageal
    echocardiography
  p. Doppler ultrasound

p. Doppler waveform
p. dose rate (PDR)
p. dye laser therapy
p. electron paramagnetic imaging
p. infrared laser
p. L-band ESR spectrometry
p. magnetization transfer MR
  imaging
p. metal vapor laser
p. mode
p. nuclear magnetic resonance
p. pump
p. therapeutic low-intensity
  ultrasound
p. wave
p. wave Doppler ultrasonography
pulsed-dye
  p.-d. laser
  p.-d. laser lithotripsy
pulsed-electron paramagnetic NMR
pulsed-gradient
  p.-g. spin echo (PGSE)
  p.-g. spin-echo echo-planar pulse
    sequence
  p.-g. spin-echo technique
pulsed-mode operation
pulsed-wave
  p.-w. Doppler
  p.-w. Doppler echocardiography
  p.-w. Doppler recording
  p.-w. spectral color Doppler signal
pulse-echo
  p.-e. distance measurement
  p.-e. method
pulse-height analyzer (PHA)
pulse-inversion
  p.-i. harmonic imaging (PIHI)
  p.-i. harmonic ultrasound
  p.-i. imaging
PulseMaster laser
Pulse-Spray
  P.-S. injector
  P.-S./PRO infusion catheter
  P.-S. pulsed infusion system
pulse-spray technique
pulsing current
pulsion diverticulum
Pulsolith laser lithotripter
pulsus
  p. alternans
  p. paradoxus

NOTES

P

pulverized
>p. plaque
>p. plaque particulate matter

pulvinar
>p. hip joint
>p. hyperintensity
>p. sign
>p. sign of vCJD
>p. of thalamus

pump
>AutoCAT intraaortic balloon p.
>balloon p.
>gradient p.
>implantable infusion p.
>intraaortic balloon p. (IABP)
>intraarterial chemotherapy p.
>ion p.
>p. lung
>pulmonary artery balloon p. (PABP)
>pulsed p.

punch
>Sweet sternal p.

punched-out
>p.-o. appearance
>p.-o. area
>p.-o. bony defect
>p.-o. lytic bone lesion
>p.-o. ulcer

punch-through
puncta (*pl. of* punctum)
punctata
>chondrodysplasia p.
>rhizomelic chondrodysplasia p.

punctate
>p. calcification
>p. enhancement
>p. hyperintense focus
>p. infiltrate
>p. lesion
>p. necrosis
>p. ulcer
>p. white matter hyperintensity

punctation
punctum, pl. **puncta**
puncture
>antegrade p.
>cisternal p.
>CT-directed p.
>diagnostic p.
>direct needle p.
>fine-needle p.
>p. fracture
>p. guidance
>lumbar p. (LP)
>maxillary sinus p.
>nephrostomy p.

>p. path
>retrograde nephrostomy p.
>stereotactic p.
>p. transducer
>p. ulcer
>ultrasound-guided nephrostomy p.
>p. wound osteomyelitis

pupillary
>p. constrictor muscle
>p. sign

pupillometer
>Pupilscan II p.

Pupilscan II pupillometer
purging
>bone marrow p.
>immunomagnetic p.

purinoceptor
>myocyte membrane p.

purity
>radiochemical p.
>radioisotopic p.
>radionuclide p.
>radiopharmaceutical p.

Purkinje fiber
purpose
>Low Energy All P. (LEAP)

purse-stringing effect
purulent
>p. lesion
>p. pleurisy
>p. pneumonia
>p. salpingitis
>p. synovitis

push maneuver
push-pull
>p.-p. ankle stress view
>p.-p. hip view

pustulotic arthroosteitis
putamen, pl. **putamina**
putaminal hemorrhage
putty kidney
PUV
>posterior urethral valve

PUVA
>posterior urethrovesical angle
>psoralen and ultraviolet A
>>PUVA radiation
>>PUVA therapy

PV
>pulmonic valve

PVA
>polyvinyl alcohol
>>PVA particle

PVB
>polyvinyl butyral

PVC
>polyvinyl chloride

premature ventricular contraction
pulmonary venous congestion
   PVC catheter
PVD
peripheral vascular disease
PVE
periventricular echogenicity
PVG
periventricular gray
   PVG matter
PVI
protracted venous infusion
PVL
periventricular leukomalacia
PVM
parallel virtual machine
PVP
polyvinylpyrrolidone
portal venous-dominant phase
portal venous phase
portal venous pressure
   PVP image
PVR
peripheral vascular resistance
perspective volume rendering
pulmonary vascular resistance
pulse volume recording
   PVR fly-through viewing
PVRI
pulmonary vascular resistance index
PVS
peritoneovenous shunt
PVST
   PVST shadow
PW
posterior wall
pulse width
P wave to QRS wave ratio (P/QRS)
PWI
perfusion-weighted imaging
PWP
pulmonary wedge pressure
PWT
posterior wall thickness
PXA
pleomorphic xanthoastrocytoma
pyarthrosis, pl. **pyarthroses**
pycnodysostosis
pyelectasia
pyelectasis
   fetal p.

pyelitis
   p. cystica
   emphysematous p.
pyelocaliceal, pyelocalyceal
   p. diverticulum
   p. system
pyelocaliectasis
pyelofluoroscopy
pyelogenic cyst
pyelogram
   dragon p.
   hydrated p.
   infusion p.
pyelographic appearance time
pyelography
   air p.
   antegrade p.
   ascending p.
   drip infusion p.
   p. by elimination
   excretion p.
   excretory intravenous p.
   p. imaging
   infusion p.
   intravenous p. (IVP)
   lateral p.
   needle p.
   percutaneous antegrade p.
   rapid-sequence intravenous p.
   respiration p.
   retrograde p.
   washout p.
pyelolymphatic backflow
pyelolysis
pyelonephritis
   acute suppurative p.
   atrophic p.
   chronic atrophic p.
   emphysematous p. (EPN)
   suppurative p.
   xanthogranulomatous p.
pyeloplasty
pyelorenal backflow
pyeloscopy
pyelostogram
pyelotomy
   Davis intubated p.
pyelotubular backflow
pyeloureteritis cystica
pyeloureterography
pyeloureterostomy
pyelovenous backflow

NOTES

P

pyemic embolus
pygopagus twin
Pyle
    P. disease
    P. dysplasia
pyloric
    p. antrum
    p. canal
    p. cap
    p. channel
    p. channel length
    p. channel ulcer
    p. diameter
    p. hypertrophy
    p. index
    p. insufficiency
    p. lymph node
    p. muscle
    p. orifice
    p. outlet
    p. outlet obstruction
    p. ring
    p. sphincter
    p. stenosis
    p. stricture
    p. teat
    p. valve
    p. volume
pyloroduodenal
    p. junction
    p. obstruction
pyloroplasty
pylorospasm
    infantile p.
    persistent p.
pylorus
    hypertrophic p.
    torus p.
pyocele
pyocephalus
pyoderma granulosa
pyogenic
    p. brain abscess
    p. cholangitis
    p. liver
    p. liver abscess
    p. osteomyelitis
    p. pneumonia

pyometra
pyomyositis
pyonephrosis
pyopneumothorax
pyosalpinx
pyothorax
pyothorax-associated pleural lymphoma
pyoureter ectopic ureterocele
PYP
    pyrophosphate
        PYP imaging
        PYP technetium myocardial scan
pyramid
    medullary p.
    p. method for ventricular volume
    petrous p.
    renal medullary p.
pyramidal
    p. bone
    p. eminence
    p. fracture
    p. hemorrhagic zone
    p. layer of cerebral cortex
    p. lobe
    p. neuron
    p. sign
    p. system
    p. tract
pyridine
    ACS-grade p.
pyridone derivative
pyriform (*var. of* piriform)
pyriformis (*var. of* piriformis)
pyrimidine
    p. analog
    halogenated p.
pyrogen testing
PYROLITE kit
pyrophosphate (PYP)
    p. arthropathy
    p. crystal
    p. imaging
    p. scintigraphy
    stannous p.
    ^{99m}Tc p.
    p. technetium myocardial scan
    tetrasodium p. (TSPP)

Q
    cardiac output
    quotient
        Q angle
        Q space
QCA
    quantitative coronary angiography
    quantitative coronary arteriography
Q-catheter catheterization recording system
Q-complex
    myocardial perfusion imaging Q-c.
QCSI
    quantitative chemical shift imaging
QCT
    quantitative computed tomography
        QCT bone densitometry system
        QCT imaging
QCT 3000 system for bone densitometry
QDA
    quadratic discriminant analysis
QDE
    quantum detection efficiency
QEEG
    quantitative electroencephalography
QF
    quality factor
QGS
    quantitative gated SPECT
QHS
    quantitative hepatobiliary scintigraphy
QM
    quantization matrix
qMRI, QMRI
    quantitative magnetic resonance imaging
QO$_2$
    oxygen consumption
QPD
    quadrature phase detector
QR pattern
QRS
    Q. interval
    Q. score
    Q. synchronized shock
    Q. vector
QRST angle
Q-switched
    Q-s. Nd:YAG laser
    Q-s. ruby laser
Q-switching
QUAD
    Q. 7000, 12000 high-field open MRI scanner
quadrangle cartilage

quadrangulation of Frouin
quadrant
    q. of death
    q. energy
    left lower q. (LLQ)
    left upper q. (LUQ)
    lower inner q. (LIQ)
    lower outer q. (LOQ)
    lower right q. (LRQ)
    outer upper right q. (OURQ)
    right lower q. (RLQ)
    right upper q. (RUQ)
    upper inner q. (UIQ)
    upper left q. (ULQ)
    upper outer q. (UOQ)
    upper right q. (URQ)
quadrantal
quadrate
    q. gyrus
    q. ligament
    q. lobe of liver
    q. muscle
quadratic
    q. dependence
    q. discriminant analysis (QDA)
    q. phase gain
quadrature
    q. body coil
    q. cervical spine coil
    q. detection
    q. excitation
    q. phase detector (QPD)
    q. phase detector artifact
    q. radiofrequency receiver coil
    q. setting
    q. surface coil MRI system
    q. terminal latency surface coil
    q. transmit/receive head coil
quadratus
    q. femoris
    q. femoris fascia
    q. lumborum
    pronator q.
quad resonance NMR probe circuit
quadriceps
    q. apron
    q. femoris
    q. femoris tendon reflex test
    q. muscle
    q. tendon
    q. tendon tear
quadricuspid
    q. aortic valve
    q. pulmonary valve

quadrigeminal
  q. plate
  q. plate cistern
  q. segment of posterior cerebral
    artery
  q. vein
quadrigeminy
quadrilateral
  q. bone
  q. brim
  q. plate
  q. retinoblastoma
  q. space syndrome
quadrilocular
quadripartite
quadriplegia
quadriplegic
quadripolar
  q. nucleus
  q. signal broadening
quadripole
quadrisect
quadrisection
quadritubercular
quadrupole moment
Quain fatty degeneration of heart
qualitative
  q. analysis
  q. assessment
  q. index
  q. study
quality
  q. factor (QF)
  image q.
quanta (*pl. of* quantum)
quantification
  acoustic q.
  automated q.
  flow q.
  rapid fluid q.
  shunt q.
quantimeter
quantitative
  q. amniotic fluid volume
  q. analysis
  q. brain imaging
  q. cardiac perfusion
  q. chemical shift imaging (QCSI)
  q. computed tomography (QCT)
  q. coronary angiography (QCA)
  q. coronary arteriography (QCA)
  q. CT densitometry
  q. CT during expiration
  q. digital radiography
  q. Doppler assessment
  q. electroencephalography (QEEG)
  q. exercise thallium-201 variable

  q. fluorescence imaging
  q. gated SPECT (QGS)
  q. hepatobiliary scintigraphy (QHS)
  q. imaging of perfusion using a
    single subtraction (QUIPPS)
  q. imaging technique
  q. index
  q. lung perfusion imaging
  q. magnetic resonance imaging
    (qMRI, QMRI)
  q. magnetization transfer
  q. regional myocardial flow
    measurement
  q. region lung function study
  q. scan
  q. spirometrically controlled CT
  q. spirometrically controlled CT
    imaging
  q. track etch autoradiography
quantitization
  vector q.
quantity
  spectrophotometric q.
quantization
  q. error
  q. matrix (QM)
  q. matrix scaling
  sequential scalar q. (SSQ)
  wavelet scalar q. (WSQ)
quantizer-design algorithm
quantum, pl. **quanta**
  q. detection efficiency (QDE)
  q. energy
  q. limit
  q. Monorail balloon catheter
  q. mottle
  q. mottle index
  q. mottling pattern
  q. noise
  q. number
  q. sink
  q. theory
  q. unit
**Quant-X color quantification imaging
  tool**
quarter-detector offset
quartisect
quartz
  q. glass
  q. lamp
quasi-accelerated fractionation
quasiradiographic image
Queckenstedt sign
quellung reaction
Quénu-Muret sign
questionable lesion

Quick
    Q. CT9800 scanner
    Q. Spin Sephadex G-50 column
Quick-Core biopsy needle
quiescence
Quik-Prep
    Quinton Q.-P.
Quimby implant system
Quinby classification of pelvic fracture
Quincke
    Q. sign
    Q. spinal needle
quinti
    abductor digiti q. (ADQ)
    extensor digiti q.

Quinton
    Q. PermCath
    Q. Quik-Prep
QUIPPS
    quantitative imaging of perfusion using a
    single subtraction
Quotane
quotient (Q)
    amnionic head q. (AHQ)
    Rayleigh q.
QUS-2 calcaneal ultrasonometer
Q-wave myocardial infarct
QX/I CT scanner

NOTES

R

radius

resistance

roentgen

root

R1

longitudinal relaxivity

R2

transverse relaxivity

r

roentgen

RA

right atrium

rotational angiography

rotational atherectomy

Integris 3D RA

Ra

radium

²²⁶Ra

radium-226

²²⁶Ra needle

RAA

right atrial appendage

Raaf Cath vascular catheter

RAB

remote afterloading brachytherapy

rabbit ear strand

racemose

r. aneurysm

r. cyst

racetrack microtron accelerator

rachioscoliosis

rachischisis of atlas

rachitic

r. pelvis

r. rosary

RAD

reactive airway disease

right axis deviation

rad

radian

radiation adsorbed dose

radarkymography

radiability

radiable

radiad

radial

r. anular tear

r. aplasia

r. artery to cephalic vein fistula

r. blurring

r. bone

r. breast scar

r. bursa

r. collateral ligament

r. deviation

r. digital artery

r. drift

r. epiphyseal displacement

r. facing of metacarpal head

r. fossa

r. glial fiber

r. head

r. head fracture

r. head subluxation

r. height

r. inclination

r. length

r. metacarpal ligament

r. neck fracture

r. neck groove

r. plane

r. ray anomaly

r. ray defect

r. ridge

r. scar

r. scar-like mammographic
appearance

r. sclerosing lesion

r. shift

r. sigmoid notch

r. split tear

r. styloid fracture

r. styloid process

r. technique

r. tuberosity

r. vascular thermal injury

r. width

radialis

flexor carpi r.

r. sign

radialized

radian (rad)

radiant energy

radiate sternocostal ligament

radiation

adjuvant r.

r. adsorbed dose (rad)

afterloading r.

alpha r.

annihilation r.

background r.

backscattered r.

r. barrier

r. beam

r. beam monitor

beta r.

r. biology

bone injury r.

braking r.

radiation *(continued)*
- bremsstrahlung r.
- r. burn
- r. carcinogenesis
- r. cataract
- Cerenkov r.
- characteristic r.
- r. chemistry
- r. chimera
- corpuscular r.
- cosmic r.
- r. counter
- cyclotron r.
- r. cystitis
- r. detector
- diagnostic r.
- direct r.
- dose equivalent r.
- r. dose perturbation
- r. dosimetry
- r. dosimetry calculation
- r. dosimetry of 18F-fluorocholine
- r. effect
- electromagnetic r.
- r. energy
- r. enhancement
- r. enteritis
- r. enteropathy
- r. erythema
- r. exposure
- external beam r.
- fatal dose of r.
- r. fistula
- fractionated r.
- gamma r.
- r. gastritis
- r. of Gratiolet
- r. hepatitis
- heterogeneous r.
- high linear energy transfer r.
- homogeneous r.
- r. hormesis
- Huldshinsky r.
- hyperfractionated r.
- hysterectomy and r. (H&R)
- infrared r.
- r. injury
- r. intensity
- r. interrogation
- interstitial r.
- intracoronary artery r.
- ionization r.
- ionizing r.
- K r.
- r. leakage
- man-made environmental r.
- Maxwell theory of r.
- megavoltage r.
- monochromatic synchrotron r.
- monoenergetic r.
- r. myelitis
- r. myelopathy
- natural r.
- r. necrosis
- r. nephritis
- r. nephropathy
- neutron r.
- nonionizing r.
- nuclear radiationoccupational r.
- r. oncogenesis
- r. oncology
- optic r.
- r. osteitis
- r. osteonecrosis
- photon theory of r.
- r. physics
- r. pneumonia
- r. pneumonitis
- r. poisoning
- polychromatic r.
- r. port
- r. portal
- prenatal r.
- primary r.
- r. proctopathy
- r. protection
- protracted r.
- PUVA r.
- radiofrequency r.
- recoil r.
- rectum r.
- remnant r.
- r. response (RR)
- r. risk
- Rollier r.
- scatter r.
- scattered r.
- secondary r.
- r. seed
- r. sensitivity testing
- r. sensitizer
- r. sickness
- solar r.
- specific r.
- spontaneous r.
- r. stenosis
- stray r.
- superficial r.
- supervoltage r.
- synchrotron r.
- r. synovectomy
- terrestrial r.
- therapeutic external r.
- r. therapy (RT)

r. therapy planning (RTP)
r. therapy planning system
r. therapy sequela
r. therapy system (RTS)
thermal r.
thorny bone r.
tissue tolerance to r.
r. treatment planning (RTP)
ultraviolet r.
useful-beam r.
r. warning symbol
r. weighting factor
white r.
whole-body r. (WBR)
r. window
radiation-associated papillary tumor
radiation-attenuating surgical glove
radiation-induced
r.-i. carcinoma
r.-i. cerebral atrophy
r.-i. change
r.-i. colitis
r.-i. fibrosis (RIF)
r.-i. ischemia
r.-i. leukoencephalopathy
r.-i. liver disease (RILD)
r.-i. necrosis (RIN)
r.-i. pericarditis
r.-i. peripheral nerve tumor
r.-i. pulmonary toxicity
r.-i. sarcoma
r.-i. sclerosing adenosis
r.-i. skin injury
r.-i. ulcer
r.-i. upregulation
radiation oncology
radiation-related
r.-r. ischemia
r.-r. ischemic change
r.-r. optic neuropathy (RON)
radiation-treated astrocytoma
radical
free r.
heterocyclic free r.
leucine r.
nitroxide-stable free r.
organic free r.
r. parametrectomy
stable free r.
r. vulvectomy
radices (*pl. of* radix)
radiciform

radicular
r. artery
r. compression
r. cyst
r. vessel
radiculomedullary artery
radiculomeningeal fistula
radiculomyelitis
radiculopathy
cervical spondylotic r.
radiculospinal artery
radiferous
RADIFOCUS
R. Glidecath
R. Glidewire
R. hydrophilic coated guidewire
radii (*pl. of* radius)
Radinyl
radioactive
r. aerosol
r. atom
r. bolus
r. brain scan
r. cancer-specific targeting agent
r. cobalt
r. colloid
r. constant (Λ)
^{11}C palmitic acid r.
r. cyanocobalamin
r. decay
r. disintegration
r. effluents
r. element
r. emission
r. equilibrium
r. fallout
r. fibrinogen imaging
r. fibrinogen scan
r. gallium
r. gas
r. half-life
r. iodide conversion ratio
r. iodinated serum albumin (RISA)
r. iodinated serum albumin scan
r. iodine
r. iodine ablation
r. iodine scan
r. iodine uptake (RAIU)
r. iron
r. isotope
r. isotope imaging agent
r. label

NOTES

radioactive *(continued)*
   r. labeling
   r. lead
   r. material
   r. metal
   r. nuclide
   r. phosphorus
   r. radon
   r. renogram test
   r. seeding
   r. series
   r. sodium
   r. source
   r. string marker
   r. strontium
   r. sulfur
   r. tag
   r. thorium
   r. tracer
   r. xenon clearance
   r. xenon gas inhalation
radioactively tagged
radioactivity
   artificial r.
   r. detection
   r. distribution
   induced r.
   natural r.
   r. per volume
   unit of r.
radioactor
radioaerosol
   r. clearance
   r. imaging study
radioanaphylaxis
radioassay
radioautogram
radioautograph
radioautography
radiobe
radiobioassay
radiobiologic, radiobiological
radiobiologist
radiobiology
radiocalcium
radiocapitellar
   r. articulation
   r. joint
   r. joint ganglion
   r. line
radiocarbon
radiocarcinogenesis
radiocardiogram
radiocardiography
radiocarpal
   r. angle
   r. articulation

   r. compartment
   r. dislocation
   r. joint
   r. ligament
   r. portal
radioccipital
radiocephalic
radiocephalpelvimetry
radiocesium
radiochemical
   r. purity
   r. study
radiochemistry
radiochemotherapy
radiochemy
radiochlorine
radiocholangiography
radiocholecystography
radiocholesterol scanning
radiochroism
radiochromatography
radiochromic
   r. dosimetry medium
   r. film
radiocineangiocardiography
radiocineangiography
radiocinematograph
radiocinematography
radiocobalt
radiocolloid
   r. lymphoscintigraphy
   r. mapping
radiocontaminant
radiocontrast
radiocontrast-associated
radiocontrast-induced
   r.-i. injury
   r.-i. nephropathy
radiocurability
radiocurable
radiode
radiodense lesion
radiodensity area
radiodermatitis
radiodermatography
radiodiagnosis
radiodiagnostics
radiodiaphane
radiodigital
radioelectrocardiogram
radioelectrocardiograph
radioelectrocardiography
radioelement
   r. solution
   surface application of r.
radioencephalogram
radioencephalography

radioenzyme
radioepidermitis
radioepithelitis
radiofibrinogen uptake scan
radiofluorinated
radiofluorine
radiofrequency (RF, rf)
  r. ablation (RFA)
  r. ablation therapy
  r. absorption
  r. balloon
  r. catheter ablation (RFCA)
  r. coil
  r. electromagnetic field
  r. energy
  r. excitation pulse
  r. gangliolysis
  gaussian r.
  r. generator
  r. hyperthermia
  r. lesion
  r. magnetic shield
  r. modification transcatheter
  r. overflow artifact
  r. percutaneous myocardial
    revascularization (RF-PMR)
  r. period
  r. pulse
  r. radiation
  r. radiogenic leukopenia
  r. radiogold
  r. radiographic control
  r. radiographic hallmark
  r. saturation band
  r. screen
  sinc-Hanning r.
  r. spatial distribution problem
    reconstruction artifact
  r. spin-echo
  r. spoiled 3D GRE sequence
  r. spoiled Fourier-acquired steady
    state (RF-FAST, RF-spoiled FAST)
  r. spoiling
  r. subsystem
  r. thermal ablation
  r. tongue base reduction
  r. transmitter-receiver coil
  r. wave
radiogallium
radiogenesis
radiogenic leukopenia

radiogold
  r. colloid
  radiofrequency r.
radiogram
radiogrammetry
radiograph (*See* radiography)
  axial r.
  biplane r.
  bitewing r.
  cephalometric r.
  Code and Carlson r.
  coned-down r.
  contact r.
  conventional r.
  decubitus r.
  digital abdominal r.
  digital chest r.
  digitally reconstructed r. (DRR)
  double-contrast r.
  dual-energy r. (DER)
  erect lateral flexion/extension r.
  extraoral r.
  frontal cephalometric r.
  internal oblique r.
  intraoral r.
  lateral cephalometric r.
  lateral decubitus r.
  lateral flexion/extension r.
  lateral oblique jaw r.
  lateral ramus r.
  lateral skull r.
  maxillary sinus r.
  mortise r.
  oblique r.
  occlusal r.
  outlet view r.
  panoramic r.
  periapical r.
  phantom r.
  plain r.
  scout digital r.
  soft tissue r.
  spot r.
  submentovertex r.
  supine r.
  survey r.
  Trendelenburg r.
  tunnel r.
  Waters view r.
radiographer
radiographic
  r. baseline

NOTES

radiographic *(continued)*
- r. blurring
- r. cephalometry
- r. contrast
- r. contrast media-induced nephropathy
- r. control
- r. criterion
- r. density
- r. distention
- r. effect
- r. image
- r. interpretation
- r. mottle
- r. noise
- r. parallel line shadow
- r. pathology
- r. pelvimetry
- r. penetration
- r. pincushion distortion
- r. projection
- r. spiculation
- r. stability of lesion

radiographically
- r. firm synostosis
- r. normal imaging
- r. occult fracture

radiographic-dense breast

radiography
- advanced multiple-beam equalization r. (AMBER)
- air-gap r.
- barium r.
- bedside r.
- biomedical r.
- body section r.
- cardiac r.
- computed r. (CR)
- computed dental r. (CDR)
- computerized r.
- contrast r.
- dental r.
- diagrammatic r.
- digital r. (DR)
- digital video gastrointestinal r.
- direct digital r.
- double-contrast r.
- electron r.
- filmless r.
- flexion-extension r.
- gamma r.
- high-resolution, low-speed r.
- horizontal-beam r.
- interventional r.
- intraoperative r.
- intraoral periapical r.
- magnification r.

- mobile r.
- moving slot r.
- mucosal relief r.
- musculoskeletal r.
- neonatal r.
- neutron r.
- pan-oral r.
- panoramic r.
- photostimulable phosphor computed r.
- photostimulable phosphor dental r.
- plain abdominal r. (PAR)
- portable r.
- postrelease r.
- postvoid r.
- quantitative digital r.
- rapid serial r.
- scanned projection r. (SPR)
- scanning equalization r.
- sectional r.
- selective r.
- selenium r.
- serial r.
- slit r.
- soft-copy computed r.
- specimen r.
- spot film r.
- stereoscopic r.
- stress r.
- video digital gastrointestinal r.

radioguided
- r. laparotomy
- r. parathyroidectomy
- r. surgery

radiohepatographic

radiohumeral
- r. articulation
- r. bursitis
- r. meniscus

radioimmunity

radioimmunoassay (RIA)
- r. method
- scintillation proximity r.

radioimmunoconjugate

radioimmunodetection (RAID)

radioimmunodiffusion

radioimmunoguided surgery (RIGS)

radioimmunoimaging

radioimmunolocalization

radioimmunoluminography

radioimmunoprecipitation test

radioimmunoscintigraphy

radioimmunosorbent

radioimmunotherapy

radioinduced sarcoma

radioinduction

radioiodide
radioiodinated serum albumin (RISA)
radioiodination
  direct r.
  electrophilic r.
radioiodine
  r. test
  r. uptake
radioiron
  r. oral absorption
  r. red cell utilization
radioisotope
  r. calibrator
  r. camera
  carrier-free r.
  cistern r.
  r. cisternography
  r. cisternography imaging
  r. delivery system (RDS)
  r. gallium imaging
  Gd-DTPA r.
  r. indium-labeled white blood cell
    imaging
  r. labeling
  r. lung scan
  r. renogram test
  r. scanner
  r. scanning
  r. scintigraphy
  r. stent
  r. synovectomy
  r. technetium imaging
  transplutonium r.
  trapping of r.
  r. uptake
  r. voiding cystogram
radioisotopic purity
radiokymography
radiolabel
radiolabeled
  r. antibody
  r. antibody imaging
  r. anti-CEA
  r. antisense oligonucleotide
  r. compound
  r. estrogen analog
  r. fibrinogen
  r. marker substrate
  r. MoAb
  r. MoAb imaging agent
  r. peptide alpha-M^2
  r. platelet

  r. water study
  r. WBCs
radiolabeling
  area of increased r.
radiolead
radiolesion
radioligand
  PET r.
radiologic
  r. anatomy
  r. diagnosis
  r. guidance
  r. percutaneous gastrostomy
  r. stigmata
  r. technology
radiological contrast medium
radiologic-anatomic correlation
radiologic-histopathologic study
radiologic-pathologic
  r.-p. concordance
  r.-p. correlation
  r.-p. discordance
radiology
  cardiovascular r.
  chest r.
  computed r. (CR)
  dental r.
  diagnostic r.
  intraoral r.
  neurointerventional r.
  oral r.
  r. outcomes data
  pediatric r.
  percutaneous interventional r.
  polytomographic r.
  radionuclide r.
  skeletal r.
  storage phosphor r.
  r. telephone access system
  therapeutic r.
radiolucency
  linear band of maximal r.
  prominent rim of r.
  relative r.
  soap-bubble r.
radiolucent
  r. area
  r. cleft
  r. crescent line
  r. density
  r. fat
  r. fat halo

radiolucent *(continued)*
- r. focus
- r. gallstone
- r. joint space
- r. lesion
- r. linear filling defect
- r. medium
- r. operating room table extension
- r. plastic occluder
- r. pneumomediastinum
- r. roll
- r. spine frame
- r. stone

radiolunate articulation
radiolunotriquetral ligament
radiolymphoscintigraphy
- intraoperative r.

radiolysis
radiomedullary artery ·
radiometallography
radiometer
- pastille r.
- photographic r.

radiometric
- r. analysis
- r. assay

radiomicrometer
radiomimetic
radiomuscular
radiomutation
radion
radionecrosis
- cerebral r.

radioneuritis
Radionics CRW stereotactic head frame
radionitrogen
radionuclear venography
radionucleotide
- positron emitting r.

radionuclide
- absorption of r.
- r. angiocardiography
- r. angiogram (RNA)
- r. angiography
- r. blood flow study
- r. bone scan
- r. bone scintigraphy
- r. camera
- r. cardiography
- r. carrier
- carrier added r.
- carrier free r.
- r. carrier system
- r. cerebral angiogram
- r. cholescintigraphy
- r. cineangiography
- r. cisternography

- concentration of r.
- r. contamination
- r. cystogram
- r. cystography
- r. ejection fraction
- r. emission tomography
- r. esophageal dead time
- r. esophagram
- r. flow scan
- r.-gated blood pool imaging
- r.-gated blood pool scan
- r. generator
- gold-195m r.
- r. inflammation
- inhaled r.
- r. injection
- r. label
- r. liver scan
- lung perfusion r.
- r. mammography
- metastable r.
- r. milk imaging
- r. milk scan
- no-carrier-added r.
- parent r.
- r. production
- r. purity
- r. radiology
- renal r.
- r. renal imaging
- r. renography imaging
- r. scanning
- r. shuntogram
- r. signal
- r. stenosis
- r. stroke volume
- r. synovectomy
- r. table
- r. testicular scintigraphy
- r. therapy
- r. thyroid imaging
- r. thyroid scan
- uptake of r.
- r. venography
- ventilation r.
- r. ventriculogram (RNV, RVG)
- r. voiding cystourethrography
- r. voiding study

radiopacity
- linear r.

radiopaque
- r. bone cement
- r. density
- r. distal tip
- r. drain
- r. fluid extravasation
- r. foreign body

r. gold marker
r. imaging agent
r. lesion
r. medium
r. medium thorium dioxide
r. pellet
r. pseudocapsule
r. urine
r. vesical calculus
r. wire of counteroccluder
  buttonhole
r. xenon gas
radioparency
radioparent
radiopathology
radiopelvimetry
radiopharmaceutical
r. ablation
r. agent
brain imaging r.
r. chemistry
r. dacryocystography
diagnostic r.
r. dosimetry
r. localization
PET r.
r. production
r. purity
r. quality control
r. synovectomy
^{99m}Tc-ECD r.
^{99m}Tc-HMPAO r.
^{99m}Tc-iminodiacetic acid
  derivative r.
^{99m}Tc-MAG3 r.
^{99m}Tc-MIBI r.
^{99m}Tc polyphosphate compound r.
technetium-99m isonitriles r.
r. therapy
trace amount of r.
r. tracer
r. uptake
r. voiding cystogram
r. volume-dilution technique
radiopharmacy
radiophobia
radiophosphate
radiophosphorus
radiophotography
radiophylaxis
radiopotassium
radiopotentiation

radioprotectant
radioprotective agent
radioprotector
radiopulmonography
radioreaction
radioreceptor
radioresistance
radioresistant
radioresponsiveness
radioscaphocapitate ligament
radioscaphoid
r. articulation
r. joint
r. ligament
radioscapholunate ligament
radioscintigraphy
radioscopy
radiosensibility
radiosensitiveness
radiosensitive tumor
radiosensitivity
fibroblast r.
radiosensitization
radiosensitizer
carbogen r.
halogenated thymidine analog r.
nicotinamide r.
radiosodium
radiospirometry
radiostereoscopy
radiostrontium
radiostyloid process
radiosulfur
radiosurgery
Bragg peak r.
charged-particle r.
dynamic stereotactic r.
gamma knife r.
heavy-charged particle Bragg
  peak r.
image-guided r.
interstitial r.
LINAC r.
modified linear accelerator r.
multiarc LINAC r.
stereotactic r. (SRS)
Winston-Lutz for LINAC-based r.
radiotellurium
radiotherapeutic agent
radiotherapist
radiotherapy, radiation therapy (RT)
arc r.

NOTES

radiotherapy *(continued)*
    AVM r.
    computerized r.
    contact r.
    continuous hyperfractionated
      accelerated r.
    dynamic r.
    electron-beam intraoperative r.
      (EBIORT)
    extended-field r.
    external beam r.
    fast neutron r.
    r. field placement
    fractionated stereotactic r. (FSR)
    hemibody r.
    high-dose r.
    high-voltage r.
    hyperfractionated r.
    iceberg r.
    interstitial r.
    intracavitary r.
    intraoperative r.
    inverted Y field r.
    large-field r.
    r. localization
    locoregional field r.
    mantle r.
    megavoltage r.
    neoadjuvant r.
    orthovoltage r.
    r. port
    postoperative r. (PORT)
    preoperative r.
    rotational r.
    short-distance r.
    skeletal targeted r. (STR)
    split-course accelerated r.
    stereotactic r.
    supervoltage r.
    teletherapy r.
    three-dimensional conformal r.
    whole-body r.
    whole-brain r. (WBRT)
    r. with hyperthermia
    r. without hyperthermia
radiothermy
radiothorium
radiothyroidectomy
radiothyroxin
radiotomy
radiotoxemia
radiotoxicity
radiotracer
    r. accumulation
    r. activity
    decreased uptake of r.
    r. deposition

    r. foil method
    increased uptake of r.
    ^{99m}Tc-HMPAO r.
    r. technique
    r. uptake
radiotransparency
radiotransparent
radiotropic
radioulnar
    r. articulation
    r. joint
    r. subluxation
    r. surface
radioulnarproximodistal translation
radium (Ra)
    r. beam therapy
    r. emanation
    intracavitary r.
    r. necrosis
    r. radioactive source
radium-226 (^{226}Ra)
radius, pl. **radii (R)**
    Bohr r.
    r. of curvature
    r. hypoplasia
    sigmoid cavity of r.
radix, pl. **radices**
radix-two algorithm
RadNet radiology information system
radon (Rn)
    r.-222 (^{222}Rn, Rn-222)
    r. progeny
    radioactive r.
    r. seed implantation
RadStat hemostasis device
RADstation radiology workstation
radwaste radioactivity detection
RAE
    right atrial enlargement
Raeder paratrigeminal syndrome
RAEL cell
RAGE
    rapid gradient echo
ragged urethra
ragpicker's disease
RAID
    radioimmunodetection
Raider triangle
RAILL test
railroad
    r. track appearance
    r. track calcification
    r. track ductus arteriosus
    r. track pattern
    r. track sign
railway spine

raiser
> stress r.

RAIU
> radioactive iodine uptake

rake ulcer

RAM
> reduced-acquisition matrix

Raman spectroscopy

Ramesh and Pramod algorithm

rami (*pl. of* ramus)

ramification

ramify

ramp
> r. down
> r. filter
> folded step r.
> maximum slew rate r.
> r. reconstruction
> r. time
> r. up

ramp-filtered back projection

ramping

Ramsay
> R. Hunt cerebellar myoclonic dyssynergia
> R. Hunt syndrome

ramus, pl. rami
> dorsal primary r.
> inferior pubic r.
> r. intermedius artery
> r. intermedius artery branch
> ischiopubic r.
> r. of ischium
> r. of lateral sulcus
> mandibular r.
> r. medialis artery
> r. medialis artery branch
> pubic r.
> superior r.
> superior pubic r.
> ventral primary r.

Randall plaque

Rand microballoon

random
> r. coincidence event
> r. count
> r. error
> r. motion
> r. point

range
> absorbed dose r.
> r. ambiguity artifact

> dynamic r.
> emission r.
> frequency r.
> gray-scale r.
> normal r.
> positron r.
> reference r.
> r. resolution
> slew r.
> therapeutic r.
> water r.

range-gated
> r.-g. Doppler spectral flow analysis
> r.-g. pulsed Doppler

ranging
> echo r.

ranine vein

rank
> Spearman r.

Ranke
> R. angle
> R. complex

ranula

Ranvier
> R. groove
> R. node

RAO
> right anterior oblique

RAP
> right atrial pressure

raphe
> abdominal r.
> amnionic r.
> anococcygeal r.
> anogenital r.
> longitudinal r.
> median r.
> palpebral r.
> penile r.
> pterygomandibular r.
> scrotal r.
> tendinous r.
> unicusp with central r.

RAPI
> resting ankle pressure index

rapid
> r. acquisition computed tomography
> r. acquisition spin echo (RASE)
> r. acquisition with relaxation enhancement (RARE)
> r. axial MR imaging
> r. biplane angiocardiography

NOTES

R

rapid (continued)
  r. deceleration injury
  r. dephasing
  r. dissolution formula
  r. distribution
  r. early repolarization phase
  r. exchange (RX)
  r. filling (RF)
  r. filling period
  r. filling wave (RFW)
  r. film changer
  r. fluid expansion
  r. fluid quantification
  r. gradient echo (RAGE)
  r. gradient reversal
  r. half-Fourier T2-weighted image
  r. image transfer
  r. inspiratory flow rate
  r. oscillatory motion
  r. pull-through technique (RPT)
  r. scan technique
  r. screen
  r. sequential CT scan
  r. serial radiography
  r. telephone access system (RTAS)
  r. thoracic compression technique
  r. tracer washout
  R. Transit catheter
  R. Transit microcatheter
  r. ventricular filling phase
  r. ventricular rate
  r. ventricular response
rapid-excitation MR imaging
Rapid-Scan spectrometery
RapidScreen RS-2000 x-ray equipment
rapid-sequence
  r.-s. imaging
  r.-s. intravenous pyelography
  r.-s. IVP
Rappaport classification
RAR
  renal-aortic ratio
RARE
  rapid acquisition with relaxation
  enhancement
    RARE technique
RARE-derived pulse sequence
rare-earth
  r.-e. scintillator
  r.-e. screen
rarefaction
  bony r.
  r. of cortex
  fluffy r.
  osseous r.
rarefied area

RAS
  renal artery stenosis
RASE
  rapid acquisition spin echo
Rashkind
  R. double umbrella device
  R. occluder
Rasmussen mycotic aneurysm
raster
  r. frequency
  r. line
  r. period
  r. spacing error
rat-bite erosion
rate
  ACR r.
  r. analysis
  atrial r. (AR)
  count r.
  digital sampling r.
  dipole-dipole relaxation r.
  disintegration r.
  exogenous glucose r.
  flow r.
  glomerular filtration r. (GFR)
  gradient slew r.
  high-dose r. (HDR)
  high frame r.
  inspiratory flow r.
  instantaneous enhancement r.
  intraoperative high dose r.
    (IOHDR)
  lipid fraction relaxation r.
  low frame r.
  LVOT flow r.
  magnet r.
  maximum midexpiratory flow r.
    (MMFR)
  maximum predicted heart r.
    (MPHR)
  mean circumferential fiber
    shortening r. (MCFSR)
  r. meter (R-meter)
  oscillatory shear r.
  oxygen extraction r. (OER)
  patency r.
  peak filling r. (PFR)
  plasma radioiron disappearance r.
  plasma radioiron turnover r.
  predicted target heart r.
  proliferation r.
  pulsed dose r. (PDR)
  rapid inspiratory flow r.
  rapid ventricular r.
  relaxation r.
  shear strain r.

Solomon-Bloembergen theory of dipole-dipole relaxation r.
specific absorption r. (SAR)
spirometer flow r.
standby r.
stroke ejection r.
time-to-peak filling r. (TPFR)
transverse relaxation r.
ultra-low dose r. (ULDR)
valley-to-peak dose r.
variable response r.
ventricular r.

ratemeter

Rathke
R. cleft cyst
R. duct
R. pouch
R. pouch tumor

ratio
adenoidal-nasopharyngeal r. (AN)
adrenal-to-spleen r. (ASR)
ankle-brachial pressure r.
aortic root r.
aortic valve opening to aortic valve closing r. (AO/AC)
apnea-bradycardia r.
artery-aortic velocity r.
artery bronchus r. (ABR)
bicaudate r.
blank-to-trues r.
blood-to-fat contrast r.
blood-to-myocardium contrast r.
bone age r.
bone and limb growth velocity r.
brain-to-background r.
branching r.
bronchus-to-pulmonary artery r.
cardiothoracic r. (CTR)
carpal content r.
carpal height r.
r. of caudate to right hepatic lobe
cerebral blood volume to cerebral blood flow r. (CBV/CBF)
chemical shift r.
compression r.
conduction r.

conversion r.
cord subarachnoid space r.
CT r.
diaphyseal bone length r.
diastolic velocity r.
differential uptake r.
distention r.
dome-to-neck r.
dose nonuniformity r. (DNR)
E/A wave r.
end-systolic pressure to end-systolic volume r. (ESP/ESV)
end-systolic wall index to end-systolic volume r.
escape-peak r.
Evans r.
false-negative r.
false-positive r.
flattening r. (FR)
gray-to-white matter activity r.
gray-to-white matter contrast r.
gray-to-white matter utilization r.
grid r.
gyromagnetic r.
head circumference-to-abdominal circumference r. (HC/AC)
heart count-to-mediastinum count r. (H/M)
heart-to-background r.
heart-to-lung r. (HLR)
hilar height r.
Holdaway r.
inferior-anterior count r.
infundibular systolic/diastolic r.
infundibular-to-bulb r.
Insall r.
Insall-Salvati r.
inspiratory to expiratory r. (I/E)
inverse inspiratory-expiratory time r.
iodine-to-particle r.
isotopic r.
kidney length to body height r. (KBR)
kidney-to-background r.
L/A peak r.

NOTES

ratio *(continued)*

left atrium-aortic root r. (LA/AR)
left ventricular systolic time interval r.
lesion-to-background r.
lesion-to-brain r. (L/B)
lesion-to-countersite r. (L/C)
lesion-to-muscle r.
lesion-to-nonlesion count r.
lesion-to-normal tissue r.
likelihood r. (LR)
limb bone length r.
Lindegaard r.
liver-to-aorta peak r.
liver-to-liver peak r. (L/LP)
liver-to-muscle contrast r.
LQ r.
magnetization transfer r. (MTR)
magnetogyric r.
maximum diameter to minimum diameter r.
metatarsal length r.
myocardium-to-abdomen count r.
myoinositol-creatine r. (Mi/Cr)
nasal-to-plasma radioactivity r.
off-axis r. (OAR)
off-center r. (OCR)
optional target-to-background r.
orifice-to-anulus r.
PASP/SASP r.
patellar ligament-patellar r.
peak systolic and diastolic r.
perimeter-area r. (P/A)
peroneal-to-anterior compartment r.
phase sampling r. (PSR)
r. of photoelectric to Compton absorption
pitch r.
Poisson r.
power r.
proportional r.
pulmonary artery-bronchus r.
pulmonic-systemic flow r.
P wave to QRS wave r. (P/QRS)
radioactive iodide conversion r.
renal-aortic r. (RAR)
repetition time to echo time r. (TR/TE)

right ventricular to left ventricular systolic pressure r. (RVP/LVP)
scatter-air r. (SAR)
scatter-maximum r. (SMR)
scatter-to-primary r.
sensitizer enhancement r.
septal-to-free wall r.
signal intensity r.
signal-to-clutter r.
signal-to-noise r. (SNR, S/N)
SI joint-to-sacrum r.
spleen-to-liver r.
standardized uptake r. (SUR)
stroke count r.
stroke volume r.
systolic-diastolic r. (S/D)
systolic velocity r.
target-to-background r.
target-to-nontarget r.
thallium-to-scalp r.
thermal enhancement r. (TER)
thickness-to-diameter of ventricle r.
tissue-air r. (TAR)
tissue-maximum r. (TMR)
tissue-phantom r. (TPR)
TME r.
r. transformer
trapezium-metacarpal eburnation r.
tumor-to-normal brain r.
unfavorable neutron-to-proton r.
uptake r. (UR)
ventilation-perfusion r.
ventricle-to-brain r. (VBR)

Ratliff avascular necrosis classification

rat-tail

r.-t. common bile duct
r.-t. esophagus

rature

r. detector
r. surface coil system

Rau

apophysis of R.

Rauchfuss triangle

rave

fracture en r.

Raw

airway resistance

ray
  actinic r.
  alpha r.
  r. amputation
  anode r.
  beta r.
  Bucky r.
  r. casting technique
  cathode r.
  central r. (CR)
  chemical r.
  corresponding r.
  delta r.
  digital r.
  direct r.
  fluorescent r.
  gamma r.
  glass r.
  grenz r.
  H r.
  hard r.
  hypermobile first r.
  incident r.
  indirect r.
  infrared r.
  infraroentgen r.
  intermediate r.
  keV gamma r.
  long axis r.
  Niewenglowski r.
  parallel r.
  r. pattern
  pollicized r.
  positive r.
  primary r.
  reflected r.
  roentgen r.
  scattered r.'s
  secondary r.
  soft r.
  r. sum
  r. therapeutic
  r. tracing
  ultraviolet r.
  vertical r.
  W r.
ray-casting method
Rayleigh
  R. noise
  R. quotient
  R. scattering
  R. scattering law

Rayleigh-Tyndall scattering
Raymond-Cestan syndrome
Raynaud
  R. phenomenon
  R. syndrome
ray-sum
  r.-s. projection
  r.-s. view
Ray-Tec x-ray detectable surgical sponge
Rb
  rubidium
^{82}Rb, Rb-82
  rubidium-82
^{82}Rb-based cardiac imaging
RBBB
  right bundle-branch block
RBC
  red blood cell
    labeled RBC
    ^{99m}Tc-labeled RBC
    ^{99m}Tc-tagged RBC
    UltraTag RBC
RBE
  relative biological effectiveness
RB-ILD
  respiratory bronchiolitis-associated interstitial lung disease
RBL
  Reid baseline
RC
  retrograde cystogram
RCA
  retained cortical activity
  right coronary angiography
  right coronary artery
  rotational coronary atherectomy
rCBF
  regional cerebral blood flow
    rCBF PET scan
rCBV
  regional cerebral blood volume
  relative cerebral blood volume
RCM
  red cell mass
rCMRO$_2$
  regional cerebral metabolic rate for oxygen
rCPP
  regional cerebral perfusion pressure
Rd
  rutherford

NOTES

RDF
rotary door flap
RDPA
right descending pulmonary artery
RDS
radioisotope delivery system
respiratory distress syndrome
RDS-like surfactant deficiency
RDX coronary radiation catheter delivery system
RE
reflux esophagitis
Biafine RE
Re
rhenium
generator-produced ^{188}Re
^{186}Re
rhenium-186
^{188}Re
rhenium-188
reabsorption
r. atelectasis
bony r.
sodium r.
reaccumulation
reactance
capacitive r.
inductive r. (XL)
reaction
allergic r.
alloxan-Schiff r.
anaphylactic r.
anaphylactoid r.
annihilation r.
arrest r.
biomolecular r.
chemotoxic r.
choriodecidual r.
complex periosteal r.
Crohn-like lymphoid r.
desmoplastic r.
dystonic r.
Eisenmenger r.
endoergic r.
exoergic r.
extrapyramidal r.
first-order r.
flare r.
fluffy periosteal r.
hair-on-end periosteal r.
hexokinase r.
hilar r.
hypersensitivity r.
idiosyncratic anaphylactoid r.
inflammatory r.
interrupted periosteal r.
Jones-Mote r.

lamellar periosteal r.
multilamellar periosteal r.
non-idiosyncratic anaphylactoid r.
nuclear r.
onionskin periosteal r.
periosteal r.
photonuclear r.
pleural r.
positron matter-antimatter annihilation r.
quellung r.
r. recovery time
sarcoid-like r.
scar tissue r.
Schultz r.
shell-type of periosteal r.
soft tissue r.
solid periosteal r.
sunburst periosteal r.
symmetric periosteal r.
thermonuclear r.
vasomotor r.
vasovagal r.
r. vial
reactivation tuberculosis
reactive
r. airway disease (RAD)
r. airway dysfunction syndrome
r. arteriole
r. arthritis
r. bone sclerosis
r. cyst cord
r. disease of smooth muscle
r. fibrosis
r. fibrous lesion
r. fibrovascular arachnoid proliferation
r. follicular hyperplasia
r. gliosis
r. hyperemia
r. interface
r. lymphadenopathy
r. lymphoid hyperplasia
r. lymphoid lesion
r. marrow edema
r. remodeling
r. spinal cyst
reactivity
bronchial r.
reactor
breeder r.
fast-breeder r.
reader
AC 3 plate r.
Immuno-mini NJ-2300 microplate r.
microplate r.

R. paratrigeminal syndrome
plate r.

reading

postradiotherapy implant survey r.
pressure r.
wet r.

readout

r. delay
echo planar r.
r. gradient
steady-state projection imaging with dynamic echo-train r. (SPIDER)
r. wavelength

reagent

lanthanide shift r. (LSR)
shift r.
splenic r.

REAL

Revised European American Lymphoma
REAL classification

REAL classification

realignment

intrarun r.
patellofemoral r.

real signal

real-time

r.-t. assessment
r.-t. biplanar needle tracking
r.-t. chirp Z transformer
r.-t. color Doppler imaging
r.-t. compression
r.-t. CT fluoroscopy
r.-t. 2D blood flow imaging
r.-t. display
r.-t. Doppler
r.-t. echocardiography
r.-t. echo-planar image
r.-t. enhancement
r.-t. format converter
r.-t. magnetic resonance imaging tracking
r.-t. phase-contrast flow
r.-t. position management (RPM)
r.-t. respiratory feedback
r.-t. scan
r.-t. scan ultrasound
r.-t. sector scanning
r.-t. sonogram
r.-t. sonography
r.-t. two-dimensional Doppler flow-imaging system

r.-t. ultrasonography
r.-t. volume rendering

rear

r. endoluminal view
r. projection screen

rearfoot varus

rebleeding of aneurysm

rebound

r. excitation
r. sign

rebreathing ventilation scan

recalcitrant

recall

multiplanar gradient r. (MPGR)

recanalization

endovascular photo acoustic r. (EPAR)
fallopian tube r.
r. technique

recanalized

r. artery
r. ductus

recapture

mobile with r.
mobile without r.
stuck with r.
stuck without r.

receive-only circular surface coil

receiver

r. coil
r. dead time
Medtronic radiofrequency r.
r. operating characteristic (ROC)
r. operating characteristic curve
r. operating characteristic method

recent dislocation

receptor

r. binding
r. expression
r. imaging
muscarinic r.

recess

attic r.
azygoesophageal r.
Baumgarten r.
cecal r.
cerebellopontine r.
cochlear r.
costodiaphragmatic r.
costomediastinal r.
costophrenic r.
duodenojejunal r.

NOTES

recess *(continued)*
    epitympanic r. (EPR)
    hepatorenal r.
    ileocecal r.
    inferior duodenal r.
    infraglenoid r.
    intersigmoid r.
    lacrimal r.
    lateral r.
    lumbosacral lateral r.
    mild r.
    optic r.
    paraduodenal r.
    peritoneal r.
    pharyngeal r.
    piriform r.
    pleural r.
    popliteal r.
    posterior pleural r.
    prestyloid r.
    rectouterine r.
    rectovesical r.
    retrocecal r.
    retroduodenal r.
    sacciform r.
    sphenoethmoidal r.
    splenorenal r.
    step-like r.
    sublabral r.
    subphrenic r.
    subscapularis r.
    superior azygoesophageal r.
    superior duodenal r.
    twining r.
recession
    nasion r.
    rib r.
reciprocal
    r. agonist-antagonist relaxation
    r. change
    r. depression
    r. rhythm
reciprocating conduction
recirculation peak
RECIST
    Response Evaluation Criteria in Solid
    Tumors
Recklinghausen
    R. disease of bone
    R. tumor
reclining position
recoarctation of aorta
recognizer
    exposure data r. (EDR)
recoil
    r. atom
    r. electron

    r. energy
    r. pressure
    r. radiation
recombinant
    r. thyrotropin contrast agent (rTSH)
    r. tissue plasminogen activator
recon pitch
reconstitution
    artery r.
    r. of blood flow in artery
    r. via profunda artery
reconstructed
    3D acquired/2D r.
    r. image
    r. radiographic imaging
reconstruction
    ACV r.
    adaptive cardiac volume r.
    r. algorithm
    analytic r.
    r. of aorta
    aortic r.
    aortobifemoral r.
    r. artifact
    coronal r.
    curved r.
    curvilinear r.
    3D r.
    3D image r.
    Dor r.
    external gamma dose r.
    fan-beam r.
    Fourier transformation r.
    Fourier two-dimensional
      projection r.
    r. from projections imaging
    gated 3D r.
    image r.
    r. interval
    iterative r.
    magnitude r.
    MIP r.
    multiplanar r. (MPR)
    oblique-angle r.
    one-sided image r.
    patch graft r.
    phase-preserving r.
    ramp r.
    renovascular r.
    respiration gated 3D r.
    sagittal r.
    segmental correction using spine r.
    single pixel r.
    spatial r.
    r. study
    transanular patch r.

r. view
zygomaticomalar r.
reconstructive imaging
reconstructor
dynamic planar r. (DPR)
dynamic spatial r. (DSR)
recording
color Doppler r.
continuous-wave Doppler r.
pullback pressure r.
pulsed-wave Doppler r.
pulse volume r. (PVR)
segmental limb pressure r.
simultaneous r.
split-screen r.
recovery
arrhythmia-insensitive flow-sensitive
alternating inversion r. (A-FAIR)
cardiac r.
3D turbo fluid-attentuated
inversion r.
fast short tau inversion r.
fluid-attenuated inversion r.
(FLAIR)
inversion r. (IR)
myocardial r.
r. period of myocardium
postischemic r.
saturation r. (SR)
selective saturation r.
shape r.
short-inversion-time inversion r.
(STIR)
short tau inversion r. (STIR)
short TI inversion r.
short T1 inversion r. (STIR)
silver r.
r. time (RT)
r. time image
total saturation r. (TSR)
turbo short tau inversion r.
turbo short tau/TI inversion r.
recrudescence
recrudescent tuberculosis
recruitment potential
recta
vasa r.
rectal
r. ampulla
r. balloon
r. carcinoma
r. contrast medium

r. dilatation
r. distention
r. duplication cyst
r. endoscopic ultrasonography
r. endosonography
r. fascia
r. fisting
r. fistula
r. fold
r. intussusception
r. lesion
r. lymph node
r. multiplane transducer
r. muscle cuff
r. narrowing
r. obstruction
r. orifice
r. penetration
r. plexus
r. polyp
r. pouch
r. prolapse
r. radiation injury
r. sheath hematoma
r. shelf
r. stenosis
r. stump
r. tear
r. tip
r. valve
r. vault
rectangular
r. disk
r. field of view
r. phalanx
r. section profile
recti (*pl. of* rectus)
rectification
four-valve-tube r.
full-wave r.
rectifier
full-wave r.
silicon-controlled r. (SCR)
r. subblock
r. tube
rectilinear
r. biphasic waveform for external
defibrillation
r. bone scan
r. bone scan imaging
r. scanner

NOTES

rectilinear *(continued)*
    r. thyroid scan
    r. tomography
rectocele
rectogenital septum
rectosigmoid
    r. carcinoma
    r. function
    r. index
    r. junction
    r. manometry
    r. polypoid lesion
rectouterine
    r. fold
    r. fossa
    r. pouch
    r. recess
rectovaginal
    r. fistula
    r. pouch
    r. septum
rectovaginouterine pouch
rectovesical
    r. fistula
    r. pouch
    r. recess
    r. septum
rectum
    benign lymphoma of r.
    Hartmann closure of r.
    r. radiation
rectus, pl. **recti**
    ampulla recti
    r. femoris
    r. femoris tendon
    gyrus recti
    r. muscle
    r. position
    r. sheath
    r. sheath pocket
recumbency
recumbent
    r. lateral projection
    r. position
    r. view
recurrence
    ipsilateral breast tumor r. (IBTR)
    local r. (LR)
    no evidence of r. (NER)
    r. pattern
    tumor r.
recurrent
    r. artery of Heubner
    r. bronchiectasis
    r. canal
    r. digital fibroma
    r. dislocation

    r. embolus
    r. fleeting infiltrate
    r. high-grade malignant glioma
    r. hyperparathyroidism
    r. laryngeal nerve
    r. lateral patellar subluxation
    r. lesion
    r. lymphoma
    r. meningeal nerve
    r. multifocal osteomyelitis
    r. pneumonia
    r. pneumothorax
    r. pyogenic cholangitis
    r. pyogenic hepatitis
    r. respiratory papillomatosis
    r. sialadenitis
    r. stricture
    r. ulcer
    r. vermian oligoastrocytoma
recursive
    r. partitioning
    r. partitioning analysis
recurvatum
    r. deformity
    genu r.
    pectus r.
red
    r. blood cell (RBC)
    r. blood cell iron turnover
    r. cell ghost
    r. cell mass (RCM)
    r. infarct
redirection of inferior vena cava
redistributed thallium scan
redistribution
    blood flow r.
    flow r.
    pulmonary blood flow r.
    pulmonary vascular r.
    r. study
    r. thallium-201 imaging
    vascular r.
Redi-Vu teleradiology system
red-out
REDS
    remote endoscopic digital spectroscopy
reduced
    r. acquisition
    r. alveolar ventilation
    r. circulation
    r. compliance of chamber
    r. filling
    r. lung volume
    r. plasma volume
    r. prominence of pulmonary vessel
    r. pulmonary compliance
    r. signal intensity

R

r. stroke volume
r. subluxation
r. systemic cardiac output
r. ventricular filling period
reduced-acquisition
r.-a. matrix (RAM)
r.-a. matrix FAST
reducing stent
reduction
anatomic r.
blood viscosity r.
closed r.
concentric r.
congruent r.
r. deformity
3D field echo acquisition with short repetition time and echo r. (3D FASTER)
electrolytic r.
fracture r.
gradient moment r. (GMR)
limb r.
open r.
postural r.
radiofrequency tongue base r.
stable r.
redundancy
r. of interposed colon segment
phase-angle display r.
redundant
r. aortic valve leaflet
r. capsule
r. carotid artery
r. mitral valve leaflet
r. scallop of posterior anulus
r. ureter
reefing
capsular r.
r. of medial retinaculum of knee
reelin mutation
reentrant
r. loop
r. well chamber
reentry
bundle-branch r. (BBR)
r. circuit
functional r.
intraatrial r.
r. point
sinus nodal r.

reexpansion
lung r.
r. pulmonary edema
reexploration
reference
chemical shift r.
r. compound
r. coordinate system
distal line of r. (DLR)
r. dose
r. image
r. line
r. phantom
plane of r.
r. range
rotating frame of r.
r. site
r. standard
sternospinal r.
r. wave
referral teleradiology
refill
capillary r.
Refinity Coblation System
reflectance-guided laser selection
reflected
r. edge of Poupart ligament
r. inguinal ligament
r. ray
reflection
r. coefficient
pleuroparenchymal r.
second-order r.
vascular r.
reflectivity
echo r.
high r.
reflectometer tuning unit
reflector
diffuse r.
specular r.
reflex
r. arc
conditioned r. (CR)
genitourinary r.
r. ileus
stapedius r.
r. sympathetic dystrophy
r. sympathetic dystrophy syndrome
refluoromyelography
reflux
acid r.

NOTES

reflux *(continued)*
- r. activity
- r. atrophy
- r. of barium
- bile r.
- congenital vesicoureteral r.
- cortical venous r.
- duodenobiliary r.
- duodenogastric r. (DGR)
- duodenogastroesophageal r.
- duodenopancreatic r.
- esophageal r.
- r. esophagitis (RE)
- free r.
- r. gastritis
- gastroesophageal r. (GER)
- gonadal vein r.
- r. grades (I–V)
- hepatojugular r.
- r. ileitis
- intrarenal r.
- nasopharyngeal r.
- r. nephropathy
- piston-like r.
- pudendal vein r.
- r. regurgitation
- uretero-ureteral r.
- vesicoureteral r. (VUR)
- vesicoureteric r.

refluxing spastic neurogenic bladder

refocus
- multiplanar gradient r.

refocusing

reformat

reformation
- curved planar r.
- DentaScan multiplanar r.
- image r.
- multiplanar r. (MPR)
- multiplanar volume r. (MPVR)

reformatted T1 magnetic resonance image

reformatting
- cardiac oblique r.
- 3D r.
- multiplanar r.

refraction

refractive shadowing

refractory
- r. congestive heart failure
- r. hypertension
- r. period of myocardium
- r. TLE
- r. to treatment
- r. tumor

refractured bone

regeneration
- imperfect r.
- nodular liver r.
- osteoblastic bone r.
- r. of tissue

regenerative
- r. chondrocyte
- r. gastric polyp
- r. liver nodule

region
- r. of activation
- Broca r.
- dark r.
- distention of the esophagogastric r.
- esophagogastric r.
- hyperechoic r.
- hypermetabolic r.
- hypervariable r.
- insular r.
- r. of interest (ROI)
- r. of interest fluoroscopy
- r. of interest imaging technique
- isthmic r.
- laterocervical r.
- limbic r.
- outer-air r.
- paratracheal r.
- parietooccipital r.
- patulous esophagogastric r.
- periauricular r.
- perihilar r.
- photodeficient r.
- photopenic r.
- pineal r.
- r. of protection
- subpial r.

regional
- r. asynergy
- r. cerebral blood flow (rCBF)
- r. cerebral blood flow response
- r. cerebral blood volume (rCBV)
- r. cerebral metabolic rate for oxygen (rCMRO$_2$)
- r. cerebral oxygen saturation
- r. cerebral perfusion
- r. cerebral perfusion pressure (rCPP)
- r. colitis
- r. contractile reserve
- r. differences in aeration
- r. dyskinesia
- r. dyssynergia
- r. ejection fraction
- r. enteritis
- r. granulomatous lymphadenitis
- r. hypokinesis
- r. hypokinetic wall motion

r. ileitis
r. left ventricular function
r. lymph node
r. mean transit time (rMTT)
r. migratory osteoporosis
r. myocardial blood flow
r. myocardial dysfunction
r. myocardial function
r. myocardial ischemia
r. myocardial mass distribution
r. oxygen extraction fraction
   (rOEF)
r. perfusion abnormality
r. pulmonary perfusion
r. spread
r. tracer uptake
r. transient osteoporosis
r. transmural ischemia
r. tumor confinement
r. vascular perfusion
r. ventilation
r. wall motion assessment
r. washout measurement

registration
r. and alignment of 3D image
combined anatomic r.
2D portal image r.
feasibility of image r.
image r.
intermodality image r.
landmark r.
robust r.
spastic r.
spatial r.
surface r.

Regnauld degeneration of MTP joint
Regnauld-type great toe degeneration
regressed cyst
regression
r. analysis
caudal r.
plaque r.
polynomial stepwise multilinear r.
spontaneous r.
stepwise r.

regressive remodeling
regridding algorithm
regrowth delay
regular
r. connective tissue
r. wedge delay

regulation
volume r.
regurgitant
r. flow delay
r. fraction
r. jet
r. lesion
r. lesion delay
r. orifice
r. orifice area (ROA)
r. pandiastolic flow
r. pocket
r. stream
r. stroke volume (RSV)
r. systolic flow
r. valve
r. velocity
regurgitation
aortic r. (AR)
congenital aortic r.
congenital mitral r. (CMR)
Dexter-Grossman classification of
   mitral r.
Doppler tricuspid r.
factitious r.
Grossman scale for r.
ischemically mediated mitral r.
massive aortic r.
mitral r. (MR)
mitral valve r.
pansystolic mitral r.
paravalvular r.
physiologic r.
pulmonic r. (PR)
pulmonic valve r.
reflux r.
semilunar aortic valve r.
semilunar pulmonic valve r.
silent r.
syphilitic aortic r.
transient tricuspid r.
tricuspid orifice r.
tricuspid valve r.
valvular r. (VR)
Reichert
R. canal
R. flexible sigmoidoscope
**Reichert-Mundinger-Fischer stereotactic
   frame**
Reid
R. baseline (RBL)

NOTES

Reid *(continued)*
   R. line
   R. lobule
Reil
   R. band
   R. island
reimplantation
   r. lung response
   r. technique
reinfarction
reinjection thallium stress examination
Reinke space
reinnervation
   motor r.
reintimalization
reirradiation
Reisseisen muscle
Reiter
   R. syndrome
   R. syndrome arthritis
relapse
   bone marrow r.
   solitary r.
   testicular r.
relapsing
   r. course
   r. polychondritis
relation
   end-diastolic pressure-volume r.
   end-systolic pressure-volume r.
   force-frequency r.
   force-length r.
   force-velocity r.
   Frank-Starling r.
   phase r.
relationship
   atlantoaxial r.
   complex anatomic r.
   dentoskeletal r.
   dose-time r.
   dose-volume r.
   globe-orbit r.
   Karplus r.
   Reynolds r.
   tumor cell-host bone r.
relative
   r. biological effectiveness (RBE)
   r. cerebral blood flow
   r. cerebral blood volume (rCBV)
   r. conversion factor
   r. error
   r. hypoxia
   r. mitral stenosis
   r. peak height
   r. radiolucency
   r. refractory period (RRP)
   r. regional blood flow (rrBF)

   r. shunt flow
   r. value scale
relativistic mass
relaxation
   absent lower esophageal
    sphincter r.
   r. atelectasis
   r. enhancement technique
   esophageal sphincter r.
   ferromagnetic r.
   incomplete lower esophageal
    sphincter r.
   isovolumetric r.
   longitudinal r.
   molecular weight dependence of r.
   multiexponential r.
   multispin r.
   nuclear electric quadripole r.
   nuclear reactornuclear r.
   paramagnetic shift r.
   r. probe
   proton r.
   r. rate
   r. rate frequency dependence
   reciprocal agonist-antagonist r.
   sinusoidal r.
   spin-lattice r.
   spin-spin r.
   r. time
   tissue-based T2 r.
   transverse r.
   T2 star r.
relaxed lower esophageal sphincter
relaxivity
   r. data
   longitudinal r. (R1)
   transverse r. (R2)
relaxometer
   Bruker PC-10 r.
   Bruker TC-10 r.
   IBM field-cycling research r.
relaxometry
   time-efficient T2 r.
   tissue r.
releasing factor
relief pattern
reloading
   anode tube r.
REM
   roentgen equivalent man
remasking
remineralization
remitting course
remnant
   cystic duct r.
   ductal r.
   gastric r.

heart r.
notochord r.
omphalomesenteric r.
r. radiation
thyroglossal duct r.
remodeling
balloon r.
bone r.
bony r.
cord r.
coronary r.
craniofacial r.
intimal r.
neural foramen r.
osseous r.
paraarticular bone r.
plaque r.
reactive r.
regressive r.
stress-induced r.
r. technique
thrombus r.
remote
r. afterloading brachytherapy (RAB)
r. afterloading system
r. endoscopic digital spectroscopy (REDS)
r. ischemia
r. lower motor neuron lesion
remote-controlled
r.-c. implantation of radioactive source
r.-c. production
removal
brachytherapy implant r.
REMP
remyelinization
Renaissance 3D workstation
renal
r. r.
r. abscess
r. adenocarcinoma
r. agenesis
r. allograft
r. allograft necrosis
r. amyloidosis
r. angiography
r. angiography imaging
r. angiomyolipoma
r. anomaly
r. anticoagulant-related bleeding
r. aortography

r. arteriography
r. arteriosclerosis
r. artery
r. artery aneurysm
r. artery fibromuscular dysplasia
r. artery hypertension
r. artery stenosis (RAS)
r. artery stenosis screening MR
r. artery transplant thrombosis
r. axis
r. calcification
r. calculus
r. calix
r. capsule
r. carbuncle
r. carcinoma
r. carcinosarcoma
r. cholesterol embolus
r. choristoma
r. clearance
r. colic
r. collecting structure
r. collecting system
r. collecting system atony
r. column
r. cortex
r. cortical adenoma
r. cortical isotope scanning agent
r. cortical necrosis
r. cortical nephrocalcinosis
r. CT imaging
r. cystic disease
r. cyst imaging
r. cyst study
r. Doppler
r. duplex imaging
r. duplex scan
r. duplication
r. dwarfism
r. dysfunction
r. edema
r. failure
r. fascia
r. flow curve
r. function differential
r. function impairment
r. function study
r. fungal infection
r. fungus ball
r. gallium scintigraphy
r. hamartoma
r. helical CT

NOTES

renal *(continued)*
   r. hemangiopericytoma
   r. hilar vessel
   r. hilum
   r. image
   r. impression
   r. infarct
   r. inflammation
   r. injury
   r. insufficiency
   r. isthmus
   r. labyrinth
   r. leiomyoma
   r. length measurement
   r. lithiasis
   r. lymphoma
   r. malrotation
   r. mass lesion
   r. medulla
   r. medullary pyramid
   r. metastasis
   r. obstruction
   r. osteodystrophy
   r. outline
   r. papilla
   r. papillary necrosis
   r. parenchyma
   r. parenchymal blush
   r. parenchymal disease
   r. parenchymal malakoplakia
   r. pelvic fibrolipomatosis
   r. pelvis
   r. perfusion
   r. pouch
   r. pseudotumor
   r. radionuclide
   r. reflux atrophy
   r. resistive index
   r. scarring
   r. sclerosis
   r. shadow
   r. shutdown
   r. sinus
   r. sinus complex
   r. sinus cyst
   r. sinus echo
   r. sinus fat
   r. sinus lipomatosis
   r. sinus mass
   r. size
   r. stone
   r. stone mineral composition
   r. surface
   r. transplant
   r. transplant GI tract perforation
   r. transplant hypertension
   r. transplant lymphocele

   r. transplant pseudoaneurysm
   r. transplant urine extravasation
   r. trauma
   r. tuberculosis
   r. tubular degeneration
   r. tubular dysgenesis
   r. tubular ectasia
   r. tubular necrosis
   r. tubular osteomalacia
   r. tubule
   r. tumor
   r. ultrasonography imaging
   r. ultrasound
   r. vascular anatomy
   r. vascular damage
   r. vascular hypertension (RVH)
   r. vein
   r. vein renin assay
   r. vein thrombosis (RVT)
   r. vein transplant thrombosis
   r. venogram
   r. venography
   vertebral, anal, tracheal,
     esophageal, r. (VATER)
renal-aortic ratio (RAR)
rendering
   3D surface r.
   r. parameter
   perspective volume r. (PVR)
   real-time volume r.
   shaded surface r. (SSR)
   transparent r.
   volume r.
Renegade microcatheter
reniform
   r. contour
   r. mass
   r. pelvis
renin-angiotensin-dependent outer cortex
reninculus
reninoma
renin-secreting tumor
ren lobatus
renocystogram
Renografin-76
Renografin-60 imaging agent
renogram
   Captopril r.
   r. curve
   diuresis r.
   F-15 r.
   r. imaging
   isotope r.
renography
   ACE inhibition r.
   acetazolamide r.
   diuretic r.

DTPA r.
emission r.
enalaprilat-enhanced r.
exercise r.
Lasix r.
technetium-99m MAG3 r.
Reno-M-30
Reno-M-60
Renotec imaging agent
renovascular
r. disease
r. hypertension
r. reconstruction
r. stent
Renovist
R. II imaging agent
R. II injector
Renovue-65 imaging agent
Renovue-Dip imaging agent
rent
fascial r.
reocclusion
postthrombolytic coronary r.
reordering
MRA using 3D k-space r.
r. of phase encoding
REP
roentgen equivalent-physical
repair
endovascular r.
paraanastomotic aneurysmal r.
reparative giant cell granuloma
repeated free-induction decay
reperfused
r. artery
r. myocardium
reperfusion
r. injury of postischemic lung
r. lung edema
r. therapy
repetition
r. time (RT)
r. time to echo time ratio
(TR/TE)
time-to-r. (TR)
repetitive
r. anterior subluxation of the tibia
r. microtrauma
r. pulse sequence
r. seizures
r. strain injury (RSI)
r. stress injury (RSI)

rephased transverse magnetization
rephasing
echo r.
even-echo r.
field-echo sequence with even-echo r. (FEER)
field-even echo r. (FEER)
r. gradient
gradient moment r. (GMR)
gradient motion r. (GMR)
replacement
aortic root r.
aortic valve r. (AVR)
bipolar hip r.
r. bone
r. fibrosis
hip r.
low-signal-intensity r.
mitral valve r. (MVR)
orthotopic total heart r.
prosthetic r.
spongiosa r.
valve r.
replacing oblique view
replantable amputation
replantation of finger
replanted digit
repolarization
ventricular r.
reporting
structured r. (SR)
structured platform-independent data entry and r. (SPIDER)
reproducibility index
reproducible baseline
reproduction
colorimetric color r.
reproductive tract embryology
reprogramming therapy
requirement
increased myocardial oxygen r.
rerotation
varus r.
reroute
resampling
volumetric r.
rescue
autologous bone marrow r.
bone marrow r.
resectability

NOTES

resectable
  r. colorectal carcinoma
  r. lesion
resecting fracture
resection
  absolute curative r.
  absolute noncurative r.
  atrial septal r.
  r. cavity
  colosigmoid r.
  computer-assisted stereotactic r.
  en bloc r.
  extraarticular r.
  r. of mobile aortic arch atheroma
  pulmonary r.
  rim r.
  subtotal gastric r.
  transurethral r. (TUR)
  wedge r.
reserve
  blood flow r.
  brain perfusion r.
  cardiac r.
  r. cardiac function
  contractile r.
  coronary flow r. (CFR)
  diastolic r.
  r. force
  left ventricular systolic functional r.
  myocardial perfusion r. (MPR)
  poor vascular r.
  preload r.
  pulmonary vascular r.
  regional contractile r.
  stenotic flow r. (SFR)
  systolic r.
  vascular r.
  ventricular r.
reservoir
  r. effect
  ICV r.
  shunt r.
residual
  r. aneurysmal sac
  r. barium
  r. cement
  r. ductal tissue
  fibrocalcific r.
  fibrocystic r.
  fibrotic r.
  r. focus
  gastric r.
  r. gradient
  r. imaging agent
  r. interstitial change
  r. limb-shaped change
  r. luminal narrowing

  r. magnetization
  r. metal fragment shaving
  r. nucleus
  r. plaque
  r. stone
  r. stress analysis
  r. urine
  r. urine accumulation
  r. volume (RV)
  r. volume/total lung capacity
    (RV/TLC)
residue
  fecal r.
residuum morphology
resilient artery
resin
  IRA-400 r.
  r. sphere
resistance (R)
  acquired radiation r.
  airway r. (Raw)
  arteriolar r.
  r. blood flow
  calculated r.
  coronary vascular r.
  decreased peripheral vascular r.
  decreased systemic r.
  drug-induced drug r.
  efferent arteriolar r.
  end organ r.
  expiratory r.
  fixed pulmonary valvular r.
  increased cerebrovascular r.
  increased outflow r.
  increased peripheral r.
  increased pulmonary vascular r.
  index of runoff r.
  nasal airway r.
  peripheral vascular r. (PVR)
  pulmonary arteriolar r.
  pulmonary vascular r. (PVR)
  systemic vascular r. (SVR)
  total peripheral r. (TPR)
  total pulmonary r. (TPR)
  vascular systemic r.
  r. wire heater
  Wood units index of r.
resistive
  r. exercise table
  r. index (RI)
  r. index angiography
  r. magnet
resistivity
  conductor r.
resistor
resolution
  anatomic r.

angle variation r.
anisotropic r.
axial r.
contrast r.
depth r.
r. element
energy r.
fibrotic r.
high temporal r.
image spatial r.
in-plane spatial r.
interval r.
intrinsic energy r.
isotropic r.
lateral r.
range r.
spatial r.
r. stage
temporal r.
Resolve non-locking draining catheter
resolving
    r. ischemic neurologic defect
    r. pneumonia
    r. power
    r. time
resonance
    bandbox r.
    biphasic magnetic r. (BP MR)
    r. capture
    computerized
      tomography/magnetic r. (CT/MR)
    cough r.
    cracked-pot r.
    electron paramagnetic r. (EPR)
    electron spin r. (ESR)
    fast-scan magnetic r.
    focused nuclear magnetic r.
    r. frequency
    gated inflow magnetic r.
    r. generator
    high-resolution magnetic r. (HR-
      MR)
    lactate r.
    r. line
    localized magnetic r. (LMR)
    low-field magnetic r.
    magnetic r. (MR)
    mobile magnetic r.
    nuclear magnetic r. (NMR)
    r. offset
    r. phenomenon
    proton magnetic r.

pulsed nuclear magnetic r.
skodaic r.
tagging cine magnetic r.
topical magnetic r. (TMR)
T1-weighted magnetic r.
velocity-encoded cine magnetic r.
  (VEC-MR)
resonant
    r. frequency
    r. frequency of oscillation
resonator
    bird-cage r.
    bridged loop-gap r.
    detunable elliptic transmission
     line r.
    Faraday shielded r.
    flexible surface-coil-type r. (FSCR)
    250 MHz crossed-loop r.
    multicoupled loop-gap r.
resorbable
    r. pin
    r. plate
    r. rod
    r. screw
resorcinol spray
resorption
    r. atelectasis
    bone r.
    cortical bone r.
    dependent edema fluid r.
    fluid r.
    r. lacuna
    osteoclastic r.
    osteoclast-mediated bone r.
    periosteal r.
    periprosthetic bone r.
    r. phase of healing
    subarticular bone r.
    subchondral bone r.
    subperiosteal bone r.
    terminal tuft r.
    total r.
    trabecular bone r.
resorptive atelectasis
Resovist MR contrast medium
respiration
    cardiac-gated r.
    r. gated 3D reconstruction
    r. pyelography
respiratory
    r. atrium
    r. bronchiolar dilatation

NOTES

respiratory *(continued)*
r. bronchiole
r. bronchiolitis
r. bronchiolitis-associated interstitial lung disease (RB-ILD)
r. burst
r. burst product
r. capacity
r. chain complex I–VI
r. compensation
r. compromise
r. decompensation
r. diaphragm
r. distress syndrome (RDS)
r. distress syndrome-like deficiency
r. disturbance of acid base
r. effort
r. embarrassment
r. failure
r. frequency
r. gated imaging
r. gating
r. insufficiency
r. modulation of vascular impedance
r. motion
r. motion artifact
r. muscle weakness
r. ordered phase encoding (ROPE)
r. sorted phase encoding
r. spasm
r. system
r. tract
r. tract infection
r. tract obstruction
r. trigger
r. triggered fast SE technique
r. triggering
r. volume
r. zoonosis
respiratory-esophageal fistula
response
abnormal ejection fraction r.
autoimmune r.
blood flow r.
blood pressure r.
cardioinhibitory r.
clinical complete r.
clinical partial r.
controlled ventricular r.
deconditioned exercise r.
desmoplastic r.
end-organ r.
R. Evaluation Criteria in Solid Tumors (RECIST)
graft-versus-tumor r.
healing flare r.

hemodynamic r.
high-rate ventricular r.
immune r.
line of r. (LOR)
magnet r.
metabolic r.
pain provocation r.
radiation r. (RR)
rapid ventricular r.
regional cerebral blood flow r.
reimplantation lung r.
slow ventricular r.
synovial inflammatory r.
therapeutic r.
vasoactive r.
vasoconstrictor r.
vasodepressor r.
vasodilatory r.
ventricular r.
whole-body inflammatory r.
responsiveness
airway r.
rest
cervical r.
glial r.
r. injection
knee r.
r. left ventricular function
r. magnetization
r. myocardial perfusion imaging
r. redistribution examination
r. redistribution imaging
r. right ventricular function
r. thallium-201 myocardial imaging
rest-and-exercise-gated nuclear angiography
restenosis
in-stent r.
postangioplasty r.
restiform body
restiformia
corpora r.
resting
r. ankle pressure index (RAPI)
r. echocardiography
r. electrocardiogram
r. end-systolic wall stress
r. energy expenditure
r. forefoot supination angle
r. heart
r. left ventricular ejection fraction
r. lower esophageal sphincter
r. MUGA imaging
r. perfusion
r. phase of cardiac action potential
r. pulse
r. regional myocardial blood flow

r. regional myocardial hypoperfusion

resting-redistribution thallium-201 scintigraphy

restoration
r. algorithm
r. of flow

restraint
r. calipers
foam-padded Velcro r.

restricted
r. diffusion
r. water diffusion

restriction
cortical diffusion r.
intrauterine growth r.
unilateral flow r.

restrictive
r. abnormality
r. bulboventricular foramen
r. cardiomyopathy
r. hemodynamic syndrome
r. lung disease
r. myocardial disease
r. pattern
r. pulmonary emphysema
r. ventilatory defect

restrictor
beam r.

restructuring

result
concordant r.
false-negative r.
false-positive r.
negative EMA r.
negative mucin r.
suboptimal r.
true-positive r.

retained
r. barium
r. common bile duct stone
r. cortical activity (RCA)
r. dead fetus
r. fetal lung fluid
r. foreign body
r. gallstone
r. gastric antrum
r. placenta
r. root
r. secretion
r. urine

retardation (*See* IUGR)
asymmetric intrauterine growth r.
fetal growth r.
growth r.
intrauterine growth r. (IUGR)

rete, pl. **retia**
r. mirabile
r. peg
r. ridge
r. testis

retention
r. of barium
CO_2 r.
r. colon polyp
r. cyst
r. enema
fluid r.
r. of food
r. meal
r. of secretion
r. stomach polyp
r. of stool
uptake and r.
water r.

retentivity
magnetic r.

retia (*pl. of* rete)

reticula (*pl. of* reticulum)

reticular
r. activating formation
r. activating substance
r. connective tissue
r. formation (RF)
r. formation of the brainstem
gray r.
r. infiltrate
r. interstitial disease pattern
r. lung pattern
r. opacity
r. type
r. varicosities

reticularis
livedo r.
zona r.

reticulated bone

reticulation
r. artifact
chronic diffuse r.
coarse lung r.
diffuse fine lung r.
lower lobe r.
r. with hilar adenopathy

R

NOTES

reticule
reticulocortical pathway
reticuloendothelial
r. imaging
r. imaging agent
r. system
r. tumor
reticuloendotheliosis
reticulogranular
r. appearance
r. pattern
r. pulmonary density
reticulohistiocytic granuloma
reticulohistiocytosis
multicentric r.
reticuloid
actinic r.
reticulonodular
r. infiltrate
r. lung disease
r. pattern
reticulosis
mast cell r.
midline malignant r.
reticulospinal tract
reticulum, pl. reticula
r. bone cell sarcoma
r. brain cell sarcoma
hematopoietic r.
retina
angiomatosis of r.
retinacular
r. disruption
r. ligament
retinaculum, pl. retinacula
avulsed r.
cubital tunnel r.
retinacula cutis
extensor r.
flexor r.
free-floating r.
inferior extensor r.
inferior peroneal r.
inferior quadriceps r.
patellar r.
peroneal r.
superior extensor r.
superior peroneal r. (SPR)
retinal
r. angiomatosis
r. anlage tumor
r. artery
r. astrocytoma
r. degeneration
r. dysplasia
r. embolus

r. hemangioblastoma
r. microaneurysm
retinalis
retinoblastoma
r. hereditary human carcinoma
quadrilateral r.
trilateral r.
retinocerebellar angiomatosis
retinochoroiditis
retinocortical time
retinocytoma
retinoma
retinopathy
retracted
r. rib
r. stoma
retractile
r. mesenteritis
r. testis
retraction
chest wall r.
clot r.
costa r.
fiber r.
inspiratory r.
intercostal r.
late systolic r.
leaflet r.
mediastinal r.
midsystolic r.
mild subcostal r.
musculotendinous r.
nipple r.
postrheumatic cusp r.
sternocleidomastoid r.
sternum r.
substernal r.
superior r.
suprasternal r.
systolic r.
upward r.
retractor
external r.
retrieval
microvascular r.
oocyte r.
transvaginal oocyte r.
transvesical oocyte r.
retroaortic
r. lymph node
r. renal vein
retroappendiceal fossa
retroareolar
r. density
r. dysplasia
retroauricular lymph node

retrobulbar
- r. fat
- r. hemorrhage
- r. mass

retrocalcaneal
- r. bursa
- r. bursitis
- r. exostosis
- r. spur

retrocardiac
- r. area
- r. density
- r. infiltrate
- r. mass
- r. space

retrocaval ureter

retrocecal
- r. appendix
- r. lymph node
- r. recess

retrocerebellar
- r. arachnoid cyst
- r. CSF collection

retrochiasmal lesion

retroclavicular

retrococcygeal air study

retrocrural
- r. adenopathy
- r. air
- r. lymphadenopathy
- r. node
- r. space

retrodiskal
- r. temporomandibular joint pad inflammation
- r. tissue

retrodisplaced fracture

retroduodenal recess

retroesophageal
- r. aorta
- r. arch
- r. right subclavian artery
- r. vessel

retrofenestral otosclerosis

retroflexed
- r. uterus
- r. view

retroflexion
- uterine r.

retrogasserian target

retrogastric space

retroglandular lesion

retrograde
- r. angiocardiography
- r. arteriography
- r. atherectomy
- r. atrial activation mapping
- r. block
- r. blood flow across valve
- r. blood velocity
- r. cannulation
- r. cardiac perfusion
- r. cardioangiography
- r. cholangiogram
- r. coronary sinus infusion
- r. cystogram (RC)
- r. cystography
- r. cystourethrography
- r. degeneration
- r. embolus
- r. femoral aortography
- r. femoral arterial approach
- r. femoral artery catheterization
- r. filling
- r. flow of gastric content
- r. injection
- r. jejunoduodenogastric intussusception
- r. left ventriculogram
- r. nephrostomy puncture
- r. pancreatocholangiogram
- r. pancreatography
- r. peristalsis
- r. pyelography
- r. refractory period
- r. systolic flow
- r. transaxillary aortography
- r. transfemoral aortography
- r. translumbar aortography
- r. transurethral prostatic urethroplasty
- r. ureteral pseudodiverticulum
- r. ureterogram
- r. ureterography
- r. ureteropyelogram
- r. urethrocystography
- r. urethrogram (RUG)
- r. urogram (RU)
- r. urography
- r. venous route
- r. ventriculoatrial conduction

retrohepatic vena cava

retroileal appendix

retroiliac ureter

NOTES

retrolental fibroplasia
retrolisthesis
    vertebral body r.
retromalleolar
    r. groove
    r. sulcus
retromammary
    r. fascia
    r. fat
    r. space
    r. space view
retromandibular
retromedullary arteriovenous
  malformation
retromembranous hematoma
retromolar trigone carcinoma
retronuchal muscle
retroorbital space
retropancreatic tunnel
retroparotid space
retropectoral mammary implant
retroperfusion
    coronary sinus r.
    synchronized r.
retroperitoneal
    r. actinomycosis
    r. adenopathy
    r. air
    r. air study
    r. area
    r. calcification
    r. cavity
    r. cyst
    r. drain
    r. fat stripe displacement
    r. fibrosis (RPF)
    r. fistula
    r. gas insufflation
    r. hematoma
    r. hemorrhage
    r. infection
    r. leiomyosarcoma
    r. liposarcoma
    r. lymphadenopathy
    r. lymphangioma
    r. lymphoma
    r. mass
    r. node
    r. organ
    r. pneumography
    r. pneumoradiography
    r. space
    r. tumor
    r. tunnel
    r. viscus
retroperitoneum

retropharyngeal
    r. abscess
    r. hematoma
    r. hemorrhage
    r. lymph node
    r. narrowing
    r. soft tissue
    r. space
    r. space mass
retroplacental
    r. hematoma
    r. hemorrhage
retropneumoperitoneum
retropulsed fracture fragment
retropulsion
    vertebral body r.
retropyloric node
retrorectal
    r. cystic hamartoma
    r. lymph node
retrosomatic cleft
retrospective
    r. respiratory gating
    r. review
    r. synchronization
retrosphenoidal space
retrosternal
    r. airspace
    r. area
    r. mass
    r. soft tissue
    r. space
    r. thyroid
retrotorsion
    femoral r.
retrotracheal
    r. adenoma
    r. goiter
    r. soft tissue
    r. vessel
retrovascular goiter
retroversion
    r. of acetabular cup
    femoral r.
retrovertebral plexus
retroverted uterus
retrovesical
    r. septum
    r. space
retrovestibular neural pathway
retrusion
    midface r.
Rett syndrome
return
    anomalous pulmonary venous r.
    arterial r.
    r. to baseline

impaired venous r.
infracardiac-type total anomalous
venous r.
interatrial transposition of venous r.
paracardiac-type total anomalous
venous r.
partial anomalous pulmonary
venous r. (PAPVR)
pulmonary venous r.
supracardiac total anomalous
venous r.
systemic venous r.
total anomalous pulmonary
venous r. (TAPVR)
venous r.

Retzius
R. foramen
R. ligament
line of R.
space of R.
R. system
R. vein

REV
room's eye view
revalidation
revascularization
cerebral r.
coronary ostial r.
endosteal r.
foot r.
graft r.
infragenicular r.
infrainguinal r.
myocardial r.
r. procedure
radiofrequency percutaneous
myocardial r. (RF-PMR)
robotic coronary r.
transmyocardial r. (TMR)
revascularized tissue
reverberating flow pattern
reverberation
r. artifact
r. echo
reversal
r. of cervical lordosis
end-systolic r.
gradient r.
mirror image r.
rapid gradient r.
shunt r.
r. sign

reverse
r. Barton fracture
r. Colles fracture
r. 3 configuration
r. distribution
r. fast imaging with steady-state
free precession (PSIF)
r. Hill-Sachs lesion
r. Monteggia fracture
r. pattern of signal intensity
r. peripheral bat-wing infiltrate
r. pivot shift (RPS)
r. Segond fracture
r. S sign
r. tennis elbow
r. transport
r. Trendelenburg position
r. Waters plane
r. Waters position
reversed
r. coarctation
r. coarctation of aorta
r. ductus arteriosus
r. greater saphenous vein
r. peristalsis
r. shunt
r. Stenvers projection
r. vein graft
r. vertebral blood flow
reversible
r. airway disease
r. bronchiectasis
r. ischemic defect
r. ischemic neurologic deficit
r. myocardial ischemia
r. posterior leukoencephalopathy
syndrome (RPLS)
r. temporary myocardial dysfunction
r. vasogenic edema
review
retrospective r.
**Revised European American Lymphoma
(REAL)**
revolving Ge-68 pin
Reynolds
R. number
R. relationship
REZ
root exit zone
RF
radiofrequency
rapid filling

NOTES

RF *(continued)*
    reticular formation
        RF coil
        RF pulse
        RF shielding
        RF spin echo
        RF spoiling
rf
    radiofrequency
RFA
    radiofrequency ablation
RFCA
    radiofrequency catheter ablation
R&F camera
RF-FAST, RF-spoiled FAST
    radiofrequency spoiled Fourier-acquired
      steady state
RF-PMR
    radiofrequency percutaneous myocardial
      revascularization
RF-shielded cupboard
RF-spoiled FAST *(var. of* RF-FAST*)*
RFW
    rapid filling wave
Rh
    rhodium
rhabdoid
    r. suture
    r. tumor
rhabdomyoblast
rhabdomyolysis
    exertional r.
rhabdomyoma
    cardiac r.
    r. of heart
rhabdomyosarcoma (RMS)
    alveolar r.
    bladder-prostate r.
    botryoid r.
    cardiac r.
    chest wall r.
    childhood r.
    embryonal r.
    extremity r.
    female genital tract r.
    genitourinary r.
    metastatic r.
    ocular r.
    orbital r.
    parameningeal r.
    paratesticular r.
    pleomorphic r.
    primary r.
    truncal r.
rhabdosarcoma
rhebosis
rhenium (Re)

    r.-188 (^{188}Re)
    r. imaging agent
    r. isotope
rhenium-186 (^{186}Re)
    rhenium-186 etidronate
    rhenium-186 HEDP
rheography
    light reflection r.
rheologic pattern
Rhese
    R. projection
    R. view
    R. view of orbit
rheumatic
    r. adherent pericardium
    r. aortic insufficiency
    r. aortic valvular stenosis
    r. granuloma
    r. heart disease
    r. heart valve
    r. lesion
    r. mitral stenosis
    r. tricuspid stenosis
    r. valvular disease
rheumatica
    polymyalgia r.
    synovitis in active polymyalgia r.
rheumatism
    articular r.
    desert r.
    hydroxyapatite r.
rheumatoid
    r. arthritis
    r. factor
    r. lung disease
    r. nodule
    r. pneumoconiosis
    r. spondylitis
rheumatologist
rhinencephalic mamillary body
rhinoplasty
rhinoscintigraphy
    ^{99m}Tc MAA r.
rhinoscleroma
rhinosinusitis
rhizolysis
rhizomelia
rhizomelic
    r. chondrodysplasia punctata
    r. dysplasia
rhizotomy
    trigeminal r.
rhm
    roentgen(s) (per) hour (at one) meter
rhodium (Rh)
    r. anode

r. filter
r. isoimmunization
rhodium-rhodium target filter combination (Rh-Rh)
rhombencephalitis
rhombencephalon
rhombencephalosynapsis
rhombic lip
rhomboid
r. fossa
r. ligament
r. major
r. of Michaelis
r. minor
rhomboideus major muscle
rho° transformation
Rh-Rh
rhodium-rhodium target filter combination
RHV
right hepatic vein
rhythm
atrial bigeminal r.
atrioventricular nodal r.
bisferious pulse r.
escape-capture r.
idioventricular r. (IVR)
mu r.
nodal r.
normal sinus r.
reciprocal r.
sinus r.
transitional r.
ventricular r.
rhythmeur
rhythmic
r. paradoxical eruption
r. segmentation
RI
resistive index
RIA
radioimmunoassay
rib
angle of r.
beaded r.
bed of r.
bicipital r.
bifid r.
bone lesion of the r.
cervical r.
r. contusion
cough fracture of r.

dense r.
r. detail
double-exposed r.
false r.
fifth r.
first r.
floating r.
r. fracture
fused r.
guillotine r.
gumma of r.
head of r.
hyperlucent r.
hypoplastic horizontal r.
inferior margin of superior r.
jail-bar r.
r. lesion
lumbar r.
minced r.
neck of r.
r. notching
overlapping r.
penciling of r.
periosteum of r.
r. recession
retracted r.
rudimentary r.
r. shadowing
shaft of r.
short r.
slipping r.
sternal r.
Stiller r.
superior border of r.
superior margin of inferior r.
true r.
r. tubercle
twisted ribbon-like r.
vertebral r.
vertebrocostal r.
vertebrosternal r.
r. view
wide r.
rib-bearing vertebra
Ribbing disease
ribbon
r. application
r. bowel
hollow r.
^{192}Ir r.
r. muscle

NOTES

ribbon *(continued)*
  seed r.
  r. uterus
ribonucleic acid (RNA)
ribosyl
ribothymidine
ribulose
rib-vertebral angle difference
rice joint body
rice-like muscle calcification
Richter
  R. hernia
  R. syndrome
Richter-Monroe line
rickets classification
rickettsial lung infection
rider's
  r. bone
  r. muscle
  r. tendon
ridge
  alveodental r.
  alveolar r.
  apical ectodermal r. (AER)
  basal r.
  bisagittal r.
  bony r.
  broad maxillary r.
  buccogingival r.
  bulbar r.
  cerebral r.
  cranial r.
  cutaneous r.
  dental r.
  dorsal r.
  epicondylar r.
  epidermal r.
  epipericardial r.
  fibrocartilaginous r.
  fibromuscular r.
  ganglion r.
  gastrocnemial r.
  genital r.
  gluteal r.
  humeral r.
  interarticular r.
  interosseous r.
  intertrochanteric r.
  interureteric r.
  longitudinal r.
  marginal r.
  mylohyoid r.
  oblique r.
  palatine r.
  Passavant r.
  pectoral r.
  petrous r.

  radial r.
  rete r.
  sagittal r.
  semicircular r.
  septal r.
  sphenoid r.
  supraaortic r.
  supracondylar r.
  supracoronary r.
  supraorbital r.
  tentorial r.
  transverse r.
  triangular r.
  ulnar r.
  urethral r.
ridged-convoluted villus
riding
  r. embolus
  r. stomach
Ridley sinus
Riedel
  R. lobe
  R. struma
  R. thyroiditis
Rieder
  R. cell
  R. cell leukemia
Riemann classification
Rieux hernia
RIF
  radiation-induced fibrosis
right
  r. anterior oblique (RAO)
  r. anterior oblique position
  r. anterior oblique position
    ventriculogram
  r. anterior oblique projection
  r. anterior oblique view
  r. aortic arch
  r. aortic arch with mirror image
    branching
  r. atrial appendage (RAA)
  r. atrial chamber
  r. atrial cuff
  r. atrial enlargement (RAE)
  r. atrial extension of uterine
    leiomyosarcoma
  r. atrial hypertrophy
  r. atrial pressure (RAP)
  r. atrial sarcoma
  r. atrium (RA)
  r. atrium oxygen saturation
  r. auricle
  r. axis deviation (RAD)
  r. border of heart
  r. brain
  r. bundle branch

r. bundle-branch block (RBBB)
r. cardiophrenic angle mass
r. colon
r. colonic flexure
r. coronary angiography (RCA)
r. coronary artery (RCA)
r. coronary cusp
r. coronary plexus
r. crus
r. descending pulmonary artery (RDPA)
r. dominant coronary anatomy
r. femoral artery
r. gutter
r. heart catheterization
r. hemisphere
r. hepatic duct
r. hepatic vein (RHV)
r. hilar lymph node
r. ileocolic artery
r. inferior epigastric artery
r. internal iliac artery
r. internal jugular artery
r. lateral decubitus view
r. and left ankle index
r. and left atrial phasic volumetric function
r. or left lateral decubitus film
r. lobe bronchus
r. lobe of liver
r. lower lobe (RLL)
r. lower lobe lesion
r. lower quadrant (RLQ)
r. lung
r. mainstem bronchus
r. mediastinum
r. middle lobe (RML)
r. middle lobe lingula
r. middle lobe syndrome
r. ovarian artery
r. paratracheal stripe
r. posterior oblique (RPO)
r. posterior oblique position
r. posterior oblique projection
r. primary bronchus
r. pulmonary artery (RPA)
r. pulmonary vein (RPV)
r. subclavian central venous (RSCVP)
r. triangular ligament
r. upper lobe (RUL)
r. upper lobe lesion

r. upper quadrant (RUQ)
r. ventricle
r. ventricle of heart
r. ventricle-pulmonary artery conduit
r. ventricle-to-ear time
r. ventricular apex (RVA)
r. ventricular apical electrogram
r. ventricular assist device (RVAD)
r. ventricular branch of right coronary artery
r. ventricular cardiomyopathy
r. ventricular chamber
r. ventricular coil
r. ventricular conduction defect
r. ventricular diastolic pressure
r. ventricular dilatation
r. ventricular dimension (RVD)
r. ventricular dysfunction (RVD)
r. ventricular dysplasia
r. ventricular ejection fraction (RVEF)
r. ventricular electrogram
r. ventricular end-diastolic pressure
r. ventricular end-diastolic volume (RVEDV)
r. ventricular end-systolic volume (RVESV)
r. ventricular enlargement (RVE)
r. ventricular failure
r. ventricular hypertrophy (RVH)
r. ventricular infarct
r. ventricular inflow view
r. ventricular infundibulum
r. ventricular internal diameter (RVID)
r. ventricular to left ventricular systolic pressure ratio (RVP/LVP ratio, RVP/LVP ratio)
r. ventricular to main pulmonary artery pressure gradient
r. ventricular mass (RVM)
r. ventricular outflow obstruction
r. ventricular outflow tract (RVOT)
r. ventricular overload
r. ventricular peak systolic pressure
r. ventricular pressure (RVP)
r. ventricular strain
r. ventricular strain pattern
r. ventricular stroke volume
r. ventricular stroke work (RVSW)

NOTES

right (*continued*)
    r. ventricular stroke work index (RVSWI)
    r. ventricular systolic/diastolic function
    r. ventricular volume pressure

right-angle chest tube

right-angled
    r.-a. isosceles triangle board
    r.-a. telescopic lens

right-handedness
    ventricular r.-h.

right-sided
    r.-s. angiocardiography
    r.-s. arch
    r.-s. cardiomyopathy
    r.-s. empyema
    r.-s. heart failure
    r.-s. heart pressure
    r.-s. pneumonia

right-sidedness
    bilateral r.-s.

right-side-down decubitus position

right-to-left
    r.-t.-l. shift
    r.-t.-l. shunting of blood

rightward

rigid
    r. endofluoroscopy
    r. manipulation
    r. ureter

rigidity
    lead-pipe r.

rigidus
    hallux r.

RigiScan Plus rigidity assessment system

Rigler
    R. sign
    R. triad
    R. triad of small bowel obstruction

RIGS
    radioimmunoguided surgery

RIGScan CR49 imaging agent

RILD
    radiation-induced liver disease

Riley-Day syndrome

rim
    r. apophysis
    bony glenoid r.
    r. of capsule
    r. of cartilage
    dark signal intensity r.
    r. degeneration
    dorsal r.
    r. enhancement
    r. of fascia

    glenoid r.
    high-density r.
    hypoechoic r.
    intercartilaginous r.
    low-density r.
    nephrogram r.
    r. nephrogram
    orbital r.
    r. resection
    sclerotic r.
    r. sign
    signal intensity r.
    volar r.

rim-enhancing lesion

rim-like calcium distribution

RIN
    radiation-induced necrosis

rind
    pleural r.

rind-like thickening

ring
    abdominal r.
    amnion r.
    anorectal r.
    r. apophysis
    r. apophysis calcification
    arc r.
    r. badge
    R. biliary drainage catheter
    r. blush on cerebral arteriography
    Carpentier r.
    Carpentier-Edwards r.
    cartilaginous r.
    ciliary r.
    common tendinous r.
    congenital r.
    constriction r.
    r. detector
    distal esophageal r.
    double-populated detector r.
    drop-lock r.
    Duran r.
    echogenic r.
    r. enhancement
    r. epiphysis
    esophageal mucosal r.
    esophageal muscular r.
    external inguinal r.
    femoral r.
    fibrous r.
    r. finger
    r. fracture
    R. guidewire
    half-r.
    halo r.
    Ilizarov r.
    inguinal r.

R

internal abdominal r.
internal inguinal r.
Kayser-Fleischer r.
r. lesion
r. ligament
low-density r.
lower esophageal mucosal r.
r. man shoulder
mitral valve r.
mucosal r.
multiple concentric GI r.'s
pelvic r.
perichondral r.
pyloric r.
r. scanner
Schatzki r.
r. shadow
r. sign
Silastic r.
silicone elastomer r.
sodium iodide r.
stereotactic r.
sugar r.
superficial inguinal r.
supravalvular r.
symptomatic vascular r.
tracheal r.
trophoblastic r.
tubal r.
umbilical r.
valve r.
vascular r.
r. of Vieussens
Waldeyer r.
Wimberger r.
ring-and-arc calcification
ring-disrupting fracture
ring-down
r.-d. artifact
r.-d. echo
ring-enhancing
r.-e. brain lesion
r.-e. mass
ringing
edge r.
ring-like
r.-l. appearance
r.-l. configuration
r.-l. contraction
r.-l. lesion
r.-l. pattern
r.-l. structure

Ring-McLean sump drainage set
ring-of-bone concept
ring-shaped form
ring-type
r.-t. imaging
r.-t. imaging system
ring-wall lesion
Riolan
R. arch
R. artery
R. muscle
R. ossicle
Riordan
R. club hand classification
R. finger pollicization
ripple voltage
RISA
radioactive iodinated serum albumin
radioiodinated serum albumin
**Riseborough-Radin intercondylar
fracture classification**
rise time
risk
radiation r.
risk-adapted CSI
Risser
R. sign
R. stage
Ritchie index
Rivero-Carvallo maneuver
Rivinus
R. canal
R. duct
RLL
right lower lobe
RLQ
right lower quadrant
R-meter
rate meter
RML
right middle lobe
RMS
rhabdomyosarcoma
rMTT
regional mean transit time
Rn
radon
^{222}Rn, Rn-222
radon-222
RNA
radionuclide angiogram

NOTES

RNA *(continued)*
   ribonucleic acid
      gated RNA
RNV
   radionuclide ventriculogram
R/O
   rule out
ROA
   regurgitant orifice area
road mapping
road-mapping
      r.-m. mode
      r.-m. technique
Roadrunner NaviGuide guidewire
Robert ligament
robertsonian translocation
Roberts syndrome
Robin
      R. anomalad
      R. sequence
Robinow syndrome
robotic
      r. coronary revascularization
      r. mitral valve surgery
robotics-controlled stereotactic frame
Robson
      R. modification of Flocks-Kadesky system
      R. staging classification
robust
      r. registration
      r. registration technique
ROC
   receiver operating characteristic
      ROC curve
      ROC method
rocker-bottom
      r.-b. foot
      r.-b. foot deformity
rocker deformity
rocking
      r. curve measurement
      r. precordial motion
Rockwood acromioclavicular injury classification
rod
      Alta reconstruction r.
      Alta tibial/humeral r.
      r. eyelet
      Harrington r.
      Hopkins r.
      IM r.
      Isolar r.
      Luque r.
      medullary r.
      orthopedic r.
      resorbable r.

      r. source
      thermoluminescent dosimeter r.
      TLD r.
rodding
      IM r.
      intramedullary r.
rodent ulcer
RODEO
   rotating delivery of excitation off-resonance
      3D RODEO
rod-shaped calcification
Roederer obliquity
rOEF
   regional oxygen extraction fraction
roentgen (R, r)
      r. equivalent man (REM)
      r. equivalent-physical (REP)
      r. knife
      r. kymography
      r. meter
      r.'s per second (R/s)
      r. ray
      r. stereophotogrammetric
      r. stereophotogrammetric analysis (RSA)
      r. tube
      r. unit (RU)
roentgen-equivalent-physical
roentgenkymogram
roentgenkymograph
roentgenkymography
roentgenogram
roentgenographic
      r. change
      r. control
      r. diagnosis
      r. finding
      r. silhouette
roentgenographically occult
roentgenography
      abdominal r.
      double-contrast r.
      magnification r.
      mucosal relief r.
      sectional r.
      selective r.
roentgenologic
roentgenological
roentgenologist
roentgenology
roentgenometer
roentgenoscope
roentgenotherapy
roentgen(s) (per) hour (at one) meter (rhm)

roentgentherapy
    intraoral r.
    intravaginal r.
Rogan teleradiology system
Roger
    R. disease
    maladie de R.
    R. system
    R. ventricular septal defect
ROI
    region of interest
Rokitansky
    R. diverticulum
    R. lobe
    R. nodule
    R. pelvis
Rokitansky-Aschoff sinus
Rokitansky-Cushing ulcer
Rokitansky-Mayer-Küster-Hauser
  syndrome
Rokus view
rolandic
    r. artery
    r. cortex
    r. fissure
    r. sulcus
Rolando
    R. angle
    R. area
    fissure of R.
    R. fracture
    R. line
    R. point
    R. tubercle
    R. zone
rolandoparietal glioma
roll
    radiolucent r.
rolled
    r. edge deformity
    r. view
roller mark artifact
Rollet stroma
Rollier radiation
rolling
    r. hiatal hernia
    r. membrane
    r. membrane Wallstent cobalt-based
      alloy balloon-expandable stent
Romano-Ward syndrome
Romberg sign
Romberg-Wood syndrome

Romhilt-Estes score for left ventricular
  hypertrophy
ROMI
    rule out myocardial infarct
RON
    radiation-related optic neuropathy
R-on-T phenomenon
roof
    acetabular r.
    r. of fourth ventricle
    r. of insula
    intercondylar r.
roofless fourth ventricle diverticulum
room
    r. eye view (REV)
    r. shielding
root (R)
    anatomic r.
    aortic r.
    cervical nerve r.
    cochlear r.
    r. compression
    coronary sinus r.
    cranial r.
    dental r.
    dilacerated tooth r.
    dilated aortic r.
    r. end granuloma
    r. entry zone
    r. entry-zone lesion
    r. exit zone (REZ)
    extrathecal nerve r.
    facial r.
    insula r.
    intradural nerve r.
    intrathecal r.
    lateral r.
    left atrium/aortic r.
    lingual r.
    lumbar nerve r.
    lung r.
    r. of mesentery
    motor r.
    nerve r.
    palatine r.
    r. of penis
    retained r.
    sensory r.
    spinal r.
    ventral r.
    ventricle r.

NOTES

rootlet
    intradural r.
root-mean-squared gradient measurement
ROPE
    respiratory ordered phase encoding
rope-like cord
ropy
Rosai-Dorfman disease
rosary
    r. bead configuration
    r. beading
    r. beading bone scintigraphy
    r. beading esophagus
    r. bead pattern
    rachitic r.
Rosch-Uchida needle
rose
    r. bengal dye
    r. bengal ^{131}I radioactive agent
    r. bengal sodium I-131 biliary
        imaging
Rose-Bradford kidney
Rosenbach sign
Rosen curved guidewire
Rosenmüller
    fossa of R.
    R. node
    R. valve
Rosenthal
    basal vein of R. (BVR)
    R. canal
rosette shape
rostral
    r. body of corpus callosum
    r. brainstem ischemia
    r. cervical nerve
    r. connection
    r. hypothalamus
    r. medulla
    r. pons
    r. spinal cord
    r. terminus
rostrocaudal extent signal abnormality
rostrum
    r. of corpus callosum
    r. sphenoidale
Rotablator thrombectomy system
rotary
    r. ankle instability
    r. deviation
    r. door flap (RDF)
    r. subluxation of scaphoid
    r. thoracolumbar scoliosis
rotatable pigtail catheter
rotated
    abducted and externally r. (ABER)
    r. craniocaudal view

rotate-rotate scan
rotate-stationary scan
rotating
    r. anode
    r. anode tube
    r. delivery of excitation off-
        resonance (RODEO)
    r. delivery of excitation off-
        resonance MR imaging
    r. disk oxygenator
    r. endoprobe
    r. frame
    r. frame imaging
    r. frame of reference
    r. gamma camera
    r. Ge-68 rod source
    r. hemostatic valve
    r. raw cine data
    r. tomographic projection
    r. ultra-fast imaging sequence
        (RUFIS)
rotating-frame zeugmatography
rotation
    360° r.
    r. angle
    anisotropic r.
    r. anomaly
    axial r.
    degree of head r.
    gantry r.
    instantaneous axis of r. (IAR)
    internal femoral r.
    medial r.
    organoaxial r.
    r.'s per minute (rpm)
    placenta r.
    pronation-external r.
    SPECT center of r.
    r. therapy
    tibiotalar r.
    tube position r.
rotational
    r. alignment
    r. angiography (RA)
    r. atherectomy (RA)
    r. atherectomy system
    r. burst fracture
    r. contact lithotripsy
    r. coronary atherectomy (RCA)
    r. correlation time
    r. deformity
    r. dislocation
    r. displacement
    r. field
    r. force
    r. frequency
    r. instability

r. malalignment
r. method
r. motion
r. radiotherapy
r. scanography
r. therapy technique
r. tomography
rotationally invariant imaging
rotation-shearing injury
rotator
r. cuff
r. cuff arthropathy
r. cuff lesion
r. cuff muscle
r. cuff tear
r. interval
rotatory
r. instability
r. load
r. load on spine
Rotch sign
Roth spot
Rotograph Plus panoramic dental tomography imaging system
rotography
Rotor syndrome
rotoscoliosis
rotoscoliotic deformity
rototomography
Rotter node
rotundum
foramen r.
Rouget muscle
roughened
r. articular surface
r. cartilage
r. state of pericardium
rough zone
round
r. bone-cell tumor
r. cancer of the breast
r. cell sarcoma
r. heart
r. ligament
r. ligament of uterus
r. lucent lesion
r. muscle
r. pneumonia
r. pronator
r. shift
r. shoulder deformity
r. ulcer

roundback deformity
round-cell tumor
rounded
r. appearance
r. atelectasis
r. border of lung
r. convex border
r. lesion
r. opacity
Rous
R. sarcoma
R. tumor
route
hematogenous r.
retrograde venous r.
thoracic duct r.
translumbar aortic r.
urinary excretory r.
routine magnification view
Rouviere
R. ligament
R. node
Roux-en-Y
R.-e.-Y. limb
R.-e.-Y. procedure
Roux loop
Rovighi sign
Rovsing sign
row
carpal r.
distal carpal r.
first carpal r.
proximal carpal r.
Rowasa enema
Rowe calcaneal fracture classification
Rowe-Lowell fracture-dislocation classification
row-mode sinogram imaging
Royal Flush 4F pigtail catheter
RPA
right pulmonary artery
RPF
retroperitoneal fibrosis
RPLS
reversible posterior leukoencephalopathy syndrome
RPM
real-time position management
RPM tracking system
rpm
rotations per minute

R

NOTES

RPO
    right posterior oblique
RPS
    reverse pivot shift
RPT
    rapid pull-through technique
RPV
    right pulmonary vein
RP X-OMAT processor
RR
    radiation response
rrBF
    relative regional blood flow
RRP
    relative refractory period
R/s
    roentgens per second
RSA
    roentgen stereophotogrammetric analysis
RSCVP
    right subclavian central venous
RSI
    repetitive strain injury
    repetitive stress injury
RSV
    regurgitant stroke volume
RT
    radiation therapy
    radiotherapy
    recovery time
    repetition time
        RT 3200 Advantage ultrasound
        RT 3200 Advantage ultrasound
            scanner
        RT 6800 ultrasound
        RT 6800 ultrasound scanner
RTAS
    rapid telephone access system
R-to-R imaging
RTP
    radiation therapy planning
    radiation treatment planning
        3D RTP
        RTP system
RTS
    radiation therapy system
        MammoSite RTS
rTSH
    recombinant thyrotropin contrast agent
RU
    retrograde urogram
    roentgen unit
Ru
    ruthenium

rubber
    r. drain
    r. vessel loop
rubidium (Rb)
    r.-82 (^{82}Rb, Rb-82)
    r. chloride imaging agent
Rubratope-57 imaging agent
Rudick red flag
rudimentary
    r. bone
    r. lung
    r. organ
    r. outlet chamber
    r. pronephron
    r. rib
    r. sinus
    r. ventricle
    r. ventricular chamber
Ruedi-Allgower
    R.-A. tibial plafond fracture
    R.-A. tibial plafond fracture
        classification
ruffled border formation
RUFIS
    rotating ultra-fast imaging sequence
RUG
    retrograde urethrogram
ruga, pl. **rugae**
    gastric rugae
rugal
    r. fold
    r. pattern
rugger
    r. jersey appearance
    r. jersey sign
    r. jersey spine
    r. jersey vertebra
rugose, rugous
RUL
    right upper lobe
rule
    Buffalo malleolar r.
    modified Simpson r.
    OAR malleolar r.
    r. of 3
    Ottawa ankle r.
    r. out (R/O)
    r. out myocardial infarct (ROMI)
rule-based scheme
ruler
    endocatheter r.
Rumstrom view
run
    high-frame-rate r.
    low-frame-rate r.
Rundles-Falls syndrome

runner's
- r. bump
- r. knee

runoff
- absent r.
- aortic r.
- aortofemoral r.
- arterial r.
- r. arteriography
- digital r.
- distal r.
- r. film
- inadequate r.
- peripheral r.
- r. resistance index
- single-vessel r.
- suboptimal r.
- three-vessel r.
- two-vessel r.
- vessel r.

Runström projection
Runyon classification
rupture
- Achilles tendon r.
- amnion r.
- aneurysmal r.
- aortic r.
- appendix r.
- arch r.
- arterial dilatation and r.
- Berry aneurysm r.
- bladder r.
- breast prosthesis r.
- bronchial r.
- buttonhole r.
- cardiac r.
- chordae tendineae r.
- chordal r.
- complex extraperitoneal r.
- contained aneurysmal r.
- contained aortic r.
- delayed splenic r.
- diaphragmatic r.
- esophageal r.
- extraperitoneal bladder r.
- forniceal r.
- frank r.
- hemidiaphragm r.
- hepatic capsular r.
- hernia r.
- interventricular septal r.
- intramural esophageal r.

- intraperitoneal r.
- intratendinous r.
- mesenteric r.
- myocardial r.
- r. of myocardium
- myotendinous junction r.
- nodal r.
- papillary muscle r.
- plantaris r.
- plaque r.
- pregnant uterus r.
- premature uterine membrane r.
- silicone implant r.
- simple extraperitoneal r.
- splenic r.
- tendon r.
- testicular r.
- tracheobronchial r.
- traumatic aortic r.
- urinary bladder r.
- ventricular free wall r.
- ventricular septal r.
- vessel r.

ruptured
- r. aneurysm
- r. aortic cusp
- r. capillary
- r. chordae tendineae
- r. disk
- r. ectopic pregnancy
- r. emphysematous bleb
- r. follicle
- r. hollow viscus
- r. spleen
- r. thoracic duct
- r. ulcer

RUQ
- right upper quadrant

Rusch catheter
rush
- peristaltic r.

Russell
- R. body
- R. effect

Russell-Rubinstein cerebrovascular malformation classification
Russell-Silver
- R.-S. dwarfism
- R.-S. syndrome

ruthenium (Ru)
rutherford (Rd)
- r. unit

NOTES

Rutner balloon dilatation helical stone extractor set
Ruvalcaba-Myhre-Smith syndrome
Ruysch
  R. disease
  R. muscle
RV
  residual volume
RVA
  right ventricular apex
    RVA electrogram
RVAD
  right ventricular assist device
RVD
  right ventricular dimension
  right ventricular dysfunction
RVE
  right ventricular enlargement
RVEDV
  right ventricular end-diastolic volume
RVEF
  right ventricular ejection fraction
RVESV
  right ventricular end-systolic volume
RVG
  radionuclide ventriculogram

RVH
  renal vascular hypertension
  right ventricular hypertrophy
RVID
  right ventricular internal diameter
RVM
  right ventricular mass
RVOT
  right ventricular outflow tract
RVP
  right ventricular pressure
RVP/LVP ratio
  right ventricular to left ventricular
    systolic pressure ratio
RVSW
  right ventricular stroke work
RVSWI
  right ventricular stroke work index
RVT
  renal vein thrombosis
RV/TLC
  residual volume/total lung capacity
RX
  rapid exchange
    RX stent delivery system
RX400

S

    S contour
    S distortion
    S number
    S shape
    S sign of Golden
    S value

S670

    S. over-the-wire coronary stent
    S. stent

^{35}S, S-35

    sulfur-35

S7 AVE stent

SA

    sarcoma
    serratus anterior
    sinoatrial
    splenic artery
    subcarinal angle
       SA node

SAAV

    simultaneous acquisition of artery and
    vein

SAB

    sinoatrial block

saber-sheath trachea

saber-shin

    s.-s. appearance
    s.-s. deformity

sabot

    coeur en s.
    s. heart

Sabouraud-Noiré instrument

Sabouraud pastille

sac

    abdominal s.
    air s.
    alveolar s.
    amnionic s.
    s. of aneurysm
    aneurysmal s.
    aortic s.
    bursal s.
    chorionic s.
    common dural s.
    cystic s.
    decidual s.
    dental s.
    double decidual s.
    dural s.
    embryonic s.
    empty gestational s.
    endolymphatic s.
    enterocele s.
    false s.

    fluid-filled s.
    gestational s. (GS)
    greater peritoneal s.
    heart s.
    hernia s.
    hydronephrotic s.
    indirect hernia s.
    intrauterine s.
    lacrimal s.
    lesser peritoneal s.
    lymphatic s.
    narrowing of thecal s.
    pericardial s.
    peritoneal s.
    pleural s.
    primary yolk s.
    primitive yolk s.
    pseudogestational s.
    residual aneurysmal s.
    sacral s.
    secondary yolk s.
    spinal s.
    terminal air s.
    thecal s.
    tight dural s.
    wide-mouth s.
    wrapped aneurysmal s.
    yolk s. (YS)

sacciform

    s. aneurysm
    s. kidney
    s. recess

saccular

    s. bronchiectasis
    s. cerebral aneurysm
    s. collection
    s. dilatation
    s. ectasia
    s. formation
    s. malformation
    s. mass
    s. outpouching
    s. pseudoaneurysm

sacculated pleurisy

sacculation

saccule

sacculocochlear canal

sacculoutricular canal

Sack-Barabas syndrome

sac-like

    s.-l. cavity
    s.-l. space

sacral

    s. agenesis
    s. ala

sacral *(continued)*
  s. aneurysm
  s. bone
  s. bone tumor
  s. canal
  s. chordoma
  s. crest
  s. cyst
  s. dysgenesis
  s. foramen
  s. gutter
  s. hyperintensity
  s. insufficiency fracture (SIF)
  s. lymph node
  s. meningocele
  s. nerve
  s. osteolysis
  s. osteomyelitis
  s. osteosarcoma
  s. plexus
  s. process
  s. promontory
  s. sac
  s. spine
  s. vertebra
sacralization
sacralized transverse process
sacrococcygeal
  s. chordoma
  s. inferior pubic point (SCIPP)
  s. inferior pubic point line
  s. joint
  s. remnant tumor
sacrococcyx
sacrodural ligament
sacrogenital fold
sacrohorizontal angle
sacroiliac (SI)
  s. articulation
  s. disease
  s. fracture
  s. infection
  s. joint
  s. joint fusion
  s. joint widening
  s. sprain
  s. subluxation
sacrolumbar dysgenesis
sacropubic diameter
sacrosciatic
  s. foramen
  s. notch
sacrospinalis muscle
sacrospinous ligament
sacrotuberous ligament
sacrouterine
sacrovertebral angle

sacrum
  cornu of s.
  tilted s.
SACT
  sinoatrial conduction time
saddle
  s. coil
  s. embolus
  s. joint
  s. lesion
  s. peristalsis ureter
  s. point
saddle-shaped
  s.-s. uterine fundus
  s.-s. uterus
SADIA
Sadowsky breast marking system
SAE
  stimulated acoustic emission
SAECG, SaECG
  signal-averaged electrocardiogram
Saemisch ulcer
Saethre-Chotzen acrocephalosyndactyly
SAFHS
  sonic-accelerated fracture-healing system
  Exogen 2000 SAFHS
  SAFHS 2000 sonic accelerated
    fracture healing system
Saf-T-Intima integrated IV catheter
Sage-Salvatore classification of
  acromioclavicular joint injury
sagging brain
sagittal
  s. canal diameter (SCD)
  s. celloidin section
  s. and coronal reconstruction view
  s. cranial suture
  s. fast spin-echo T2-weighted MR
    imaging
  s. fat-suppressed T1-weighted 3D
    spoiled gradient-echo image
  s. fontanelle
  s. gradient-echo imaging
  s. groove
  s. HR-MR
  s. localization
  s. magnetization transfer view
  s. oblique imaging
  s. orientation
  s. paraffin section
  s. plane
  s. plane fault
  s. plane loop
  s. plane vectorcardiography
  s. porta hepatis
  s. reconstruction
  s. ridge

s. roll spondylolisthesis
s. scan
s. scout image
s. sinus
s. slice
s. synostosis
s. thrombosis
s. tomogram
s. transabdominal imaging
s. T1-weighted MR image
s. ultrasound

SAH

subarachnoid hemorrhage

Sahara

S. clinical bone sonometer
S. portable bone densitometer

sail-like tricuspid valve
sail sign
Saint triad
**Sakellarides classification of calcaneal
fracture**
Saldino-Noonan syndrome
Salem sump tube
saline

s. implant
s. infusion sonohysterography (SIS)
s. solution
s. torch

saline-enhanced

s.-e. MR arthrography
s.-e. MR imaging
s.-e. RF tissue ablation

salivary

s. calculus
s. gland
s. gland carcinoma
s. gland dysfunction
s. gland function study
s. gland infection
s. gland lymphoepithelioma
s. gland scan
s. gland scintigraphy
s. stone

salmon-patch hemorrhage
salpinges (*pl. of* salpinx)
salpingitis

chronic interstitial s.
follicular s.
hemorrhagic s.
interstitial s.
s. isthmica nodosa
pseudofollicular s.

purulent s.
tuberculous s.

salpingogram
salpingography

selective osteal s.

salpingopharyngeus
salpinx, pl. **salpinges**
salt-and-pepper

s.-a.-p. chromatin pattern
s.-a.-p. duodenal erosion

saltans

coxa s.
hallux s.

Salter-Harris

S.-H. classification of epiphyseal
fracture 1–5
S.-H. growth plate injury
classification

**Salter-Harris-Rang epiphyseal fracture
classification**
salt-losing nephritis
Saltzman anatomy
salvage

s. of myocardium
s. therapy

salvo of echoes
SAM

scanning acoustic microscope
systolic anterior motion

samarium (Sm)

s. imaging agent
s. scintigraphy

samarium-153 (^{153}Sm, Sm-153)

s. ethyl-
enediaminetetramethylenephosphonic
acid therapy

same-day

s.-d. exercise-rest Tc-99m
tetrofosmin myocardial perfusion
scintigraphy
s.-d. microsurgical arthroscopic
lateral-approach laser-assisted
fluoroscopic diskectomy

sampling

angular s.
asymmetric data s.
s. error
Gibbs s.
length-biased s.
nonlinear s.
partial k-space s.

NOTES

sampling *(continued)*
    s. window
    zonal s.
SAN
    sinoatrial node
Sanchez-Perez cassette changer
sanctuary
    s. organ
    s. site
sandal-gap deformity
sandbagging fracture
sandbag hazard
Sanders sign
sand-like lucency
Sand process
sand tumor
sandwich
    s. appearance
    s. configuration
    s. configuration adenopathy
    s. patch closure
    s. sign
    s. technique
    s. vertebra
Sanfilippo syndrome
sanguifacient
sanguiferous
sanguification
sanguineous, sanguinous
San Joaquin Valley fever
Sansom sign
Sansregret method
Santiani-Stone classification of pancreatitis
Santorini
    S. canal
    S. duct
    S. ligament
    S. muscle
    S. papilla
SAPA
    spatial average-pulse average
saphenofemoral junction
saphenous
    s. nerve
    s. system
    s. varix
    s. vein
    s. vein bypass graft
    s. vein incompetence
    s. vein mapping
    s. vein stenosis
SAPHO
    synovitis, acne, pustolosis, hyperostosis, osteitis
SAPHO syndrome
saponated cresol solution

Sappey
    S. inferior vein
    S. ligament
    S. line
saprophytic
    s. aspergillosis
    s. colonization
SAR
    scatter-air ratio
    specific absorption rate
sarcocarcinoma
sarcofetal pregnancy
sarcohysteric pregnancy
sarcoid
    s. granuloma
    lung s.
sarcoid-like reaction
sarcoidosis
    acinar s.
    alveolar s.
    bone s.
    cardiac s.
    endobronchial s.
    hepatic s.
    musculocutaneous s.
    orbital s.
    osteosclerosis vertebral s.
    pulmonary s.
    spinal cord s.
    spleen s.
sarcoma (SA)
    African Kaposi s.
    alveolar soft-part s. (ASPS)
    ameloblastic s.
    angiolithic s.
    bone-forming s.
    botryoid s.
    breast s.
    cardiac s.
    cerebellar s.
    cervical s.
    chloroma granulocytic s.
    clear cell s.
    diaphragmatic s.
    embryonal liver s.
    endobronchial Kaposi s.
    endometrial stromal s.
    epithelioid s.
    Ewing s.
    extraosseous Ewing s.
    fascicular s.
    giant cell s.
    granulocytic s.
    hemangioendothelial bone s.
    hemangioendothelial liver s.
    hepatic anaplastic s.
    high-grade surface osteogenic s.

intracortical osteogenic s.
intrathoracic Kaposi s.
juxtacortical osteogenic s.
Kaposi s. (KS)
Kupffer cell s.
low-grade central osteogenic s.
lymphatic s.
malignant myeloid s.
meningeal s.
mesenterial s.
mesodermal s.
mixed cell s.
multicentric osteogenic s.
multiple idiopathic hemorrhagic s.
neurogenic s.
orbital granulocytic s.
osteogenic s.
parosteal osteogenic s.
periosteal s.
pleomorphic s.
postirradiation osteogenic s.
primary s.
pulmonary artery s.
pulmonary Kaposi s.
radiation-induced s.
radioinduced s.
reticulum bone cell s.
reticulum brain cell s.
right atrial s.
round cell s.
Rous s.
sclerotic osteogenic s.
soft tissue s.
synovial s.
telangiectatic osteogenic s.
tendosynovial s.
undifferentiated liver s.
vascular s.
vasoablative endothelial s. (VABES)

sarcomatode
sarcomatoid
sarcomatosis
diffuse s.
sclerosing osteogenic s.
sarcomatous
sarcomere
sartorius
s. insertion
s. muscle
s. tendon
SAS
supravalvular aortic stenosis

SA-SD bursitis
Sassouni analysis
SATA
spatial average-temporal average
satellite
s. cartilaginous focus
s. lesion
s. metastasis
s. node
s. nodule
s. structure
satellitosis
Sat Pad
satumomab
s. pendetide imaging agent
s. pentetide
saturated potassium iodide solution (SSKI)
saturation
s. analysis
aortic oxygen s.
arterial oxygen s.
s. band
s. current
fat s.
frequency-selective fat s.
gaussian line s.
s. index (SI)
s. inversion projection (SIP)
jugular venous oxygen s.
line s.
lorentzian line s.
mixed venous s.
MT s.
off-resonance s.
oxygen s.
partial s. (PS)
progressive spin s.
s. pulse
s. recovery (SR)
s. recovery image
s. recovery sequence
s. recovery technique
regional cerebral oxygen s.
right atrium oxygen s.
selective s.
spatial-spectral prepulses for fat s.
spectral s.
s. stripe
systemic oxygen s.
s. transfer

S

NOTES

saturation *(continued)*
> T1-weighted axial image with
> > fat s.

saucerization of vertebra
saucer-shaped excavation
sausage
> s. digit
> s. finger
> s. segment effect

sausage-shaped appearance
sausaging of vein
Sauvage filamentous velour graft
SAVANT
> surgical anatomy visualization and
> navigation tools
> > SAVANT imaging system

sawtooth
> s. appearance
> s. configuration
> s. edge
> s. excretory pattern
> s. irregularity of bowel contour
> s. sign
> s. ureter

sawtooth-like thickening
SBDX
> scanning-beam digital x-ray

SBE
> small bowel enteroscopy

SBF
> systemic blood flow

SBFT
> small bowel follow-through

SBO
> small bowel obstruction
> spina bifida occulta

SBP
> solitary bone plasmacytoma

SBPA
SBS
> shaken baby syndrome

SBSP
> simultaneous bilateral spontaneous
> pneumothorax

Sc
> scandium

⁴⁷Sc, Sc-47
> scandium-47

SCA
> single-channel analyzer
> superior cerebellar artery

scabbard trachea
SCAD
> spontaneous coronary artery dissection

scalar
> s. coupling
> s. effect

scalariform
scale
> abbreviated injury s. (AIS)
> Bloch s.
> color-flame s.
> digital gray s.
> expanded-disability status s. (EDSS)
> false color s.
> Flint colon injury s.
> Glasgow outcome s.
> gray s.
> Hunt and Hess subarachnoid
> > hemorrhage s.
> injury severity s. (ISS)
> relative value s.
> Scandinavian Stroke s.

scalene
> s. fat pad
> s. maneuver
> s. musculature
> s. node
> s. triangle
> s. tubercle

scalenus
> s. anterior
> s. anterior muscle
> s. anticus muscle hypertrophy
> s. anticus syndrome
> s. medius
> s. minimus

scaler
> s. counter
> decade s.

scaling
> s. device
> quantization matrix s.

scalloped
> s. appearance
> s. appearance of white matter
> s. border
> s. bowel lumen
> s. commissure
> s. luminal configuration

scalloping
> bone tumor s.
> s. contour
> cortical s.
> endosteal s.
> s. of margin of vertebral body
> s. osteolysis
> petrous pyramid s.
> posterior vertebral s.
> vertebral s.

scalp
> s. branch of external carotid artery
> s. hematoma

s. hypothermia
s. vein needle
scalpel
s. cut
interactive electronic s.
ultrasonically activated s.
scan (*See* scanning)
A s.
abdominal CT s.
adrenal s.
aerosol ventilation s.
A-mode amplitude modulation s.
attenuation s.
axial s.
axial unenhanced CT s.
B s.
Becton Dickinson FAC s.
bile duct s.
biphasic helical CT s.
blank s.
blood pool radionuclide s.
B-mode brightness modulation s.
bone marrow s.
brain s.
bremsstrahlung s.
brightness modulation s.
C s.
capillary blockade perfusion C-
mode s.
cardiac s.
CE-FAST s.
cerebral perfusion SPECT s.
cine CT s.
cine view in MUGA s.
clearance phase ventilation s.
^{11}C-methionine PET s.
coincidence detection s.
colloid shift on s.
color-flow duplex s.
computed tomography s.
contiguous s.
s. converter
coregistered s.
coronal s.
coronary artery s. (CAS)
CT s.
s. decrement
s. defect
dental s.
DEXA s.
diffusion s.
diuretic renal s.

dot s.
double helical CT s.
2D sector s.
dual-phase s.
dynamic CT s.
dynamic emission s.
elbow coronal s.
electromagnetic interference s.
enhanced CT s.
equilibrium MUGA s.
^{18}FDG PET s.
flow portion of bone s.
fluorescent s.
full-body CT s.
^{67}Ga bone s.
gadolinium s.
gallium s.
gamma s.
gastric emptying s.
gated blood pool s.
Heart CT s.
helical thin-section CT s.
hepatobiliary s.
hepatoiminodiacetic acid s.
HIDA s.
ictal PET s.
^{125}I fibrinogen s.
indium-111-labeled white blood
cell s.
infarct s.
In-111 pentetreotide s.
interictal SPECT s.
intravenously enhanced CT s.
iodine-131 whole-body s.
isotope bone s.
isotopic lung s.
kidney s.
krypton s.
labeled leukocyte s.
lacrimal s.
left-side-down decubitus s.
left ventricular gated blood pool s.
liver s.
liver-lung s.
liver-spleen s.
longitudinal s.
lung s.
mechanical compound s.
Meckel s.
medronate s.
MET-PET s.
MIBG SPECT s.

S

NOTES

scan *(continued)*

M-mode time motion s.
MUGA s.
multi-detector row CT s.
multiple gated acquisition s.
multiple gated blood pool s.
multiple line s. (MLS)
multislice full line s.
myocardial perfusion s.
NMR s.
noncontrast CT s.
nonenhanced CT s.
nongated CT s.
nuclear magnetic resonance s.
nucleotide s.
octreotide tumor localization s.
oral-enhanced CT s.
s. orientation
pancreatic s.
panoramic CT s.
para-isopropyl-iminodiacetic acid
  technetium-99m hepatobiliary s.
s. parameter
pelvic ultrasound CT s.
pentetreotide tumor localization s.
perfusion lung s.
PET s.
PIPIDA s.
s. pitch
s. pitch pit
planar thallium s.
s. plane
portal-phased spiral CT s.
postgadolinium s.
postictal cerebral blood flow s.
postinjection attenuation s.
postmetrizamide CT s.
precontrast s.
preoperative resting MUGA s.
ProstaScint s.
proton-density axial MR s.
PYP technetium myocardial s.
pyrophosphate technetium
  myocardial s.
quantitative s.
radioactive brain s.
radioactive fibrinogen s.
radioactive iodinated serum
  albumin s.
radioactive iodine s.
radiofibrinogen uptake s.
radioisotope lung s.
radionuclide bone s.
radionuclide flow s.
radionuclide-gated blood pool s.
radionuclide liver s.
radionuclide milk s.

radionuclide thyroid s.
rapid sequential CT s.
rCBF PET s.
real-time s.
rebreathing ventilation s.
rectilinear bone s.
rectilinear thyroid s.
redistributed thallium s.
renal duplex s.
rotate-rotate s.
rotate-stationary s.
sagittal s.
salivary gland s.
scintillation s.
sector s.
segmental lung defect s.
segmenting dual-echo MR head s.
selective excitation line s.
s. sequence
serial duplex s.
single-pass s.
single-photon emission-computed
  tomography technetium
  sestamibi s.
single sweep s.
spatially normalized PET and
  SPECT s.
spin-echo s.
spiral CT s.
spleen s.
splenic perfusion measurement by
  dynamic CT s.
s. spot
stacked s.
static emission s.
stereotactic CT s.
stimulation s.
stress thallium s.
strip s.
sulfur colloid s.
suppression s.
survey s.
^{99m}Tc HMPAO-labeled leukocyte
  total-body s.
^{99m}Tc-labeled macroaggregated
  albumin s.
TcO_4 thyroid s.
^{99m}Tc WBC s.
teboroxime cardiac s.
technetium-99m hepatoiminodiacetic
  acid s.
technetium-99m phytate s.
thallium-201 s.
thallium myocardial s.
thallium single-photon emission
  computed tomography s.
thorium-201 SPECT s.

three-head s.
three-phase bone s.
thyroid stimulation s.
thyroid suppression s.
thyroid whole-body s.
s. time
transaxial CT s.
transaxial joint s.
transaxial PET s.
transmission s.
transverse s.
triple-phase bone s.
T2-weighted s.
unenhanced magnetic resonance
  imaging s.
uniform phantom s.
venous s.
ventilation lung s.
ventilation-perfusion lung s.
s. volume
volumetric s.
V/Q lung segment s.
washout phase ventilation s.
water path s.
water signal on magnetic resonance
  imaging s.
whole-body bone s.
whole-body PET s.
whole-body transmission s.
s. with contrast enhancement
ZeroRad MRI s.
Scandinavian Stroke scale
Scanditronix
  S. 1024-7B camera
  S. MLC system
  S. PET scanner
scandium (Sc)
scandium-47 (^{47}Sc, Sc-47)
Scanmaster DX x-ray film digitizer
  scanner
scannable tumor
scanned
  s. focal point (SFP)
  s. projection radiography (SPR)
scanned-slot detector system
scanner
  Acuson 128EP s.
  Acuson XP 10 s.
  Advanced NMR Systems s.
  Agfa Medical s.
  All-Tronics s.
  Aloka ultrasound linear s.

Aloka ultrasound sector s.
American Shared-CuraCare s.
ANMR Insta-scan MR s.
Aquilion plus V-detector CT s.
Artoscan MRI s.
ATL Mark 600 real-time sector s.
ATL Neurosector real-time s.
Aura Laser helical s.
Aurora MR breast imaging
  system s.
BioSpec MR imaging system s.
biplane sector s.
Bruel-Kjaer ultrasound s.
Bruker s.
Canon s.
Cardio Data MK3 Holter s.
cardiovascular computed
  tomographic s. (CVCT)
Cencit surface s.
charge-coupled device s.
cine CT s.
C-150 LXP EBT s.
coincidence imaging s.
C-PET s.
CT9000, 9800 s.
CT body s.
CTI 933/04 ECAT s.
CTI 931 PET s.
CT Max 640 s.
dedicated head s.
dedicated PET s.
Delarnette s.
Diasonics ultrasound s.
Discovery LS, ST^4 PET/CT s.
Dornier s.
DSR s.
3D surface digitizer s.
dual-probe rectilinear s.
duplex s.
DuPont s.
Eastman Kodak s.
EBT s.
Echospeed Signa LX 1.5 T s.
electron beam CT s.
8000-element linear array CCD s.
Elscint Excel 905 s.
Elscint MR s.
Elscint Twin CT s.
EMED s.
EMI 7070 s.
EMI brain s.
EMI CT 500 s.

S

NOTES

scanner *(continued)*
    Esaote extremity s.
    Evolution XP s.
    FONAR-360 MRI s.
    full ring s.
    Galen Scan s.
    gamma ray s.
    Gammex RMI s.
    gated CT s.
    GE Advance PET s.
    GE CT Advantage s.
    GE CTI 9800 s.
    GE CTI single detector s.
    GE CT Max s.
    GE CT Pace s.
    GE 8800 CT/T s.
    GE CT/T7 s.
    GE CT/T 8800 s.
    GE Genesis CT s.
    GE GN 500-MHz s.
    GE 9800 high-resolution CT s.
    GE HiSpeed Advantage helical
      CT s.
    GE HiSpeed single detector s.
    GE Lightspeed CT s.
    GE MR Max s.
    GE MR Signa s.
    GE MR Vectra s.
    GE Omega 500-MHz s.
    GE Pace CT s.
    GE QE 300-MHz s.
    GE Signa 4.7 MRI s.
    GE Signa 1.5-T s.
    GE Signa 5.2 with SR-230 three-
      axis EPI gradient upgrade s.
    GE Spiral CT s.
    GE Vectra MR s.
    Gyroscan ACS-NT MRI s.
    Gyroscan ACS-NT 1.5 T MR s.
    Gyroscan Interna s.
    Gyroscan S15 s.
    Harvard multidetector s.
    helical CT s.
    Hewlett-Packard s.
    high-field open MRI s.
    high-field-strength s.
    HiLight Advantage System CT s.
    HiSpeed Advantage helical s.
    HiSpeed Advantage System CT s.
    Hitachi CT s.
    Hitachi MR s.
    Hitachi Open MRI system s.
    Hitachi 0.3-T unit s.
    Hologic 2000 s.
    Hologic QDR 1000W dual-energy
      x-ray absorptiometry s.
    Horizon LX s.

Howtek Scanmaster DX s.
IDSI s.
Imatron C-100 EBT s.
Imatron C-150L EBCT s.
Imatron C-1000 UFCT s.
Imatron C-100 Ultrafast CT s.
Imatron C-150XL CT s.
Imatron C-100XP CT s.
Imatron Fastrac C-100 cine x-ray
  CT s.
Indomitable s.
Innervision MR s.
InstaScan s.
Integris 3000 s.
Irex Exemplar ultrasound s.
IRIS s.
Konica s.
large-bore 0.6-T, 1,5-T imaging
  system s.
LightSpeed multidetector CT s.
LightSpeed QX/i s.
low-field MR s.
Lumiscan LS 85 s.
Lumisys 20 digital x-ray s.
Lunar s.
LymphoScan nuclear imaging
  system s.
3M s.
Magna-SL s.
Magnes 2500 whole-blood s.
Magnetom SP63 s.
Magnetom 1.5-T s.
Magnetom Vision s.
Magnex MR s.
Mallinckrodt s.
Malvern 2600 Sizer laser
  diffraction s.
Max Plus MR s.
mechanical sector s.
MedImage s.
Medison s.
Medspec MR imaging system s.
Medspec 30/80 tesla MR s.
Medx s.
microCT-20 s.
Microtek ScanMaker 9600XL s.
midget MRI s.
mobile spiral computed
  tomography s.
modified electron-beam CT s.
mPower PET s.
MR catheter imaging and
  spectroscopy system s.
multidetector CT s.
multidetector helical s.
multiple jointed digitizer s.

multisensor structured light-range
digitizer s.
multislice CT s.
neurodiagnostic s.
NeuroFOCUS s.
neurSector s.
NewTom CT s.
Nishimoto Sangyo s.
Norland pQCT XCT2000 s.
nuclear s.
Ohio Nuclear Delta 50 FS,
2000 s.
Olympus endoscopic ultrasound s.
Oxford 2-T large-bore imaging
system s.
Pace Plus System s.
Park Medical Systems s.
partial-ring bismuth germanate-
crystal s.
Perception s.
PET/CT s.
PET full-ring s.
PETite s.
PETT VI PET s.
Pfizer 200 FS, 400 s.
phased-array s.
Philips Gyroscan ACS, NT, NT5,
NT15, S5, T5 s.
Philips 1.5-T NT MR s.
Philips Tomoscan 350, SR 6000
CT s.
Philips 4.7-T small-bore system s.
Picker MR s.
Picker PQ 5000 helical CT s.
Picker PQ 2000 spiral CT s.
Picker PRISM 3000 PET s.
Picker Synerview 600 s.
4096 Plus PET s.
Posicam HZ PET s.
PQCT s.
PQ 5000 CT s.
ProSpeed CT s.
QUAD 7000, 12000 high-field
open MRI s.
Quick CT9800 s.
QX/I CT s.
radioisotope s.
rectilinear s.
ring s.
RT 3200 Advantage ultrasound s.
RT 6800 ultrasound s.
Scanditronix PET s.

Scanmaster DX x-ray film
digitizer s.
scintillation s.
SCU-1200, -2200 digital color
ultrasound s.
sector s.
SFP s.
Shimadzu CT s.
Shimadzu MR s.
Siemens DRH CT s.
Siemens Magnetom GBS II s.
Siemens Magnetom SP 4000 s.
Siemens Magnetom 1.5-T s.
Siemens Magnetom Vision s.
Siemens One Tesla s.
Siemens Somaform 512 CT s.
Siemens Somatom DR2, DR3
whole-body s.
Siemens Somatom Plus CT s.
Siemens Sonoline Elegra
ultrasound s.
Signa Horizon LX SR 77
gradients 1.5-T MR s.
Signa MRI s.
Signa 1.5T s.
Signa VH/i3.0-T MR s.
single-detector helical s.
single-detector row s.
small-bore s.
SmartPrep s.
Somatom DR CT s.
Somatom Plus-S CT s.
spiral CT, XCT s.
supercam scintillation s.
Swissray s.
TCT900S helical CT s.
Technicare Delta 2020 s.
Tecmag Libra-S16 system s.
1.5 T Magnetom Symphony whole-
body s.
tomographic multiplane s.
Tomoscan AVEU spiral CT s.
Tomoscan SR 7000 s.
Toshiba MR s.
Toshiba 900S helical CT s.
Toshiba 900S/XII s.
Toshiba TCT-80 CT s.
Toshiba Xpress SX helical CT s.
Toshiba X-Vigor s.
Toshiba Xvision s.
Trionix s.
4T whole-body GI Signa MRI s.

NOTES

scanner *(continued)*
    ultrafast computed tomography s.
    Ultramark 9 s.
    UM 4 real-time sector s.
    Varian CT s.
    Vidar s.
    Vision Ten V-scan s.
    Vision 1.5 T Siemens MRI s.
    whole-body 1.5 Tesla s.
    whole-body 3T MRI system s.
    whole-body 1.5-T Siemens
      Vision s.
    Xpress/SW helical CT s.
    Xpress/SX helical CT s.
    X-Vigor s.
scanning *(See scan)*
    s. acoustic microscope (SAM)
    s. arm
    s. beam digital system
    body s.
    breath-hold s.
    close-space thin-section s.
    collimation s.
    combined ^{99m}Tc-DMSA and ^{99m}Tc-
      DTPA s.
    continuous s.
    contrast material-enhanced s.
    delayed phase s.
    diagnostic radioiodine s. (DxRaI)
    diffusion-weighted s.
    discontinuous s.
    dual isotope s.
    electrical impedance s. (EIS)
    s. electron microscope (SEM)
    s. equalization radiography
    external s.
    full-line s.
    gamma s.
    gated equilibrium blood pool s.
    high-resolution ultrasound s.
    IDA s.
    interleaved BOLD-fMRI s.
    laser diffraction s.
    s. laser ophthalmoscopy
    light s.
    line s. (LS)
    linear s.
    s. locus
    M-mode s.
    multiplanar s.
    nuclear s.
    parasternal s.
    paravertebral s.
    point s.
    positron s.
    s. power
    radiocholesterol s.

    radioisotope s.
    radionuclide s.
    real-time sector s.
    sector s.
    sensitive point s.
    spiral CT s.
    spot s.
    suprasternal s.
    ^{99m}Tc (V) DMSA s.
    s. technique
    total body s.
    transabdominal s.
    triplex s.
    whole-body ^{29}FDG s.
    wide-beam s.
    xenon CT s.
scanning-beam digital x-ray (SBDX)
scanogram imaging
scanography
    rotational s.
    slit s.
    spot s.
3-Scape real-time 3D imaging
scaphocapitate
    s. joint
    s. syndrome
scaphocephalic head shape
scaphocephaly
scaphoid
    s. bone
    congenital bipartite s.
    s. facet
    s. fat stripe
    s. hand fracture
    s. pole
    s. projection
    rotary subluxation of s.
    s. shape
    s. stomach
scapholunate (SL)
    s. advanced collapse (SLAC)
    s. arthritic collapse
    s. dislocation
    s. dissociation
    s. joint
    s. ligament (LSS)
    s. space
    s. widening
scaphotrapeziotrapezoid (STT)
    t. joint
scaphotriquetral ligament
scapula, pl. **scapulae**
    body of s.
    high-riding s.
    inferior tip of s.
    margin of s.

swallowtail malformation of s.
winged s.

scapulae
incisura s.
levator s.

scapular
s. angle
s. body
s. bone
dorsal s.
s. flap
s. margin
s. notch
s. winging

scapuloclavicular articulation
scapulocostal syndrome
scapulothoracic
s. joint
s. motion

scapulovertebral border
scar (*See* scarring)
s. band
s. carcinoma
central pancreatic lesion s.
s. contracture
dense s.
s. emphysema
femoral physeal s.
fibrocartilaginous s.
s. formation
infarcted s.
s. lesion
lung starfish s.
myocardial s.
nonviable s.
s. ossification
ossified s.
pulmonary s.
radial s.
radial breast s.
s. tissue
s. tissue entrapment
s. tissue reaction
tumor of liver s.
well-demarcated s.

scarification of pleura
scarified duodenum
Scarpa
canal of S.
S. fascia
S. ganglion
ligament of S.

method of S.
S. triangle

scarred
s. duodenum
s. kidney

scarring (*See* scar)
apical s.
basilar pleural s.
fibrotic s.
glial s.
interstitial s.
parenchymal s.
parietal pleural s.
pleural s.
postbiopsy s.
postinflammatory s.
postnecrotic s.
postpyelonephritis cortical s.
renal s.
selective s.
valvular s.

scatter
s. activity
s. compensation
s. correction
s. degradation factor
s. dose
s. fraction
s. graph
low-frequency s.
s. radiation
s. and veiling glare (SVG)

scatter-air ratio (SAR)
scattered
s. air bronchogram
s. coincidence event
s. count
s. radiation
s. rays

scatterer
s. depth
echogenicity s.

scattergram
scattering
broad-beam s.
classical s.
coherent s.
collimator s.
Compton s.
s. foil
s. foil compensator
forward-angle light s.

S

NOTES

scattering *(continued)*
    image-degrading s.
    low-angle s.
    Rayleigh s.
    Rayleigh-Tyndall s.
    side s.
    small-angle multiple s.
    s. system
    Thomson s.
scatter-maximum ratio (SMR)
scatterplot
scatter-to-primary ratio
scavenging system
SCD
    sagittal canal diameter
scene
    s. coordinate system
    s. domain
    s. intensity
scene-based
    s.-b. interpolation
    s.-b. visualization
Sceratti goniometer
SCFE
    slipped capital femoral epiphysis
Scharff-Bloom-Richardson
    S.-B.-R. grade
    S.-B.-R. histologic grade system
Schatzker fracture classification
Schatzki
    S. ring
    S. view
Schaumann body
Scheibe dysplasia
Scheie syndrome
scheme
    6-ablation, 14-ablation s.
    computer-aided diagnosis s.
    cylindrical-ablation s.
    decay s.
    gradient s.
    rule-based s.
    single-ablation s.
    zero-filling interpolation s.
schemic injury (SE)
Schepelmann sign
Scheuermann
    S. disease
    S. juvenile kyphosis
    S. nodule
Schick sign of tuberculosis
Schiff-Sherrington phenomenon
Schilder disease
Schiller-Duval body
schistosomal bladder carcinoma
schistosomiasis
schizencephaly

Schlemm
    S. canal
    S. ligament
Schlesinger
    S. sign
    S. vein
Schmid disease
Schmid-like metaphyseal
    chondrodysplasia
Schmidt optics system
Schmid-type metaphyseal dysplasia
Schmincke tumor
Schmorl
    S. disease
    S. node
    S. nodule
Schneider
    S. enteral stent
    S. Guider catheter
schneiderian
    s. carcinoma
    s. papilloma
Schoemaker line
Schonander film changer
Schönlein-Henoch syndrome
Schroedinger equation
Schüller
    S. position
    S. projection
    S. view
Schultze
    S. bundle
    S. placenta
Schultz reaction
Schumacher criterion
Schwann
    S. cell
    S. cell of myelin sheath
    S. tumor
schwannoma
    acoustic s.
    facial s.
    geniculate ganglion s.
    jugular foramen s.
    orbital s.
    s. trigeminal
    vestibular s.
Schwartz
    S. criterion
    S. test for patency of deep
      saphenous veins
Schwartze sign
Schwartz-Jampel syndrome (SJS)
SCI
    spinal cord injury
sciatic
    s. endometriosis

s. notch
s. plexus
scimitar
s. deformity
shadow s.
s. sign
s. syndrome
s. vein
scimitar-shaped
s.-s. flap
s.-s. shadow
scintiangiography
scinticisternography
Scinticore multicrystal scintillation camera
scintigram
parallel-hole s.
pinhole s.
spatial resolution s.
^{99m}Tc MDP skeletal s.
scintigraphic
s. angiography
s. balloon
s. balloon topography
s. evidence
s. perfusion defect
s. scan imaging
s. study
scintigraphy
ACE inhibition s.
adrenal s.
antifibrin s.
s. artifact
bleeding s.
blood pool s.
bone marrow s.
brain perfusion s.
Captopril-enhanced renal s.
cardiac s.
cerebral s.
cholesterol-based s.
cold defect renal s.
combined ventilation-perfusion s.
cortical s.
dipyridamole thallium-201 s.
dual intracoronary s.
dynamic antral s.
dynamic radionuclide renal s.
early bone s.
exercise myocardial perfusion s.
exercise stress-redistribution s.
exercise thallium s.

four-phase bone s.
functional radioiodine s.
^{67}Ga citrate s.
gallium bone s.
gallium lung s.
gallium tumor s.
gastrointestinal s.
gated blood pool s.
GI tract s.
heart s.
hepatobiliary s.
^{123}I metaiodobenzylguanidine s.
^{111}In antimyosin s.
In-pentetreotide s.
iodine s.
iodine-131 whole-body s.
iodomethyl-norcholesterol-59 s.
isotope s.
labeled free fatty acid s.
lacrimal s.
liver s.
long segmental diaphyseal uptake bone s.
lung s.
lymphoma gallium s.
marrow agent bone s.
MIBG s.
microsphere perfusion s.
morphine sulfate s.
myocardial perfusion s.
NEFA s.
^{59}NP s.
nuclear renal s.
octreotide paraganglioma s.
oropharyngoesophageal s. (OPES)
osteomyelitis s.
parathyroid s.
pediatric s.
perfusion s.
peritoneal s.
pertechnetate s.
photon-deficient lesion bone s.
planar diagnostic 1231 s.
planar exercise thallium-201 s.
pulmonary s.
pyrophosphate s.
s. quality control
quantitative hepatobiliary s. (QHS)
radioisotope s.
radionuclide bone s.
radionuclide testicular s.
renal gallium s.

S

NOTES

scintigraphy *(continued)*
resting-redistribution thallium-201 s.
rosary beading bone s.
salivary gland s.
samarium s.
same-day exercise-rest Tc-99m
tetrofosmin myocardial
perfusion s.
sestamibi parathyroid s. (SPS)
single-photon planar s. (SPPS)
soft tissue uptake bone s.
somatostatin receptor s. (SRS)
source of artifact s.
SPECT brain perfusion s.
SPECT thallium s.
splenic s.
split-function s.
stress perfusion s.
sulfur colloid s.
^{99m}Tc depreotide s.
^{99m}Tc-DMSA s.
^{99m}Tc HIG s.
^{99m}Tc human polyclonal
immunoglobulin G s.
^{99m}Tc human serum albumin s.
Tc-labeled red blood cell s.
^{99m}Tc-labeled white blood cell s.
^{99m}Tc-methoxyisobutylisonitrile s.
TcO$_4$ MIBI subtraction s.
^{99m}Tc-PYP s.
technetium-99m heat-denatured RBC
splenic s.
technetium-99m (V) DMSA s.
thallium-201 myocardial s.
thallium perfusion s.
three-phase bone s. (TPBS)
thyroid s.
thyroidal lymph node s.
time course fracture s.
transit s.
ventilation s.
ventilation-perfusion pulmonary s.
vesicoureteral s.
white blood cell with indium-
111 s.
scintillascope
scintillation
s. camera
s. camera field uniformity
s. camera geometry
s. camera linearity
s. camera linearity differential
s. camera uniformity differential
s. counter
s. counting technique
s. crystal
s. detector

s. imaging
migrainous s.
s. probe
s. proximity radioimmunoassay
s. scan
s. scanner
s. spectrometer
s. spectrometry
scintillator
cesium iodide s.
rare-earth s.
scintillometer
scintimammography (SMM)
technetium-99m
methoxyisobutylisonitrile s.
scintiphoto
combined transmission-emission s.
scintiphotograph
scintiphotography
liver s.
scintirenography
scintiscan
scintiscanner
Scintiview nuclear computer system
Scintron IV nuclear computer system
SCIPP
sacrococcygeal inferior pubic point
scirrhous
s. breast carcinoma
s. infiltrating adenocarcinoma
s. lesion
s. tumor
scission
double-strand s.
single-strand s.
scissoring of legs
SCIWORA
spinal cord injury without radiographic
abnormality
SCL
sinus cycle length
SCLBCL
secondary cutaneous large B-cell
lymphoma
SCLC
small-cell lung carcinoma
scleral canal
sclerocystic ovary
scleroderma
complicated s.
diffuse s.
s. of esophagus
ScleroLaser laser system
scleroma
ScleroPLUS HP laser system
sclerosed temporal bone

sclerosing
- s. adenitis
- s. adenosis
- s. agent
- s. basal cell carcinoma
- s. cholangitis
- s. duct hyperplasia
- s. hemangioma
- s. hepatic carcinoma (SHC)
- s. inflammation
- s. injection
- s. lesion
- s. lipogranuloma
- s. mediastinitis
- s. mesenteritis
- s. myeloma
- s. nonsuppurative osteomyelitis
- s. osteogenic sarcomatosis
- s. osteosarcoma
- s. panencephalitis

sclerosis, pl. **scleroses**
- aortic s.
- arterial s.
- arteriocapillary s.
- arteriolar s.
- Baló concentric s.
- bony s.
- calcified s.
- chronic subperitoneal s.
- congenital hippocampal s.
- coronary s.
- cyst s.
- diaphyseal s.
- diffuse CNS s.
- diffuse myelinoclastic s.
- disseminated s.
- endocardial s.
- endplate s.
- esophageal variceal s.
- focal bone s.
- gastric s.
- hepatic s.
- hepatoportal s.
- hippocampal s.
- idiopathic hypertrophic subaortic s. (IHSS)
- incisural s.
- Krabbe diffuse s.
- laser s.
- lobar s.
- marginal s.
- marked s.
- medial calcific s.
- mesenteric s.
- mesial temporal s.
- multifocal subperitoneal s.
- multiple s.
- pedicle s.
- photothermal s.
- posterolateral s.
- progressive systemic s.
- pulmonary and cardiac s.
- reactive bone s.
- renal s.
- segmental vein s.
- subchondral low-signal-intensity s.
- subendocardial s.
- systemic s.
- temporal bone s.
- thick rind s.
- tuberous s. (TS)
- tumefactive multiple s.
- unilateral mesial temporal s.
- valvular s.
- variceal s.
- vascular s.
- venous s.

sclerostenosis

sclerotherapy
- percutaneous ethanol s.
- talc s.

sclerotic
- s. area
- s. border
- s. calvarial patch
- s. calvarium bone island
- s. coronary artery
- s. degeneration
- s. kidney
- s. lesion
- s. margin
- s. osteogenic sarcoma
- s. pattern
- s. plaque
- s. rim
- s. stomach

sclerotomy
- ab-externo laser s.
- ab-interno laser s.

SCM
- spinal cord malformation

SCNB
- stereotactic core needle biopsy

S

NOTES

scoliosis
    adolescent idiopathic s. (AIS)
    Aussies-Isseis unstable s.
    Cobb measurement of s.
    dextrorotary s.
    Dwyer correction of s.
    Fergusson method for measuring s.
    fixation of s.
    functional s.
    idiopathic s.
    King classification of thoracic s.
    King-Moe s.
    levorotary s.
    lumbar s.
    rotary thoracolumbar s.
    S-shaped s.
    thoracic s.
    thoracolumbar s.
    uncompensated rotary s.
    Winter-King-Moe s.
scoliotic
    s. pelvis
    s. spine
Scopix Laser film
scorbutic white line
score
    Agatston s.
    biophysical profile s. (BPS)
    coronary artery calcium s. (CACS)
    densitometry z s.
    electron-beam CT-derived CAC s.
    fetal biophysical profile s.
    injury severity s. (ISS)
    late effect of normal tissues s.
    late effect toxicity s.
    LENT s.
    Mallampati s.
    mean wall motion s.
    QRS s.
    stroke scale s.
    thallium SPECT s.
    total calcium s. (TCS)
    volume s.
    wall motion s.
scored cartilage
scoring
    calcium s.
scotograph
scotometry
scottie, scotty
    s. dog appearance
    s. dog fracture
    s. dog view
scout
    s. digital radiograph
    s. film
    s. image

    s. imaging
    s. sequence
    s. view
SCP
    supracristal plane
SCR
    silicon-controlled rectifier
scrambled image
screen
    s. craze artifact
    fluorescent s.
    guilt s.
    intensifying s.
    Kodak Min-R s.
    Lanex medium s.
    s. oxygenator
    radiofrequency s.
    rapid s.
    rare-earth s.
    rear projection s.
    s. type film
    Ultra Vision Rapid s.
screen-film
    s.-f. contact
    s.-f. mammography
screening
    biplane s.
    breast cancer s.
    s. mammography
    s. technique
screening-detected abnormality
screen-intensifying factor (IF)
screenless mammography film
screw
    bicortical s.
    bone s.
    cancellous s.
    compression plate and s.
    DHS s.
    s. fixation
    interference s.
    lag s.
    metallic s.
    orthopedic s.
    resorbable s.
    transfixing s.
    unicortical s.
scroll bone
scrotal
    s. abscess
    s. anatomy
    s. area
    s. calcification
    s. fasciitis
    s. fibroma
    s. gas
    s. hematocele

s. hernia
s. histiocytoma
s. mass
s. pearl
s. raphe
s. vein
s. wall thickening
scrotum, pl. **scrota, scrotums**
acutely symptomatic s.
SCT
Sertoli cell tumor
star-cancellation test
SCTA
spiral computed tomography
arteriography
SCU-1200, -2200 digital color ultrasound scanner
Scully tumor
scyphoid
SD
septal defect
SDD
surfactant deficiency disorder
SDH
subdural hemorrhage
succinate dehydrogenase
S/D ratio
systolic/diastolic ratio
SDRI
small, deep, recent infarct
SE
schemic injury
spin-echo
SE proton-density weighted image
⁷⁵Se, Se-75
selenium-75
⁷⁵Se selenomethionine radioactive
agent
SEA
spinal epidural abscess
seagull
s. joint
s. sign
seal
water s.
sealed
mechanically s.
seal-fin deformity
seam
osteoid s.

seatbelt
s. fracture
s. injury
sea urchin granuloma
sebaceous
s. adenoma
s. carcinoma
s. cyst
s. gland calcification
sebaceum
adenoma s.
SEBI
stereotactic external-beam irradiation
Sebileau muscle
second
s. branchial arch
s. branchial cleft cyst
s. cranial nerve
s. cuneiform bone
cycles per s. (cps)
s. diagonal branch
S. Look CAD system
s. malignant neoplasm (SMN)
meters per s. (mps)
s. order subtraction
s. portion of duodenum
roentgens per s. (R/s)
s. ventricle of cerebrum
secondary
s. achalasia
s. acquired cholesteatoma
s. amyloidosis
s. archnoid cyst
s. atelectasis
s. axillary adenopathy
s. axillary lymphadenopathy
s. biliary cirrhosis
s. brain lymphoma
s. bronchus
s. calcification
s. cartilaginous joint
s. center of ossification
s. chondromatosis
s. coccidioidomycosis
s. collimation
s. contracture
s. cutaneous large B-cell lymphoma (SCLBCL)
s. degeneration
s. electron
s. electron production
s. extravasation

NOTES

secondary *(continued)*
s. fracture
s. gliosis
s. hydrocele
s. hydrocephalus
s. hyperparathyroidism
s. hypoparathyroidism
s. hypothyroidism
s. intracranial hypertension (SIH)
s. lesion
s. lymphangiectasis
s. malignancy
s. myeloid metaphysis
s. obstruction
s. osteosarcoma
s. ovarian tumor
s. peristalsis
s. pleurisy
s. pneumonia
s. pulmonary lobule
s. radiation
s. ray
s. retroperitoneal fibrosis
s. retroperitoneal organ
s. sclerosing cholangitis
s. sequestrum
s. sonographic finding
s. teeth
s. ulcer
s. union
s. venous insufficiency
s. wave
s. yolk sac
second-degree
s.-d. AV block
s.-d. heart block
second-echo image
second-harmonic imaging
second-look arthroscopy
second-order
s.-o. chorda
s.-o. compensation
s.-o. correction
s.-o. reflection
second-trimester
s.-t. gestational dating
s.-t. placenta
secretin-enhanced dynamic MRCP
secretion
adrenocortical s.
bowel s.
gastric s.
hyperdense sinus s.
inspissated s.
mineralocorticoid s.
retained s.
retention of s.

sinonasal s.
tubular kidney s.
secretion-filled bronchus
secretory
s. adenocarcinoma
s. calcification
s. capacity
s. carcinoma
s. component
s. phase endometrium
section
axial celloidin s.
celloidin s.
contiguous interleaved axial s.
coronal s.
cross s.
distal leg cross s.
flood s.
frontal s.
hip muscle cross s.
midfrontal plane coronal s.
paramedian s.
penultimate s.
sagittal celloidin s.
sagittal paraffin s.
serial s.
serpiginous s.
step s.
s. timing correction
tomographic s.
transverse s.
sectional
s. radiography
s. roentgenography
s. segmental anatomy
section-select
s.-s. flow compensation
s.-s. pulse
section-sensitivity profile
sector
2D s. scan
lower field visual s.
2.5-, 5-MHz s. transducer
nipple s.
nonnipple s.
s. scan
s. scanner
s. scanning
Sommer s.
s. transducer
sector-scan echocardiography imaging
secular equilibrium
secundum
s. atrial septal defect
ostium s.
septum s.
sedimented calcium

seed
    encapsulated radioactive s.
    gold s.
    I-Plant brachytherapy s.'s
    PharmaSeed palladium-103 s.'s
    s. point
    radiation s.
    s. ribbon
    Symmetra I-125 brachytherapy s.'s
    s. voxel

seeding
    intracranial s.
    metastatic s.
    perichondral cell s.
    peritoneal s.
    prostate s.
    radioactive s.
    subarachnoid s.
    subependymal s.
    TheraSeed s.
    tumor s.

seeker
    bone s.

seen on end

seesaw peristalsis ureter

Seessel pouch

see-through image

segment
    aganglionic s.
    akinetic s.
    angulated s.
    anterobasal s.
    anterolateral s.
    aortic s.
    aperistaltic distal ureteral s.
    apical s.
    apicoposterior s.
    arterial s.
    atretic s.
    atretic aortic s.
    blind s.
    bronchopulmonary s.
    cardiac s.
    coarcted s.
    contiguous s.
    diaphragmatic s.
    distal s.
    s. distraction
    diversity s.
    duodenal s.
    expansile aortic s.
    hypokinetic s.

    infarcted lung s.
    inferoapical s.
    inferobasal s.
    inferoposterior s.
    intercalated s.
    interleaved inversion-readout s.
    interposed colon s.
    intradiaphragmatic aortic s.
    intramuscular aortic s.
    ischemic s.
    joint s.
    liver s.
    meatal s.
    nonfilling venous s.
    noninfarcted s.
    occlusal s.
    posterior apical s.
    posterobasal s.
    posterolateral s.
    proximal s.
    pulmonary s.
    redundancy of interposed colon s.
    septal wall s.
    superior s.
    tail-like s.
    variable s.
    vaterian s.
    venous s.
    view per s. (VPS)

segmental
    s. alveolar pattern
    s. asynergy
    s. biliary obstruction
    s. bone defect
    s. bone loss
    s. bowel infarct
    s. branch of artery
    s. bronchus
    s. bronchus consolidation
    s. bronchus defect
    s. bronchus fracture
    s. bronchus ischemia
    s. bronchus lesion
    s. bronchus lower extremity
      Doppler pressure
    s. bronchus narrowing
    s. bronchus orifice
    s. bronchus perfusion abnormality
    s. bronchus plethysmography
    s. bronchus renal artery waveform
    s. bronchus symptom

S

NOTES

segmental *(continued)*
    s. correction using spine reconstruction
    s. correction using x-ray measurement
    s. demyelination
    s. dyssynergia
    s. k-space turbo gradient-echo breath-hold sequence imaging
    s. limb pressure recording
    s. liver anatomy
    s. lung defect scan
    s. lung density
    s. necrotizing glomerulonephritis
    s. nephrogram
    s. neurofibromatosis
    s. omental infarct
    s. pneumonia
    s. portal hypertension
    s. pressure measurement
    s. renal artery branch
    s. resorption atelectasis
    s. spinal dysgenesis (SSD)
    s. stenosis
    s. vein
    s. vein sclerosis
    s. wall motion

segmentation
    anatomy-oriented colon s. (AOCS)
    s. anomaly
    automatic lumen edge s.
    barium s.
    GM s.
    inside-to-outside s.
    lung s.
    s. method
    s. method for real-time display
    MRI s.
    outer-air s.
    outside-to-inside s.
    s. procedure
    rhythmic s.
    semiautomated cerebrospinal fluid s.
    time-resolved imaging by automatic data s. (TRIADS)
    vascular s.

segmented
    s. echo-planar imaging (SEPI)
    s. k-space cardiac tagging
    s. k-space data acquisition
    s. k-space time-of-flight MR angiography

segmenting
    s. dual-echo MR head scan
    s. dual-echo MR imaging

Segond fracture
Segre chart

SEH
    spinal epidural hemorrhage
SEI
    subendocardial infarct
Seidelin body
Seidlitz powder test
Seinsheimer classification of femoral fracture
seizure
    absence s.
    generalized s.
    grand mal s.
    s. localization
    partial complex s.
    s. pattern
    petit mal s.
    s. phenomenon
    repetitive s.'s
    s. threshold
SELCA
    smooth excimer laser coronary angioplasty
Seldinger
    S. angiography
    S. catheterization
    S. needle
    S. percutaneous technique
select
    bimodal slice s. (BOSS)
Selecta 7000 laser
selection
    s. bias
    coil s.
    delay time s.
    gradient s.
    guidance system s.
    reflectance-guided laser s.
    slice s.
selective
    s. angiocardiography
    s. arterial injection
    s. arterial magnetic resonance angiography
    s. cannulation
    s. cerebral arteriography
    s. coronary arteriography
    s. coronary arteriography view
    s. coronary cineangiography
    s. excitation
    s. excitation line scan
    s. excitation method
    s. excitation projection reconstruction imaging
    s. hole burning
    s. laser sintering (SLS)
    s. occlusion of aneurysmal neck
    s. osteal salpingography

s. partial inversion-recovery (SPIR)
s. population inversion (SPI)
s. population transfer (SPT)
s. presaturation MR angiography
s. pulse
s. radiography
s. reduction of pregnancy
s. roentgenography
s. saturation
s. saturation method
s. saturation recovery
s. scarring
s. separation
s. test occlusion
s. venography
s. venous magnetic resonance angiography
s. visceral aortography
s. visceral arteriography
s. visualization

selectivity
spatial s.

Selectron system

selenium
amorphous s.
s. imaging agent
s. plate
s. radiography

selenium-75 (^{75}Se, Se-75)
selenium-based digital chest system
selenium-drum-detector system
selenium-labeled bile acid imaging
selenomethylcholesterol
self-aspirating cut-biopsy needle
self-expandable metal stent
self-expanding
s.-e. metallic endoprosthesis
s.-e. tulip sheath
8 (x) 50 mm s.-e. Easy Wallstent
self-quenched counter tube
self-reinforced polyglycolide
self-retaining Cope loop pigtail catheter
self-scattering
self-sealing latex balloon
self-selection bias
self-shielding
sella, pl. **sellae**
ballooned s.
decalcified dorsum s.
diaphragma s.
dorsum s.
empty s.

s. enlargement
J-shaped s.
tuberculum s.
s. turcica
s. turcica calcification
s. turcica diaphragm
sella-nasion plane
sellar
s. destruction
s. floor
s. tomography
SEM
scanning electron microscope
semialdehyde
succinic s.
semiautomated cerebrospinal fluid segmentation
semiautonomous nodule
semiaxial
s. anteroposterior projection
s. position
s. transcranial projection
semicircular
s. canal
s. canal hydrops
s. ridge
semicommitted mode
semiconductor
complementary metal oxide s. (CMOS)
s. detector
semicoronal plane
semidynamic splint
semierect
s. film
s. position
semiflexed MTP
semi-Fowler position
semihorizontal heart
semiinvasive aspergillosis
semilateral position
semiliquid feces
semilobar holoprosencephaly
semilunar
s. aortic valve regurgitation
s. bone
s. bone formation
s. calcification
s. cartilage
s. fold
s. indentation
s. line

S

NOTES

semilunar *(continued)*
- s. notch
- s. pulmonic valve regurgitation
- s. valve
- s. valve cusp

semilunaris
- hiatus s.
- linea s.

semimembranosus
- s. bursa
- s. tendon

semimembranosus-tibial collateral ligament bursa

semimembranous muscle

seminal
- s. colliculus
- s. tract
- s. vesicle
- s. vesicle atrophy
- s. vesicle cyst
- s. vesicle hypoplasia
- s. vesicle invasion (SVI)
- s. vesiculography

seminiferous
- s. tubular damage
- s. tubular ectasia
- s. tubule

seminoma
- extragonadal s.
- mediastinal s.
- s. mediastinum
- testicular s.

seminomatous tumor

semiopaque

semiovale
- centrum s.

semiquantitative
- s. measurement
- s. technique

semirecumbent position

semispinal muscle

semisupine position

semitendinosus tendon

semitendinous muscle

semiupright
- s. position
- s. view

semivertical heart

^{77}Se MRI spectroscopy

send-receive phased-array extremity coil

senescence
- premature placental s.

senescent
- s. aortic stenosis
- s. change

Sengstaken-Blakemore tube

senile
- s. amyloidosis
- s. ankylosing hyperostosis
- s. arteriosclerosis
- s. change
- s. degeneration
- s. emphysema
- s. fibroma
- s. myocardium
- s. nephrosclerosis
- s. osteomalacia
- s. osteoporosis
- s. plaque
- s. subcapital fracture

senilis
- coxa s.

Senning
- S. operation
- S. procedure

senograph

Senographe
- S. 2000D digital mammography system
- S. DMRt mammography system
- S. 500T, 600T, 700T, 800T mammography

senography

SenoScan full field mammography system

Sens-A-Ray dental imaging system

SENSE
- sensitivity encoding
- SENSE method

sensing
- s. coil
- s. error

sensitive
- s. plane
- s. plane projection reconstruction imaging
- s. point
- s. point scanning
- s. volume

sensitivity
- s. analysis
- contrast s.
- s. encoding (SENSE)
- s. encoding method
- index of s.
- line-shape s.
- percussion s.
- plane s.
- point s.
- poor s.
- spectral s.
- uniform s.

sensitization
    protracted exposure s.
sensitizer
    s. enhancement ratio
    radiation s.
sensitizing gradient
sensitometer
    electroluminescent s.
sensitometric
    s. curve
    s. strip
sensitometry
    processor s.
sensor
    PressureWire s.
    temperature s.
sensorimotor
    s. cortex
    s. gyrus
sensory
    s. ganglion
    s. impairment
    s. nucleus
    s. paralytic bladder
    s. root
    s. strip
    s. tract
sentinel
    s. clot sign
    s. fold
    s. fracture
    s. loop
    s. loop sign
    s. lymph node (SLN)
    s. node dissection
    s. node localization and biopsy
    s. pile
    s. transoral hemorrhage
SEP
    systolic ejection period
separation
    acromioclavicular joint s.
    aortic cusp s.
    atlantoaxial s.
    atlantooccipital s.
    s. of bowel loop
    carrier-free s.
    chorioamnionic s.
    chromatographic s.
    collagen fiber s.
    costochondral junction s.
    E point to septal s. (EPSS)

fat/water signal s.
fracture fragment s.
frequency s.
s. of ghosts
leaflet s.
meniscocapsular s.
meniscotibial s.
mitral valve septal s.
selective s.
septal s.
shoulder s.
small bowel s.
separator tube
Sephadex bead
SEPI
    segmented echo-planar imaging
    spiral EPI
septal
    s. accessory pathway
    s. amplitude
    s. arcade
    s. area
    s. asymmetry
    s. band
    s. bone
    s. cartilage plate
    s. cirrhosis
    s. cusp
    s. cusp of calve
    s. defect (SD)
    s. deviation
    s. dip
    s. hyperperfusion
    s. hypertrophy
    s. hypokinesis
    s. hypoperfusion
    s. leaflet
    s. line
    s. malformation
    s. myocardial infarct
    s. necrosis
    s. notch
    s. papillary muscle
    s. perforating branch
    s. perforation
    s. perforator
    s. perforator artery
    s. placenta cyst
    s. ridge
    s. separation
    s. thickening
    s.-to-free wall ratio

NOTES

septal *(continued)*
 s. tricuspid anulus
 s. vein
 s. wall
 s. wall motion
 s. wall segment
 s. wall thickness
septate
 s. appearance
 s. hypertrophy
septation
 gallbladder s.
 s. septal defect
septic
 s. arthritis
 s. bursitis
 s. cholangitis
 s. diskitis
 s. lung
 s. necrosis
 s. pleurisy
 s. pneumonia
 s. pulmonary embolus
 s. pulmonary infarct
 s. thrombosis
septomarginal
 s. band
 s. trabecula
septooptic dysplasia
septostomy
 atrial s.
 balloon atrial s.
septum
 alveolar s.
 anal intermuscular s.
 anteroapical trabecular s.
 aortic s.
 aortopulmonary s.
 atrial s.
 atrioventricular nodal s.
 s. band
 s. of Bertin
 bronchial s.
 bulbar s.
 canal s.
 cartilaginous s.
 s. cavum vergae
 conal s.
 connective tissue s.
 conus s.
 crural s.
 distal bulbar s.
 dyskinetic s.
 epirenal s.
 femoral s.
 fibrous s.
 gingival s.

infundibular s.
intact ventricular s.
interatrial s. (IAS)
interhaustral s.
interlobar s.
interlobular lung s.
intermuscular s.
internal intermuscular s.
interventricular s.
intraventricular s.
Kürner s.
lipomatous hypertrophy of the
 interatrial s.
low-signal-intensity fibrous s.
median s.
mediastinal s.
membranous s.
muscular atrioventricular s.
myometrial s.
nasal s.
parietal extension of infundibular s.
s. pellucidum
s. pellucidum cavity
perirenal s.
placental s.
posterior median s.
s. primum
rectogenital s.
rectovaginal s.
rectovesical s.
retrovesical s.
s. secundum
sinus s.
subarachnoid s.
thickened s.
s. transversum
s. transversum defect
ventricular s. (VS)
sequela, pl. **sequelae**
 late normal tissue s.
 post ECT sequelae
 radiation therapy s.
 significant s.
 tissue s.
sequence
 amnion rupture s.
 breath-hold fast-recovery fast SE
  pulse s.
 breath-hold gradient-recalled echo s.
 s. bypass graft
 cardiac-gated PGSE s.
 Carr-Purcell s.
 Carr-Purcell-Meiboom-Gill s.
 cine-FFE breath-hold s.
 cine gradient-echo s.
 conventional pulse s.
 CP s.

CPMG s.
DANTE s.
3D gadolinium s.
diffusion pulse s.
diffusion-sensitive s.
diffusion-weighted pulse s.
double inversion recovery s.
3D spoiled gradient-recalled
 echo s.
3D time-of-flight magnetic
 resonance angiographic s.
3D transesophageal
 echocardiographic s.
dual-echo s.
dual gradient-recalled echo pulse s.
dysplasia-carcinoma s.
s. echo-planar imaging
echo-planar pulse s.
fast FLAIR s.
fast gradient-echo s.
FAST pulse s.
fat-suppressed T2-weighted fast
 spin-echo s.
fat-suppression pulse s.
field-echo pulse s.
FISP pulse s.
flow-compensated gradient-echo s.
gradient-echo imaging s.
gradient-echo pulse s.
GRASS pulse s.
Hahn spin-echo s.
high-resolution volumetric s.
hypervariable s.
in-phase s.
interleaved GRE s.
inversion recovery s.
IRSE s.
Klippel-Feil s.
long-echo-train fast spin-echo s.
long TR/TE s.
magnetization-prepared rapid
 acquisition gradient-echo s.
Meiboom-Gill s.
missing pulse steady-state free
 precession s.
s. monophasic shock
multiecho s.
multiplanar gradient refocused s.
multislice spin-echo s.
nuclear magnetic resonance
 scanning s.
oblique sagittal s.

s. obstruction
opposed-phase s.
partial saturation pulse s.
peristaltic s.
phase-encode time-reduced
 acquisition s.
point-resolved spectroscopy s.
 (PRESS)
postenhancement s.
Potter s.
preenhancement s.
s. processor
pulse s.
pulsed arterial spin labeling s.
pulsed-gradient spin-echo echo-
 planar pulse s.
s. quantitative MR imaging
radiofrequency spoiled 3D GRE s.
RARE-derived pulse s.
repetitive pulse s.
Robin s.
rotating ultra-fast imaging s.
 (RUFIS)
saturation recovery s.
scan s.
scout s.
Shine-Dalgamo s.
short repetition time s.
short TI inversion recovery
 pulse s.
single breath-hold s.
single-echo versus multiple-echo s.
SL-GRE s.
spin-echo imaging s.
spin-echo pulse s.
spin-warp pulse s.
spiral-pulse s.
spoiled gradient echo pulse s.
steady-state free precession s.
STEAM s.
STIR s.
susceptibility-sensitive s.
three-point Dixon water-fat
 separation s.
s. time
TONE s.
turboFLASH s.
turbo inversion recovery s.
turbo IR s.
turbo pulse s.
turbo SE s.
T2-weighted combination s.

NOTES

sequence *(continued)*
    T1-weighted coronal fat-suppressed
      fast spin-echo s.
    T2-weighted fat-saturated s.
    T2-weighted pulse s.
    T2-weighted spin-echo s.
    twin-reversed arterial perfusion s.
    ultrafast FLASH 2D s.
    velocity-encoded s.
    VIBE s.
    voiding s.
    water suppression pulse s.
sequencing
    2D TOF pulse s.
sequential
    s. balloon inflation
    s. circulator
    s. determinant
    s. extraction-radiotracer technique
    s. films
    s. first pass imaging
    s. image acquisition
    s. line imaging
    s. mode
    s. paired opposed plaque (SPOP)
    s. plane imaging
    s. point imaging
    s. postcontrast MR image
    s. quantitative MR imaging
    s. scalar quantization (SSQ)
sequestered
    s. disk
    s. lobe
    s. lobe of lung
sequestra (*pl. of* sequestrum)
sequestral
sequestration
    bronchopulmonary s.
    disk s.
    extralobar s.
    extrapulmonary s.
    fluid s.
    intralobar s.
    labeled red blood cell s.
    pulmonary s. (PS)
    s. system
    third-space s.
sequestrum, pl. **sequestra**
    associated s.
    bony s.
    kissing s.
    necrotic s.
    primary s.
    secondary s.
    tertiary s.
sequoiosis
serendipity view

serial
    s. change
    s. cholangiogram
    s. contrast MR imaging
    s. CT slice
    s. cut film technique
    s. diffusion-weighted MR imaging
      and proton MR spectroscopy
    s. duplex imaging
    s. duplex scan
    s. dynamic imaging
    s. film changer
    s. injection
    s. lesion
    s. radiographic survey
    s. radiography
    s. section
    s. splinting
    s. subtraction film
serialoangiocardiography
serialogram
serialograph
serialography imaging
sericite pneumoconiosis
series, pl. **series**
    abdominal s.
    acute abdominal s. (AAS)
    basophilic s.
    cardiac s.
    decay s.
    diagnostic skull s.
    dynamic s.
    factor analysis of dynamic s.
      (FADS)
    FCS s.
      full cervical spine series
    gallbladder s. (GBS)
    gallbladder-gastrointestinal s.
    gastrointestinal s.
    GB-GI s.
    intubated small bowel s.
    Kempe s.
    lumbosacral s.
    metabolic bone s.
    motor meal barium GI s.
    radioactive s.
    sinus s.
    small bowel s.
    upper gastrointestinal s.
seriograph
seriography
serioscopy
SER-IV
    supination-external rotation IV
    SER-IV fracture
serofibrinous pericardial effusion
serofibrous pleurisy

serohemorrhagic fluid
seroma
    mediastinal s.
    perigraft s.
    postoperative s.
seromuscular layer
serosa
    cecal s.
serosal
    s. endometrial implant
    s. myoma
    s. surface
    s. tear
serosanguineous fluid
serous
    s. adenocarcinoma
    s. carcinoma
    s. cystadenocarcinoma
    s. cystadenoma
    s. effusion
    s. intraparenchymatous cyst
    s. ligament
    s. membrane
    s. ovarian tumor
    s. pericardium
    s. pleurisy
serpentine
    s. aneurysm
    s. appearance
    s. asbestos
    s. enhancement
    s. signal void
    s. structure
serpiginosum
    angioma s.
serpiginous
    s. band
    s. low signal intensity border
    s. luminal filling defect
    s. section
    s. ulcer
serrated
    s. appearance
    s. suture
serration
    esophageal margin s.
    marginal s.
serratus
    s. anterior (SA)
    s. anterior muscle
Sertoli cell tumor (SCT)
Sertoli-Leydig cell tumor

Servelle vein
server
    AquariusNET 2D/3D medical
      imaging s.
servomotor
    magnetic s.
servo power amplifier
Servox amplifier
sesamoid
    s. bone
    s. complex
    fibular hallux s.
    s. injury
    s. ligament
    s. migration
    tibial hallux s.
sesamoidometatarsal joint
sesamophalangeal ligament
sessile
    s. adenoma
    s. filling defect
    s. hydatid
    s. lesion
    s. nodular carcinoma
    s. plaque
    s. polyp
    s. tumor
sestamibi
    s. imaging agent
    s. parathyroid scintigraphy (SPS)
    s. polar map
    s. stress scan imaging
    ^{99m}Tc s.
    s. ^{99m}Tc with dipyridamole stress
      test
    s. technetium-99m
set
    access s.
    Amplatz dilator s.
    s. angle
    coaxial micropuncture needle s.
    Curry intravascular retriever s.
    3D anatomic data s.
    data s.
    3D MRI data s.
    foreshortened image data s.
    Greene biopsy s.
    Hawkins accordion catheter
      drainage s.
    Hawkins inside-out nephrostomy s.
    Huisman percutaneous drainage s.
    image s.

NOTES

set *(continued)*
    McNamara coaxial catheter
      infusion s.
    minimally invasive access s.
    Neff percutaneous access s.
    Ring-McLean sump drainage s.
    Rutner balloon dilatation helical
      stone extractor s.
    telescopic bougie s.
    Van Sonnenberg chest drain s.
    volumetric data s.

Sethotope radioactive imaging agent

seton

Settegast
    S. method
    S. position
    S. projection

setting
    discriminator s.
    quadrature s.
    simulation-aided field s.
    soft tissue window s.
    wide window s.
    window/level s.

setting-sun sign

Sever disease

SEW
    slice excitation wave

sextuplet pregnancy

SF$_6$
    sulfur hexafluoride

SFA
    superficial femoral artery

SFD
    source-film distance

SFP
    scanned focal point
      SFP scanner

SFR
    stenotic flow reserve

SFTP
    solitary fibrous tumor of the pleura

SGE
    spoiled gradient echo

shaded
    s. surface display
    s. surface display imaging
    s. surface rendering (SSR)

shading
    s. appearance
    image s.

shadow *(See* shadowing*)*
    acoustic s.
    band-like s.
    batwing s.
    bony s.
    s. box

    breast s.
    butterfly breast s.
    calcific s.
    cardiac s.
    cardiomediastinal s.
    cardiothymic s.
    cardiovascular s.
    centrilobular s.
    clean s.
    companion s.
    concatenation of s.'s
    cortical signet ring s.
    discoid s.
    double-arc gallbladder s.
    double-bubble s.
    dumbbell-shaped s.
    edge s.
    effusion s.
    fusiform s.
    gloved-finger s.
    heart s.
    hilar s.
    iliopsoas muscle s.
    kidney s.
    large thymus s.
    line s.
    linear s.
    mitral configuration of cardiac s.
    nipple s.
    overlap s.
    overlying bowel s.'s
    psoas s.
    PVST s.
    radiographic parallel line s.
    renal s.
    ring s.
    s. scimitar
    scimitar-shaped s.
    snowstorm s.
    soft tissue s.
    sound s.
    spindle-shaped s.
    summation of s.'s
    superimposition of bowel s.
    thymic s.
    toothpaste s.'s
    tramline s.
    tumor-like s.
    vascular s.
    wall-echo s. (WES)
    widened heart s.

shadowgram

shadowgraph

shadowgraphy

shadowing
    dirty acoustic s.
    hyperechoic structure with s.

hypointense signal s.
interstitial s.
lateral wall refractive s.
marked hypoechogenicity s.
paraspinal soft tissue s.
posterior acoustic s.
refractive s.
rib s.
s. stone

shaft

bone s.
femoral s.
s. flange
s. fracture
middle third s.
ministem s.
proximal third s.
s. of rib

shag

aortic s.

shagging of cardiac border

shaggy

s. esophagus
s. heart border
s. lung nodule
s. pericardium

shaken baby syndrome (SBS)

shallow

s. inspiration
s. inspiratory effort

shank bone

shape

aneurysm with simple s.
baseball bat s.
brachycephalic head s.
cardiac s.
cricket bat s.
dumbbell s.
exponential s.
gaussian line s.
gooseneck s.
half-moon s.
head s.
heat s.
horseshoe s.
hourglass s.
ice cream cone s.
irregular s.
line s.
lobulated s.
S. Maker system
mesocephalic head s.

mushroom s.
oval s.
ovoid s.
peak s.
pulse s.
s. recovery
rosette s.
S s.
scaphocephalic head s.
scaphoid s.
sickle s.
spherical s.
spheroid s.
vertebral body s.
wine glass s.

shaper

beam s.

shaping

heat s.

shared coronary artery

sharp

s. border of lung
s. carina
s. dissection
s. lateral margin

Sharpey fiber

Sharplan SilkTouch Flashscan surgical laser

sharply demarcated circumferential lesion

sharpness

image s.

Sharp-Purser test

shattered

s. kidney
s. spleen

Shaver disease

shaving

femoral condylar s.
patellar s.
residual metal fragment s.

SHC

sclerosing hepatic carcinoma

shear

s. fracture
s. interface
s. strain
s. strain rate
s. stress

shearing

axonal s.
s. force

NOTES

shearing *(continued)*
   s. of white matter
   s. white matter injury
shear-strain deformation
sheath
   Amplatz Teflon s.
   angioplasty s.
   anterior rectus s.
   ArrowFlex s.
   arterial s.
   axillary s.
   bicipital synovial s.
   bicipital tendon s.
   carotid s.
   catheter s.
   caudal s.
   Check-Flo s.
   check-valve s.
   Colapinto s.
   common synovial flexor s.
   Cordis s.
   crural s.
   dentinal s.
   dural s.
   extensor carpi ulnaris s.
   fascial s.
   femoral s.
   fenestrated s.
   fibrous s.
   flexor tendon s.
   giant cell tumor of the tendon s.
   guiding s.
   Henle s.
   intratendon s.
   s. ligament
   muscle s.
   myelin s.
   s. needle
   nerve root s.
   neural s.
   peel-away s.
   periarteriolar lymphoid s.
   periradicular s.
   pilar s.
   plicated dural s.
   posterior rectus s.
   rectus s.
   Schwann cell of myelin s.
   self-expanding tulip s.
   s. and side-arm
   Spectranetics laser s. (SLS)
   synovial s.
   tendon s.
   transseptal s.
   tulip s.
   unplicated s.
   vascular s.

   venous s.
   working s.
sheathing canal
Shebele physician reporting workstation
Sheehan syndrome
sheet
   amnionic s.
sheet-like
   s.-l. dysplasia
   s.-l. growth pattern
Sheffield gamma unit
shelf, pl. **shelves**
   Blumer rectal s.
   buccal s.
   dental s.
   lateral s.
   medial s.
   mesocolic s.
   palatine s.
   patellar s.
   rectal s.
   synovial s.
shell
   acetabular s.
   K s.
   L s.
   M s.
   s. nephrogram
   O s.
shelling off of cartilage
shell-like demarcation
shell-of-bone appearance
shell-type of periosteal reaction
Shelton femur fracture classification
shelves (*pl. of* shelf)
shelving edge of Poupart ligament
Shenton line
shepherd
   s. crook configuration
   s. crook deformity
   S. fracture
Shepp-Logan filter function
SHG
   sonohysterography
Shibley sign
shibuol
shield
   acrylic syringe s.
   AME PinSite s.
   apron s.
   Faraday s.
   lead apron s.
   lead eye s.
   lead gonad s.
   radiofrequency magnetic s.
   Tungsten eye s.
   Tungsten syringe s.

shielded gradient coil
shielding
    active s.
    faulty radiofrequency s.
    gonadal s.
    magnetic s.
    passive s.
    RF s.
    room s.
shift
    anterior capsular s.
    aromatic solvent-induced s. (ASIS)
    chemical s.
    colloid s.
    diamagnetic s.
    distal s.
    Doppler frequency s.
    flow-related phase s.
    s. of the heart
    intracranial s.
    lanthanide-induced s.
    left-to-right s.
    mediastinal s.
    midline s.
    motion-induced phase s.
    navigator s.
    neonate mediastinal s.
    paramagnetic s.
    phase s.
    pineal gland s.
    pivot s.
    plantar s.
    s. probe
    proximal brain s.
    radial s.
    s. reagents
    reverse pivot s. (RPS)
    right-to-left s.
    round s.
    simple s.
    square brain s.
    ST-segment s.
    superior frontal axis s.
    tracheal s.
    velocity-induced phase s.
    s. of ventricle
    ventricular s.
shim
    s. coil
    s. placement
Shimadzu
    S. CT scanner

    S. HeadTome Set-031 camera
    S. HeadTome system
    S. MR scanner
shimmed magnet
shimmering
    visual s.
shimming
    active s.
    localized s.
    passive s.
shin bone
Shine-Dalgamo sequence
Shiner radiopaque tube
Shinnar-LeRoux algorithm
Shirmer test
shish
    s. kabob esophagus
    s. kabob pattern
shiver
    esophageal s.
shock
    bowel s.
    cardiac s.
    circulation s.
    distributive s.
    hypovolemic s.
    joule s.
    lung s.
    nephrogram s.
    QRS synchronized s.
    sequence monophasic s.
shockwave pressure
shoemaker's breast
Shone
    S. anomaly
    S. syndrome
shoot-through lateral x-ray film
Shope fibroma
short
    s. acquisition window
    s. axis acquisition
    s. axis image
    s. axis parasternal view
    s. axis plane
    s. axis slice
    s. axis view echocardiography
    s. bone
    s. echo point resolved
        spectroscopic sequence spectrum
    s. esophagus-type hiatal hernia
    s. gut syndrome
    s. half-life

NOTES

S

short *(continued)*
s. head
s. head of biceps
s. insular gyrus
s. inversion recovery imaging
s. limb dysplasia
s. muscle
s. oblique fracture
s. radiolunate ligament
s. repetition time sequence
s. rib
s. rib-polydactyly syndrome
s. scale contrast
s. tau inversion recovery (STIR)
s. tau inversion recovery image
s. TE proton MR spectroscopy
s. TI inversion recovery
s. TI inversion recovery imaging
s. TI inversion recovery pulse
sequence
s. T1 inversion recovery (STIR)
s. T1 relaxation time
s. TR/TE

short-bore magnet
short-cannula coaxial method
short-distance
s.-d. radiation therapy
s.-d. radiotherapy

short-echo time
short-echo-time proton spectroscopy
shortened
fat-suppressed acquisition with TE
and TR times s.

shortening
Achilles tendon s.
circumferential s.
s. fraction
fractional s. (FS)
fractional myocardial s.
left ventricular functional s.
(LVFS)
leg s.
phalangeal s.
skeleton s.
suboccipital s.
systolic fractional s.
T1 s.
T2 s.
tendon s.
T2-weighted s.

short-increment sensitivity index
short-inversion-time inversion recovery
(STIR)
short-range isotope
short-segment Barrett esophagus (SSBE)
short-term patency

shot
cusp s.
fast low-angle s. (FLASH)
fluid-attenuated inversion recovery-
fast low-angle s.
guiding s.
multiple echo single s. (MESS)
pocket s.
turbo fast low-angle s.
(turboFLASH)

shoulder
s. ankylosis
arthrotomography of s.
baseball s.
curvilinear threshold s.
s. dislocation
s. dome
double-contrast arthrotomography
of s.
drooping s.
drop s.
dynamic ultrasound of s. (DUS)
s. dystocia
flail s.
frozen s.
s. girdle
s. of heart
s. immobilizer
s. impingement
s. impingement syndrome
intrathoracic dislocation of s.
s. isocenter
s. joint
s. joint instability
knocked-down s.
s. labral capsular complex
Little Leaguer s.
loose s.
s. muscle
s. pointer
s. presentation
ring man s.
s. separation
subcoracoid dislocation of s.
subglenoid dislocation of s.
s. surface coil
swimmer's s.
tennis s.

shoulder-hand syndrome
shower
s. of echoes
embolic s.
s.'s of microemboli

Shprintzen velocardiofacial syndrome
shrapnel
Shrapnell membrane

shrinkage
  brain s.
  graft s.
  tumor s.
shriveled kidney
shrunken
  s. bladder
  s. folia
  s. gallbladder
  s. liver
  s. lung
SH U 508A contrast agent
shudder
  carotid s.
shunt
  barium-sulfate impregnated s.
  bidirectional s.
  biliopancreatic s.
  Blalock s.
  Blalock-Taussig s.
  cardiac atrial s.
  cardiovascular s.
  cerebral s.
  Cimino AV s.
  Cimino dialysis s.
  cystoatrial s.
  Davidson s.
  Denver s.
  dialysis s.
  distal splenorenal s.
  esophageal s.
  s. evaluation
  s. fraction
  gastrorenal s.
  Glenn s.
  indwelling nonvascular s.
  jejunoileal s.
  JI s.
  mesocaval s.
  net s.
  s. patency
  peritoneovenous s. (PVS)
  s. placement
  portacaval s.
  portopulmonary s.
  portosystemic s.
  Potts s.
  s. quantification
  s. reservoir
  s. reversal
  reversed s.
  small bowel s.

  splenorenal s.
  s. thrombosis
  transjugular intrahepatic
    portosystemic s. (TIPS)
  s. tube
  VA s.
  s. valve
  ventriculoatrial s.
  ventriculoperitoneal s.
  VP s.
  Waterson s.
  Waterson-Cooley s.
  s. with normal left atrium
shunted
  s. blood
  s. hydrocephalus
  s. tracer
shunting
  s. circuit
  lumboperitoneal s.
  peritoneal s.
  pleural s.
  syringosubarachnoid s.
  s. of tracer to the bone marrow
shuntogram
  s. imaging
  radionuclide s.
shuntography
shutdown
  renal s.
shuttering
  white s.
Shwachman syndrome
SI
  sacroiliac
  saturation index
  signal intensity
  sinus irregularity
  stroke index
    SI joint
    SI joint-to-sacrum ratio
S/I
  superior/inferior
Si
  silicon
    Si (Li) detector
sialadenitis (*var. of* sialoadenitis)
sialadenitis
  acute suppurative s.
  autoimmune s.
  chronic recurrent s.

NOTES

sialadenitis *(continued)*
    myoepithelial s.
    recurrent s.
sialadenography
sialangiography
sialectasis
sialoadenitis, sialadenitis
sialogram
sialography
    CT s.
    s. imaging
    magnetic resonance s.
    s. needle
    parotid gland s.
    submaxillary s.
sialolithiasis
sialometaplasia
sialometry
sialosis
siboroxime
    technetium-99m s.
Sibson
    S. fascia
    S. groove
    S. muscle
sickle shape
sickle-shaped fold
sickling
    intravascular s.
sickness
    decompression s.
    radiation s.
sick sinus node
SID
    source-to-image receptor distance
side
    s. branch
    s. effect
    s. lobe artifact
    s. scattering
side-arm
    sheath and s.-a.
sideband
    total suppression of s. (TOSS)
side-branch occlusion
side-by-side
    s.-b.-s. object
    s.-b.-s. transposition of great artery
side-exiting
    s.-e. coaxial needle system
    s.-e. coaxial system
    s.-e. guide
side-firing probe
side-hole cannulated probe
side-lying position
sideplate
Sideris buttoned double-disk device

sideropenic dysphagia
siderotic
    s. nodule in the spleen
    s. splenomegaly
sideswipe fracture
sidewall
    s. impingement
    pelvic s.
Sidewinder catheter
SIE
    stroke in evolution
Siemens
    S. AG system
    S. DRH CT scanner
    S. gamma camera
    S. HICOR/BICOR x-ray system
    S. ICON
    S. Lithostar lithotripter
    S. Magnetom GBS II scanner
    S. Magnetom SP 4000 scanner
    S. Magnetom 1.5-T scanner
    S. Magnetom Vision scanner
    S. Mevatron 74 linear accelerator
    S. One Tesla scanner
    S. Orbiter large-field-of-view camera
    S. Satellite CT evaluation console
    S. Somaform 512 CT scanner
    S. Somatom DR2, DR3 whole-body scanner
    S. Somatom nonhelical unit
    S. Somatom Plus CT scanner
    S. Somatom Plus-4 CT system
    S. Sonoline Elegra ultrasound scanner
    S. 1.5-T system
SieScape ultrasound
sieve bone
sievert (Sv)
SIF
    sacral insufficiency fracture
sigma filter
sigmoid
    s. carcinoma
    s. cavity
    s. cavity of radius
    s. cavity of ulna
    s. colon
    s. colon volvulus
    s. density curve
    s. diverticulitis
    s. diverticulum
    s. flexure
    s. fold
    s. hair pattern
    s. kidney
    s. loop

s. lymph node
s. mesocolon
s. notch
s. omentum
s. polyp
s. pseudostenosis
s. sinus
s. sulcus
s. valve
sigmoidoscope
Reichert flexible s.
sigmoidoscopy
sigmoid-shaped configuration
sign
Aaron s.
Abrahams s.
absent bow-tie s.
absent diaphragm s.
accordion s.
air crescent s.
Allis s.
Amoss s.
angel-wing s.
antecedent s.
anterior drawer s.
aortic nipple s.
apical cap s.
arrowhead s.
banana s.
Battle s.
B6 bronchus s.
beaded septum s.
beak s.
Beevor s.
Bergman s.
blade of grass s.
Blumberg s.
bowler hat s.
bowstring s.
bow-tie s.
Bozzolo s.
Bragard s.
Braunwald s.
brim s.
bronchial cuff s.
bronchus s.
Brudzinski s.
Bryant s.
bubble s.
C s.
calcium s.
Cantelli s.

cardinal s.
cardiorespiratory s.
Carman s.
Carnett s.
carotid string s.
Carvallo s.
catheter coiling s.
Chaddock s.
Chilaiditi s.
Claybrook s.
clockwise whirlpool s.
cobblestone s.
Codman s.
Cogan lid twitch s.
cogwheel s.
coiled spring s.
collapsing cord s.
collar s.
Collier s.
colon cutoff s.
comb s.
comet-tail s.
commemorative s.
Comolli s.
continuous diaphragm s.
contralateral s.
Coopernail s.
cord s.
Corrigan s.
cortical rim s.
cortical vein s.
Courvoisier s.
cranial nerve s.
crescent s.
crescent-in-doughnut s.
Cullen s.
cupola s.
cutoff s.
dagger s.
Dance s.
David Letterman s.
Dawbarn s.
deep sulcus s.
Dejérine s.
Delbet s.
delta s.
Demianoff s.
de Musset s.
dense MCA s.
d'Eśpine s.
Dorendorf s.
double-bleb s.

S

NOTES

sign *(continued)*

double-bubble s.
double decidual sac s.
double density s.
double diaphragm s.
double duct s.
double-halo s.
double lesion s.
double line s.
double-ring esophageal s.
double track s.
double wall s.
doughnut s.
drooping lily s.
Drummond s.
Duchenne s.
duct-penetrating s.
Dupuytren s.
Duroziez s.
Ebstein s.
Erichsen s.
Ewart s.
extrapleural s.
falciform ligament s.
fallen lung s.
false localizing s.
fan s.
fat-blood interface s.
fat pad s.
FBI s.
feeding vessel s.
figure-3 s.
Finkelstein s.
Fischer s.
fissure s.
fleck s.
Fleischner s.
flipped meniscus s.
floppy-thumb s.
flush-tank s.
focal neurologic s.
football s.
Friedreich s.
Froment s.
frontal lobe s.
Frostberg s.
Gaenslen s.
Galeazzi s.
garland s.
Gerhardt s.
geyser s.
Glasgow s.
gloved-finger s.
Goldthwait s.
Gordon s.
Gottron s.
Gowers s.

Grey Turner s.
Griesinger s.
Grocco s.
Gunn crossing s.
half-moon s.
halo s.
Hamman s.
harlequin s.
hatchet s.
Hawkins s.
hay-fork s.
Heim-Kreysig s.
hilar s.
Hildreth s.
Hill s.
Hirschberg s.
Hoffmann s.
Hoover s.
Horner s.
hot nose s.
Howship-Romberg s.
hyperdense middle cerebral
  artery s.
iliopsoas s.
insular ribbon s.
interface s.
interrupted duct s.
intradecidual s.
inverted teardrop s.
inverted-V s.
Jaccoud s.
Jackson s.
Kanavel s.
Kantor string s.
Karplus s.
Kehr s.
Kellock s.
Kernig s.
Klemm s.
Kussmaul s.
Lachman s.
Lancisi s.
Landolfi s.
Lasègue s.
lateralizing s.
Lazarus s.
Leichtenstern s.
lemon s.
leptomeningeal ivy s.
Leri s.
Livierato s.
localizing s.
long tract s.
luftsichel s.
Macewen s.
Maisonneuve s.
Mannkopf s.

Martorell s.
McGinn-White s.
melting s.
Meltzer s.
meniscus s.
Mennell s.
metacarpal s.
Minor s.
Morquio s.
Mulder s.
Müller s.
Musset s.
Myerson s.
Naffziger s.
naked-facet s.
Napoleon hat s.
Neer impingement s.
Nicoladoni-Branham s.
obturator s.
Oliver-Cardarelli s.
open bronchus s.
Oppenheim s.
Ortolani s.
Osler s.
Payr s.
Perez s.
peritoneal s.
peroneal s.
piano key s.
Pins s.
Piotrowski s.
pivot-shift s.
Plummer s.
Potain s.
premonitory s.
psoas s.
puddle s.
pulvinar s.
pupillary s.
pyramidal s.
Queckenstedt s.
Quénu-Muret s.
Quincke s.
radialis s.
railroad track s.
rebound s.
reversal s.
reverse S s.
Rigler s.
rim s.
ring s.
Risser s.

Romberg s.
Rosenbach s.
Rotch s.
Rovighi s.
Rovsing s.
rugger jersey s.
sail s.
Sanders s.
sandwich s.
Sansom s.
sawtooth s.
Schepelmann s.
Schlesinger s.
Schwartze s.
scimitar s.
seagull s.
sentinel clot s.
sentinel loop s.
setting-sun s.
Shibley s.
signet ring s.
silhouette s.
Sister Mary Joseph s.
Skoda s.
slim carotid artery s.
sonographic Murphy s.
Spalding s.
spinal s.
spine s.
Spurling s.
steeple s.
Steinberg s.
stepladder s.
Sternberg s.
Stewart-Holmes s.
Stierlin s.
string s.
string-of-beads s.
string-of-pearls s.
stripe s.
Strümpell s.
Strunsky s.
Sumner s.
superior triangle s.
tail s.
target s.
Terry Thomas s.
thread-and-streaks s.
Thurston Holland s.
thymic sail s.
tibialis s.
Tinel s.

S

NOTES

sign *(continued)*
    Traube s.
    tree-in-bud s.
    triple-bubble s.
    triple track s.
    Troisier s.
    trolley-track s.
    trough s.
    Trousseau s.
    Turyn s.
    twin peak s.
    Uhthoff s.
    Vanzetti s.
    Waddell s.
    Wartenberg s.
    Wegner s.
    Weill s.
    Weiss s.
    Westermark s.
    whirl s.
    whirlpool s.
    white cerebellum s.
    Wimberger s.
    windsock s.

Signa
    S. Advantage system
    S. Horizon LX MRI system
    S. Horizon LX SR 77 gradients
      1.5-T MR scanner
    S. MR imaging system
    S. MRI scanner
    1.5T S. MR unit
    S. 1.5T scanner
    1.5T S. whole-body
      imager/spectrometer
    S. VH/i3.0-T MR scanner

signal
    abnormal bright s.
    s. acquisition
    s. attenuation
    s. average
    s. blooming
    BOLD s.
    bright s.
    s. change
    s. characteristic
    color Doppler s.
    composite s.
    D s.
    s. dephasing
    s. depth
    differential s.
    Doppler blood flow velocity s.
    Doppler ovary s.
    s. drop-out artifact
    s. enhancement
    s. fallout

flow velocity s.
fluid s.
free induction decay s.
gamma s.
high-intensity s.
high-intensity transient s. (HITS)
high-pitched s.
hyperintense s.
hypointense s.
imaginary s.
increased echo s.
s. intensity (SI)
s. intensity inhomogeneity
s. intensity measurement
s. intensity ratio
s. intensity rim
s. intensity time curve
isointense s.
s. joint
linear low s.
lipid s.
s. loss
magnetic resonance s.
s. magnification
mosaic jet s.
navigable echo s.
NMR s.
s. node
nuclear s.
ovarian Doppler s.
periventricular bright s.
power Doppler s.
s. processing
pulsed-wave spectral color
  Doppler s.
radionuclide s.
real s.
s. sonographic feature analysis
s. source
SSFP s.
stimulus-correlated water s.
superimposition of s.
s. suppression
symmetric abnormal increased s.
s. time course
s. transducer
s. transduction
turbulent s.
T2-weighted s.
unsuppressed water s.
velocity-encoded color Doppler s.
s. void
weak s.
signal-averaged electrocardiogram
  (SAECG, SaECG)
signaling molecule
signal-to-clutter ratio

signal-to-noise
> s.-t.-n. calculation
> s.-t.-n. ratio (SNR, S/N)
> s.-t.-n. threshold

signature
> echo s.
> gut s.
> tissue s.
> tumor s.

signet
> s. ring cell carcinoma
> s. ring pattern
> s. ring sign

significance level

significant
> s. axis deviation
> s. residual deficit
> s. sequela

SIH
> secondary intracranial hypertension

Silastic
> S. collar-reinforced stoma
> S. finger joint
> S. ring

silence
> electrocerebral s. (ECS)

silent
> s. area of brain
> s. cerebral embolus
> s. gallstone
> s. ischemic episode
> s. mitral stenosis
> s. myocardial infarct
> s. myocardial ischemia
> s. patent ductus arteriosus
> s. regurgitation
> s. sinus syndrome

silhouette
> cardiac s.
> cardiothymic s.
> cardiovascular s.
> enlarged cardiac s.
> heart s.
> s. imaging
> S. laser system
> luminal s.
> pericardial s.
> roentgenographic s.
> s. sign
> s. sign of Felson
> s. technique
> widened cardiac s.

silhouetted out

silhouetting

silicate pneumoconiosis

silicon (Si)
> amorphous s.
> s. diode array
> s. diode dosimeter
> S. Graphics Reality Engine system

silicon-controlled rectifier (SCR)

silicone
> s. elastomer band
> s. elastomer ring
> s. elastomer rubber ball implant
> s. fluid
> s. granuloma
> s. implant leakage
> s. implant rupture
> s. injection
> s. microsphere
> s. oil
> s. stent
> s. wrist implant

silicoproteinosis
> acute s.

silicosis
> accelerated s.
> chronic simple s.
> complicated s.
> Liverpool s.
> nonnodular s.
> simple s.

silicotic
> s. fibrosis of lung
> s. nodule
> s. visceral pleura

silicotuberculosis

silk
> s. aesthetic laser system
> s. suture
> s. tuft

SilkLaser
> 2040 erbium S.

Sillence classification of osteogenesis imperfecta

sillimanite pneumoconiosis

silo-filler's
> s.-f. disease
> s.-f. lung

silver
> s. finisher's lung
> s. fork fracture
> Grocott methenamine s.

NOTES

silver *(continued)*
  s. halide film
  s. iodide
  s. polisher's lung
  s. recovery
  S. Speed 0.010-inch guidewire
  s. wire effect
simian griffe
Simmond disease
Simmons catheter
Simon
  S. focus
  S. Nitinol vena cava filter
Simonart
  S. band
  S. ligament
SIM/Plant
simple
  s. block
  s. bolus
  s. bone cyst
  s. breast cyst
  s. capillary lymphangioma
  s. cortical renal cyst
  s. dislocation
  s. extraperitoneal rupture
  s. goiter
  s. mechanical obstruction
  s. meningocele
  s. shift
  s. silicosis
  s. skull fracture
  s. ureterocele
simplex
  carcinoma s.
  xanthoma tuberosum s.
SimpliCT interventional guidance system
Simpson
  S. atherectomy
  S. Coronary AtheroCath (SCA)
  system
  S. directional atherectomy catheter
  S. rule method for ventricular
  volume
  S. white line
Sims position
simulated
  s. annealing
  s. annealing method
  s. annealing method projection
  s. echo
  s. equilibrium factor study
simulation
  s. of converging port
  s. film
  MCPT s.

  Monte Carlo photon transport s.
  s. of tangential portal
simulation-aided field setting
simulator
  AcQsim CT s.
  magnetic resonance s.
  Maxwell 3D field s.
  virtual reality s.
  Ximatron s.
simultaneous
  s. acquisition of artery and vein
  (SAAV)
  s. balloon inflation
  s. bilateral spontaneous
  pneumothorax (SBSP)
  s. fluoroscopy
  s. MSDI
  s. multifilm tomography
  s. multislice acquisition
  s. recording
  s. slice
  s. volume imaging
sincalide
  s. cholescintigraphy
  s. imaging agent
sinc-Hanning radiofrequency
sinc interpolation
sincipital cephalocele
Sinding-Larsen-Johansson disease (SLJD)
sine wave
singer's
  s. node
  s. nodule
Singh osteoporosis index
single
  s. atrium
  s. axis
  s. breath-hold
  s. breath-hold dynamic subtraction
  CT with multidetector row helical
  technology
  s. breath-hold sequence
  s. collision energy loss
  s. colonic filling defect
  s. fill/void technique
  s. functioning kidney
  s. isocenter
  s. label
  s. peak
  s. photon/maximum intensity
  s. pixel reconstruction
  s. pleurisy
  s. polyp
  s. port
  s. section 2D image
  s. suture synostosis
  s. sweep scan

s. umbilical artery
s. umbilical artery spectrum
s. ventricle
s. voxel proton brain spectroscopy
imaging
s. voxel proton MR spectroscopy
(1H-MRS)
s. voxel stimulated echo acquisition
mode MR spectroscopy
s. voxel in vivo proton spectrum
s. x-ray dosimetry
single-ablation scheme
single-breath view
single-cannula atrial cannulation
single-cavity cochlea
single-channel analyzer (SCA)
single-contrast
s.-c. arthrography
s.-c. barium enema
s.-c. study
single-crystal endoprobe
single-curved Cobra catheter
single-detector
s.-d. CTA
s.-d. helical CT
s.-d. helical scanner
s.-d. row scanner
single-dose gadolinium imaging
single-echo
s.-e. diffusion imaging
s.-e. versus multiple-echo sequence
**single-energy x-ray absorptiometer
(SXA)**
single-field hyperthermia technique
single-headed instrument
single-head rotating gamma camera
single-hole collimator
single-lumen silicone breast implant
single-needle biopsy technique
single-outlet heart
single-pass scan
single-phase current
single-photon
s.-p. absorptiometry (SPA)
s.-p. counting system
s.-p. densitometer
s.-p. emission-computed tomography
(SPECT)
s.-p. emission-computed tomography
technetium sestamibi scan
s.-p. emission CT

s.-p. emission tomography (SPET)
s.-p. planar scintigraphy (SPPS)
single-plane angiography
single-pole double-throw (SPDT)
single-sample
s.-s. clearance
s.-s. technique
single-shot
s.-s. embolization of micro-AVM
s.-s. fast spin echo (SSFSE)
s.-s. gradient echo-planar imaging
s.-s. imaging technique
s.-s. MR cholangiogram
single-slice
s.-s. CTA
s.-s. gradient-echo image
s.-s. helical CT
s.-s. long-axis tomogram
single-stick system
single-strand scission
single-stripe colitis (SSC)
single-vessel
s.-v. disease
s.-v. runoff
single-view oblique mammography
**single-voxel proton brain examination
(PROBE-SV)**
single-wall needle
sinistral portal hypertension
sinistrum
atrium s.
sink
s. effect
quantum s.
sink-trap malformation
sinoatrial (SA)
s. block (SAB)
s. branch
s. bundle
s. conduction time (SACT)
s. exit block
s. nodal reentry tachycardia
s. node (SAN)
s. node artery
s. node dysfunction
s. node infarct
sinoauricular node
sinodural plate
Sinografin imaging agent
sinogram
sinography

NOTES

sinonasal
- s. carcinoma
- s. cavity
- s. lesion
- s. lymphoma
- s. polyposis
- s. psammomatoid ossifying fibroma
- s. secretion
- s. tumor

sinotubular junction
sinovaginal bulb
sintering
- selective laser s. (SLS)

sinus
- accessory s.
- alternating s.
- aortic valve s.
- s. arrest
- artery of inferior cavernous s. (AICS)
- basilar s.
- branchial s.
- bronchial s.
- carotid s.
- cavernous s.
- s. cavity
- cerebral venous s.
- cervical s.
- circular s.
- cloudy s.
- coccygeal s.
- coronary s. (CS)
- costomediastinal s.
- costophrenic s.
- cranial s.
- s. cycle length (SCL)
- dilated intercavernous s.
- distal coronary s. (DCS)
- dorsal dermal s.
- dorsal enteric s.
- draining s.
- dural venous s.
- dura mater venous s.
- endodermal s.
- s. of epididymis
- ethmoid s.
- frontal s.
- frontalis s.
- granulomatous lesion of s.
- Guérin s.
- s. histiocytosis
- s. hyperplasia
- hypoechoic renal s.
- s. hypoplasia
- inferior sagittal s. (ISS)
- intercavernous s.
- s. irregularity (SI)

- lactiferous s.
- lateral s.
- s. lateralis
- left coronary s.
- s. lipomatosis
- lumbosacral dermal s.
- lymph node s.
- manual pressure over carotid s.
- marginal s.
- mastoid s.
- maxillary s.
- s. mechanism
- medullary s.
- middle coronary s. (MCS)
- s. of Morgagni
- nasal s.
- s. nodal artery
- s. nodal reentry
- s. node
- s. node automaticity
- s. node depression
- s. node dysfunction
- s. node electrogram
- s. node exit block
- s. node recovery time (SNRT)
- noncoronary s.
- oblique pericardial s.
- occipital s.
- osteomyelitic s.
- paranasal s.
- s. pattern
- s. pause
- pericardial s.
- s. pericranii
- perineal s.
- Petit s.
- petrosal s.
- pilonidal s.
- piriform s.
- precoronal sagittal s.
- prostatic s.
- pulmonary s.
- s. of pulmonary trunk
- renal s.
- s. rhythm
- s. rhythm mapping
- Ridley s.
- Rokitansky-Aschoff s.
- rudimentary s.
- sagittal s.
- s. septum
- s. series
- sigmoid s.
- s. slowing
- sphenoid s.
- sphenoparietal s.
- straight s.

subeustachian s.
superior petrous s. (SPS)
superior sagittal s. (SSS)
tarsal s.
s. tarsi syndrome
thickened s.
s. thrombosis
s. tract
s. tract imaging
s. tract study
transverse pericardial s.
urachal s.
urogenital s.
s. of Valsalva
s. of Valsalva aneurysm
s. of vena cava
s. venosus
s. venosus atrial septal defect
venous s.
vertebral articular s.

sinusitis
acute s.
allergic s.
bacterial s.
bronchiectasis-ethmoid s.
s. cerebritis
chronic s.
mycotic s.
paranasal s.
sphenoidal s.

sinusography
cerebral s.

sinusoid
hepatic s.
s. reference function

sinusoidal
s. capillary
s. histiocyte
s. lesion
s. relaxation
s. vascular space
s. waveform

sinusoidalization
sinuvertebral nerve of Luschka
SIP
saturation inversion projection

siphon
carotid s.

Sipple syndrome
sirenomelia
SIS
saline infusion sonohysterography

SISCOM
Subtraction ictal SPECT coregistered to
MRI

SISCO spectrometer
Sister
S. Mary Joseph node
S. Mary Joseph nodule
S. Mary Joseph sign

site
anastomotic s.
binding s.
bleeding s.
catheter exit s.
cellular binding s.
donor s.
extraadrenal s.
extranodal s.
fracture s.
implantation s.
ipsilateral antegrade s.
s. of maximal intensity
metastatic s.
reference s.
S. Rite sonographic guide
sanctuary s.
termination s.
unknown primary s.

site-specific labeling
sitting-up
s.-u. view
s.-u. view angiography

situ
adenocarcinoma in s.
carcinoma in s.
ductal carcinoma in s. (DCIS)
in s.
intracystic breast papillary
carcinoma in s.
lobular carcinoma in s. (LCIS)

situs
atrial s.
s. atrialis solitus
s. concordance
D-loop ventricular s.
s. inversus
L-loop ventricular s.
s. perversus
s. transversus
s. viscerum inversus

Sitzmarks
S. capsule
S. radiopaque marker

NOTES

S

sixth

    s. compartment
    s. nucleus
    s. ventricle

size

    abnormal placental s.
    borderline heart s.
    decreased placenta s.
    effective focal spot s.
    embryo s.
    s. estimation error
    gallbladder s.
    kernel s.
    kidney s.
    matrix s.
    ovarian s.
    renal s.
    s. of spinal cord
    top normal limits of s.
    uterine s.
    ventricular s.
    vertebral body s.
    voxel s.
    x-ray beam s.

Sjögren syndrome

SJS

    Schwartz-Jampel syndrome
    Swyer-James syndrome

skeletal

    s. amyloidosis
    s. bed
    s. biopsy
    s. disruption
    s. dysplasia
    s. emphysema
    s. hyperostosis
    s. hypoplasia
    s. lesion
    s. lymphoma
    s. maturation
    s. metastasis
    s. muscle
    s. muscle fiber
    s. neoplasm
    s. radiology
    s. survey
    s. system
    s. targeted radiotherapy (STR)
    s. tuberculosis

skeletally

    s. immature
    s. mature

skeletography

skeletology

skeleton

    appendicular s.
    s. appendiculare

    articulated s.
    axial s.
    s. axiale
    bony s.
    cardiac s.
    fibrous s.
    gill arch s.
    laryngeal s.
    peripheral s.
    s. shortening
    spidering s.
    spiky s.
    sulcal s.
    s. thoracis
    visceral s.

skeletonizing

skeletopia

skeletopy

skiagram

skiagraph

skiagraphy

skier's

    s. fracture
    s. injury
    s. thumb

ski jump view

Skillern fracture

skimming of magnetic field

skin

    s. bridge
    s. calcification
    s. carcinoma
    s. crease artifact
    s. depth
    s. dose
    s. effect
    s. fold
    s. fold artifact
    s. lesion artifact
    s. line
    s. staple
    s. thickening

Skinner line

skinny needle

skin-rolling scapular tenderness

skin-sparing effect

skip

    s. aganglionosis
    s. area
    s. lesion
    s. metastasis
    s. tomography

skodaic resonance

Skoda sign

skull

    abnormally thin s.

anterior cerebral artery crawling
under the s.
s. asymmetry
base of s. (BOS)
beaten brass s.
beaten silver appearance of s.
button sequestrum s.
cloverleaf s.
dentate suture of s.
s. film
s. fracture
geographic s.
hair-on-end of s.
hammered-silver s.
hammer-marked s.
hot-cross bun s.
s. hyperostosis
indented fracture of s.
inner table of s.
lacunar s.
lytic lesion of s.
map-like s.
molding of s.
natiform s.
occipital view of s.
s. osteolysis
outer table of s.
s. plate
sonolucent s.
suture of s.
synchondrosis of s.
thin s.
West-Engstler s.
West lacuna s.

skull-base
s.-b. approach
s.-b. foramen
s.-b. tumor

SKYLight gantry-free nuclear medicine gamma camera

skyline
s. projection
s. view
s. view of patella

SL
scapholunate
structured light
SL joint
SL technique

slab
coronal s.
3D MRA s.

interleaved axial s.
s. thickness

slab-MIP

SLAC
scapholunate advanced collapse
SLAC wrist

slant hole collimator

SLAP
superior labral anterior to posterior
SLAP lesion
SLAP tear

sleeve
conjoined root s.
s. fracture
s. lobectomy
nerve root s.
Smitt s.
thoracic root s.

SLE 2000 ventilator

slew range

SL-GRE
spin lock gradient-echo
SL-GRE sequence

slice
angled s.
apical short-axis s.
axial s.
basal short-axis s.
contiguous s.
coronal s.
cross s.
digitized CT s.
direct s.
2D sequential s.
s. excitation wave (SEW)
s. format
s. fracture
gated stress myocardial perfusion s.
s. geometry
horizontal long axis s.
s. interference
intermediate CT s.
long-axis s.
midventricular short-axis s.
nonattenuation-corrected s.
nonplanar s.
oblique s.
s. orientation
s. overlap artifact
plurality of s.'s
s. profile artifact
sagittal s.

NOTES

slice *(continued)*
    s. select gradient (SS)
    s. selection
    s. sensitivity profile (SSP)
    serial CT s.
    short axis s.
    simultaneous s.
    STIR s.
    texture s.
    s. thickness
    tissue s.
    tomographic s.
    transaxial s.
    transverse s.
    vertical long-axis s.
    s. volume
slice-of-sausage breast pattern
slice-point MRS
slice-selective excitation
slicing plane
slider crank theory
sliding
    s. hiatal hernia
    s. thin-slab maximum intensity projection (STS-MIP)
    s. thin-slab maximum intensity projection image
    s. thin-slab minimum intensity projection technique
sliding interleaved Ky (SLINKY)
slim carotid artery sign
sling
    cardiac s.
    s. muscle fiber
    pulmonary s.
    s. ring complex
    tendon s.
    vascular s.
SLINKY
    sliding interleaved Ky
slip
    s. angle
    diaphragmatic s.
    muscular s.
    s. of tendon
slip-angle spondylolisthesis
slip-in connection
slippage
    epiphyseal s.
    film s.
slipped
    s. capital femoral epiphysis (SCFE)
    s. tendon
    s. upper femoral epiphysis (SUFE)
slipping
    s. rib
    s. rib syndrome

slip-ring
    s.-r. camera
    s.-r. CT
    s.-r. gantry system
    s.-r. imaging
    s.-r. technology
slit
    s. collimator
    s. hemorrhage
    s. radiography
    s. scanography
    s. ventricle
    s. ventricle syndrome
slit-lamp biomicroscopy
slit-like
    s.-l. lumen
    s.-l. orafice
    s.-l. residual lucency
slit-shaped vessel lumen
sliver
    bone s.
SLJD
    Sinding-Larsen-Johansson disease
SLL
    spinolaminar line
SLN
    sentinel lymph node
slope
    acromial s.
    s. blot analysis
    closing s.
    decreased E-to-F s.
    disappearance s.
    downward s.
    D-to-E s.
    E-to-F s.
    flat diastolic s.
    flattened E-to-F s.
    mitral deceleration s.
    normalized plateau s.
    opening s.
    palmar s.
    ST/HR s.
        ST segment/heart rate slope
    triquetrohamate helicoid s.
    valve opening s.
slot-scanning detector
sloughed
    s. mucosa
    s. papilla
    s. urethra syndrome
sloughing ulcer
slow
    s. exchange soft tissue
    s. filling wave
    s. neutron

s. stroke
s. ventricular response
slow-channel blocking drug
slow-flow
s.-f. lesion
s.-f. vascular anomaly
s.-f. vascular malformation
slow-flowing giant saccular aneurysm
slowing
background s.
sinus s.
slowly
s. developing atelectasis
s. developing lesion
slow-twitch muscle
slow-wave activity
SLP
subluxation of patella
SLS
selective laser sintering
Spectranetics laser sheath
SLS laser
sludge
aggregated s.
s. ball
biliary s.
blood s.
gallbladder s.
tumefactive s.
tumefactive biliary s.
sludge-like intraluminal echo
sludging of retinal vein
sluggish flow
Sm
samarium
¹⁵³Sm, Sm-153
samarium-153
SMA
spinal muscular atrophy
superior mesenteric artery
Doppler sonography of the SMA
SMAI
superior-medial acetabular index
small
s. adrenal tumor
s. airway
s. airway dysfunction
s. aorta syndrome
s. B-cell lymphoma
s. bowel
s. bowel adenocarcinoma
s. bowel adenoma

s. bowel atresia
s. bowel benign tumor
s. bowel carcinoma
s. bowel cavitary lesion
s. bowel content
s. bowel delayed transit
s. bowel disease
s. bowel diverticulum
s. bowel duplication cyst
s. bowel enema
s. bowel enteroscopy (SBE)
s. bowel filling defect
s. bowel fold anatomy
s. bowel folds atrophy
s. bowel follow-through (SBFT)
s. bowel gas
s. bowel hemangioma
s. bowel hemorrhage
s. bowel infarct
s. bowel leiomyoma
s. bowel leiomyosarcoma
s. bowel loop
s. bowel malignant tumor
s. bowel malrotation
s. bowel meal
s. bowel metastasis
s. bowel motility
s. bowel mucosal pattern
s. bowel multiple ulcer
s. bowel obstruction (SBO)
s. bowel peristalsis
s. bowel pseudodiverticula
s. bowel pseudotumor
s. bowel separation
s. bowel series
s. bowel shunt
s. bowel transit time
s. bowel volvulus
s. bowel wall thickening
s. cardiac vein
s. colonic J-pouch
s., deep, recent infarct (SDRI)
s. feminine aorta
s. field-of-view MR imaging
s. gallbladder
s. for gestational age fetus
s. gut
s. internal auditory canal
s. intestine
s. intestine carcinoma
s. intestine mesentery
s. left colon syndrome

NOTES

S

small *(continued)*
    s. LITT applicator
    s. lymphocytic T-cell lymphoma
    s. part of fetus
    s. pelvis
    s. round cell carcinoma
    s. saphenous vein
    s. spleen
    s. vertebral body
    s. water-hammer pulse
small-angle multiple scattering
small-bore scanner
small-cell
    s.-c. cribriform carcinoma
    s.-c. lung carcinoma (SCLC)
    s.-c. osteosarcoma
    s.-c. undifferentiated carcinoma
small-droplet fatty liver
small-lunged emphysema
small-step distraction
small-vessel stroke
small-volume tissue ablation
small-voxel acquisition
SMAP
    systemic mean arterial pressure
SmartBeam IMRT
SmartNeedle
SMART Nitinol self-expandable stent
SmartPrep
    S. imaging agent
    S. scanner
SmartScore CT imaging
SmartSPOT high-resolution digital imaging system
SMAS
    superior mesenteric artery syndrome
smear fragment
Smelloff-Cutter valve
SMI
Smith
    S. dislocation
    S. fracture
    S. orthogonal hole test
    S. sesamoid position classification
Smith-Lemli-Opitz syndrome
Smith-Petersen nail
Smith-Robinson bone graft
Smitt sleeve
SMM
    scintimammography
SMN
    second malignant neoplasm
smoked glass image
smoke-like echo
smoker's
    s. bronchiolitis
    s. lung

smooth
    s. border
    s. brain
    s. contour
    s. esophageal narrowing
    s. excimer laser coronary angioplasty (SELCA)
    s. hyperplasia
    s. muscle
    s. muscle hypertrophy
    s. muscle tumor
    s. tapered appearance
    s. thickened mucosal fold
smooth-bordered
smoothed curve fit
smoothing
    gaussian s.
    spatial s.
    temporal s.
smooth-walled bladder
SMR
    scatter-maximum ratio
smudged papilla
SMV
    superior mesenteric vein
S/N *(var. of* SNR*)*
Sn
    stannum
    tin
^{113}**Sn**
    tin-113
snake
    s. graft
    s. head appearance
snapping
    s. fascia lata
    s. hip
    s. hip syndrome
    s. triceps syndrome
snapshot
    contrast-enhanced dynamic s.
    dynamic s.
    s. fashion
snare
    Amplatz Goose Neck s.
sneaker osteomyelitis
Sneddon syndrome
Sneppen fracture of talus
sniff test
Sniper Elite hydrophilic guidewire
snowboarder fracture
snowflake-like calcification
snowflake pattern
snowman
    s. abnormality
    s. appearance of heart

s. configuration
s. deformity
snowplow
s. effect
s. occlusion
snowstorm
s. breast pattern
s. shadow
SNR, S/N
signal-to-noise ratio
SNRT
sinus node recovery time
snuffbox
anatomic s.
Snyder classification
soap
calcium bile s.
soap-bubble
s.-b. appearance
s.-b. nephrogram
s.-b. radiolucency
SOC
sum of cylinder
socket-stump interface
SOCRATES telementoring system
sodium
acetrizoate s.
s. and/or methylglucamine diatrizoate contrast agent
s. bicarbonate imaging agent
s. chloride imaging agent
s. diatrizoate imaging agent
^{18}F s. fluoride imaging agent
fluorescein s.
s. imaging
s. iodide (NaI)
s. iodide detector
s. iodide iodine-131
s. iodide ring
s. iodide ring imaging agent
iodohippurate s.
s. iodohippurate imaging agent
iothalamate s.
s. iothalamate imaging agent
ioxaglate s.
ipodate s.
s. ipodate imaging agent
liothyronine s.
s. meglumine ioxaglate contrast agent
s. metrizoate acid contrast agent
s. pertechnetate

s. pertechnetate imaging agent
s. phosphate (P-32)
s. phosphate ^{32}P
radioactive s.
s. reabsorption
s. sodium imaging agent
technetium-99m pertechnetate s.
tetrabromophenolphthalein s.
s. tetradecyl sulfate
tetraiodophenolphthalein s.
total exchangeable s. (TENa)
tyropanoate s.
s. tyropanoate imaging agent
warfarin s.
ytterbium pentetate s.
sodium-23 (^{23}Na)
sodium-24 (^{24}Na)
sodium-2-mercaptoethane sulfonate
sodium-potassium ATPase dependent exchange mechanism
Soemmerring
S. ligament
S. muscle
soft
s. disk herniation
s. food dysphagia
s. infiltrate
s. palate carcinoma
s. papilloma
s. photon
s. pigment stone
s. ray
S.-Tip catheter
s. tissue
s. tissue ablation
s. tissue abnormality
s. tissue abscess
s. tissue attenuation value
s. tissue canal encroachment
s. tissue chondroma
s. tissue contracture
s. tissue contrast
s. tissue contusion
s. tissue convexity
s. tissue defect
s. tissue density
s. tissue density mass
s. tissue density structure
s. tissue derangement
s. tissue distraction
s. tissue entrapment
s. tissue envelope

S

NOTES

855

soft *(continued)*
- s. tissue fibroma
- s. tissue ganglion
- s. tissue gas
- s. tissue hemangioma
- s. tissue injury
- s. tissue interposition
- s. tissue kernel
- s. tissue lesion classification
- s. tissue lipoma
- s. tissue lipomatosis
- s. tissue necrosis
- s. tissue neoplasm
- s. tissue ossification
- s. tissue osteochondroma
- s. tissue osteoma
- s. tissue pathoanatomy in melorheostosis
- s. tissue radiograph
- s. tissue reaction
- s. tissue sarcoma
- s. tissue shadow
- s. tissue stranding
- s. tissue stroma
- s. tissue swelling
- s. tissue uptake bone scintigraphy
- s. tissue window
- s. tissue window setting
- S. Torque uterine catheter

softball sliding injury
soft-copy computed radiography
softening
- s. of brain
- s. of cartilage

Softouch catheter
SoftScan laser mammography system
Soft-Vu angiographic catheter
software
- BrainVoyager interactive s.
- CT Perfusion 2 s.
- DecThreads s.
- FuncTool s.
- GammaPlan s.
- GE Viewer s.
- HeartView cardiac reconstruction s.
- image-processing s.
- IP-plus image processing s.
- Kodak s.
- linear combination model s.
- LX 8.3 s.
- magnetic resonance user interface s.
- modified vessel image processor s.
- MRUI s.
- multigated spectral Doppler analysis s.
- multiplanar gradient-echo s.

- NeuroEcho s.
- Neuro Lobe s.
- Neuro SPGR s.
- P-LINK s.
- Plug n View 3D medical imaging s.
- SPARC s.
- SPOT mobile 3D ultrasound system and s.
- Starlink s.
- StereoPlan stereotactic planning software
- Three-Dimensional Perfusion/Motion Map s.
- VERT s.
- ViewMax s.
- Voxel-Man s.
- VoxelView s.

software-controlled internal hardware filter
SOG
- supraorbital groove

sojourn time
solar
- s. plexus
- s. radiation

solarization
soldier's
- s. heart
- s. patches of pericardium
- s. spot

soleal
- s. line
- s. vein

sole cluster of microcalcification
solenoid surface coil
soleus
- s. muscle
- s. syndrome

solid
- s. bolus challenge
- s. bone
- s. bony union
- s. circumscribed breast carcinoma
- s. component
- s. consolidation
- s. and cystic pancreatic tumor
- s. DCIS
- s. echo
- s. edema
- s. edema of lung
- s. food dysphagia
- s. lesion spleen
- s. lesion thymus
- s. mass
- s. matrix
- s. organ transplant (SOT)

s. ovarian teratoma
s. ovarian tumor
s. and papillary pancreatic
carcinoma
s. pattern
s. periosteal reaction
s. pilocytic astrocytoma
s. primary tumor
s. splenic lesion
s. thymic lesion
s. viscus
s. viscus injury
solidifying agent
solid-phase extraction tube
solid-pseudopapillary tumor
solid-rod ureteroscope
solid-state
s.-s. manometry catheter
s.-s. nuclear track detector
solitary
s. adenoma
s. bone cyst
s. bone myeloma
s. bone plasmacytoma (SBP)
s. cold lesion
s. collapsed vertebra
s. dilated duct
s. fibrous tumor of the pleura
(SFTP)
s. gallstone
s. left IVC
s. lymph node
s. mass
s. metastatic lung nodule
s. osteosclerosis
s. osteosclerotic lesion
s. plasmacytoma
s. pleura tumor
s. pulmonary necrobiotic nodule
s. pulmonary nodule (SPN)
s. rectal ulcer
s. rectal ulcer syndrome
s. relapse
s. rib hot spot
s. rib lesion
s. small bowel filling defect
s. sternal lesion
s. sternal metastasis
solitus
abdominal situs s.
atrial situs s.
cardiac situs s.

situs atrialis s.
visceral situs s.
Solomon-Bloembergen
S.-B. equation
S.-B. theory of dipole-dipole
relaxation rate
Solomon syndrome
solubilize
solution
aqueous s.
Blancophor FFG, SV s.
Carnoy s.
Hartmann s.
hundredth-normal s.
hyperosmotic s.
hypertonic s.
isosmotic water s.
lidocaine-adrenaline s.
MACRO-P s.
Melrose s.
molal s.
Phosphotope oral s.
radioelement s.
saline s.
saponated cresol s.
saturated potassium iodide s.
(SSKI)
**Solutrast 200, 250, 300, 370 contrast
medium**
solvent
s. suppression
s. water TI frequency dependence
SOM
supraorbital margin
somatic muscle
Somatom
S. DR CT scanner
S. Plus-S CT scanner
S. Volume Zoom CT system
somatosensory cortex
somatostatin
s. imaging agent
s. receptor scintigraphy (SRS)
^{99m}Tc-labeled s.
somatostatinoma
Sommer sector
Sonablate 200 ultrasound system
sonar
sonarography
Sonata imager
Sonazoid contrast agent

NOTES

S

Sones
    S. cineangiography technique
    S. selective coronary arteriography
Song covered duodenal stent
sonic-accelerated fracture-healing system
  (SAFHS)
sonicated
    s. albumin microbubbles
    s. dextrose albumin imaging agent
    s. saline contrast medium
Sonicath Ultra imaging catheter
sonication
Sonicator portable ultrasound
sonic effect
SonicWAVE phacoemulsification system
Sonifer sonicating system
SONK
    spontaneous osteonecrosis of knee
Sonnenberg classification of erosive
  esophagitis
SONOACE 6000 II ultrasound system
sonoangiogram
SonoCT real-time compound imaging
Sonocut ultrasonic aspirator
sonodynamic therapy
sonofluoroscopy
sonogram
    dual transverse linear-array s.
    fatty meal s. (FMS)
    real-time s.
    transabdominal s.
sonographer
sonographic
    s. assessment
    s. detection
    s. diagnosis
    s. echo
    s. feature analysis
    s. guidance
    s. hip type
    s. measurement of subtalar joint
      instability
    s. Murphy sign
    s. parameter
    S. Planning of Oncology Treatment
      (SPOT)
sonography
    abdominal s.
    Acuson computed s.
    Acuson transvaginal s.
    breast s.
    carotid s.
    color-coded duplex s.
    color-coded real-time s.
    color Doppler s. (CDS)
    color-flow Doppler s.
    color power transcranial Doppler s.

    compression s.
    contrast-enhanced transrectal s.
    Doppler s.
    duplex s. (DS)
    duplex-pulsed Doppler s.
    dynamic s.
    endoanal s.
    endoluminal s.
    endoscopic s.
    endovaginal s.
    fatty meal s.
    fetal s.
    follow-up duplex Doppler s.
    freehand interventional s.
    graded compression s.
    gray-scale s.
    hysterosalpingo-contrast s.
    intraaortic endovascular s.
    intraoperative s. (IOS)
    obstetric s.
    pelvic s.
    penile s.
    power Doppler s. (PDS)
    real-time s.
    TCD s.
    thoracic s.
    tissue harmonic s.
    transabdominal color Doppler s.
    transcranial color-coded s.
    transcranial color-coded Doppler s.
    transcranial color-coded duplex s.
      (TCCS)
    transcranial real-time color-flow
      Doppler s.
    transrectal s.
    transvaginal s. (TVS)
    triplex mode Doppler s.
    s. unit
    velocity-encoded color Doppler s.
    whole-breast s.
SonoHeart ELITE personal hand-carried
  ultrasound system
sonohysterography (SHG)
    saline infusion s. (SIS)
Sonolayer model SSA-270A ultrasound
Sonoline
    S. Elegra ultrasound system
Sonolith Praktis lithotripter
sonolucent
    s. area
    s. cystic lesion
    s. cystic mass
    s. doughnut
    s. halo
    s. layer
    s. skull
    s. zone

sonometer
> Omnisense 7000S bone s.
> Sahara clinical bone s.
> SoundScan 2000 bone s.
> SoundScan Compact bone s.
> UBIS 5000 ultrasound bone s.

SonoRx oral ultrasound contrast agent
Sonos
> S. 2000 ultrasound unit

SonoSite
> S. digital ultrasound
> S. pulsed wave Doppler
> S. 180 ultrasound system

Sonotron electronic therapeutic device
SonoVue
Sopha DSX1 camera
SOPHY
> S. camera

Sophy programmable valve
Sorbie calcaneal fracture classification
sorbitol 70% imaging agent
Sorbol heel
sorption
> s. kinetics
> s. potential

sorter
> FACSVantage cell s.
> fluorescence-activated cell s.
>   (FACScan)

Sos Pulse-Vu Bloodless Entry Needle
SOT
> solid organ transplant

Sotos syndrome
souffle
> funic s.
> placental s.
> systolic mammary s.

sound
> s. beam
> bowel s.
> heart s.
> palpable aortic ejection s.
> palpable pulmonic ejection s.
> pericardial knock s.
> s. shadow
> speed of s.
> s. transmission
> s. wave

SoundScan
> S. 2000 bone sonometer
> S. Compact bone sonometer

source
> americium radioactive s.
> s. of artifact scintigraphy
> cobalt radioactive s.
> ^{137}Cs point s.
> diagnostic x-ray camera and
>   imaging s.
> discrete bleeding s.
> dummy s.
> s. of emission
> external heat generating s.
> fiberoptic light s.
> flood s.
> gold radioactive s.
> heat-generating s.
> s. imaging
> interstitial heat-generating s.
> intracavitary radiation s.
> intrastitial radiation s.
> iodine radioactive s.
> radioactive s.
> radium radioactive s.
> remote-controlled implantation of
>   radioactive s.
> rod s.
> rotating Ge-68 rod s.
> signal s.
> yttrium radioactive s.

source-film distance (SFD)
source-skin distance (SSD)
source-surface distance (SSD)
source-to-image receptor distance (SID)
source-tray distance (STD)
SP6 camera
SPA
> single-photon absorptiometry

SPACE
> spatial and chemical-shift encoded
>   excitation

space (*See* spacing)
> abdominal s.
> acromioclavicular s.
> action s.
> alveolar dead s.
> anatomic dead s.
> antecubital s.
> anterior clear s.
> anterior pararenal s. (APS)
> arachnoid s.
> axillary s.
> Bogros s.
> Bowman s.

NOTES

space *(continued)*
    buccal s.
    capsular s.
    carotid s.
    cartilage joint s.
    cavitary s.
    cisternal s.
    coracoclavicular s.
    Crookes s.
    CY color s.
    dead s.
    s. deficit
    disk s.
    Disse s.
    dorsal subaponeurotic s.
    dorsal subcutaneous s.
    echo s.
    echo-free s.
    enlarged presacral s.
    enlargement of the
       subarachnoidal s.
    epicardial s.
    epidural s.
    episcleral s.
    epitympanic s.
    extraaxial s.
    extracellular s.
    extradural s.
    extrapleural s.
    fifth intercostal s.
    fluid s.
    foraminal s.
    fourth intercostal s.
    free pericardial s.
    gingival s.
    hip joint s.
    Holzknecht s.
    hyperintense marrow s.
    increased lateral joint s.
    infraglottic s.
    inframesocolic s.
    intercellular s.
    intercondylar joint s.
    intercostal s.
    interlobar s.
    intermetatarsal s.
    interosseous s.
    interpeduncular s.
    interpleural s.
    interstitial fluid s.
    intervertebral disk s.
    intrathecal s.
    intravascular s.
    joint s.
    lateral joint s.
    left intercostal s. (LICS)
    masticator s.

medial joint s.
midpalmar s.
orbital s.
paralaryngeal s.
parapharyngeal s.
pararenal s.
patellofemoral joint s.
pelvic s.
peribronchial alveolar s.
pericardial s.
peridental s.
perihepatic s.
perineal s.
perinephric s.
perirenal s.
perisinusoidal s.
peritoneal s.
perivascular s.
pleural s.
popliteal s.
portacaval s.
portal s.
posterior cervical s.
posterior septal s.
predental s.
preepiglottic s.
premasseteric s.
presacral s.
prevertebral s.
Prussak s.
pulp s.
Q s.
radiolucent joint s.
Reinke s.
retrocardiac s.
retrocrural s.
retrogastric s.
retromammary s.
retroorbital s.
retroparotid s.
retroperitoneal s.
retropharyngeal s.
retrosphenoidal s.
retrosternal s.
retrovesical s.
s. of Retzius
s. of Retzius abscess
sac-like s.
scapholunate s.
sinusoidal vascular s.
spatial frequency s.
subacromial s.
subarachnoid s.
subdural s.
subhepatic s.
subperitoneal s.
subphrenic s.

subpulmonic pleural s.
subumbilical s.
supralevator s.
supratentorial s.
Talairach stereotaxic s.
thenar s.
tissue s.
ventricular s.
Virchow-Robin perivascular s.
visceral s.
widened joint s.

space-occupying
s.-o. intracranial lesion
s.-o. mass
s.-o. process

spacing
gray-level s.
interecho s.
multiple-beam interface s.
parallel-line equal s. (PLES)

spade
s. field
s. finger

spade-like
s.-l. appearance
s.-l. hand

spade-shaped valvotome
Spalding sign
spall
spallation product
SPAMM
SPAMM technique

span
levator s.
liver s.
ventricular s.

SPARC software
sparing
arytenoid s.
fatty s.

spark
s. chamber
s. gap generator

sparkling appearance of myocardium
SPARS
spatially resolved spectroscopy

sparsity of bone formation
spasm
arterial s.
bowel s.
bronchial smooth muscle s.
catheter-induced coronary artery s.

colonic s.
coronary artery s. (CAS)
diffuse arteriolar s.
diffuse esophageal s. (DES)
esophageal s.
hemifacial s.
inspiratory s.
intermittent diffuse esophageal s.
muscle s.
postbypass s.
respiratory s.
vascular s.
venous s.

spasmodic stricture
spastic
s. bowel syndrome
s. colon
s. electron paramagnetic resonance
imaging
s. equinovarus deformity
s. esophagus
s. heart
s. hindfoot valgus deformity
s. ileus
s. mapping
s. pseudosclerosis
s. registration

spastica
dysphagia s.

spatial
s. average-pulse average (SAPA)
s. average-pulse average intensity
s. average-temporal average (SATA)
s. average-temporal average
intensity
s. and chemical-shift encoded
excitation (SPACE)
s. distribution
s. dose distribution
s. encoding
s. filter
s. frequency
s. frequency domain
s. frequency error
s. frequency space
s. localization procedure
s. mapping
s. misregistration artifact
s. modulation of magnetization
s. modulation of magnetization
image
s. normalization

NOTES

S

spatial *(continued)*
- s. offset image artifact
- s. orientation
- s. origin
- s. peak-temporal average (SPTA)
- s. peak-temporal average intensity
- s. position
- s. presaturation
- s. presaturation band
- s. reconstruction
- s. registration
- s. resolution
- s. resolution scintigram
- s. selectivity
- s. smoothing
- s. vectorcardiography

spatially
- s. localized spectroscopy
- s. normalized PET and SPECT scan
- s. resolved spectroscopy (SPARS)
- s. selective inversion pulse

spatial-spectral prepulses for fat saturation

SPDT
- single-pole double-throw

Spearman
- S. correlation coefficient
- S. rank
- S. rank test

spear tackler's spine

special bolus

specific
- s. absorption rate (SAR)
- s. activity
- s. modulation
- s. radiation

specified
- not otherwise s. (NOS)

specimen radiography

specious finding

speck finger

speckled pattern

speckling
- heterogeneous color s.

SPECT
- single-photon emission-computed tomography
- acetazolamide-enhanced SPECT
- brain perfusion SPECT
- SPECT brain perfusion scintigraphy
- SPECT center of rotation
- cerebral SPECT
- dual-head SPECT
- dual-isotope SPECT
- dynamic volumetric SPECT
- electrocardiogram-gated SPECT

- FDG SPECT
- ^{67}Ga SPECT
- GE SPECT
- ictal ^{99m}Tc HMPAO brain SPECT
- SPECT imaging
- interictal brain SPECT
- methoxyisobutyl isonitrile SPECT
- SPECT perfusion pattern
- pharmacologic stress dual-isotope myocardial perfusion SPECT
- SPECT quality control
- quantitative gated SPECT (QGS)
- ^{99m}Tc-HMPAO SPECT
- ^{99m}Tc red blood cell SPECT
- technetium-99m somatostatin analog SPECT
- SPECT thallium scintigraphy
- Trionix SPECT
- SPECT uniformity

spectamine
- s. brain imaging
- ^{123}I brain imaging s.

spectography
- nuclear magnetic resonance s.

spectra *(pl. of* spectrum)

spectral
- s. analysis
- s. broadening
- s. diffusion
- s. Doppler
- s. Doppler imaging
- s. editing
- s. emission
- s. line
- s. noise distribution
- s. pattern
- s. saturation
- s. sensitivity
- s. ultrasound
- s. waveform
- s. width
- s. window

spectral-spatial
- s.-s. fat suppression
- s.-s. image

Spectranetics
- S. excimer laser
- S. laser sheath (SLS)

spectrin

Spectris
- S. MR-compatible injector
- S. power injector

SPECTRO-20000 2.OT

spectrofluorometry

spectrometer
- beta-ray s.
- Bragg s.

Bruker AMX 300 NMR s.
Compton suppression s.
EDXRF s.
gamma ray s.
GE GN300 7.05-T/89-mm bore
  multinuclear s.
GE NMR s.
IBM NMR s.
liquid scintillation s.
mass s.
Mossbauer s.
Nicolet NMR s.
NMR s.
nuclear magnetic resonance s.
Rapid-Scan s.
scintillation s.
SISCO s.
Varian Associates 11.7-T, 51-mm
  bore s.
Varian NMR s.
VT multinuclear s.
x-ray s.

spectrometry
accelerator mass s. (AMS)
Fourier transform NMR s.
inductively coupled plasma atomic
  emission s. (ICP-AES)
liquid scintillation s.
PROBE-SV s.
pulsed L-band ESR s.
scintillation s.

spectrophotofluorometer
spectrophotometer
absorption s.
F-1200, 2000, 4500 fluorescence s.
U-1100 UV-Vis s.

spectrophotometric
s. calculation
s. quantity

spectrophotometry
atomic absorption s.
ultraviolet s.

spectroscope
direct vision s.

spectroscopic voxel
spectroscopy
atomic absorption s.
brain proton magnetic resonance s.
carbon-13 s.
circular dichroism s.
COSY H-1 MR s.
CSI s.

depth-resolved surface s. (DRESS)
diffusion s.
2D J-resolved 1H MR s.
double-spin echo proton s.
3D proton MR s.
elastic scattering s.
electrospray ionization mass s.
flame emission s. (FES)
fluorescence s.
fluorine-19 s.
Fourier transform infrared s.
Fourier transform Raman s.
glutamate s.
H-1 MR s.
hydrogen-1, -2, -3 MR s.
image-selected in vivo s.
INVOS 2100 optical s.
ISIS s.
laser correlational s. (LCS)
localized H1 s.
localized proton magnetic
  resonance s.
long TE MR s.
magnetic resonance s. (MRS)
MR proton s.
near infrared s. (NIRS)
nonresonance Raman s.
nuclear magnetic resonance s.
oxygen-17 NMR s.
^{31}P s.
phosphorus magnetic resonance s.
  (P-MRS)
phosphorus-31 magnetic
  resonance s.
photon correlation s.
plasma emission s.
proton nuclear magnetic
  resonance s.
Raman s.
remote endoscopic digital s.
  (REDS)
^{77}Se MRI s.
serial diffusion-weighted MR
  imaging and proton MR s.
short-echo-time proton s.
short TE proton MR s.
single voxel proton MR s. (1H-
  MRS)
single voxel stimulated echo
  acquisition mode MR s.
spatially localized s.
spatially resolved s. (SPARS)

NOTES

spectroscopy *(continued)*
    surface coil rotating-frame s.
    in vivo optical s. (INVOS)
    in vivo proton MR s.
spectrum, pl. **spectra, spectrums**
    absorption x-ray s.
    artery s.
    chromatic s.
    color s.
    continuous x-ray s.
    Dandy-Walker s.
    S. DG-P pediatric cradle
    Doppler frequency s.
    electromagnetic s.
    energy s.
    excitation s.
    frequency s.
    gamma ray s.
    infinitesimal Z s.
    infrared s.
    invisible s.
    localized single-voxel proton s.
    midsystolic notching of velocity s.
    nuclear magnetic resonance s.
    proton nuclear magnetic
      resonance s.
    pulmonary sequestration s.
    short echo point resolved
      spectroscopic sequence s.
    single umbilical artery s.
    single voxel in vivo proton s.
    thermal s.
    ultraviolet s.
    VACTERLS s.
    velocity s.
    water-suppressed proton s.
    Wiener s.
    x-ray s.
specular
    s. echo
    s. reflector
speech area
speed
    film s.
    s. of sound
Spence
    axillary tail of S.
    tail of S.
Spengler fragment
Spens syndrome
spent phase
spermatic
    s. artery
    s. calculus
    s. cord
    s. cord torsion

    s. vein
    s. venography
spermatocele
spermatogonia
sperm granuloma
SPET
    single-photon emission tomography
SPGR
    spoiled GRASS
S-phase
    S-p. analysis
    S-p. fraction
    S-p. fractionation
sphenocephaly
sphenoethmoidal
    s. encephalocele
    s. recess
    s. suture
sphenofrontal suture
sphenoid
    s. angle
    s. bone
    s. bone fracture
    s. dysplasia
    s. fontanelle
    s. ridge
    s. ridge meningioma
    s. ridge tumor
    s. sinus
    s. sinus metastasis
    s. wing
    s. wing meningioma
sphenoidal
    s. encephalocele
    s. fossa
    s. sinusitis
    s. turbinated bone
sphenoidale
    planum s.
    pneumatosis s.
    rostrum s.
sphenomalar suture
sphenomandibularis muscle
sphenomandibular ligament
sphenomaxillary
    s. encephalocele
    s. suture
sphenooccipital
    s. chordoma
    s. suture
    s. synchondrosis
sphenoorbital
    s. encephalocele
    s. meningioma
    s. suture
sphenopalatine
    s. canal

s. foramen
s. ganglion
s. neuralgia
sphenoparietal
s. sinus
s. sulcus
s. suture
sphenopetrosal suture
sphenopharyngeal
s. canal
s. encephalocele
s. meningoencephalocele
sphenosquamous suture
sphenotemporal suture
sphenovomerine suture
sphenozygomatic suture
sphere
s. organelle
resin s.
spherical
s. disk
s. kernel
s. lesion
s. map
s. mass
s. neoplasm
s. shape
s. structure
spheroid
s. shape
tumor s.
spherule
sphincter
antral s.
s. atony
basal s.
bicanalicular s.
s. of bile duct
Boyden s.
canalicular s.
cecal s.
choledochal s.
colic s.
cricopharyngeal s.
duodenal s.
duodenojejunal s.
s. dysfunction
external anal s.
external urethral s.
extrinsic s.
first duodenal s.
functional s.

hypertensive lower esophageal s.
s. incompetence
inferior esophageal s. (IES)
lower esophageal s. (LES)
s. of Oddi
s. of Oddi manometry
pancreatic duct s.
pancreaticobiliary s.
pharyngoesophageal s.
physiologic s.
prepyloric s.
s. preservation
pyloric s.
relaxed lower esophageal s.
resting lower esophageal s.
tonically contracted s.
upper esophageal s. (UES)
sphincteric mechanism
sphingomyelin lipidosis
sphygmography
SPI
selective population inversion
spicular
s. density
s. protrusion
spiculated
s. border
s. carcinoma
s. distortion
s. margin
s. mass
s. scirrhous lesion
spiculation
radiographic s.
spicule
bony s.
SPIDER
steady-state projection imaging with
dynamic echo-train readout
structured platform-independent data
entry and reporting
spider
s. angioma
s. finger
s. pelvis
stainless steel s.
s. x-ray view
spidering skeleton
spider-like
s.-l. calix
s.-l. pelvocaliceal system

S

NOTES

spiderweb
    s. appearance
    s. circulation
spigelian
    s. fascia
    s. hernia
    s. lobe
spike
    s. averaging
    s. loading
    s. staple
    sterile vent s.
spike-related functional MR imaging
spiking
    interictal s.
spiky skeleton
spill
    ileal s.
spin
    s. coupling
    s. density
    s. density weighted
    s. dephasing
    s. diffusion
    s. echo
    electron s.
    s. exchange
    s. flip
    flowing s.
    high s.
    incoherent s.
    s. lock gradient-echo (SL-GRE)
    nuclear s.
    s. quantum number
    stationary s.
    s. tagging
    transverse relaxation of proton s.
    uncoupled s.
    unsaturated s.
    s. vector
spina, pl. **spinae**
    s. bifida
    s. bifida aperta
    s. bifida occulta (SBO)
    erector spinae
    s. ventosa
spinal
    s. accessory lymph node
    s. accessory nerve
    s. angiogram
    s. angulation
    s. anomaly
    s. arteriography
    s. artery
    s. axis
    s. axis tumor
    s. capillary hemangioblastoma

    s. chordoma
    s. column stabilization
    s. concussion
    s. cord
    s. cord angiography
    s. cord atrophy
    s. cord caliber
    s. cord canal
    s. cord cleft
    s. cord compression
    s. cord decompression
    s. cord depression
    s. cord diameter
    s. cord ependymoma
    s. cord glioma
    s. cord hemisection
    s. cord infarct
    s. cord injury (SCI)
    s. cord injury without radiographic abnormality (SCIWORA)
    s. cord laceration
    s. cord lesion
    s. cord malformation (SCM)
    s. cord metastasis
    s. cord parenchyma
    s. cord sarcoidosis
    s. cord stroke
    s. cord syrinx
    s. cord transsection
    s. cord tumor
    s. degeneration
    s. dermoid
    s. diastematomyelia
    s. dorsal horn
    s. dural arteriovenous fistula
    s. dural AVF
    s. empyema
    s. endplate change
    s. epidural abscess (SEA)
    s. epidural hemorrhage (SEH)
    s. epidural lymphoma
    s. fixation
    s. fixation device
    s. fluid
    s. fracture
    s. fusion
    s. ganglion
    s. growth
    s. hemiplegia
    s. hydatid cyst
    s. infection
    s. inflammation
    s. instability
    s. integrity
    s. lordosis
    s. medulla
    s. meningioma

s. muscular atrophy (SMA)
s. needle
s. nerve plexus
s. nerve root avulsion
s. osteochondrosis
s. osteomyelitis
s. osteophyte
s. pedicle
s. plasma cell myeloma
s. root
s. sac
s. sign
s. stenosis
s. subarachnoid hemorrhage
s. subdural hemorrhage (SSH)
s. syndesmophyte
s. teratoma
s. tuberculosis
s. vascular malformation
ventral derotating s. (VDS)
s. videofluoroscopy
spindle
aortic s.
s. colonic groove
His s.
muscle s.
ureteral s.
spindle-shaped
s.-s. aneurysm
s.-s. muscle
s.-s. shadow
spindling
spine
alar s.
s. angioreticuloma
angulation of s.
anterior column of s.
anterior-inferior iliac s.
anterior maxillary s.
anterior-superior iliac s. (ASIS)
anteroposterior iliac s.
arachnoid loculation of the s.
bamboo s.
basilar s.
biomechanically normal s.
caroticojugular s.
cervical fusion of s.
Charcot s.
cleft s.
coccygeal s.
dendritic s.
dens view of cervical s.

dorsal s.
dysraphic s.
epidermoid s.
extension injury of s.
fetal s.
functional units of s.
s. hyperflexion
iliac s.
intermaxillary s.
ischial s.
kinetic cervical s.
kissing s.
s. lipoma
lumbar s.
lumbarized s.
lumbosacral s. (LS)
maxillary s.
mental s.
microcystic lumbar s.
midthoracic s.
s. morphology
nasal s.
s. ossification
poker s.
posterior column of s.
posterior inferior s.
posterior inferior iliac s.
railway s.
rotatory load on s.
rugger jersey s.
sacral s.
scoliotic s.
s. sign
spear tackler's s.
static cervical s.
thin-plate s.
thoracic s.
thoracolumbar s.
tibial s.
trochanteric s.
vertebral s.
wedge fracture of s.
spin-echo (SE)
axial single shot fast s.-e.
s.-e. cardiac imaging
dual-echo turbo s.-e.
fast s.-e. (FSE)
half-Fourier acquisition single-shot
turbo s.-e. (HASTE)
s.-e. imaging sequence
inversion recovery s.-e. (IRSE)
s.-e. magnetic resonance imaging

NOTES

spin-echo *(continued)*
    s.-e. pilot image
    s.-e. pulse sequence
    radiofrequency s.-e.
    s.-e. scan
    s.-e. technique
    s.-e. train
    turbo s.-e. (TSE)
    T1-weighted conventional s.-e.
    s.-e. T1-weighted image
    s.-e. T1-weighted transaxial MR
      imaging
    s.-e. using repeated gradient echoes
spin-label
    s.-l. method
    s.-l. technique
spin-lattice
    s.-l. relaxation
    s.-l. relaxation time
spin-lock
    s.-l. imaging technique
    s.-l. and magnetization transfer
      imaging
    s.-l. prepulse
spin-lock-induced T1-rho weighted
  image
spin-locking
    off-resonance s.-l.
spinning
    variable-angle s. (VAS)
spinning-top
    s.-t. test
    s.-t. urethra
spinocerebellar
    s. degeneration
    s. tract
spinoglenoid
    s. ligament
    s. notch
spinogram
spinographic
    s. angle
    s. line
spinography
    digitized s.
spinolaminar line (SLL)
spinoreticular tract
spinosum
    foramen s.
spinothalamic tract
spinous
    s. foramen
    s. plane
    s. process
    s. process avulsion
    s. process fracture
    s. tarsus ligament

spin-phase
    s.-p. graph
    s.-p. phenomenon
spin-spin
    s.-s. coupling
    s.-s. relaxation
    s.-s. relaxation time
spintharicon
spinthariscope
spin-warp
    s.-w. imaging
    s.-w. method
    s.-w. pulse sequence
SPIO
    superparamagnetic iron oxide
SPIO-enhanced MR imaging
spiperone
SPIR
    selective partial inversion-recovery
spiral
    s. appearance
    s. arthrosis
    s. band of Gosset
    s. computed tomography
    s. computed tomography
      arteriography (SCTA)
    s. CT pitch
    s. CT pitch pit
    s. CT scan
    s. CT scanning
    s. CT, XCT scanner
    s. dissection
    s. echo-planar technique
    s. EPI (SEPI)
    s. flow pattern
    s. fold
    s. imaging method
    s. k-space coverage
    s. ligament
    s. multidetector CT
    s. oblique fracture
    s. scanning technique
    s. valve
    s. volumetric CT
    s. x-ray computed tomography
      (SVCT, SXCT)
spiral-pulse sequence
spirometer flow rate
spirometric
    s. acquisition
    s. gating
spirometrically
    s. controlled CT lung densitometry
spirometry
    full-volume loop s.
splanchnapophysis

splanchnic
    s. aneurysm
    s. AV fistula
    s. blood
    s. vascular imaging
    s. vasculature
    s. venous system
    s. vessel
splanchnography
splanchnoskeleton
SPLATT
    split anterior tibial tendon
splayed cranial suture
splayfoot deformity
splaying
    s. of frontal horn
    s. of pedicles
spleen
    aberrant s.
    absence of s.
    accessory s.
    s. angiosarcoma
    delayed rupture s.
    s. density
    s. diameter
    s. dimension
    ectopic s.
    epithelial s.
    floating s.
    hamartoma s.
    hyperdense s.
    increased density s.
    s. inflammation
    inflammatory s.
    s. laceration
    large s.
    s. lesion
    liver, kidneys, and s. (LKS)
    long axis of s.
    malpighian body of the s.
    microabscess of the s.
    multiple accessory s.
    nonvisualization of s.
    s. peliosis
    primary cyst of s.
    prolapse of s.
    ruptured s.
    s. sarcoidosis
    s. scan
    shattered s.
    siderotic nodule in the s.
    small s.

    solid lesion s.
    tail of the s.
    tip of s.
    s. ultrasonography imaging
    wandering s.
spleen-to-liver ratio
splenatrophy
splenauxe
splenculus
splenectasis
splenectopia
splenelcosis
spleneolus
splenia (*pl. of* splenium)
splenial branch of posterior cerebral artery
splenic
    s. abscess
    s. amyloidosis
    s. angle
    s. arteriography
    s. artery (SA)
    s. artery aneurysm
    s. artery pseudoaneurysm
    s. AV fistula
    s. B-cell lymphoma
    s. bleeding
    s. bump
    s. calcification
    s. capsule
    s. cleft
    s. congestion
    s. epidermoid cyst
    s. flexure
    s. flexure carcinoma
    s. hamartoma
    s. hemangioma
    s. hilum
    s. hyperplasia
    s. infarct
    s. lesion
    s. lobule
    s. lymph node
    s. metastasis
    s. microabscess
    s. notch
    s. perfusion measurement by dynamic CT scan
    s. portal venography
    s. portography
    s. pseudocyst
    s. reagent

NOTES

splenic *(continued)*
s. rupture
s. scintigraphy
s. torsion
s. trauma
s. vein
s. vein thrombosis
s. vessel
spleniculus, pl. **spleniculi**
splenium, pl. **splenia**
s. of corpus callosum
splenization
splenobronchial fistula
splenocaval
splenocolic ligament
splenogastric omentum
splenogonadal fusion
splenography
splenoma
splenomalacia
splenomedullary
splenomegaly
congenital s.
congestive s.
Egyptian s.
fibrocongestive s.
Gaucher s.
hemolytic s.
infectious s.
myelophthisic s.
Opitz thrombophlebitic s.
persistent s.
postcardiotomy lymphocytic s.
siderotic s.
splenomyelomalacia
splenoncus
splenonephric
splenopancreatic
splenophrenic
splenoportal
s. junction
s. venography
splenoportogram
splenoportography
direct s.
s. imaging
percutaneous s.
splenorenal
s. anastomosis
s. angle
s. arterial bypass graft
s. ligament
s. recess
s. shunt

splenosis
abdominal s.
thoracic s.
splenunculus, pl. **splenunculi**
spline curve
splint
bird-cage s.
semidynamic s.
thigh s.
splintered
s. bone
s. fracture
splinting
serial s.
Spli-Prest
S.-P. latex
S.-P. negative control
S.-P. plate
S.-P. positive control
split
s. anterior tibial tendon (SPLATT)
s. atlas
s. brain
s. compression fracture
s. cranium
s. foot deformity
s. image artifact
s. notochord syndrome
s. peroneus brevis
s. renal function decrease
s. spinal cord
s. spinal cord malformation
(SSCM)
split-brain
s.-b. imaging
s.-b. study
split-cord syndrome
split-course
s.-c. accelerated radiotherapy
s.-c. hyperfractionated radiation
therapy
s.-c. technique
split-function scintigraphy
split-heel fracture
split-screen recording
splitter
beam s.
splitting
s. fracture
plaque s.
sternal s.
zero-field s.
SPN
solitary pulmonary nodule
SPOCS
Surgical Planning and Orientation
Computer System

spoiled
  s. gradient echo (SGE)
  s. gradient echo pulse sequence
  s. gradient-recalled
  s. GRASS (SPGR)
spoiler
  s. gradient pattern
  lucite beam s.
spoiling
  radiofrequency s.
  RF s.
  surface s.
spoke bone
spoked wheel pattern
spondylarthritis
spondylitic
  s. change
  s. deformity
spondylitis
  ankylosing s.
  cryptococcal s.
  s. deformans
  diskovertebral s.
  juvenile ankylosing s.
  lung ankylosis s.
  rheumatoid s.
  staphylococcal diskovertebral s.
  tuberculous s.
spondyloarthritis, pl. **spondyloarthritides**
spondyloarthropathy
  destructive s.
  juvenile s.
spondylocostal dysplasia
spondylodiskitis drainage
spondyloepiphyseal dysplasia
spondylolisthesis
  degenerative s.
  isthmic s.
  sagittal roll s.
  slip-angle s.
  spondylolytic s.
  traumatic s.
spondylolisthetic pelvis
spondylolysis
  traumatic s.
spondylolytic spondylolisthesis
spondylomalacia
spondylosis
  cervical spine s.
  s. deformans
  degenerative s.

  diffuse s.
  Nurick classification of s.
spondylosyndesis
spondylothoracic dysplasia
spondylotic myelopathy
sponge
  blood-filled bone s.
  gelatin s.
  Ivalon s.
  s. kidney
  medullary s.
  Ray-Tec x-ray detectable
   surgical s.
  surgical s.
  Vistec x-ray detectable s.
spongiform
  s. change
  s. degeneration
  s. leukoencephalopathy
spongioblastoma
spongiocytoma
spongiosa
  s. of mitral valve
  s. replacement
spongiosis
spongiosum
  corpus s.
  osteoma s.
spongy
  s. appearance
  s. bone
  s. osteoma
  s. white matter degeneration
spontaneous
  s. carotid dissection
  s. closure of defect
  s. conversion
  s. coronary artery dissection
   (SCAD)
  s. detorsion
  s. disintegration
  s. drainage
  s. echo contrast
  s. fetal movement
  s. fracture
  s. hematoma
  s. hemodialysis catheter fracture
   and embolization
  s. infantile ductal aneurysm
  s. intracranial hypotension
  s. involution
  s. lesion

S

NOTES

spontaneous *(continued)*
    s. osteonecrosis
    s. osteonecrosis of knee (SONK)
    s. perforation
    s. perforation of common bile duct
    s. pneumomediastinum
    s. radiation
    s. regression
    s. renal hemorrhage
    s. tension pneumothorax
    s. transient vasoconstriction
    s. urinary extravasation
spoon-like
    s.-l. protrusion
    s.-l. protrusion of leaflet
spoon-shaped nail
SPOP
    sequential paired opposed plaque
    SPOP technique
sporadic
    s. Burkitt lymphoma
    s. colorectal carcinoma
    s. tumor
SPOT
    Sonographic Planning of Oncology
    Treatment
spot
    blooming focal s.
    capitate soft s.
    Carleton s.
    cold s.
    s. compression
    s. compression image
    s. compression magnification
      mammography
    s. compression paddle
    s. compression view
    cotton-wool s.
    EIS s.
    s. film
    s. film device
    s. film fluorography
    s. film radiography
    flying focal s.
    focal s. (FS)
    focal liver hot s.
    hematocystic s. (HCS)
    hot-s.
    hyperechoic splenic s.
    s. magnification
    pelvic s.
    pituitary bright s.
    s. radiograph
    Roth s.
    scan s.
    s. scanning
    s. scanography

    soldier's s.
    solitary rib hot s.
    thermal hot s.
    tree-shaped s.
spot-film
spot-magnification image
SPOT mobile 3D ultrasound system
    and software
spotted nephrogram
SPPS
    single-photon planar scintigraphy
SPR
    scanned projection radiography
    superior peroneal retinaculum
sprain
    acute s.
    chronic s.
    eversion s.
    s. fracture
    inversion s.
    sacroiliac s.
    syndesmosis s.
spray
    pulse fashion pulse s.
    resorcinol s.
spread
    s. Bragg peak
    distant s.
    hematogenous s.
    intraocular s.
    lymphatic tumor s.
    pattern of s.
    perineural tumor s.
    regional s.
    subependymal s.
    s. suture
    transfascial s.
    s. of tumor
Sprengel deformity
spring
    s. ligament
    s. onion ureter
spring-driven system
Springer fracture
spring-loaded biopsy needle
sprinter's fracture
SPRINT fixed-detector research system
sprodiamide imaging agent
SPS
    sestamibi parathyroid scintigraphy
    superior petrous sinus
SPT
    selective population transfer
SPTA
    spatial peak-temporal average
SPTL-1b vascular lesion laser

spur

 acromial s.
 anterior s.
 bone s.
 bronchial s.
 calcaneal s.
 calcific s.
 degenerative s.
 drum s.
 s. formation
 heel s.
 impingement s.
 inferior s.
 marginal s.
 medial traction s.
 osteoarthritic s.
 plantar calcaneal s.
 posterior s.
 prominent s.
 retrocalcaneal s.
 traction s.
 uncovertebral s.

spuriae

 costae s.
 vertebra s.

spurious

 s. aneurysm
 s. ankylosis
 s. finding
 s. pregnancy

Spurling sign

spurring

 bony s.
 degenerative s.
 hypertrophic marginal s.
 marginal s.
 osteophytic s.
 ulnar traction s.

SQFT

 subcutaneous quadriceps fat thickness

squamosal suture

squamosomastoid suture

squamosoparietal suture

squamososphenoid suture

squamous

 s. metaphysis
 s. metaplasia
 s. metaplasia white epithelium
 s. odontogenic tumor
 s. part of frontal bone
 s. part of occipital bone

 s. part of temporal bone
 s. suture

square

 s. brain shift
 least s. (LS)
 s. wave

squared

 s. patella
 s. vertebral body

squared-off

 s.-o. heart
 s.-o. thorax

squatting

 s. facet
 s. maneuver
 s. position

Squibb system

SQUID

 superconducting quantum interference
 device

SR

 saturation recovery
 structured reporting

Sr

 strontium
  Sr 87m

^{90}Sr

 strontium-90

^{89}Sr

 strontium-89
  ^{89}Sr bracelet

^{90}Sr-loaded eye applicator

SRO 2550 x-ray tube

SRS

 somatostatin receptor scintigraphy
 stereotactic radiosurgery

SS

 slice select gradient

SSBE

 short-segment Barrett esophagus

SSC

 single-stripe colitis

SSCM

 split spinal cord malformation

SSD

 segmental spinal dysgenesis
 source-skin distance
 source-surface distance
 surface shaded display
  SSD algorithm
  SSD imaging

NOTES

SSFP
    steady-state free precession
      SSFP magnetization
      SSFP process
      SSFP signal

SSFSE
    single-shot fast spin echo

SSH
    spinal subdural hemorrhage

S-shaped
    S-s. gallbladder
    S-s. pouch
    S-s. scoliosis

SSKI
    saturated potassium iodide solution

SSP
    slice sensitivity profile
    stereotactic surface projection

SSPE
    subacute sclerosing panencephalitis

SSQ
    sequential scalar quantization

SSR
    shaded surface rendering

SSS
    superior sagittal sinus

stability
    bony s.
    s. of fracture
    magnet s.

stabilization
    electronic s.
    s. plate
    spinal column s.

stabilizer
    dynamic s.
    static s.

stabilizing bullet

stable
    s. cavitation
    s. fracture
    s. free radical
    s. isotope
    s. reduction
    s. Xenon CT

stable-state tuberculosis

stacked
    s. ovoid lesion
    s. scan
    s. tomogram

stacked-coin appearance
stacked-foil technique
stacked-metaphor workstation
stacked-scan imaging
stack mode display
stack-of-coins mucosal fold
Stafne idiopathic bone cavity

stage
    resolution s.
    Risser s.
    s. 4S neuroblastoma

stage-matched
    s.-m. intervention
    s.-m. intervention on repeat
      mammography

staghorn
    s. calculus
    s. stone

staging
    distraction-flexion s. (DFS)
    Ficat s.
    invasive surgical s. (ISS)
    Kadish s.
    lymphoma s.
    malignant melanoma s.
    neuraxis s.
    neuroblastoma s.
    nodal s.
    preslip s.

stagnant-loop syndrome
stag wound
stain
    Bielschowsky s.
    hematoxylin and eosin s.
    mucicarmine s.

stained-glass appearance
staining
    immunocytochemical s.
    tumor s.

stainless
    s. steel coil
    s. steel mesh stent
    s. steel microsphere
    s. steel plate
    s. steel spider

staircase phenomenon
stairstep
    s. air-fluid level
    s. artifact
    s. fracture

stalk
    body s.
    fibrovascular s.
    infundibular s.
    pituitary s.
    polyp s.
    tumor s.
    yolk s.

standard
    ACR teleradiology s.
    s. atlas
    criterion s.
    s. deviation
    s. exchange wire

s. fixed core guidewire
international s. (IS)
s. LITT applicator
s. multiecho
reference s.
s. single echo
s. uptake value (SUV)
standard-dose enhanced conventional T1 weighted image
standardized uptake ratio (SUR)
standby rate
standing
s. dorsoplantar view
s. false profile view
s. lateral view
s. post void view
s. wave
s. weightbearing view
standoff
standstill
atrial s.
cardiac s.
ventricular s.
Stanford
S. aortic dissection classification
S. type B aortic dissection
S. type B dissection closure
S. and Wheatstone stereoscope
Stanley cervical ligament
stannosis
stannous
s. chloride
s. pyrophosphate
stannum (Sn)
stapedes (*pl. of* stapes)
stapedial
s. artery
s. nerve anatomy
s. otosclerosis
stapedius reflex
stapes, pl. **stapedes**
staphylococcal diskovertebral spondylitis
staphyloma
staple
metallic s.
orthopedic s.
skin s.
spike s.
stone s.
surgical s.
star
s. artifact

s. effect
s. pattern
s. test pattern
Starcam camera
star-cancellation test (SCT)
Starling curve
Starlink software
STARRT falloposcopy system
star-shaped vessel lumen
start test pattern
stasis, pl. **stases**
antral s.
bile s.
bladder s.
s. of blood flow
chronic venous s.
circulation s.
s. cirrhosis
complete vascular s.
s. edema
s. esophagitis
s. gallbladder
intrahepatic biliary s.
s. liver
s. ulcer
ureteral s.
urinary s.
vascular s.
venous s.
state
cardiac steady s.
chronic constrictive s.
contrast-enhanced Fourier-acquired steady s. (CE-FAST)
double-mode steady s.
s. equilibrium
fast adiabatic trajectory in steady s. (FATS)
Fourier-acquired steady s. (FAST)
gradient-recalled acquisition in the steady s. (GRASS)
ground s.
high-output s.
hypoperfused s.
inducibility basal s.
metastable s.
oxidation s.
post Diamox s.
radiofrequency spoiled Fourier-acquired steady s. (RF-FAST, RF-spoiled FAST)
Statham electromagnetic flowmetry

S

NOTES

static
- s. bone phase
- s. cervical spine
- s. coupling
- s. 3D FLASH imaging
- s. emission scan
- s. foot deformity
- s. image
- s. image display
- s. lung
- s. magnetic field
- s. rCBF tracer
- s. stabilizer
- s. view

station
- oscilloscope tuning s.

stationary
- s. anode
- s. field
- s. focus
- s. spin
- s. zero-order motion

statistical noise
Stauffer syndrome
Staunig position
STD
- source-tray distance

STE
- stimulated echo

steady-state
- s.-s. coherent
- s.-s. free precession (SSFP)
- s.-s. free precession imaging
- s.-s. free precession magnetization
- s.-s. free precession sequence
- s.-s. gradient-echo imaging
- s.-s. projection imaging with dynamic echo-train readout (SPIDER)

steal
- arterial s.
- s. effect
- false s.
- pelvic s.
- s. phenomenon
- subclavian s.
- s. syndrome
- transmural s.

STEAM
- stimulated echo acquisition mode STEAM sequence

steatosis
- hepatic s.
- liver s.

Stecher position
steel coil

steep
- s. left anterior oblique projection
- s. left anterior oblique view
- s. Towne projection
- s. Trendelenburg position

steeple sign
steerable guide wire system
steering
- beam s.
- coaxial s.
- electronic independent beam s.

steganography
Steinberg
- S. classification
- S. sign

Steinbrocker rheumatoid arthritis classification
Steinert epiphyseal fracture classification
Stein-Leventhal syndrome
Steinstrasse calculus
Stejskal-Tanner gradient
stellate
- s. abnormality
- s. border breast lesion
- s. configuration
- s. confluence
- s. crease
- s. defect
- s. granuloma
- s. ligament
- s. mass
- s. pattern
- s. skull fracture
- s. tear
- s. undepressed fracture

stem
- s. base plate
- brain s.
- bronchus s.
- straight s.

stem-loop structure
Stener lesion
stenion
stenocardia
stenogyria
steno-obstructive lesion
stenosed aortic valve
stenosing
- s. ring of left atrium
- s. tenosynovitis

stenosis, pl. stenoses
- acquired aortic valve s.
- acquired mitral s.
- acquired spinal s.
- ampullary s.
- anal s.
- anastomotic s.

antral s.
s. of aorta
aortic s. (AS)
aortoiliac s.
aqueduct s.
aqueductal s.
s. area
arterial s.
atheromatous s.
atherosclerotic s.
atypical aortic valve s.
benign papillary s.
benign tracheobronchial s.
bicuspid valvular aortic s.
bilateral carotid s.
bowel s.
branch pulmonary artery s.
bronchial s.
buttonhole mitral s.
calcific bicuspid valvular s.
calcific senile aortic valvular s.
canal s.
carotid artery s.
central canal s.
central spinal s.
cerebral artery s.
cervical s.
choledochoduodenal junctional s.
circumferential venous s.
common pulmonary vein s.
concentric hourglass s.
coronary artery s.
coronary luminal s.
coronary ostial s.
critical coronary s.
critical valvular s.
cross-sectional area s.
culprit s.
s. diameter
diffuse s.
discrete focal s.
discrete subaortic s.
discrete subvalvular aortic s.
  (DSAS)
duodenal hourglass s.
dynamic subaortic s.
eccentric s.
s. encroachment
esophageal s.
external iliac s.
femoropopliteal atheromatous s.
fibromuscular subaortic s.

fishmouth mitral s.
fixed-orifice aortic s.
flow-limiting s.
focal eccentric s.
foraminal s.
graft s.
granulation s.
hemodialysis-related venous s.
hemodynamically significant s.
hepatic artery s.
high-grade proximal s.
hourglass s.
hypercalcemic supravalvular
  aortic s.
hypertrophic infundibular
  subpulmonic s.
hypertrophic pyloric s. (HPS)
hypertrophic pyloric string sign s.
hypertrophic pyloric target sign s.
hypertrophic subaortic s.
idiopathic hypertrophic subaortic s.
ileal s.
iliac artery s.
iliofemoral venous s.
infrainguinal bypass s.
infrarenal s.
infundibular pulmonary s.
infundibular subpulmonic s.
innominate artery s.
in-stent s.
intragraft s.
intrarenal s.
intrinsic vein graft s.
iris-like s.
juxtaanastomotic s.
lateral recess s.
linear s.
lumbar spinal s.
luminal s.
membranous subaortic s.
membranous subvalvular aortic s.
midgraft s.
mitral s. (MS)
mitral valve s. (MVS)
multifocal short s.
multiple small bowel s.
muscular subaortic s.
napkin-ring anular s.
native kidney renal artery s.
neoplastic s.
noncalcified coronary s.
noncritical s.

S

NOTES

stenosis *(continued)*
nonrheumatic valvular aortic s.
ostial renal artery s.
papillary bile duct s.
papilla of Vater s.
pelvic venous s.
peripheral pulmonary artery s.
(PPAS)
petrous carotid canal s.
postangioplasty s.
postoperative s.
post PTCA residual s.
preangioplasty s.
pulmonary s.
pulmonary artery s.
pulmonary valve s.
pulmonary vein s.
pulmonic s.
pulmonic valvular s.
pyloric s.
radiation s.
radionuclide s.
rectal s.
relative mitral s.
renal artery s. (RAS)
rheumatic aortic valvular s.
rheumatic mitral s.
rheumatic tricuspid s.
saphenous vein s.
segmental s.
senescent aortic s.
silent mitral s.
spinal s.
stomal s.
string-sign s.
subaortic s.
subclavian artery s.
subglottic s.
subinfundibular s.
subsonic s.
subvalvular aortic s.
subvalvular pulmonary s.
supraaortic s.
supraclavicular aortic s.
suprarenal s.
supravalvular aortic s. (SAS,
SVAS)
supravalvular mitral s.
supravalvular pulmonary s.
tapering s.
tendon sheath s.
TOCU for internal carotid artery s.
tracheal s.
tricuspid s.
true mitral s.
truncal renal artery s.
tubular s.

tunnel subaortic s.
tunnel subvalvular aortic s.
uncomplicated supraclavicular s.
unicuspid aortic valve s.
unilateral carotid s.
ureteral s.
valvular aortic s.
valvular pulmonic s.
vein graft s.
vertebral artery s.

stenotic
s. change
s. coronary artery
s. esophagogastric anastomosis
s. flow reserve (SFR)
s. gradient
s. isthmus
s. lesion
s. plaque
s. tricuspid valve

Stensen
S. canal
S. duct
S. foramen
S. gland

stent
AneuRx s.
AVE bridge stainless steel balloon-
expandable s.
biliary s.
biodegradable s.
Cary-Coon biliary s.
C-flex s.
cobalt alloy s.
coil vascular s.
compliance matching s. (CMS)
Corinthian stainless steel balloon-
expandable s.
Cragg s.
Dacron s.
deployed s.
s. deployment
double-helix prostatic s.
double-J ureteral s.
Easy Wallstent s.
Esophacoil s.
esophageal s.
s. expansion
Flamingo s.
Gianturco s.
Gianturco-Rosch biliary s.
gold-marked s.
Hemobahn s.
indwelling s.
internal biliary s.
internal ureteral s.
IntraCoil s.

intravascular s.
[192]Ir-loaded s.
kissing s.
Luminexx biliary s.
Mac-Loc Ultrathane Cope
  nephroureterostomy s.
MEGALINK s.
Memotherm Nitinol self-
  expandable s.
s. mesh
metallic s.
s. migration
Miller double mushroom biliary s.
ML-Ultra balloon s.
30-mm-long Palmaz s.
nephroureteral s.
nephroureterostomy s.
Ni-Ti alloy s.
Nitinol Symphony s.
Palmaz PS 424 s.
Palmaz P 394 stainless steel
  balloon-expandable s.
pancreatic duct s.
Passager Nitinol self-expandable s.
patent s.
Percuflex s.
percutaneous s.
Perflex stainless steel balloon-
  expandable s.
pigtail s.
platinum-marked s.
polyethylene s.
Polyflex s.
polyurethane s.
porous metallic s.
prostatic s.
s. proximity
PTFE s.
radioisotope s.
reducing s.
renovascular s.
rolling membrane Wallstent cobalt-
  based alloy balloon-expandable s.
S670 s.
S7 AVE s.
Schneider enteral s.
self-expandable metal s.
silicone s.
SMART Nitinol self-expandable s.
Song covered duodenal s.
S670 over-the-wire coronary s.
stainless steel mesh s.

straight s.
Strecker Nitinol self-expandable s.
Strecker tantalum balloon-
  expandable s.
s. strut
Symphony Nitinol self-
  expandable s.
tandem s.
tantalum s.
Temp Tip ureteral s.
s. thrombosis
transhepatic biliary s.
T-tube s.
Ultraflex s.
Ultrathane Amplatz ureteral s.
urethral metallic s.
urinary s.
U-tube s.
vascular s.
Wallgraft cobalt-based alloy
  balloon-expandable s.
Wallstent s.
XT radiopaque coronary s.
ZA-stent Nitinol self-expandable s.
Zenith stainless steel self-
  expandable s.
zigzag s.
Zilver s.

stent-graft
AneuRx s.-g.
Cragg EndoPro s.-g.
endovascular s.-g.
Excluder s.-g.
FreeFlo s.-g.
Hemobahn PTFE-covered s.-g.
Jomed peripheral s.-g.
OPTA balloon s.-g.
Wallgraft endoprosthesis s.-g.

stenting
antegrade ureteral s.
brachiocephalic artery s.
bronchial s.
carotid artery s.
colon s.
endobiliary s.
iliac artery s.
innominate artery s.
intracoronary s.
intravascular s.
pulmonary artery s.
subclavian artery s.
tracheobronchial s.

S

NOTES

stenting *(continued)*
    ureteral s.
    venous s.
stentless porcine aortic valve
stent-mounted
    s.-m. allograft valve
    s.-m. heterograft valve
stent-related artifact
stent-vessel wall contact
Stenver
    S. position
    S. projection
    S. view
step
    modality performed procedure s.
      (MPPS)
    phase-encoding s.
    s. section
    s. wedge
step-and-shoot
    s.-a.-s. mode
    s.-a.-s. technique
step-down transformer
stepladder
    s. appearance
    s. sign
step-like recess
step-oblique mammography
stepoff
    s. of fracture
    orbital rim s.
stepping-source position
stepping-table MRA
step-up transformer
stepwise
    s. regression
    s. regression analysis
stercora
stercoraceous
stercoral ulcer
stercoroma
stercorous
stercus
stereo
    s. mammography
    s. right lateral projection
stereocinefluorography
stereoencephalotomy
stereofluoroscopy
stereogram
stereograph
stereographic projection
stereography
StereoGuide
    LORAD S.
    S. prone breast biopsy system
    S. stereotactic needle core biopsy

stereolithography
StereoLoc upright biopsy system
stereologic method of volume estimation
stereomammography
stereometry
stereomicroradiography
stereophotogrammetric
    roentgen s.
StereoPlan stereotactic planning system
stereoradiogram
stereoradiography
stereoroentgenogram
stereoroentgenography
stereoroentgenometry
stereosalpingography
stereoscope
    binocular s.
    Stanford and Wheatstone s.
stereoscopic
    s. radiography
    s. view
    s. vision
    s. zonography
stereoscopy
stereoskiagraphy
stereotactic, stereotaxic
    s. ablation
    s. apparatus
    s. automated technique
    s. breast biopsy
    s. breast biopsy system
    s. cerebral angiography
    s. core needle biopsy (SCNB)
    s. CT scan
    s. data
    s. device
    s. external-beam irradiation (SEBI)
    s. head frame
    s. localization
    s. localization frame
    s. mammography
    s. percutaneous lumbar diskectomy
    s. percutaneous needle biopsy
    s. procedure
    s. puncture
    s. radiation therapy
    s. radiosurgery (SRS)
    s. radiotherapy
    s. ring
    s. surface projection (SSP)
    s. surgery
    s. tractotomy
    s. vacuum-assisted biopsy
stereotaxically guided interstitial laser therapy
stereotaxis
    computer-assisted volumetric s.

imaging-based s.
volumetric minimally invasive s.

stereotaxy

frameless s.

sterile vent spike

sterna (*pl. of* sternum)

sternal

s. abscess
s. angle
s. angle of Louis
s. apex
s. border
s. cartilage
s. clip
s. edge
s. joint
s. lesion
s. lift
s. marrow
s. notch
s. part of diaphragm
s. rib
s. splitting
s. suture
s. vertebra
s. view

Sternberg

S. myocardial insufficiency
S. sign

Sterner lesion

sterni

corpus s.

sternochondral junction

sternoclavicular

s. angle
s. dislocation
s. hyperostosis
s. joint
s. joint disk
s. ligament

sternocleidomastoid

clavicular head of s.
s. muscle
s. muscle border
s. retraction
s. tumor

sternocostal

s. joint
s. part of diaphragm
s. surface of heart

sternohyoid muscle

sternomanubrial joint

sternopericardial ligament

sternospinal reference

sternothyroid muscle

sternotomy wire

sternoxiphoid plane

sternum, pl. **sterna**

anterior bowing of s.
osteitic lesion of the s.
s. retraction
tie s.

stethoscope

ultrasound s.

Steward-Milford fracture classification

Stewart-Hamilton equation

Stewart-Holmes sign

Stewart-Treves syndrome

ST/HR slope

Stickler syndrome

Stieda

S. fracture
S. process

Stierlin sign

stiff

s. guidewire
s. lung syndrome
s. man syndrome
s. noncompliant lung

stiffness

aortic s.
s. coefficient
lung s.
ventricular s.

stigmata

radiologic s.

Still disease

Stiller rib

Stilling canal

Stimucath continuous nerve block catheter

stimulated

s. acoustic emission (SAE)
s. echo (STE)
s. echo acquisition mode (STEAM)
s. echo artifact
s. echo-tagging technique

stimulation

alternating hemifield s.
cardiosynchronous s.
electric s.
high-voltage s. (HVS)
high-voltage pulsed galvanic s. (HVPGS)

NOTES

stimulation *(continued)*
    intraoperative electrocortical s.
      (IOECS)
    magnetic s.
    s. mode
    noninvasive programmed s. (NIPS)
    percutaneous electrical nerve s.
    s. scan
    vagus nerve s. (VNS)
stimulator
    AME bone growth s.
    bone growth s.
    DTU-215 cardiac digital s.
    transcutaneous electrical nerve s.
stimulus-correlated
    s.-c. water signal
stippled
    s. appearance
    s. calcification
    s. mineralization
    s. soft tissue
stippling of lung field
STIR
    short-inversion-time inversion recovery
    short tau inversion recovery
    short T1 inversion recovery
      fast STIR
      STIR imaging
      STIR sequence
      STIR slice
      STIR technique
stirrup bone
Stoerck loop
Stokes theorem
stoma, pl. **stomata**
    abdominal s.
    anastomotic s.
    bowel s.
    diverting s.
    gastroenterostomy s.
    gastrointestinal s.
    permanent s.
    prolapsed s.
    retracted s.
    Silastic collar-reinforced s.
stomach
    aberrant umbilical s.
    s. adenocarcinoma
    air contrast view of the s.
    angulus of s.
    antrum of s.
    s. atony
    s. bed
    bilocular s.
    body of the s.
    s. bubble
    s. calculus

canal of s.
cardiac s.
cascade s.
cobblestone appearance s.
contrast-filled s.
convex border of s.
coronary artery of s.
cup-and-spill s.
s. curvature
s. defect incisura
distal blind s.
distended s.
s. diverticulum
dumping s.
s. filling defect
s. fundus
greater curvature of s.
hourglass s.
intrathoracic s.
J-shaped s.
leather bottle s.
s. leiomyoma
s. leiomyosarcoma
lesser curvature of s.
s. margin
miniature s.
mucous lake of s.
s. narrowing
nonvisualization of fetal s.
pit of s.
s. pneumatosis
riding s.
scaphoid s.
sclerotic s.
thoracic s.
trifid s.
s. tube
s. ulcer
upside-down s.
s. varioliform erosion
s. varix
s. volvulus
s. wall
waterfall s.
water-trap s.
wet s.
stomal
    s. edema
    s. intussusception
    s. stenosis
stomata (*pl. of* stoma)
stone
    barrel-shaped s.
    bile duct s.
    biliary tract s.
    bilirubinate s.
    black faceted s.

bladder s.
bosselated s.
common bile duct s.
cystic duct remnant s.
cystine s.
dropped s.
s. extraction
extrahepatic s.
fecal s.
gallbladder s.
gas-containing s.
s. heart
high-attenuation s.
impacted urethral s.
s. impaction
intrahepatic s.
intraluminal s.
intravesical s.
kidney s.
lung s.
metabolic s.
multiple s.'s
nonopaque s.
nonradiopaque s.
opaque s.
pigment s.
pituitary s.
pulp s.
radiolucent s.
renal s.
residual s.
retained common bile duct s.
salivary s.
shadowing s.
soft pigment s.
staghorn s.
s. staple
ureteral s.
urinary bladder s.
vein s.
womb s.
stone-like calculus
stony mass
stool
retention of s.
stool-tagging agent
stop
crimp s.
s. test
stop-action
s.-a. image
s.-a. imaging

stopcock
Accel s.
three-way s.
stopping power
storage
digital s.
magnetic tape s.
s. phosphor-based technique
s. phosphor imaging
s. phosphor radiology
s. phosphor system
storiform pattern
storiform-pleomorphic
s.-p. malignant fibrous histiocytoma
s.-p. MFH
s.-p. pattern
storm
thyroid s.
Storz thoracoscope
stoved finger
STR
skeletal targeted radiotherapy
strabismus convergens alternans
straddle
s. fracture
s. injury
straddling
chondroblastoma s.
s. embolus
straight
s. anterior vertebral border
s. AP pelvic injection
s. chest tube
s. cord
s. end-hole catheter
s. guidewire
s. interposition graft
s. lateral projection
s. side-hole catheter
s. sinus
s. stem
s. stent
s. tubule
s. ureter
strain
adductor muscle s.
s. fracture
left ventricular hypertrophy with s.
ligamentous s.
lumbosacral spine s.
muscle s.
myotendinous s.

NOTES

S

strain *(continued)*
    s. pattern
    right ventricular s.
    shear s.
strain-gauge plethysmography
strain-rate MR imaging
strand
    s.'s of increased density
    rabbit ear s.
stranding
    fascial s.
    fat s.
    glial s.
    mesenteric fat s.
    soft tissue s.
strangulated
    s. bowel
    s. inguinal hernia
    s. obstruction
    s. viscus
strangulating obstruction
strangulation necrosis
strap muscle
strata *(pl. of* stratum)
stratification
    mural s.
stratified
stratiform
stratigraphy
Stratis II MRI system
stratum, pl. **strata**
strawberry gallbladder
strawberry-shaped head
stray
    s. neutron field
    s. radiation
streak
    s. artifact
    s. of atelectasis
    atherosclerotic fatty s.
    fatty intima s.
    s. of increased density
    primitive s.
streak-like
    s.-l. artifact
    s.-l. configuration
stream
    electron s.
    regurgitant s.
streaming
    tram-track s.
Strecker
    S. Nitinol self-expandable stent
    S. tantalum balloon-expandable
    stent
Streeter dysplasia

strength
    air-kerma s.
    diffusion encoding s.
    field s.
    high gradient field s.
    magnetic field s.
streptavidin peroxidase technique
stress
    adduction s.
    biomechanical s.
    s. Broden view
    s. cystogram
    s. echocardiography
    s. endpoint
    s. eversion view
    s. film
    s. fracture
    hoop s.
    s. incontinence
    s. injury
    s. inversion view
    mediolateral s.
    s. perfusion and rest function
    s. perfusion scintigraphy
    pharmacologic s.
    s. projection
    s. radiography
    s. raiser
    resting end-systolic wall s.
    shear s.
    s. thallium image
    s. thallium-201 myocardial imaging
    s. thallium scan
    torque s.
    torsion s.
    s. ulcer
    valgus s.
    varus s.
    wall shear s.
stress-and-rest image
stress-gated blood pool cardiac
    examination
stress-induced
    s.-i. ischemia
    s.-i. left ventricular dilatation
    s.-i. remodeling
stress-injected
stress-only perfusion imaging
stress-redistribution
    s.-r. examination
    s.-r. imaging
stress-rest reinjection examination
stress-strain curve
stretched
    s. lung
    s. out ligament
stria, pl. **striae**

s. medullaris thalami
s. vascularis ductus cochlearis
striatal
s. lesion
s. output pathway
striate
s. cortex
s. hemorrhage
s. vein
striated
s. angiographic nephrogram
s. muscle
striation
fiber-bundle s.
intermediate signal s.
paint brush s.
urothelial s.
striation across image
striatonigral degeneration
striatothalamic groove
striatum
corpus s.
Strichman SME-810 camera
Strickler method
stricture
anal s.
anastomotic s.
antral s.
anular esophageal s.
benign biliary s.
benign peptic s.
bile duct s.
biliary s.
bronchial s.
choledochojejunostomy s.
cicatricial s.
colonic s.
common bile duct s.
congenital urethral s.
contractile s.
duodenal s.
enteric s.
esophageal peptic s.
gastroesophageal junction s.
irritable s.
longitudinal esophageal s.
peptic s.
pyloric s.
recurrent s.
spasmodic s.
tracheal s.

ureteral s.
urethral s.
string
s. cell carcinoma
s. guideline
navel s.
s. sign
string-like bands of fibrous tissue
string-of-beads
s.-o.-b. appearance
s.-o.-b. sign
string-of-pearls
s.-o.-p. appearance
s.-o.-p. nuclear arrangement
s.-o.-p. sign
string-sign stenosis
strip
primary motor s.
s. scan
sensitometric s.
sensory s.
stripe
aortopulmonary mediastinal s.
central high-signal intensity s.
central intraluminal saturation s.
endometrial s.
esophageal-pleural s.
flank s.
Gennari s.
paraspinal pleural s.
paratracheal tissue s.
pleural s.
pleuroesophageal s.
properitoneal flank s.
psoas s.
right paratracheal s.
saturation s.
scaphoid fat s.
s. sign
tracheal s.
tracheal wall s.
vertebral s.
striping
horizontal s.
stripped atom
stripping
fibrin sleeve s.
stroke
cardiogenic embolic s.
cerebrovascular s.
completed s.
s. count image

NOTES

S

stroke *(continued)*
    s. count ratio
    s. ejection rate
    embolic s.
    s. in evolution (SIE)
    s. force
    hemisphere s.
    hemorrhagic s.
    hyperacute s.
    hypertensive s.
    incomplete s.
    s. index (SI)
    lacunar s.
    s. output
    s. power
    progressive s.
    s. scale score
    slow s.
    small-vessel s.
    spinal cord s.
    thromboembolic s.
    vertebrobasilar distribution s.
    s. volume (SV)
    s. volume image
    s. volume index (SVI)
    s. volume ratio
stroke-work index (SWI)
stroma, pl. **stromata**
    bone marrow s.
    cartilage s.
    cervical s.
    extralobular s.
    fibrocollagenous s.
    gonadal s.
    Rollet s.
    soft tissue s.
    vascular s.
stromal
    s. carcinoid tumor of ovary
    s. cell tumor
    s. matrix
    s. necrosis
    s. pattern of breast
strongyloidiasis
strontium (Sr)
    s. isotope
    radioactive s.
    s. with yttrium 90
strontium-89 (^{89}Sr)
    s. chloride
    s. imaging agent
strontium-90 (^{90}Sr)
structural
    s. abnormality
    s. anomaly
    s. epilepsy
    s. lesion

    s. pulmonary immaturity
    s. weakness
structurally immature lung
structure
    biliary s.
    bony s.
    brain s.
    branching linear s.
    branching tubular s.
    calcified density s.
    central hilar s.
    cervical s.
    collagenous s.
    cord s.
    cystic s.
    demineralized bony s.
    denture-supporting s.
    3D shape of neuroanatomic s.
    elongated s.
    extracolonic s.
    high-density s.
    hilar s.
    hollow s.
    hypoechoic s.
    intracranial s.
    intratumoral s.
    labyrinthine s.
    linear s.
    low-contrast s.
    low-density s.
    mediastinal s.
    midline cystic s.
    noncolonic s.
    nuclear s.
    opaque branching s.
    organoid s.
    osseous s.
    ossification of cartilaginous s.
    parcellation of s.
    periappendiceal s.
    prominent ductal vascular s.
    renal collecting s.
    ring-like s.
    satellite s.
    serpentine s.
    soft tissue density s.
    spherical s.
    stem-loop s.
    superior mediastinal s.
    supraglottic s.
    target parenchymal s.
    test tube s.
    thin linear s.
    tree-like airway s.
    tuboreticular s.
    tubular s.
    vascular s.

structured
  s. coil electromagnet
  s. light (SL)
  s. noise
  s. platform-independent data entry
    and reporting (SPIDER)
  s. reporting (SR)
  s. water
struma, pl. **strumae**
  Riedel s.
Strümpell sign
Strunsky sign
strut
  bone s.
  s. chorda
  corticocancellous s.
  s. fracture
  optic s.
  stent s.
  s. thickness
  tricuspid valve s.
  valve outflow s.
Struthers
  S. arcade
  S. ligament
struvite calculus
Stryker
  S. frame
  S. notch projection
  S. notch view
ST segment/heart rate slope (ST/HR slope)
ST-segment shift
STS-MIP
  sliding thin-slab maximum intensity
    projection
STT
  scaphotrapeziotrapezoid
  STT joint
stuck
  s. without recapture
  s. with recapture
studded fissure
study
  air contrast s.
  anatomopathologic s.
  anisotropic volume s.
  antegrade pressure s.
  barium meal s.
  biplane pelvic oblique s.
  bladder contractility s.
  blood flow s.

bone density s.
bone length s.
bone mineral content s.
brain activation s.
cardiac-gated s.
carotid duplex s.
cerebral blood flow s.
cerebral perfusion s.
cine s.
complete stress/rest s.
compressibility and phasicity s.
conventional s.
cornflake esophageal motility s.
correlative Doppler s.
Doppler flow probe s.
double-contrast barium s.
double-probe pH s.
DPTA CSF flow s.
dual-contrast s.
dynamic contrast-enhanced
  subtraction s.
dynamic supine s.
efficacy s.
electromagnetic blood flow s.
endovascular flow wire s.
factor analysis of dynamic s.
first-pass s.
fistula tract s.
flow s.
gallbladder s.
gas ventilation s.
gated imaging s.
gated planar s.
Gd-DOTA-enhanced subtraction
  dynamic s.
horizontal beam s.
ictal phase s.
imaging s.
inhalation s.
interictal PET FDG s.
interictal SPECT s.
intervention s.
iodized oil s.
isotopic 3D s.
isotopic volume s.
kidney function s.
kinematic MRI s.
lumbar flexion and extension s.
marker transit s.
minute-sequence s.
morphine-augmented s.
motility s.

S

NOTES

study *(continued)*
    MR flow quantification s.
    MRI CSF flow s.
    multibreath washout s.
    multitracer s.
    musculoskeletal imaging s.
    noble gas in magnetic resonance s.
    noninvasive imaging s.
    paleopathologic and radiologic s.
    paramagnetic contrast-enhanced
      MR s.
    perfusion s.
    peripheral small airway s.
    perirenal air s.
    phantom s.
    phonation s.
    postcaptopril radioisotope s.
    precaptopril radioisotope s.
    pressure perfusion s.
    pullback s.
    pulmonary blood flow s.
    pulmonary quantitative differential
      function s.
    qualitative s.
    quantitative region lung function s.
    radioaerosol imaging s.
    radiochemical s.
    radiolabeled water s.
    radiologic-histopathologic s.
    radionuclide blood flow s.
    radionuclide voiding s.
    reconstruction s.
    redistribution s.
    renal cyst s.
    renal function s.
    retrococcygeal air s.
    retroperitoneal air s.
    salivary gland function s.
    scintigraphic s.
    simulated equilibrium factor s.
    single-contrast s.
    sinus tract s.
    split-brain s.
    technetium albumin s.
    three-phase technetium s.
    thymidine suicide s.
    tracer s.
    transmission electron microscopic s.
    T1-weighted s.
    ureteral reflux s.
    urodynamic pressure-flow s.
    ventilation s.
    videotape s.
    in vivo disposition s.
    voiding s.
    wall motion s.
    wash-in/wash-out s.

    washout s.
    xenon washout s.
stump
    appendiceal s.
    bulbous s.
    s. carcinoma
    cystic duct s.
    duodenal s.
    gastric s.
    s. pregnancy
    s. pressure
    rectal s.
stunned myocardium
stunning
    myocardial s.
    postexercise s.
    poststress s.
    thyroid s.
stunted fetus
Sturge-Weber
    S.-W. syndrome
    S.-W. telangiectasia
Sturge-Weber-Dimitri syndrome
Stylet esophageal MRI coil
styloglossus muscle
stylohyoid
    s. ligament
    s. muscle
styloid
    s. process
    s. prominence
    ulnar s.
styloidium
    os s.
stylomandibular ligament
stylomastoid foramen
stylomaxillary ligament
stylopharyngeus
subacromial
    s. bursa
    s. bursal adhesion
    s. bursitis
    s. enthesophyte
    s. space
subacromial-subdeltoid
    s.-s. bursa
    s.-s. septic bursitis
subacute
    s. bacterial endocarditis
    s. bronchopneumonia
    s. cardiac tamponade
    s. combined spinal cord
      degeneration
    s. denervation atrophy
    s. encephalitis
    s. extrinsic allergic alveolitis
    s. granulomatous

s. hemorrhage
s. hepatic necrosis
s. inflammation
s. ischemic brain infarct
s. myocardial infarct
s. myositis ossificans
s. necrotizing encephalomyelopathy
s. necrotizing myelitis
s. necrotizing myelopathy
s. renal vein thrombosis
s. sclerosing panencephalitis (SSPE)
s. subdural hematoma
s. testicular torsion
s. thyroiditis
subadditivity
subadventitial
s. fibrosis
s. hyperplasia
s. plane
s. tissue
subanular
s. calcification
s. placement
subaortic
s. curtain
s. gland
s. muscle
s. stenosis
subapical bronchus
subaponeurotic abscess
subarachnoid
s. cavity
s. cistern
s. clot
s. cyst
s. hemorrhage (SAH)
s. hemorrhage Fisher grade 1–4
s. injection
s. instillation
s. metastatic disease
s. nerve block
s. phenol block
s. seeding
s. septum
s. space
s. space disease
subareolar
s. breast density
s. carcinoma
s. duct
s. lesion

s. mass
s. plexus
subarticular
s. bone resorption
s. cyst
s. pseudocyst
subastragalar dislocation
subastrocytic tumor
subatheromatous ulcer
subatmospheric pressure
subband
wavelet s.
subblock
rectifier s.
subcallosal gyrus
subcapital fracture
subcapsular
s. bleed
s. hepatic necrosis
s. renal hematoma
subcardinal vein
subcarina
subcarinal
s. angle (SA)
s. lymph node
subcecal appendix
subcentimeter node
subchondral
s. bone
s. bone plate
s. bone resorption
s. collapse
s. cyst
s. cystic cavity
s. fracture
s. fracture line
s. lesion
s. low-signal-intensity sclerosis
s. marrow edema
s. marrow hyperemia
s. microfracture
s. osteosclerosis
s. trabecular compression
subchorionic
s. hematoma
s. hemorrhage
subclavian
s. aneurysm
s. arteriography
s. artery
s. artery obstruction
s. artery occlusion

NOTES

subclavian *(continued)*
- s. artery stenosis
- s. artery stenting
- s. flap
- s. flap aortoplasty
- s. line
- s. loop
- s. steal
- s. turndown technique
- s. vein
- s. vein occlusion
- s. vein thrombosis
- s. vessel
- s. vessel thrombosis

subclavicular

subclavius

subcollateral gyrus

subcoracoid
- s. bursitis
- s. dislocation of shoulder

subcortical
- s. arteriosclerotic encephalopathy
- s. atherosclerotic encephalopathy
- s. CNS hamartoma
- s. cyst
- s. defect
- s. infarct
- s. intracerebral hemorrhage
- s. intracranial lesion
- s. ischemic vascular dementia
- s. low-intensity lesion
- s. Sudeck osteoporotic atrophy
- s. tumor

subcostal
- s. artery
- s. branch
- s. four-chamber view
- s. long-axis view
- s. margin
- s. nerve
- s. plane
- s. short-axis view
- s. short-axis view echocardiography
- s. window

subcritical narrowing

subcutaneous
- s. air
- s. array electrode
- s. arterial bypass graft
- s. connective tissue
- s. edema
- s. emphysema
- s. fascia
- s. fat
- s. fat line
- s. fat necrosis
- s. fibroma
- s. fracture
- s. hemangioma
- s. implanted injection port
- s. infiltrate
- s. infusion
- s. injection of contrast artifact
- s. nodule
- s. patch
- s. pocket
- s. quadriceps fat thickness (SQFT)
- s. sacrococcygeal myxopapillary ependymoma
- s. tissue gas
- s. tumor
- s. tunnel
- s. vein

subdeltoid
- s. bursa
- s. bursal adhesion
- s. bursal effusion
- s. bursitis
- s. fat plane obliteration

subdiaphragmatic
- s. abscess
- s. fat

subdural
- s. abscess
- s. blood
- s. button
- s. cavity
- s. clot
- s. contrast injection
- s. effusion
- s. empyema
- s. hemorrhage (SDH)
- s. hygroma
- s. interhemispheric hematoma
- s. space
- s. window

subendocardial
- s. infarct (SEI)
- s. injury
- s. ischemia
- s. myocardial infarct
- s. necrosis
- s. sclerosis

subendometrial halo

subependymal
- s. cyst
- s. germinolysis
- s. giant cell astrocytoma
- s. hamartoma
- s. hemorrhage
- s. heterotopia
- s. oligodendroglioma
- s. seeding

s. spread
s. vein
subependymal/subpial focus
subependymoma
subepicardial fat
suberosis
subeustachian sinus
subfalcine herniation
subfascial
s. hematoma
s. transposition
subfascially
subfrontal meningioma
subgaleal
s. abscess
s. cerebrospinal fluid
s. hematoma
s. hemorrhage
subglenoid dislocation of shoulder
subglottic
s. area
s. carcinoma
s. edema
s. hemangioma
s. narrowing
s. stenosis
subglottis
subgluteus
s. maximus bursa
s. medius bursa
subhepatic
s. abscess
s. area
s. cecum
s. space
subinfundibular stenosis
subinsular mass
subintimal
s. cleavage plane
s. dissection
s. fibrosis
s. filling
subject
s. contrast
s. placement
sublabral
s. foramen
s. recess
subligamentous
s. disk herniation
s. extension
s. vertebral osteomyelitis

sublimis tendon
sublingual
s. gland
s. varix
sublux
subluxation
anterior tibial s.
s. articulation
atlantoaxial s.
s. complex
distal radioulnar s.
element s.
forward s.
lateral s.
occult s.
s. of patella (SLP)
patellar s.
peroneal tendon s.
posterior s.
posterolateral rotatory s.
radial head s.
radioulnar s.
recurrent lateral patellar s.
reduced s.
sacroiliac s.
tendon s.
unilateral facet s.
subluxed
s. facet joint
s. vertebra
subluxing patella
submandibular
s. duct
s. duct calculus
s. ganglion
s. gland
s. lymph node
s. triangle
submassive
s. hemorrhage
s. hepatic necrosis
s. pulmonary embolus
submaxillary
s. gland
s. sialography
s. view
submembranous placental hematoma
submental
s. lymph node
s. vertex view
submentovertex
s. position

S

NOTES

submentovertex (*continued*)
  s. projection
  s. radiograph
submentovertical
  s. view
submerged segment of the esophagus
submetatarsal bursa
submicron
  s. magnetic particles
submucosal
  s. circular fold
  s. colon tumor
  s. esophageal tumor
  s. fibroid
  s. hemorrhage
  s. lesion
  s. lymphangiectasis
  s. thickening
  s. venous plexus
submucous myoma
suboccipital shortening
suboccipitobregmatic diameter
suboptimal
  s. detail
  s. effort
  s. examination
  s. film
  s. result
  s. runoff
  s. visualization
suboptimally visualized
subpectoral
  s. implant
  s. pocket
subperiosteal
  s. abscess
  s. bone resorption
  s. cortical abrasion
  s. cortical defect
  s. desmoid
  s. fracture
  s. hematoma
  s. hemorrhage
  s. infection
  s. new bone
  s. osteoid osteoma
subperitoneal space
subphrenic
  s. abscess
  s. biloma
  s. fluid
  s. recess
  s. space
subpial
  s. arteriovenous malformation
  s. lipoma
  s. region

subpleural
  s. air cyst
  s. bleb
  s. curvilinear line
  s. dot
  s. effusion
  s. lymphatic
  s. micronodule
  s. pulmonary arcade
subpubic arch
subpulmonic
  s. effusion
  s. fluid
  s. obstruction
  s. outflow
  s. pleural space
subpyloric node
subrectus obstruction
subsartorial
  s. canal
  s. tunnel
subscapular
  s. artery
  s. bursa
  s. echocardiographic view
  s. fossa
  s. lymph node
subscapularis
  s. muscle
  s. recess
  s. tendon
subsecond FLASH imaging
subsegmental
  s. bibasilar atelectasis
  s. bronchus
  s. lower lobe atelectasis
  s. perfusion abnormality
  s. perfusion defect
  s. renal artery branch
subsegment of lung
subselective cannulation
subseptus
  uterus s.
subserosal
  s. fibroid
  s. fibrosis
  s. hemorrhage
  s. layer
  s. lymphangiectasis
  s. tumor
subsite
subsonic stenosis
subspinous dislocation
substance
  bone s.
  brain s.

diamagnetic s.
reticular activating s.
substantia
s. nigra
s. propria
substernal
s. angle
s. goiter
s. retraction
s. thyroid
s. thyroid gland
substitute
bone s.
oxygenated perfluorocarbon blood s.
substrate
main energy s.
radiolabeled marker s.
subsystem
radiofrequency s.
subtalar
s. angle
s. articulation
s. axis
s. instability
s. joint
s. varus
s. view
subtendinous bursa
subtentorial lesion
subthalamus
subtle
s. gradation
s. haziness
s. malalignment
s. microcalcification
subtotal
s. gastric exclusion
s. gastric resection
s. lesion
s. occlusion
s. overframing
subtracted image
subtraction
s. angiography
background s.
s. cloning
complex s.
computer-assisted blood
background s. (CABBS)
digital s.
dual-energy s.
energy s.

s. film
S. ictal SPECT coregistered to
MRI (SISCOM)
s. image
s. imaging
quantitative imaging of perfusion
using a single s. (QUIPPS)
second order s.
s. technique
vector s.
s. venography
subtractive noise
subtrochanteric
s. fracture
s. varus deformity
subumbilical space
subungual
s. abscess
s. fibroma
s. glomus tumor
subunit
functional s. (FSU)
subvalvular
s. aneurysm
s. aortic obstruction
s. aortic stenosis
s. diffuse muscular obstruction
s. gradient
s. pulmonary stenosis
subvesical duct
subxiphoid
s. implantation
s. view
succenturiate placental lobe
succimer
succinate dehydrogenase (SDH)
succinic semialdehyde
sucking
s. muscle
s. pneumothorax
Sucquet-Hoyer
S.-H. anastomosis
S.-H. canal
sucralfate
gadolinium s.
sucrose
s. dosimeter
s. polyester imaging agent
suction tube
sudden
s. blockage of coronary artery
s. cardiac death

NOTES

Sudeck
- S. atrophy
- S. dystrophy
- S. point

SUFE
- slipped upper femoral epiphysis

suffocative goiter

sugar
- s. ring
- s. tumor

suit
- MAST s.

sulcal
- s. atrophy
- s. dilatation
- s. enhancement
- s. enlargement
- s. marking
- s. pattern
- s. skeleton

sulcation

sulcocommissural
- s. artery
- s. branch

sulcus, pl. **sulci**
- s. angle
- angularis s.
- atrioventricular s.
- basilar s.
- blunted posterior s.
- s. calcanei
- calcarine s.
- callosal s.
- carotid s.
- central s.
- cerebral s.
- s. chiasmaticus
- cingulate s.
- collateral s.
- coronary s.
- cortical s.
- costal s.
- costophrenic s.
- s. dilatation
- dilatation of s.
- s. effacement
- frontal s.
- Harrison s.
- hippocampal s.
- hypothalamic s.
- lateral femoral s.
- lateral occipital s.
- lip of lateral s.
- mapping of cerebral s.
- occipitotemporal s.
- olfactory s.
- parietooccipital s.

- perilabral s.
- pontomedullary s.
- postcentral s.
- posterior interventricular s.
- precentral s.
- pulmonary s.
- ramus of lateral s.
- retromalleolar s.
- rolandic s.
- sigmoid s.
- sphenoparietal s.
- superior frontal s.
- superior pulmonary s.
- superior temporal s.
- supracallosal s.
- s. talus
- temporal s.
- ulnar s.
- widened s.

sulfasalazine-induced pulmonary infiltrate

sulfate
- barium s. (BaSO4)
- barium lead s.
- barium strontium s.
- manganese s.
- sodium tetradecyl s.
- tetradecyl s.

sulfobromophthalein imaging agent

sulfonate
- sodium-2-mercaptoethane s.

sulfur
- s. colloid
- colloidal s.
- s. colloid imaging agent
- s. colloid scan
- s. colloid scintigraphy
- s. hexafluoride (SF_6)
- radioactive s.

sulfur-35 (^{35}S, S-35)

sum
- s. of cylinder (SOC)
- field-echo s.
- s. peak coincidence
- ray s.

summation
- s. shadow artifact
- s. of shadows

summing correction

summit
- ventricular septal s.

Sumner sign

sump
- s. drain
- s. drainage catheter

sum-peak method

sun
>Brett s.
>s. lamp
>S. SPARCstation system
>S. workstation

sunburst
>s. appearance
>s. brain vascularity
>s. gyral pattern
>s. nephrogram
>s. periosteal reaction

sun-ray appearance

sunrise
>s. projection
>s. view

sunset view

Super
>S. Angiorex model G DSA system
>S. 50 CP high-voltage generator

superabsorbent polymer embolic material

superacute

supercam scintillation scanner

superciliary arch

superconducting
>s. magnet
>s. open-magnet system
>s. quantum interference device (SQUID)

superconductive
>s. magnet
>s. MR system

superconductor
>niobium/titanium s.

superdominant left anterior descending artery

Superdup'r SD6891 left heart system

superfecundation

superfetation

superficial
>s. angioma
>s. basal cell carcinoma
>s. depressed carcinoma
>s. diffuse nephroblastomatosis
>s. dorsal sacrococcygeal ligament
>s. external pudendal artery
>s. femoral artery (SFA)
>s. femoral artery occlusion
>s. femoral vein
>s. hyperthermia treatment
>s. inguinal lymph node
>s. inguinal pouch

>s. inguinal ring
>s. lesion
>s. lymphadenopathy
>s. lymphatic vessel
>s. muscle
>s. necrosis
>s. palmar arterial arch
>s. palmaris longus tendon
>s. perineal pouch
>s. plexus
>s. pneumonia
>s. posterior compartment
>s. posterior sacrococcygeal ligament
>s. radiation
>s. spreading esophageal carcinoma
>s. spreading stomach carcinoma
>s. temporal artery
>s. temporalis fascia
>s. temporoparietal fascia
>s. tendo-Achilles bursa
>s. transverse metacarpal ligament
>s. transverse metatarsal ligament

superficialis
>s. arcade
>flexor digitorum s.
>s. tendon

superimage

superimposed
>s. acute partial tear
>s. bowel gas
>s. fungal infection

superimposition
>s. artifact
>s. of bowel shadow
>s. of signal

superincumbent spinal curve

superior
>apertura pelvis s.
>s. articular facet
>s. articulating process
>s. aspect
>s. azygoesophageal recess
>s. bilateral vena cava
>s. border
>s. border of heart
>s. border of rib
>s. bronchial artery
>s. caval defect
>s. cerebellar artery (SCA)
>s. cervical ganglion
>s. colliculus
>s. costal facet

NOTES

superior *(continued)*
  s. costotransverse ligament
  s. duodenal fold
  s. duodenal recess
  s. epigastric artery
  s. extensor retinaculum
  s. frontal axis shift
  s. frontal gyrus
  s. frontal sulcus
  s. genicular artery
  s. gluteal vessel
  s. hypogastric plexus
  s. intercostal artery
  s. intercostal vein
  s. jugular vein bulb
  s. labral anterior posterior
  s. labral anterior to posterior
    (SLAP)
  s. labral anterior-posterior injury
  s. labral anterior-posterior lesion
  s. labral anterior to posterior tear
  s. lobe
  s. lobe bronchus
  s. lobe of lung
  s. longitudinal fasciculus
  s. marginal defect
  s. margin of inferior rib
  s. maxillary foramen
  s. mediastinal structure
  s. mediastinum
  s. mesenteric
  s. mesenteric arteriography
  s. mesenteric artery (SMA)
  s. mesenteric artery syndrome
    (SMAS)
  s. mesenteric ganglion
  s. mesenteric plexus
  s. mesenteric vein (SMV)
  s. oblique
  s. occipitofrontal fasciculus
  s. olivary complex
  s. ophthalmic vein
  s. ophthalmic vein thrombosis
  s. orbital fissure
  s. orbital fissure anatomy
  s. parietal lobule gyrus
  s. peroneal retinaculum (SPR)
  s. peroneal retinaculum disruption
  s. petrosal sinus catheterization
  s. petrous sinus (SPS)
  s. phrenic branch
  s. pole
  s. pubic ligament
  s. pubic ramus
  s. pulmonary artery
  s. pulmonary sulcus
  s. pulmonary sulcus tumor

  s. pulmonary vein
  s. ramus
  s. rectal vein
  s. retraction
  s. sagittal sinus (SSS)
  s. sagittal sinus thrombosis
  s. segment
  s. segmental bronchus
  s. temporal gyrus
  s. temporal sulcus
  s. thoracic aperture
  s. thyroid artery
  s. transverse rectal fold
  s. transverse scapular ligament
  s. triangle sign
  s. turbinated bone
  s. vena cava (SVC)
  s. vena cava obstruction (SVCO)
  s. vena cava pressure
  s. vena cava syndrome
  zygapophysis s.
superior/inferior (S/I)
superior-inferior flow direction
superioris
superior-medial acetabular index
  (SMAI)
supernormal
  s. artery
  s. excitation
supernumerary
  s. digit
  s. kidney
  s. parathyroid gland
  s. sesamoid bone
  s. teeth
superoinferior
  s. heart
  s. projection
  s. view
superolateral
  s. aspect
  s. displacement
superolaterally
superomedial
  s. margin
  s. portal
  s. surface
superoxide dismutase
superparamagnetic
  s. agent iron oxide
  s. iron oxide (SPIO)
  s. iron oxide blood pool agent
  s. iron oxide imaging agent
  s. iron oxide MR imaging
  s. iron oxide particle
  s. microsphere
Superpump System SPS3891

Superscan
superselective
    s. angio-CT
    s. angiography
    s. infusion
    s. mesenteric artery catheterization
    s. microcatheter placement
super-stiff guidewire
supersystemic pulmonary artery
  pressure
supervoltage
    s. generator
    s. radiation
    s. radiotherapy
    s. technique
supinate
supination
    s. deformity
    s., external rotation type IV
      fracture
supination-adduction
    s.-a. fracture
    s.-a. injury
supination-eversion fracture
supination-external
    s.-e. rotation injury
    s.-e. rotation IV (SER-IV)
supination-outward rotation injury
supinator
supine
    s. bicycle stress echocardiography
    s. film
    s. full view
    s. position
    s. radiograph
supplemental beam filtration
supply
    accessory blood s.
    arterial scrotum s.
    collateral blood s.
    dual blood s.
    indirect blood s.
    lenticulostriate s.
    longitudinal blood s.
    pudendal blood s.
    three-phase voltage s.
    tumor blood s.
    vascular s.
support
    biventricular s. (BVS)
    elevated leg s.
    lateral lumbar s.

    ligamentous s.
    wedge-shaped s.
suppressed tissue
suppression
    chemsat fat s.
    Cytomel s.
    DIET method of fat s.
    double-echo three-point Dixon
      method fat s.
    drug-induced bone marrow s.
    fat signal s.
    FSE-T2 with fat s.
    s. of heart pulsation artifact
    overdrive s.
    paradoxical s.
    s. scan
    signal s.
    solvent s.
    spectral-spatial fat s.
suppuration
suppurative
    s. ascending cholangitis
    s. inflammation
    s. pancreatitis
    s. pleurisy
    s. pneumonia
    s. pyelonephritis
    s. thyroiditis
supraanal fascia
supraanular constriction
supraaortic
    s. lesion
    s. ridge
    s. stenosis
supracallosal
    s. gyrus
    s. sulcus
supracardiac total anomalous venous
  return
supracardinal vein
supraceliac aorta
supracervical hysterectomy
supraclavicular
    s. aortic stenosis
    s. fossa
    s. lymph node
    s. node involvement
    s. triangle
supraclinoid
    s. carotid aneurysm
    s. ICA
    s. portion

S

NOTES

supraclinoid · suprasyndesmotic

supraclinoid *(continued)*
  s. segment of internal carotid artery
supracolic compartment
supracollicular spike of cortical bone
supracondylar
  s. femoral fracture
  s. humeral fracture
  s. plate
  s. process
  s. ridge
  s. Y-shaped fracture
supracondyloid process
supracoronary ridge
supracricoid interval
supracristal
  s. plane (SCP)
  s. ventricular septal defect
supradditivity
supradiaphragmatic
  s. aorta
  s. extension
supraepicondylar
supraepitrochlear
supraglenoid tubercle
supraglottic
  s. carcinoma
  s. edema
  s. laryngectomy
  s. larynx
  s. narrowing
  s. structure
supraglottis
suprahepatic
  s. caval cuff
  s. hypertension
  s. vena cava
suprahisian block
suprahyoid
suprailiac aortic mesenteric graft
suprainterparietal bone
supralevator
  s. fistula
  s. space
supraligamentous disk herniation
supramalleolar open amputation
supramarginal gyrus
supramesocolic compartment
supranaviculare
  os s.
supranuclear lesion
supraoccipital bone
supraorbital
  s. artery
  s. canal
  s. fissure
  s. foramen
  s. groove (SOG)
  s. margin (SOM)
  s. ridge
suprapancreatic obstruction
suprapatellar
  s. bursa
  s. plica
  s. pouch
suprapharyngeal bone
suprapubic
  s. area
  s. transabdominal ultrasound
suprapyloric node
suprarenal
  s. aortic aneurysm
  s. extension of aneurysm
  s. gland
  s. impression
  s. stenosis
suprascapular
  s. ligament
  s. nerve entrapment
  s. notch syndrome
suprasellar
  s. adenoma
  s. aneurysm
  s. atypical teratoma
  s. capsule
  s. extension
  s. extension of tumor
  s. hemorrhagic germinoma
  s. low-density lesion
  s. mass
  s. mass calcification
  s. meningioma
  s. subarachnoid cistern
suprasphincteric fistula
supraspinatus
  s. muscle
  s. musculotendinous junction
  s. nerve
  s. tendinosis
  s. tendon
supraspinous
  s. ligament
  s. ligament disruption
suprasternal
  s. bone
  s. bulge
  s. notch
  s. notch plane
  s. notch view
  s. retraction
  s. scanning
  s. window
suprasyndesmotic fixation

supratentorial
  s. astrocytoma
  s. brain tumor
  s. cerebral blood flow
  s. flow compensation
  s. glioma
  s. gray matter
  s. lesion
  s. neoplasm
  s. primitive neuroectodermal tumor
  s. space
  s. volume
  s. white matter
suprathreshold
supratip nasal tip deformity
supratrochlear
  s. artery
  s. node
supratubercular ridge of Meyer
supravalvular
  s. aortic stenosis (SAS, SVAS)
  s. aortography
  s. mitral stenosis
  s. pulmonary stenosis
  s. ring
supravaterian duodenum
supraventricular
  s. crest (SVC)
  s. level
  s. tachyarrhythmia
  s. tachycardia
  s. venous echo
supraventricularis
  crista s.
supravesical obstruction
supreme turbinate bone
SUR
  standardized uptake ratio
sural nerve
SureStart contrast tracking
surface
  acromial articular s.
  anterolateral s.
  anteromedial s.
  s. application of radioelement
  apposing articular s.
  articular s.
  articulating s.
  arytenoidal articular s.
  attenuated cortical s.
  auricular s.
  axial s.

basal s.
bone s.
bosselated s.
buccal s.
calcaneal articular s.
carpal articular s.
cartilaginous joint s.
cerebral s.
s. coil
s. coil localization
s. coil method
s. coil NMR
s. coil rotating-frame spectroscopy
colic s.
s. configuration
contiguous articular s.
s. convexity pattern
corrugated fat pad s.
costal s.
cuboidal articular s.
diaphragmatic s.
distal s.
s. distance
s. dose variation
endosteal s.
endothelial s.
epicardial s.
s. epithelium
erosion of articular s.
fibular articular s.
gastric s.
glenoid s.
grooving of articular s.
immunostained s.
joint articular s.
s. matching technique
mediastinal lung s.
s. nodularity
occlusal s.
opposing articular s.'s
opposing pleural s.'s
s. osteosarcoma
s. ovarian epithelium tumor
palmar s.
parallelism of articular s.
pelvic peritoneal s.
plantar s.
posterior s.
s. projection
s. radioelement application
radioulnar s.
s. registration

NOTES

S

surface *(continued)*
    renal s.
    roughened articular s.
    serosal s.
    s. shaded display (SSD)
    s. spoiling
    superomedial s.
    synovial s.
    s. tension of lung
    s. variable-attenuation correction
    ventral s.
    weightbearing s.
surfactant
    s. deficiency
    s. deficiency disorder (SDD)
surfer's
    s. knot
    s. nodule
surgery
    coronary artery bypass s. (CABS)
    CT-guided stereotactic s.
    gastric bypass s. (GBS)
    image-guided s.
    radioguided s.
    radioimmunoguided s. (RIGS)
    robotic mitral valve s.
    stereotactic s.
    telecollaboration s.
surgical
    s. anatomy visualization and
      navigation tools (SAVANT)
    s. angle
    s. artifact
    s. decompression
    s. emphysema
    s. endarterectomy
    s. inspection
    s. neck
    s. neck fracture
    s. neck of humerus
    S. Planning and Orientation
      Computer System (SPOCS)
    s. simulation CT
    s. sponge
    s. staple
    s. venous interruption
    s. wound
surgically
    s. corrected transposition of the
      great artery
    s. created resection cavity
Surgilase
    S. 150 high-powered CO_2 laser
    S. Nd:YAG laser
SurgiScope
Surgitron portable radiosurgical unit

Surgi-Vision MRI coil
surveillance
    endoscopic s.
    imaging s.
survey
    bone s.
    s. film
    four-view wrist s.
    isotopic skeletal s.
    joint s.
    long bone s.
    metabolic bone s.
    metastatic bone s.
    osseous s.
    postimplant radiation s.
    preloading radiation s.
    s. radiograph
    s. scan
    serial radiographic s.
    skeletal s.
    traumatic bone s.
    s. view
survival
    failure-free s.
susceptibility
    s. artifact
    bulk magnetic s. (BMS)
    s. contrast-weighted MRI
    diamagnetic s.
    s. effect
    magnetic s.
    s. mapping
susceptibility-sensitive sequence
susceptibility-weighted MR imaging
suspended
    s. heart
    s. inspiration
suspension
    barium s.
    s. characteristic
    chromic phosphate s.
    colloidal s.
    Definity injectable s.
    Enecat CT concentrated rectal s.
    E-Z-Paque barium s.
    fast exchange-cellular s.
    galactose-based s.
    s. of kidney
    liquid barium s.
    perflutren lipid microsphere
      injectable s.
suspensory
    s. ligament
    s. ligament of ovary
    s. ligament of penis
    s. muscle of duodenum

suspicious
>s. lesion
>s. mass

sustained
>s. anterior parasternal motion
>s. apical impulse
>s. left ventricular heave

sustentacular trauma

sustentaculi
>os s.

sustentaculum
>s. lienis
>s. tali

sutural
>s. bone
>s. calcification
>s. ligament
>s. marking

suture
>anterior palatine s.
>apical s.
>basilar s.
>bioabsorbable Dexon s.
>biparietal s.
>bony s.
>bregmatomastoid s.
>coronal s.
>cranial s.
>delayed closure of s.
>dentate s.
>denticulate s.
>diastasis of s.
>diastatic lambdoid s.
>ethmoidolacrimal s.
>ethmoidomaxillary s.
>false s.
>flat s.
>frontal s.
>frontoethmoidal s.
>frontolacrimal s.
>frontomalar s.
>frontomaxillary s.
>frontonasal s.
>frontoparietal s.
>frontosphenoid s.
>frontozygomatic s.
>Gillies s.
>Gruber s.
>incisive s.
>infiltration s.
>infraorbital s.
>intermaxillary s.

internasal s.
interpalatine s.
interparietal s.
jugal s.
lacrimoconchal s.
lacrimoethmoidal s.
lacrimomaxillary s.
lacrimoturbinal s.
lambdoid s.
lambdoidal cranial s.
limbus s.
s. line
s. line carcinoma
longitudinal s.
malomaxillary s.
mamillary s.
mastoid s.
median palatine s.
metallic s.
metopic s.
middle palatine s.
nasal s.
nasofrontal s.
nasomaxillary s.
nonfusion of cranial s.
occipital s.
occipitomastoid s.
occipitoparietal s.
occipitosphenoid s.
opaque wire s.
overlapping s.
palatine s.
palatoethmoidal s.
palatomaxillary s.
parietal s.
parietomastoid s.
parietooccipital s.
parietotemporal s.
persistent metopic s.
petrobasilar s.
petrosphenobasilar s.
petrosphenooccipital s.
petrosquamosal s.
petrosquamous s.
plane s.
posterior palatine s.
prematurely closed s.
premaxillary s.
rhabdoid s.
sagittal cranial s.
serrated s.
silk s.

S

NOTES

suture *(continued)*
    s. of skull
    sphenoethmoidal s.
    sphenofrontal s.
    sphenomalar s.
    sphenomaxillary s.
    sphenooccipital s.
    sphenoorbital s.
    sphenoparietal s.
    sphenopetrosal s.
    sphenosquamous s.
    sphenotemporal s.
    sphenovomerine s.
    sphenozygomatic s.
    splayed cranial s.
    spread s.
    squamosal s.
    squamosomastoid s.
    squamosoparietal s.
    squamososphenoid s.
    squamous s.
    sternal s.
    temporal s.
    temporomalar s.
    temporozygomatic s.
    true s.
    wide s.
    zygomaticofrontal s.
    zygomaticotemporal s.
SUV
    standard uptake value
SV
    stroke volume
Sv
    sievert
SVAS
    supravalvular aortic stenosis
SVC
    superior vena cava
    supraventricular crest
SVCO
    superior vena cava obstruction
SVCT
    spiral x-ray computed tomography
SVG
    scatter and veiling glare
SVI
    seminal vesicle invasion
    stroke volume index
SvO$_2$
    systemic vascular resistance index
SVR
    systemic vascular resistance
SVRI
    systemic vascular resistance index
swallow
    barium s.

    dry s.
    Gastrografin s.
    Hypaque s.
    ice-water s.
    video barium s.
    water-soluble contrast esophageal s.
    wet s.
swallowing
    s. artifact
    s. center
    s. dysfunction
    fetal s.
    s. function
    s. mechanism
swallowtail
    s. configuration
    s. malformation of scapula
swamp-static artifact
Swan-Ganz balloon catheter
swan-neck
    s.-n. finger deformity
    s.-n. shape of ventricular outflow
    s.-n. tubular lesion
Swanson finger joint
sweat
    s. duct adenoma
    s. gland carcinoma
sweep
    duodenal s.
    whole-body s.
    widened duodenal s.
Sweet
    S. method
    S. sternal punch
swelling
    ankle s.
    blennorrhagic s.
    brain s.
    bulbar s.
    s. of cartilage
    congestive brain s.
    fusiform s.
    joint s.
    periumbilical s.
    prevertebral soft tissue s.
    soft tissue s.
Swenson pull-through procedure
SWI
    stroke-work index
swimmer's
    s. position
    s. projection
    s. shoulder
    s. view
swimming pool granuloma
swinging heart

swirling
> s. motion
> s. smokelike echoes

Swiss
> S. Alps appearance
> S. cheese air bronchogram
> S. cheese appearance
> S. cheese nephrogram
> S. cheese ventricular septal defect
> S. lithoclast intracorporeal
> lithotripter
> S. roll technique

Swissray scanner
switchable coil
swollen
> s. brain hemisphere
> s. tissue

Swyer-James-Macleod syndrome
Swyer-James syndrome (SJS)
Swyer syndrome
SXA
> single-energy x-ray absorptiometer

SXCT
> spiral x-ray computed tomography

Syed-Neblett template
**Syed-Puthawala-Hedger esophageal
   applicator**
Syed template
sylvian
> s. aqueduct
> s. aqueduct syndrome
> s. candelabra
> s. cistern
> s. fissure
> s. operculum
> s. point
> s. triangle

sylvian-rolandic junction
Sylvius
> aqueduct of S.
> cistern of S.
> S. fossa
> S. ventricle

symbol
> radiation warning s.

Syme ankle disarticulation amputation
Symington body
Symmers fibrosis
Symmetra I-125 brachytherapy seeds
symmetric
> s. abnormal increased signal
> bilaterally s.

> s. chest
> s. confluent high signal intensity
> s. consolidation
> s. distribution
> s. echo
> s. heart hypertrophy
> s. IUGR
> s. loss of DAT
> s. narrowing
> s. pattern of radiotracer uptake
> s. periosteal reaction
> s. phased array
> s. pulmonary congestion
> s. thorax

symmetry
> architectural s.
> bilateral s.
> inverse s.

sympathetic
> s. block
> s. chain
> s. denervation
> s. discharge
> s. dystrophy
> s. ganglia tumor
> s. ganglion
> s. innervation
> s. nervous tissue
> s. vascular instability

sympathicoblastoma
sympathicogonioma
sympathicolysis
> MR-guided lumbar s.

sympathoblastoma
sympathogonia
sympathogonioma
Symphony
> S. MR imaging system
> S. Nitinol self-expandable stent

symphyseal
symphysis, pl. **symphyses**
> s. cartilage joint
> s. of the mandible
> s. manubriosternalis
> s. ossium pubis
> pubic s.
> s. pubica

symptom
> constellation of s.'s
> constitutional s.
> segmental bronchus s.
> vasomotor s.

NOTES

symptomatic
    s. coarctation of aorta
    s. gallstone
    s. lateral synovial plica
    s. metastatic spinal cord
      compression
    s. obstructive hydrocephalus
    s. vascular ring

synaptic
    s. cleft
    s. dopamine concentration
    s. pathway
    s. vesicle

sync
    V sync

syncephalus

synchondrosis, pl. **synchondroses**
    cartilaginous s.
    disruption of the cartilaginous s.
    low signal intensity s.
    s. manubriosternalis
    neurocentral s.
    posterior intraoccipital s.
    s. of skull
    sphenooccipital s.
    s. xiphosternalis

synchronicity

synchronization
    s. device
    prospective s.
    retrospective s.

synchronized retroperfusion

synchronous
    s. carotid arterial pulse
    s. disease
    s. lesion
    s. transitional cell carcinoma

synchrony
    ventricular s.

synchrotron
    monochromatic s.
    s. radiation

synclitic

syncliticism

synclitism

syncytium
    circular s.

syndactylization of digit

syndactyly in fetus

syndesmophyte
    marginal s.
    spinal s.

syndesmosis, pl. **syndesmoses**
    distal tibiofibular s.
    s. sprain
    tibiofibular s.
    s. tympanostapedialis

syndesmotic
    s. diastasis
    s. impingement
    s. ligament
    s. ligament complex

syndrome (*See* disease, phenomenon)
    abdominal muscle deficiency s.
    acquired adult Fanconi s.
    acquired immunodeficiency s.
    (AIDS)
    acute central cord s.
    acute chest s.
    acute compartment s.
    acute radiation s.
    acute respiratory distress s.
    (ARDS)
    acute retroviral s.
    Adams-Stokes s.
    adductor insertion avulsion s.
    adrenogenital s.
    adult respiratory distress s. (ARDS)
    afferent loop s.
    Aicardi s.
    Alagille s.
    Albright s.
    Albright-McCune-Sternberg s.
    Alibert-Bazin s.
    Alpers-Huttenlocher s. (AHS)
    amnionic band s.
    angiomatous s.
    angioosteohypertrophy s.
    anterior compartment s.
    anterior cord s.
    anterior impingement s.
    anterior spinal artery s.
    anterior tarsal tunnel s.
    anterolateral impingement s.
    aortitis s.
    apallic s.
    apple-peel s.
    Arnold-Chiari s.
    Asherson s.
    atherosclerotic occlusive s.
    autoerythrocyte sensitization s.
    Avellis s.
    axonopathic neurogenic thoracic
      outlet s.
    Ayerza s.
    Bäfverstedt s.
    Balint s.
    Bannayan-Riley-Ruvalcaba s.
    Banti s.
    Barlow s.
    Barré-Lieou s.
    Bartter s.
    basal cell nevus s.
    basilar artery s.

Bazex s.
Beckwith-Wiedemann s.
Behr s.
Berdon s.
Bernard-Horner s.
Bernard-Soulier s.
Bertolotti s.
Beuren s.
biliary obstruction s.
Bing-Horton s.
Blackfan-Diamond s.
Bland-Garland-White s.
Blesovsky s.
blind loop s.
blind pouch s.
blueberry muffin s.
blue-digit s.
blue rubber-bleb nevus s.
blue-toe s.
Boerhaave s.
Bouveret s.
Brissaud s.
Brown-Séquard s.
Brugada s.
Budd-Chiari s.
Caffey s.
Caffey-Kempe s.
capillary leak s.
Caplan s.
carcinoid s.
cardiocutaneous s.
cardiosplenic s.
Carney s.
carotid blowout s.
carotid sinus s. (CSS)
carpal tunnel s.
cauda equina s. (CES)
caudal regression s.
cavernous sinus s.
Cayler s.
Ceelen-Gellerstedt s.
celiac artery compression s.
celiac axis s.
central cervical cord s.
cerebellar s.
cerebral steal s.
cerebrohepatorenal s. (CHRS)
cervical disk s.
cervical pain s.
cervical rib s.
Cestan-Chenais s.
Chédiak-Steinbrinck-Higashi s.

Chilaiditi s.
CHILD s.
chronic overuse s.
Churg-Strauss s.
Clarke-Hadefield s.
Claude s.
cleft face s.
Clerc-Levy-Cristico s.
COACH s.
coarctation s.
Cobb s.
Cockayne s.
Collet-Sicard s.
compartment s.
compression s.
congenital adrenogenital s.
congenital pulmonary venolobar s.
congenital vascular-bone s. (CVBS)
Conn s.
Conradi-Hünermann s.
constriction band s.
coronary artery steal s.
coronary-subclavian steal s.
costoclavicular s.
Courvoisier-Terrier s.
Cowden s.
craniofacial pain s.
craniomandibular s.
craniosynostosis s.
CREST s.
cri-du-chat s.
Cronkhite-Canada s.
Crouzon s.
Crow-Fukase s.
crush s.
cubital tunnel s.
Cushing s.
Cyriax s.
Dandy-Walker s.
Davies-Colley s.
defibrination s.
Degos s.
de Lange s.
Demons-Meigs s.
de Morsier s.
Denys s.
Diamond-Blackfan s.
DiGeorge s.
Di Guglielmo s.
disseminated intravascular
   coagulation s.
distal intestinal obstruction s.

S

NOTES

syndrome *(continued)*

Down s.
Drash s.
Dressler s.
Dubin-Johnson s.
dumping s.
Dyke-Davidoff-Masson s.
dysarthria clumsy hand s.
Eagle-Barrett s.
ectopic ACTH s.
ectrodactyly-ectodermal dysplasia-
  clefting s.
Edwards s.
Ehlers-Danlos s.
Eisenmenger s.
Ellis-van Creveld s.
empty sella s.
encephalotrigeminal s.
enlarged vestibular vascular
  aqueduct s.
excessive lateral pressure s. (ELPS)
facet s.
facioauriculovertebral s.
failed back s. (FBS)
failed back surgery s. (FBSS)
Fallot s.
familial adenomatous polyposis s.
Fanconi s.
Fanconi-Hegglin s.
fat embolism s. (FES)
Felty s.
feminizing testes s.
fetal alcohol s.
fetal cardiosplenic s.
Feuerstein-Mims s.
fibrocystic breast s.
Fiessinger-Leroy s.
Fiessinger-Leroy-Reiter s.
Fitz-Hugh and Curtis s.
floppy valve s.
Foix-Alajouanine s.
Foix-Chavany-Marie s.
Forney s.
functional bowel s.
Gaisböck s.
Gardner bone s.
gas-bloat s.
Gasser s.
gastrocardiac s.
generalized lymphadenopathy s.
Gerstmann s.
Gianotti-Crosti s.
Goldenhar s.
Goodpasture s.
Gorlin s.
Gorlin-Goltz s.
Graham-Burford-Mayer s.

Grisel s.
Gsell-Erdheim s.
Haglund s.
Hajdu-Cheney s.
Hallermann-Streiff-François s.
Hamman-Rich s.
Hare s.
Hegglin s.
hemisensory s.
hemolyticuremic s.
Hennekam s.
hepatorenal s. (HRS)
hereditary flat adenoma s.
Hermansky-Pudlak s.
heterotaxy s.
holiday heart s.
Holmes s.
Holt-Oram s.
Horner s.
Howell-Evans s.
Hughes-Stovin s.
Hurler s. (HS)
Hurley-Schele s.
Hutchinson s.
Hutchinson-Gilford s.
Hutinel-Pick s.
hyperabduction s.
hypoplastic left heart s. (HLHS)
hypoplastic left parietal s.
hypoplastic right heart s.
ileocecal s.
iliotibial band friction s.
immature lung s.
s. of impending thrombosis
impingement s.
inferior vena cava s.
infrapatellar contracture s. (IPCS)
inguinal ligament s.
inhibitory s.
innominate artery compression s.
intermediate coronary s.
intestinal Behçet s.
intestinal hypoperistalsis s.
irritable bowel s.
Ivemark CHD s.
Jadassohn-Lewandowsky s.
Jaffe-Campanacci s.
Jarcho-Levin s.
Jeune s.
Joubert s.
jugular foramen s.
juvenile polyposis s. (JPS)
Kallmann s.
Kartagener s.
Kasabach-Merritt s.
Kast s.
Katayama s.

Kearns-Sayre s.
Kimmelstiel-Wilson s.
Kinsbourne s.
Kleffner-Landau s.
Klippel-Feil s.
Klippel-Trenaunay s.
Klippel-Trenaunay-Weber s.
Lady Windermere s.
Lambert-Eaton myasthenic s.
Landau-Kleffner s.
Larsen s.
lateral recess s.
Laubry-Pezzi s.
leaky lung s. (LLS)
left heart s.
Lennox-Gastaut s.
Leriche s.
Leri-Weill s.
Lesch-Nyhan s.
Lhermitte-Duclos s.
Lightwood s.
linear sebaceous nevus s.
locked-in s.
Löffler s.
Löfgren s.
Louis-Bar s.
low back s.
low-flow s.
Lown-Ganong-Levine s. (LGL)
luteinized unruptured follicle s.
Lutembacher s.
luxury perfusion s.
lymphadenopathy s.
lymph node s.
Macleod s.
Maffucci s.
male Turner s.
Mallory-Weiss s.
Marchiafava-Micheli s.
Marcus Gunn s.
Marfan s.
Marine-Lenhart s.
Maroteaux-Lamy s.
Martorell aortic arch s.
Mayer-Rokitansky-Küster-Hauser s.
May-Thurner s.
Mazabraud s.
McCune-Albright s.
McKusick-Kaufman s.
Meadows s.
Meckel s.
Meckel-Gruber s.

meconium aspiration s.
meconium plug s.
medial tibial stress s.
megacystis-microcolon-intestinal
  hypoperistalsis s.
Meigs s.
Meigs-Cass s.
Meigs-Salmon s.
Melnick-Needles s.
Mendelson s.
Mèniére s.
Menkes s.
mermaid s.
metastatic carcinoid s.
midaortic s.
middle aortic s.
middle fossa s.
middle lobe s.
Mikity-Wilson s.
Mikulicz s.
milk-alkali s.
milk leg s.
Milkman s.
Miller-Dieker s.
Milwaukee shoulder s.
Minot-von Willebrand s.
Mirizzi s.
Mohr s.
Morgagni s.
Morgagni-Adams-Stokes s.
Morquio s.
Morquio-Brailsford s.
Mosse s.
Mounier-Kuhn s.
moyamoya s.
Moynahan s.
MSA s.
mucocutaneous lymph node s.
  (MCLS)
mucosal prolapse s.
Muir-Torre s.
multiple endocrine neoplasia s.
multiple mucosal neuroma s.
multiple pterygium s.
multiple system atrophy s.
myofascial pain-dysfunction s.
nail-patella s.
Naumoff s.
Nelson s.
nephrotic s.
neurocutaneous s.
nevoid basal cell carcinoma s.

S

NOTES

syndrome *(continued)*

Nievergelt s.
Noonan s.
Nothnagel s.
nutcracker s.
Ogilvie s.
Omenn s.
orbital apex s.
organic brain s. (OBS)
orodigitofacial s.
Ortner s.
Osler-Libman-Sacks s.
Osler-Weber-Rendu s.
os peroneum s.
os trigonum s.
ovarian hyperstimulation s.
ovarian remnant s.
ovarian vein s.
Paget-von Schroetter s.
painful osmotic demyelination s.
Pancoast s.
pancreatic cholera s.
pancreaticohepatic s.
pancytopenia-dysmelia s.
Papillon-Léfevré s.
paraneoplastic s.
Parinaud s.
Parkes-Weber s.
Patau s.
Pearson s.
pectoralis major s.
pelvic congestion s.
Pena Shokeir s.
Pendred s.
Pepper s.
Peutz-Jeghers s.
Pfeiffer s.
Pfoundler-Hurler s.
phantom limb s.
Pierre Robin s.
pinch-off s.
plica s.
Plummer-Vinson s.
POEMS s.
Poland s.
polycystic ovary s. (PCOS)
polysplenia s.
popliteal artery entrapment s.
postcardiac injury s. (PCIS)
postembolization s.
posterior column s.
posterior impingement s.
posterior joint s.
posterior reversible
  encephalopathy s. (PRES)
postmaturity s.
postmyocardial infarction s.

postpericardiotomy s.
postpolio s.
Potter s.
Proteus s.
proximal loop s.
prune belly s.
pseudothrombophlebitis s.
pseudo-Turner s.
pseudo-Zollinger-Ellison s.
quadrilateral space s.
Raeder paratrigeminal s.
Ramsay Hunt s.
Raymond-Cestan s.
Raynaud s.
reactive airway dysfunction s.
Reader paratrigeminal s.
reflex sympathetic dystrophy s.
Reiter s.
respiratory distress s. (RDS)
restrictive hemodynamic s.
Rett s.
reversible posterior
  leukoencephalopathy s. (RPLS)
Richter s.
right middle lobe s.
Riley-Day s.
Roberts s.
Robinow s.
Rokitansky-Mayer-Küster-Hauser s.
Romano-Ward s.
Romberg-Wood s.
Rotor s.
Rundles-Falls s.
Russell-Silver s.
Ruvalcaba-Myhre-Smith s.
Sack-Barabas s.
Saldino-Noonan s.
Sanfilippo s.
SAPHO s.
scalenus anticus s.
scaphocapitate s.
scapulocostal s.
Scheie s.
Schönlein-Henoch s.
Schwartz-Jampel s. (SJS)
scimitar s.
shaken baby s. (SBS)
Sheehan s.
Shone s.
short gut s.
short rib-polydactyly s.
shoulder-hand s.
shoulder impingement s.
Shprintzen velocardiofacial s.
Shwachman s.
silent sinus s.
sinus tarsi s.

Sipple s.
Sjögren s.
slipping rib s.
slit ventricle s.
sloughed urethra s.
small aorta s.
small left colon s.
Smith-Lemli-Opitz s.
snapping hip s.
snapping triceps s.
Sneddon s.
soleus s.
solitary rectal ulcer s.
Solomon s.
Sotos s.
spastic bowel s.
Spens s.
split-cord s.
split notochord s.
stagnant-loop s.
Stauffer s.
steal s.
Stein-Leventhal s.
Stewart-Treves s.
Stickler s.
stiff lung s.
stiff man s.
Sturge-Weber s.
Sturge-Weber-Dimitri s.
superior mesenteric artery s.
  (SMAS)
superior vena cava s.
suprascapular notch s.
Swyer s.
Swyer-James s. (SJS)
Swyer-James-Macleod s.
sylvian aqueduct s.
synovitis, acne, pustulosis,
  hyperostosis, osteitis s.
systemic inflammatory response s.
TAR s.
tarsal tunnel s.
Taussig-Bing s.
Taussig-Snellen-Alberts s.
terminal reservoir s.
tethered cord s. (TCS)
thoracic inlet s.
thoracic outlet s. (TOS)
thrombocytopenia-absent radius s.
Tietze s.
tight filum terminale s.
Tolosa-Hunt s.

Torre s.
Touraine-Solente-Golé s.
transient bone marrow edema s.
Treacher Collins s.
trisomy 8 s.
trisomy D, E s.
Trousseau s.
Turcot s.
Turner s.
twiddler's s.
twin embolization s.
twin-to-twin transfusion s. (TTTS)
ulnar impaction s.
ulnar tunnel s.
ulnolunate impaction s.
uncal herniation s.
unroofed coronary sinus s.
urethral s.
VACTERL s.
van Buchem s.
Van der Hoeve s.
vanishing lung s.
vanishing testes s.
vascular leak s.
venolobar s.
venous statis s.
Verner-Morrison s.
vertebral artery s.
vertebrobasilar artery s.
vestibular aqueduct s. (VAS)
Villaret-Mackenzie s.
von Hippel-Lindau s.
Waardenburg s.
Wallenberg lateral medullary s.
Weil s.
Weill-Marchesani s.
Wermer s.
Werner s.
Wernicke-Korsakoff s.
West s.
wet lung s.
Widal s.
Wiedemann-Beckwith s.
Wilkie s.
Williams s.
Williams-Beuren s.
Williams-Campbell s.
Wilson-Mikity s.
s. with multiple cortical renal cyst
Wolff-Parkinson-White s.
Wolf-Hirschhorn s.
Wolfram s.

S

NOTES

syndrome *(continued)*
 Wyburn-Mason s.
 s. X
 XY s.
 Yunis-Varon s.
 Zellweger s.
 Zieve s.
 Zollinger-Ellison s. (ZES)
synechia, pl. **synechiae**
 uterine s.
 s. vulvae
synergic muscle
Synergy ultrasound system
syngeneic
 s. bone marrow transplant
 s. tissue
syngraft
synkinesis
synophridia
synophrys
synostosis, synosteosis, pl. **synostoses**
 bicoronal s.
 cervical s.
 congenital radioulnar s.
 coronal suture s.
 cranial s.
 craniofacial s.
 lambdoid s.
 metatarsal s.
 multiple-suture s.
 nonsyndromic bicoronal s.
 nonsyndromic unicoronal s.
 premature suture s.
 radiographically firm s.
 sagittal s.
 single suture s.
 terminal s.
 tibiofibular s.
 unicoronal s.
synostotic posterior plagiocephaly
synovectomy
 radiation s.
 radioisotope s.
 radionuclide s.
 radiopharmaceutical s.
synovial
 s. bursa
 s. cavity
 s. chondromatosis
 s. cyst
 s. diarthroidal joint
 s. diffuse lipoma
 s. envelope
 s. fluid
 s. fringe
 s. gutter
 s. hemangioma

 s. herniation pit
 s. inflammatory response
 s. ligament
 s. membrane
 s. osteochondromatosis
 s. pannus
 s. plica
 s. proliferation
 s. sarcoma
 s. sheath
 s. shelf
 s. surface
 s. thickening
 s. tissue
synoviogram
synovioma
synoviorthesis
synovitis
 s., acne, pustolosis, hyperostosis, osteitis (SAPHO)
 s., acne, pustulosis, hyperostosis, osteitis syndrome
 s. in active polymyalgia rheumatica
 boggy s.
 brucellar s.
 intraarticular localized nodular s.
 nodular s.
 pan s.
 peripheral s.
 pigmented villonodular s.
 purulent s.
 toxic s.
 transient s.
 s. tumor
synovium
 boggy s.
 exuberant s.
 hyperplastic s.
 opaque s.
 pannus of s.
synovium-filled degenerative cyst
synovium-lined fascicle
synpneumonic empyema
synspondylism
 cervical s.
synthesizer
 frequency s.
synthetic
 s. bone implant
 s. graft bypass to ankle
 s. valve
 s. vascular bypass graft
syntropy
syphilis
 bone s.
 tertiary s.

syphilitic
> s. aortic aneurysm
> s. aortic regurgitation
> s. node

syringe
> electric s.
> Isovue prefilled s.
> Isovue-370 prefilled s.
> tuberculin s.
> Ultraject prefilled s.

syringes (*pl. of* syrinx)
syringobulbia
syringocarcinoma
syringocele
syringoencephalia
syringoencephalomyelia
syringohydromyelia
> holocord s.

syringohydromyelic cavity
syringoma
> chondroid s.

syringomeningocele
syringomyelia
> ape hand of s.
> cervical s.
> Chiari-associated s.
> communicating s.
> posttraumatic s.

syringopontia
syringosubarachnoid shunting
syrinx, pl. **syringes**
> s. cavity
> central spinal cord s.
> fusiform s.
> posttraumatic central spinal cord s.
> spinal cord s.
> traumatic s.

syrup
> diet cola and metoclopramide s.

syssarcosic
syssarcosis
syssarcotic
system (*See also* device, machine, scanner, unit)
> ABBI s.
> Ablatherm HIFU s.
> AbMap electrophysiologic imaging s.
> accuDEXA bone mineral density assessment s.
> ACIST contrast delivery injection s.

Acuson 128XP ultrasound s.
Add-On Bucky image acquisition s.
Advantx-E Legacy s.
Advantx LC+ cardiovascular imaging s.
AEGIS sonography management s.
AESOP Hermes-Ready s.
Agfa ADC 70 storage phosphor s.
Agfa CR, PACS s.
air-filtration s.
AIRIS II MR s.
Alexa 1000 s.
Aloka SSD ultrasound s.
ALT ultrasound s.
American Medical Association Ligament Injury Classification S.
Amplatz Anchor S.
AneuRx bifurcated stent-graft s.
Angioflow meter s.
Angiomat 3000, 6000 contrast delivery s.
Angiomat ILLUMENA injector s.
AngioRad radiation s.
Angio-Seal s.
AngioSURF s.
anterolateral s.
aortoiliac inflow s.
Apogee CX100, CX200 echocardiography s.
Apogee RX400 diagnostic ultrasound s.
Apollo DXA bone densitometry s.
AquaSens FMS 1000 fluid monitoring s.
archival s.
arrhythmia mapping s.
arterial port catheter s.
ArthroCare Coblation-based cosmetic surgery s.
ArthroProbe laser s.
Artoscan MRI s.
Ashhurst fracture classification s.
Aspen digital ultrasound s.
Aspire continuous imaging s.
Atlas 2.0 diagnostic ultrasound s.
ATL HDI 3000, 3500, 4000, 5000 ultrasound s.
Aurora dedicated breast MRI s.
Aurora diode-based dental laser s.
automated angle-encoder s.
automated biopsy s.

S

NOTES

system *(continued)*

automated cellular imaging s. (ACIS)
automated infusion s.
autonomic nervous s.
Avera breast imaging s.
Aviva mammography s.
BAK interbody fusion s.
Bard CPS s.
Bard percutaneous cardiopulmonary support s.
BAT s.
Batson vertebral brain s.
Beta-Cath s.
Biad SPECT imaging s.
biliary s.
biograph molecular imaging s.
Biosound AU3, AU4, AU5 s.
BioSpec MR imaging s.
BioZ s.
biplane s.
BrainLAB VectorVision neuronavigation s.
Brasfield scoring s.
Breast cancer s. 2100
Breast Imaging Reporting and Data S. (BI-RADS)
Bremer Halo Crown s.
Broselow-Luten Pediatric S.
Brown-Roberts-Wells stereotactic s.
Bruker CSI Omega MR s.
BRW stereotactic s.
CAAS QCA s.
CADx SecondLook s.
caliceal s.
cardiopulmonary support s.
cardiovascular s.
cardiovascular angiography analysis s. (CAAS)
C-arm DSA s.
carrier-mediated transport s.
cartesian reference coordinate s.
CARTO EP navigation s.
cascade s.
catenary s.
CathTrack catheter locator s.
CDRPan digital x-ray s.
Cemax/Icon PACS s.
Centauri Er:YAG dental laser s.
central nervous s. (CNS)
CerASPECT s.
CGR biplane angiographic s.
Checkmate s.
Chemo-Port vascular access s.
circumflex s.
collateral s.
collecting s.

collimating s.
COMPASS stereotactic s.
Compton suppression s.
computer information s.
Computerized Thermal Imaging s.
continuous-wave Doppler ultrasound s.
continuous-wave laser s.
Cordis endovascular s.
Coroskop Plus cardiac angiography s.
Cotrel-Dubousset s.
CRYOguide ultrasound guidance s.
CryoHit tumor ablation s.
CrystalEYES video s.
Curix Capacity Plus film processing s.
CVIS information s.
CyberKnife stereotactic radiosurgery s.
Cyberware 3D scanning s.
data-acquisition s. (DAS)
data collection s.
da Vinci surgical s.
dedicated mammography s.
Delta 32 digital stereotactic s.
DELTAmanager MedImage s.
Delta 32 TACT three-dimensional breast imaging s.
detector s.
16-detector PET s.
digestive s.
Digital Add-On-Bucky radiographic detector image acquisition s.
digital chest imaging s.
Digital Equipment s.
digital holography s.
digital mammographic s.
Digital Medical S.
digital selenium-based chest imaging s.
Digital Traumex s.
Digitron digital subtraction imaging s.
DirectView CR 900 imaging s.
Discovery LS imaging s.
display s.
display coordinate s.
DOBI s.
dryer s.
DryView laser imaging s.
dual-head coincidence detection s.
duplicated renal collecting s.
3D-VIEWNIX software s.
dye laser s.
dynamic optical breast imaging s. (DOBI)

DynaRad portable x-ray s.
E.CAM dual-head emission
imaging s.
ECAT Reveal PET/CT imaging s.
Eccocee CS ultrasound s.
EchoEye ultrasound imaging s.
Eclipse MR S.
electrostatic imaging s.
Elscint Prestige MRI s.
endovascular s.
EndoVasix EPAR laser s.
EPAR laser s.
EP2000 electrophysiology
imaging s.
Evans-D'Angio staging s.
ExAblate 2000 ultrasound s.
excimer laser s.
Exogen 2000+ low-intensity,
ultrasound fracture healing s.
Explorer X70 intraoral
radiography s.
extracranial carotid s.
extrapyramidal s.
femoropopliteal s.
femtosecond laser s.
fetal musculoskeletal s.
Ficat and Axlet staging s.
fiducial alignment s.
FilmFax teleradiology s.
flexible over-wire s.
Flocks and Kadesky s.
FluoroPlus real-time digital
imaging s.
fluoroptic thermometry s.
FluoroTrak fluoroscopy-based
surgical navigation s.
flying spot excimer laser s.
FONAR Standing Ovation MRI s.
Fuji AC2 storage phosphor
computed radiology s.
Fuji FCR9000 computed
radiology s.
full-field digital mammography s.
Galen teleradiology s.
Galileo intravascular radiotherapy s.
gasless laparoscopic s.
gated s.
GE CT HiSpeed Advantage CT s.
generation 6 integrated
radiotherapy s.
generator s.
GentleLASE Plus laser s.

GE Senographe 2000D digital
mammography s.
GE Voluson 730 4D ultrasound s.
Given diagnostic imaging s.
GliaSite radiotherapy s.
gradient s.
GRASS s.
greater saphenous s.
Gyrus endourology s.
HDI 1000, 3000, 3500, 4000,
5000 ultrasound imaging s.
Helios laser s.
hepatic artery s.
hepatic ductal s.
hepatic venous s.
HERMES s.
Hewlett-Packard phased-array
ultrasound imaging s.
high-field s.
Hi-Star MRI s.
Hitachi Altaire Open MRI s.
Hitachi EUB-555 diagnostic
ultrasound s.
Hitachi four-head s.
Hitachi rotating detector array s.
homonuclear spin s.
House grading s.
HP SONOS 5500 ultrasound
echocardiography s.
Hunt and Hess aneurysm
grading s.
Hydra Vision Plus DR, ES, HP
urological imaging s.
hydrodynamic thrombectomy s.
Hyperion LTK s.
HyperPACS teleradiology s.
IDIS angiography s.
IDXrad radiology information s.
image analysis s.
image-forming s.
image intensifier s.
image recording s.
IMPAX PACS s.
implantable drug delivery s.
Indigo LaserOptic treatment s.
infrared navigational s.
InnerVasc vascular access s.
integrated clinical information s.
(ICIS)
Integris III-V DSA s.
Integris V 3000 digital
subtraction s.

S

NOTES

system *(continued)*
    intensified radiographic imaging s. (IRIS)
    internal carotid s.
    Intrabeam intraoperative radiotherapy s.
    intramedullary skeletal kinetic distractor s.
    Intra-Op autotransfusion s.
    intrarenal collecting s.
    INVOS 3100, 3100A cerebral oximeter monitoring s.
    iON IntraOperative Navigation S.
    ISKD s.
    Isocam scintillation imaging s.
    Isocam SPECT imaging s.
    Jackson staging s.
    Kadish staging s.
    Kaplan PenduLaser 115 laser s.
    Kelly-Goerss COMPASS stereotactic s.
    Kretztechnik ultrasound s.
    Krigel staging s.
    Lagios classification s.
    Laitinen CT guidance s.
    laser s.
    LaTIS endovascular laser s.
    left iliac s.
    left ventricular support s.
    Leksell stereotactic s.
    LENT scoring s.
    lesser saphenous s.
    Liebel-Flarsheim CT 9000 contrast delivery s.
    LightSpeed Ultra CT s.
    limbic s.
    linear compartmental s.
    lipophilic sequestration s.
    LocaLisa cardiac navigation s.
    LORAD full-field digital mammography s.
    lower pole collecting s.
    low-field MRI s.
    LPI laser s.
    LTX3000 lumbar rehabilitation s.
    Luxtec fiberoptic s.
    LVs s.
    LX EchoSpeed 1.5T CV/i, NVi MR s.
    LymphoScan nuclear imaging s.
    Magnes biomagnetometer s.
    Magnetic Surgery S.
    Magnetom Open s.
    Magnetom Sonata 1.5T MR s.
    Magnetom Trio 3T unlimited MRI s.
    Magnetom Vision 1.5T MR imaging s.
    Magnex Alpha MR s.
    mamillary s.
    MAMMEX TR computer-aided mammography diagnosis s.
    Mammo Plus mammography s.
    MammoReader computer-aided dectection s.
    MammoReader mammography s.
    Mammotest breast biopsy s.
    Mammotome ultrasound s.
    Manchester LDR implant s.
    Marex MRI s.
    Massachusetts (General Hospital) Utility Multiprogramming S.
    MEDDARS cardiac catheterization analysis s.
    Medilase angioscope-laser delivery s.
    Medi-tech ureteral stent s.
    Medspec MR imaging s.
    Med Tec Vac Loc immobilization s.
    Medweb clinical reporting s.
    microSelectron rapid delivery s.
    microwave cardiac ablation s.
    Mini-Balloon s.
    MIR s.
    Mitsuyasu staging s.
    Mobetron electron beam s.
    Mobetron intraoperative radiation therapy treatment s.
    mobile artery and vein imaging s. (MAVIS)
    mucosal mass collecting s.
    multicrystal BGO ring s.
    multidetector s.
    multigated pulsed Doppler flow s.
    multileaf collimating s.
    multiple-side-hole infusion s.
    Multistar Top Plus DSA s.
    musculoskeletal s.
    Navi Ball guidance s.
    Navigus cranial electrode s.
    Navitrack computer-assisted surgery s.
    nephroureteral stent s.
    NeuroLink II data acquisition s.
    NeuroSector ultrasound s.
    Nidek EC-5000 excimer laser s.
    nondilated s.
    Novacor left ventricular assist s.
    Novalis radiosurgery s.
    nuclear medicine information s.
    object coordinate s.
    OctreoScan s.

ocular magnification s.
OEC Series 9600 cardiac s.
Olympus EU-M30 s.
one-stick s.
Opdima digital mammography s.
OPD-Scan optical path difference
  scanning s.
open-architecture s.
open-configuration magnetic
  resonance s.
open MRI s.
OpenPACS s.
Opmilas 144 Plus laser s.
Optistar MR contrast delivery s.
OR1 electronic s.
OSCAR ultrasonic bone cement
  removal s.
OsteoView desktop hand x-ray s.
OsteoView 2000 digital imaging s.
Ostreg spinal marker s.
Ovation falloposcopy s.
Packard Merlin life-monitoring s.
parasympathetic nervous s.
Paris ultrasound s.
Paterson-Parker s.
Peacock s.
pelvocaliceal s.
PenRad mammography clinical
  reporting s.
Pentax-Hitachi FG32UA
  endosonographic s.
Perclose PVS suture s.
Performa mammography s.
peripheral nervous s.
PFA-100 s.
Philips DVI 1 s.
Philips Integris 5000 digital
  subtraction angiography s.
PhorMax CR desktop
  workstation s.
photoelectric s.
Photon cataract removal s.
Photon Radiosurgery S. (PRS)
Photopic Imaging ultrasound s.
Picker s.
picture archiving and
  communication s. (PACS)
Pinnacle$_3$ radiotherapy planning s.
PMT robotic fulcrumless
  tomographic s.
polar coordinate s.
polypoid fibroma collecting s.

portal vein s.
PortalVision radiation oncology s.
port-catheter s.
pressure-gradient wire s.
PrinceStar electrophysiologic
  imaging study s.
PRISM three-head s.
Probe balloon dilatation s.
Profile mammography s.
Prostalase laser s.
pulmonary venous s.
Pulse-Spray pulsed infusion s.
pyelocaliceal s.
pyramidal s.
Q-catheter catheterization
  recording s.
QCT bone densitometry s.
quadrature surface coil MRI s.
Quimby implant s.
radiation therapy s. (RTS)
radiation therapy planning s.
radioisotope delivery s. (RDS)
radiology telephone access s.
radionuclide carrier s.
RadNet radiology information s.
rapid telephone access s. (RTAS)
rature surface coil s.
RDX coronary radiation catheter
  delivery s.
real-time two-dimensional Doppler
  flow-imaging s.
Redi-Vu teleradiology s.
reference coordinate s.
Refinity Coblation S.
remote afterloading s.
renal collecting s.
respiratory s.
reticuloendothelial s.
Retzius s.
RigiScan Plus rigidity
  assessment s.
RIGS s.
ring-type imaging s.
Robson modification of Flocks-
  Kadesky s.
Rogan teleradiology s.
Roger s.
Rotablator thrombectomy s.
rotational atherectomy s.
Rotograph Plus panoramic dental
  tomography imaging s.
RPM tracking s.

NOTES

S

system *(continued)*
RTP s.
RX stent delivery s.
Sadowsky breast marking s.
SAFHS 2000 sonic accelerated
 fracture healing s.
saphenous s.
SAVANT imaging s.
Scanditronix MLC s.
scanned-slot detector s.
scanning beam digital s.
scattering s.
scavenging s.
scene coordinate s.
Scharff-Bloom-Richardson histologic
 grade s.
Schmidt optics s.
Scintiview nuclear computer s.
Scintron IV nuclear computer s.
ScleroLaser laser s.
ScleroPLUS HP laser s.
Second Look CAD s.
Selectron s.
selenium-based digital chest s.
selenium-drum-detector s.
Senographe 2000D digital
 mammography s.
Senographe DMRt mammography s.
SenoScan full field
 mammography s.
Sens-A-Ray dental imaging s.
sequestration s.
Shape Maker s.
Shimadzu HeadTome s.
side-exiting coaxial s.
side-exiting coaxial needle s.
Siemens AG s.
Siemens HICOR/BICOR x-ray s.
Siemens Somatom Plus-4 CT s.
Siemens 1.5-T s.
Signa Advantage s.
Signa Horizon LX MRI s.
Signa MR imaging s.
Silhouette laser s.
Silicon Graphics Reality Engine s.
SilkLaser aesthetic laser s.
SimpliCT interventional guidance s.
Simpson Coronary AtheroCath
 (SCA) s.
single-photon counting s.
single-stick s.
skeletal s.
slip-ring gantry s.
SmartSPOT high-resolution digital
 imaging s.
SOCRATES telementoring s.
SoftScan laser mammography s.

Somatom Volume Zoom CT s.
Sonablate 200 ultrasound s.
sonic-accelerated fracture-healing s.
 (SAFHS)
SonicWAVE phacoemulsification s.
Sonifer sonicating s.
SONOACE 6000 II ultrasound s.
SonoHeart ELITE personal hand-
 carried ultrasound s.
Sonoline Elegra ultrasound s.
SonoSite 180 ultrasound s.
spider-like pelvocaliceal s.
splanchnic venous s.
spring-driven s.
SPRINT fixed-detector research s.
Squibb s.
STARRT falloposcopy s.
steerable guide wire s.
StereoGuide prone breast biopsy s.
StereoLoc upright biopsy s.
stereotactic breast biopsy s.
storage phosphor s.
Stratis II MRI s.
Sun SPARCstation s.
Super Angiorex model G DSA s.
superconducting open-magnet s.
superconductive MR s.
Superdup'r SD6891 left heart s.
Surgical Planning and Orientation
 Computer S. (SPOCS)
Symphony MR imaging s.
Synergy ultrasound s.
systemic venous s.
TCD100M digital transcranial
 Doppler s.
Tecmag Libra-S16 s.
TEGwire ST s.
thermal dosimetry s.
three-compartment s.
three-head gamma camera-based
 SPECT s.
three-phase s.
Thrombex PMT s.
tibioperoneal runoff s.
time-of-flight PET imaging s.
Tomolex tomographic s.
Tomomatic five-slice SPECT
 imaging s.
Tomomatic three-slice SPECT
 imaging s.
Tomomatic two-slice SPECT
 imaging s.
Total Recall digital imaging s.
Transonics s.
TransScan TS2000 electrical
 impedance breast scanning s.
treatment planning s. (TMS)

Trex digital mammography s.
(TDMS)
Triad SPECT imaging s.
TRON 3 VACI cardiac imaging s.
trumpet-like pelvocaliceal s.
1.5T whole-body MR imaging s.
two-channel phased-array RF
receiver coil s.
two-compartment s.
UltraFine Erbium laser s.
UltraPACS diagnostic imaging s.
ultrasound s.
UltraSTAR computer-based
ultrasound reporting s.
UltraSure DTR-one imaging
ultrasound s.
UMC-I microwave delivery s.
University of Florida staging s.
Univision echocardiographic s.
s. unsharpness
uPACS picture archiving s.
upper pole collecting s.
USCI Probe balloon-on-a-wire
dilatation s.
Vac-Lok patient immobilization s.
vacuum cassette s.
Varian brachytherapy s.
Varian MLC s.
VasoView balloon dissection s.
VAX 4100 s.
Vbeam pulsed dye laser s.
ventricular s.
VentTrak monitoring s.
Versatome D8 Perioperative
Doppler S.
vertebral artery s.
vertebrobasilar s.
VEST s.
Viatronix, Inc. virtual
colonoscopy s.
view shadow projection
microtomographic s.
Vingmed CFM ultrasound s.
virtual retinal display s.
Virtuoso portable 3D imaging s.
Vision high-performance gradient s.
Vision MR imaging s.
VISX Star S2 excimer laser s.
VISX WaveScan Wavefront S.
Vitrea 3D s.
VNUS closure s.
VoxelView s.

widened collecting s.
xenon trap s.
Xillix LIFE-GI fluorescence
endoscopy s.
Xillix LIFE-Lung fluorescence
endoscopy s.
XKnife stereotactic radiosurgery s.
Xplorer 1000 digital imaging s.
x-ray shadow projection
microtomographic s.
Yaglazr s.
Zeus s.
Zlatkin grading s.

systematic
s. error
s. noise
s. relaxation effect
s. ultrasound-guided biopsy

systemic
s. adjuvant therapy
s. arterial circulation
s. arterial hypertension
s. arterial vasoconstriction
s. arteriolar resistance index
s. blood flow (SBF)
s. brain lymphoma
s. diastolic blood pressure
s. disorder
s. erythematosus lupus
s. granulomatous disease
s. heart
s. hypoperfusion
s. inflammatory response syndrome
s. juvenile rheumatoid arthritis
s. lesion
s. mastocytosis
s. mean arterial pressure (SMAP)
s. micrometastasis
s. nodular panniculitis
s. output
s. output flow
s. output index
s. oxygen saturation
s. sclerosis
s. vascular resistance (SVR)
s. vascular resistance index (SvO$_2$,
SVRI)
s. vein
s. venous
s. venous hypertension
s. venous return
s. venous system

S

NOTES

systole

  atrial s.
  cervical CSF s.
  CSF ventricular s.
  end s. (ES)
  end of atrial s.
  left ventricular internal dimension
    at end s. (LVIDs)
  left ventricular internal end s.
  ventricular s.

systolic

  s. acceleration time
  s. anterior motion (SAM)
  s. anterior motion of mitral valve
  s. anterior movement
  s. atrial volume
  s. ejection fraction
  s. ejection period (SEP)
  s. fractional shortening
  s. function
  s. gating

  s. gradient
  s. heart failure
  s. hypertension
  s. impulse
  left ventricular s. (LVs)
  s. mammary souffle
  s. pressure-time index
  s. prolapse
  s. prolapse of mitral valve leaflet
  s. reserve
  s. retraction
  s. retraction of apex
  s. S wave
  s. toe/brachial index
  s. upstroke time
  s. velocity ratio
  s. velocity-time integral
  s. ventricular overload

systolic-diastolic blood pressure
systolic/diastolic ratio (S/D)

γ-T
  gamma tocopherol
T
  temperature
  temporal
  tesla
  thoracic
  tocopherol
  torque
    T artifact
    T axis
    T condylar fracture
    T configuration
    T fracture
    T loop
    1.5 T Magnetom Symphony whole-
      body scanner
    3T MRI
    1.0T, 1.5T superconducting magnet
    T tubogram
    T vector
    1.5T whole-body MR imaging
      system
T1
    T1 shortening
    T1, T2 relaxation time
    T1, T2 value
T2
    T2 dephasing effect
    T2 image
    T2 PRE
    T2 proton relaxation enhancement
      (T2 PRE)
    T2 quantitative MRI
    T2 shortening
    T2 star relaxation
    T2 time constant
T-1824
T₄
  thyroxine
Tₑ
  echo train echo time
t
  transformer
T1-contamination artifact
T2-gradient refocused image
T4 uptake
Ta
  tantalum
¹⁸²Ta
  tantalum-182
¹⁷⁸Ta
  tantalum-178
Tabar pattern

tabes
    burned-out t.
    t. dorsalis
table
    binary opacity t.
    critical dose t.
    dual lookup t.
    Hydradjust IV t.
    inner t.
    MobiTrak automated t.
    MobiTrak moving t.
    t. movement
    pivoting t.
    radionuclide t.
    resistive exercise t.
    tilt t.
tabletop
    auxiliary CT t.
TACE
    transarterial chemoembolization
    transcatheter arterial chemoembolization
tachyarrhythmia
    supraventricular t.
tachycardia
    atrial ectopic automatic t.
    atrioventricular nodal reentry t.
    nodoventricular t.
    noninducible t.
    paroxysmal auricular t.
    sinoatrial nodal reentry t.
    supraventricular t.
    ventricular paroxysmal t.
tachycardia-induced cardiomyopathy
tachypnea
    transient t.
tackler's exostosis
tactile disk
TAD steerable guidewire
taenia tissue
tag
    t. of cartilage
    t. image file format (TIFF)
    t. plane
    radioactive t.
**Tagarno 3SD cine projector for
  angiography**
tagged
    t. atom
    radioactively t.
    t. red cell
tagging
    barium-based fecal t.
    bolus t.
    cine magnetic resonance t.
    t. cine magnetic resonance

T

919

tagging *(continued)*
  myocardial t.
  t. pattern
  segmented k-space cardiac t.
  spin t.
tail
  t. bone
  t. of breast
  dural t.
  t. of epididymis
  hippocampal head, body, and t.
  long dural t.
  t. of pancreas
  t. sign
  t. of Spence
  t. of the spleen
  t. vertebra
  wool t.
tailgut cyst
tail-like segment
tailored
  t. excitation
  t. pulse
tailor's
  t. ankle
  t. muscle
Takayasu
  T. aortitis
  T. arteritis
  T. disease
takeoff
  t. of artery
  t. of vessel
Talairach
  T. coordinate
  T. stereotaxic space
talar
  t. avulsion fracture
  t. beaking
  t. body fusion
  t. dome
  t. dome articular cartilage
  t. dome cyst
  t. dome fracture
  t. dome ischemia
  t. dome osteochondral injury
  t. impingement
  t. neck fracture
  t. osteochondral fracture
  t. tilt angle
talc
  t. plaque
  t. pneumoconiosis
  t. sclerotherapy
talcosis
  lung t.
  pulmonary t.

Talent stent graft
tali (*pl. of* talus)
talipes
  t. arcuatus
  t. calcaneus
  t. calcaneus calcaneocavus
  t. cavovalgus
  t. cavus
  t. cavus calcaneocavus
  t. equinovarus
  t. valgus
  t. varus
talocalcaneal
  t. angle
  anteroposterior t. (APTC)
  t. articulation
  t. coalition
  t. index
  t. index classification
  t. joint
  lateral t. (LATC)
  t. ligament
talocalcaneonavicular
  t. articulation
  t. joint
talocrural
  t. angle
  t. fusion
  t. joint
talofibular
  t. impingement
  t. joint
  t. ligament
  t. ligament injury
  posterior t. (PTF)
Talo horizontal angle
talometatarsal angle
talonavicular
  t. angle
  t. articulation
  t. beaking
  t. capsule
  t. joint
  t. ligament
talus, pl. **tali**
  beaking of head of t.
  t. bone
  Cedell fracture of t.
  congenital vertical t.
  flat-top t.
  t. foot deformity
  lateral process of the t.
  neck of t.
  Sneppen fracture of t.
  sulcus t.
  sustentaculum tali
  vertical t.

tam-o-shanter appearance
Tamp catheter
tamponade
> balloon t.
> cardiac t.
> chronic t.
> esophagogastric t.
> ferromagnetic t.
> florid cardiac t.
> full-blown cardiac t.
> heart t.
> low-pressure cardiac t.
> pericardial chyle with t.
> subacute cardiac t.

tandem
> t. applicator
> external beam with t.
> Fletcher-Suit-Delclos t.
> t. ICA/MCA occlusion
> t. lesion
> MIR intrauterine t.
> t. and ovoid
> t. stent
> t. technique
> t. transplant

tangential
> t. breast field
> t. constriction
> t. cut
> t. layer of hand
> t. port
> t. projection
> t. scapular view

tangentially
tangle
> intraneuronal neurofibrillary t.
> neurofibrillary t.

tanned red cell (TRC)
tannex
> bisacodyl t.

tantalate
> lutetium t.

tantalum (Ta)
> t. bronchogram
> t. imaging agent
> t. mesh
> t. powder
> t. stent
> t. tracer

tantalum-178 (^{178}Ta)
> t. contrast medium

tantalum-182 (^{182}Ta)

taper
> fiberoptic t.

tapered
> t. core guidewire
> t. finger

tapered-tip guidewire
tapering
> t. border
> t. dose
> t. occlusion
> t. stenosis

tapetal
tapetoretinal dysplasia
tapetum
tapeworm
tapiroid
tapir's mouth
TAPVD
> total anomalous pulmonary venous
> drainage

TAPVR
> total anomalous pulmonary venous return

TAR
> tissue-air ratio
> TAR syndrome

tar
> coal t.

tarda
> osteogenesis imperfecta t.

tardive
tardus-parvus waveform
target
> angiographic t.
> t. appearance
> t. arch
> t. bone
> t. calcification
> t. canal
> t. coalition
> t. depth
> 3D reconstructed t.
> gas t.
> internal cyclotron t.
> t. lung lesion
> t. material
> metal technetium t.
> minimal deformation t. (MDT)
> molybdenum t.
> t. navicular
> t. organ
> t. parenchymal structure
> t. point

NOTES

target *(continued)*
    retrogasserian t.
    t. sign
    t. tissue
    tungsten t.
targeted
    t. contrast agent
    t. EIS
target-film distance (TFD)
target-filter combination
targeting
    angiographic t.
    t. bead
    B-mode acquisition and t. (BAT)
targetoid growth
target-skin distance (TSD)
target-to-background ratio
target-to-nontarget
    t.-t.-n. ratio
    t.-t.-n. ratio for myocardial imaging
Tarlov cyst
TARP
    total atrial refractory period
Tarrant position
tarsal
    t. arch
    t. bone
    t. canal
    t. coalition
    t. cyst
    t. joint
    t. ligament
    t. navicular
    t. plate
    t. sinus
    t. tunnel
    t. tunnel syndrome
tarsoepiphyseal aclasis
tarsometatarsal
    t. angle
    t. articulation
    t. joint
    t. ligament
tartrate
    thorium t.
task
    block motor t.
task-rest pattern
taurodontism
TAUS
    transabdominal ultrasound
Taussig-Bing
    T.-B. anomaly
    T.-B. congenital malformation of
    heart
    T.-B. syndrome
Taussig-Snellen-Alberts syndrome

tautography
taut pericardial effusion
TAV
    transcutaneous aortovelography
Taveras injector
Tawara atrioventricular node
Taylor-Blackwood mechanism
Taylor position
TB
    tuberculosis
      HIV-related TB
TBI
    tracheobronchial injury
    traumatic brain injury
TBNA
    transbronchial needle aspiration
TBT
    transcervical balloon tuboplasty
TBV
    total brain volume
TBW
    total body water
TC
    thoracic circumference
Tc
    technetium
^{99m}Tc, Tc-99m
    technetium-99m
      ^{99m}Tc aggregated albumin imaging
      agent
      ^{99m}Tc albumin colloid imaging
      agent
      ^{99m}Tc albumin microspheres
      imaging agent
      ^{99m}Tc biciromab imaging agent
      ^{99m}Tc bicisate imaging agent
      ^{99m}Tc Ceretec
      ^{99m}Tc Ceretec bind
      denatured ^{99m}Tc-RBC
      ^{99m}Tc depreotide
      ^{99m}Tc depreotide scintigraphy
      ^{99m}Tc dimer captosuccinic acid
      imaging agent
      ^{99m}Tc disofenin imaging agent
      ^{99m}Tc-DMSA scintigraphy
      ^{99m}Tc ECD
      ^{99m}Tc-ECD radiopharmaceutical
      ^{99m}Tc exametazime imaging agent
      ^{99m}Tc furifosmin imaging agent
      ^{99m}Tc galactosyl human serum
      albumin imaging agent
      ^{99m}Tc glucarate imaging agent
      ^{99m}Tc gluceptate imaging agent
      ^{99m}Tc glucoheptanoate
      ^{99m}Tc-GSA imaging agent
      heat-damaged ^{99m}Tc-RBC

^{99m}Tc hexamethylpropylene amine oxime
^{99m}Tc-HIG scintigraphy
^{99m}Tc HMPAO
^{99m}Tc-HMPAO cerebral perfusion SPECT imaging
^{99m}Tc-HMPAO hyperfixation
^{99m}Tc HMPAO-labeled leukocyte total-body scan
^{99m}Tc-HMPAO radiopharmaceutical
^{99m}Tc-HMPAO radiotracer
^{99m}Tc-HMPAO SPECT
^{99m}Tc-HMPAO uptake
^{99m}Tc HSA
^{99m}Tc human polyclonal immunoglobulin G scintigraphy
^{99m}Tc human serum albumin imaging agent
^{99m}Tc human serum albumin scintigraphy
^{99m}Tc-iminodiacetic acid derivative radiopharmaceutical
^{99m}Tc-labeled anti-E-selectin Fab fragment
^{99m}Tc-labeled antigranulocyte antibody
^{99m}Tc-labeled cerebral perfusion imaging agent
^{99m}Tc-labeled denatured autologous RBC imaging
^{99m}Tc-labeled iminodiacetic acid
^{99m}Tc-labeled ligand
^{99m}Tc-labeled macroaggregated albumin scan
^{99m}Tc-labeled phosphate analog
^{99m}Tc-labeled RBC
^{99m}Tc-labeled somatostatin
^{99m}Tc-labeled WBC
^{99m}Tc-labeled white blood cell scintigraphy
^{99m}Tc lidofenin imaging agent
^{99m}Tc MAA
^{99m}Tc-MAA rhinoscintigraphy
^{99m}Tc-MAG3 radiopharmaceutical
^{99m}Tc-MDP skeletal scintigram
^{99m}Tc-MDP uptake
^{99m}Tc mebrofenin imaging agent
^{99m}Tc medronate imaging agent
^{99m}Tc mercaptoacetythiglycine
^{99m}Tc mertiatide imaging agent
^{99m}Tc methoxyisobutylisonitrile scintigraphy

^{99m}Tc-MIBI radiopharmaceutical
^{99m}Tc microaggregated albumin imaging agent
^{99m}Tc Myoview myocardial perfusion imaging
^{99m}Tc-N-NOEt neutral myocardial perfusion imaging agent
^{99m}Tc-labeled octreotide
^{99m}Tc oxidronate imaging agent
^{99m}Tc pentetate calcium trisodium imaging agent
^{99m}Tc pentetate sodium imaging agent
^{99m}Tc pertechnetate thyroid
^{99m}Tc phosphate
^{99m}Tc polyphosphate compound radiopharmaceutical
^{99m}Tc polyphosphate imaging agent
^{99m}Tc-PYP
^{99m}Tc-PYP scintigraphy
^{99m}Tc pyrophosphate
^{99m}Tc pyrophosphate imaging agent
^{99m}Tc red blood cell SPECT
^{99m}Tc sestamibi
^{99m}Tc sestamibi imaging agent
^{99m}Tc sodium pertechnetate imaging agent
^{99m}Tc succimer imaging agent
^{99m}Tc sulfur colloid
^{99m}Tc sulfur colloid imaging agent
^{99m}Tc-tagged RBC
^{99m}Tc teboroxime imaging agent
^{99m}Tc tetrofosmin imaging agent
^{99m}Tc (V) DMSA
^{99m}Tc (V) DMSA scanning
^{99m}Tc WBC scan

TCA
  tentorium cerebelli attachment
  transcondylar axis
TCAT
  transmission computer-assisted tomography
TCBF
  total cerebral blood flow
TCC
  transitional cell carcinoma
TCCS
  transcranial color-coded duplex sonography
TCD
  transcranial Doppler
  transverse cerebellar diameter

T

NOTES

TCD (*continued*)
    TCD measurement
    TCD sonography
    TCD ultrasound
    TCD velocity
TCD100M digital transcranial Doppler system
TCD-detectable turbulence
^{99m}Tc-DTPA
    technetium-99m diethylenetriamine pentaacetic acid
T-cell
    T.-c. acute lymphoblastic leukemia
    T.-c. lymphoblastic lymphoma
    T.-c. neoplasm
    T.-c.-type acute lymphoblastic leukemia
T4-cell
^{99m}Tc-ethyl cysteinate dimer (EDC)
TCF
    time correlation function
TcHIDA
^{99m}Tc-labeled
    technetium-99m-labeled
Tc-labeled red blood cell scintigraphy
Tc-99m (*var. of* ^{99m}Tc)
TcO^{4-}
    technetium pertechnetate
TcO$_4$
    TcO$_4$ MIBI subtraction scintigraphy
    TcO$_4$ thyroid scan
T-configuration
TCP/IP
    transmission control protocol/Internet protocol
tcPO$_2$
    transcutaneous oxygen pressure measurement
TCS
    tethered cord syndrome
    total calcium score
TCT900S helical CT scanner
TD
    transition delay
    trigger delay
TDD
    teardrop distance
TDE
    two-dimensional echocardiography
TDE-derived epsilonþ and epsilonm
TDLU
    terminal ductal lobular unit
TDMS
    Trex digital mammography system
TE
    echo delay time
    echo time

thromboembolic
time delay between excitation and echo maximum
tracheoesophageal
    TE fistula
teacup
    t. breast calcification
    t. fracture
teacup-shaped calcification
Teale amputation
tear
    anular t.
    attritional t.
    Bateman classification of full-thickness t.'s
    bowstring t.
    bucket-handle meniscus t.
    buttonhole t.
    cleavage t.
    complete t.
    concentric anular t.
    degenerative horizontal cleavage t.
    dural t.
    entry t.
    esophageal t.
    fishtail t.
    flap t.
    full-thickness t.
    high-grade partial t.
    iatrogenic dural t.
    interstitial meniscal t.
    intimal t.
    intrasubstance cleavage t.
    Johnson-Jahss classification of posterior tibial tendon t.
    ligament t.
    Mallory-Weiss esophageal t.
    Mallory-Weiss mucosal t.
    meniscus t.
    mesenteric t.
    micro t.
    parrot-beak labral t.
    parrot-beak meniscus t.
    partial bursal surface t.
    partial thickness split t.
    peripheral meniscocapsular t.
    posterior longitudinal ligament t.
    quadriceps tendon t.
    radial anular t.
    radial split t.
    rectal t.
    rotator cuff t.
    serosal t.
    SLAP t.
    stellate t.
    superimposed acute partial t.

superior labral anterior to
  posterior t.
tendon t. (types I–IV)
teres minor tendon t.
tibial tendon t.
transverse anular t.
traumatic aortic t.
tricorn bucket-handle t.
vertical split nondetached t.

teardrop
  t. appearance
  t. bladder
  t. burst fracture
  t. distance (TDD)
  t. heart
  t. pelvic anatomy
  t. ventriculomegaly

teardrop-shaped
  t.-s. flexion-compression fracture
  t.-s. lesion

tearing
  plaque t.

teat
  pyloric t.

teboroxime
  t. cardiac scan
  t. imaging agent
  t. resting washout (TRW)

TEC-2100 postioning laser
Technegas
Techneplex imaging agent
techneScan
  t. Gluceptate
  T. HDP, MAA, MAG3, PYP
    imaging agent
  T. HIDA
  T. MDP
  T. Sulfur Colloid

technetium (Tc)
  t. albumin study
  hydrolyzed t.
  t. imaging agent
  t. polyphosphonate
  t. stannous pyrophosphate
  t. stannous pyrophosphate imaging
  t. Tc 99m pyrophosphate imaging
  t. Tc99m venography

technetium-99m (^{99m}Tc, Tc-99m)
  t. albumin microsphere
  t. antibody labeling
  t. anti-CEA Fab murine
    monoclonal antibody imaging

t. antimony trisulfide colloid
t. antimyosin Fab fragment
t. depreotide
t. dextran
t. diethylenetriamine pentaacetic
  acid (^{99m}Tc-DTPA)
t. dimer captosuccinic acid
t. disofenin
t. DMSA, DTPA
t. DTPA aerosol
t. ethyl cysteinate dimer
t. etidronate
t. ferpentetate
t. generator
t. heat-denatured erythrocyte
t. heat-denatured RBC splenic
  scintigraphy
t. hepatoiminodiacetic acid scan
t. Hepatolite
t. hexamethylpropylene amine
  oxime
t. HMPAO mixed leukocyte
  LeukoScan
t. human albumin microsphere
t. human immune globulin
t. IDA analog
t. Infecton imaging
t. iron-ascorbate-DTPA
t. isonitriles radiopharmaceutical
^{99m} t. L-ethyl cysteinate dimer
  (^{99m}Tc ECD)
t. leukocyte
t. MAG3 renography
t. mercaptoacetyltriglycine
t. mertiatide
t. methoxyisobutylisonitrile
  scintimammography
t. minimicroaggregated albumin
t. minimicroaggregated albumin
  colloid
t. nanocolloid
t. pertechnetate GI bleed
t. pertechnetate sodium
t. phytate scan
t. PIPIDA
sestamibi t.
t. sestamibi dual-phase technique
t. sestamibi parathyroid
t. siboroxime
t. somatostatin analog SPECT

T

NOTES

technetium-99m (continued)
  t. sulfur colloid GI bleed
  t. tetrofosmin exercise-rest SPECT
    myocardial perfusion imaging
  t. (V) DMSA scintigraphy
technetium-99m-labeled (^{99m}Tc-labeled)
technetium-sulfur colloid
technetium-tagged
  t.-t. Cardiolite
  t.-t. RBC labeling
  t.-t. red blood cell
technetium-thallium subtraction imaging
Technicare
  T. camera
  T. Delta 2020 scanner
technique
  acquisition t.
  add-on t.
  adiabatic fast scanning t.
  AEC t.
  afterloading t.
  air-gap t.
  algebraic reconstruction t. (ART)
  Amplatz t.
  antialiasing t.
  antiradial t.
  autoradiographic t.
  axial multiplanar reformation t.
  background subtraction t.
  balanced-gradient t.
  bayesian t.
  best-guess t.
  black blood t.
  blended beam t.
  bolus chase t.
  bougienage t.
  brain surface matching t.
  bread loaf t.
  breast mammographic t.
  breath-hold t.
  Brown-Roberts-Wells t.
  bull's eye t.
  cardiovascular imaging t.
  catheter-securing t.
  cerebral flow image t.
  chemical shift imaging t.
  chemical shift selective
    suppression t.
  chromatographic-fluorometric t.
  computer subtraction t.
  concentric circle t.
  contralateral subtraction t.
  contrast-enhanced CT with saline
    flush t.
  coronal oblique t.
  Cr-chromate-labeled red cell t.
  cress-correlation t.

Cr-labeled red blood cell t.
cross-correlation t.
cut-film t.
2D t.
3D t.
deblurring t.
deconvolution t.
dephase-rephase magnitude
  subtraction t.
depth-pulse t.
destructive interference t.
3D gradient echo acquisition t.
digital subtraction t.
diskographic t.
2D multiplanar reformatted t.
DNA microinjection t.
double-contrast t.
double-freeze t.
double-umbrella t.
double-wire atherectomy t.
drip infusion t.
driven equilibrium Fourier
  transform t.
2D time-of-flight t.
dual-isotope subtraction t.
3D volume t.
3D volume-rendering t.
dye injection t.
dynamic bolus tracking t.
echo-tagging t.
ejection fraction by first-pass t.
Eklund t.
endofluoroscopic t.
endovascular t.
enzyme-multiplied immunoassay t.
Epistar perfusion t.
equilibrium radionuclide
  angiocardiography t.
esophageal balloon t.
exclusion-HPLC t.
external looping t.
FAST t.
fast-FLAIR t.
Fast Imaging Employing Steady-
  State Acquisition t.
fat-suppressed T2-weighted FSE t.
fat suppression t.
field-fitting t.
FIESTA imaging t.
first-pass t.
FLAK t.
flow cytometry t.
flow mapping t.
fluoroscopic pushing t.
fluoroscopic road-mapping t.
four-field t.
Fourier-acquired steady state t.

Fourier imaging t.
FRODO t.
FSPGR t.
full-column t.
gadolinium-enhanced venographic t.
gated inflow t.
graded compression sonography t.
gradient-echo cine t.
gradient-echo recall t.
grasping t.
GRE t.
grid t.
Grüntzig PTCA t.
guidewire exchange t.
half-Fourier three-dimensional t.
half-Fourier transformation t.
half-wedged field t.
Hampton t.
hanging-block t.
HARC-C wavelet compression t.
helical t.
high-kV t.
high-resolution bone algorithm t.
hybridization-subtraction t.
hybrid subtraction t.
immersion t.
inhalation t.
intercomparison measurement t.
interleaved phase contrast t.
intraoperative scanning t.
intravascular MRI catheter-based t.
inverse radiotherapy t.
inversion-recovery t.
Judkins t.
jugular t.
kinematic MR t.
kissing atherectomy t.
kissing-balloon t.
Klein t.
large-core t.
loading t.
localization t.
low-angle shot t.
low-dose film mammographic t.
low-dose screen-film t.
magnetic resonance hydrographic t.
magnetization transfer t.
mammographic t.
mammography t.
Markov chain Monte Carlo t.
Monte Carlo t.

motion artifact suppression t. (MAST)
moving table t.
MPGR t.
MP-RAGE t.
MSCT t.
multiline scanning t.
multimodal image fusion t.
multiphasic multislice MRI t.
multiphasic multislice spin-echo imaging t.
multislice spin-echo t.
navigator echo motion correction t.
nonaxial beam t.
noncoplanar arc t.
noncoplanar arch t.
noncoplanar beam t.
noninvasive t.
packing, extraction, and calculation t.
Papillon t.
partial flip-angle fast-scan t.
partial Fourier t.
partial saturation t.
percutaneous retrograde transfemoral t.
percutaneous transluminal coronary recanalization t.
perfusion measurement t.
pinhole t.
point-resolved spectroscopy localization t.
presaturation t.
pressure-controlled intermittent coronary occlusion t.
pressure half-time t.
projection-reconstruction t.
pulsed-gradient spin-echo t.
pulse-echo t.
pulse-spray t.
quantitative imaging t.
radial t.
radiopharmaceutical volume-dilution t.
radiotracer t.
rapid pull-through t. (RPT)
rapid scan t.
rapid thoracic compression t.
RARE t.
ray casting t.
recanalization t.
region of interest imaging t.

NOTES

technique *(continued)*
  reimplantation t.
  relaxation enhancement t.
  remodeling t.
  respiratory triggered fast SE t.
  road-mapping t.
  robust registration t.
  rotational therapy t.
  sandwich t.
  saturation recovery t.
  scanning t.
  scintillation counting t.
  screening t.
  Seldinger percutaneous t.
  semiquantitative t.
  sequential extraction-radiotracer t.
  serial cut film t.
  silhouette t.
  single-field hyperthermia t.
  single fill/void t.
  single-needle biopsy t.
  single-sample t.
  single-shot imaging t.
  SL t.
  sliding thin-slab minimum intensity projection t.
  Sones cineangiography t.
  SPAMM t.
  spin-echo t.
  spin-label t.
  spin-lock imaging t.
  spiral echo-planar t.
  spiral scanning t.
  split-course t.
  SPOP t.
  stacked-foil t.
  step-and-shoot t.
  stereotactic automated t.
  stimulated echo-tagging t.
  STIR t.
  storage phosphor-based t.
  streptavidin peroxidase t.
  subclavian turndown t.
  subtraction t.
  supervoltage t.
  surface matching t.
  Swiss roll t.
  tandem t.
  technetium-99m sestamibi dual-phase t.
  Tesla system imaging t.
  test bolus t.
  three-point Dixon t.
  time-of-flight t.
  tissue characterization t.
  tourniquet t.
  transcatheter t.

  transgluteal CT-guided t.
  trephine t.
  triple pass t.
  trocar-cannula t.
  turbo spin-echo t.
  two-balloon t.
  two-needle biopsy t.
  two-step t.
  upgated t.
  ureteral compression t.
  in vivo t.
  volume rendering t.
  volumetric mapping t.
  water-suppression t.
  wedged-pair t.
  Welin t.
  xeroradiographic t.
technology
  acoustic response t.
  adaptive focusing t. (AFT)
  amorphous silicon filmless digital x-ray detection t.
  ARTMA virtual patient t.
  CellSeek t.
  computer automated scan t. (CAST)
  fused image t.
  noncontact imaging t.
  radiologic t.
  single breath-hold dynamic subtraction CT with multidetector row helical t.
  slip-ring t.
  ultrasound imaging t.
Technovit 7210 VLC contact glue
Techtides
Tecmag
  T. Libra-S16 system
  T. Libra-S16 system scanner
tecta (*pl. of* tectum)
tectal
  t. beaking
  t. cyst
  t. glioma
  t. lesion
  t. plate
tectocerebellar dysraphia
tectoral ligament
tectospinal tract
tectum, pl. **tecta**
  t. commissure
TED
  thromboembolic disease
TEDE
  total effective dose equivalent
Tedlar bag

TEE
> transesophageal echocardiography

teeth
>> connate t.
>> floating t.
>> Hutchinson t.
>> incisor t.
>> milk t.
>> molar t.
>> premolar t.
>> primary t.
>> secondary t.
>> supernumerary t.
>> wisdom t.

TEF
> tracheoesophageal fistula

Teflon
>> T. catheter
>> T. fascial dilator
>> T. probe

Teflon-coated guidewire

tegmental tract

tegmentum
>> t. of brainstem
>> medullary t.
>> midbrain t.
>> t. of pons
>> pontine t.

tegmen tympani

TEGwire ST system

Teichholz
>> T. ejection fraction
>> T. equation
>> T. equation for left ventricular volume

TEK
> total exchangeable potassium

T1EL
> type I endoleak

T2EL
> type II endoleak

tela choroidea

telangiectasia
>> ataxia t.
>> t. brain capillary
>> capillary t.
>> Osler-Weber-Rendu t.
>> pulmonary t.
>> Sturge-Weber t.

telangiectasis
>> bilateral juxtafoveal t.

telangiectatic
>> t. angioma
>> t. carcinoma
>> t. fibroma
>> t. lesion
>> t. osteogenic sarcoma
>> t. osteosarcoma
>> t. vessel

telangiectaticum

Telebrix contrast medium

telecobalt
>> t. therapy

telecollaboration surgery

telecord

telecurietherapy

telefluoroscopy

telemammography

telemetry

telencephalic
>> t. malformation
>> t. ventriculofugal artery

telencephalon

TelePACS

Telepaque imaging agent

teleradiogram

teleradiography

teleradiology
>> diagnostic t.
>> referral t.
>> t. videoconferencing

teleradium therapy

teleroentgenogram

teleroentgenography

teleroentgentherapy

telescopic
>> t. aerial dilator
>> t. bougie set

teletherapy
>> C-60 t.
>> t. radiotherapy

telognosis

telomere repeat amplification protocol

Telos radiographic stress device

Temno II cutting needle

Temp
>> T. Tip drainage catheter
>> T. Tip ureteral stent

temperature (T)
>> t. distribution measurement
>> firing t.
>> mean perfusate t.

NOTES

temperature *(continued)*
    Neel t.
    t. sensor
template
    deformable t.
    Syed t.
    Syed-Neblett t.
Tempofilter vena cava filter
temporal (T)
    t. aliasing
    t. artery
    t. artery tap maneuver
    t. average intensity
    t. bone
    t. bone anatomy
    t. bone fracture
    t. bone sclerosis
    t. bone tomogram
    t. bone tumor
    t. canal
    t. diameter
    t. filter
    t. fossa
    t. granulomatous arteritis
    t. gyrus
    t. horn
    t. horn atrophy
    t. horn of lateral ventricle
    t. instability artifact
    t. isthmus
    t. limb of the anterior commissure
    t. lobe
    t. lobe epilepsy (TLE)
    t. lobe herniation
    t. lobe infarct
    t. lobe lesion
    t. lobe tumor
    t. meningioma
    t. orientation
    t. peak (TP)
    t. peak intensity
    t. phase delay
    t. plane
    t. pole
    t. predominance
    t. process
    t. resolution
    t. sawtooth pattern
    t. smoothing
    t. space infection
    t. sulcus
    t. suture
temporalis muscle
temporally
temporary
    t. atrial pacing wire

    t. interstitial implant
    t. pacing catheter
temporoinsular astrocytoma
temporomalar suture
temporomandibular
    t. joint (TMJ)
    t. joint arthrography
    t. joint destruction
    t. joint disk
    t. joint osteolysis
    t. ligament
temporooccipital
    t. artery
    t. glioma
    t. junction
temporoparietooccipital junction
temporopontine tract
temporozygomatic suture
TENa
    total exchangeable sodium
Tenckhoff catheter
tenderness
    skin-rolling scapular t.
tendineae
    ruptured chordae t.
tendines (*pl. of* tendo)
tendinitis (*var. of* tendonitis)
tendinopathy
    patellar t.
tendinosis
    angiofibroblastic t.
    common extensor t.
    patellar t.
    supraspinatus t.
tendinous
    t. attachment
    t. band
    t. insertion
    t. part of epicranius muscle
    t. raphe
tendo, pl. **tendines**
    t. Achilles
    t. calcaneus
tendo-Achilles bursa
tendon
    abductor digiti quinti t.
    abductor hallucis t.
    abductor pollicis brevis t.
    abductor pollicis longus t.
    accessory communicating t.
    Achilles t.
    adductor hallucis t.
    adductor pollicis brevis t.
    adherent profundus t.
    anchoring t.
    anterior tibial t.
    t. aponeurosis

aponeurotic t.
t. attenuation
attrition rupture of t.
biceps brachialis t.
biceps brachii t.
biceps femoris t.
bicipital t.
bifid biceps t.
boomerang t.
bowing of t.
brachialis t.
brachial plexus t.
brachioradialis t.
brevis t.
calcaneal t.
carpi radialis brevis t.
carpi radialis longus t.
central perineal t.
common t.
conjoined t.
coronary t.
cricoesophageal t.
digital extensor t.
digital flexor t.
digiti quinti proprius t.
elbow extensor t.
extensor carpi radialis brevis t.
extensor carpi radialis longus t.
extensor carpi ulnaris t.
extensor digiti minimi t.
extensor digiti quinti t.
extensor digitorum brevis t.
extensor digitorum communis t.
extensor digitorum longus t.
extensor hallucis longus t.
extensor indicis proprius t.
extensor pollicis brevis t.
extensor pollicis longus t.
extensor quinti t.
flexor carpi radialis t.
flexor carpi ulnaris t.
flexor digitorum communis t.
flexor digitorum longus t.
flexor digitorum profundus t.
flexor digitorum sublimis t.
flexor digitorum superficialis t.
flexor hallucis brevis t.
flexor hallucis longus t.
flexor pollicis brevis t.
flexor pollicis longus t.
flexor profundus t.
flexor sublimis t.

gastrocnemius t.
gastrocnemius-soleus t.
Golgi t.
goose foot t.
gracilis t.
hamstring t.
t. of Hector
heel t.
hilus of t.
iliopsoas t.
t. inflammation
infrapatellar t.
infraspinatus t.
interosseous t.
t. irregularity
t. laceration
long head biceps t.
longitudinal split biceps t.
longitudinal tear of the brevis t.
lumbrical t.
membranaceous t.
midpatellar t.
t. nodularity
t. nodule
obturator internus t.
palmaris longus t.
patellar t.
patelloquadriceps t.
peroneal brevis t.
peroneal longus t.
peroneus brevis t.
peroneus longus t.
peroneus tertius t.
plantaris t.
t. plate
pollicis longus t.
popliteal t.
popliteus t.
posterior tibial t. (PTT)
profundus t.
pronator teres t.
proprius t.
quadriceps t.
rectus femoris t.
rider's t.
t. rupture
sartorius t.
semimembranosus t.
semitendinosus t.
t. sheath
t. sheath giant cell tumor
t. sheath space infection

T

NOTES

tendon *(continued)*
 t. sheath stenosis
 t. sheath thickening
 t. shortening
 t. sling
 slip of t.
 slipped t.
 split anterior tibial t. (SPLATT)
 sublimis t.
 t. subluxation
 subscapularis t.
 superficialis t.
 superficial palmaris longus t.
 supraspinatus t.
 t. tear (types I–IV)
 thumb extensor t.
 thumb flexor t.
 tibial t.
 tibialis anterior t.
 tibialis posterior t.
 t. tissue
 toe extensor t.
 triceps brachii t.
 t. of Zinn
tendonitis, tendinitis
 calcific t.
 popliteal t.
tendonosis
tendon-to-bone attachment
tendosynovial sarcoma
tenesmus
tennis
 t. elbow
 t. leg
 t. shoulder
 t. toe
tenocyte hyperplasia
tenodesis
 band t.
tenography
tenonavicular
tenosynovial osteochondromatosis
tenosynovitis
 flexor t.
 LHBT t.
 peroneal t.
 stenosing t.
 tibialis posterior t.
 tuberculous t.
tense fontanelle
tensile
 t. force
 t. injury
tension
 t. cyst
 diffusion t. (DT)
 t. endothorax

 epicardial t.
 t. fracture
 intraventricular systolic t.
 t. pneumothorax
tension-time index (TTI)
tensor
 diffusion t. (DT)
 t. diffusion-weighted MR image
 t. fasciae latae
 t. tympani
 t. veli palatini muscle
tented up
tenth-value layer
tenting
 baseline t.
 t. of diaphragm
 t. of hemidiaphragm
tentorial
 t. edge
 t. meningioma
 t. notch herniation
 t. ridge
 t. traversal
tentorium
 t. cerebelli
 t. cerebelli attachment (TCA)
 t. keyhole configuration
TER
 thermal enhancement ratio
 time of formation of RF spin-echo when
  adjusted to be different from gradient
  spin-echo
teratoblastoma of ovary
teratocarcinoma
 mediastinum t.
 t. of ovary
 pineal gland t.
teratogenic effect
teratogenicity of contrast agent
teratoid
 t. mediastinum
 t. tumor
teratoma, pl. **teratomata**
 atypical brain t.
 benign t.
 cardiac t.
 CNS t.
 cystic t.
 embryonal ovary t.
 immature ovarian t.
 malignant t.
 mature mediastinum t.
 mature ovarian cystic t.
 mediastinum t.
 neck t.
 orbital t.
 ovarian systic t.

pineal t.
solid ovarian t.
spinal t.
suprasellar atypical t.
testicular t.
teratomatous mass
teres
ligamentum t.
t. major
t. minor
t. minor tendon tear
pronator t. (PT)
terminad
terminal
t. air sac
t. airspace
t. aorta
t. bile duct
t. bronchiole
t. carcinoma
t. cistern
t. crest
t. ductal lobular unit (TDLU)
t. edema
t. head
t. ileitis
t. ileum
t. inversion
t. pneumonia
t. reservoir syndrome
t. segment of posterior cerebral
artery
t. synostosis
t. thrombosis
t. tuft
t. tuft resorption
t. ventricle
t. web
t. zone of the Yakolev
terminale
fatty filum t.
filum t.
os t.
persistent ossiculum t.
tight filum t.
terminalis
cistern of lamina t.
terminatio, pl. **terminationes**
termination
early-phase t.
late-phase t.

t. site
underdrive t.
terminus
duodenal t.
intrapapillary t.
rostral t.
terrestrial radiation
territory
posterior circulation t.
Terry Thomas sign
tertiary
t. collimation
t. hyperparathyroidism (tHPT)
t. hypothyroidism
t. sequestrum
t. syphilis
t. wave
Terumo guidewire
tesla (T)
t. field
T. magnetic resonance imager
T. superconductive magnet unit
T. system imaging technique
Teslascan
tessellated
test (*See* testing)
abduction stress t.
acetazolamide vasodilator t.
Alcock t.
aluminum ion breakthrough t.
attached proton t. (APT)
axial manual traction t.
t. balloon occlusion
balloon occlusion tolerance t.
Barlow hip instability t.
t. bolus
bolus challenge t.
t. bolus technique
chlormerodrin accumulation t.
^{14}C lactose breath t.
coin t.
colorimetric t.
conglutinating complement
absorption t.
contraction stress t. (CST)
costoclavicular t.
Dicopac t.
dipyridamole handgrip t.
duplex screening t.
dye reduction spot t.
exercise tolerance t. (ETT)
fat absorption t.

NOTES

test (*continued*)
 fetal stress t.
 film screen contact t.
 flat-hand t.
 gallbladder function t.
 gastrointestinal protein loss t.
 Heaf t.
 t. injection
 internal carotid balloon t.
 intrinsic field uniformity t.
 Kruskal-Wallis t.
 Leclercq t.
 Linsman water t.
 log-rank t.
 lung connectivity t.
 McMurray t.
 t. meal
 Mecholyl t.
 molybdenum-99 breakthrough t.
 Moschcowitz t.
 Müller t.
 NMR LipoProfile t.
 nonstress t. (NST)
 nonstress fetal t.
 O'Connor finger dexterity t.
 Ortolani t.
 Osteo-Gram bone density t.
 pelvic steal t.
 perchlorate washout t.
 peritoneal-venous shunt patency t.
 positive washout t.
 pulmonary function t.
 quadriceps femoris tendon reflex t.
 radioactive renogram t.
 radioimmunoprecipitation t.
 radioiodine t.
 radioisotope renogram t.
 RAILL t.
 Seidlitz powder t.
 sestamibi ^{99m}Tc with dipyridamole
  stress t.
 Sharp-Purser t.
 Shirmer t.
 Smith orthogonal hole t.
 sniff t.
 Spearman rank t.
 spinning-top t.
 star-cancellation t. (SCT)
 stop t.
 Triboulet t.
 triple-marker screening t.
 t. tube structure
 ultrasound t.
 ultrasound dilution t.
 ureteral perfusion t.
 USP XX t.
 vasodilatory hemodynamic stress t.

 washout t.
 Wetzel t.
 Whitaker t.
 Whitfield t.
 Wilcoxon signed-rank t.
 Yergason t.
testes (*pl. of* testis)
testicle
 undescended t.
testicular
 t. abscess
 t. adrenal rest tissue
 t. appendage torsion
 t. artery
 t. artery avulsion
 t. carcinoma
 t. choriocarcinoma
 t. cyst
 t. cystic lesion
 t. degeneration
 t. ectopia
 t. feminization
 t. gland
 t. infarct
 t. ischemia
 t. metastasis
 t. microlithiasis
 t. parenchyma
 t. posttraumatic edema
 t. relapse
 t. rupture
 t. seminoma
 t. stromal cell tumor
 t. teratoma
 t. torsion appendage
 t. trauma
 t. tubular adenoma
 t. vein
 t. vein embolization
 t. venography
testiculoma
testing (*See* test)
 bronchial provocation t.
 Doppler ultrasound segmental blood
  pressure t.
 nuclear gated blood pool t.
 perimetry t.
 pyrogen t.
 radiation sensitivity t.
testis, pl. **testes**
 appendix t.
 burned-out tumor of t.
 t. carcinoma
 dilated rete t.
 t. dysfunction
 t. dysplasia
 echo-poor t.

ectopic t.
efferent ductule of t.
t. fracture
t. germ cell tumor
hypoechoic t.
infarcted t.
maldescended t.
malpositioned t.
mediastinum t.
occult primary tumor of t.
rete t.
retractile t.
torsed t.
torsion of t.
tubular ectasia of rete t.
undescended t.
test-retest precision
Tesuloid
tethered
t. cord syndrome (TCS)
t. small bowel fold
t. spinal cord
tethering
tetraazacyclododecanetetraacetic acid (DOTA)
tetrabromophenolphthalein sodium
tetrad
Fallot t.
tetradecyl sulfate
tetradiploid tumor
tetrahedron chest
tetrahydrobiopterin
tetrahydrouridine
tetraiodophenolphthalein
t. contrast medium
t. sodium
tetralogy
t. of Fallot (TOF)
pink t.
tetraphocomelia
tetraploid tumor
tetrasodium-meso-tetra
manganese tetrasodium-meso-t. (Mn-TPPS$_4$)
tetrasodium pyrophosphate (TSPP)
tetrofosmin
Teutleben ligament
texaphyrin
gadolinium t. (Gd-Tex)
textiloma
texture
echo t.

ground-glass t.
inhomogeneous echo t.
t. mapping
t. slice
TFA
thigh-foot angle
tibiofemoral angle
T1-FAST
T-fastener
T.-f. delivery needle
T.-f. device
TFC
threaded fusion cage
triangular fibrocartilage
TFCC
triangular fibrocartilaginous complex
TFD
target-film distance
T1FS
T1-weighted fat-suppressed image
TGA
transposition of great artery
TGG
thalamogeniculate group
THAD
transient hepatic attenuation difference
thalamectomy
thalami (*pl. of* thalamus)
thalamic
t. edema
t. fracture
t. fracture of calcaneus
t. glioma
t. hemorrhage
t. infarct
t. lesion
t. plane
t. syndrome of Dejérine-Roussy
t. vein
thalamic-hypothalamic mass
thalamocaudate artery
thalamogeniculate
t. artery
t. group (TGG)
thalamoperforating
t. artery
t. branch
thalamostriate vein
thalamotegmental involvement
thalamotomy
anterior t.

T

NOTES

thalamotomy *(continued)*
   dorsomedial t.
   parafascicular t.
thalamus, pl. **thalami**
   intralaminar t.
   pulvinar of t.
thallium
   t. debris
   t. imaging agent
   t. myocardial perfusion imaging
   t. myocardial scan
   t. myocardial scan with SPECT
      imaging
   t. perfusion scintigraphy
   t. redistribution phase
   t. rest-redistribution imaging
   t. scintography imaging
   t. single-photon emission computed
      tomography scan
   t. SPECT score
   t. stress imaging
thallium-201 (^{201}Tl)
   t. chloride
   t. imaging
   t. myocardial scintigraphy
   t. scan
   t. single-photon emission CT
   t. uptake and distribution
thallium-activated
   t.-a. sodium iodide
   t.-a. sodium iodine detector
thallium-to-scalp ratio
thallous chloride imaging agent
Thal-Quick chest tube
thanatophoric
   t. dwarfism
   t. dysplasia
Thayer-Doisy unit
THC
   transhepatic cholangiogram
THC:YAG laser
thebesian
   t. circulation
   t. foramen
   t. valve
   t. vein
theca, pl. **thecae**
   t. externa
   t. interna
theca-cell ovarian tumor
thecal
   t. abscess
   t. sac
   t. whitlow
theca-lutein ovarian cyst
The Closer arterial puncture site
   closure device

thecoma of ovary
Theile
   T. canal
   T. muscle
thenar
   t. eminence
   t. muscle
   t. space
   t. space abscess
theophylline attenuation
theorem
   Bayes t.
   Nyquist sampling t.
   Stokes t.
theory
   Bohr t.
   crystal field t.
   Culiner t.
   density matrix t.
   electron t.
   Fourier optical t.
   t. of fuzzy connectedness
   fuzzy set t.
   Kubelka-Munk t.
   Planck quantum t.
   quantum t.
   slider crank t.
therapeutic
   t. amniocentesis
   t. angiography
   t. barium enema
   t. chemoembolization
   t. cordocentesis
   t. embolus
   t. external radiation
   t. gain factor
   t. index
   t. intervention
   t. pneumothorax
   t. radiology
   t. range
   ray t.
   t. response
   t. thrombosis
therapy *(See* radiotherapy)
   ablative laser t.
   adjunctive t.
   adjuvant t.
   antiestrogen radiologic t.
   antitubercular t.
   arc t.
   beam t.
   beta-ray ophthalmic plaque t.
   boost t.
   brisement t.
   catheter-directed thrombolytic t.
   Chaoul t.

compartmental radioimmunoglobulin t.
computer-controlled conformal radiation t. (CCRT)
concomitant boost radiation t.
conformal neutron and photon radiation t.
conformal radiation t. (CRT)
contact radiation t.
continuous hyperfractionated accelerated radiation t.
conventionally fractionated stereotactic radiation t.
coronary radiation t. (CRT)
craniospinal axis radiation t.
crossfire radiation t.
3D conformal radiation t.
deep roentgen ray t.
dynamic conformal t.
dynamic radiation t.
electron arc t.
electron beam t.
embolization transcatheter t.
endocrine ablative t.
enzyme replacement t.
enzyme supplementation t.
Exogen 2000+ noninvasive ultrasound t.
extended-field irradiation t.
external beam radiation t. (EBRT)
external x-ray t.
eye-view 3D conformal radiation t.
fast-neutron radiation t.
fibrinolytic t.
first-line t.
Fletcher-Suit system for radium t.
fluoroscopy-guided subarachnoid phenol block t.
four-fiber t.
fractionated external beam radiation t.
fractionated stereotactic radiation t.
fragmentation t.
gamma ray t.
gamma-ribbon radiation t.
gene t.
grid t.
hadron t.
half-body radiation t.
heavy particle t.
high-dose t.

high-dose-rate intracavitary radiation t.
high-voltage roentgen t.
hyperfractionated accelerated radiation t. (HART)
hypofractionated radiation t.
hysterectomy and radiation t.
^{131}I t.
I-B1 radiolabeled antibody injection radiation t.
image-guided t.
indicator dilution t.
induction t.
infusion transcatheter t.
intensity-modulated arc t.
intensity-modulated radiation t. (IMRT)
interferential current t.
internal radiation t.
interstitial radiation t.
interstitial radioactive colloid t.
interstitial radium t.
intraarticular radiopharmaceutical t.
intracavitary radiation t.
intracavitary radioactive colloid t.
intracoronary radiation t. (ICRT)
intracoronary thrombolytic t.
intraoperative radiation t.
intraoperative red light t. (IRLT)
intravascular radiopharmaceutical t.
^{192}Ir seed t.
large-field radiation t.
lens-sparing external beam radiation t. (LSRT)
light t.
low-intensity laser t. (LILT)
MammoSite Radiation T.
megavolt t.
megavoltage grid t.
megavoltage radiation t.
megavoltage x-ray t.
microwave t.
MRI-guided periradicular nerve root infiltration t.
multimodality t.
neoadjuvant hormonal t.
neodymium:YAG laser t.
neuraxis radiation t.
neutron t.
neutron/gamma transmission t.
nonsurgical ablative t.
ocular radiation t. (ORT)

NOTES

therapy *(continued)*
orthovoltage radiation t.
palliative radiation t.
pamidronate t.
partial-brain radiation t.
particle-beam radiation t.
percutaneous ethanol injection t.
percutaneous microwave
coagulation t.
percutaneous transcatheter t.
peroral cone radiation t.
photodynamic t. (PDT)
photon-neutron mixed-beam
radiation t.
PhotoPoint photodynamic t.
plesiocurie t.
postmenopausal estrogen t.
postorchiectomy paraaortic
radiation t.
pulsed dye laser t.
PUVA t.
radiation t. (RT)
radiofrequency ablation t.
radionuclide t.
radiopharmaceutical t.
radium beam t.
reperfusion t.
reprogramming t.
rotation t.
salvage t.
samarium-153 ethyl-
enediaminetetramethylenephosphonic
acid t.
short-distance radiation t.
sonodynamic t.
split-course hyperfractionated
radiation t.
stereotactic radiation t.
stereotaxically guided interstitial
laser t.
systemic adjuvant t.
telecobalt t.
teleradium t.
thrombolytic t.
tiered t.
timed-sequential t.
total androgen suppression t.
transcatheter t.
triple t. (TT)
triple-H t.
ultra-early thrombolytic t.
ultrasound ablative t.
ultrasound-guided percutaneous
microwave coagulation t.
updraft t.
upper mantle radiation t.
virus-directed enzyme/prodrug t.
virus-mediated gene t.
whole-body radiation t.
whole-brain radiation t. (WBRT)
wide-field radiation t. (WFRT)
x-ray t.
Y-90 silicate t.
yttrium-90 silicate t.
t. zone

TheraSeed
T. imaging agent
T. seeding

thermal
t. ablation
t. bioeffect
t. compression
t. conductivity
t. convection pattern
t. diffusion
t. dosimetry system
t. effect
t. energy
t. enhancement ratio (TER)
t. equilibrium
t. hot spot
t. insult
t. modeling
t. neutron
t. noise
t. occlusion
t. radiation
t. relaxation time
t. shape memory
t. spectrum
t. treatment parameter

Thermex
Direx T.

thermistor plethysmography
thermoactinomyces vulgaris
thermocoagulation
thermodilution
t. cardiac output
t. ejection fraction
t. method of cardiac output
measurement
t. stroke volume

thermodynamics
thermogram
thermograph
continuous scan t.

thermography
blood vessel t.
infrared t.
laser-induced t. (LITT)
liquid crystal t. (LCT)
liquid crystal contact t.

thermoluminescence dosimetry

thermoluminescent
    t. dosimeter (TLD)
    t. dosimeter rod
thermometry
    invasive t.
    noninvasive t.
thermomostography
thermonic emission
thermonuclear reaction
thermophilic actinomycetes
thermoplacentography
thermoradiosensitization
thermotherapy
    laser-induced t. (LITT)
    laser-induced interstitial t. (LITT)
    MR-guided laser-induced t.
    MRI-guided laser-induced
    interstitial t.
thermotolerance
thermovision
thesaurosis
THI
    tissue harmonic imaging
thick
    t. bone
    t. echo
    t. rind sclerosis
    t. slab 3D multiplanar reformatted
    image
thickened
    t. airway wall
    t. aortic valve
    t. bladder
    t. bladder wall
    t. bowel loop
    t. duodenal fold
    t. esophageal fold
    t. gallbladder wall
    t. gastric fold
    t. heel pad
    t. hypoechoic tissue
    t. irregular endometrium
    t. irregular small bowel fold
    dilatation
    t. nodular irregular small bowel
    fold
    t. septum
    t. sinus
    t. smooth small bowel fold
    dilatation
    t. stomach fold
    t. straight small bowel fold

thickening
    anterior joint capsule t.
    antral mucosal t.
    aortic valve t.
    aortic wall t.
    apical pleural t.
    asbestos-related pleural t.
    beaded septal t.
    breast skin t.
    bronchial wall t.
    capsular t.
    cecal t.
    circumferential t.
    diffuse gallbladder wall t.
    diffuse intimal t.
    diffuse pleural t.
    disproportionate upper septal t.
    facial t.
    focal cecal apical t.
    focal gallbladder wall t.
    focal intimal t.
    t. fraction
    fusiform t.
    gastric wall t.
    heel pad t.
    inner table t.
    interlobular septal t.
    interstitial t.
    intimal t.
    intralobular interstitial t.
    irregular gallbladder wall t.
    joint capsule t.
    ligamentous t.
    ligamentum flavum t.
    mediastinal t.
    minimal interstitial t.
    mottled t.
    mucosal t.
    mural t.
    myocardial t.
    nuchal skin t.
    optic excrescentic t.
    optic nerve fusiform t.
    outer table t.
    partial t.
    peribronchial t.
    pleural t.
    postlumpectomy skin t.
    rind-like t.
    sawtooth-like t.
    scrotal wall t.
    septal t.

NOTES

T

thickening *(continued)*
>skin t.
>small bowel wall t.
>submucosal t.
>synovial t.
>tendon sheath t.
>trabecular t.
>urinary bladder wall t.
>valve t.
>wall t.

thickness
>antropyloric muscle t. (APT)
>arterial wall t.
>bladder wall t.
>effective section t.
>endometrial t.
>full t.
>image slice t.
>increased skull t.
>interventricular septal t. (IVST)
>intimal-medial t. (IMT)
>patellar cartilage t.
>posterior wall t. (PWT)
>postmenopausal endometrial t.
>preacinar arterial wall t.
>septal wall t.
>slab t.
>slice t.
>strut t.
>subcutaneous quadriceps fat t.
> (SQFT)
>urethral t. (UT)
>ventricular free wall t.
>wall t.

thickness-to-diameter of ventricle ratio
thick-septa collimator
thick-slice imaging
thick-walled
>t.-w. cyst
>t.-w. gallbladder
>t.-w. ventricle

thigh
>t. bone
>t. muscle
>t. muscle cross-section
>t. splint

thigh-foot angle (TFA)
thin
>t. border
>t. cylindrical uniform field volume
>t. fibrous cap
>t. film analysis
>t. linear structure
>t. skull

thin-collimation
>t.-c. image
>t.-c. imaging

thin-cut axial CT image
thin-film transistor array
thinned
>t. cartilage
>t. myocardium

thinning
>apical t.
>cortical t.
>parietal bone t.
>pulmonary interstitial t.
>white matter t.

thin-plate spine
thin-section
>t.-s. axial image
>t.-s. CT

thin-septa collimator
thin-slab minimum intensity projection
thin-slice
>t.-s. CT
>t.-s. imaging

thin-walled
>t.-w. atrium
>t.-w. catheter
>t.-w. cyst
>t.-w. gallbladder
>t.-w. lung cavity

thiol
>t. augmentation
>t. modification

thiosemicarbazide
third
>t. branchial arch
>t. cardiac mogul
>t. inflow
>t. intercondylar tubercle of Parsons
>t. portion of duodenum
>t. projection of Chausse
>t. ventricle
>t. ventricle of cerebrum
>t. ventricle tumor
>t. ventricular hemangioblastoma

third-degree
>t.-d. AV block
>t.-d. heart block

third-order chorda
third-space sequestration
third-trimester
>t.-t. gestational dating
>t.-t. placenta

Thom method
**Thompson-Epstein femoral fracture
 classification**
Thompson ligament
Thomson scattering
thoracentesis
>misplaced t.

thoraces (*pl. of* thorax)
thoracic (**T**)
    t. adenopathy
    t. angiography
    t. aorta
    t. aortic aneurysm
    t. aortic coarctation
    t. aortic dissection
    t. arch aortography
    t. asymmetry
    t. bone
    t. cage configuration
    t. cavity
    t. circumference (TC)
    t. crush
    t. deformity
    t. disk
    t. disk herniation
    t. duct
    t. duct-cutaneous fistula
    t. duct cyst
    t. duct imaging
    t. duct ligation
    t. duct route
    t. dysplasia
    t. empyema
    t. esophagus
    t. gas volume
    t. gibbus
    t. index
    t. inlet
    t. inlet lesion
    t. inlet soft tissue
    t. inlet syndrome
    t. joint
    t. kidney
    t. kyphosis
    t. lordosis
    t. myelography
    t. OPLL
    t. outlet
    t. outlet syndrome (TOS)
    t. paraganglioma
    t. plane
    t. pulsion diverticulum
    t. root sleeve
    t. root sleeve diverticulum
    t. scoliosis
    t. sonography
    t. spinal cord
    t. spinal neoplasm
    t. spine

    t. spine anatomy
    t. spine curve
    t. spine fracture
    t. splenosis
    t. stomach
    t. vent
    t. vertebra
    t. view
    t. wall
thoracis
    skeleton t.
thoracoabdominal
    t. aorta
    t. aortic aneurysm
    t. diaphragm
    t. duplication
    t. gradient
    t. venous collateral circulation
    t. wall
thoracoacromial artery
thoracodorsal artery
thoracoepigastric vein
thoracofemoral conversion
thoracolumbar
    t. burst fracture
    t. fascia
    t. junction fracture
    t. kyphosis
    t. scoliosis
    t. spine
    t. spine column
    t. vertebral disk
thoracoomphalopagus
thoracopagus twins
thoracoplasty
Thoracoport
thoracoscope
    Storz t.
thoracoscopic poudrage
thoracoscopy
    video-assisted t. (VAT)
thoracostomy
    tube t.
    t. tube
thoracotomy
Thoramat
Thoravision selenium x-ray detector
thorax, pl. **thoraces**
    t. articulation
    asymmetric t.
    bell-shaped t.
    bony t.

T

NOTES

thorax *(continued)*
    cylindrical t.
    squared-off t.
    symmetric t.
Thoreau filter
Thorel
    T. bundle
    T. pathway
thorium
    t. compound
    t. dioxide granuloma
    t. dioxide imaging agent
    t. emanation
    radioactive t.
    t. tartrate
    t. X
thorium-201 SPECT scan
thorn ulcer
thorny bone radiation
Thorotrast
    T. accumulation
    T. imaging agent
thorotrastosis
Thorpe plastic lens
tHPT
    tertiary hyperparathyroidism
thread-and-streaks
    t.-a.-s. sign
    t.-a.-s. vascular channel
threaded fusion cage (TFC)
threatened vessel closure
three-axis gradient coil
three-chambered heart
three-column injury
three-compartment
    t.-c. arthrography
    t.-c. system
    t.-c. wrist angiography
three-dimensional (3D) *(See* 3D)
    t.-d. analysis
    t.-d. conformal radiotherapy
    t.-d. contrast-enhanced (3DCE)
    t.-d. digital subtraction angiography (3D-DSA)
    t.-d. Fourier transform (3DFT)
    t.-d. Fourier transform volume image
    t.-d. magnetic resonance angiography (3D MRA)
    T.-d. Perfusion/Motion Map software
three-head
    t.-h. gamma camera-based SPECT system
    t.-h. scan
three-level Haar wavelet decomposition
three-part fracture

three-phase
    t.-p. bone scan
    t.-p. bone scintigraphy (TPBS)
    t.-p. current
    t.-p. generator
    t.-p. imaging
    t.-p. system
    t.-p. technetium study
    t.-p. voltage supply
    t.-p. whole-body bone imaging (TPWBBI)
three-point
    t.-p. Dixon technique
    t.-p. Dixon water-fat separation sequence
three-quarters prone position
three-stopcock manifold
three-vessel
    t.-v. coronary disease
    t.-v. multiple projection biplane angiography
    t.-v. runoff
    t.-v. umbilical cord
three-way stopcock
threshold
    above-selected t. (AST)
    alpha t.
    attenuation t.
    t. body
    CACS t.
    cell-dose t.
    count-density t.
    detection t.
    erythema t.
    t. erythema dose
    t. of Firooznia
    fracture t.
    malignancy t.
    seizure t.
    signal-to-noise t.
    ultrasound t.
thresholding
    t. algorithm
    diffusion anisotropy t.
    gray-level t.
    t. method
thrombectomy
    t. device
    mechanical t.
Thrombex PMT system
thrombi (*pl. of* thrombus)
thrombin
    t. formation
    human t.
thromboangiitis obliterans
thromboaspiration
thrombocythemia

thrombocytopenia-absent radius syndrome
thromboelastogram
thromboelastograph
thromboelastography
thromboembolic (TE)
    t. disease (TED)
    t. lung disease
    t. pontine infarct
    t. stroke
thromboembolism
    aortic t.
    chronic lung t.
    mesenteric t. (MTE)
    paraneoplastic t.
    Prolyse in acute cerebral t. (PROACT)
    pulmonary t.
thromboembolization
    catheter-induced t.
    deep venous t.
    pulmonary t.
    venous t.
thromboembolus
thrombogenic coil
thrombokinesis
thrombolysis
    brachiocephalic artery t.
    t. in brain ischemia flow grade
    catheter-directed extremity t.
    clot removal by laser t.
    intracerebral t.
    mechanical t.
    t. in myocardial infarct (TIMI)
    venous t.
thrombolytic therapy
thrombopathy
thrombopenia
thrombophlebitis
    breast t.
    cerebral t.
    venography-related t.
thromboplastinogen
thromboresistance
ThromboScan
    T. imaging
    T. molecular recognition unit
    T. MRU
thrombosed
    t. giant vertebral artery aneurysm
    t. intraaortic artery
thrombosis, pl. **thromboses**

abdominal aorta t.
acute renal vein t.
aortic t.
aortoiliac t.
arterial t.
ascending medullary vein t.
atrial t.
atrophic t.
axillary vein traumatic t.
axillosubclavian vein t.
calf vein t.
capsular t.
cardiac t.
catheter-induced subclavian vein t.
central splanchnic venous t. (CSVT)
cerebral venous t.
chronic renal vein t.
coronary t. (CT)
cortical vein t.
deep venous t. (DVT)
dural venous sinus t.
effort t.
femoropopliteal t.
hepatic artery t.
hepatic vein t.
iliofemoral t.
infective t.
intentional reversible t.
intervillous placental t.
intraarterial t.
intracranial sinus t.
intravascular t.
jugular vein t.
large-vessel t.
luminal t.
mesenteric arterial t.
mesenteric venous t.
native kidney renal vein t.
necrotizing t.
ovarian vein t.
pelvic vein t.
portal vein t.
portomesenteric venous t.
portosplenic t.
postangioplasty mural t.
pulmonary t.
renal artery transplant t.
renal vein t. (RVT)
renal vein transplant t.
sagittal t.
septic t.

NOTES

thrombosis *(continued)*
    shunt t.
    sinus t.
    splenic vein t.
    stent t.
    subacute renal vein t.
    subclavian vein t.
    subclavian vessel t.
    superior ophthalmic vein t.
    superior sagittal sinus t.
    syndrome of impending t.
    terminal t.
    therapeutic t.
    transverse sinus t.
    vein graft t.
    venous sinus t.
thrombospondin
thrombostasis
Thrombotest
thrombotic
    t. aneurysm
    t. endocarditis
    t. infarct
    t. microangiopathy
    t. obstruction
    t. occlusion
    t. pulmonary artery (TPA)
thrombus, pl. thrombi
    adherent t.
    anechoic t.
    ball-valve t.
    blood plate t.
    t. calcification
    calcified t.
    coral t.
    echogenic intraluminal t.
    t. embolus
    t. extension
    t. formation
    iliocaval t.
    intraaneurysmal t.
    intraarterial t.
    intraatrial t.
    intracardiac t.
    intraluminal t.
    intramural t.
    intravascular tumor t.
    laminated intraluminal t.
    laser desiccation of t.
    mobile t.
    mural t.
    t. nidus
    obstructive t.
    occlusive arterial t.
    pedunculated t.
    percutaneous dissolution of t.
    pericatheter t.

    peroneal t.
    platelet-rich t.
    primary t.
    t. remodeling
    tibial obliterative t.
    traumatic t.
    tumor t.
through
    barium meal and follow t. (BaFT)
through-and-through
    t.-a.-t. fracture
    t.-a.-t. guidewire
    t.-a.-t. injury
through-plane flow
through-sound transmission
through-the-scope
through-transfer imaging
through-transmission
thrower's
    t. elbow
    t. fracture
throwing arm injury
thrush breast heart
thrusting ventricle
thulium thumbprinting
thumb
    adducted t.
    adductor sweep of t.
    basal joint of t.
    base of t.
    bowler's t.
    cortical t.
    t. extensor tendon
    t. flexor tendon
    floating t.
    gamekeeper's t.
    hypoplastic t.
    pouce t.
    skier's t.
    triphalangeal t.
    t. web
thumb-in-palm deformity
thumbprint appearance
thumbprinting
    t. appearance of the colon
    gastric t.
    thulium t.
thump
    wall t.
Thurston
    T. Holland fracture
    T. Holland sign
thymectomy
thymic
    t. agenesis
    t. carcinoid
    t. carcinoma

t. cyst
t. dysplasia
t. enlargement
t. hyperplasia
t. index
t. lymphoma
t. mass
t. neoplasm
t. sail sign
t. shadow
thymidine
t. labeling index (TLI)
t. phosphorylase (TP)
t. suicide study
tritiated t. (TT)
thymion
thymokesis
thymokinetic
thymolipoma
thymoma
benign t.
t. of heart
malignant t.
noninvasive t.
thymotoxic
thymus
congenital absence of t.
diffuse enlargement of the t.
ectopic t.
t. gland
mass t.
solid lesion t.
t. weight
thyroarytenoid
thyrocardiac disease
thyrocervical
t. trunk
t. trunk of subclavian artery
thyroepiglottic ligament
thyroglossal
t. duct
t. duct cyst
t. duct remnant
thyrohyoid ligament
thyroid
t. abscess
t. acropachy
t. adenoma
t. adenoma calcification
t. adenoma nodule
t. artery
t. capsule

t. carcinoma
t. cartilage
cold nodule t.
t. colloid nodule
t. cyst
t. cystadenoma
cystic area t.
t. degeneration
discordant nodule t.
t. disease
t. dysgenesis
t. eminence
t. follicle
t. gland
t. gland inflammation
t. goiter
t. hyperplasia
t. insufficiency
intrathoracic t.
iodine-123, -131 t.
t. isthmus
lingual t.
t. lobe
t. lymph node
t. lymphoma
t. mass
multinodular t.
t. orbitopathy
t. organification defect
t. psammoma body
t. radioiodine treatment
t. radioiodine uptake
retrosternal t.
t. scintigraphy
t. stimulation scan
t. storm
t. stunning
substernal t.
t. suppression scan
^{99m}Tc pertechnetate t.
t. trapping defect
t. ultrasonography imaging
t. uptake measurement
t. whole-body scan
thyroidal lymph node scintigraphy
thyroiditis
acute suppurative t.
chronic lymphocytic t.
de Quervain t.
Hashimoto t.
painless t.
Riedel t.

T

NOTES

thyroiditis *(continued)*
    subacute t.
    suppurative t.
thyrotoxicosis medicamentosa
thyrotroph cell adenoma
thyroxine (T$_4$)
Thyrx timer
TI
    inversion time
    time following inversion pulse
    tricuspid incompetence
    tricuspid insufficiency
TIA
    transient ischemic attack
      carotid distribution TIA
      crescendo TIA
      ipsilateral hemispheric carotid TIA
tibarius
    torsus t.
tibia, pl. **tibiae**
    anterior bowing t.
    t. bone
    t. bone marrow development
    focal fibrocartilaginous dysplasia
      of t.
    malleolus tibiae
    posteromedial t.
    proximal t.
    repetitive anterior subluxation of
      the t.
    t. vara
tibial
    t. artery
    t. artery disease
    t. bending fracture
    t. collateral ligament
    t. collateral ligament bursa
    t. condyle
    t. condyle fracture
    t. crest
    t. diaphyseal fracture
    t. epiphysis
    t. flare
    t. hallux sesamoid
    t. intercondylar eminence
    t. medullary canal
    t. node
    t. obliterative thrombus
    t. open fracture
    t. pilon fracture
    t. plafond
    t. plafond fracture
    t. plateau
    t. plateau depression
    t. plateau fracture
    t. pseudoarthrosis

    t. sesamoid bone
    t. sesamoid ligament
    t. sesamoid position
    t. shaft fracture
    t. spine
    t. tendon
    t. tendon tear
    t. torsion
    t. translation
    t. triplane fracture
    t. tubercle
    t. tubercle ossification center
    t. tubercle prominence
    t. tuberosity
    t. tuberosity fracture
    t. varus
    t. vein
tibialis
    t. anterior
    t. anterior tendon
    t. posterior
    t. posterior tendon
    t. posterior tenosynovitis
    t. sign
tibiocalcaneal
    t. angle
    t. fusion
    t. joint complex
    t. ligament
tibiofemoral
    t. angle (TFA)
    t. joint dislocation
tibiofibular
    t. articulation
    t. diastasis
    t. fracture
    t. joint
    t. ligament
    t. syndesmosis
    t. synostosis
tibioligamentous fascicle
tibionavicular ligament
tibioperoneal
    t. occlusive disease
    t. runoff system
    t. trunk
tibiotalar
    t. angle
    t. joint
    t. rotation
tibiotalocalcaneal fusion
tibiotarsal dislocation
TIC
    time intensity curve
TICA
    traumatic intracranial aneurysm

tidal
t. inspiratory flow volume
t. wave of carotid arterial pulse
tiered therapy
tie sternum
Tietze syndrome
TIFF
tag image file format
tight
t. dural sac
t. filum terminale
t. filum terminale syndrome
t. lesion
t. spinal canal
tigroid
t. demyelination
t. pattern
tile mode display
Tillaux-Chaput fracture
Tillaux fracture
Tillaux-Kleiger fracture
tilt
bent-knee pelvic t.
caudal t.
gantry t.
infundibular t.
lunate t.
palmar t.
patellar t.
t. table
valgus t.
varus t.
volar t.
tilted
t. optimized nonsaturating excitation (TONE)
t. sacrum
tilting-disk valve
time
acceleration t. (AT)
acquisition t.
activated partial thromboplastin t.
arm-lung t.
asymmetric appearance t.
atrial activation t.
atrioventricular t.
bolus arrival t. (BAT)
calculated clearance t.
capillary filling t.
carotid ejection t.
cerebral circulation t.
chromoscopy t.

circulation t. (CT)
colonic transit t.
concentration times t. (C x T)
t. constant
corrected sinus node recovery t.
correlation t.
t. correlation function (TCF)
t. course fracture scintigraphy
cycle t.
data acquisition t.
dead t.
decay t.
deceleration t.
t. delay between excitation and echo maximum (TE)
delayed transit t.
diastolic perfusion t.
diffusion t.
t. domain
echo t. (TE)
echo delay t. (TE)
echo train echo t. (T_E)
effective transverse relation t.
efficient relaxation t.
ejection t. (ET)
emptying t.
esophageal transit t.
fixing t.
t. following inversion pulse (TI)
t. of formation of RF spin-echo when adjusted to be different from gradient spin-echo (TER)
gantry rotation t.
gastric transit t.
image-acquisition t.
image-reconstruction t.
imaging t.
increased left ventricular ejection t.
t. intensity curve (TIC)
interpulse t.
inversion t. (TI)
ischemic t.
isovolumetric contraction t.
isovolumic relaxation t. (IVRT)
lattice relaxation t.
left ventricular ejection t. (LVET)
left ventricular fast filling t.
left ventricular slow filling t.
longitudinal recovery t.
longitudinal relaxation t.
maximum inflation t.
mean circulating t.

NOTES

time *(continued)*
> mean circulation t. (MCT)
> mean examination t.
> mean pulmonary transit t. (MTT)
> mean transit t. (MTT)
> membrane closure t.
> t. motion (TM)
> myocardial contrast appearance t. (MCAT)
> perfusion t.
> phasing-in t.
> t. to PME (tPME)
> t. point
> prolonged ejection t.
> proton spin-lattice relaxation t.
> pulse reappearance t.
> pulse repetition t.
> pulse transit t. (PTT)
> pyelographic appearance t.
> radionuclide esophageal dead t.
> ramp t.
> reaction recovery t.
> receiver dead t.
> recovery t. (RT)
> regional mean transit t. (rMTT)
> relaxation t.
> repetition t. (RT)
> resolving t.
> retinocortical t.
> right ventricle-to-ear t.
> rise t.
> rotational correlation t.
> scan t.
> sequence t.
> short-echo t.
> short T1 relaxation t.
> sinoatrial conduction t. (SACT)
> sinus node recovery t. (SNRT)
> small bowel transit t.
> sojourn t.
> spin-lattice relaxation t.
> spin-spin relaxation t.
> systolic acceleration t.
> systolic upstroke t.
> thermal relaxation t.
> transit t.
> transverse relaxation t.
> trigger delay t.
> T1, T2 relaxation t.
> t. velocity integral
> venous filling t. (VFT)
> venous refill t. (VRT)
> venous return t.
> ventricular activation t. (VAT)
> ventricular isovolumic relaxation t.

time-action analysis
time-activity curve

time-attenuation curve
time-averaged flow
time-compensated gain
timed
> t. bolus delivery
> t. imaging

time-density curve
time-dependent
> t.-d. metabolic cascade
> t.-d. xenon concentration

timed-sequential therapy
time-efficient T2 relaxometry
time-gain compensation
time-insensitive
time-lapse quantitative computed tomography lymphography
time-of-flight (TOF)
> t.-o.-f. echo-planar imaging
> t.-o.-f. effect
> t.-o.-f. enhancement
> t.-o.-f. flow measurement
> t.-o.-f. magnetic resonance angiography (TOF-MRA)
> t.-o.-f. method
> t.-o.-f. PET imaging system
> t.-o.-f. signal loss
> t.-o.-f. technique
> two-dimensional t.-o.-f. (2D TOF)

time-out
> ventriculoatrial t.-o.

time-proportional phase incrementation (TPPI)
timer
> Thyrx t.

time-resolved
> t.-r. imaging by automatic data segmentation (TRIADS)
> t.-r. imaging of contrast kinetics (TRICKS)

times (x)
time-sensitive
time-to-distant failure
time-to-local failure
time-to-peak
> t.-t.-p. activity
> t.-t.-p. contrast (TPC)
> t.-t.-p. filling rate (TPFR)
> t.-t.-p. intensity (TTP)
> t.-t.-p. value (TTP)

time-to-treatment
> t.-t.-t. bias
> t.-t.-t. failure (TTF)

time-varied
> t.-v. gain (TVG)
> t.-v. gain control

time-varying magnetic field
time-velocity measurement

time-weighted average
TIMI
    thrombolysis in myocardial infarct
timing
        bolus t.
        gradient t.
        t. parameter
tin (Sn)
        t. oxide inhalation
        t. with indium 113m
tin-113 (^{113}Sn)
Tinel sign
tiny ventricle
tip
        t. angle
        catheter t.
        conus t.
        t. deflector
        t. dispersion characteristic
        hockey-stick appearance of
            catheter t.
        mitral valve leaflet t.
        occipital t.
        petrous t.
        pole t.
        radiopaque distal t.
        rectal t.
        t. of spleen
        valve t.
tip-deflecting guidewire
TIPS
        transjugular intrahepatic portosystemic
        shunt
        TIPS failure
        TIPS imaging
tissue
        aberrant t.
        abnormal t.
        t. adhesive
        adipose t.
        adventitial t.
        aerated t.
        anisotropic t.
        apical t.
        areolar connective t.
        bony t.
        breast t.
        bronchus-associated lymphoid t.
            (BALT)
        cancellous t.
        t. capsule
        cartilaginous t.

        cavernous t.
        t. characterization
        t. characterization technique
        chondroid t.
        chorionic t.
        collagenous t.
        t. conductivity
        connective t.
        t. contrast
        t. cooling
        cortical t.
        crushed t.
        dartoic t.
        dead t.
        t. deficit compensator
        degenerated t.
        dense connective t.
        t. density
        destruction of t.
        devitalized t.
        disk t.
        t. Doppler imaging
        ectopic endometrial t.
        ectopic thyroid t.
        edematous t.
        engorged t.
        escape of air into lung
            connective t.
        extraadrenal chromaffin t.
        extralobular connective t.
        exuberant granulation t.
        fast exchange-soft t.
        fatty prostatic t.
        fetal lymphoid t.
        t. of fetus
        fibroadipose t.
        fibroareolar t.
        fibrocartilaginous t.
        fibrocollagenous connective t.
        fibrofatty breast t.
        fibroglandular t.
        fibromuscular t.
        fibrosing t.
        fibrotic t.
        fibrous connective t.
        fibrous scar t.
        fibrovascular t.
        t. flow
        gangrenous t.
        gastrointestinal-associated
            lymphoid t.
        gelatinous t.

NOTES

T

949

tissue *(continued)*

granulation t.
grumous t.
gut-associated lymphoid t. (GALT)
t. harmonic imaging (THI)
t. harmonic sonography
hyalinized fibrocollagenous t.
hyperplastic t.
hypertrophic t.
hypervascular granulation t.
hypoechoic t.
t. imprint
indurated t.
t. inhomogeneity factor
interlobular t.
interstitial t.
intertrabecular soft t.
intralobular connective t.
island of t.
t. island
isointense soft t.
isotropic t.
joint t.
late effect of normal t. (LENT)
lipomatous t.
loose mesenchymal t.
lymphatic t.
lymph node t.
lymphoid t.
lymphoreticular t.
mammary t.
t. mass
mediastinal thyroid t.
mesenchymal t.
mesenteric t.
t. migration
mucosa-associated lymphoid t.
  (MALT)
muscle t.
necrotic t.
neoplastic t.
neural crest t.
nodal t.
noncontractile scar t.
noncritical soft t.
nonviable t.
osseous tumor of soft t.
osteocartilaginous t.
t. outflow valve
t. oxygenation
paraffin-embedded t.
paratracheal soft t.
paravaginal soft t.
parenchymal t.
passively congested lung t.
t. perfusion
periarticular t.

peribronchial connective t.
perilobular connective t.
peritumoral t.
t. plate
postcricoid soft t.
postoperative scar t.
postpharyngeal soft t.
preepiglottic soft t.
prevertebral soft t.
proliferation of fibrous t.
regeneration of t.
regular connective t.
t. relaxometry
residual ductal t.
reticular connective t.
retrodiskal t.
retropharyngeal soft t.
retrosternal soft t.
retrotracheal soft t.
revascularized t.
scar t.
t. sequela
t. signature
t. slice
slow exchange soft t.
soft t.
t. space
stippled soft t.
string-like bands of fibrous t.
subadventitial t.
subcutaneous connective t.
suppressed t.
swollen t.
sympathetic nervous t.
syngeneic t.
synovial t.
taenia t.
target t.
tendon t.
testicular adrenal rest t.
thickened hypoechoic t.
thoracic inlet soft t.
t. tolerance dose (TTD)
t. tolerance to radiation
tongue of t.
tuberculosis granulation t.
underlying t.
vascular t.
vascularized granulation t.
t. veil
ventricular soft t.
t. viability
visceral adipose t. (VAT)
t. water content
t. weighting factor
white cotton-like fibrous t.

tissue-air ratio (TAR)

tissue-based T2 relaxation
tissue-equivalent detector
tissue-maximum ratio (TMR)
tissue-phantom ratio (TPR)
tissue-specific imaging agent
tissue-type plasminogen activator
titanate
    barium t.
titanium
    t. compound
    t. dioxide
    t. plate
Titterington position
TIV
    total intracranial volume
TKA
    total knee arthroplasty
Tl-201
    Cardiolite T.
²⁰¹Tl
    thallium-201
        ²⁰¹Tl chloride
        LDD-gated SPECT with ²⁰¹Tl
TLA
    translumbar aortography
        TLA needle
TLB
    transjugular liver biopsy
TLD
    thermoluminescent dosimeter
        TLD rod
TLE
    temporal lobe epilepsy
        refractory TLE
TLI
    thymidine labeling index
TM
    time motion
        TM ultrasound
TMA
    transmetatarsal amputation
    true metatarsus adductus
TME
    trapezium-metacarpal eburnation
        TME ratio
TMJ
    temporomandibular joint
TMR
    tissue-maximum ratio
    topical magnetic resonance
    transmyocardial revascularization

TMS
    treatment planning system
TN
    true negative
to-and-fro flow
tobacco
    t. heart
    t. nodule
tocolysis
tocopherol (T)
    alpha t.
    gamma t. (gamma-T, γ-T)
TOCU
    transoral carotid ultrasonography
        TOCU for internal carotid artery
        stenosis
Todani classification
Todani-type cyst
Todaro triangle
Todd cirrhosis
toddler's fracture
TODE
    total organ dose equivalent
Tod muscle
toe
    base of t.
    t. extensor tendon
    Morton t.
    overriding t.
    tennis t.
TOF
    tetralogy of Fallot
    time-of-flight
        2D TOF
            two-dimensional time-of-flight
        2D TOF pulse sequencing
        TOF imaging
        TOF signal loss
TOF-MRA
    time-of-flight magnetic resonance
    angiography
Toldt
    white line of T.
tolerance
    drug t.
    Fletcher rule of irradiation t.
    irradiation t.
    narrow gating t.
Tolosa-Hunt syndrome
tombstone
    t. pelvis
    t. pelvis configuration

T

NOTES

Tomocat imaging agent
tomogram
blurred-image t.
plain t.
sagittal t.
single-slice long-axis t.
stacked t.
temporal bone t.
tomograph
Heidelberg retina t. II (HRT II)
tomographic
t. cut
t. imaging
t. modality
t. multiplane scanner
t. section
t. skull immobilizer
t. slice
t. view
tomography (*See* CT, PET, PETT, SPECT)
automated computed axial t. (ACAT)
axial transverse t.
^{11}C-methionine positron emission t. (MET-PET)
coincidence detection positron emission t.
computed t. (CT)
computed transmission t.
computerized axial t. (CAT)
computerized cranial t.
computerized transverse axial t. (CTAT)
contrast-enhanced computed t.
contrast enhanced computed t. (CECT)
conventional t.
cranial computed t. (CCT)
direct imaging of local gradients by group echo selection t. (DIGGEST)
dual-phase helical computed t. (DHCT)
dynamic computed t. (DCT)
dynamic computerized t.
electrical impedance t. (EIT)
electrocardiogram-gated t.
electron-beam t. (EBT)
electron-beam computed t. (EBCT)
emission t.
emission computed t. (ECT)
emission computer-assisted t.
emission computerized axial t. (ECAT)
endoscopic optical coherence t. (EOCT)

exercise thallium-201 t.
expiratory computed t.
FDG positron emission t.
^{18}F-fluorodeoxyglucose positron emission t. (FDG-PET)
flow mode ultrafast computed t.
fluoride ion-positron emission t. (F-18-PET)
fluorine-18 fluorodeoxyglucose-positron emission t.
fluorodeoxyglucose positron emission t. (FDG-PET)
focal plane t.
focused appendix computed t. (FACT)
gated single-photon emission-computed t. (GSPECT)
helical biphasic computed t.
high-resolution computed t. (HRCT)
high-resolution 3D microcomputed t.
high spatial resolution cine computed t. (HSRCCT)
high-temporal-resolution cine computed t. (HTRCCT)
hypercycloidal t.
hypocycloidal t.
indirect computed t.
intravascular contrast-enhanced computed t.
kidney t.
lateral t.
limited-slice computed t.
linear t.
longitudinal section t.
magnetic resonance t. (MRT)
metrizamide-assisted computed t. (CTMM)
multidetector computed t.
multiphasic renal computerized t.
multislice computed t.
myocardial perfusion t.
nonenhanced computed t. (NECT)
nuclear magnetic resonance t.
optical coherence t. (OCT)
panoramic t.
peripheral quantitative computed t. (pQCT)
plesiosectional t.
polycycloidal t.
polydirectional t.
positron emission t. (PET)
positron emission transaxial t. (PETT)
positron emission transverse t. (PETT)
process t. (PT)

quantitative computed t. (QCT)
radionuclide emission t.
rapid acquisition computed t.
rectilinear t.
rotational t.
sellar t.
simultaneous multifilm t.
single-photon emission t. (SPET)
single-photon emission-computed t. (SPECT)
skip t.
spiral computed t.
spiral x-ray computed t. (SVCT, SXCT)
transmission computed t.
transmission computer-assisted t. (TCAT)
transversal t.
trispiral t.
two-phase helical computed t.
ultrafast computed t. (UFCT)
ultrafast CT electron beam t.
ultrasonic t.
ultrasound computed t. (UCT)
ultrasound diffraction t.
volumetric computed t.
water-contrast computed t.
whole-body computed t.
wide-angle t.
xenon computed t. (XeCT)
xenon-enhanced computed t.
x-ray computed t. (XCT)

Tomolex tomographic system
Tomomatic
T. five-slice SPECT imaging system
T. three-slice SPECT imaging system
T. two-slice SPECT imaging system

tomomyelography
Tomoscan
T. AVEU spiral CT scanner
T. SR 7000 scanner

tomoscintigraphy
tomoscopy
tomosynthesis
digital t.

TomTec
TONE
tilted optimized nonsaturating excitation
TONE sequence

tone
440-Hz t.
vascular t.

tongue
t. carcinoma
t. fasciculation
t. fracture
t. stud artifact
t. of tissue
venous malformation of the t.

tongue-shaped villus
tongue-type intraarticular fracture
tonically contracted sphincter
tonography
carotid compression t.

tonometric blood pressure monitor
tonsil
adenoid t.
buried t.
t. carcinoma
cerebellar t.
eustachian t.
faucial t.
lingual t.
pharyngeal t.
t. of torus tubarius
tubal t.

tonsillar
t. carcinoma
t. ectopia
t. herniation
t. pillar

tonus
arterial t.

tool
Quant-X color quantification imaging t.
surgical anatomy visualization and navigation t.'s (SAVANT)

tooth
fibroosteoma of the t.

toothed vertebra
toothpaste shadows
top
t. of carotid T occlusion
t. normal limits of size

Topaz CO$_2$ laser
tophaceous gout
tophus, pl. **tophi**
t. formation
gouty t.

T

NOTES

topical
    t. magnetic resonance (TMR)
    t. water-soluble contrast medium
topodermatography
topogram
topographic
    t. identification
    t. measurement
topography
    arterial t.
    balloon t.
    ocular globe t.
    scintigraphic balloon t.
    vessel t.
    x-ray t.
torch
    saline t.
Torcon blue catheter
torcula
torcular herophili
torcular-lambdoid inversion
tori (*pl. of* torus)
Tornado coil
torn meniscotibial ligament
Tornwaldt
    T. bursitis
    T. cyst
torque (T)
    t. control guidewire
    high t.
    t. stress
Torre syndrome
torr pressure
torsed
    t. ovarian mass
    t. testis
torsion
    t. abnormality
    acute testicular t.
    adnexal t.
    t. alignment
    t. attenuating diameter guidewire
    chronic testicular t.
    t. deformity
    external tibial t.
    extravaginal testicular t.
    t. fracture
    t. of fracture fragment
    gallbladder t.
    t. impaction force
    internal tibial t. (ITT)
    internal tibiofibular t.
    intravaginal t.
    lung t.
    missed testicular t.
    ovarian t.
    spermatic cord t.

    splenic t.
    t. stress
    subacute testicular t.
    testicular appendage t.
    t. of testis
    tibial t.
    t. wedge nonunion
torso phased-array coil (TPAC)
torsus tibarius
torticollis
tortuosity
    t. of cervical vessel
    elongation and t.
    t. of ureter
    vessel t.
tortuous
    t. aorta
    t. aortic arch
    t. emptying
    t. esophagus
    t. vein
    t. vein dilatation
    t. vessel
toruloma
torus, pl. **tori**
    t. fracture
    t. hyperplasia
    t. mandibularis
    t. pylorus
    t. tubarius
TOS
    thoracic outlet syndrome
Toshiba
    T. Aspire continuous imaging
    T. GGA 9300 camera
    T. MR scanner
    T. 900S helical CT scanner
    T. 900S/XII scanner
    T. TCT-80 CT scanner
    T. Xpress SX helical CT scanner
    T. X-Vigor scanner
    T. Xvision scanner
TOSS
    total suppression of sideband
total
    t. ablation
    t. androgen suppression therapy
    t. anomalous pulmonary venous connection
    t. anomalous pulmonary venous drainage (TAPVD)
    t. anomalous pulmonary venous return (TAPVR)
    t. artificial heart
    t. atrial refractory period (TARP)
    t. body scan imaging
    t. body scanning

t. body water (TBW)
t. brain volume (TBV)
t. calcium score (TCS)
t. cerebral blood flow (TCBF)
t. condylar depression fracture
t. effective dose equivalent (TEDE)
t. exchangeable potassium (TEK)
t. exchangeable sodium (TENa)
t. image noise
t. intracranial volume (TIV)
t. knee arthroplasty (TKA)
t. knee implant
t. lesion
t. lung capacity
t. necrosis
t. occlusion
t. organ dose equivalent (TODE)
t. peripheral resistance (TPR)
t. placenta previa
t. pulmonary resistance (TPR)
T. Recall digital imaging system
t. reference air kerma (TRAK)
t. resorption
t. saturation recovery (TSR)
t. stroke volume (TSV)
t. suppression of sideband (TOSS)
totipotential stem cell
toto
in t.
Touraine-Solente-Golé syndrome
tourniquet
caval t.
t. technique
towering cerebellum
Towne
T. position
T. projection
T. view
toxic
t. adenoma
t. cardiomyopathy
t. cirrhosis
t. leukoencephalopathy
t. lung disease
t. megacolon
t. multinodular goiter
t. nodular goiter
t. nodule
t. pneumonia
t. synovitis
toxicity
bone marrow t.

dose-limiting t.
radiation-induced pulmonary t.
toxin
bacterial t.
toxoabscess
toxoplasmosis
cerebral t.
CNS t.
t. encephalitis
Toynbee muscle
TP
temporal peak
thymidine phosphorylase
true positive
TPA
thrombotic pulmonary artery
TPAC
torso phased-array coil
TPBS
three-phase bone scintigraphy
TPC
time-to-peak contrast
TPFR
time-to-peak filling rate
tPME
time to PME
T-portagram
TPPI
time-proportional phase incrementation
TPR
tissue-phantom ratio
total peripheral resistance
total pulmonary resistance
TPWBBI
three-phase whole-body bone imaging
TR
time-to-repetition
ultralong TR
variable TE, TR
trabecula, pl. **trabeculae**
septomarginal t.
trabecular
t. architecture
t. bone
t. bone resorption
t. carcinoma
t. degeneration
t. destruction
t. disruption
t. fracture
t. microfracture
t. osteoma

NOTES

T

trabecular *(continued)*
- t. pattern
- t. thickening
- t. weakening

trabeculated
- t. atrium
- t. bone
- t. bone lesion
- t. osteolysis
- t. outline

trabeculation
- endocardial t.

trabeculectomy
- argon laser t. (ATL)

trabeculoplasty

trace
- t. amount of radiopharmaceutical
- t. edema
- t. element distribution
- t. map

tracer
- t. abnormality
- t. accumulation
- t. activity
- t. bolus
- delayed transport of t.
- deposition of t.
- diffusible t.
- t. dose
- focal pooling of t.
- gold-195m t.
- t. horseradish peroxidase
- ^{13}N ammonia radioactive t.
- neutron-rich biomedical t.
- patchy distribution of t.
- t. principle
- radioactive t.
- radiopharmaceutical t.
- shunted t.
- static rCBF t.
- t. study
- tantalum t.
- transependymal uptake of t.
- tumor-specific t.
- t. uptake

trachea, pl. tracheae
- anular ligament of t.
- carina of t.
- carrot-shaped t.
- intrathoracic t.
- lunate-shaped t.
- napkin-ring t.
- saber-sheath t.
- scabbard t.

tracheal
- t. anastomosis
- t. aspiration
- t. band
- t. B button
- t. bifurcation
- t. bifurcation angle
- t. bronchus
- t. caliber
- t. cartilage
- t. deviation
- t. displacement
- t. diverticulosis
- t. fracture
- t. granuloma
- t. lumen
- t. lymph node
- t. mass effect
- t. narrowing
- t. ring
- t. shift
- t. stenosis
- t. stricture
- t. stripe
- t. triangle
- t. tube
- t. tumor
- t. wall stripe

tracheobiliary fistula

tracheobronchial
- t. angle
- t. fistula
- t. foreign body
- t. hypersensitivity
- t. injury (TBI)
- t. lymph node
- t. mucosal necrosis
- t. papillomatosis
- t. rupture
- t. stenting
- t. tree

tracheobronchoesophageal fistula

tracheobronchography
- CT t.

tracheobronchomalacia
- acquired t.

tracheobronchomegaly
- congenital t.

tracheobronchoscopy
- CT-based virual t.

tracheocele

tracheoesophageal (TE)
- t. fistula (TEF)
- t. junction

tracheomalacia
- congenital t.

tracheopathia

tracheostomy tube

tracing
- carotid pulse t.

electrocardiogram t.
pulmonary capillary wedge t.
ray t.
vessel t.

track

t. cone length
deep white matter t.
t. dilatation
t. etching
ionization t.
nephrostomy t.
t. of pin
t. valve

Tracker

T. 10 catheter
T. Excel catheter
T. 10 microcatheter

tracking

abnormal t.
anterior t.
automatic peak t. (APT)
bolus t.
focal spot t.
t. limit
magnetic bolus t.
magnetic resonance needle t.
periportal t.
presaturation bolus t.
real-time biplanar needle t.
real-time magnetic resonance
  imaging t.
SureStart contrast t.
vessel t.

tract

aerodigestive t.
alimentary t.
anterior corticospinal t.
anterior spinocerebellar t.
anterior spinothalamic t.
apple-peel appearance of GI t.
ascending t.
atriofascicular t.
atrio-His bypass t.
atrioventricular nodal bypass t.
biliary t.
brainstem pyramidal t.
bronchial t.
bulbar t.
carcinoid GI t.
central tegmental t. (CTT)
cerebellar t.
corticobulbar t. (CBT)

corticopontine t.
corticorubral t.
corticospinal t. (CST)
cuneocerebellar t.
dentatothalamic t.
dermal sinus t.
descending t.
digestive t.
dorsal spinocerebellar t.
dorsolateral t.
extrapyramidal t.
fascial t.
fasiculoventricular bypass t.
fetal urogenital t.
fistulous t.
flow t.
frontopontine t.
frontotemporal t.
gastrointestinal t.
geniculocalcarine t.
genital t.
genitourinary t.
GI t.
hepatic outflow t.
hypothalamohypophysial t.
ileal inflow t.
iliotibial t.
intermediolateral t.
intersegmental t.
intestinal t.
intrahepatic biliary t.
lateral corticospinal t.
lateral lemniscus t.
lateral spinothalamic t.
left ventricular outflow t. (LVOT)
Lissauer t.
long t.
lower t.
mesencephalic t.
motor t.
nucleus of the solitary t.
occipitopontine t.
olfactory t.
outflow t.
pancreaticobiliary t.
pilonidal t.
posterior spinocerebellar t.
pyramidal t.
respiratory t.
reticulospinal t.
right ventricular outflow t. (RVOT)
seminal t.

T

NOTES

tract *(continued)*
   sensory t.
   sinus t.
   spinocerebellar t.
   spinoreticular t.
   spinothalamic t.
   tectospinal t.
   tegmental t.
   temporopontine t.
   trigeminothalamic t.
   upper aerodigestive t.
   upper gastrointestinal t.
   urinary t.
   urogenital t.
   ventral spinocerebellar t.
   ventral spinothalamic t.
   ventricular outflow t.
   vestibulospinal t.
traction
   t. anchor
   breast t.
   bronchiectasis t.
   t. bronchiolectasis
   t. diverticulum
   t. epiphysis
   t. exostosis
   t. fracture
   t. spur
tractogram
tractography
tractotomy
   stereotactic t.
tragus
train
   echo t.
   spin-echo t.
trajectory
   k-space t.
TRAK
   total reference air kerma
Trak Back pullback device
tramline
   t. cortical calcification
   t. effect in the liver
   t. shadow
trampoline fracture
tram-track
   t.-t. appearance
   t.-t. ductus arteriosus calcification
   t.-t. gyral calcification
   t.-t. pattern
   t.-t. renal cortical necrosis
   calcification
   t.-t. streaming
transabdominal
   t. cholangiography
   t. color Doppler sonography

   t. imaging
   t. left lateral retroperitoneal
   maneuver
   t. pneumoperitoneum
   t. scanning
   t. sonogram
   t. ultrasound (TAUS)
transanular patch reconstruction
transaortic
   t. radiofrequency ablation
   t. systolic gradient
transapical endocardial ablation
transarterial chemoembolization (TACE)
transaxial
   t. annihilation photon pair
   t. CT scan
   t. fat-saturated 3D image
   t. imaging
   t. joint scan
   t. maximum-intensity projection
   t. PET scan
   t. scan plane
   t. slice
   t. thoracic inlet
transaxillary lateral view
transbrachial arch aortogram
transbronchial
   t. lung biopsy
   t. needle aspiration (TBNA)
transcaphoid fracture
transcapitate fracture
transcarpal amputation
transcatheter
   t. ablation
   t. arterial chemoembolization
   (TACE)
   t. filter placement
   t. hepatic arterial
   chemoembolization
   t. oily chemoembolization
   radiofrequency modification t.
   t. stent-graft treatment
   t. technique
   t. therapy
transcerebral medullary vein
transcervical
   t. balloon tuboplasty (TBT)
   t. catheterization of fallopian tube
   imaging
   t. femoral fracture
transchondral talar fracture
transcondylar
   t. amputation
   t. axis (TCA)
   t. fracture
   t. line
transcoronal STIR image

transcortical
transcranial
    t. color-coded Doppler
    t. color-coded Doppler sonography
    t. color-coded duplex sonography
     (TCCS)
    t. color-coded duplex ultrasound
    t. color-coded sonography
    t. Doppler (TCD)
    t. Doppler ultrasound
    t. Doppler velocity
    t. examination
    t. lateral view
    t. real-time color Doppler imaging
    t. real-time color-flow Doppler
     sonography
transcutaneous
    t. angiogenesis gene delivery
    t. aortovelography (TAV)
    t. broadband sector transducer
    t. crush injury
    t. electrical nerve stimulator
    t. extraction catheter atherectomy
    t. oxygen pressure measurement
     (tcPO$_2$)
transducer
    Acuson linear array t.
    Acuson V5M multiplane
     transesophageal
     echocardiographic t.
    Acuson 128 XP t.
    Aloka SSD-1700 t.
    anular array t.
    ART t.
    t. beam pattern
    biopsy t.
    biplanar t.
    broadband t.
    catheter-borne sector t.
    diffracting Doppler t.
    electronic linear array t.
    end-fire t.
    end-viewing t.
    epicardial Doppler flow sector t.
    Gaeltec catheter-tip pressure t.
    Gould Statham pressure t.
    high-frequency t.
    high-resolution linear array t.
    linear array t.
    Logic 700 MR t.
    magnetic resonance imaging-guided
     focused ultrasound sector t.

    7.5-MHz linear t.
    12- to 5-MHz linear array t.
    2.5-, 5-MHz sector t.
    Millar catheter-tip t.
    M-mode sector t.
    Mountain View t.
    MRI-guided focused ultrasound t.
    multiplanar t.
    phased-array t.
    piezoelectric t.
    PSH-25GT transcranial imaging t.
    puncture t.
    rectal multiplane t.
    sector t.
    signal t.
    transcutaneous broadband sector t.
    transesophageal t.
    Ultramark 8 t.
    ultrasound t.
    V510B Biplane TEE t.
    V5M Multiplane t.
transducer-skin interface
transducer-tipped catheter
transduction
    signal t.
transduodenal
    t. endoscopic decompression
    t. endosonography
    t. fiberscopic duct injection
transdural fistula
transection (*var. of* transsection)
transependymal uptake of tracer
transepiphyseal fracture
transesophageal
    t. Doppler color flow imaging
    t. echocardiography (TEE)
    t. echocardiography probe
    t. transducer
transethmoidal encephalocele
transfascial spread
transfemoral
    t. arteriography
    t. cerebral angiography
transfer
    energy t.
    Fourier t.
    gradient echo MR with
     magnetization t.
    His-Haas muscle t.
    t. imaging
    interhemispheric t.
    inversion t.

T

NOTES

transfer *(continued)*
    t. lesion
    linear energy t. (LET)
    magnetization t. (MT)
    quantitative magnetization t.
    rapid image t.
    saturation t.
    selective population t. (SPT)
    ultrafast video t.
    ultrasound guidance during
        embryo t.
transferrin
    indium t.
transfibular fusion
transfixing screw
transforaminal
    t. examination
    t. insonation
    t. window
transform
    automated Hough t.
    cosine t.
    2D Fourier t. (2DFT)
    discrete cosine t. (DCT)
    discrete Fourier t. (DFT)
    driven equilibrium Fourier t.
    fast Fourier t. (FFT)
    fast inversion-recovery Fourier t.
        (FIRFT)
    Fourier t. (FT)
    Hough t. (HT)
    t. imaging
    inverse Fourier t. (IFT)
    partially relaxed Fourier t. (PRFT)
    three-dimensional Fourier t. (3DFT)
    water eliminated Fourier t. (WEFT)
    wavelet t.
transformation
    blastic t.
    cavernous portal vein t.
    t. constant
    enthesopathic t.
    Fourier discrete t.
    hemorrhagic t.
    malignant t.
    t. matrix
    nuclear magnetic resonance
        Fourier t.
    photo t.
    rho° t.
    vascular t.
    t. zone
transformer (t)
    closed core t.
    Coolidge t.
    distribution t.

doughnut t.
t. equation
filament t.
high-voltage t.
t. law
t. loss
ratio t.
real-time chirp Z t.
step-down t.
step-up t.
transfusional iron overload
transgastric
    t. echocardiographic view
    t. endosonography
transgluteal CT-guided technique
transgression
    cortical t.
transhamate fracture
transhepatic
    t. biliary stent
    t. cholangiogram (THC)
    t. drainage
    t. portography
transhiatal esophagectomy
transient
    t. AV block
    t. bone marrow edema
    t. bone marrow edema syndrome
    t. cavitation
    t. cerebral ischemia
    t. chyle leak
    t. equilibrium
    t. gallbladder hydrops
    t. hepatic attenuation difference
        (THAD)
    t. hiatal hernia
    t. intussusception
    t. ischemic attack (TIA)
    t. ischemic carotid insufficiency
    t. left ventricular dilatation
    t. myocardial ischemia
    t. osteoporosis of hip
    t. perfusion defect
    t. peritumoral enhancement
    t. pleural effusion
    t. punctate cortical hyperintensities
        on T1-weighted image
    t. regional osteoporosis
    t. shunt obstruction
    t. sinus arrest
    t. symmetric pulmonary infiltrate
    t. synovitis
    t. synovitis of hip
    t. tachypnea
    t. tricuspid regurgitation
transiliac fracture

transillumination
> t. of head
> multispectral diffuse t.

transit
> biliary-to-bowel t.
> bolus t.
> delayed small bowel t.
> impaired tubular t.
> parenchymal t.
> t. scintigraphy
> small bowel delayed t.
> t. time
> tubular t.
> t. volume

transition
> allowed beta t.
> beta t.
> t. delay (TD)
> t. electron
> isobaric t.
> isomeric t.
> t. metal
> t. ureteral cell carcinoma
> t. zone

transitional
> t. cell carcinoma (TCC)
> t. cell neoplasm
> t. kidney cell carcinoma
> t. meningioma
> t. rhythm
> t. urethral cell papilloma
> t. urinary bladder cell carcinoma
> t. vertebra
> t. zone fissure

transjugular
> t. cholangiogram
> t. intrahepatic portosystemic shunt (TIPS)
> t. intrahepatic portosystemic shunt gradient
> t. intrahepatic portosystemic shunt imaging
> t. liver biopsy (TLB)
> t. portography
> t. portosystemic stent shunt placement
> t. venography

translation
> condylar t.
> parallel mean t.
> perpendicular mean t.

> radioulnarproximodistal t.
> tibial t.

translational
> t. diffusion
> t. motion

translation-invariant filter
translesional gradient
translocation
> t. of coronary artery
> robertsonian t.

translucency
> first-trimester nuchal t.
> nuchal t.

translucent
> t. depression
> t. silicone tube

translumbar
> t. amputation
> t. aortic route
> t. aortography (TLA)
> t. aortography needle

transluminal
> t. atherectomy
> t. balloon angioplasty
> t. coronary artery angioplasty complex
> t. dilatation
> t. endarterectomy
> t. endograft implantation
> t. endovascular stent-graft placement

transluminally placed stented graft
transmalleolar
> t. ankle
> t. axis-thigh angle

transmantle dysplasia
transmedial plane
transmesenteric plication
transmetallation assessment
transmetatarsal amputation (TMA)
transmetatarsal-thigh angle
transmissible venereal tumor
transmission
> airborne t.
> t. block
> t. computed tomography
> t. computer-assisted tomography (TCAT)
> t. control protocol/Internet protocol (TCP/IP)
> t. data
> direct-contact t.
> t. dosimetry

T

NOTES

transmission *(continued)*
    t. electron microscopic study
    indirect-contract t.
    t. scan
    sound t.
    through-sound t.
transmitral
    t. flow
    t. gradient
transmit-receive coil
transmitter coil
transmural
    t. colitis
    t. fibrosis
    t. inflammation
    t. invasion
    t. match
    t. myocardial infarct
    t. necrosis
    t. steal
transmyocardial
    t. perfusion pressure
    t. revascularization (TMR)
transnasal
transnasally
transonic
Transonics
    T. flow probe
    T. system
transoral carotid ultrasonography (TOCU)
transorally
transorbital window
transosseous venography
transpapillary placement
transparent rendering
transpedicular
    t. decompression
    t. vertebroplasty
transperineal
    t. implant
    t. ultrasound
transphyseal bone bridge
transplant
    allogeneic bone marrow t.
    allogeneic peripheral cell t.
    antigen-modulated mini-stem cell t.
    arteriovenous fistula t.
    autologous bone marrow t.
    bone marrow t.
    cadaveric renal t.
    enteric-drained pancreas t.
    heart t.
    heart-lung t.
    hepatic t.
    kidney t.
    kidney-pancreas t.

    liver t.
    lung t.
    marrow t.
    organ t.
    pancreas t.
    renal t.
    solid organ t. (SOT)
    syngeneic bone marrow t.
    tandem t.
transplantation
    autologous stem-cell t.
transplutonium radioisotope
transporionic axis
transport
    forward t.
    iodide t.
    Monte Carlo photon t. (MCPT)
    reverse t.
transporter
    dopamine t.
    vesicular amine t.
transposed
    t. adnexa
    t. aorta
transposition
    atrial t.
    carotid-subclavian t.
    t. cipher
    t. complex
    congenitally corrected t.
    gastric t.
    t. of great artery (TGA)
    great vessel t.
    t. of great vessel
    inferior vena cava t.
    t. of inferior vena cava
    Jatene t.
    t. of ovary
    subfascial t.
    ventricular t.
transpulmonary pressure (Ptp)
transpulmonic gradient
transpyloric plane
transradial styloid perilunate dislocation
transradiancy
transradiant
    t. air
    t. zone
transrectal
    t. echography
    t. sonography
    t. ultrasound (TRUS)
    t. ultrasound-guided biopsy of the prostate
transrenal ureteric occlusion
transsacral fracture

TransScan TS2000 electrical impedance breast scanning system
transscaphoid
    t. dislocation fracture
    t. perilunate dislocation
transscapular view
transsection, transection
    aortic t.
    spinal cord t.
    t. of spinal cord
    traumatic aortic t.
transseptal
    t. angiocardiography
    t. angiography
    t. perforation
    t. radiofrequency ablation
    t. sheath
transsphincteric anal fistula
transstenotic gradient
transsyndesmotic screw fixation
transtemporal
    t. insonation
    t. window
transtentorial herniation
transtentorially
transthoracic
    t. esophagectomy
    t. imaging
    t. needle aspiration biopsy (TTNAB)
    t. projection
    t. three-dimensional echocardiography
    t. ultrasound
    t. view
transthyretin
transtracheal aspiration
transtricuspid valve diastolic gradient
transtriquetral fracture
transtubercular plane (TTP)
transudate
transudation of fluid
transudative
    t. pericardial fluid
    t. pleural effusion
transumbilical plane (TUP)
transureteroureterostomy
transurethral
    t. incision of prostate
    t. needle ablation (TUNA)
    t. resection (TUR)
    t. resection of bladder

    t. resection of prostate (TURP)
    t. ultrasound-guided laser-induced prostatectomy (TULIP)
transvaginal
    t. cone
    t. echography
    t. hysterosonography (TVHS)
    t. implant
    t. oocyte retrieval
    t. sonography (TVS)
    t. ultrasound (TVUS)
    t. ultrasound-guided drainage
transvalvular pressure gradient
transvenous
    t. digital subtraction angiography
    t. implantation
    t. occlusion
transversalis fascia
transversal tomography
transversarium
    foramen t.
transverse
    t. acoustic wave
    t. anular tear
    t. aortic arch
    t. atlantal ligament
    t. band
    t. breath-hold gradient-echo cine magnetic resonance imaging
    t. carpal ligament
    t. cerebellar diameter (TCD)
    t. cervical ligament
    t. colon
    t. colon carcinoma
    t. colon loop
    t. comminuted fracture
    t. cord lesion
    t. costal facet
    t. cranial area
    t. crural ligament
    t. diameter between ischia
    t. ECD brain SPECT image
    t. esophageal fold
    t. genicular ligament
    t. heart
    t. humeral ligament
    t. hypoplasia
    t. intertarsal ligament
    t. lie
    t. ligament of atlas
    t. lucent metaphyseal line
    t. magnetization

NOTES

T

transverse *(continued)*
   t. maxillary fracture
   t. mesocolon
   t. metacarpal ligament
   t. metatarsal ligament
   t. myelitis
   t. orientation
   t. oval pelvis
   t. pelvic diameter
   t. pericardial sinus
   t. perineal ligament
   t. plane
   t. plane alignment
   t. plane force
   t. plane vectorcardiography
   t. presentation
   t. process
   t. process fracture
   t. process of vertebra
   t. relaxation
   t. relaxation of proton spin
   t. relaxation rate
   t. relaxation time
   t. relaxivity (R2)
   t. ridge
   t. scan
   t. section
   t. section imaging
   t. sinus thrombosis
   t. slice
   t. suture of Krause
   t. tarsal joint
   t. temporal gyrus
   t. testicular ectopia
   t. tibiofibular ligament
   t. ultrasound
   t. view
transversely oriented endplate
  compression fracture
transverse/neutral view
transverse-plane PET image
transversum
   septum t.
transversus
   t. abdominis muscle
   situs t.
transvesical oocyte retrieval
Transwell membrane
trap
   duodenum water t.
   metastable t.
TrapEase
   T. inferior vena cava filter
   T. vena cava filter
trapezia (*pl. of* trapezium)
trapeziometacarpal joint
trapezioscaphoid joint

trapeziotrapezoid joint
trapezium, pl. **trapezia**
   t. bone
   t. fracture
trapezium-metacarpal
   t.-m. eburnation (TME)
   t.-m. eburnation ratio
trapezius muscle
trapezoid
   t. body
   t. bone
   t. bone of Henle
   t. bone of Lyser
   t. ligament
trapping
   air t.
   t. of aneurysm
   gas t.
   t. of radioisotope
   t. thyroid defect
Traube
   T. heart
   T. sign
trauma
   abdominal blunt t.
   acoustic t.
   asphyxial renal t.
   bladder contusion t.
   blunt chest t.
   blunt gastrointestinal t.
   blunt pancreatic t.
   cardiothoracic t.
   carotid artery dissection t.
   chest wall t.
   eye t.
   focused abdominal sonography
    for t. (FAST)
   gallbladder t.
   genitourinary tract t.
   GI tract t.
   head t.
   hepatic t.
   high-energy t.
   hypovolemia t.
   kidney t.
   ligamentous t.
   liver t.
   multiple t.
   t. oblique
   ocular t.
   osseous t.
   pancreatic t.
   pelvic vascular t.
   penetrating t.
   t. register image
   renal t.
   splenic t.

sustentacular t.
testicular t.
urethral t.
urinary bladder t.
vascular t.
vessel t.

traumatic
t. amputation
t. aortic disruption
t. aortic injury
t. aortic pseudoaneurysm
t. aortic rupture
t. aortic tear
t. aortic transsection
t. arthritis
t. avulsion
t. bone cyst
t. bone survey
t. brain injury (TBI)
t. clinodactyly
t. degeneration
t. diaphragmatic hernia
t. dislocation
t. emphysema
t. fat necrosis
t. head injury
t. infarct
t. intracranial aneurysm (TICA)
t. lipid cyst
t. lung cyst
t. meningeal hemorrhage
t. meningocele
t. osteoarthritis
t. pneumatocele
t. pneumomediastinum
t. pneumonia
t. pneumothorax
t. rupture of the diaphragm (TRD)
t. spondylolisthesis
t. spondylolysis
t. syrinx
t. thrombus
t. tricuspid incompetence

traumatogenic occlusion
traversal
tentorial t.
traverse
traversing the fracture
TRAX catheter
tray
Müller t.

TRC
tanned red cell
TRD
traumatic rupture of the diaphragm
penetrating TRD
Treacher Collins syndrome
treatment
allocation of t.
cobalt-60 gamma knife
radiosurgical t.
crossfire t.
early endovascular t.
t. energy
equivalent t.
ferromagnetic microembolization t.
fibrinolytic t.
intensity-modulated radiotherapy t.
(IMRT)
interstitial hyperthermia t.
intracavitary hyperthermia t.
iodine-131 antiferritin t.
low-energy radiofrequency
conduction hyperthermia t.
microwave hyperthermia t.
microwave nonsurgical t.
percutaneous tumor t.
t. planning system (TMS)
t. port
refractory to t.
Sonographic Planning of
Oncology T. (SPOT)
superficial hyperthermia t.
thyroid radioiodine t.
transcatheter stent-graft t.
ultrasound hyperthermia t.

tree
airway t.
arterial t.
t. artifact
bile t.
biliary t.
bronchial t.
coronary artery t.
hepatobiliary t.
iliocaval t.
intrahepatic biliary t.
lower extremity arterial t.
tracheobronchial t.
tree-barking kidney
tree-in-bud
t.-i.-b. bronchiole
t.-i.-b. opacity

NOTES

T

tree-in-bud *(continued)*
  t.-i.-b. pattern
  t.-i.-b. sign
tree-in-winter bile duct appearance
tree-like airway structure
tree-shaped spot
trefoil
  t. appearance
  t. deformity
Treitz
  T. fossa
  T. hernia
  ligament of T.
  T. muscle
Trendelenburg
  T. position
  T. radiograph
trephine technique
treppe phenomenon
Trerotola thrombectomy device
Trevor disease
**Trex digital mammography system
  (TDMS)**
triad
  acute compression t.
  Beck t.
  Carney t.
  Charcot t.
  Currarino t.
  Cushing t.
  Garland t.
  Kartagener t.
  O'Donoghue unhappy t.
  Osler t.
  portal t.
  Rigler t.
  Saint t.
  T. SPECT imaging system
  wall-echo shadow t.
  Whipple t.
TRIADS
  time-resolved imaging by automatic data
    segmentation
trial
  carotid revascularization
    endarterectomy stent t.
  Malmo mammographic screening t.
  PROACT I, II t.
triamine
triangle
  aponeurotic t.
  auricular t.
  axillary t.
  Bolton t.
  Bryant t.
  Burger scalene t.
  Calot t.

t. of Capener
cardiohepatic t.
carotid t.
cephalic t.
cervical t.
clavipectoral t.
Codman t.
t. configuration
crural t.
cysticohepatic t.
deltoideopectoral t.
digastric t.
Einthoven t.
facial t.
femoral t.
Garland t.
Gerhardt t.
Grynfeltt t.
Henke t.
Hesselbach t.
iliofemoral t.
inguinal t.
insular t.
internal jugular t.
Kager t.
Koch t.
Korányi-Grocco t.
Labbé t.
t. of Laimer
Langenbeck t.
Lesgaft t.
Livingston t.
lumbocostoabdominal t.
mandibular t.
mesenteric t.
paramedian t.
Pawlik t.
posterior cervical t.
Raider t.
Rauchfuss t.
scalene t.
Scarpa t.
submandibular t.
supraclavicular t.
sylvian t.
Todaro t.
tracheal t.
urogenital t.
vertebrocostal t.
Ward t.
triangular
  t. area of dullness
  t. bone
  t. defect
  t. disk
  t. external ankle fixation
  t. fibrocartilage (TFC)

t. fibrocartilaginous complex (TFCC)
t. fontanelle
t. ligament
t. muscle
t. ridge
triangulation method
triatrial heart
triatriatum
cor t.
Triboulet test
tributary
t. collateral
extrahepatic portal vein t.
large venous t.
tricarboxylic acid cycle
triceps
t. brachii
t. brachii tendon
trichinous embolus
trichloroacetic acid
trichobezoar
trichoptysis
trichorhinophalangeal (TRP)
TRICKS
time-resolved imaging of contrast kinetics
tricompartmental chondromalacia of the knee
tricorn bucket-handle tear
tricuspid
t. aortic valve
t. incompetence (TI)
t. insufficiency (TI)
t. orifice
t. orifice regurgitation
t. stenosis
t. valve (TV)
t. valve anomaly
t. valve anulus
t. valve area
t. valve atresia
t. valve closure
t. valve cusp
t. valve deformity
t. valve dysplasia
t. valve flow
t. valve gradient
t. valve prolapse
t. valve regurgitation
t. valve strut
t. vertebra

trident
t. hand
t. pelvis
Tridrate bowel preparation
trifascicular block
trifid
t. precordial motion
t. stomach
triflanged nail
trifurcation
t. of artery
patency t.
popliteal artery t.
trigeminal
t. cavernous fistula
t. cavity
t. cistern
t. ganglion
t. hemangioma
t. nerve anatomy
t. pattern
t. rhizotomy
schwannoma t.
t. trigeminy
t. trigonal hypertrophy
trigeminothalamic tract
trigeminy
trigeminal t.
ventricular t.
trigger
t. delay (TD)
t. delay time
ECG t.
electrocardiogram t.
t. finger
t. finger deformity
respiratory t.
triggered-flow mode
triggered pacing mode
triggering
electrocardiograph t.
navigator echo-based real-time respiratory gating and t.
respiratory t.
trigona (*pl. of* trigonum)
trigonal
t. hypertrophy
t. muscle
t. process
trigone
angles of t.
t. of bladder

T

NOTES

967

trigone *(continued)*
    collateral t.
    deltoideopectoral t.
    fibrous t.
    Henke t.
    hypertrophied t.
    hypoglossal t.
    inguinal t.
    lateral ventricle t.
    Lieutaud t.
    Pawlik t.
    t. of ventricle
    vertebrocostal t.
trigonocephaly
trigonum, pl. trigona
    t. calcis
    os t.
    unfused os t.
triiodinated imaging agent
triiodobenzoic
    t. acid
    t. acid contrast medium
triiodothyronine
trilaminar appearance
trilateral retinoblastoma
trilayer appearance
trileaflet aortic valve
trilinear interpolation
trilobate
trilobed
trilobulation
trilocular heart
trilogy of Fallot
trimalleolar
    t. ankle fracture
triode tube
triolein
    iodine-131 t.
Trionix
    T. camera
    T. scanner
    T. SPECT
Trionix-Triad camera
Triosil contrast medium
tripartite duodenal carcinoma
triphalangeal
    t. thumb
    t. thumb deformity
triphasic
    t. spiral CT
    t. waveform
Triphasix generator
triphenyltetrazolium chloride (TTC)
triphosphate
    adenosine t.
    arabinsylguanosine t.

cyclic guanosine t.
nucleoside t. (NTP)
triplane fracture
triple
    t. label
    t. match
    t. pass technique
    t. therapy (TT)
    t. track sign
triple-bubble sign
triple-dose
    t.-d. gadolinium-enhanced MR
        imaging without MT
    t.-d. gadolinium imaging
triple-head gamma camera
triple-H therapy
triple-leaf collimator
triple-marker screening test
triple-peak cerebellum configuration
triple-phase
    t.-p. bone scan
    t.-p. bone scan imaging
triple-resonance NMR probe circuit
triplet
    t. gestation
    ghost reduction by equalized
        acquisition t.'s (GREAT)
triple-voiding
    t.-v. cystogram
    t.-v. cystography
triplex
    t. mode Doppler sonography
    t. scanning
tripod
    t. fracture
    t. position
tripoint bullet
Tripter
    Direx T.
triquetral
    t. bone
    t. fracture
    t. impingement
triquetrohamate
    t. helicoid slope
    t. joint
    t. ligament
triquetrolunate dislocation
triquetropisiform articulation
triquetroscaphoid
    t. fascicle
    t. ligament
triquetrotrapezoid fascicle
triquetrum
triradiate cartilage
trisacryl gelatin microsphere

trisodium
  gadofosveset t.
  mangafodipir t.
trisomic fetus
trisomy
  t. D, E syndrome
  t. 8 syndrome
TriSpan aneurysm neck-bride device
trispiral tomography
tristimulus
  t. value
  t. value flip
tritiated
  t. thymidine (TT)
  t. thymidine labeling index
tritium
triton tumor
trocar-cannula technique
trochanter
  greater t.
  lesser t.
trochanteric
  t. bursa
  t. bursitis
  t. flare
  t. spine
trochlea, pl. trochleae
  peroneal t.
trochlear
  t. defect
  t. groove
  t. nerve
  t. nerve neoplasm
  t. notch
  t. process
trochleocapitellar groove
troika
  aponeurotic t.
Troisier
  T. node
  T. sign
troland
Trolard
  vein of T.
trolley-track sign
TRON 3 VACI cardiac imaging system
Tronzo intertrochanteric fracture classification
trophedema
trophic
  t. fracture
  t. lesion

trophoblastic
  t. material
  t. ring
tropical
  t. pancreatitis
  t. ulcer osteoma
tropic ulcer
tropism
  facet t.
tropolone
tropomyosin
trough
  t. line
  t. sign
  t. of venous pulse
  X t.
  Y t.
trousers
  military antishock t. (MAST)
Trousseau
  T. sign
  T. syndrome
TRP
  trichorhinophalangeal
TR/TE
  repetition time to echo time ratio
  long T.
  short T.
true
  t. aortic aneurysm
  t. back muscle
  t. channel
  t. conjugate measurement
  t. dynamic joint imaging
  t. event
  t. fast imaging with steady-state
    precession (TrueFISP)
  t. heart aneurysm
  t. hermaphroditism
  t. histiocytic lymphoma
  t. intersex
  t. lateral view
  t. lumen
  t. metatarsus adductus (TMA)
  t. mitral stenosis
  t. negative (TN)
  t. pelvis
  t. porencephaly
  t. positive (TP)
  t. rib
  t. suture
  t. umbilical cord knot

T

NOTES

true *(continued)*
>   t. ventricular aneurysm
>   t. vertebra
>   t. vocal cord

TrueFISP
>   true fast imaging with steady-state precession
>>   blood-to-myocardium contrast of T.

true-negative
>   t.-n. lesion
>   t.-n. mammogram

true-positive result

Trümmerfeld
>   T. line
>   T. zone

trumpet-like pelvocaliceal system

truncal
>   t. artery
>   t. instability
>   t. renal artery stenosis
>   t. rhabdomyosarcoma
>   t. valve

truncated
>   t. arch index
>   t. atrial appendage
>   t. NMR probe

truncation
>   t. band artifact
>   t. phenomenon

truncus arteriosus

trunk
>   aortopulmonary t.
>   arterial brachiocephalic t.
>   atrioventricular t.
>   bifurcation of t.
>   brachiocephalic t.
>   bronchomediastinal lymph t.
>   celiac t.
>   celiomesenteric t.
>   cord-like t.
>   costocervical t.
>   dilated pulmonary t.
>   joints of t.
>   lumbosacral t.
>   lymphatic t.
>   meningohypophyseal t.
>   nerve t.
>   neuromeningeal t.
>   posterior vagal t.
>   pulmonary t.
>   sinus of pulmonary t.
>   thyrocervical t.
>   tibioperoneal t.
>   twin t.
>   vagal t.

Trunkey fracture classification

TRUS
>   transrectal ultrasound

TRW
>   teboroxime resting washout

TS
>   tuberous sclerosis

T-Scan 2000

T-score measurement of bone mineral density

TSD
>   target-skin distance

TSE
>   turbo spin-echo
>>   TSE image

TSE-relaxometry

T-shaped
>>   T-s. fracture
>>   T-s. uterus

TSPP
>   tetrasodium pyrophosphate
>>   TSPP imaging

TSR
>   total saturation recovery

T-stage

TS2000 TransScan 2000

TSV
>   total stroke volume

TT
>   triple therapy
>   tritiated thymidine

TTC
>   triphenyltetrazolium chloride
>   T-tube cholangiogram

TTD
>   tissue tolerance dose

TTF
>   time-to-treatment failure

TTI
>   tension-time index

TTNAB
>   transthoracic needle aspiration biopsy

TTP
>   time-to-peak intensity
>   time-to-peak value
>   transtubercular plane

TTTS
>   twin-to-twin transfusion syndrome

T-tube
>>   T-t. cholangiogram (TTC)
>>   T-t. cholangiography
>>   French T-t.
>>   T-t. stent

tubal
>   t. canal
>   t. fimbrial opening
>   t. insufflation
>   t. mass

t. obstruction
t. occlusion
t. pregnancy
t. ring
t. tonsil

tubarius
tonsil of torus t.
torus t.

tube
Angio-Seal carrier t.
angled pleural t.
anode t.
anteroposterior t.
apically directed chest t.
atretic t.
auditory t.
bilateral pleural t.
blocked shunt t.
bronchial t.
calix t.
Cantor t.
capillary t.
carrier t.
cathode ray t. (CRT)
Celestin t.
Chaoul voltage x-ray t.
chest t.
collecting t.
Coolidge x-ray t.
corneal t.
Crookes t.
cuffed endotracheal t.
t. current
t. decompression
decompression t.
Dennis t.
t. device
dialysis t.
digestive t.
discharge t.
Dotter t.
t. drainage
electron multiplier t.
endobronchial t.
endotracheal t.
eustachian t.
fallopian t.
feeding t.
fenestrated t.
field emission t.
fMR t.
Frederick-Miller t.

functional MR t.
gastrostomy t.
Geiger-Müller t.
t. geometry module
glow modular t.
Herring t.
high-heat-capacity x-ray t.
hot cathode x-ray t.
image intensifier t.
interstitial afterloading nylon t.
intestinal t.
J-shaped t.
large-caliber t.
Lenard ray t.
Levine t.
mediastinal t.
metallic distal end of t.
MIC gastroenteric t.
MIC jejunal t.
microfocal direct magnification in
vitro x-ray t.
Miller-Abbott t.
Minnesota t.
molybdenum target t.
Moss gastrostomy t.
muscular t.
nasogastric (NG) t.
nasojejunal feeding t.
nasotracheal t.
neural t.
Newvicon camera t.
obstructed shunt t.
Olshevsky t.
oroendotracheal t.
orogastric t.
Orthicon t.
overcouch t.
pharyngotympanic t.
photomultiplier t. (PMT)
pickup t.
pleural t.
polyethylene t.
t. position rotation
pull-type gastrostomy t.
rectifier t.
right-angle chest t.
roentgen t.
rotating anode t.
Salem sump t.
self-quenched counter t.
Sengstaken-Blakemore t.
separator t.

T

NOTES

tube *(continued)*
    Shiner radiopaque t.
    shunt t.
    solid-phase extraction t.
    SRO 2550 x-ray t.
    stomach t.
    straight chest t.
    suction t.
    Thal-Quick chest t.
    t. thoracostomy
    thoracostomy t.
    tracheal t.
    tracheostomy t.
    translucent silicone t.
    triode t.
    uterine t.
    vacuum t.
    valve t.
    Vidicon camera t.
    t. voltage waveform
    Westergren t.
    x-ray t.

tuber
    brain t.
    t. cinereum
    t. cinereum hamartoma
    cortical t.

tubercle
    accessory t.
    acoustic t.
    adductor t.
    amygdaloid t.
    articular t.
    auricular t.
    calcaneal t.
    carotid t.
    Chaput t.
    conoid t.
    corniculate t.
    costal t.
    crown t.
    cuneiform t.
    darwinian t.
    dental t.
    dissection t.
    dorsal t.
    epiglottic t.
    fibrous t.
    genial t.
    Gerdy t.
    Ghon t.
    greater t.
    iliac t.
    intercondylar t.
    jugular t.
    lesser t.
    Lister t.

    Lower t.
    t. of Morgagni
    noncaseating t.
    Parsons t.
    peroneal t.
    prominent t.
    pubic t.
    rib t.
    Rolando t.
    scalene t.
    supraglenoid t.
    tibial t.
    ulnar t.

tubercula (*pl. of* tuberculum)
tuberculate
tuberculated
tuberculation
tuberculin syringe
tuberculoid
tuberculoma
    brain t.
    calcified myocardial t.
    intracranial t.
    intraparenchymal t.
    lung t.

tuberculosis (TB)
    acinar t.
    adrenal t.
    airway t.
    anorectal t.
    anthrocotic t.
    atypical t.
    basal t.
    bone t.
    cavitary t.
    cestodic t.
    t. cutis indurativa
    t. cutis lichenoides
    cystic t.
    Delmege sign of t.
    disseminated t.
    endobronchial t.
    extrapulmonary t.
    exudative t.
    fibroproductive t.
    fulminant t.
    genitourinary t.
    GI tract t.
    t. granulation tissue
    GU tract t.
    hematogenous t.
    inhalation t.
    t. lichenoides
    meningeal t.
    mesenteric t.
    miliary pulmonary t.
    multidrug-resistant t.

neural t.
open t.
postprimary pulmonary t.
primary pulmonary t.
progressive primary t.
pulmonary t.
reactivation t.
recrudescent t.
renal t.
Schick sign of t.
skeletal t.
spinal t.
stable-state t.
t. verrucosa cutis
tuberculous
t. arthritis
t. bone
t. bronchiectasis
t. bronchopneumonia
t. cystitis
t. dactylitis
t. effusion
t. empyema
t. granuloma
t. infiltrate
t. lesion
t. mediastinal adenopathy
t. nodule
t. osteomyelitis
t. peritonitis
t. pneumonia
t. pneumothorax
t. salpingitis
t. spondylitis
t. tenosynovitis
tuberculum, pl. **tubercula**
t. sella
t. sellae meningioma
tuberosis
tuberositas
tuberosity
bicipital t.
calcaneal t.
coracoid t.
costal t.
deltoid t.
femoral t.
greater t.
iliac t.
infraglenoid t.
ischial t.
lesser t.

navicular t.
omental t.
radial t.
tibial t.
ulnar t.
unguicular t.
tuberous sclerosis (TS)
tubing (*See* tube)
tuboabdominal pregnancy
tubogram
T t.
tuboligamentary pregnancy
tuboovarian
t. abscess
t. mass
t. pregnancy
tuboplasty
balloon t.
transcervical balloon t. (TBT)
ultrasound transcervical t.
tuboreticular structure
tubotympanic canal
tubouterine pregnancy
tubular
t. aneurysm
t. aortic hypoplasia
t. bone
t. breast carcinoma
t. bronchiectasis
t. cavity
t. dilatation
t. dysgenesis
t. ectasia
t. ectasia of rete testis
t. fertility index
t. fluid-density adnexal mass
t. function
t. gas pattern
t. hiatal hernia
t. kidney secretion
t. lesion
t. lung density
t. magnet
t. necrosis
t. nephrogram
t. opacity
t. polyp
t. stenosis
t. structure
t. transit
t. ventricle
t. wire mesh

T

NOTES

tubule
    collecting t.
    connecting t.
    convoluted t.
    dentinal t.
    discharging t.
    distal convoluted t.
    proximal convoluted t.
    renal t.
    seminiferous t.
    straight t.
tubuloacinar
tubulointerstitial nephritis
tubulovillous
    t. colon adenoma
    t. polyp
Tuffier inferior ligament
tuft
    t. fracture
    osteolysis t.
    osteosclerosis t.
    penciling of terminal t.
    silk t.
    terminal t.
    ungual t.
    vascular t.
tularemic pneumonia
TULIP
    transurethral ultrasound-guided laser-induced prostatectomy
tulip
    t. bulb aorta
    t. sheath
tumefactive
    t. biliary sludge
    t. multiple sclerosis
    t. sludge
tumor
    abdominal wall desmoid t.
    t. ablation
    Abrikosov t.
    acidophilic pituitary t.
    acinic cell t.
    acoustic nerve sheath t.
    ACTH-producing t.
    acute splenic t.
    adenoid t.
    adenomatoid odontogenic t.
    adipose t.
    adrenal t.
    adrenocortical t.
    amelanotic t.
    ameloblastic adenomatoid t.
    ampulla t.
    amyloid t.
    anaplastic t.
    androgen-producing t.

    angiogenesis t.
    angiomatoid t.
    aortic body t.
    apple-core t.
    Askin thoracopulmonary neuroepithelial t.
    astrocytic t.
    astroglial t.
    Azzopardi t.
    ball-valve t.
    basiocciput t.
    B-cell t.
    t. bed
    Bednar t.
    benign congenital Wilms t.
    benign duodenal t.
    benign fibrous bone t.
    benign lung t.
    benign lymphoepithelial parotid t.
    benign ovarian t.
    benign small bowel t.
    benign teratoid mediastinum t.
    benign urethral t.
    biphasic breast t.
    bladder t.
    t. blood supply
    blood vessel t.
    t. blush
    t. blush on angiography
    bone t.
    bone-forming bone t.
    t. boundary
    brain t.
    Braun t.
    breast phyllode t.
    Brenner t.
    bright-signal-intensity t.
    bronchial carcinoid t.
    Brooke t.
    brown t.
    bulky t.
    t. burden
    burned-out t.
    Buschke-Löwenstein t.
    calcified amorphous t.
    t. capillary permeability
    t. capsule
    carcinoid t.
    cardiac t.
    carotid body t.
    cartilage-containing giant cell t.
    cartilage-forming bone t.
    cartilaginous soft-tissue t.
    catecholamine-producing t.
    cavernous t.
    cell t.
    t. cell-host bone relationship

cellular t.
central nervous system t.
cerebellopontine angle t.
cervical t.
chondrogenic t.
chondroid-origin t.
chromaffin t.
t. cleavage plane
clivus meningioma t.
CNS ghost t.
CNS multifocal t.
Codman t.
collision t.
colloid cystic t.
congenital cardiac t.
connective tissue fibrous t.
cranial nerve sheath t.
cystic t.
deep t.
deep-seated t.
t. defect
t. d'emblee mycosis fungoides
Denys-Drash t.
dermal duct t.
dermoid t.
desmoid t.
desmoplastic small round-cell t.
  (DSRCT)
destructive t.
discrete t.
t. dormancy
drug-resistant t.
ductectatic mucinous t.
dumbbell t.
duodenum malignant t.
dysembryoplastic neuroepithelial t.
  (DNET)
echogenic t.
eighth nerve t.
t. embolus
embryonic t., embryonal tumor
endobronchial t.
endocrine t.
endodermal sinus ovarian t.
endodermal sinus testis t.
endolymphatic sac t.
endometrioid t.
t. entity
epidermoid t.
epithelial t.
Erdheim t.
t. erosion

esophageal t.
essential t.
estrogen-producing t.
Ewing t.
t. extension
t. extirpation
extraaxial t.
extracompartmental t.
extradural t.
extrahepatic primary malignant t.
extramedullary t.
extratesticular t.
exuberant t.
fatty soft tissue t.
fecal t.
feign t.
feminizing adrenal t.
fetal mesenchymal t.
fibroid t.
fibrous connective tissue t.
finger of t.
flocculonodular t.
focal t.
focus of t.
fourth ventricle t.
friable t.
frontal lobe t.
fungating t.
galeal extension of t.
ganglion cell t.
gastroesophageal junction t.
gastrointestinal stromal t. (GIST)
gestational trophoblastic t.
giant cell t.
Glazunov t.
glial brain t.
globular t.
glomus body t.
glomus bone t.
glomus jugulare t.
glomus jugulotympanicum t.
glomus neck t.
Godwin t.
gonadal stromal t.
granulosa-theca cell t.
Grawitz t.
gross t.
Gubler t.
heart t.
hepatic t.
high-grade t.
highly vascular t.

T

NOTES

tumor *(continued)*
    hilar t.
    Hodgkin t.
    hourglass t.
    HPV16-associated t.
    HPV18-associated t.
    hypervascular pancreatic t.
    hypodiploid t.
    hypoechogenic t.
    hypoechoic solid t.
    hypopharyngeal t.
    hypothalamus t.
    t. hypoxia
    t. imaging
    t. implant
    incomplete t.
    t. inflammation
    inflammatory myofibroblastic t.
    infratentorial Lindau t.
    infundibular t.
    t. of infundibulum
    inoperable brain t.
    intestinal carcinoid t.
    intraaxial brain t.
    intracavitary extension of t.
    intracerebral t.
    intracompartmental t.
    intracranial t.
    intraductal mucin-producing t.
    intraductal papillary mucinous t.
      (IPMT)
    intradural extramedullary t.
    intradural intramedullary t.
    intramedullary spinal cord t.
    intramural t.
    intraosseous desmoid t.
    intraparenchymal lung t.
    intrasellar t.
    intraspinal t.
    intraventricular brain t.
    invasive malignant sheath t.
    islet cell t.
    jugular bulb t.
    juxtaglomerular t.
    Klatskin t.
    Krukenberg t.
    Leydig cell t. (LCT)
    lipogenic t.
    lipomatous t.
    t. of liver scar
    lobulated t.
    localized pleura t.
    locally invasive t.
    low-signal-intensity t.
    lung t.
    lymphocyte-rich t.
    lymphoepithelial parotid t.

    lymphoid t.
    main t.
    malignant duodenal t.
    malignant mediastinum teratoid t.
    malignant ovarian germ cell t.
    malignant ovarian teratoma t.
    malignant small bowel t.
    t. margin
    t. marker
    masculinizing t.
    t. mass
    t. matrix
    mediastinal teratoid t.
    melanotic neuroectodermal t.
    meningeal cell t.
    mesenchymal t.
    metastatic myocardial t.
    metasynchronous t.
    microcystic pancreatic t.
    micropapillary t.
    mucinous ovarian t.
    mucosal esophageal t.
    müllerian mucinous borderline t.
    multicentric carcinoid t.
    multifocal brain t.
    musculoskeletal t.
    napkin-ring anular t.
    neck germ-cell t.
    t. necrosis
    necrotic t.
    t. neovascularity
    t. neovasculature
    nerve root t.
    nerve sheath t.
    neural origin bone t.
    neuroectodermal t.
    neuroendocrine t.
    neurogenic t.
    neuroglial t.
    neuronal cell origin t.
    t. nidus
    nonechogenic t.
    nonfunctioning islet cell t.
    nonneoplastic t.
    nonseminomatous germ cell t.
    occult phosphaturic mesenchymal t.
    odontogenic t.
    optic complex t.
    oral cavity t.
    orbital childhood t.
    osteoblastic t.
    osteocartilaginous t.
    t. osteoid
    osteoid-origin t.
    ovarian mesonephroid t.
    ovary germ cell t.
    Pancoast t.

pancreatic islet cell t.
papillary t.
paracardiac t.
parasellar dermoid t.
parasympathetic ganglia t.
paratesticular t.
parathyroid t.
parotid t.
paucilocular t.
pearly CNS t.
pediatric primary brain t.
pediatric solid t.
pedunculated vesical t.
Pepper t.
periampullary duodenal t.
perineural fibroblastoma t.
peripheral neuroectodermal t.
peritoneum desmoid t.
phantom breast t.
phantom lung t.
phosphaturic t.
phosphaturic-inducing t.
phyllode t.
pilar t.
pilocytic t.
Pindborg t.
pineal germ-cell t.
pineal gland t.
pineal parenchymal t.
pineal region t.
pituitary t.
placenta t.
pontine angle t.
poorly circumscribed t.
poorly differentiated t.
posterior fossa t.
Pott puffy t.
pregnancy t.
primary benign liver t.
primary implanted t.
primary intracranial germ cell t.
primary malignant liver t.
primary renal t.
primitive neuroectodermal t.
  (PNET)
primitive neuroepithelial t.
prolapsed t.
pseudomalignant t.
pseudoorbital t.
pulmonary t.
radiation-associated papillary t.
radiation-induced peripheral nerve t.

radiosensitive t.
Rathke pouch t.
Recklinghausen t.
t. recurrence
refractory t.
renal t.
renin-secreting t.
Response Evaluation Criteria in
  Solid T.'s (RECIST)
reticuloendothelial t.
retinal anlage t.
retroperitoneal t.
rhabdoid t.
round bone-cell t.
round-cell t.
Rous t.
sacral bone t.
sacrococcygeal remnant t.
sand t.
scannable t.
Schmincke t.
Schwann t.
scirrhous t.
Scully t.
secondary ovarian t.
t. seeding
seminomatous t.
serous ovarian t.
Sertoli cell t. (SCT)
Sertoli-Leydig cell t.
sessile t.
t. shrinkage
t. signature
sinonasal t.
skull-base t.
small adrenal t.
small bowel benign t.
small bowel malignant t.
smooth muscle t.
solid and cystic pancreatic t.
solid ovarian t.
solid primary t.
solid-pseudopapillary t.
solitary pleura t.
sphenoid ridge t.
t. spheroid
spinal axis t.
spinal cord t.
sporadic t.
spread of t.
squamous odontogenic t.
t. staining

NOTES

tumor *(continued)*
t. stalk
sternocleidomastoid t.
stromal cell t.
subastrocytic t.
subcortical t.
subcutaneous t.
submucosal colon t.
submucosal esophageal t.
subserosal t.
subungual glomus t.
sugar t.
superior pulmonary sulcus t.
suprasellar extension of t.
supratentorial brain t.
supratentorial primitive
neuroectodermal t.
t. of surface epithelium
surface ovarian epithelium t.
sympathetic ganglia t.
synovitis t.
temporal bone t.
temporal lobe t.
tendon sheath giant cell t.
teratoid t.
testicular stromal cell t.
testis germ cell t.
tetradiploid t.
tetraploid t.
theca-cell ovarian t.
third ventricle t.
t. thrombus
t.-to-normal brain ratio
tracheal t.
transmissible venereal t.
triton t.
turban t.
ulcerative t.
umbilical t.
unilocular t.
urethral t.
urinary bladder t.
uroepithelial t.
vaginal t.
vanishing lung t.
t. vascularity
t. vascularization
vascular origin bone t.
vasoactive intestinal polypeptide t.
(VIPoma)
ventricular t.
vertebral body bone t.
villous t.
t. volume
t. volumetry
von Hippel retina t.
Warthin t.

well-circumscribed t.
well-differentiated polycystic
Wilms t.
Wharton t.
yolk sac ovary t.
Zollinger-Ellison t.
tumoral
t. calcification
t. calcinosis
t. callus
t. fat
t. invasion
tumor-angiogenesis factor
tumor-associated tissue eosinophilia
tumor-bearing bone
tumorigenesis
mammary t.
tumorigenic
tumorlet
tumor-like
t.-l. lesion
t.-l. shadow
tumor-mimicking breast lesion
tumorous
tumor-related spontaneous bleed
tumor-specific tracer
TUNA
transurethral needle ablation
tungstate
calcium t.
tungsten (W)
t. anode
t. carbide pneumoconiosis
T. eye shield
T. syringe shield
t. target
tungsten-188 (^{188}W)
tunica, pl. **tunicae**
t. albuginea cyst
t. intima
t. medium
t. propria
t. vaginalis
tunicary
tunicate
tunnel
aortic-left ventricular t.
baffled t.
carpal t.
cubital t.
fibroosseous t.
intramural t.
t. projection
t. radiograph
retropancreatic t.
retroperitoneal t.
t. subaortic stenosis

subcutaneous t.
subsartorial t.
t. subvalvular aortic stenosis
tarsal t.
t. view
tunneled catheter
Tuohy aortography needle
Tuohy-Borst introducer
TUP
transumbilical plane
TUR
transurethral resection
turban tumor
turbidimetric detection
turbinate
t. bone
nasal t.
paradoxical middle t.
turbo
t. fast low-angle shot
(turboFLASH)
t. gradient-refocused echo
(turboGRE)
t. inversion recovery sequence
t. IR sequence
t. pulse sequence
t. SE sequence
t. short tau inversion recovery
t. short tau/TI inversion recovery
t. spin-echo (TSE)
t. spin-echo technique
turboFLAIR
t. imaging
turboFLASH
turbo fast low-angle shot
turboFLASH imaging
turboFLASH sequence
turboGRE
turbo gradient-refocused echo
turboSTIR image
turbulence
TCD-detectable t.
turbulent
t. blood flow
t. intraluminal flow
t. signal
turcica
sella t.
Turcot syndrome
turn
insufficient cochlear t.
turned-up pulp deformity

Turner
T. marginal gyrus
T. syndrome
turnover
bone t.
erythrocyte iron t.
plasma iron t.
red blood cell iron t.
TURP
transurethral resection of prostate
turret exostosis
turricephaly
Turyn sign
tutamen
TV
tricuspid valve
TVG
time-varied gain
TVHS
transvaginal hysterosonography
TVS
transvaginal sonography
TVUS
transvaginal ultrasound
T-wave
asymmetric negative T-w.
T1-weighted
T1-w. acquisition
T1-w. axial image
T1-w. axial image with fat
saturation
T1-w. axial localizer
T1-w. conventional spin-echo
T1-w. coronal fat-suppressed fast
spin-echo sequence
T1-w. coronal image
T1-w. coronal imaging
T1-w. FAST
T1-w. fat-suppressed gadolinium-
enhanced SE image
T1-w. fat-suppressed image (T1FS)
T1-w. gadolinium-enhanced SE
image
T1-w. image (T1WI)
T1-w. magnetic resonance
T1-w. sagittal imaging
T1-w. spin echo
T1-w. study
T2-weighted
T2-w. axial image
T2-w. fast spin-echo coronal
oblique

T

NOTES

T2-weighted *(continued)*
    T2-w. fat-saturated sequence
    T2-w. image (T2WI)
    T2-w. pulse sequence
    T2-w. sagittal oblique image
    T2-w. scan
    T2-w. shortening
    T2-w. signal
    T2-w. spin-echo image
    T2-w. spin-echo sequence
    T2-w. turbo SE image
T2-weighted combination sequence
T1WI
    T1-weighted image
T2WI
    T2-weighted image
twiddler's syndrome
twig
    t. of artery
    cutaneous t.
    muscular t.
twin
    conjoined t.
    craniopagus t.
    dichorionic-diamniotic t.
    discordant t.
    dizygotic t.
    donor t.
    t. ectopic pregnancy
    t. embolization syndrome
    fraternal t.
    ischiopagus t.
    monochorionic-monoamniotic t.
    monozygotic t.
    omphalopagus t.
    t. peak sign
    perfused t.
    t. pregnancy discordant growth
    pygopagus t.
    thoracopagus t.
    t. trunk
    vanishing t.'s
twin-beam CT
twining
    t. line
    T. position
    t. recess
    T. view
twinkling artifact
twin-peaked pulse
twin-reversed arterial perfusion sequence
twin-to-twin transfusion syndrome (TTTS)
twist
    myocardial t.

twisted
    t. ankle
    t. body habitus
    t. ribbon-like rib
    t. small bowel ribbon appearance
twister gradient
two-balloon technique
two-bellied muscle
two-chamber echocardiography
two-channel phased-array RF receiver coil system
two-column injury
two-compartment system
two-dimensional (2D)
    t.-d. echocardiography (TDE)
    t.-d. magnetic resonance digital subtraction angiography (2D MRDSA)
    t.-d. time-of-flight (2D TOF)
two-dye method
two-element phased-array coil
two-frame gated imaging
two-loop ileal J pouch
two-needle biopsy technique
two-part fracture
two-phase
    t.-p. computed tomographic imaging
    t.-p. CT imaging
    t.-p. helical computed tomography
    t.-p. helical CT
two-plane
    t.-p. fluorometry
    t.-p. view
two-stage
    t.-s. amputation
    t.-s. fusion
    t.-s. venous cannulation
two-staged stent implantation
two-step
    t.-s. procedure
    t.-s. technique
two-vessel
    t.-v. runoff
    t.-v. umbilical cord
two-view
    t.-v. chest x-ray
    t.-v. film-screen mammography
tylectomy
tylosis, pl. **tyloses**
tympani
    tegmen t.
    tensor t.
tympanic
    t. bone
    t. cavity
    t. plexus

tympanicum
  glomus t.
tympanography
tympanosclerosis
type
  t. A carotid cavernous fistula
  t. A–C right ventricular
  hypertrophy
  centrocyte-like t.
  collagen defect t. I, II
  diffuse fibrosis t.
  glutaric aciduria t. I, II
  t. I endoleak (T1EL)
  t. II collagen C-telopeptide
  t. II endoleak (T2EL)
  t. I, II muscle fiber
  t. II (infracristal) ventricular septal
  defect
  t. I (supracristal) ventricular septal
  defect
  t. IV (muscular) ventricular septal
  defect

  MPS t.'s I–IV
  mucopolysaccharidosis t.'s I–IV
  t. 1, 2 neurofibromatosis
  odontoid fracture t.'s I–III
  pleomorphic t.
  reticular t.
  sonographic hip t.
type-MHRE/72
typhoid
  t. nodule
  t. pleurisy
typhus nodule
typical
  t. cobblestone pattern
  t. medullary carcinoma
tyropanoate
  t. sodium
Tyropaque imaging agent
tyrosinase
tyrphostin radiotracer for PET
T-zone lymphoma

NOTES

T

U
  unit
  uranium
U-1100 UV-Vis spectrophotometer
U1-NA cephalometric measurement
UA
  umbilical artery
    UA velocimetry
UAE
  uterine artery embolization
UAL
  ultrasound-assisted lipoplasty
UBIS 5000 ultrasound bone sonometer
UBM
  ultrasound backscatter microscopy
  ultrasound biomicroscopy
    UBM imaging
UBO
  unidentified bright object
UC
  ulcerative colitis
UCG
  ultrasonic cardiogram
UCL
  ulnar collateral ligament
UCLA imaging protocol
U-clips
    nitinol U-c.
UCT
  ultrasound computed tomography
UE
  angle electron
  upper extremity
UES
  upper esophageal sphincter
UFCT
  ultrafast computed tomography
UFE
  uterine fibroid embolization
U-fiber damage
UGI
  upper gastrointestinal
Uhl
    U. anomaly
    U. disease
UHMM
  ultra-high magnification mammography
Uhthoff sign
UI
  urethral inclination
UIP
  usual interstitial pneumonia
  usual interstitial pneumonia of Liebow
UIQ
  upper inner quadrant

UL
  upper lobe
  urethral length
ulcer
    acid peptic u.
    active duodenal u.
    acute peptic u.
    anastomotic u.
    anterior wall antral u.
    antral u.
    aortic penetrating u.
    aphthoid u.
    aphthous stomach u.
    apical duodenal u.
    arteriolar ischemic u.
    atheromatous u.
    atherosclerotic aortic u.
    Barrett u.
    u. base
    bear's claw u.
    benign gastric u.
    bleeding u.
    bulbar peptic u.
    channel pyloric u.
    chronic peptic u.
    collar-button u.
    colonic u.
    u. crater
    crater-like u.
    Cruveilhier u.
    Curling u.
    Cushing u.
    Cushing-Rokitansky u.
    decubitus u.
    u. disease
    duodenal u.
    esophageal u.
    flask-shaped u.
    focal u.
    frontier u.
    gastric u. (GU)
    gastrointestinal u.
    giant duodenal u.
    giant peptic u.
    greater curvature u.
    healed gastric u.
    healing u.
    Hunner u.
    hypertensive ischemic u.
    indolent radiation-induced rectal u.
    intestinal u.
    intractable u.
    ischemic u.
    jejunal u.
    juxtapyloric u.

U

ulcer *(continued)*
    kissing u.
    Kocher dilatation u.
    lesser curvature u.
    linear u.
    malignant gastric u.
    marginal u.
    Martorell hypertensive u.
    minute bleeding u.
    mucosal u.
    multiple small bowel u.'s
    necrotic u.
    u. osteoma
    patchy colonic u.
    penetrating aortic u.
    penetrating atherosclerotic u.
    peptic u.
    perforated u.
    u. perforation
    phagedenic u.
    postbulbar u.
    postsurgical recurrent u.
    prepyloric u.
    punched-out u.
    punctate u.
    puncture u.
    pyloric channel u.
    radiation-induced u.
    rake u.
    recurrent u.
    rodent u.
    Rokitansky-Cushing u.
    round u.
    ruptured u.
    Saemisch u.
    secondary u.
    serpiginous u.
    sloughing u.
    small bowel multiple u.
    solitary rectal u.
    stasis u.
    stercoral u.
    stomach u.
    stress u.
    subatheromatous u.
    thorn u.
    tropic u.
    urinary u.
    venous u.
    V-shaped u.
    u. with heaped-up edges
ulcerated
    u. atheromatous plaque
    u. carotid artery plaque
ulcerating
    u. adenocarcinoma
    u. granuloma of pudenda

ulcerative
    u. colitis (UC)
    u. esophageal carcinoma
    u. jejunitis
    u. jejunoileitis
    u. lesion
    u. lymphoma
    u. tumor
ULDR
    ultra-low dose rate
Ullmann line
ulna, pl. **ulnae**
    capitulum ulnae
    coronoid of u.
    fetal biometry u.
    sigmoid cavity of u.
ulnar
    u. bone
    u. bursa
    u. chondromalacia
    u. collateral ligament (UCL)
    u. deviation
    u. deviation view
    u. digital artery
    u. drift deformity
    u. extensor
    u. facing of metacarpal head
    u. fracture
    u. groove
    u. hand
    u. head
    u. impaction syndrome
    u. inclination
    u. nerve entrapment
    u. nerve lesion
    u. notch
    u. ridge
    u. sesamoid bone
    u. styloid
    u. styloid process
    u. styloid process index (USPI)
    u. sulcus
    u. traction spurring
    u. translocation of the carpus
    u. tubercle
    u. tuberosity
    u. tunnel syndrome
    u. variance
ulnaris
    extensor carpi u.
    flexor carpi u.
ulnocarpal ligament
ulnolunate
    u. impaction syndrome
    u. impingement
    u. ligament

ulnotriquetral
> u. distance
> u. ligament

ULP
> ultra-low profile

ULQ
> upper left quadrant

ultimobranchial pouch

Ultra
> U. ICE 9F/9 MHz catheter
> U. Tag kit
> U. Vision Rapid screen

UltraCision ultrasonic knife

Ultracranio T

ultra-early thrombolytic therapy

UltraEase ultrasound pad

ultrafast
> u. computed tomography (UFCT)
> u. computed tomography scanner
> u. contrast-enhanced MRA
> u. CT
> u. CT electron beam tomography
> u. CT imaging
> u. 3D MR digital subtraction
> angiography
> u. FLASH 2D sequence
> u. MRI
> u. video transfer

ultrafiltration

UltraFine Erbium laser system

Ultraflex stent

Ultra-Fluid
> 70–50% Lipiodol U.-F.

ultra-high
> u.-h. magnification
> u.-h. magnification mammography
> (UHMM)

ultrahigh-resolution, parallel-hole collimator

Ultraject prefilled syringe

ultralong TR

ultra-low
> u.-l. dose rate (ULDR)
> u.-l. profile (ULP)

Ultramark
> ATL U. 8, 9
> U. 9 scanner
> U. 8 transducer
> U. 4 ultrasound

UltraPACS diagnostic imaging system

UltraPulse CO$_2$ laser

ultrascan
> B-mode u.

Ultraseed brachytherapy

ultrasmall superparamagnetic iron oxide (USPIO)

UltraSoft
> 2/3-cm U. GDC
> 2/6-cm U. GDC
> U. GDC

ultrasonic
> u. aortography
> u. aspiration
> u. assessment
> u. assessment of injury
> u. atherolysis
> u. attenuation
> u. cardiogram (UCG)
> u. cardiography
> u. cephalometry
> u. guidance
> u. hysterography
> u. hysterosalpingography
> u. lithotripsy
> u. lithotripter cannula
> u. probe
> u. tomographic image
> u. tomographic imaging
> u. tomography
> u. wave

ultrasonically activated scalpel

ultrasonogram

ultrasonographic
> u. echo
> u. finding
> u. modeling

ultrasonographically guided injection

ultrasonography (US)   (*See* ultrasound)
> axillary u.
> compression u.
> endovascular u.
> infant cranial Doppler u.
> intracaval endovascular u.
> intraductal u.
> intraportal endovascular u. (IPEUS)
> laparoscopic contact u. (LCU)
> periorbital directional Doppler u.
> pulsed wave Doppler u.
> real-time u.
> rectal endoscopic u.
> transoral carotid u. (TOCU)
> venous u.

U

NOTES

ultrasonography *(continued)*
    vertebrobasilar transcranial color-coded duplex u.
ultrasonometer
    QUS-2 calcaneal u.
ultrasonometry
ultrasound (US)
    abdominal u.
    u. ablative therapy
    ACM u.
    Acuson 128 Doppler u.
    ADR Ultramark 4 u.
    AI 5200 diagnostic u.
    Aloka linear u.
    Aloka sector u.
    A-scan u.
    u. augmented mammography
    automated cardiac flow measurement u.
    u. backscatter microscopy (UBM)
    u. backscatter microscopy imaging
    u. biomicroscopy (UBM)
    BladderScan u.
    B-mode u.
    breast u.
    Bruel-Kjaer u.
    carotid duplex u.
    color-coded duplex u.
    color-coded real-time u.
    color Doppler u. (CDUS)
    color duplex u.
    color power transcranial Doppler u.
    u. computed tomography (UCT)
    contact B-scan u.
    contrast-enhanced u.
    cranial u.
    CT-guided u.
    1D u.
    2D B-mode u.
    3D freehand u.
    u. diagnosis
    diagnostic range u.
    u. diagnostic yield
    Diasonics u.
    diathermy u.
    u. diffraction tomography
    u. dilution
    u. dilution test
    Doppler u.
    duplex u. (DU)
    duplex B-mode u.
    duplex carotid u.
    duplex Doppler u.
    duplex-pulsed Doppler u.
    u. echocardiography
    EchoGen-enhanced u.
    u. echogenicity

    endoanal u.
    endorectal u. (ERU, ERUS, EUS)
    endoscopic u. (EUS)
    endovaginal u. (EVUS)
    endovascular u.
    FDI u.
    fetal u.
    FloWire Doppler u.
    focused u.
    freehand interventional u.
    full bladder u.
    gallbladder u.
    gastrointestinal endoscopic u.
    u. gel
    graded compression u.
    gray-scale u.
    gray-scale endorectal u.
    u. guidance during embryo transfer
    Hewlett-Packard u.
    high-frequency Doppler u.
    high-frequency therapeutic u.
    high-intensity focused u. (HIFU)
    high-resolution u.
    Hitachi u.
    u. hyperthermia treatment
    hypoechoic area of u.
    u. imaging technology
    immersion B-scan u.
    intracoronary u. (ICUS)
    intraluminal u. (ILUS)
    intraoperative u. (IOUS)
    intrarectal u.
    intravascular u. (IVUS)
    Irex Exemplar u.
    laparoscopic u. (LapUS, LUS)
    laparoscopic intracorporeal u. (LICU)
    level I obstetric u.
    limitation of u.
    low frequency u. (LFUS)
    low-intensity pulsed u.
    M-mode u.
    u. monitoring
    multiplanar endorectal u.
    neonatal adrenal u.
    neonatal transfontanellar brain u.
    NeuroSector u.
    noninvasive u.
    obstetric u.
    Olympus endoscopic u.
    u. pad
    pancreaticobiliary u.
    pelvic u.
    photoacoustic u.
    power Doppler u.
    PowerVision u.
    u. probe

ProSound SSD-5500 u.
pulsed Doppler u.
pulsed therapeutic low-intensity u.
pulse-inversion harmonic u.
real-time scan u.
renal u.
RT 6800 u.
RT 3200 Advantage u.
sagittal u.
SieScape u.
Sonicator portable u.
Sonolayer model SSA-270A u.
SonoSite digital u.
spectral u.
u. stethoscope
suprapubic transabdominal u.
u. system
TCD u.
u. test
u. threshold
TM u.
transabdominal u. (TAUS)
u. transcervical tuboplasty
transcranial color-coded duplex u.
transcranial Doppler u.
u. transducer
transperineal u.
transrectal u. (TRUS)
transthoracic u.
transvaginal u. (TVUS)
transverse u.
Ultramark 4 u.
u. venography
Vingmed u.
ultrasound-assisted lipoplasty (UAL)
ultrasound-based strain rate and strain imaging
ultrasound-guided
u.-g. anterior subcostal liver biopsy
celiac plexus neurolysis, endoscopic u.-g.
u.-g. core biopsy
u.-g. cyst aspiration
u.-g. large core-needle biopsy
u.-g. nephrostomy puncture
u.-g. percutaneous cholecystostomy
u.-g. percutaneous interstitial laser ablation
u.-g. percutaneous microwave coagulation therapy
u.-g. pseudoaneurysm compression

u.-g. reduction of a spigelian hernia
u.-g. stereotactic biopsy
u.-g. transthoracic needle aspiration
u.-g. vacuum-assisted biopsy
UltraSTAR computer-based ultrasound reporting system
ultrastructural abnormality
UltraSure DTR-one imaging ultrasound system
UltraTag RBC
Ultrathane Amplatz ureteral stent
ultratherm
Ultrathin Diamond balloon
ultraviolet
u. A, B, C
extravital u.
u. fluorescent dosimeter
intravital u.
u. lamp
psoralen and u. A (PUVA)
u. radiation
u. ray
u. spectrophotometry
u. spectrum
Ultravist 150, 240, 300, 370 contrast agent
umbau zone
umbilical
u. artery (UA)
u. artery velocimetry
u. canal
u. cord
u. cord anatomy
u. cord angiomyxoma
u. cord cyst
u. cord edema
u. cord hemangioma
u. cord hematoma
u. cord lesion
u. cord pseudocyst
u. fissure
u. granuloma
u. hernia
u. ligament
u. mass
u. plane
u. portography
u. ring
u. tumor
u. vein
u. vein varix

U

NOTES

umbilicovesical fascia
umbilicus
umbo, pl. umbones
umbonate
UMC-I microwave delivery system
UM 4 real-time sector scanner
unattached fraction
unbalanced hemivertebra
uncal
> u. gyrus
> u. herniation
> u. herniation syndrome

uncalcified pleural plaque
uncertainty principle
unciform bone
uncinate
> u. aura
> u. gyrus
> u. process
> u. process fracture
> u. process mass
> u. process of pancreas

uncoiling
> u. ascending aorta
> u. descending aorta
> u. of the great vessels

uncommitted metaphyseal lesion
uncompensated rotary scoliosis
uncomplicated
> u. myocardial infarct
> u. myoma
> u. pneumothorax
> u. supraclavicular stenosis

uncoupled spin
uncoupler
> mitochondrial u.

uncovering
> lateral meniscal u.

uncovertebral
> u. joint
> u. spur

uncus
> arachnoid of u.
> u. corporis
> u. of temporal lobe

undefined lymphoma
undepressed skull fracture
undercorrection
underdamping
underdetection
underdrainage
underdrive
> u. mode
> u. termination

under-filled submentovertical projection
underinflation
> lung u.

underloading
> ventricular u.

underlying
> u. disorder
> u. tissue

underperfusion
under-scan
> u.-s. method
> u.-s. method projection

undersurface
> u. of liver
> u. of patella

underventilated lung
underventilation
undescended
> u. testicle
> u. testis

undifferentiated
> u. liver sarcoma
> u. nasopharyngeal carcinoma
> u. non-Hodgkin lymphoma

undifferentiation
undisplaced fracture
Undritz anomaly
undulant impulse
undulating
> u. contour
> u. course

unenhanced
> u. magnetic resonance imaging scan
> u. MR imaging

unequal pulmonary blood flow
uneven
> u. air expansion
> u. recruitment of alveolar populations
> u. ventilation

unfavorable neutron-to-proton ratio
unfused
> u. os trigonum
> u. physis

ungual
> u. fibroma
> u. tuft

unguicular tuberosity
uniaxial
unibasal
unicaliceal kidney
unicameral
> u. bone cyst
> u. brain

unicentral
unicentric angiofollicular lymph node hyperplasia
unicollis
unicommissural aortic valve

unicondylar fracture
unicornis unicollis uterus
unicornous
unicornuate uterus
unicoronal synostosis
unicortical screw
unicuspid
    u. aortic valve stenosis
    u. with aortic valve
unicusp with central raphe
unidentified bright object (UBO)
unidirectional
    u. block
    u. current
    u. lead configuration
unifascicular block
unifocal
unifocalization
uniform
    u. attenuation coefficient
    u. distribution
    u. loading
    u. phantom scan
    u. sensitivity
    u. TR excitation
    u. uptake
uniformity
    differential u.
    extrinsic field u.
    field u.
    image u.
    intervertebral disk space u.
    intrinsic field u.
    scintillation camera field u.
    SPECT u.
uniformly hyperechoic
Uni-Fuse infusion catheter
uniglandular
unigravida
unilateral
    u. adrenal mass
    u. bronchogram
    u. carotid stenosis
    u. consolidation
    u. diaphragmatic elevation
    u. facet dislocation
    u. facet subluxation
    u. fetal chest mass
    u. flow restriction
    u. fracture
    u. fragmentation
    u. hallux valgus

    u. hydrocephalus
    u. hyperlucent lung
    u. hypertrophy
    u. interfacetal dislocation
    u. intrafacetal dislocation
    u. kidney mass
    u. large smooth kidney
    u. lesion
    u. lobar emphysema
    u. locked facet injury
    u. lung perfusion
    u. megalencephaly
    u. mesial temporal sclerosis
    u. occlusion
    u. ossification
    u. overinflation
    u. pleural effusion
    u. pulmonary agenesis
    u. pulmonary edema
    u. Raynaud phenomenon
    u. small kidney
unilobar
unilobular cirrhosis
unilocular
    u. cyst
    u. cystic lesion
    u. disk
    u. osteolysis
    u. tumor
    u. well-demarcated bone defect
      expansile lesion
unimalleolar fracture
uninfected infarct
uninhibited bladder
union
    bony u.
    delayed fracture u.
    faulty u.
    fibrous u.
    u. of fracture fragment
    nonbony u.
    osseous u.
    secondary u.
    solid bony u.
unipapillary kidney
unipara
unipediculate approach
unipennate muscle
uniphasic imaging agent
unipolar pacing mode
unirhinal phantosmia

U

NOTES

uniseptate
unit (U)
adapted standard mammography u.
add-on stereotactic u.
AdvanTeq II TENS u.
Ångström u.
Aspen sonography u.
atomic mass u. (amu)
Bart abdominoperipheral
angiography u.
Behnken u.
Bethesda u.
BICAP u.
biplane DSA u.
British thermal u.
burst-forming u.
C-arm portable x-ray u.
cobalt 60 beam therapy u.
colony-forming u.
Cox sterilizer and incinerator u.
CT u.
DENT-X intraoral x-ray u.
depicted Hounsfield u.
dry heat sterilizer and
incinerator u.
Eclipse TENS u.
electromagnetic u. (emu)
EMI u.
gamma u.
gray u.
Gyroscan ACS-NT MR u.
Hampson u.
heat u. (HU)
Hercules 7000 mobile x-ray u.
Holzknecht u. (H)
Hounsfield u. (H, HU)
Hounsfield calcium density
measurement u.
Intelect Legend Combo stimulator
and ultrasound u.
JACE-STIM electrotherapy u.
Kienböck u. (X)
Leksell gamma u.
linear accelerator u.
Magnetom Vision MR u.
Mammotest u.
Maxima II TENS u.
molecular recognition u. (MRU)
monitor u.
Multistar angiographic u.
musculotendinous u.
Odelca camera u.
Optiplanimat automated u.
Orbix x-ray u.
Orthopantomograph-panoramic digital
radiography u.
ostiomeatal u.

photodisplay u.
pilosebaceous u.
Plasma 1000 ICP-AES u.
pressor u.
quantum u.
u. of radioactivity
reflectometer tuning u.
roentgen u. (RU)
rutherford u.
Sheffield gamma u.
Siemens Somatom nonhelical u.
sonography u.
Sonos 2000 ultrasound u.
Surgitron portable radiosurgical u.
terminal ductal lobular u. (TDLU)
Tesla superconductive magnet u.
Thayer-Doisy u.
ThromboScan molecular
recognition u.
1.5T Signa MR u.
video display u. (VDU)
u. of wavelength
whole-body u.
Wood u.
X u.
x-ray u.
uniting canal
univentricular heart
University
U. of Florida linear accelerator
U. of Florida staging system
Univision echocardiographic system
Unix/X11 workstation
unknown
u. primary
u. primary site
unleveling
pelvic u.
unloading
bone u.
unmitigated
unmodulated radiofrequency current
unmyelinated nerve fiber
unneurulated neural placode
unopacified bowel loop
unopposed image
unossified cartilage
unpaired
u. parietal branch
u. visceral branch
unplicated sheath
unraveling
digital u.
unresectable
u. colorectal carcinoma
u. lesion
unresolved pneumonia

unroofed coronary sinus syndrome
unruptured follicle
unsaturated
 u. compound
 u. spin
unsegmented vertebral bar
unsharp
 u. masking
 u. mask-type contrast
unsharpness
 absorption u.
 geometric u.
 motion u.
 system u.
unshunted hydrocephalus
unstable
 u. fracture
 u. joint
 u. lesion
unsuppressed
 u. examination
 u. imaging
 u. water signal
untethered
untransformed nadir
ununited fracture
unusual
 u. fetal lie
 u. interstitial pneumonitis
 u. marrow distribution
unwinding of aorta
unwrapping
 Dixon method of phase u.
UOQ
 upper outer quadrant
up
 ramp u.
 tented u.
UP7 film
uPACS picture archiving system
updraft therapy
upfront delay
upgated technique
uphill varix
UPJ
 ureteropelvic junction
upper
 u. aerodigestive tract
 u. airway obstruction
 u. esophageal sphincter (UES)
 u. extremity (UE)
 u. gastrointestinal (UGI)

 u. gastrointestinal endoscopy
 u. gastrointestinal hemorrhage
 u. gastrointestinal series
 u. gastrointestinal tract
 u. GI with small bowel follow-
 through
 u. inner quadrant (UIQ)
 u. jaw bone
 u. left quadrant (ULQ)
 u. limits of normal
 u. lobe (UL)
 u. lobe vein prominence
 u. lung disease
 u. lung field
 u. mantle radiation therapy
 u. moiety ureter
 u. motor neuron
 u. motor neuron lesion
 u. outer quadrant (UOQ)
 u. pole
 u. pole collecting system
 u. pole moiety
 u. pole of ureter
 u. pulmonary lobe atelectasis
 u. rate interval
 u. respiratory tract disease
 u. right quadrant (URQ)
 u. sternal border
 u. thoracic esophagus
 u. thoracic spine fracture
upregulated AQP4 expression
upregulation
 radiation-induced u.
upright
 u. chest film
 u. compression spot film
 u. position
 u. postvoid view
UPSC
 uterine papillary serous carcinoma
upscanning
upside-down stomach
up-sloping curve of kidney
upstairs-downstairs heart
upstream blood
upstroke
 carotid pulse u.
 u. phase of cardiac action potential
 weak carotid u.
uptake
 absence of u.
 absent radiotracer u.

U

NOTES

uptake *(continued)*

asymmetric limb u.
bilateral diffuse increased u.
bilateral reduction of tracer u.
u. in bone marrow
cell preparation bone marrow u.
contrast u.
decreased thyroid radiotracer u.
diffuse lung u.
dye u.
u. and excretion
extracardiac focal u.
extracerebral soft tissue u.
extraosseous u.
extraskeletal u.
^{18}F 2-deoxyglucose u.
FDG u.
fluorescein u.
focal decreased radiotracer u.
focal pulmonary u.
Ga-67 u.
Ga 67 u.
gallium u.
hepatocyte tracer u.
heterogeneous u.
incidental lung u.
increased isotope u.
increased thyroid u.
increased tracer u.
intense u.
iodine u.
isotope u.
laryngeal musculature
    fluorodeoxyglucose u.
localized u.
mediastinal u.
metabolic tracer u.
mottled hepatic u.
mottled liver u.
muscle u.
myocardial u.
^{13}N ammonia u.
near-normal radiotracer u.
normal variant of Ga-67 u.
observed maximal u.
predicted maximal u.
progressive u.
prominent u.
radioactive iodine u. (RAIU)
u. of radioactive material
radioiodine u.
radioisotope u.
u. of radionuclide
radiopharmaceutical u.
radiotracer u.
u. ratio (UR)
regional tracer u.

u. and retention
symmetric pattern of radiotracer u.
T4 u.
^{99m}Tc HMPAO u.
^{99m}Tc MDP u.
thyroid radioiodine u.
tracer u.
uniform u.
variable u.
V-like pattern of u.

uptilted cardiac apex
upward

u. and backward dislocation
u. lens dislocation
u. retraction

UR

uptake ratio

urachal

u. abnormality
u. anomaly
u. carcinoma
u. cyst
u. diverticulum
u. ligament
u. sinus

urachus

patent u.

uracil
uranium (U)

^{235}u., u.-235
u. imaging agent

urate

u. arthropathy
u. calculus
u. nephropathy

urceiform
urceolate
uremic amaurosis
ureter

atonic u.
beaded u.
bifid u.
champagne glass u.
circumcaval u.
u. cobra head
cobra-head u.
corkscrew u.
curlicue u.
u. deviation
u. diameter
dilatation of u.
dilated u.
ectopic u.
extravesical infrasphincteric
    ectopic u.
hockey-stick appearance of the u.
hood-shaped u.

intestinal u.
intramural portion of distal u.
intravesical u.
J-hook deformity of distal u.
J-shaped u.
kinked u.
lower moiety u.
lower pole u.
moderately dilated u.
notching u.
orthotopic u.
pipestem u.
postcaval u.
redundant u.
retrocaval u.
retroiliac u.
rigid u.
saddle peristalsis u.
sawtooth u.
seesaw peristalsis u.
spring onion u.
straight u.
tortuosity of u.
upper moiety u.
upper pole of u.
ureteral
    u. achalasia
    u. adenomyosis
    u. bud
    u. bud bifurcation
    u. calculus
    u. carcinoma
    u. compression technique
    u. dilatation
    u. distention
    u. division
    u. duplication
    u. endometriosis
    u. filling
    u. filling defect
    u. fistula
    u. jet
    u. notching
    u. occlusion
    u. orifice
    u. perforation
    u. perfusion test
    u. reflux study
    u. renal transplant obstruction
    u. seesaw peristalsis
    u. spindle
    u. stasis

    u. stenosis
    u. stenting
    u. stone
    u. stricture
ureterectasis
ureteric
    u. clipping
    u. jet
    u. kinking
ureteritis cystica
ureterocele
    ectopic u.
    orthotopic u.
    pyoureter ectopic u.
    simple u.
ureterocutaneous fistula
ureterocystography
ureterogram
    retrograde u.
ureterography
    bulb u.
    retrograde u.
ureterohydronephrosis
ureteroileostomy
ureterointestinal fistula
ureterolysis
ureteroneocystostomy
ureteropelvic
    u. junction (UPJ)
    u. junction obstruction
ureteroperitoneal fistula
ureteropyelogram
    retrograde u.
ureteropyelography
ureteropyelostomy
ureterorenal junction
ureterorenoscopy
ureteroscope
    solid-rod u.
ureteroscopy
ureterostomy
ureteroureteral anastomosis
uretero-ureteral reflux
ureterovaginal fistula
ureterovesical
    u. junction
    u. junction obstruction
urethra
    angle of inclination of u.
    anterior u.
    bulbous u.
    cavernous u.

U

NOTES

urethra *(continued)*
    female u.
    male u.
    membranous u.
    pendulous u.
    penile u.
    posterior u.
    prostatic u.
    ragged u.
    spinning-top u.

urethral
    u. amyloidosis
    u. angle
    u. atresia
    u. calculus
    u. crest
    u. diverticulum
    u. gland
    u. groove
    u. inclination (UI)
    u. length (UL)
    u. metallic stent
    u. obstruction
    u. orifice
    u. papilla
    u. ridge
    u. straddle injury
    u. stricture
    u. syndrome
    u. thickness (UT)
    u. trauma
    u. tumor
    u. uterus
    u. valve
    u. warming

urethritis
urethrocystogram
urethrocystography
    u. imaging
    retrograde u.
    voiding u.
urethrocystometry
urethrogram
    normal fold u.
    retrograde u. (RUG)
urethrography
urethroplasty
    prostatic u.
    retrograde transurethral prostatic u.
urethroscopy
urethrotome
urethrotomy
    internal u.
urethrovaginal fistula
urethrovesical angle (UVA)

uric
    u. acid calculus
    u. acid nephropathy
urinary
    u. bladder adenocarcinoma
    u. bladder atony
    u. bladder calculus
    u. bladder capacity
    u. bladder contusion
    u. bladder diverticulum
    u. bladder exstrophy
    u. bladder extrinsic mass
    u. bladder fundus
    u. bladder hemangioma
    u. bladder leiomyoma
    u. bladder lymphoma
    u. bladder rupture
    u. bladder stone
    u. bladder trauma
    u. bladder tumor
    u. bladder wall calcification
    u. bladder wall mass
    u. bladder wall thickening
    u. blunt trauma bladder
    u. conduit
    u. diversion
    u. excretion
    u. excretory route
    u. extravasation
    u. fistula
    u. glucosyl-galactosyl-pyridinoline
    u. obstruction
    u. stasis
    u. stent
    u. tract
    u. tract anomaly
    u. tract calculus
    u. tract fibroepithelioma
    u. tract gas
    u. ulcer
urine
    u. ascites
    postvoid residual u.
    radiopaque u.
    residual u.
    retained u.
urinoma
urinothorax
uriposia
urodynamic
    u. pressure-flow study
uroepithelial
    u. malignancy
    u. tumor
urogenital
    u. canal
    u. diaphragm

u. embryology
u. malignancy
u. sinus
u. tract
u. triangle
Urografin imaging agent
urogram
constant infusion excretory u.
diuresis u.
excretory u.
retrograde u. (RU)
urographic density
urography
antegrade u.
ascending u.
cystoscopic u.
descending u.
diuretic radionuclide u.
drip infusion u.
excretion u.
excretory u. (EU)
excretory urethrogram drip
  infusion u.
u. imaging
intravenous u. (IVU)
magnetic resonance u. (MRU)
oral u.
percutaneous antegrade u.
retrograde u.
urokinase
catheter-directed u.
u. imaging agent
urokymography
Urolase
U. fiber laser
U. fiber laser ablation
urolithiasis
Uromiro contrast medium
uropathy
chronic obstructive u.
obstructive u.
uroradiology
Uroselectan
urostealith calculus
urothelial
u. carcinoma
u. striation
urothelium
Urovision
Urovist
U. Cysto imaging agent

U. Meglumine imaging agent
U. Sodium imaging agent
URQ
upper right quadrant
urticate
urtication
US
ultrasonography
ultrasound
USCI
U. PET balloon
U. probe
U. Probe balloon-on-a-wire
  dilatation system
useful beam
useful-beam radiation
USPI
ulnar styloid process index
USPIO
ultrasmall superparamagnetic iron oxide
  USPIO imaging agent
USP XX test
usual
u. interstitial pneumonia (UIP)
u. interstitial pneumonia of Liebow
  (UIP)
u. interstitial pneumonitis
UT
urethral thickness
uteri (*pl. of* uterus)
uteric fold
uterine
u. adenomyosis
u. agenesis
u. anatomy
u. artery
u. artery embolization (UAE)
u. artery pseudoaneurysm
u. artery waveform
u. blood volume flow
u. body
u. canal
u. cavity
u. cervical ganglion
u. cervix
u. cervix carcinoma
u. cirsoid aneurysm
u. contraction
u. corpus carcinoma
u. didelphia
u. didelphys
u. duplication anomaly

U

NOTES

uterine *(continued)*
    u. fibroid
    u. fibroid embolization (UFE)
    u. fibroid polyp
    u. fundus
    u. horn
    u. hypoplasia
    u. insufficiency
    u. isthmus
    u. leiomyoma
    u. ligament
    u. mass
    u. myoma
    u. myometrium
    u. opacity
    u. papillary serous carcinoma
    (UPSC)
    u. retroflexion
    u. sarcoma metastasis
    u. size
    u. synechia
    u. tube
    u. venography
    u. wry neck
utero
    fetal death in u.
    fetal echocardiography in u.
    in u.
uteroabdominal pregnancy
uterocervical canal
uterogram
uterography
uteropelvic
uteroplacental
    u. circulation
    u. insufficiency
uterosacral ligament
uterosalpingogram
uterosalpingography
uterotubal pregnancy
uterotubography
uterovaginal
    u. canal
    u. plexus
uterovesical
    u. fossa
    u. junction
    u. ligament
    u. pouch
uterus, pl. uteri
    adenocarcinoma of u.
    anteflexed u.
    anteverted u.
    aplastic u.
    arcuate u.
    u. arcuatus
    bicameral u.

    bicornis u.
    bicornuate u.
    biforate u.
    bilocular u.
    bipartite u.
    bleeding u.
    body of u.
    cervix uteri
    cochleate u.
    cornu of u.
    corpus uteri
    Couvelaire u.
    didelphic u.
    double u.
    double-mouthed u.
    duplex u.
    empty u.
    enlargement of u.
    fetal u.
    fibroid u.
    fundus uteri
    gas gangrene of u.
    gravid u.
    heart-shaped u.
    horn of u.
    infantile u.
    isthmus of u.
    large-for-dates u.
    nonpregnant horn of bicornuate u.
    outer border of u.
    pear-shaped u.
    pregnant u.
    prostatic u.
    pubescent u.
    retroflexed u.
    retroverted u.
    ribbon u.
    round ligament of u.
    saddle-shaped u.
    u. subseptus
    T-shaped u.
    unicornis unicollis u.
    unicornuate u.
    urethral u.
utilization
    radioiron red cell u.
utricle
    large u.
utriculosaccular canal
utriculus
U-tube
    U-t. stent
UVA
    urethrovesical angle
uveitis
    granulomatous u.
uviometer

uvioresistant
uviosensitive
uvula, pl. uvuli
    u. of bladder
    cerebellar u.

    musculus u.
    u. palatina
uvulopalatoplasty
    laser-assisted u. (LAUP)

NOTES

U

V
  lung volume
  vanadium
  ventricular
    V pattern
    V peak of jugular venous pulse
    V sync
V4
  fourth ventricle
v
  volt
V510B Biplane TEE transducer
V5M Multiplane transducer
VA
  alveolar ventilation
  ventriculoatrial
  vertebral artery
    VA shunt
va
  volt-ampere
VABES
  vasoablative endothelial sarcoma
Vac-Lok patient immobilization system
VACTERL
  vertebral, anal, cardiac, tracheal,
    esophageal, renal, limb
    VACTERL syndrome
VACTERLS spectrum
vacuolated
vacuole
vacuolization
vacuum
  v. arthrography
  v. cassette system
  v. cleft
  v. disk phenomenon
  v. extraction
  facet joint v.
  v. tube
vacuum-assisted
  v.-a. biopsy
  v.-a. core biopsy
vagale
  glomus v.
vagal trunk
vagatomy effect
vagi (*pl. of* vagus)
vagina, pl. **vaginae**
  anterior fornix of v.
  azygos artery of v.
  double v.
  vestibule of v.
vaginal
  v. agenesis
  v. canal

v. carcinoma
v. cuff
v. cylinder
v. endosonography
v. fistula
v. fornix
v. fundus
v. intraepithelial neoplasm
v. ligament
v. orifice
v. plexus
v. tumor
v. wall
vaginalis
  portio v.
  processus v.
  tunica v.
  vestigium processus v.
vaginitis emphysematosa
vaginogram
vaginography
  barium v.
vaginoperineoplasty
vagotomy
vagus, pl. **vagi**
  v. nerve
  v. nerve stimulated functional MRI
    (VNS-fMRI)
  v. nerve stimulation (VNS)
  v. nerve stimulation-synchronized
    blood oxygen level-dependent
    functional MRI (VNS-synchronized
    BOLD fMRI)
Valdini method
valence
  v. band
  v. bond
  electron v.
  ionic polar v.
valgus
  adolescent hallux v.
  anatomic genu v.
  v. angulation
  bilateral hallux v.
  v. carrying angle
  cubitus v.
  v. deviation
  digitus v.
  v. foot
  hallux v. (HV)
  v. heel deformity
  hindfoot v.
  v. index
  metatarsus v.
  pes malleus v.

V

valgus *(continued)*
    v. stress
    talipes v.
    v. tilt
    unilateral hallux v.
valgus-external rotation injury
vallecula, pl. **valleculae**
    v. cerebelli
vallecular
    v. dysphagia
    v. narrowing
valley-to-peak dose rate
Valsalva
    coronary sinus of V.
    V. maneuver
    V. muscle
    sinus of V.
valsalviana
    dysphagia v.
value
    ADCav v.
    attenuation v.
    bright pixel v.
    comparative v.
    CT attenuation v.
    dark pixel v.
    echo-train v.
    v. flip
    negative predictive v.
    pixel v.
    positive predictive v. (PPV)
    S v.
    soft tissue attenuation v.
    standard uptake v. (SUV)
    time-to-peak v. (TTP)
    tristimulus v.
    T1, T2 v.
    velocity encoding v. (VENC)
    venous blood gas v.
valve
    absent v.
    Ahmed glaucoma v.
    anterior semilunar v.
    v. anulus
    aortic v. (AoV)
    aortocoronary v.
    v. area
    artificial cardiac v.
    atrioventricular nodal v.
    v. attenuation
    ball-occluder v.
    ball-type v.
    Bauhin v.
    Beall v.
    bicommissural aortic v.
    bicuspid aortic v.
    bicuspid atrioventricular v.

    bileaflet v.
    billowing mitral v.
    biological tissue v.
    Björk-Shiley heart v.
    blunting of v.
    Braunwald-Cutter v.
    Bunsen-type v.
    calcified aortic v.
    capillary v.
    Carbomedics v.
    cardiac v.
    caval v.
    C-C heart v.
    central caged ball occluder v.
    central caged disk occluder v.
    v. cinefluoroscopy
    cleft mitral v.
    v. closure
    Codman Medos programmable v.
    v. commissure
    competent ileocecal v.
    composite aortic v.
    conduit v.
    congenital absence of pulmonary v.
    congenital anomaly of mitral v.
      (CAMV)
    convexoconcave heart v.
    coronary sinus v.
    C-to-E amplitude of mitral v.
    v. cusp
    v. dehiscence
    v. diameter
    disk-type v.
    doming of v.
    dysplastic pulmonary v.
    early opening of v.
    eccentric monocuspid disk v.
    echo-dense v.
    ectatic aortic v.
    E-to-F slope of v.
    eustachian v.
    failed v.
    fibroelastoma of heart v.
    fishmouth configuration of
      mitral v.
    flail mitral v.
    flap-like v.
    floppy mitral v.
    flow-controlled v.
    foramen ovale v.
    frenulum of v.
    globular v.
    gradient across v.
    Harken v.
    heart v.
    v. of Heister

hockey-stick deformity of
  tricuspid v.
v. of Houston
hypoplastic v.
ileocecal v.
incompetent ileocecal v.
v. leaflet
leaky v.
low-profile mitral v.
lymphatic v.
v. malformation
mechanical v.
Medos Hakim programmable v.
midsystolic buckling of mitral v.
miniaturized mitral v.
mitral v.
monocusp v.
monocuspid tilting disk v.
M-shaped pattern of mitral v.
mural leaflet of mitral v.
narrowed v.
native aortic v.
v. of navicular fossa
neoaortic v.
nonfunctioning heart v.
notching of pulmonic v.
Omniscience v.
v. opening slope
v. outflow strut
parachute deformity of mitral v.
v. plane
v. pocket
posterior urethral v. (PUV)
premature mid diastolic closure of
  mitral v.
preservation of native aortic v.
pressure-activated safety v. (PASV)
programmable ventricular shunt v.
v. prolapse
prolapse of aortic v.
prolapsed mitral v. (PMV)
prosthetic heart v.
prosthetic mitral v.
pullback across aortic v.
pulmonary v.
pulmonic v. (PV)
pyloric v.
quadricuspid aortic v.
quadricuspid pulmonary v.
rectal v.
regurgitant v.
v. replacement

retrograde blood flow across v.
rheumatic heart v.
v. ring
Rosenmüller v.
rotating hemostatic v.
sail-like tricuspid v.
semilunar v.
shunt v.
sigmoid v.
Smelloff-Cutter v.
Sophy programmable v.
spiral v.
spongiosa of mitral v.
stenosed aortic v.
stenotic tricuspid v.
stentless porcine aortic v.
stent-mounted allograft v.
stent-mounted heterograft v.
synthetic v.
systolic anterior motion of
  mitral v.
thebesian v.
thickened aortic v.
v. thickening
tilting-disk v.
v. tip
tissue outflow v.
track v.
tricuspid v. (TV)
tricuspid aortic v.
trileaflet aortic v.
truncal v.
v. tube
unicommissural aortic v.
unicuspid with aortic v.
urethral v.
v. vegetation
venous v.
Vieussens v.
v. wrapping
xenograft v.

valviform
valvoplasty, valvuloplasty
  balloon mitral v.
valvotome
  spade-shaped v.
valvotomy
  balloon v.
valvula, pl. **valvulae**
valvular
  v. aortic insufficiency
  v. aortic stenosis

NOTES

1001

valvular *(continued)*
    v. apparatus
    v. atresia
    v. cardiac defect
    v. damage
    v. disease (VD)
    v. dysfunction
    v. efficiency
    v. heart disease
    v. incompetence
    v. leaflet calcification
    v. opening
    v. orifice
    v. pneumothorax
    v. pulmonic stenosis
    v. regurgitant lesion
    v. regurgitation (VR)
    v. scarring
    v. sclerosis
valvuloplasty *(var. of* valvoplasty)
van
    V. Aman pulmonary pigtail catheter
    v. Buchem disease
    v. Buchem syndrome
    V. de Graaf generator
    V. der Hoeve syndrome
    V. Nuys Prognostic Index for DCIS
    V. Rosen view
    V. Sonnenberg chest drain set
    V. Sonnenberg sump catheter
vanadium (V)
vanishing
    v. bone disease
    v. lung syndrome
    v. lung tumor
    v. testes syndrome
    v. twins
Vanzetti sign
vaporization
    plaque v.
Vaquez disease
vara
    Blount tibia v.
    coxa v.
    epiphyseal coxa v.
    tibia v.
variability
    anatomic v.
    beat-to-beat v.
    interpretive v.
    peak flow v.
variable
    v. cerebral dysplasia
    v. energy
    v. flip-angle excitation

    v. intensity
    v. projection (VARPRO)
    quantitative exercise thallium-201 v.
    v. response rate
    v. segment
    v. stiffness guidewire
    v. TE, TR
    v. tube current
    v. tube potential
    v. uptake
variable-angle
    v.-a. gamma camera
    v.-a. spinning (VAS)
    v.-a. uniform signal excitation (VUSE)
Varian
    V. accelerator
    V. Associates 11.7-T, 51-mm bore spectrometer
    V. brachytherapy system
    V. CT scanner
    V. LINAC
    V. MLC system
    V. NMR spectrometer
variance
    v. image
    ulnar v.
variant
    anatomic bile duct v.
    blastic v.
    congenital mediastinal arterial v.
    v. of Creutzfeldt-Jacob disease (vCJD)
    Dandy-Walker v.
    electrocardiographic v.
    fibrosarcoma v.
    Heidenhain v.
    labral v.
    mediastinal arterial v.
    normal v.
    ossification v.
    pancreaticobiliary function v.
variation
    anatomic v.
    area/hemidiameter v.
    B_O field v.
    circadian v.
    coefficient of v. (c.v.)
    v. in density
    exposure v.
    field v.
    interobserver v.
    intraobserver v.
    low interobserver v.
    normal anatomic v.
    observer v.
    positional v.

pulse width v.
surface dose v.
view-to-view v.
Varibar oral contrast agent
varication
variceal
v. column
v. decompression
v. hemorrhage
v. sclerosis
v. wall
varices (*pl. of* varix)
varicocele
idiopathic v.
varicography
varicoid esophageal carcinoma
varicose
v. aneurysm
v. bronchiectasis
v. vein
varicosity
paraovarian v.
reticular v.'s
variegated pattern
variocele tumor of breast
varioliform erosion
VariTone
Varivas loop graft
varix, pl. **varices**
v. of aneurysm
arterial v.
arteriovenous v.
colonic v.
Dagradi classification of
esophageal v.
downhill v.
duodenal v.
esophageal v.
gastric v.
intraaxial v.
lung v.
Okuda transhepatic obliteration
of v.
orbital v.
paraesophageal v.
pericholedochal v.
pulmonary v.
saphenous v.
stomach v.
sublingual v.
umbilical vein v.
uphill v.

VARPRO
variable projection
varum
genu v.
varus
v. angulation
cubitus v.
v. deformity
v. deviation
digitus v.
v. foot
hallux v.
v. heel
mechanical genu v.
v. metatarsophalangeal angle
metatarsus v.
pes v.
rearfoot v.
v. rerotation
v. stress
v. stress laxity
subtalar v.
talipes v.
tibial v.
v. tilt
varus-valgus
v.-v. instability
v.-v. plane
varying degrees of obliquity
VAS
variable-angle spinning
vestibular aqueduct syndrome
vas, pl. **vasa**
vascular
v. abdominal calcification
v. abnormality
v. access device
v. and airway modeling
v. anomaly
v. assessment
v. band
v. bed
v. blood
v. blood pool
v. blush
v. bone
v. brachytherapy
v. brain occlusion
v. bud
v. bundle
v. bypass graft
v. catastrophe

V

NOTES

vascular *(continued)*
v. cell adhesion molecule-1 (VCAM-1)
v. channel
v. cirrhosis
v. colon ectasia
v. compartment
v. compromise
v. congestion
v. contour
v. cord damage
v. encasement
v. esophageal compression
v. fibrous polyp
v. flask
v. flow imaging
v. goiter
v. groove
v. hamartoma
v. hemangioma
v. hydraulic conductivity
v. hydraulics
v. impedance
v. insufficiency
v. insult
v. invasion
v. jejunization
v. kidney anatomy
v. leak syndrome
v. leiomyoma
v. lesion
v. lumen
v. malformation
v. marking
v. MR contrast enhancement
v. myxoma
v. necrosis
v. network
v. obstruction
v. occlusive disease
v. origin bone tumor
v. patency
v. pedicle
v. perforation
v. phase
v. plexus
v. protrusion
v. pterygoid attachment
v. redistribution
v. reflection
v. renal anatomy
v. reserve
v. ring
v. sarcoma
v. sclerosis
v. segmentation

v. segmentation and extraction
v. shadow
v. sheath
v. sling
v. smooth muscle
v. space of the placenta
v. spasm
v. stasis
v. stent
v. stroma
v. structure
v. supply
v. systemic resistance
v. tissue
v. tone
v. tracheal compression
v. transformation
v. trauma
v. tuft
v. villous atrophy
v. wall
v. xenograft
v. zone
vascularity
decreased pulmonary v.
femoral head v.
increased pulmonary v.
moyamoya v.
overcirculation v.
pulmonary v.
sunburst brain v.
tumor v.
vascularization
hand v.
tumor v.
vascularized granulation tissue
vasculature
cardiac v.
cerebral v.
depiction of v.
extracranial cerebral v.
increased pulmonary v.
interlobular v.
peripheral v.
pruned appearance of pulmonary v.
pulmonary v.
splanchnic v.
vasculitic lesion
vasculitis
mesenteric v. (MV)
vasculopathy
lenticulostriate v. (LSV)
vas deferens
vasoablative endothelial sarcoma (VABES)

vasoactive
> v. intestinal polypeptide tumor
> (VIPoma)
> v. response

vasoconstriction
> hypoxic pulmonary v.
> peripheral circulatory v.
> peripheral cutaneous v.
> pulmonary arteriolar v.
> spontaneous transient v.
> systemic arterial v.

vasoconstrictor response
vasodepressor response
vasodilating agent
vasodilation
> breakthrough v.

vasodilator administration
vasodilatory
> v. capacity
> v. effect
> v. hemodynamic stress test
> v. response

vasoepididymography
vasogenic
> v. edema
> v. impotence

vasography
vasomotor
> v. change
> v. reaction
> v. symptom

vasoocclusive angiotherapy (VAT)
vasoreactivity
> cerebral v.
> pulmonary v.

vasoregulation
vasorelaxation of epicardial vessel
vasorum
> aortic vasa v.
> vasa v.

VasoSeal ES, VHD arterial puncture site closure device
vasospasm
> cerebral v.
> primary v.

vasospastic vessel
vasovagal reaction
VasoView balloon dissection system
vastus
> v. intermedius
> v. lateralis
> v. medialis

> v. medialis advancement (VMA)
> v. medialis muscle

VAT
> vasoocclusive angiotherapy
> ventricular activation time
> video-assisted thoracoscopy
> visceral adipose tissue

VATER
> vertebral, anal, tracheal, esophageal, renal
> > V. association
> > V. complex

Vater
> ampulla of V.
> V. diverticulum
> V. duct
> V. fold
> papilla of V.

vaterian segment
vault
> cranial v.
> plantar v.
> rectal v.

Vaxcel peripherally inserted catheter
VAX 4100 system
VB
> virtual bronchoscopy

Vbeam pulsed dye laser system
VBI
> vertebrobasilar insufficiency

VBR
> ventricle-to-brain ratio

VC
> vital capacity

VCA
> vertical-center-anterior

VCAM-1
> vascular cell adhesion molecule-1

VCB
> ventricular capture beat

VCF
> ventricular contractility function

VCG
> vectorcardiogram

vCJD
> variant of Creutzfeldt-Jacob disease
> > pulvinar sign of vCJD

VCMG
> videocystometrography

VCU, VCUG
> voiding cystourethrogram
> voiding cystourethrography

V

NOTES

VCUG
   vesicoureterogram
   voiding cystourethrogram
VD
   valvular disease
Vd
   apparent volume of distribution
VDI
   venous distensibility index
(V)-dimer captosuccinic acid (DMSA)
VDS
   ventral derotating spinal
     VDS implant
VDU
   video display unit
VE
   voluntary effort
VEA
   ventricular ectopic activity
VEB
   ventricular ectopic beat
VEC
   velocity-encoded cine
VEC-MR
   velocity-encoded cine magnetic
   resonance
vectocardiogram
vectocardiography
vector
   bulk magnetization v.
   expression v.
   v. loop
   v. loop vectorcardiography
   macroscopic magnetization v.
   mean cardiac v.
   net magnetization v.
   nonviral v.
   QRS v.
   v. quantitization
   spin v.
   v. subtraction
   T v.
vectorcardiogram (VCG)
vectorcardiography
   Frank v.
   frontal plane v.
   v. imaging
   sagittal plane v.
   spatial v.
   transverse plane v.
   vector loop v.
vegetation
   dendritic v.
   friable v.
   heart valve v.
   valve v.
vegetative lesion

veil
   tissue v.
veiling glare
vein
   absent peripheral v.
   accessory cephalic v.
   accessory hemiazygos v.
   accessory hepatic v.
   accessory saphenous v.
   accessory vertebral v.
   accompanying v.
   adrenal v.
   anal v.
   anastomotic v.
   aneurysmal v.
   angular v.
   anonymous v.
   antebrachial v.
   antecubital v.
   anterior cardiac v.
   anterior internal vertebral v.
   (AIVV)
   anterior jugular v.
   anterior terminal v. (ATV)
   aplasia of deep v.
   appendicular v.
   aqueous v.
   arciform v.
   arcuate v.
   arterial v.
   v., artery, nerve
   ascending lumbar v.
   auditory v.
   auricular v.
   autogenous v.
   axillary v.
   azygos v.
   basal placenta v.
   basilic v.
   basivertebral v.
   blind percutaneous puncture of
   subclavian v.
   Boyd perforating v.
   brachial v.
   brachiocephalic v.
   brain bridging v.
   branches of v.
   bronchial v.
   bulb of v.
   Burrow v.
   cannulated central v.
   capacious v.
   capillary v.
   cardiac v.
   cardinal v.
   carotid v.
   caudate v.

cavernous transfer of portal v.
cavernous transformation of
  portal v.
central v.
cephalic v.
cerebral v.
cervical v.
choroid v.
chronic insufficiency of v.
ciliary v.
circumaortic left renal v.
circumflex v.
colic v.
common basal v.
common cardinal v.
common facial v.
common femoral v.
communicating v.
companion v.
condylar emissary v.
congenital stenosis of pulmonary v.
conjunctival v.
coronary v.
cortical v.
costoaxillary v.
cutaneous v.
cystic v.
deep v.
digital v.
v. dilatation
dilated collateral v.
diploic v.
distended v.
dorsal penile v.
dorsispinal v.
duodenal v.
embryonal v.
embryonic umbilical v.
emissary v.
engorged v.
epigastric v.
episcleral v.
esophageal v.
ethmoidal v.
external jugular v. (EJV)
external pudendal v.
extirpation of saphenous v.
extradural vertebral plexus of v.
facial v.
familial varicose v.
feeder v.
femoral v.

fibular v.
flat neck v.
frontal v.
v. of Galen malformation
gastric v.
gastroepiploic v.
v. graft
v. graft occlusion
v. graft stenosis
v. graft thrombosis
great cardiac v.
greater saphenous v.
harvested v.
hemiazygos v.
hemispheric v.
hepatic v.
ileocolic v.
ileofemoral v.
iliac v.
iliofemoral v.
inferior mesenteric v.
inferior ophthalmic v.
inferior pulmonary v.
inferior rectal v.
inferior thyroid v.
v. inflammation
infradiaphragmatic v.
innominate v.
intercostal v.
internal cerebral v. (ICV)
internal jugular v. (IJV)
internal thoracic v.
intraforaminal v.
intrahepatic umbilical v.
v. intussusception
jugular v.
Labbé v.
labial v.
leaking v.
left hepatic v. (LHV)
left pulmonary v. (LPV)
left retroaortic renal v.
lesser saphenous v.
lobe of azygos v.
marginal v.
Marshall v.
median antebrachial v.
mediastinal v.
medullary v.
meningeal v.
mesencephalic v.
mesenteric v.

NOTES

vein *(continued)*
    middle cardiac v.
    middle hepatic v. (MHV)
    middle rectal v.
    v. nodularity
    oblique v.
    ophthalmic v.
    orbital varix ophthalmic v.
    ovarian v.
    palmar cutaneous v.
    pancreatic v.
    parathyroid v.
    paraumbilical v.
    parent v.
    v. patency
    patency and valvular reflux of deep v.
    penile v.
    perforating v.
    pericallosal v.
    pericardiacophrenic v.
    pericardial v.
    perithyroid v.
    peroneal v.
    petrosal v.
    pontomesencephalic v.
    popliteal v.
    portal v.
    posterior auricular v.
    posterior cardinal v.
    posterior interventricular v.
    precentral cerebellar v.
    prepyloric v.
    pudendal v.
    pulmonary v.
    pulsating v.
    quadrigeminal v.
    ranine v.
    renal v.
    retroaortic renal v.
    Retzius v.
    reversed greater saphenous v.
    right hepatic v. (RHV)
    right pulmonary v. (RPV)
    saphenous v.
    Sappey inferior v.
    sausaging of v.
    Schlesinger v.
    Schwartz test for patency of deep saphenous v.'s
    scimitar v.
    scrotal v.
    segmental v.
    septal v.
    Servelle v.
    simultaneous acquisition of artery and v. (SAAV)

    sludging of retinal v.
    small cardiac v.
    small saphenous v.
    soleal v.
    spermatic v.
    splenic v.
    v. stone
    striate v.
    subcardinal v.
    subclavian v.
    subcutaneous v.
    subependymal v.
    superficial femoral v.
    superior intercostal v.
    superior mesenteric v. (SMV)
    superior ophthalmic v.
    superior pulmonary v.
    superior rectal v.
    supracardinal v.
    systemic v.
    testicular v.
    thalamic v.
    thalamostriate v.
    thebesian v.
    thoracoepigastric v.
    tibial v.
    tortuous v.
    transcerebral medullary v.
    v. of Trolard
    umbilical v.
    v. valve wrapping
    varicose v.
    vermian v.
    vertebral v.
vela (*pl. of* velum)
velamentous
    v. insertion
    v. insertion of cord
    v. placenta
velamentum
velar
veliform
vellus
velocimetry
    laser Doppler v.
    UA v.
    umbilical artery v.
velocity
    acoustic v.
    angular v.
    v. artifact
    blood flow v.
    v. calculation
    carotid v.
    closing v.
    v. compensation
    coronary blood flow v. (CBFV)

decreased closing v.
diastolic regurgitant v.
v. distribution function (F(v))
v. encoding on brain MR
  angiography
v. encoding value (VENC)
fiber-shortening v.
flow v.
forward v.
v. gradient
high v.
v. imaging
impact v.
main portal vein peak v. (MPPv)
v. mapping
maximal transaortic jet v.
mean aortic flow v.
mean posterior wall v.
mean pulmonary flow v.
midshunt peak v. (MSPv)
mitral inflow v.
modal v.
muzzle v.
neurologic sequelae
peak aortic flow v.
peak early diastolic filling v.
peak late diastolic filling v.
peak pulmonary flow v.
peak regurgitant flow v.
peak systolic v.
peak transmitted v.
portal vein v.
v. profile
regurgitant v.
retrograde blood v.
v. spectrum
TCD v.
transcranial Doppler v.
v. waveform (VWF)
velocity-compensating gradient pulse
velocity-density imaging
velocity-encoded
  v.-e. cine (VEC)
  v.-e. cine imaging (VINNIE)
  v.-e. cine magnetic resonance
    (VEC-MR)
  v.-e. cine MR imaging
  v.-e. color Doppler signal
  v.-e. color Doppler sonography
  v.-e. image
  v.-e. sequence
velocity-evaluation phantom

velocity-induced phase shift
velocity-time graph
velopharyngeal
  v. closure
  v. insufficiency
velopharynx
Velpeau
  V. axillary view
  V. deformity
velum, pl. **vela**
vena, pl. **venae**
  v. cava
  v. cava anomaly
  v. caval filter
  v. comitans
  V. Tech-LGM vena cava filter
venacavagram
venacavogram
venacavography
  inferior v. (IVCV)
venacavotony
venae (*pl. of* vena)
VENC
  velocity encoding value
venereum
  lymphogranuloma v.
venetian blind artifact
venoarterial cannulation
venobiliary fistula
venodilator
venofibrosis
venogram
  magnetic resonance v. (MRV)
  renal v.
venography
  adrenal v.
  antegrade v.
  ascending contrast v.
  cerebral CT v.
  contrast v.
  conventional v.
  descending v.
  digital free hepatic v.
  direct v.
  epidural v.
  extradural v.
  free hepatic v.
  gonadal v.
  hepatic v.
  iliac v.
  v. imaging
  impedance v.

NOTES

V

venography *(continued)*
   intraosseous v.
   isotope v.
   limb v.
   lower limb v.
   magnetic resonance v. (MRV)
   ovarian v.
   peripheral v.
   portal v.
   radionuclear v.
   radionuclide v.
   renal v.
   selective v.
   spermatic v.
   splenic portal v.
   splenoportal v.
   subtraction v.
   technetium Tc99m v.
   testicular v.
   transjugular v.
   transosseous v.
   ultrasound v.
   uterine v.
   vertebral v.
   wedged hepatic v.
venography-related
   v.-r. air embolism
   v.-r. arrhythmia
   v.-r. thrombophlebitis
venolobar syndrome
venospasm
venostasis
venosum
   foramen v.
venosus
   ductus v.
   sinus v.
venotomy
venous
   v. access device
   v. anatomy
   v. aneurysm
   v. angiocardiography
   v. angioma
   v. angioplasty
   v. anomaly
   v. aortography
   v. avulsion
   v. backflow
   v. blood
   v. blood gas value
   v. brain angiography
   v. brain angle
   v. bypass graft
   v. calcification
   v. cannulation
   v. capillary

v. circulation
v. collateral
v. contamination
v. decompression
v. defect
v. distensibility index (VDI)
v. distention
v. Doppler examination
v. drainage
v. edema
v. embolism
v. filling time (VFT)
v. fistulogram
v. groove
v. heart congestion
v. hemangioma
v. hemorrhage
v. hyperemia
v. hypertension
v. imaging
v. infarct
v. injection
v. insufficiency
v. interposition graft
v. intraplacental lake
v. intravasation
v. intussusception
v. junction
v. ligament
v. malformation of the tongue
v. motion
v. neck angle
v. network
v. obstruction
v. occlusion
v. overlay
v. oxygen content
v. plethysmography
v. plexus
v. pooling
v. pouch
v. pressure
v. refill time (VRT)
v. return
v. return time
right subclavian central v.
   (RSCVP)
v. scan
v. sclerosis
v. segment
v. sheath
v. sinus
v. sinus thrombosis
v. skull lake
v. spasm
v. stasis
v. statis syndrome

v. stenting
systemic v.
v. thromboembolic disease (VTED)
v. thromboembolization
v. thrombolysis
v. thrombosis embolus
v. ulcer
v. ultrasonography
v. valve
v. vascular malformation
v. ventricle
v. waveform
v. web

venovenous cannulation

vent

pulmonary arterial v.
thoracic v.

ventilation

airway pressure release v.
alveolar v. (VA)
v. defect
high-minute v.
v. image
v. lung scan
mask v.
maximal voluntary v. (MVV)
mechanical v.
minute v.
partial liquid v.
v. pneumonitis
pulmonary perfusion and v.
v. radionuclide
reduced alveolar v.
regional v.
v. scintigraphy
v. scintigraphy equilibrium phase
v. study
uneven v.
volume-controlled inverse ratio v.
volume-cycled v.

ventilation-perfusion (V/Q)

v.-p. defect
v.-p. imaging
impaired v.-p.
v.-p. inequality
v.-p. lung scan
v.-p. mismatch
v.-p. pulmonary scintigraphy
v.-p. ratio

ventilator

babyPAC v.
SLE 2000 v.

ventilatory

v. capacity-demand imbalance
v. dysfunction
v. effort
v. failure

venting of heart

ventosa

spina v.

ventrad

ventral

v. aorta
v. aspect
v. branch
v. bridge
v. cochlear nucleus
v. decubitus position
v. derotating spinal (VDS)
v. derotating spinal implant
v. duct of Wirsung
v. epidural abscess
v. epidural fat
v. hernia
v. hernia defect
v. horn
v. mesentery
v. muscle
v. pancreas
v. pancreatic anlage
v. pancreatic bud
v. pontine infarct
v. primary ramus
v. root
v. sacrococcygeal ligament
v. sacroiliac ligament
v. spinocerebellar tract
v. spinothalamic tract
v. surface
v. venous pressure line

ventralward

ventricle

absent v.
akinetic left v.
aortic vestibule of v.
Arantius v.
atrialized v.
augmented filling of right v.
auxiliary v.
backrush of blood into left v.
ballooned floor of v.
v. batwing appearance
batwing configuration of v.
bulb of occipital horn of lateral v.

V

NOTES

ventricle *(continued)*
  bulb of posterior horn of
    lateral v.
  cephalic v.
  cerebral v.
  colloid cyst of third v.
  compensatory enlargement of v.
  dilatation of v.
  dilated v.
  double-inlet left v.
  double-inlet single v.
  double-outlet both v.'s (DOBV)
  double-outlet left v. (DOLV)
  double-outlet right v. (DORV)
  dual v.
  v. effacement
  elongation of v.
  enlargement of v.
  fifth v.
  floor of v.
  fourth v. (V4)
  fractional shortening of left v.
  frontal horn of lateral v.
  Galen v.
  high-riding third v.
  hourglass v.
  hyperdynamic fourth v.
  hypokinetic left v.
  hypoplastic heart v.
  hypoplastic left v.
  hypoplastic right v.
  v. impedance adapter
  inflow tract of left v.
  ipsilateral lateral v.
  laryngeal v.
  v. of larynx
  lateral v.
  left v.
  loculated v.
  Morgagni v.
  morphologic left v.
  native v.
  outflow of v.
  papilloma of the fourth v.
  parchment right v.
  partial obliteration of lateral v.
  pineal v.
  primitive v.
  right v.
  roof of fourth v.
  v. root
  rudimentary v.
  shift of v.
  single v.
  sixth v.
  slit v.
  Sylvius v.

  temporal horn of lateral v.
  terminal v.
  thick-walled v.
  third v.
  thrusting v.
  tiny v.
  trigone of v.
  tubular v.
  venous v.
  Verga v.
ventricle-to-brain ratio (VBR)
ventricose
ventricular (V)
  v. aberration
  v. activation time (VAT)
  v. apex
  v. aqueduct
  v. assist device
  v. atresia
  v. atrium
  v. block
  v. branch
  v. canal
  v. capture beat (VCB)
  v. catheter blockage
  v. cavity
  v. cineangiogram
  v. cleft
  v. contractility function (VCF)
  v. contraction pattern
  v. decompensation
  v. depression
  v. disproportion
  v. D-loop
  v. drainage
  v. dysfunction
  v. dysplasia
  v. echo
  v. ectopic activity (VEA)
  v. ectopic beat (VEB)
  v. effective refractory period
    (VERP)
  v. ejection fraction
  v. electrical instability
  v. encasement
  v. end-diastolic volume
  v. endomyocardial biopsy
  v. enlargement
  v. escape mechanism
  v. failure
  v. filling
  v. free wall
  v. free wall rupture
  v. free wall thickness
  v. function curve
  v. function equilibrium image
  v. function parameter

v. gradient
v. horn
v. hypertrophy
v. index (VI)
v. intracerebral hemorrhage
v. inversion
v. irritability
v. isovolumic relaxation time
v. left-handedness
v. ligament
v. loop
v. mass
v. muscle necrosis
v. myocardium
v. myxoma
v. obstruction
v. outflow tract
v. outlet
v. output
v. paroxysmal tachycardia
v. perforation
v. preexcitation
v. premature beat (VPB)
v. premature complex (VPC)
v. premature contraction (VPC)
v. premature contraction couplet
v. premature depolarization (VPD)
v. pressure
v. pseudoperfusion beat
v. rate
v. repolarization
v. reserve
v. response
v. rhythm
v. right-handedness
v. segmental contraction
v. septal aneurysm
v. septal defect (VSD)
v. septal rupture
v. septal summit
v. septum (VS)
v. shift
v. size
v. soft tissue
v. space
v. span
v. standstill
v. stiffness
v. synchrony
v. system
v. systole
v. transposition

v. trigeminy
v. tumor
v. underloading
v. view
v. wall dilatation
v. wall motion
v. wall motion echocardiography

ventricularization of pressure
ventriculoarterial
v. conduit
v. connection

ventriculoatrial (VA)
v. block
v. conduction
v. interval
v. shunt
v. time-out

ventriculocele
ventriculocisternostomy
ventriculofugal artery
ventriculogmegaly
ventriculogram
axial left anterior oblique v.
bicycle exercise radionuclide v.
biplane v.
cine left v.
contrast v.
digital subtraction v.
dipyridamole thallium v.
exercise radionuclide v.
gated blood pool v.
gated nuclear v.
gated radionuclide v.
intraoperative v.
iohexol CT v.
left v. (LVG)
left anterior oblique projection v.
metrizamide v.
radionuclide v. (RNV, RVG)
retrograde left v.
right anterior oblique position v.
xenon-133 v.

ventriculography
cardiac v.
v. catheter
cerebral v.
first-pass radionuclide v.
isotope v.

ventriculoinfundibular fold
ventriculomegaly
ex vacuo v.

V

NOTES

ventriculomegaly *(continued)*
    fetal v.
    teardrop v.
ventriculoperitoneal (VP)
    v. diversion
    v. shunt
ventriculoradial dysplasia
ventriculotomy
    map-guided partial endocardial v.
ventriculus cordis
ventricumbent
ventriduct
ventriduction
ventriflexion
ventrimesal
ventrimeson
ventrodorsad
ventrodorsal
ventroinguinal
ventrolateral
ventromedial hypothalamic hamartoma
ventromedian
ventroposterior
ventrose
VentTrak monitoring system
Venturi effect
venule
    high endothelial v.
    postcapillary v.
venulitis
    cutaneous necrotizing v.
vera
    vertebra v.
verae
    costae v.
Verga
    V. lacrimal groove
    V. ventricle
vergae
    septum cavum v.
verge
    anal v.
vergence
    downward v.
Verluma diagnostic imaging agent
vermetoid
vermian
    v. agenesis
    v. hypoplasia
    v. medulloblastoma
    v. pseudotumor
    v. vein
vermian-cerebellar hypoplasia
vermicular
    v. appendage
    v. appendix

vermiform
    v. appendix
    v. process
verminous aneurysm
vermis
    cerebellar v.
    folium v.
    v. hypoplasia
vermography
vernal edema
Verner-Morrison syndrome
Verneuil canal
vernix membrane
Verocay body
VERP
    ventricular effective refractory period
verruciform
verruciformis
verrucose
verrucosus
    nevus v.
verrucous
    v. carcinoma
    v. hemangioma
Versadopp ultrasonic Doppler probe
VersaLight laser
VersaPulse holmium laser
Versatome D8 Perioperative Doppler System
verse
    inclination v.
versive motor
vertebra, pl. **vertebrae**
    abdominal v.
    accordion v.
    anterior scalloping of v.
    articular process of v.
    basilar v.
    beaked v.
    block v.
    body of v.
    bone-within-bone v.
    bony projection from v.
    bullet-shaped v.
    butterfly v.
    butterfly-wing v.
    caudal v.
    cervical v.
    cleft v.
    coccygeal v.
    codfish v.
    coin-on-edge v.
    coronal cleft v.
    cranial v.
    v. dentata
    displaced v.
    dorsal v.

facet surface of v.
false v.
fishmouth v.
fishtail v.
focal subluxation of vertebrae
fractured v.
fused vertebrae
great terminal v.
honeycomb v.
hooked v.
hourglass v.
H-shaped v.
ivory v.
last normal v. (LNV)
limbus v.
v. lumbales
lumbar v. (L)
v. magnum
mature v.
midbody of v.
movable v.
non-rib-bearing v.
notched v.
odontoid v.
pedicle of v.
picture frame v.
v. plana
posterior scalloping of v.
primitive v.
prominent v.
rib-bearing v.
rugger jersey v.
sacral v.
sandwich v.
saucerization of v.
solitary collapsed v.
v. spuriae
sternal v.
subluxed v.
tail v.
thoracic v.
toothed v.
transitional v.
transverse process of v.
tricuspid v.
true v.
v. vera
wedge-shaped v.

vertebral

    v., anal, cardiac, tracheal,
      esophageal, renal, limb
      (VACTERL)

v., anal, tracheal, esophageal, renal
  (VATER)
v. angiography
v. ankylosis
v. arch
v. arch ligament ossification
v. arterial dissection
v. arteriography
v. artery (VA)
v. artery fenestration
v. artery of Henry
v. artery occlusion
v. artery segment V0-V4
v. artery stenosis
v. artery syndrome
v. artery system
v. articular sinus
v. body alignment
v. body bone tumor
v. body collapse
v. body endplate
v. body fracture
v. body height
v. body index
v. body line
v. body margin
v. body marrow signal intensity
v. body ossification center
v. body overgrowth
v. body plate
v. body ratio method
v. body retrolisthesis
v. body retropulsion
v. body shape
v. body size
v. border abnormality
v. canal
v. chordoma
v. column
v. compression fracture
v. cross-section
v. disk
v. disk interspace
v. endplate abnormality
v. epiphysitis
v. expansile lesion
v. foramen
v. fusion
v. groove
v. hemangioma
v. hyperostosis
v. lamina

V

NOTES

vertebral *(continued)*
v. osteochondrosis
v. osteomyelitis
v. part of diaphragm
v. plana fracture
v. process
v. rib
v. scalloping
v. segmentation anomaly
v. spine
v. steal phenomenon
v. stripe
v. vein
v. venography
v. venous plexus
v. wedge compression fracture
v. wedging
vertebrobasilar
v. artery
v. artery occlusion
v. artery syndrome
v. circulation
v. complex
v. disease
v. distribution stroke
v. dolichoectasia
v. insufficiency (VBI)
v. ischemia
v. occlusion
v. system
v. transcranial color-coded duplex
ultrasonography
vertebrocostal
v. rib
v. triangle
v. trigone
vertebrojugular fistula
vertebromammary diameter
vertebropelvic ligament
vertebrophrenic angle
vertebroplasty
percutaneous v.
transpedicular v.
vertebrospinous process
vertebrosternal rib
vertebrovertebral fistula
vertex, pl. vertices
v. of bony cranium
V. camera
v. corneae
v. cranii
cube v.
v. presentation
vertical
v. axis
v. diameter
v. heart

v. long-axis slice
v. muscle
v. partial laryngectomy
v. plane
posterior temporal v. (PTV)
v. ray
v. shear fracture
v. split nondetached tear
v. synchronization pulse
v. talus
v. talus foot deformity
vertical-center-anterior (VCA)
v.-c.-a. angle
verticalis
vertical-long axis
vertices (*pl. of* vertex)
verticillate
verticomental
verticosubmental
v. position
v. projection
v. view
vertigraphy
VERT software
vesalian bone
vesalianum of vertebral body
Vesalius
foramen of V.
vesical
v. distention
v. diverticulum
v. fascia
v. fistula
v. injury
v. neck
v. outlet obstruction
v. stone formation
v. venous plexus
vesicancy
vesicant
vesicatory
vesicle
acoustic v.
acrosomal v.
air v.
allantoic v.
auditory v.
brain region v.
v. calculus
cerebral v.
cervical v.
encephalic v.
graafian v.
grape-like v.
malpighian v.
metanephric v.
pulmonary v.

seminal v.
synaptic v.
vesicocolic fistula
vesicorectal
vesicosacral ligament
vesicoumbilical ligament
vesicoureteral
v. reflux (VUR)
v. scintigraphy
vesicoureteric reflux
vesicoureterogram (VCUG)
vesicourethral
v. angle
v. canal
vesicouterine
v. ligament
v. pouch
vesicovaginal fistula
vesicula
vesicular
v. amine transporter
v. block
v. bronchiolitis
v. emphysema
v. lymph node
v. pattern
vesiculogram
vesiculography
v. imaging
seminal v.
vesiculosa appendix
vessel, pl. **vessels**
abdominal great v.
aberrant v.
absorbent v.
afferent lymph v.
angiographically occult v.
anomalous v.
antegrade filling of v.
arcuate v.
atraumatic occlusion of v.
axillary v.
beading of v.
blood v.
brachiocephalic v.
bronchial v.
v. caliber
capillary v.
cephalized v.
cerebral blood v.
chyle v.
chyliferous v.

circumflex v.
codominant v.
collateral v.
collecting v.
commencement of v.
complex of v.
contralateral v.
corkscrew v.
coursing v.
cranial v.
cross-pelvic collateral v.
culprit v.
curved v.
v. cutoff of contrast material
deep lymphatic v.
v. diameter
diminutive v.
disease-free v.
displacement of brain v.
v. displacement brain infection
distal runoff v.
dominant v.
eccentric v.
efferent lymph v.
end-on v.
enlarged pulmonary v.
extracranial v.
feeding v.
femoropopliteal v.
fenestrated v.
v. filling
gastroepiploic v.
great v.
hairpin v.
heart and great vessels
hilar v.
ileocolic v.
iliac v.
uncoiling of the great vessels
increased prominence of
  pulmonary v.
infrapopliteal v.
in-plane v.
intercostal v.
interlobular v.
internal pudendal v.
intimal attachment of diseased v.
intracranial v.
intradural v.
kidney v.
lacteal v.
lenticulostriate v.

NOTES

V

vessel *(continued)*
  v. loop
  lymphatic v.
  lymphocapillary v.
  mesenteric v.
  mesocolonic v.
  minute v.
  musculophrenic v.
  native v.
  nondominant v.
  occipital v.
  v. occlusion
  origin of v.
  parent v.
  patency of v.
  patent v.
  pelvic collateral v.
  penile v.
  perforator v.
  perfusate v.
  pericallosal v.
  peripelvic collateral v.
  peripheral v.
  peroneal v.
  pial v.
  plump v.
  pole of v.
  portosystemic collateral v.
  posterior lumbar v.
  proximal and distal portion of v.
  pulmonary v.
  radicular v.
  reduced prominence of
    pulmonary v.
  renal hilar v.
  v. reshaping by angioplasty
  retroesophageal v.
  retrotracheal v.
  v. runoff
  v. rupture
  splanchnic v.
  splenic v.
  subclavian v.
  superficial lymphatic v.
  superior gluteal v.
  takeoff of v.
  telangiectatic v.
  v. topography
  v. tortuosity
  tortuosity of cervical v.
  tortuous v.
  v. tracing
  v. tracking
  transposition of great v.
  v. trauma
  vasorelaxation of epicardial v.
  vasospastic v.

  vestigial v.
  v. wall abnormality
  Windkessel v.
  wraparound v.
vest
  Bremer AirFlo V.
  halo v.
vestibula (*pl. of* vestibulum)
vestibular
  v. apparatus
  v. aqueduct
  v. aqueduct syndrome (VAS)
  v. canal
  v. division of eighth cranial nerve
  v. ganglion
  v. labyrinth
  v. ligament
  v. schwannoma
  v. window
vestibule
  anatomic esophageal v.
  esophageal v.
  inner ear v.
  large v.
  laryngeal v.
  v. of larynx
  v. of vagina
vestibulocochlear nerve
vestibulogenic
vestibulospinal tract
vestibulum, pl. **vestibula**
vestige
  coccygeal v.
vestigial
  v. commissure
  v. fold
  v. left sinoatrial node
  v. vessel
vestigium, pl. **vestigia**
  v. processus vaginalis
VEST system
VFT
  venous filling time
VHL
  von Hippel-Lindau
VI
  ventricular index
viability
  myocardial tissue v.
  tissue v.
viable
  v. fetus
  v. myocardium
vial
  multidose v.
  reaction v.

VIATORR
> V. endoprosthesis
> V. transjugular intrahepatic portosystemic shunt stent graft

Viatronix, Inc. virtual colonoscopy system
VIA 7991 ventricle impedance adapter
VIBE
> volumetric interpolated breath-hold examination
> VIBE sequence

vibex, pl. **vibices**
vibrating-reed electrometer
vibration
> v. frequency
> lattice v.
> molecular v.

vibratory motion
vibrio
vicarious contrast excretion
Victoreen dosimeter
Vidar scanner
video
> v. barium swallow
> v. cystourethrography
> v. digital gastrointestinal radiography
> v. display camera
> v. display unit (VDU)
> v. electroencephalography monitoring
> v. proctogram
> v. signal generator

videoangiography
> digital v.

video-assisted thoracoscopy (VAT)
videoconferencing
> teleradiology v.

videocystometrography (VCMG)
videodensitometric
videodensitometry
videodensity curve
videofluoroscopic imaging
videofluoroscopy
> spinal v.

videognosis
videolaseroscopy
videometry
videoradiography
videotape study
videothoracoscopy

vidian
> v. artery
> v. canal
> v. nerve

vidicon
> V. camera tube
> x-ray sensitive v.

Vieussens
> ansa of V.
> V. anulus
> circle of V.
> isthmus of V.
> limbus of V.
> V. loop
> ring of V.
> V. valve

view (*See* viewing)
> abdominal v.
> afferent v.
> air-contrast v.
> Alexander v.
> amputated-foot v.
> angiographic system for unlimited rolling field-of-v.'s (angioSURF)
> angled craniocaudal v.
> anterior feet v.
> anterior-posterior, posterior-anterior v.
> anteroposterior v.
> apical lordotic v.
> apical and subcostal four-chambered v.
> AP inversion stress vagina v.
> AP supine portable v.
> Arcelin v.
> axial sesamoid v.
> axillary tail v.
> ball catcher v.
> basal short-axis v.
> base v.
> baseline v.
> beam's eye v. (BEV)
> Beath v.
> biplane orthogonal v.
> bird's eye v.
> v. box
> Broden v.
> brow-down skull v.
> brow-up skull v.
> Bucky v.
> bull's eye v.
> Caldwell occipitofrontal v.

NOTES

V

view *(continued)*
cardiac long axis v.
cardiac short axis v.
carpal tunnel v.
Carter-Rowe v.
caudal v.
caudocranial tangential v.
cephalic tilt v.
cerebellar v.
cervical spine dens v.
Chamberlain-Towne v.
Chassard-Lapiné v.
Chausse v.
Chaussier v.
chest v.
cine v.
cineradiographic v.
classic carpal tunnel v.
clenched fist v.
Cleopatra v.
closed-mouth v.
close-up v.
coalition v.
comparison v.
coned-down compression v.
cone spot compression v.
contact lateral v.
coronal bending v.
coronal reconstruction v.
couch v.
cranial angled v.
craniocaudal v.
crosstable lateral v. (CTLV)
decubitus v.
3D endoluminal v.
dens v.
dorsal v.
dorsiflexion v.
dorsoplantar v.
Dunlop-Shands v.
efferent v.
Eklund v.
endoluminal v.
en face v.
equilibrium v.
erect v.
exaggerated craniocaudal v.
expiration v.
expiratory v.
extended field of v.
extension v.
external rotation v.
fan-shaped v.
fast spin-echo v.
FCS v.
femoral v.
Ferguson v.

fetal echocardiographic v.
field of v. (FOV)
first-pass v.
Fleckinger v.
flexion and extension v.'s
fluoroscopic v.
follow-through v.
four-chamber apical v.
frogleg lateral v.
frontal v.
Fuchs odontoid v.
full cervical spine v.
full column v.
full length v.
Garth v.
gated v.
Granger v.
Grashey shoulder v.
great vessel v.
half-axial v.
Hampton v.
Harris v.
Harris-Beath axial hindfoot v.
heavily penetrated v.
Heinig v.
hemiaxial v.
hepatoclavicular v.
hip-to-ankle v.
Hobb v.
Hughston v.
ice-pick v.
infrapatellar v.
inspiration and expiration v.'s
inspiratory v.
v. insufficiency artifact
internal and external rotation v.'s
intraoperative v.
inversion ankle stress v.
Jones v.
Jude pelvic v.
Judet v.
knee v.
KUB v.
kyphotic v.
large field of v. (LFV)
lateral anterior drawer stress v.
lateral bending v.
lateral decubitus v.
lateral extension v.
lateral flexion v.
lateral oblique v.
lateral tilt stress ankle v.
lateromedial oblique v.
Laurin x-ray v.
Law v.
left anterior oblique v.
limited v.

long axial oblique v.
long axis parasternal v.
longitudinal ultrasound v.
lordotic v.
Low-Beers v.
lumbar spine v.
magnification v.
Mayer v.
medial oblique v.
mediolateral v. (MLO)
mediolateral oblique v.
Merchant v.
v. microtomography
mortise v.
MPR v.
Mukherjee-Sivaya v.
multiplanar reformatting v.
navicular v.
Neer lateral v.
Neer transscapular v.
nonforeshortened angiographic v.
nonstanding lateral oblique v.
nonweightbearing v.
normal anteroposterior v.
notch v.
oblique v.
occipital v.
odontoid v.
open-mouth odontoid v.
optimally positioned v.
orthogonal v.
outlet v.
overcouch v.
overhead oblique v.
Owen v.
panoramic v.
Panorex v.
pantomographic v.
parallax v.
parasternal long-axis v.
parasternal short-axis v.
patellar skyline v.
pelvic v.
v. per segment (VPS)
Pillar v.
plain v.
planar v.
plantar axial v.
plantar flexion stress v.
plumbline v.
portable v.
posterior skull v.

posteroanterior v.
posterooblique v.
postevacuation v.
postoperative v.
postreduction v.
postvoid v.
preliminary v.
preoperative v.
prereduction v.
profile ray v.
prone lateral v.
push-pull ankle stress v.
push-pull hip v.
ray-sum v.
rear endoluminal v.
reconstruction v.
rectangular field of v.
recumbent v.
replacing oblique v.
retroflexed v.
retromammary space v.
Rhese v.
rib v.
right anterior oblique v.
right lateral decubitus v.
right ventricular inflow v.
Rokus v.
rolled v.
room's eye v. (REV)
rotated craniocaudal v.
routine magnification v.
Rumstrom v.
sagittal and coronal
   reconstruction v.
sagittal magnetization transfer v.
Schatzki v.
Schüller v.
scottie dog v.
scout v.
selective coronary arteriography v.
semiupright v.
serendipity v.
v. shadow projection
   microtomographic system
short axis parasternal v.
single-breath v.
sitting-up v.
ski jump v.
skyline v.
spider x-ray v.
spot compression v.
standing dorsoplantar v.

V

NOTES

view *(continued)*
   standing false profile v.
   standing lateral v.
   standing post void v.
   standing weightbearing v.
   static v.
   steep left anterior oblique v.
   Stenver v.
   stereoscopic v.
   sternal v.
   stress Broden v.
   stress eversion v.
   stress inversion v.
   Stryker notch v.
   subcostal four-chamber v.
   subcostal long-axis v.
   subcostal short-axis v.
   submaxillary v.
   submental vertex v.
   submentovertical v.
   subscapular echocardiographic v.
   subtalar v.
   subxiphoid v.
   sunrise v.
   sunset v.
   superoinferior v.
   supine full v.
   suprasternal notch v.
   swimmer's v.
   tangential scapular v.
   thoracic v.
   tomographic v.
   Towne v.
   transaxillary lateral v.
   transcranial lateral v.
   transgastric echocardiographic v.
   transscapular v.
   transthoracic v.
   transverse v.
   transverse/neutral v.
   true lateral v.
   tunnel v.
   Twining v.
   two-plane v.
   ulnar deviation v.
   upright postvoid v.
   Van Rosen v.
   Velpeau axillary v.
   ventricular v.
   verticosubmental v.
   virtual endoscopic v.
   von Rosen v.
   washout v.
   Waters v.
   weeping willow v.
   weightbearing dorsoplantar v.
   West Point v.
   White leg-length v.
   whole-body imaging with
     magnified v.'s
   x-ray v.
   Zanca v.

viewbox
   v. luminance
   virtual reality v.

viewer
   dedicated v.
   Mammo Mask dedicated v.

viewing
   cine-based v.
   film-based v.
   fly-through v.
   group v.
   PVR fly-through v.
   V. Wand

ViewMax software
view-to-view variation
vignetting
vigorous achalasia
Villaret-Mackenzie syndrome
villi (*pl. of* villus)
villoglandular polyp
villotubular adenoma
villous
   v. adenoma
   v. atrophy
   v. carcinoma
   v. frond
   v. hypertrophy
   v. papilloma
   v. placenta
   v. proliferation
   v. stomach polyp
   v. tumor

villus, pl. **villi**
   anchoring v.
   arachnoid v.
   atrophic v.
   duodenal v.
   finger-like v.
   floating v.
   gallbladder v.
   hydropic v.
   intestinal v.
   leaf-like v.
   placental v.
   ridged-convoluted v.
   tongue-shaped v.

vinculum breve
Vingmed
   V. CFM ultrasound system
   V. ultrasound

VINNIE
   velocity-encoded cine imaging

violation
 articular cartilage v.
VIPoma
 vasoactive intestinal polypeptide tumor
viral
 v. esophagitis
 v. particle
 v. pleuritis
 v. vector delivery
Virchow
 V. gland
 V. hydatid
 V. law of skull growth
 V. metastasis
 V. plane
 V. psammoma
 V. sentinel node
Virchow-Robin
 V.-R. perivascular space
 V.-R. space of brain
 V.-R. space dilatation
Virchow-Troisier node
virtual
 v. arterial endoscopy
 v. bronchoscopy (VB)
 v. colonoscopy
 V. CT colonography
 v. cystoscopy
 v. endoscope
 v. endoscopic view
 v. reality imaging
 v. reality simulator
 v. reality viewbox
 v. retinal display system
Virtuoso portable 3D imaging system
virulent atherosclerosis
virus
 human immunodeficiency v. (HIV)
virus-directed enzyme/prodrug therapy
virus-mediated gene therapy
viscera (*pl. of* viscus)
visceral
 v. adipose tissue (VAT)
 v. angiography
 v. angiomatosis
 v. aortography
 v. arteriography
 v. artery
 v. catheter
 v. edema
 v. embolus
 v. heterotaxia

 v. layer
 v. lesion
 v. lymph node
 v. muscle
 v. pelvic fascia
 v. pericardial calcification
 v. pericardium
 v. peritoneum
 v. pleura
 v. pleurisy
 v. situs solitus
 v. skeleton
 v. space
 v. surface of liver
viscerocranium
 cartilaginous v.
 membranous v.
viscerography
visceromegaly
visceroparietal
visceroperitoneal
visceropleural
visceroptosis
viscerosomatic
viscid
viscosity coefficient
viscous
viscus, pl. **viscera**
 abdominal v.
 abdominopelvic v.
 hollow v.
 intraabdominal v.
 intraperitoneal v.
 mediastinal v.
 pelvic v.
 perforated hollow v.
 retroperitoneal v.
 ruptured hollow v.
 solid v.
 strangulated v.
VISI
 volar intercalated segment instability
 VISI deformity
visibility of the foramen magnum
visible
 v. anterior motion
 v. peristalsis
vision
 V. camera
 V. high-performance gradient system
 V. MR imaging system

NOTES

vision *(continued)*
  stereoscopic v.
  V. Ten V-scan scanner
  V. 1.5 T Siemens MRI scanner
Visipaque 270, 320 contrast agent
Vistec x-ray detectable sponge
visual
  v. cortex
  v. inspection
  v. laser ablation of prostate
  (VLAP)
  v. shimmering
visualization
  breakthrough v.
  delayed v.
  direct v.
  double-contrast v.
  endoluminal v.
  genital v.
  inadequate v.
  intraoperative x-ray v.
  needle v.
  object-based v.
  optimal v.
  poor v.
  scene-based v.
  selective v.
  suboptimal v.
  volume mode v.
  v. of the Z line
visualized
  suboptimally v.
Visulas Nd:YAG laser
VISX
  V. Star S2 excimer laser system
  V. WaveScan Wavefront System
vita glass
vital capacity (VC)
vitelline
  v. duct
  v. fistula
Viterbi decoding
Vitesse Cos laser
Vitrea
  V. 2 computer workstation
  V. 3D imaging
  V. 3D system
  V. workstation v. 1.1, 1.2
vitreous
  v. hemorrhage
  v. lymphoma
  primary v.
vivo
  DAI in v.
  hydrolysis in v.
  in v.
  measurement in v.

  micron-resolution retinal image
  in v.
  water diffusion in v.
Vladimiroff-Mikulicz amputation
VLAP
  visual laser ablation of prostate
V-like pattern of uptake
VM–26
VMA
  vastus medialis advancement
VMO
VNS
  vagus nerve stimulation
  VNS epoch
VNS-fMRI
  vagus nerve stimulated functional MRI
VNS-synchronized
  VNS-s. BOLD fMRI
VNUS
  V. closure system
  V. radiofrequency generator
vocal
  v. cord
  v. cord carcinoma
  v. cord paralysis
  v. ligament
  v. muscle
vocalis muscle
Vogt
  V. bone-free projection
  V. cephalosyndactyly
VOI
  volume of interest
void
  color v.
  v. determination
  flow v.
  serpentine signal v.
  signal v.
voiding
  v. cystogram
  v. cystourethrogram (VCU, VCUG)
  v. cystourethrography (VCU,
  VCUG)
  v. sequence
  v. study
  v. urethrocystography
volar
  v. angulation
  v. capsule
  v. carpal ligament
  v. dislocation
  v. inclination
  v. intercalated segment instability
  (VISI)
  v. plate
  v. radiocarpal ligament disruption

v. rim
v. rim distal radial fracture
v. tilt
v. wrist
volar-flexed intercalated segment instability
volarward
Volkmann
V. canal
V. deformity
V. fracture
V. ischemic contracture
volt (v)
billion electron v. (BEV)
electron v. (eV, ev)
kiloelectron v. (keV, kev)
million electron v. (MeV)
Volta effect
voltage
v. amplifier
operating v.
pulse v.
ripple v.
volt-ampere (va)
volume
v. acquisition
adaptive cardio v. (ACV)
adequate stroke v.
alveolar v.
amnionic fluid v.
amygdala v.
v. analysis
aortic flow v.
aqueductal CSF stroke v.
articular cartilage v.
Arvidsson dimension-length method for ventricular v.
atomic v.
atrial emptying v.
augmented stroke v.
v. averaging
back stroke v.
bladder v.
blood v.
brain v.
capillary blood v.
cardiac v.
caudate v.
cavity v.
central blood v.
cerebellar v.
cerebral blood v. (CBV)

cerebrospinal fluid v.
chamber v.
circulating blood v.
circulation v.
clinical target v. (CTV)
closing v.
v. coil
3D v.
decreased stroke v.
decreased tidal v.
determination of lung v.
diastolic atrial v.
diminished lung v.
Dodge area-length method for ventricular v.
v. element
end-diastolic v.
end-expiratory lung v.
endocardial v.
end-systolic v. (ESV)
end-systolic pressure:end-systolic v.
end-systolic residual v.
epicardial v.
v. estimation
expiratory reserve v. (ERV)
extracellular fluid v.
fetal aortic flow v.
flow v.
fluid v.
forced expiratory v.
forward stroke v. (FSV)
fractional moving blood v.
fractional vascular v.
gas v.
gland v.
gross tumor v. (GTV)
heart stroke v.
heart-to-thorax v.
hippocampal v.
v. histogram
image v.
v. imaging
v. implant calculation
increased extracellular fluid v.
inspiratory reserve v. (IRV)
v. of interest (VOI)
interstitial lung disease with increased lung v.
intracranial v.
ipsilateral lung v.
left atrial maximal v.
left ventricular chamber v.

V

NOTES

volume *(continued)*
    left ventricular end-diastolic v.
    left ventricular inflow v. (LVIV)
    left ventricular maximal v.
    left ventricular outflow v. (LVOV)
    left ventricular stroke v.
    v. loss
    low lung v.
    lung v. (V)
    mean corpuscular v.
    minimal v.
    minute v.
    v. mode
    v. mode visualization
    molar v.
    ovarian v.
    v. overload
    patient v.
    pericardial reserve v.
    ping-pong heart v.
    planning target v. (PTV)
    plasma v.
    postvoid residual urine v.
    prism method for ventricular v.
    pulmonary blood v.
    pyloric v.
    pyramid method for ventricular v.
    quantitative amniotic fluid v.
    radioactivity per v.
    radionuclide stroke v.
    reduced lung v.
    reduced plasma v.
    reduced stroke v.
    regional cerebral blood v. (rCBV)
    v. regulation
    regurgitant stroke v. (RSV)
    relative cerebral blood v. (rCBV)
    v. rendering
    v. rendering of helical CT data
    v. rendering technique
    residual v. (RV)
    respiratory v.
    right ventricular end-diastolic v.
      (RVEDV)
    right ventricular end-systolic v.
      (RVESV)
    right ventricular stroke v.
    scan v.
    v. score
    sensitive v.
    Simpson rule method for
      ventricular v.
    slice v.
    stroke v. (SV)
    supratentorial v.
    systolic atrial v.

    Teichholz equation for left
      ventricular v.
    thermodilution stroke v.
    thin cylindrical uniform field v.
    thoracic gas v.
    tidal inspiratory flow v.
    total brain v. (TBV)
    total intracranial v. (TIV)
    total stroke v. (TSV)
    transit v.
    tumor v.
    ventricular end-diastolic v.
    voxel v.
    whole-brain parenchymal v.
volume-controlled inverse ratio
    ventilation
volume-cycled ventilation
volume-mode EBCT
volume-ratio method
volume-rendered
    v.-r. CT colonography
    v.-r. 3D image
    v.-r. MR angiogram
volume-selective excitation
volumetric
    v. acquisition
    v. analysis
    v. computed tomography
    v. data set
    v. function
    v. image
    v. image data
    v. imaging
    v. interpolated breath-hold
      examination (VIBE)
    v. interstitial hyperthermia
    v. magnetic resonance brain
      mapping
    v. mapping technique
    v. minimally invasive stereotaxis
    v. multiplexed transmission
      holography
    v. resampling
    v. scan
volumetry
    CT-aided v.
    3D ultrasound v.
    hippocampal magnetic resonance v.
    tumor v.
    v. of ventilated airspace
voluming artifact
voluntary
    v. effort (VE)
    v. muscle
volute
volvulus
    cecal v.

colonic v.
gastric v.
mesenteroaxial v.
midgut v.
organoaxial v.
sigmoid colon v.
small bowel v.
stomach v.
Volz wrist
vomer bone
vomerine canal
vomerorostral canal
vomerovaginal canal
von
v. Hippel-Lindau (VHL)
v. Hippel-Lindau syndrome
v. Hippel retina tumor
v. Meyenburg complex
prefrontal bone of v. Bardeleben
v. Recklinghausen disease
v. Rosen view
v. Willebrand disease
Voorhoeve disease
vortex, pl. **vortices**
v. coccygeus
v. cordis
vorticity
Vostal radial fracture classification
VOXAR Plug n View 3D imager
voxel
adjacent v.
v. array
cubic v.
v. element
v. gradient
isotropic v.
v. localization
seed v.
v. size
spectroscopic v.
v. volume
Voxel-Man software
VoxelView
V. software
V. system
Voxgram multiple-exposure holography
VP
ventriculoperitoneal
VP shunt
VPB
ventricular premature beat

VPC
ventricular premature complex
ventricular premature contraction
VPD
ventricular premature depolarization
VPS
view per segment
V/Q
ventilation-perfusion
V/Q imaging
V/Q lung segment scan
V/Q mismatch
VR
valvular regurgitation
VRT
venous refill time
VS
ventricular septum
VScore with AutoGate cardiac imaging
VSD
ventricular septal defect
V-shaped
V-s. fracture
V-s. ulcer
V-sign of Naclerio
VTED
venous thromboembolic disease
VT multinuclear spectrometer
vulgaris
thermoactinomyces v.
vulva, pl. **vulvae**
preinvasive disease of cervix,
vagina, and v.
synechia vulvae
vulvar
v. adenoid cystic adenocarcinoma
v. carcinoma
v. intraepithelial neoplasm
v. malignancy
vulvectomy
radical v.
vulvouterine canal
vulvovaginal carcinoma
VUR
vesicoureteral reflux
VUSE
variable-angle uniform signal excitation
V0-V4
vertebral artery segment V0-V4
V-wave pressure
VWF
velocity waveform

V

NOTES

VWF *(continued)*
     Doppler VWF

W
    tungsten
188W
    tungsten-188
w
    watt
Waardenburg syndrome
Waddell sign
wafer
    w. of endocardium
    Gliadel w.
wafer-like appearance
wafer-shaped injury
Wagner line
Wagstaffe fracture
waist
    w. in balloon
    cardiac w.
waist-like constriction
waiter's tip palsy
Walcher position
Waldeyer
    W. fascia
    W. fossa
    W. ring
    W. ring lesion
    W. ring lymphoma
Walker
    W. carcinoma
    W. carcinosarcoma
    W. magnet
walking
    w. pneumonia
    w. saturation band
walking-stick appearance
wall
    aneurysmal w.
    anterior abdominal w.
    anterolateral abdominal w.
    apical w.
    arterial w.
    axial w.
    bladder w.
    body w.
    bowel w.
    bullous edema of bladder w.
    w. calcification
    capillary w.
    carotid w.
    cavity w.
    chest w.
    cystic w.
    dorsal abdominal w.
    fetal abdominal w.

w. filter
friable w.
full-thickness button of aortic w.
gallbladder w.
w. hypokinesis
inferior w.
inferoapical w.
intestinal w.
left anterior chest wall w.
left ventricular w. (LVW)
left ventricular free w. (LVFW)
left ventricular posterior w.
  (LVPW)
linear focus within cyst w.
luminal w.
midabdominal w.
w. motion
w. motion abnormality (WMA)
w. motion imaging
w. motion score
w. motion score index
w. motion study
multiple bull's eye lesions
  bowel w.
myocardial w.
nasal cavity w.
orbital w.
paraumbilical anterior abdominal w.
pelvic w.
posterior w. (PW)
posterior abdominal w.
posterior free w.
posterolateral w.
septal w.
w. shear stress
stomach w.
thickened airway w.
thickened bladder w.
thickened gallbladder w.
w. thickening
w. thickness
thoracic w.
thoracoabdominal w.
w. thump
vaginal w.
variceal w.
vascular w.
ventricular free w.
wall-echo
    w.-e. shadow (WES)
    w.-e. shadow triad
walled-off abscess
Wallenberg lateral medullary syndrome
Wallerian degeneration

W

Wallgraft
  W. cobalt-based alloy balloon-
    expandable stent
  W. endoprosthesis
  W. endoprosthesis stent-graft
Wallstent
  W. biliary endoprosthesis
  Magic S/P W.
  W. stent
  8 (x) 50 mm self-expanding
    Easy W.
Walt Disney dwarfism
Walther
  W. fracture
  W. oblique ligament
Waltman loop
wand
  programmer w.
  Viewing W.
wandering
  w. gallbladder
  w. goiter
  w. heart
  w. kidney
  w. liver
  w. spleen
Wang applicator
Wang-Binford edge detector
Warburg
  W. disease
  W. effect
Ward triangle
warfarin
  w. embryopathy
  w. sodium
warming
  urethral w.
warm nodule
Wartenberg sign
Warthin tumor
washboard effect
wash-in
  w.-i. effect
  w.-i. phase
wash-in/wash-out study
washout
  contrast medium w.
  w. curve
  delayed w.
  differential w.
  w. effect
  w. gradient
  kidney w.
  w. kinetics
  lung w.
  MIBG w.
  nitrogen w.

  w. phase
  w. phase ventilation scan
  w. pyelography
  rapid tracer w.
  w. study
  teboroxime resting w. (TRW)
  w. test
  w. view
wasp-tail deformity
**Wassel classification of thumb
  polydactyly**
wastage
  pregnancy w.
wasting
  cerebral salt w.
  muscle fiber w.
Watanabe discoid meniscus classification
watch
  Yperwatch gamma control w.
water
  w. bolus
  coexistent intravoxel fat and w.
  w. density
  w. density area
  w. density line
  diffusion characteristics of w.
  w. diffusion in vivo
  doped w.
  w. eliminated Fourier transform
    (WEFT)
  glucose w.
  heavy w.
  intracellular w.
  ion-bound w.
  w. on the brain
  w. path
  w. path scan
  w. perfusable tissue index
  polar-bound w.
  w. range
  w. retention
  w. seal
  w. selective spin-echo imaging
  w. signal on magnetic resonance
    imaging scan
  structured w.
  w. suppression pulse sequence
  total body w. (TBW)
water-bottle
  w.-b. configuration
  w.-b. heart
water-contrast computed tomography
waterfall
  w. appearance
  w. hilum
  w. stomach
WATERGATE

water-infusion catheter
water-like signal intensity
Waters
    W. position
    W. positioner
    W. projection
    W. view
    W. view radiograph
watershed
    w. area
    w. brain infarct
    w. mechanism
    w. zone in the brain
water-soluble
    w.-s. contrast enema
    w.-s. contrast esophageal swallow
    w.-s. contrast medium (WSCM)
    w.-s. iodinated imaging agent
    w.-s. myelography
    w.-s. nonionic imaging agent
Waterson-Cooley shunt
Waterson shunt
Waterston groove
water-suppressed proton spectrum
water-suppression technique
water-trap stomach
Watson-Jones tibial tubercle avulsion
  fracture classification
watt (w)
wave
    abdominal fluid w.
    acoustic w.
    aperiodic w.
    circular polarization w.
    constant tilt w.
    continuous w. (CW)
    electromagnetic w.
    energy w.
    w. of excitation
    extracorporeal shock w.
    fluid w.
    longitudinal acoustic w.
    peristaltic w.
    pressure w.
    primary peristaltic w.
    pulsed w.
    radiofrequency w.
    rapid filling w. (RFW)
    reference w.
    secondary w.
    sine w.
    slice excitation w. (SEW)

    slow filling w.
    sound w.
    square w.
    standing w.
    systolic S w.
    terahertz w.
    tertiary w.
    transverse acoustic w.
    ultrasonic w.
waveform
    apiculate w.
    arterial w.
    cerebrospinal fluid flow w.
    dampened w.
    Doppler spectral w.
    flow velocity w.
    w. generator
    gradient w.
    low-resistance spectral w.
    parvus et tardus w.
    pressure w.
    pulsed Doppler w.
    pulse volume w.
    segmental bronchus renal artery w.
    sinusoidal w.
    spectral w.
    tardus-parvus w.
    triphasic w.
    tube voltage w.
    uterine artery w.
    velocity w. (VWF)
    venous w.
wavelength (Λ)
    Compton w.
    de Broglie w.
    double-echo Broglie w.
    energy w.
    readout w.
    unit of w.
wavelet
    w. compression
    w. encoding
    w. scalar quantization (WSQ)
    w. subband
    w. transform
wavelet-encoded magnetic resonance
  imaging
WaveWire angioplasty guidewire
wax phantom
waxy liver
WBC
    white blood cell

W

NOTES

WBC *(continued)*
^{111}In WBCs
In-111 oxine WBCs
radiolabeled WBCs
^{99m}Tc-labeled WBC
WBR
whole-body radiation
WBRT
whole-brain radiation therapy
whole-brain radiotherapy
weak
w. carotid upstroke
w. signal
weakened artery
weakening
trabecular w.
weakness
respiratory muscle w.
structural w.
wear-and-tear degeneration
web
antral w.
w. contracture
duodenal w.
esophageal w.
fibrous w.
finger w.
hepatic w.
intestinal w.
laryngeal w.
lateral w.
postcricoid w.
terminal w.
thumb w.
venous w.
webbed
w. finger
w. neck
w. penis
Weber
W. C fracture
circle of W.
Weber-Christian mesentery
web-like appearance
wedge
w. arteriography
w. bond
w. compression fracture
45-degree spinal w.
55-degree tomography w.
dynamic w.
w. factor
w. filter
w. flexion-compression fracture
w. fracture of spine
w. hepatic venous pressure
(WHVP)

w. isodose angle
matchline w.
mediastinal w.
w. pressure
w. resection
step w.
wedged hepatic venography
wedged-pair
w.-p. beam
w.-p. technique
wedge-shaped
w.-s. defect
w.-s. density
w.-s. infarct
w.-s. lesion
w.-s. lobe
w.-s. mass
w.-s. support
w.-s. vertebra
w.-s. zone
wedging
anterior w.
w. deformity
vertebral w.
w. of vertebral interspace
week
gestational w.
weeping willow view
WEFT
water eliminated Fourier transform
Wegener granulomatosis
Wegner
W. line
W. sign
Weibel-Palade body
weight
body w.
estimated fetal w. (EFW)
fetal w.
normal spleen w.
thymus w.
weightbearing
w. acetabular dome
w. axis
w. bone
w. dorsoplantar view
w. film
w. joint
w. rotational injury
w. surface
weighted
spin density w.
w. spin-echo column
weighted-CT-dose index
weighting
exponential w.

human visual sensitivity w.
multislice spiral w.
Weill-Marchesani syndrome
Weill sign
Weil syndrome
Weiner spatially varying filter
Weiss sign
Weitbrecht
W. cord
W. foramen
W. ligament
Welcher basal angle
Welcker angle
weld
callus w.
welder's lung
welding
laser w.
Welin technique
well
w. counter
96-w. scanning fluorometer
well-circumscribed
w.-c. breast mass
w.-c. neoplasm
w.-c. tumor
well-circumscribed lesion
well-defined
w.-d. appearance
w.-d. border
w.-d. mass
well-defined lesion
well-demarcated scar
well-differentiated
w.-d. adenoma
w.-d. astrocytoma
w.-d. polycystic Wilms tumor
well-inflated lung
well-preserved ejection fraction
well-type ionization chamber
Wenckebach
W. AV block
W. cardioptosis
W. phenomenon
Werdnig-Hoffmann disease
Wermer syndrome
Werner
W. classification
W. syndrome
Wernicke area
Wernicke-Korsakoff syndrome
Wertheim hysterectomy

WES
wall-echo shadow
West
W. lacuna skull
W. Point view
W. syndrome
zones 1–4 of W.
Westcott needle
West-Engstler skull
Westergren tube
Westermark sign
western boot in open fracture
Westphal-Strümpell disease
Westphal zone
wet
w. bowel preparation
w. brain
w. laser imaging
w. lung
w. lung syndrome
w. pleurisy
w. reading
w. stomach
w. swallow
Wetzel test
WFRT
wide-field radiation therapy
Wharton
W. duct
W. gland
W. tumor
Wheatstone bridge
wheelchair artifact
whiplash injury
Whipple
W. disease
W. operation
W. procedure
W. triad
whirlpool
w. appearance
w. sign
whirl sign
whistling deformity
Whitacre spinal needle
Whitaker test
white
w. asbestos
black and w. (BW)
w. blood cell (WBC)
w. blood cell imaging

W

NOTES

white *(continued)*
w. blood cell with indium-111 scintigraphy
w. branching linear pattern
w. cerebellum sign
w. commissure of spinal cord
w. cotton-like fibrous tissue
w. echo writing
w. epidermoid
w. epithelium
W. leg-length view
w. light pattern projector
w. line
w. line of Toldt
w. lung
w. masking
w. matter
w. matter abnormality
w. matter commissure
w. matter demyelination
w. matter diffusivity
w. matter disease
w. matter edema
w. matter hypodensity
w. matter infarct
w. matter lambda
w. matter lesion
w. matter shearing injury
w. matter signal hyperintensity
w. matter thinning
w. matter tract direction
w. metastasis
w. noise artifact
w. pneumonia
w. point
w. radiation
w. shuttering
w. star breast lesion
Whitehead deformity
white-out
Whitfield test
whitlow
herpetic w.
melanotic w.
thecal w.
WHO
World Health Organization
WHO classification
whole-body
w.-b. bone scan
w.-b. computed tomography
w.-b. counter
w.-b. counting
w.-b. dose monitoring
w.-b. echo-planar MR imaging
w.-b. ^{29}FDG scanning
w.-b. imaging with magnified views
w.-b. inflammatory response
w.-b. nuclear physical examination
w.-b. PET scan
w.-b. radiation (WBR)
w.-b. radiation therapy
w.-b. radiotherapy
w.-b. scan imaging
w.-b. sweep
w.-b. 1.5 Tesla scanner
4T w.-b. GI Signa MRI scanner
w.-b. thallium imaging
w.-b. 3T MRI system scanner
w.-b. transmission scan
w.-b. 1.5-T Siemens Vision scanner
w.-b. unit
whole-brain
w.-b. acquisition
w.-b. magnetization transfer measurement
w.-b. parenchymal volume
w.-b. radiation therapy (WBRT)
w.-b. radiotherapy (WBRT)
whole-breast sonography
whole-lung opacity
whole-volume coil
Wholey steerable guidewire
whorl
coccygeal w.
whorled appearance
whorling
WHVP
wedge hepatic venous pressure
Wiberg
W. angle
capital epiphysis angle of W.
CE angle of W.
center-edge angle of W.
W. patellar types classification
Wickham-Miller nephroscope
Widal syndrome
wide
w. caliber
w. field lesion
w. latitude film
w. rib
w. suture
w. tortuous aorta
w. window setting
wide-angle tomography
wide-based, blunt-ended, right-sided, atrial appendage
wide-beam scanning
wide-field radiation therapy (WFRT)
widely patent
wide-mouth sac

wide-neck carotid cavernous aneurysm
widened
> w. anterior meningeal index
> w. cardiac silhouette
> w. collecting system
> w. duodenal sweep
> w. heart shadow
> w. joint space
> w. mediastinum
> w. optic canal
> w. sacroiliac joint
> w. sulcus
> w. superior orbital fissure
> w. sweep duodenum
> w. symphysis pubis
> w. teardrop distance
> w. thoracic outlet

widening
> acute mediastinal w.
> ankle mortise w.
> w. of aorta
> crural cistern w.
> growth plate w.
> infundibulum w.
> interpedicular distance w.
> interspinous w.
> joint w.
> mediastinal w.
> sacroiliac joint w.
> scapholunate w.

widespread
> w. hyperattenuating mediastinal adenopathy
> w. metastasis

width
> aryepiglottic fold w.
> collimated slice w.
> collimation w.
> contrast window w.
> intracranial w. (ICW)
> isodose w.
> line w.
> metatarsal head w. (MHW)
> prevertebral w.
> pulse w. (PW)
> radial w.
> spectral w.
> window w.

Wiedemann-Beckwith syndrome
Wiener
> W. MRI filter
> W. spectrum

Wigby-Taylor position
Wigle scale for ventricular hypertrophy
Wilcoxon signed-rank test
Wilkie syndrome
Wilkins radial fracture classification
Williams-Beuren syndrome
Williams-Campbell syndrome
Williams syndrome
Willis
> W. antrum
> arterial circle of W.
> artery of W.
> circle of W.
> W. pouch

Willisii
> chordae W.

willow fracture
Wilson
> W. block
> W. cloud chamber
> W. disease
> W. fracture
> W. muscle

Wilson-Mikity syndrome
Wiltze angle
Wimberger
> W. ring
> W. sign

Winchester disk
windblown deformity
winding
> Y w.
> zero-pitch solenoidal w.

Windkessel vessel
window
> acoustic w.
> acquisition w.
> aortic w.
> aortopulmonary w.
> apical w.
> beryllium mammography x-ray tube w.
> biologic w.
> bone w.
> brain w.
> w. center
> coincidence-resolving w.
> cortical w.
> CT bone w.
> cycle-length w.
> w. ductus
> w. efficiency

NOTES

W

window *(continued)*
    energy w.
    esophageal w.
    gastric w.
    w. level
    localization w.
    lung w.
    mediastinal w.
    oval w.
    parasternal w.
    pericardial w.
    w. period
    pulmonary parenchymal w.
    radiation w.
    sampling w.
    short acquisition w.
    soft tissue w.
    spectral w.
    subcostal w.
    subdural w.
    suprasternal w.
    transforaminal w.
    transorbital w.
    transtemporal w.
    vestibular w.
    w. width
    xenon energy w.
windowed balloon
windowing
    intensity w.
window/level setting
windsock
    w. aneurysm
    w. appearance
    w. appearance of duodenum
    w. sign
windswept
    w. deformity
    w. hand
windup injury
wine
    w. glass appearance
    w. glass pelvis
    w. glass shape
wineglass
wing
    absent greater sphenoid w.
    champagne glass iliac w.
    greater sphenoid w.
    iliac w.
    sphenoid w.
    w. of sphenoid bone
winged
    w. configuration
    w. scapula
winging
    scapular w.

Winiwarter-Buerger disease
Winquist-Hansen femoral fracture classification
Winslow
    foramen of W.
    W. ligament
Winston-Lutz for LINAC-based radiosurgery
Winter-King-Moe scoliosis
wire *(See* guidewire)
    w. fixation
    heavy-duty standard exchange w.
    0.0015-inch platinum w.
    0.00175-inch platinum w.
    ^{192}Ir w.
    iridium w.
    Kirschner w. (K-wire)
    w. localization
    pacemaker w.
    standard exchange w.
    sternotomy w.
    temporary atrial pacing w.
wire-fixation buckle
wire-loop lesion
wire-related defect
wiring
    intraosseous w.
Wirsung
    W. dilatation
    W. duct
    ventral duct of W.
wisdom teeth
Wiseman classification
wispy connection
withdrawal pressure
within-slice filtering process
within-view motion
Wits measurement
WMA
    wall motion abnormality
Wolf
    W. method
    W. Piezolith 2200 lithotripter
Wolfe
    W. breast carcinoma classification
    W. DY, NI, P1, P2 pattern
    W. mammographic parenchymal pattern
Wolff-Chaikoff effect
wolffian
    w. cyst
    w. duct
    w. duct carcinoma
Wolff law
Wolff-Parkinson-White syndrome
Wolf-Hirschhorn syndrome

Wolfram syndrome
Wolin meniscoid lesion
Wolman xanthomatosis
womb stone
Wood
W. lamp
W. light
W. unit
W. unit index
W. units index of resistance
wooden shoe configuration
woody mass
wool
w. coil
w. tail
work
left ventricular stroke w. (LVSW)
myocardial w.
right ventricular stroke w. (RVSW)
working
w. film
W. Formulation classification
w. sheath
workstation
AccuView computer w.
Advantage W. 3.1
Alpha 21064 microprocessor w.
DIMAQ integrated ultrasound w.
eNTEGRA w.
freestanding w.
Fuji QA 771 w.
image processing w.
imaging w.
ISG medical imaging w.
MacSpect real-time NMR w.
Navigator computer w.
Octane postprocessing w.
PACS w.
Pegasys w.
postprocessing w.
POWERstation LNX w.
RADstation radiology w.
Renaissance 3D w.
Shebele physician reporting w.
stacked-metaphor w.
Sun w.
Unix/X11 w.
Vitrea 2 computer w.
Vitrea w. v. 1.1, 1.2
World
W. Health Organization (WHO)

W. Health Organization
classification
worm aneurysm
wormian bone
wormy appearance
wound
w. dehiscence
exit w.
gunshot w. (GSW)
high-velocity gunshot w.
missile w.
penetrating w.
perforating w.
stag w.
surgical w.
woven bone
wrap
aortic w.
no frequency w.
wraparound
w. ghosting artifact
w. vessel
wrapped aneurysmal sac
wrapping
valve w.
vein valve w.
Wratten 6B filter
W ray
wrenched knee
wrestler's elbow
wrinkle artifact
wrinkled pleura
wrinkler muscle
Wrisberg
W. cardiac ganglion
intermediate nerve of W.
W. ligament
ligaments of Henry and W.
wrist
w. capsule
w. dislocation
w. extensor compartment
gymnast's w.
w. joint
palmar w.
w. quadrature phased-array surface
coil
SLAC w.
w. triquetrum bone
volar w.
Volz w.
wristdrop

W

NOTES

writing
    black echo w.
    white echo w.
WSCM
    water-soluble contrast medium
W-shaped ileal pouch

WSQ
    wavelet scalar quantization
Wyburn-Mason
    W.-M. arteriovenous malformation
    W.-M. syndrome

X
    Kienböck unit
    magnification
    xanthosine
        X axis
        X gradient
        syndrome X
        X trough
        X unit

x
    times
        8x. 8-pixel block

Xanar 20 Ambulase CO$_2$ laser

xanthelasma

xanthic calculus

xanthoastrocytoma
    pleomorphic x. (PXA)

xanthogranuloma
    bone x.
    juvenile x.

xanthogranulomatous
    x. cholecystitis
    x. pyelonephritis

xanthoma, pl. **xanthomata**
    Achilles tendon x.
    gastric x.
    malignant fibrous x.
    x. tuberosum simplex

xanthomatosis
    cerebrotendinous x.
    primary familial x.
    Wolman x.

xanthomatous
    x. granuloma
    x. pseudotumor

xanthosarcoma

xanthosine (X)

X-band Linac

X-CBF
    cerebral xenon-enhanced blood flow

XCCL
    exaggerated craniocaudal lateral

XCT
    x-ray computed tomography

Xe
    xenon

^{133}Xe
    xenon-133

^{127}Xe
    xenon-127

^{129}Xe
    xenon-129

XeCl excimer

XeCT
    xenon computed tomography

Xenetix 250, 300, 350 contrast medium

xenograft
    bovine heart x.
    porcine heart x.
    x. valve
    vascular x.

xenon (Xe)
    x. arch photocoagulator
    x. arc lamp
    x. computed tomography (XeCT)
    X. CT
    x. CT measurement
    x. CT scanning
    x. energy window
    x. imaging agent
    x. trap system
    x. washout study

xenon-127 (^{127}Xe)

xenon-129 (^{129}Xe)

xenon-133 (^{133}Xe)
    x. SPECT imaging
    x. ventriculogram

xenon-enhanced
    x.-e. computed tomography
    x.-e. CT

xenotransplantation

xerogram

xerography

xeromammogram
    chest wall lateral x.

xeromammography

xeroradiogram

xeroradiograph

xeroradiographic
    x. selenium plate
    x. technique

xeroradiography

xerosialography

xerotomography

x-height

Xillix
    X. LIFE-GI fluorescence endoscopy
    system
    X. LIFE-Lung fluorescence
    endoscopy system

Ximatron simulator

XIP
    x-ray in plaster

xiphicostal ligament

xiphisternal joint

xiphogus

xiphoid
    x. angle
    x. appendix
    x. bone

X

xiphoid *(continued)*
    x. cartilage
    x. ligament
    x. process
xiphopubic area
xiphosternalis
    synchondrosis x.
x-irradiation
XKnife stereotactic radiosurgery system
XL
    inductive reactance
X-linked
XOP
    x-ray out of plaster
Xplorer 1000 digital imaging system
X-Prep bowel preparation
Xpress/SW helical CT scanner
Xpress/SX helical CT scanner
XRA
    x-ray arteriography
x-radiation
x-ray
    x-r. arteriography (XRA)
    x-r. attenuation
    baseline chest x-r.
    x-r. beam
    x-r. beam size
    x-r. burn
    characteristic x-r.
    chest x-r. (CXR)
    x-r. computed tomography (XCT)
    x-r. crystallography
    x-r. detector
    x-r. diffraction
    x-r. diffraction analysis
    x-r. dosimetry
    x-r. energy
    E sign on x-r.
    x-r. film
    five-view chest x-r.
    four-view chest x-r.
    x-r. generator
    x-r. image
    inside-out x-r.

    Jude pelvic x-r.
    x-r. mammography
    x-r. microscope
    mobile mass x-r. (MMR)
    monochromatic x-r.
    x-r. out of plaster (XOP)
    peripheral dual energy x-r.
     (pDEXA)
    x-r. in plaster (XIP)
    portable x-r.
    postreduction x-r.
    prereduction x-r.
    scanning-beam digital x-r. (SBDX)
    x-r. sensitive vidicon
    x-r. shadow projection
     microtomographic system
    x-r. spectrometer
    x-r. spectrum
    x-r. therapy
    x-r. thickness gauge
    x-r. tomographic microscope (XTM)
    x-r. topography
    x-r. tube
    x-r. tube housing
    x-r. tube rating chart
    two-view chest x-r.
    x-r. unit
    x-r. view
x-ray-sensitive vidicon imaging
x-shaped guidewire
X-terminal
XTM
    x-ray tomographic microscope
XT radiopaque coronary stent
X-Vigor scanner
X-wave pressure
XY
    XY plane
    XY syndrome
xylenol
    x. orange imaging agent
xylol pulse indicator
X, Y, and Z coordinates for target
    lesion

Y

    Y axis
    Y bone plate
    Y cartilage
    Y configuration
    Y fracture
    Y trough
    Y winding

Y-50

  yttrium-50

Y-90

  yttrium-90
    Y-90 silicate therapy

YAG

  yttrium-aluminum-garnet
    YAG laser

Yaglazr system
Yakolev

    terminal zone of the Y.

Yb

  ytterbium

yellow cartilage
yellow-out
Yergason test
Yeuh centesis needle
yield

    y. comparison
    diagnostic y.
    low y.
    ultrasound diagnostic y.

yin-yang appearance
Y-jaws
YLF

  yttrium lithium fluoride

yoke
yolk

    y. sac (YS)

    y. sac diameter
    y. sac ovary tumor
    y. stalk

yo-yo

    y.-y. esophageal peristalsis
    y.-y. ureteral peristalsis

Yperwatch gamma control watch
YS

  yolk sac

Y-shaped

    Y-s. acetabulum
    Y-s. distortion
    Y-s. ligament

Y-T fracture
ytterbium (Yb)

    y. pentetate sodium

ytterbium-169 DTPA
ytterbium-90 microsphere
yttrium

    ferritin-labeled y.
    y. lithium fluoride (YLF)
    y. radioactive source

yttrium-50 (^{50}Y, Y-50)
yttrium-90 (^{90}Y, Y-90)

    y. microsphere
    y. silicate therapy

yttrium-aluminum-garnet (YAG)

    y.-a.-g. laser

yttrium-90-labeled
Y-tube
Yuge

    oculosubcutaneous syndrome of Y.

Yunis-Varon syndrome
Y-wave pressure

Y

Z

Z axis
Z axis field
Z band
Z gradient
Z line

Zaglas ligament

Zahn

Z. anomaly
pocket of Z.

Zanca view

Zanelli position

ZA-stent Nitinol self-expandable stent

Z-dependent CT

zebra

z. stripe appearance
z. stripe artifact
z. stripe image

zebra-striped pattern

Zeeman hamiltonian function

Zeiss Visulas 690s laser

Zellballen

Zellweger syndrome

Zener diode

Zenith stainless steel self-expandable stent

Zenker

Z. degeneration
Z. diverticulum
Z. necrosis
Z. pouch

zeolite pneumoconiosis

zero

z. exposure
z. filling
z. line
z. net flow
z. padding
z. phase
z. reference level
z. time of the x-ray apparatus

zero-field splitting

zero-fill

z.-f. artifact
z.-f. interpolation (ZIP)

zero-filling interpolation scheme

zero-pitch solenoidal winding

ZeroRad MRI scan

zeroth moment

ZES

Zollinger-Ellison syndrome

zetacrit

Zetafuge

zeugmatography

Fourier transformation z.
rotating-frame z.

zeugopodium

Zeus system

Z-filtering

Zickel supercondylar nail

Zielke derotation level

Zieve syndrome

zigzag stent

Zilver stent

Zimmerman

Z. arch
Z. cell

Zimmermann elementary particle

Zimmer method

zinc (Zn)

irradiated z.

zinc-65 (^{65}Zn, Zn-65)

Zinn

Z. anulus
Z. ligament
tendon of Z.

Z-interpolation algorithm

ZIP

zero-fill interpolation

zipper artifact

zirconium (Zr)

z. granuloma
z. with niobium 95

Zlatkin grading system

Z-line of esophagus

ZMC

ZMC fracture

Z-MED balloon catheter

Z-MIVE

^{123}I-labeled Z.-M.

Zn

zinc

^{65}Zn, Zn-65

zinc-65

Zollinger-Ellison

Z.-E. syndrome (ZES)
Z.-E. tumor

zona, pl. zonae

z. fasciculata
z. glomerulosa
z. orbicularis
z. reticularis

zonal

z. gastritis
z. prostate anatomy

Z

zonal *(continued)*
  z. sampling
  z. uterine anatomy
zonary
zone
  air-trapping z.
  arrhythmogenic border z.
  basal z.
  bilaminar z.
  border z.
  clear z.
  convergence z.
  cross-sectional z.
  detection z.
  dorsal root entry z. (DREZ)
  echo-free central z.
  entry z.
  epileptogenic z.
  esophageal transition z.
  focal z. (FZ)
  focal high-intensity z.
  z. focusing
  fracture z.
  Fraunhofer z.
  Fresnel z.
  high-intensity z. (HIZ)
  high-signal-intensity z.
  hypoechogenic retroplacental
    myometrial z.
  hypoechoic z.
  hypovascular z.
  ischemic z.
  junctional z.
  lipid z.
  Looser transformation z.
  lung z.
  marginal z.
  midlung z.
  z. of partial preservation (ZPP)
  patchy z.
  penumbra z.
  posterior root entry z.
  prostatic transition z.
  pyramidal hemorrhagic z.
  Rolando z.
  root entry z.
  root exit z. (REZ)
  rough z.
  z. of slow conduction
  sonolucent z.
  therapy z.
  transformation z.
  transition z.
  transradiant z.
  Trümmerfeld z.
  umbau z.

  vascular z.
  wedge-shaped z.
  z.'s 1–4 of West
  Westphal z.
zonifugal
zonipetal
zonogram
zonography
  stereoscopic z.
zonoskeleton
zonula ciliaris
zoonosis
  respiratory z.
Z-point pressure
ZPP
  zone of partial preservation
Zr
  zirconium
**Z-score in bone mineral density
  measurement**
z-stent
Zuckerguss
Zuckerkandl
  Z. body
  Z. convolution
  Z. fascia
  Z. organ
Zuska disease
zwitterion
zygal
zygapophyseal
  z. articulation
  z. joint
zygapophysis
  z. inferior
  z. superior
zygoma
zygomatic
  z. arch
  z. bone
  z. process
zygomaticofacial
  z. canal
  z. foramen
zygomaticofrontal suture
zygomaticomalar
  z. area
  z. reconstruction
zygomaticomaxillary
  z. complex
  z. fracture
zygomaticotemporal
  z. canal
  z. suture
zygomaxillary
ZY plane

Appendix 1
Anatomical Illustrations

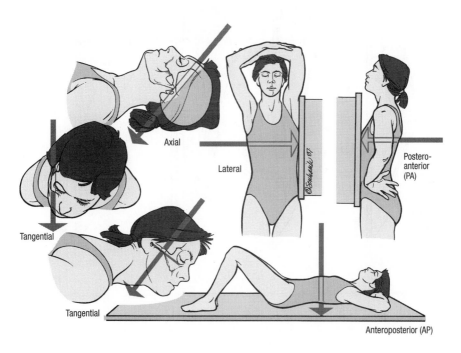

Figure 1. Radiographic projections. X-rays pass through body part with the denser structures absorbing more x-rays, resulting in the lighter areas on the radiograph.

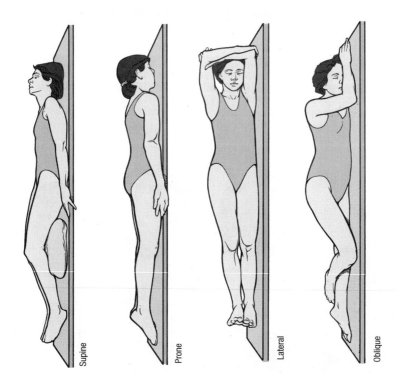

Supine

Prone

Lateral

Oblique

Figure 2. Patient positions.

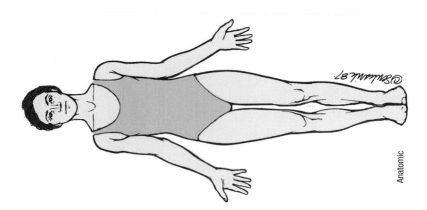

Anatomic

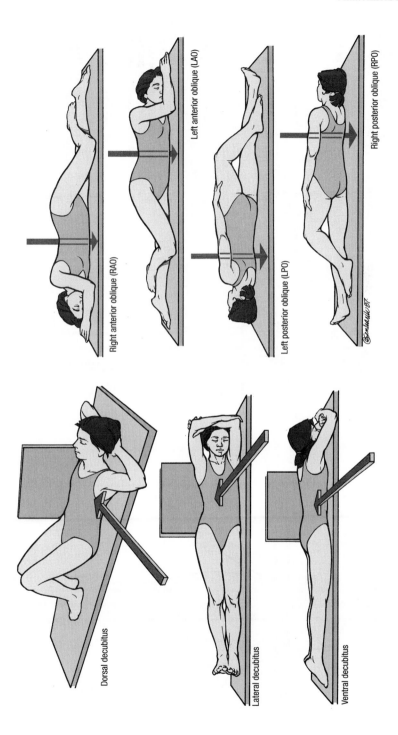

Figure 3. Patient positions.

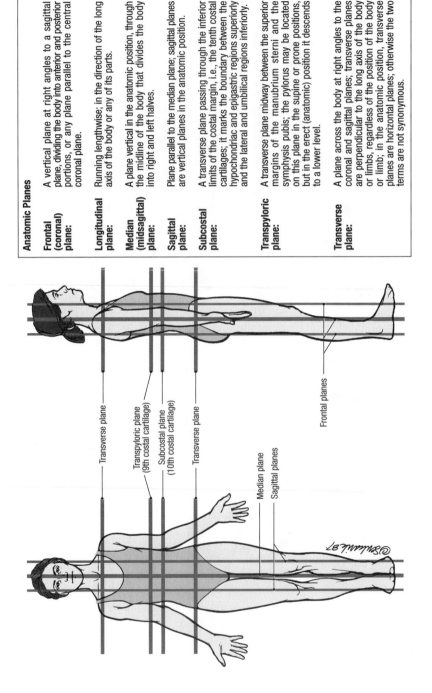

Anatomic Planes

Frontal (coronal) plane: A vertical plane at right angles to a sagittal plane, dividing the body into anterior and posterior portions, or any plane parallel to the central coronal plane.

Longitudinal plane: Running lengthwise; in the direction of the long axis of the body or any of its parts.

Median (midsagittal) plane: A plane vertical in the anatomic position, through the midline of the body that divides the body into right and left halves.

Sagittal plane: Plane parallel to the median plane; sagittal planes are vertical planes in the anatomic position.

Subcostal plane: A transverse plane passing through the inferior limits of the costal margin, i.e., the tenth costal cartilages; it marks the boundary between the hypochondriac and epigastric regions superiorly and the lateral and umbilical regions inferiorly.

Transpyloric plane: A transverse plane midway between the superior margins of the manubrium sterni and the symphysis pubis; the pylorus may be located on this plane in the supine or prone positions, but in the erect (anatomic) position it descends to a lower level.

Transverse plane: A plane across the body at right angles to the coronal and sagittal planes; transverse planes are perpendicular to the long axis of the body or limbs, regardless of the position of the body or limb; in the anatomic position, transverse planes are horizontal planes; otherwise the two terms are not synonymous.

— Transverse plane

— Transpyloric plane (9th costal cartilage)

— Subcostal plane (10th costal cartilage)

— Transverse plane

Frontal planes

Median plane
Sagittal planes

Figure 4. Terms of relationship. Anatomic planes.

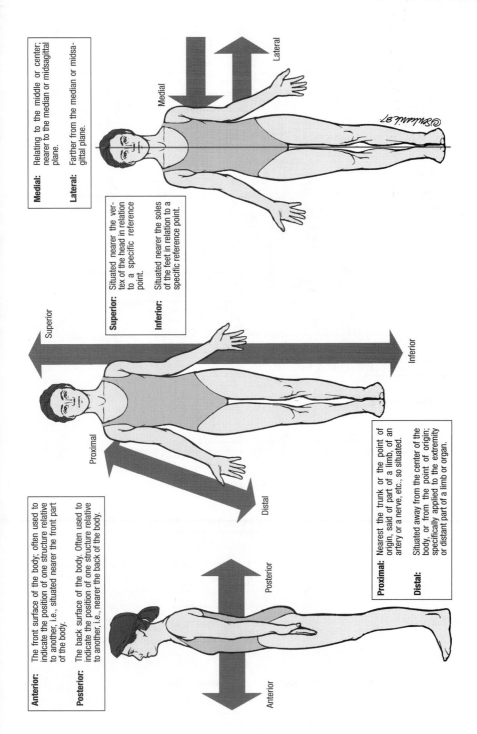

Figure 5. Terms of relationship. Body part terminology.

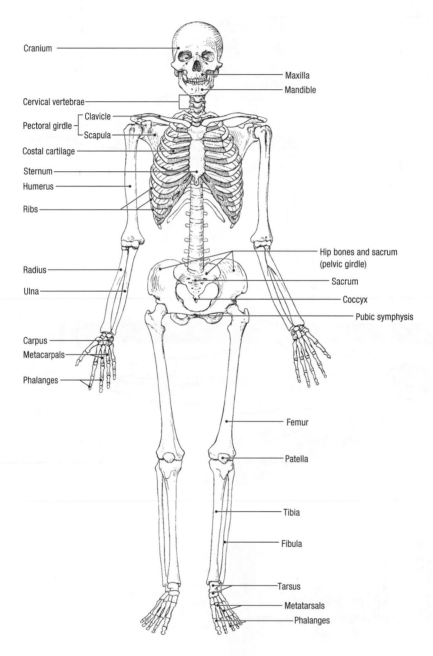

Figure 6. Skeleton, adult, anterior view.

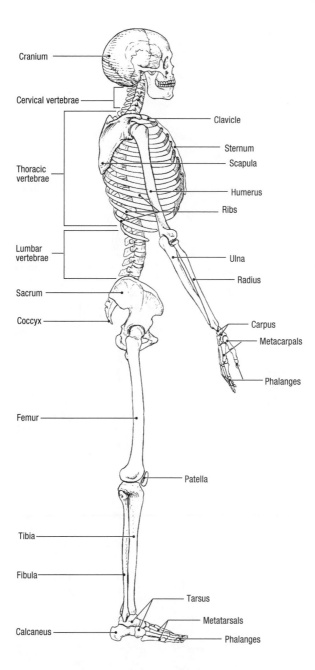

Figure 7. Skeleton, adult, lateral view.

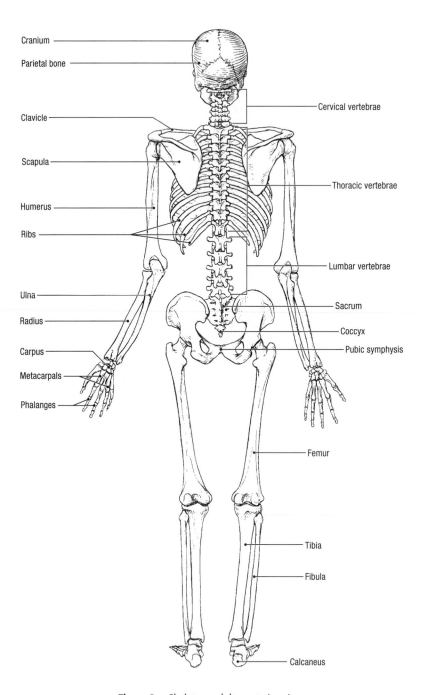

Figure 8. Skeleton, adult, posterior view.

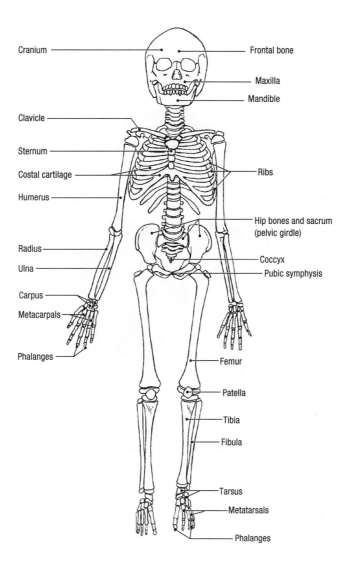

Figure 9. Skeleton, child, anterior view.

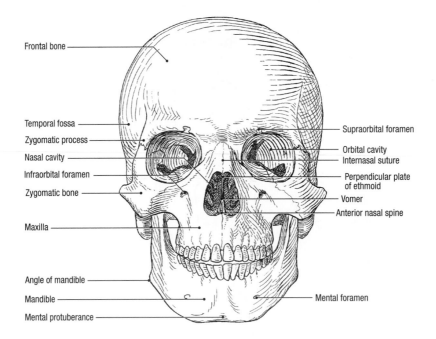

Frontal bone

Temporal fossa

Zygomatic process

Nasal cavity

Infraorbital foramen

Zygomatic bone

Maxilla

Angle of mandible

Mandible

Mental protuberance

Supraorbital foramen

Orbital cavity
Internasal suture

Perpendicular plate
of ethmoid

Vomer

Anterior nasal spine

Mental foramen

Figure 10. Skull, frontal view.

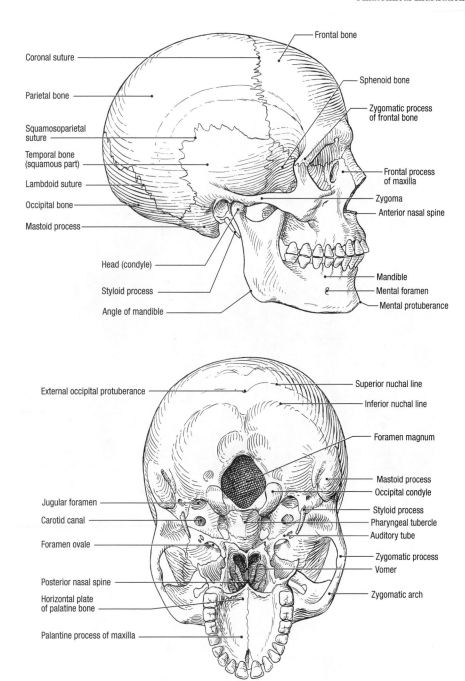

Figure 11. Skull, lateral (top) and inferior (bottom) views.

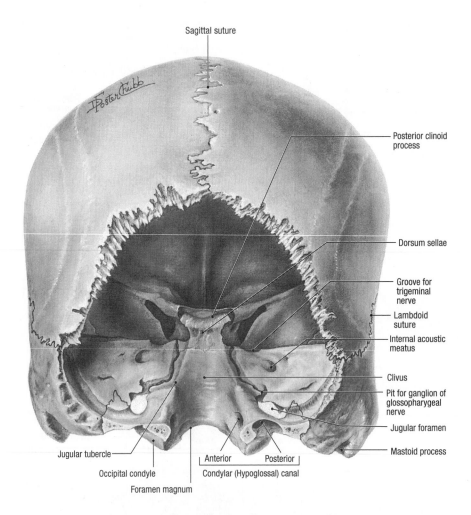

Figure 12. Skull. Bony features of posterior cranial fossa.

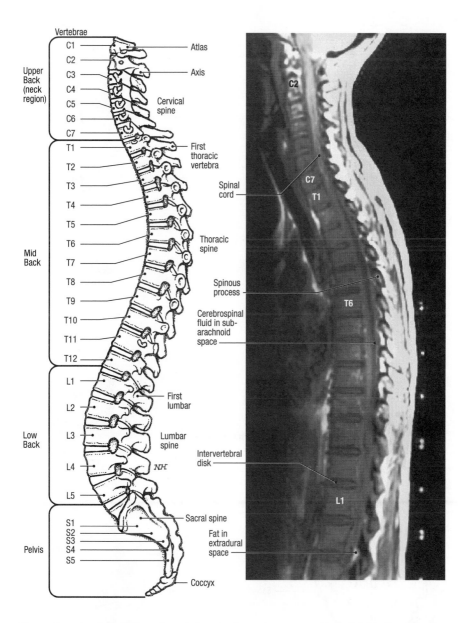

Figure 13. Vertebral column, lateral view. Radiograph courtesy of Dr. D. Salonen, University of Toronto, Toronto, Ontario, Canada.

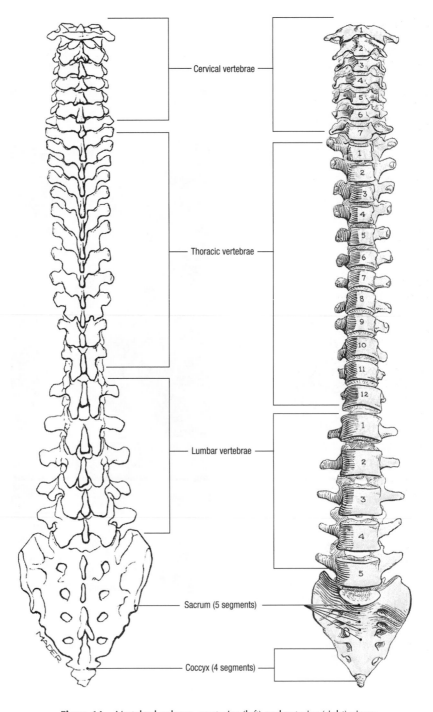

Figure 14. Vertebral column, posterior (left) and anterior (right) views.

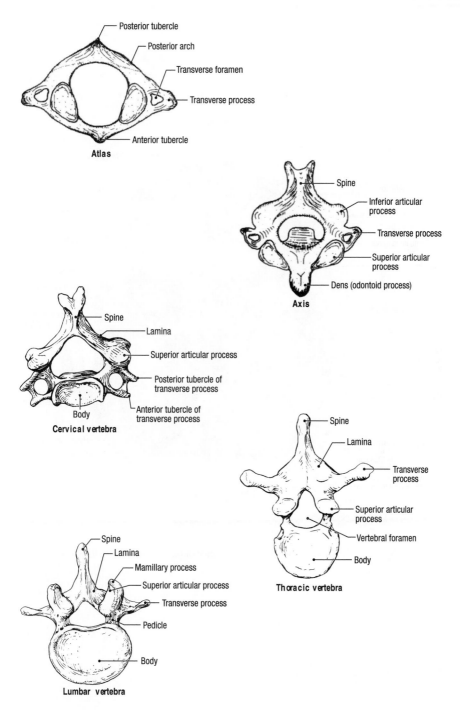

Figure 15. Typical atlas, axis, cervical, thoracic, and lumbar vertebrae.

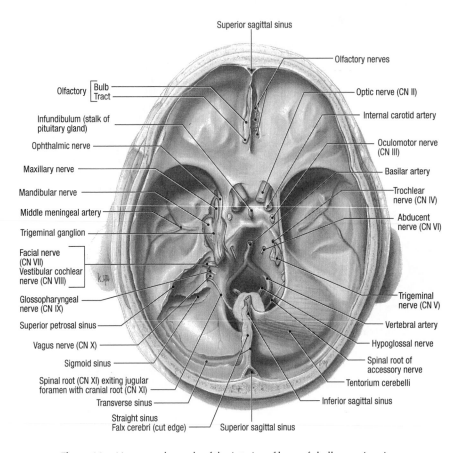

Superior sagittal sinus

Olfactory nerves

Olfactory { Bulb / Tract

Optic nerve (CN II)

Internal carotid artery

Infundibulum (stalk of pituitary gland)

Ophthalmic nerve

Oculomotor nerve (CN III)

Maxillary nerve

Basilar artery

Mandibular nerve

Trochlear nerve (CN IV)

Middle meningeal artery

Abducent nerve (CN VI)

Trigeminal ganglion

Facial nerve (CN VII) / Vestibular cochlear nerve (CN VIII)

Glossopharyngeal nerve (CN IX)

Trigeminal nerve (CN V)

Superior petrosal sinus

Vertebral artery

Vagus nerve (CN X)

Hypoglossal nerve

Sigmoid sinus

Spinal root of accessory nerve

Spinal root (CN XI) exiting jugular foramen with cranial root (CN XI)

Tentorium cerebelli

Transverse sinus

Inferior sagittal sinus

Straight sinus / Falx cerebri (cut edge)

Superior sagittal sinus

Figure 16. Nerves and vessels of the interior of base of skull, superior view.

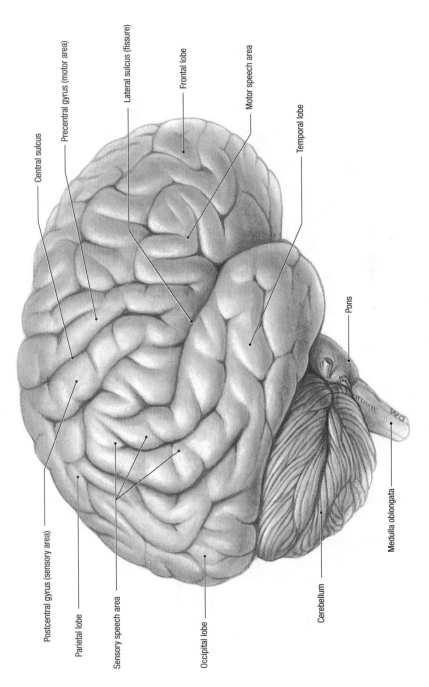

Central sulcus

Precentral gyrus (motor area)

Lateral sulcus (fissure)

Frontal lobe

Motor speech area

Temporal lobe

Pons

Postcentral gyrus (sensory area)

Parietal lobe

Sensory speech area

Occipital lobe

Cerebellum

Medulla oblongata

Figure 17. Brain, lateral view.

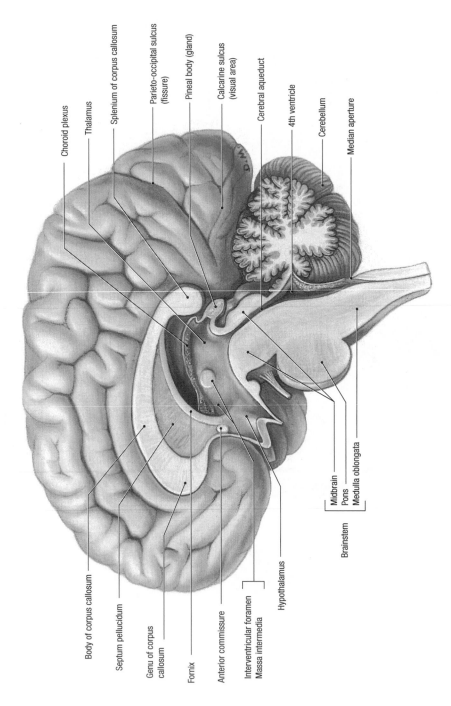

Figure 18. Brain, median section.

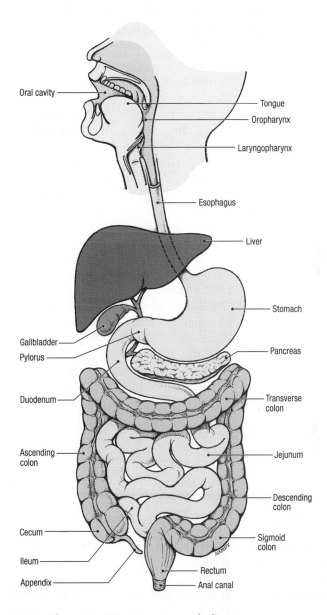

Figure 19. Digestive system and adjacent organs.

Contrast Media, Imaging Agents, and Related Substances

acetrizoate
AcuTect
Adenoscan
Altropane
AMI 121
AMI 227
amidotrizoic acid
Amipaque
Amiscan
Anatrast
Angiografin
AngioMARK
Apomate
arcitumomab
Baricon
barium sulfate
Baro-Cat
Barosperse
benzamide
benzoic acid
Biliscopin
Biloptin
bismuth
calcium 45 (^{45}Ca)
calcium 47 (^{47}Ca)
calcium ipodate
carbon 11 (^{11}C)
carbon-11 acetate
carbon-11 butanol
carbon-11 carfentanil
carbon-11 flumazenil
carbon 11-labeled
   cocaine
carbon 11-labeled fatty
   acids
carbon-11 N-
   methylspiperone
carbon-11 nomifensine
carbon-11 raclopride

carbon-11 thymidine
CardioGen-82
Cardiolite
Cardiotec
CEA-Scan
CEA-Tc 99m
   (^{99m}Tc CEA)
CentoRx
Ceretec
cerium
cesium chloride
CheeTah
Cholebrine
Choletec
Cholografin
Cholografin Meglumine
Chromitope Sodium
chromium
Clariscan
Cobatope-57
Combidex
Conray 30, 43, 400
copper
copper 64 (^{64}Cu)
^{11}Cu-TETA octreotide
cyanocobalamin
Cysto-Conray
Cysto-Conray II
Cystografin
Cystografin Dilute
d,1-HMPAO
Definity
deuterium
dextrose 5% in water
Diaginol
diatrizoate
diatrizoate meglumine
diatrizoate sodium
diatrizoic acid

diazepam
diethylenetriaminepentaa
   cetic acid (DTPA)
Digibar 190
Digital HD
Dionosil
Dionosil Oily
dobutamine
dodecafluoropentane
   (DDFP)
Dopascan
dysprosium
EchoGen
Echovist
Enecat
EneMark
Enhancer
Entero Vu
Entrobar
EntroEase
Eovist
Esopho-Cat
ethiodized oil
Ethiodol
etidronate disodium
Evans blue
exametazime
E-Z-AC
E-Z-Cat
E-Z-Cat Dry
E-Z-HD
E-Z-Paque
E-Z-Paste
F-18 fluoro-2-
   deoxyglucose
F-18 sodium fluoride
Feridex I.V.
feruglose
ferumoxsil

Fibrimage
Flo-Coat
fluorine
fluorine-18-dihydroxy-
  phenylalanine
  (^{18}F-DOPA)
fluorodeoxyglucose
  (FDG)
FS-069
furosemide
gadobenate dimeglumine
  (Gd-BOPTA)
gadobenic acid
gadobutrol
gadodiamide (Gd-DTPA-
  BMA)
gadolinium (Gd)
gadolinium chelate
gadolinium oxide
gadopentetate
  dimeglumine
  (Gd-DTPA)
gadoterate meglumine
  (Gd-DOTA)
gadoteridol (Gd-D03A)
gadoversetamide
gadoxetic acid (Gd-
  EOB-DTPA)
galactose
gallium
Gastrografin
GastroMARK
Gastromiro
Gastrovist
Gd-DTPA with mannitol
Glofil-125
glucagon
glucarate
HD 85
HD 200 Plus
Hepatolite
Hexabrix
Hippuran

holmium
human serum albumin
  (HSA)
hydrogen peroxide
hyoscine butylbromide
Hypaque-76
Hypaque-Cysto
Hypaque Meglumine
Hypaque Sodium
Imagent GI
Imavist
ImmuRAIT
indium 111 (^{111}In)
indium-111 pentetreotide
Indium-Oxine
indocyanine green (ICG)
Intropaste
iobitridol
iocetamic acid
iodamide
iodide
iodine-123 MIBG
iodine-131 MIBG
iodipamide
iodipamide meglumine
iodixanol
iodized oil
5-iodo-2-deoxyuridine
  (IUdR)
iodohippurate sodium
  I-123
iodohippurate sodium
  I-131
iodopyracet
Iodotope
ioglunide
iohexol
Iomeron 150, 250, 300,
  350
iopamidol
iopanoate
iopanoic acid
iophendylate

iopromide
iothalamate
iothalamate meglumine
iothalamate sodium
iothalamic acid
iotrolan
iotroxamide
ioversol
ioxaglate
ioxaglate meglumine
ioxaglate sodium
ioxaglic acid
ioxilan
ioxithalamate
ipodate
ipodate sodium
iridium
iridium 192 (^{192}Ir)
Isopaque
isosulfan blue
Isovue
Isovue-200, -250, -300,
  -370
Isovue-M 200, 300
Isovue Multipack-250,
  -300, -370
Kinevac
LeukoScan
LeuTech
Levovist
Lipiodol
Liqui-Coat HD
Liquid Barosperse
L-tyrosine
Lymphazurin
LymphoScan
macroaggregated
  albumin
Macrotec
magnesium
magnetite albumin
Magnevist
mangafodipir trisodium

manganese chloride
mannitol and saline
MD-76R
MD-Gastroview
MDP-Bracco
Medebar Plus
Medescan
meglumine
meglumine diatrizoate
meglumine iocarmate
meglumine iodipamide
meglumine iothalamate
meglumine iotroxate
Metastron
methyl methacrylate
methylglucamine
metrizamide
metrizoate
Micropaque
mineral oil
Miraluma
MS-325
MultiHance
Myoscint
Myoview
naloxone
NeoSpect
NeoTect
Neurolite
nicotinamide
nimodipine
Niopam
nitrogen-13 ammonia
nofetumomab
OctreoScan
octreotide
Omnipaque 140, 180,
    240, 300, 350
Omniscan
OncoScint CR/OV
OncoSeed
OptiMARK

Optiray 160, 240, 300,
    320, 350
Optison
Oragrafin Calcium
Oragrafin Sodium
Oxilan
palladium
Pantopaque
pentagastrin
pentetreotide
peppermint oil
Perchloracap
perflubron
perfluorocarbon
Persantine
pertechnetate
phosphoric acid
phosphorus
Phosphotec
Polibar
Polibar Plus
potassium
potassium perchlorate
Prepcat
ProHance
propyliodone
ProstaScint
Quadramet
radiopaque polyvinyl
    chloride
RAPID strand
Readi-Cat
Readi-Cat 2
recombinant thyrotropin
Reno-60
Renocal-76
Reno-DIP
Renografin-60
Renovist
Renovist II
Renovue-65
Renovue-Dip

rhenium
RIGScan CR49
rubidium chloride
Rubratope-57
samarium
samarium-153 ethylene-
    diamine tetramethylene
    phosphoric acid
    (^{153}Sm-EDTMP)
satumomab pendetide
selenium
sestamibi
Sethotope
sincalide
Sinografin
Sitzmarks
sodium
sodium bicarbonate
sodium chloride
sodium diatrizoate
sodium iodide
sodium iodipamide
sodium iodohippurate
sodium iothalamate
sodium ipodate
sodium meglumine
    ioxaglate
sodium methiodal
sodium metrizoate
sodium pertechnetate
sodium tartrate
sodium tyropanoate
Sol-O-Pake
Solu-Biloptin
Solutrast
somatostatin
Sonazoid
SonoRx
SonoVue
sorbitol
sprodiamide
strontium

sucrose polyester
sulfobromophthalein
sulfur colloid
tantalum
tantalum 178 (^{178}Ta)
teboroxime
Techneplex
TechneScan HDP, MAA, MAG3, PYP
technetium 99m (^{99m}Tc)
technetium-99m albumin
technetium-99m albumin aggregated
technetium-99m albumin colloid
technetium-99m albumin microspheres
technetium-99m biciromab
technetium-99m bicisate
technetium-99m depreotide
technetium-99m dimer-captosuccinic acid
technetium-99m disofenin
technetium-99m exametazime
technetium-99m furifosmin
technetium-99m galactosyl human serum albumin
technetium-99m glucarate
technetium-99m gluceptate
technetium-99m hepatoiminodiacetic acid (Tc-HIDA)
technetium-99m Hepatolite

technetium-99m human serum albumin
technetium-99m lidofenin
technetium-99m macroaggregated albumin
technetium-99m MAG 3
technetium-99m mebrofenin
technetium-99m medronate
technetium-99m mertiatide
technetium-99m oxidronate
technetium-99m N-para-isopropyl-acetanilide-iminodiacetic acid (Tc-PIPIDA)
technetium-99m pentetate
technetium-99m pentetate calcium trisodium
technetium-99m pertechnetate sodium
technetium-99m polyphosphate
technetium-99m pyrophosphate
technetium-99m sestamibi
technetium-99m siboroxime
technetium-99m sodium
technetium-99m sodium pertechnetate
technetium-99m succimer
technetium-99m sulfur colloid

technetium-99m teboroxime
technetium-99m tetrofosmin
technetium stannous pyrophosphate (TSPP)
Telebrix
Telepaque
Teslascan
tetrabromophenolph-thalein
tetraiodophenolph-thalein
thallium 201
thallous chloride
TheraSeed
thorium dioxide
Thorotrast
Tomocat
Tomocat 1000
Tonojug
Tonopaque
triiodobenzoic acid
Triosil
tyropanoate
Ultra-R
UltraTag
Ultravist 150, 240, 300, 370
uranium
Urografin
Uromiro
Urovist Cysto
Urovist Meglumine
Urovist Sodium 300
UroVysion
Varibar
Verluma
Visipaque 270, 320
Xenetix 250, 300, 350
xenon
xylenol orange

Appendix 3
Common Radiation Oncology Terms

absolute dose
adjacent field
adjuvant therapy
algorithm
alloy
alpha cradle immobilization device
amygdaloid complex
angle
simulated annealing
applicator
Aquaplast immobilization device
arc
asymmetric collimation
attenuation
backscatter
beam modifier
beam's eye view
belly board
beta radiation
betatron
bite block
block
bolus
boost
brachytherapy
breast board
buildup region
calculation
calipers
catheter
centigray (cGy)
central axis
central plane
Cerrobend
cesium
cesium teletherapy unit
cesium-137 (^{137}Cs, Cs-137)
chemoradiotherapy
chemotherapy regimen
Clinac linear accelerator

clinical target volume (CTV)
cobalt-60 (^{60}Co, Co-60)
cobalt teletherapy unit
cold spot
collimator angle
collimator leaf
compensator
composite plan
coned down
conformal radiotherapy
contour
convergence
coplanar beam arrangement
couch angle
couch kick
craniospinal irradiation
CT simulator
curative intent care
curative radiotherapy
cyclotron
decay
Delclos applicator
depth dose
desquamation
digitally composited radiograph
   (DCR)
digitally reconstructed radiograph
   (DRR)
diode
divergence
divergent beams
dose calculation
dose distribution
dose escalation
dose-volume histograms
dosimetrist
dosimetry
dwell position
dynamic multileaf collimator (DMLC)
dynamic wedge

electron
electron beam radiation therapy
electron cone
Ellis filter
equal weighting
extended distance
external beam radiation therapy (EBRT, XRT)
eye shield
facial mask
fluorodeoxyglucose positron emission tomography (FDG PET)
field arrangement
film digitizer
fluid-attenuated inversion recovery (FLAIR)
Fletcher-Suit applicator
fraction
fractionated external beam radiation therapy
frontocentral
gamma knife
gamma radiation
gantry
gap
gap calculation
geometry
gold-198 (^{198}Au, Au-198)
Gray (Gy)
gross tumor volume (GTV)
half beam block
half valve layer
half valve thickness
half-life
hand block
headrest (sizes range from A to F)
Heyman capsule
high dose
high dose rate (HDR)
high linear energy transfer (LET) radiation
high-dose-rate remote afterloading
hindbrain

hot spot
hyperfractionation
hyperthermia
image fusion
immobilization device
implant
independent collimator
informed consent
intensity modulated radiation therapy (IMRT)
interaortocaval lymphadenopathy
interpeduncular cistern
interstitial brachytherapy
interstitial implant
intracavitary irradiation
intracavitary therapy
intraluminal implant
intraoperative radiation therapy (RT)
iodine-125 (^{125}I, I-125)
ionization chamber
iridium
iridium-192 (^{192}Ir, Ir-192)
irradiated volume
irregular fields
isocenter
isocentric
isodose curve
isodose plan
isotherm
isotope
Karnofsky Performance Status (KPS)
kilovolt (kV)
laser
laser alignment system
lead
lesion length
linear accelerator (LINAC)
local-regional
low dose rate (LDR)
lucite filter
mantle field
megavolts (MV or MeV)
minimum target dose

missing tissue compensator
mold
monitor unit (MU)
mucositis
multileaf collimator
multiplanar reconstruction
neutron
noncoplanar beam arrangements
oblique
off-axis factor
orthogonal pair
orthovoltage
ovoid
palliation
palliative intent care
paraaortic field
parallel opposed fields
parenchymal hyperlucency
particle beam
particle beam treatment
penumbra
percentage depth dose (PPD)
perimesencephalic cistern
permanent implant
photon
photon beam radiation therapy
piriform sinus
planning target volume (PTV)
point calculation
port
port film
portal
portal imaging
prescription point
prostate seed implant
proton
pterygoid process
punctate foci
radiation biology
radiation field
radiation physics
radiation portal
radiation therapy, radiotherapy

radiation therapy planning
radiation therapy technologist (RTT)
radiobiology
radioimmunotherapy (RIT)
radioiodine seeds (I-125)
radiolabeled antibodies
radionuclide
radioprotector, radiation protector
radiosensitizer
radium implant
Red Journal (International Journal of
    Radiation Oncology/Biology/
    Physics)
reference depth
ribbon
rotational therapy
separation
sestamibi
shield
short tau inversion recovery (STIR)
    image
simulation
simulator
single-photon emission computed
    tomography (SPECT) imaging
source axis distance (SAD)
source film distance (SFD)
source surface distance (SSD)
spiculated margin
stereotactic head frame
stereotactic radiosurgery (SRS)
stereotactic radiotherapy (SRT)
stereotaxis
strontium 89 (^{89}Sr, Sr-89)
strontium 90 (^{90}Sr, Sr-90)
superficial machine
surface mold
systemic radiation therapy
T1 fat-saturated
tandem
target localization
tattoo
teletherapy

testicular shield
thermoluminescent dosimeter (TLD)
thermoplastic
three-dimensional conformal radiation
   therapy
three-dimensional radiotherapy
   treatment planning (3DRTP)
total body irradiation (TBI)
total skin electron (TSE) irradiation
treatment plan
treatment time

tumor volume
tungsten
two-dimensional radiotherapy
   treatment planning (2DRTP)
unequal weighting
vaginal cylinder
verification film
volumetric calculation
wedge
wing board
X-knife

Sample Reports and Dictation

Cranial PET Report

HISTORY: The patient is a 72-year-old male to assess for recurrent brain tumor versus radiation necrosis. Abnormal enhancement in the left parietal lobe is present on prior MR.

TECHNIQUE: Fusion PET CT imaging of the head was performed via the GE Discovery LS system. Serum glucose prior to the examination was 134 mg/dl. Following the IV administration of 16.5 mCi F-18 FDG, PO administration of 10 mg Valium for muscle relaxation, and a 50-minute uptake interval, cranial 3D PET imaging with CT attenuation correction was performed utilizing one bed position for 20 minutes per bed. Concordant multislice helical CT scanning was performed using low-dose technique with 5-mm collimation and 5-mm reconstruction interval, without intravenous or oral contrast. Image analysis including evaluation of fusion imaging was performed on the Entegra workstation.

COMPARISON: Pre- and postcontrast head MR.

FINDINGS: Noncontrast head CT obtained for fusion imaging with 5-mm axial images demonstrate third and lateral ventriculomegaly, which is moderate and more prominent than prior CT. Sulci and cisterns are within normal limits of size for age. Bifrontal and biparietal white matter low attenuation corresponds to abnormal FLAIR signal on recent MR. There has been a left parietal craniotomy. Within the left parietal lobe and adjacent to the cortex is a slightly higher attenuation focus surrounded by lower attenuation. This corresponds to the enhancing lesion on recent MR. This lesion shows increased PET activity compared to normal cortex. The parenchyma surrounding this high-activity lesion shows decreased activity extending to the cortex. The low cortical activity corresponds to low attenuation on CT and abnormal FLAIR signal on MR. The volume of increased PET activity is similar to the enhancement on MR.

IMPRESSIONS AND RECOMMENDATIONS:
1. Left parietal enhancing lesion peripherally on outside MR shows increased PET activity consistent with recurrent tumor. Surrounding parenchyma shows decreased cortical activity consistent with surrounding infarct versus radiation change with decreased metabolism. This is subjacent to the patient's prior craniotomy.
2. Lateral ventriculomegaly similar to prior MR, but worsened. This may represent central volume loss, possibly associated with the diffuse white matter disease seen

on MR and CT. Normal pressure hydrocephalus would be a consideration in the proper clinical setting.

CT Scan of the Chest & Adrenals with Contrast

HISTORY: Left pulmonary nodule on chest x-ray.

TECHNIQUE: Helical transaxial images, 7 mm, of the chest were obtained after the administration of oral and intravenous contrast.

FINDINGS: Patient's chest x-rays from February 24 and 25 were reviewed. There is an ill-defined opacity suggested in the left midlung zones on those studies, including oblique views.

Within the left lower lobe laterally, there is an approximately 2-cm area of parenchymal density which has the appearance of interstitial changes without findings of significant nodule or mass. This finding may relate to scarring. There is no other nodule, mass, or effusion. Within the mediastinum, there is no evidence of adenopathy seen. The heart and great vessels are normal in appearance. There is a suggestion of minimal pericardial thickening anteriorly, which is not specific. Osseous structures show degenerative changes with osteophyte formation at multiple levels in the thoracic spine.

Visualized upper abdominal structures including liver, spleen, kidneys, pancreas, aorta, and paraaortic retroperitoneum, show no specific finding. The adrenal glands are not enlarged.

IMPRESSION: Small focal area of increased parenchymal density, which has interstitial pattern. There is no significant nodule or mass. This is suggestive of scarring. There is no nodule, mass, effusion, or adenopathy seen. Consider chest x-ray followup of this lesion to assess stability.

CT Scan of the Paranasal Sinuses

HISTORY: The patient is a 37-year-old female with sinusitis.

TECHNIQUE: Coronal noncontrast CT images of the paranasal sinuses were performed.

FINDINGS: Patient is status post bilateral uncinectomies and partial ethmoidectomies and turbinectomies. Mild scattered frontal ethmoid and maxillary mucosal thickening is present. A 15-mm polyp is seen in the left sphenoid sinus. There is filling of a residual right anterior ethmoid air cell. Orbital walls are intact. Mucosal thickening is seen along the nasal septum, which is deviated to the left.

IMPRESSION

1. Scattered paranasal sinus mucosal disease including a 15-mm polyp in the left sphenoid sinus.
2. Status post bilateral uncinectomies, turbinectomies and partial ethmoidectomies.
3. Mucosal thickening along the nasal septum, which is deviated to the left.

Graded Exercise Test with Myocardial Perfusion Imaging

CLINICAL INFORMATION: Abnormal ECG, hyperlipidemia, tobacco abuse, family history of coronary artery disease.

TECHNIQUE: Resting, gated, and tomographic images were obtained with a SPECT camera following the injection of 10.5 mCi of ^{99m}Tc tetrofosmin. The patient exercised for 9 minutes and 30 seconds on a ramped Bruce protocol. Baseline heart rate was 74. Baseline blood pressure was 124/70. Heart rate at peak exercise was 155, which equaled 89% of the age-predicted maximum heart rate. Blood pressure at peak exercise was 160/80. Maximum work capacity 10.9 METS. The test was terminated due to fatigue and achievement of target heart rate. The patient did not have symptoms of chest discomfort during exercise. During exercise the patient developed approximately 2 mm of downsloping ST depression in leads II, III aVF and V4 through V6. These resolved gradually during the recovery phase. The patient's heart rate, measured one minute into the recovery phase, was 131. At peak exercise, the patient was injected with 33 mCi of ^{99m}Tc tetrofosmin and stress tomographic images were once again obtained with a SPECT camera.

IMAGING RESULTS: Analysis of resting and stress-gated and tomographic images reveal homogenous distribution of radiotracer throughout all ventricular segments. There is no evidence of ischemia or prior infarction. Global left ventricular systolic function is normal with an ejection fraction of 40% by gated analysis without evidence of regional wall motion abnormality, possibly underestimating true LV systolic function. There is no dilatation of the left ventricle cavity.

IMPRESSIONS:

1. Adequate functional capacity for age.
2. No stress-provoked angina.
3. There was 2 mm of downsloping ST depression in the inferolateral leads resolv-

ing gradually during the recovery phase, likely suggesting false positive electro-cardiographic response to exercise.
4. No exercise-induced tachyarrhythmia.
5. Mildly hypertensive blood pressure response to exercise.
6. Normal heart rate recovery of 24, measured one minute into the recovery phase.
7. Normal myocardial perfusion scan.
8. Normal gated wall motion analysis as detailed above with calculated left ventricular ejection fraction of 40% without evidence of regional wall motion abnormality, possibly underestimating true global left ventricular systolic function.

The above perfusion scan is normal without evidence of prior infarction or stress-provoked angina.

MRI of the Brain and MRA of the Brain and Neck

TECHNIQUE: T1-weighted sagittal; FSE T2-weighted axial; T1-weighted axial. TOF angiography of the intracranial and extracranial vessels is performed. Multiple reconstruction images are obtained.

FINDINGS: No intracranial tumor is present. No hydrocephalus or shift is present. No intracerebral edema is present. No acute infarct is present. The brain stem and cerebellopontine angles are normal. The pericavernous spaces are normal. The corpus callosum and tectal plate are normal.

MR angiogram of the carotid bifurcations shows the right and left carotid bifurcations to be normal. No stenosis or ulceration is present.

Intracranial MR angiogram reveals the internal carotid arteries and carotid bifurcations to be normal. The anterior and middle cerebral arteries are normal. The vertebrobasilar junction is normal. The basilar artery and basilar apex are normal. The posterior cerebral arteries are normal.

IMPRESSIONS AND RECOMMENDATIONS:
1. Normal MRI examination of the brain.
2. Normal MR angiogram of the cervical carotid bifurcations.
3. Normal MR angiogram of the intracranial circulation.

MRI of the Brain With and Without Contrast

INDICATIONS: The patient is a 50-year-old female with numbness in the left upper extremity and in both hands.

TECHNIQUE: Using an ultrafast, ultrahigh-resolution 1.5 Tesla Symphony MRI scanner with ultra gradients and Integrated Panoramic Array coil technology, the following sequences were obtained: Sagittal T1 and axial T1 and turbo spin-echo T2-weighted and turbo FLAIR and postgadolinium contrast axial T1-weighted with magnetization transfer. Total: Five sequences.

FINDINGS: The ventricles are normal in size. There is no midline shift. There is no extraaxial fluid collection. No parenchymal high or low-intensity lesion is noted. In particular, no definite white matter lesion is identified. The posterior fossa structures are unremarkable. The regions of sella and parasellar structures are unremarkable. The cerebellar tonsils are low lying without evidence for herniation or Chiari malformation. The visualized sinuses are unremarkable. There is suggestion of bilateral concha bullosa. After administration of contrast, no abnormal enhancement is identified. There is a dominant left vertebral artery with the right side appearing much smaller. Flow voids are noted in the major vessels otherwise.

IMPRESSIONS:
1. Unremarkable MRI of the brain with and without contrast.
2. A dominant left vertebral artery. Bilateral concha bullosa.

MRI of the Brain with Gadolinium

HISTORY: Hyponatremia due to resetting of her osmostat.

TECHNIQUE: Axial FLAIR and T2 and coronal T2-weighted images of the brain were performed. Sagittal and coronal T1-weighted pre- and postgadolinium images were performed through the sella and parasellar regions. The study was terminated prior to obtaining adequate postcontrast images because the patient complained of severe headache and could not tolerate further imaging.

FINDINGS: The exam was limited with postcontrast images severely degraded by motion artifact.

Images through the brain show normal sulci and ventricles. There is no mass lesion, mass effect, hemorrhage, or infarction. White matter structures have normal configuration and signal characteristics. The brain stem and cerebellum are normal.

Orbits, visualized paranasal sinuses, and mastoid air cells are normal.

Images through the sella and parasellar regions show no evidence of mass. Pituitary gland has normal size and configuration. Normal high signal of the posterior pituitary is demonstrated. Pituitary infundibulum is midline. Suprasellar cistern and optic chiasm are normal. Floor of the anterior third ventricle and region of the hypothalamus appear within normal limits.

IMPRESSION: Essentially normal MRI of the brain and pituitary. Postcontrast images are significantly degraded by patient motion artifact.

MRI of the Lumbar Spine

CLINICAL HISTORY: Lumbar radiculopathy.

PROCEDURE: Image sequences obtained include: Sagittal T1, T2 and STIR, axial T1 and T2.

FINDINGS: Multilevel degenerative spondylosis is present with loss of disc height and disc signal at several levels. Vertebral body heights in the lumbar region are preserved. There is minimal anterior wedging of T12. The conus terminates toward the upper part of L1. It appears normal.

L5–S1 level: There is loss of disc height and of disc signal. A 3-mm broad-based bulge is present with associated posterior marginal osteophytes. The central canal is normal. The S1 nerve roots appear normal. The foramina appear somewhat narrowed bilaterally and should be correlated with clinical evidence for bilateral L5 radiculopathy.

L4–5 level: The facets appear hypertrophied. There is thickening of the overlying ligamentum flavum. A 3- to 4-mm broad-based bulge is present. The central canal appears slightly narrowed at approximately 8- to 9-mm. The foramina appear adequate.

L3–4 level: The facets appear moderately prominent. A 2- to 3-mm broad-based bulge is present. The canal appears adequate at 11- to 12-mm. The foramina appear adequate.

L2–3 level: A 3- to 4-mm broad-based bulge is present. Anteroposterior dimension of the central canal is borderline at 1 cm. The foramina appear adequate.

L1–2 level: A 3-mm broad-based bulge is present. The central canal appears adequate. The foramina appear adequate.

T12–L1 level: A 2- to 3-mm bulge is present. The central canal appears to be adequate.

IMPRESSIONS AND RECOMMENDATIONS:
1. Slight anterior wedging of T12.
2. Preservation of normal vertebral body heights and alignment in the lumbar region.
3. Multilevel degenerative spondylosis as described at each level above.
4. The central canal appears stenotic at the L4–5 level.
5. The foramina at L5-S1 appear to be narrowed.
6. The foramina elsewhere appear to be adequate.

MRI of the Pelvis

Clinical History: The patient has intermittent but consistent sharp pain in the general area of the left ovary. This has been ongoing for the past five to six years. The patient has had multiple transvaginal and transabdominal pelvic ultrasounds in the past. These have only shown uterine fibroids. The patient is noted to have a history of moderately elevated CA-125.

TECHNIQUE: Sagittal T2 FSE as well as T1 spin-echo images were obtained through the pelvis. Axial T2 FSE images as well as T1 spin-echo images were also obtained. Coronal T2 FSE images were also obtained.

FINDINGS: Sagittal T2-weighted sequence is moderately degraded by motion artifact. This is the ideal sequence to evaluate the junctional zone of the uterus. However, the junctional zone is felt to be within normal limits in size. There is only a questionable low-signal mass identified on the T2-weighted sequence within the posterior body of the uterus. This possibly represents the patient's known uterine fibroid. It measures approximately 1.5 cm in maximum diameter.

Both ovaries are thought to be identified. On the left, there are two tiny ovarian cysts. These measure up to approximately 1.8 cm in maximum diameter. The right ovarian cyst is also identified. It also measures approximately 1.8 cm in maximum diameter. No other pelvic masses are identified. There is no pelvic free fluid.

Incidental note is made in the L4 and L5 vertebral body zones of abnormal marrow signal. Each of these zones have narrow zones of transition. Each zone is roughly ovoid in shape. The L5 zone measures approximately 2.1 cm in maximum diameter. The L4 vertebral body zone measures approximately 1.8 cm in maximum diameter. These are of increased signal intensity on the T2-weighted sequences. The L5 lesion is of intermediate signal intensity on the T1 spin-echo sequence. The L4 lesion is not included on the T1 spin-echo sequence. L5-S1 degenerative disc bulging is noted.

IMPRESSIONS AND RECOMMENDATIONS:

1. Bilateral small ovarian cysts.
2. Possible uterine fibroid identified.
3. L4 and L5 vertebral body lesions. These may represent atypical hemangioma. Other considerations including secondary neoplasm cannot be excluded, however. Recommend dedicated MRI of the lumbar spine for further evaluation.
4. Otherwise normal MRI of the pelvis.

Thoracic Aortogram with Cerebral Angiography

HISTORY: The patient is an 82-year-old man with thoracic aneurysm and carotid stenosis.

TECHNIQUE: A 20-minute consultation was utilized explaining risks, benefits, and alternatives of angiography. All the patient's questions were answered, and he had given informed consent prior to the procedure. The patient was premedicated with IM Demerol and Phenergan. Buffered lidocaine was used for local anesthesia. Sedation was not required.

A 5-French pigtail catheter was advanced into the aorta via the right femoral artery with standard Seldinger technique. With the tip of the catheter in the ascending aorta, aortogram with digital subtraction technique was obtained in the left anterior projection. AP frontal view of the intracranial circulation was also obtained from an arch injection. Catheter was then exchanged over a guide wire for a 5-French Simmons II catheter. The carotid and left vertebral artery were selectively catheterized and injected with contrast for digital subtraction filming. In the right common carotid, it was initially difficult to get stable catheter position, and various combinations of guide wires and a Simmons III catheter were used to obtain selective catheterization. After all images were reviewed, the catheter was removed, and direct pressure was applied to the puncture site until complete hemostasis was achieved.

Total contrast load was 132 cc of Isovue. Fluoroscopy time was 41.5 minutes.

FINDINGS: The ascending aorta is dilated and has a more normal diameter just after the left subclavian catheter, and then the descending thoracic aorta enlarges again. There is no evidence of intimal dissection. The origins from the arch are patent. The right carotid bifurcation is slightly irregular; however, no hemodynamically significant stenosis is observed in the right internal carotid. The right external carotid is open. The left external carotid is completely occluded. The left internal carotid has 75% reduction of its cross-sectional area near its origin. On selective injections, it is interesting to note that the right anterior cerebral artery does not fill from the right carotid injection, but both anterior cerebral arteries fill from the left carotid injection. Vertebral arteries are patent. The left vertebral artery is larger. No obvious intracranial abnormality is observed.

IMPRESSION: There is 75% stenosis of the left internal carotid. Complete occlusion, left external carotid. Very mild irregularity of the right internal carotid. Widely patent right external carotid. Both vertebral arteries are patent.

Ultrasound of the Pelvis

Images from a real-time transabdominal and transvaginal examination demonstrate the uterus to be somewhat retroverted transabdominally but normal in contour and position transvaginally. It is normal in overall size and contour. Central endometrial echoes are quite prominent, uniform but hyperechoic, ranging between 6 and 12 mm in thickness. No uterine mass or endocavitary lesion is evident. The left ovary is rather inferior and posterior, normal in size, demonstrating numerous small peripheral follicles. The right ovary is considerably enlarged at approximately 6.1 × 4.4 × 4.3 cm. It is distended by a complex, partially cystic but well-circumscribed lesion measuring approximately 4.3 × 4.2 × 3.7 cm in diameter. The posteroinferior third of the mass is filled by mildly heterogeneous, mildly hypoechoic tissue which may represent some dependent debris or solid tissue, though no discrete tumor mass is delineated. There are multiple thin and partial septations through the cystic region as well as diffuse low-level echoes. There is no disruption of the ovarian capsule and there is only a tiny amount of adjacent free fluid.

IMPRESSIONS:
1. Complex right adnexal mass, predominantly cystic. The appearance is nonspecific but, in the absence of signs of infection, most likely represents a hemorrhagic cyst or benign neoplasm.
2. Close clinical followup is recommended. Although this is unlikely to represent a malignancy, excision may be necessary if the lesion does not resolve.

Ultrasound of the Right Breast

Images from a high-resolution real-time examination were obtained in the anterior lower inner portion of the breast where an area of increased density was noted on mammography in August and September of this year. It appears sonographically as a collection of small cysts and multiple overlapping, mildly dilated ducts encompassing an area of approximately 1.0 × 1.5 cm. There is some enhanced posterior through transmission of sound from the largest cystic area, which measures roughly 5 mm in diameter. No solid mass, architectural distortion, or pathologic shadowing is demonstrated.

IMPRESSION:
1. BI-RADS Category 2: Benign findings.
2. Sonography demonstrates the mammographic opacity to represent an area of cystic ductal ectasia. In the absence of any compelling clinical findings, recommend routine bilateral mammographic followup in August of next year.

Ultrasound of the Thyroid

CLINICAL INFORMATION: Thyroid nodule.

FINDINGS: The right lobe of the thyroid measures 4.0 cm long × 1.1 cm in AP dimension. The right lobe of the thyroid contains a 1.0 × 0.75 × 1.1-cm hypoechoic solid mass in the posterior aspect of the right lobe of the thyroid adjacent to the great vessels. A second isoechoic nodule measuring 1.6 × 0.3 × 1.5 cm is seen in the right lobe of the thyroid.

The left lobe measures almost 4.0 × 1.2 cm. It contains a 0.4 × 0.4 × 0.4-cm hypoechoic nodule laterally located adjacent to the great vessels. A small 0.2 × 0.2 × 0.3-cm simple cyst is seen in the midbody of the thyroid on the left side, more anteriorly placed.

CONCLUSION
1. At least two solid nodules are seen in the right lobe of the thyroid as discussed above. In light of the patient's history of follicular thyroid carcinoma, correlation with previous ultrasound examination and nuclear medicine scan is recommended.
2. Two very small hypoechoic nodules in the left lobe of the thyroid.

Ventilation/Perfusion Lung Scan

REASON FOR STUDY: The patient is a 64-year-old female admitted with shortness of breath and chest pain. Past history of deep venous thrombosis

TECHNIQUE: Xenon 133, 20 mCi, was inhaled for the ventilation study, and 6 mCi of Tc-99m MAA was injected for the perfusion study.

FINDINGS: The ventilation study done in the anterior and posterior projections, including single-breath, equilibrium, and washout phases, shows xenon retention in the lower lung fields bilaterally. There appears to be marked cardiomegaly.

The perfusion scan demonstrates irregular areas of diminished perfusion in the lower lung fields bilaterally, corresponding to the abnormalities noted on the ventilation scan. The heart is enlarged.

CONCLUSION: Abnormal lung scan demonstrating matched defects in the lower lung fields and an enlarged heart. Low-probability lung scan for pulmonary emboli.

Whole Body Scan

STUDY PERFORMED: Whole body scan.

Coronary artery calcium scoring was performed using EKG-gated technique and demonstrates a cardiac score of 195, with a predominant calcification located within the left anterior descending artery. This is at the 75th percentile of expected for age and documents the presence of at least moderate atherosclerotic plaque formation. This means that mild coronary artery narrowing is possible or even likely, with significant narrowing being possible although somewhat unlikely. Assessment and modification of cardiac risk factors is advised, and cardiology followup is recommended.

Thin-section multidetector CT scanning of the chest was performed and demonstrates four separate and discrete, noncalcified nodules of the right middle lobe of the lung, without evidence of any calcified nodules. Although these likely represent benign and incidental granulomas of no medical significance, the lack of calcium means it is impossible to make this diagnosis with absolute certainty and, therefore, a four-month followup scan to help document stability is recommended. Two of these nodules are 3 mm in diameter and two of these nodules are 7 mm in diameter.

Thin-section multidetector CT scanning of the abdomen and pelvis demonstrates mild atherosclerotic calcification of the abdominal aorta and bilateral iliac arteries. The liver, spleen, pancreas, kidneys, and adrenal glands are otherwise normal in appearance, without other evidence of significant abnormality. If colonoscopy has not been performed in the recent past, followup evaluation by means of virtual colonoscopy is recommended as a routine screen for colon cancer.

IMPRESSION: Moderately elevated cardiac score documents moderate atherosclerotic disease of the coronary arteries. Assessment and modification of cardiac risk factors and cardiology followup is advised. There are also four tiny, noncalcified right middle lobe lung nodules. Given the history of cigarette exposure, a four-month followup scan is suggested to document stability and confirm that these are likely incidental granulomas.

Common Terms by Procedure

Cranial PET Report

attenuation
axial image
cistern
collimation
cortex
cortical activity
CT attenuation
Entegra workstation
F18-FDG
FLAIR signal
fusion PET CT imaging
GE Discovery LS system
infarct
left parietal lobe
megacurie (mCi)
magnetic resonance (MR)
multislice helical CT scanning
normal-pressure hydrocephalus
parenchyma
PET activity
radiation change
radiation necrosis
reconstruction interval
subjacent
sulci
uptake interval
Valium
ventriculomegaly
white matter

CT Scan of the Chest & Adrenals with Contrast

adenopathy
degenerative change
effusion
focal area
great vessels

helical transaxial image
interstitial changes
intravenous contrast
left lower lobe
lesion
mass
mediastinum
midlung zones
oblique view
opacity
oral contrast
osseous structures
osteophyte formation
paraaortic retroperitoneum
parenchymal density
pericardial thickening
pulmonary nodule
scarring
upper abdominal structures

CT Scan of the Paranasal Sinuses

anterior ethmoid air cell
coronal noncontrast CT image
deviated
ethmoid
ethmoidectomies
maxillary
mucosal thickening
nasal septum
noncontrast
orbital walls
paranasal sinuses
polyp
scattered
sphenoid sinus
turbinectomies
uncinectomies

Graded Exercise Test with Myocardial Perfusion Imaging

age-predicted maximum heart rate
baseline blood pressure
baseline heart rate
downsloping ST depression
exercise-induced
false positive
functional capacity
gated wall motion analysis
global left ventricular systolic function
left ventricular ejection fraction
maximum work capacity
megacurie (mCi)
metabolic equivalents (METS)
peak exercise
radiotracer
ramped Bruce protocol
recovery phase
regional wall motion abnormality
resting and stress gated and
   tomographic images
SPECT camera
stress tomographic image
stress-provoked
systolic function
tachycardia
target heart rate
^{99m}Tc tetrofosmin
tomographic image
wall motion

MRA of the Brain and MRA of the Brain and Neck

basilar apex
basilar artery
carotid bifurcation
cerebellopontine angles
corpus callosum
FSE T2-weighted axial image
hydrocephalus

intracerebral edema
intracerebral tumor
intracranial MR angiogram
intracranial tumor
pericavernous space
posterior cerebral arteries
reconstruction image
T1-weighted axial image
T1-weighted sagittal image
tectal plate
vertebrobasilar junction

MRI of the Brain With and Without Contrast

axial T1 image
cerebellar tonsils
Chiari malformation
concha bullosa
extraaxial fluid collection
flow void
gadolinium
gradients
herniation
Integrated Panoramic Array
magnetic transfer
parasellar structures
parenchymal low-intensity lesion
posterior fossa
postgadolinium contrast axial T-1
   weighted image
sagittal T1 image
sella
1.5 Tesla Symphony
turbo FLAIR image
turbo spin-echo T2-weighted image
vertebral artery
white matter lesion

MRI of the Brain with Gadolinium

axial FLAIR image
brain stem

cerebellum
configuration
coronal T2-weighted image
hemorrhage
hyponatremia
hypothalamus
infarction
mass effect
mass lesion
mastoid air cells
motion artifact
optic chiasm
orbits
osmostat
paranasal sinuses
parasellar regions
pituitary gland
pituitary infundibulum
postcontrast images
pre- and postgadolinium image
sagittal and coronal T1-weighted image
sella and parasellar regions
signal characteristics
sulci
suprasellar cistern
T2-weighted image
ventricles
white matter

MRI of the Lumbar Spine

alignment
anterior wedging
axial T1 and T2
central canal
conus
degenerative spondylosis
disc height
disc signal
facets
foramina
hypertrophied
ligamentum flavum

lumbar radiculopathy
nerve roots
osteophytes
posterior marginal osteophytes
radiculopathy
sagittal T1
stenotic
T2 and STIR
vertebral body heights

MRI of the Pelvis

abnormal marrow signal
axial T2 FSE image
CA-125
coronal T2 FSE image
degenerative disc bulging
degraded
free fluid
hemangioma
junctional zone
lesion
low-signal mass
motion artifact
neoplasm
ovarian cysts
ovoid
pelvic ultrasound
sagittal T2 FSE image
sagittal T2-weighted sequence
signal intensity
T1 spin-echo image
transabdominal pelvis ultrasound
transvaginal pelvic ultrasound
uterine fibroid
zones of transition

Thoracic Aortogram with Cerebral Angiography

anterior cerebral arteries
aortic arch
aortogram
AP frontal view

arch injection
ascending aorta
buffered lidocaine
carotid bifurcation
carotid stenosis
catheterization
common carotid artery
contrast load
Demerol
descending thoracic aorta
digital subtraction technique
external carotid artery
fluoroscopy
5-French pigtail catheter
5-French Simmons II catheter
guide wire
hemodynamically significant stenosis
hemostasis
internal carotid artery
intimal dissection
intracranial circulation
Isovue
left anterior projection
local anesthesia
Phenergan
puncture site
Seldinger technique
selective catheterization
thoracic aneurysm
vertebral arteries

Ultrasound of the Pelvis

adnexal mass
benign neoplasm
central endometrial echoes
contour
debris
discrete
distended
endocavitary lesion
endometrial echoes
free fluid
hemorrhagic cyst

heterogeneous
hyperechoic
hypoechoic
malignancy
nonspecific
ovarian capsule
peripheral follicles
real-time transabdominal examination
real-time transvaginal examination
retroverted
septation
uterine mass
well-circumscribed lesion

Ultrasound, Right Breast

architectural distortion
BI-RADS Category
density
ductal ectasia
opacity
pathologic shadowing
real-time examination
solid mass
sonography

Ultrasound of the Thyroid

AP dimension
follicular thyroid carcinoma
great vessels
hypoechoic nodule
isoechoic nodule
left lobe
mass
midbody
nuclear medicine scan
right lobe
simple cyst
thyroid nodule

Ventilation/Perfusion Lung Scan

cardiomegaly
equilibrium phase

megacurie (mCi)
pulmonary emboli
single-breath phase
technetium-99m macroaggregated
   albumin (Tc-99m MAA)
washout phase
xenon 133

Whole Body Scan
atherosclerotic calcification
atherosclerotic disease

atherosclerotic plaque
calcification
calcified nodules
cardiac risk factors
coronary artery calcium scoring
electrocardiogram (EKG)
gated technique
granulomas
noncalcified nodules
thin-section multidetector CT scanning
virtual colonoscopy